2

THE
ESSENTIAL GUIDE
TO
PRESCRIPTION
DRUGS

1997 EDITION

James J. Rybacki, Pharm. D.
James W. Long, M.D.

HarperPerennial
A Division of HarperCollinsPublishers

THE ESSENTIAL GUIDE TO PRESCRIPTION DRUGS 1997. Copyright © 1996 by James J. Rybacki and James W. Long. Copyright © 1994 by James W. Long and James J. Rybacki. Copyright © 1977, 1980, 1982, 1985, 1987, 1988, 1989, 1990, 1991, 1992, 1993 by James W. Long. All rights reserved. Printed in the United States of America. No part of this book may be used or reproduced in any manner whatsoever without written permission except in the case of brief quotations embodied in critical articles and reviews. For information address HarperCollins Publishers Inc., 10 East 53rd Street, New York, NY 10022.

HarperCollins books may be purchased for educational, business, or sales promotional use. For information please write: Special Markets Department, HarperCollins Publishers Inc., 10 East 53rd Street, New York, NY 10022.

Designed by C. Linda Dingler

Library of Congress Catalog Card Number 87–657561

ISSN 0894-7058
ISBN 0–06-271603-4   96 97 98 RRD 10 9 8 7 6 5 4 3 2 1
ISBN 0–06-273429-6 (pbk.) 96 97 98 RRD 10 9 8 7 6 5 4 3 2 1

Contents

Author's Note
for the 1997 Edition

In the past year our health care system has continued to evolve, some novel medicines gained FDA approval, and once again adverse drug reactions continue to have a huge impact on our lives. Over the last two years there has been a terrible human toll as well as more than 14 billion dollars spent treating these drug reactions in the United States alone. The fact that you've purchased this book may make the difference for you and your loved ones. If the information you find here raises any questions, bring your concerns to your doctor or pharmacist immediately. A large number of adverse medicine reactions can be minimized if they are caught early.

I personally believe that the best results or outcomes are achieved by the patient who most fully understands all their medical conditions and their appropriate treatments. This edition of *The Essential Guide* includes a completely new section called "True Breakthroughs in Medicines." Its focus is on agents that will make a difference in maintaining or returning our health. It may not highlight the latest drug advertised in consumer magazines. As in every past edition, all of the medicine profiles and tables have been updated with the latest FDA approvals as well as current research leading to potential new therapeutic uses . . . intended to help you make your medicines work for and not against you.

Still, every year I read article after article outlining permanent disability or even death resulting from misuse of or adverse reactions to prescription and nonprescription medicines. My own father had a serious reaction to one of his heart medications—I know enough to prevent that now, yet it's too late for him. So when I read about other reactions now, I find myself taking them personally, wondering if that life is another one I could have saved if I had only been there. Remember, the decision to use

every prescription and nonprescription medicine is based on the balance between benefit and risk. Capital letters once again define more important benefits and highlight critical risks of medicines included in this book. In the last few years a rash of new nonprescription medicines have come on the market that just recently were available by prescription only. Always remember to ask your pharmacist or doctor **before** you combine any medicines.

"The Leading Edge" brings you news of medicines which offer great promise and are waiting just over the next horizon. Many of the medicines from last year's section have since gained FDA approval and are covered in detail in their own drug profiles. I've also broadened information contained in the "Conditions Requiring Dosing Adjustments" where appropriate, to tell you how medication dose or frequency should be adjusted for people with certain chronic conditions such as kidney or liver compromise. I believe that this is another way to help us avoid dangerous and unnecessary toxic drug reactions.

Be an active participant in your health care. Rybacki's first recommendation: "It's always better to prevent a disease or condition than to have to treat it." Be aware of both your family history and any current conditions, and attempt to find out about available vaccines or nutrition patterns that can protect you from other serious illnesses. As difficult as it can be to give up any habit you enjoy—from smoking too much to daily double-scoop ice cream cones—try to decrease ongoing risk. If a disease or condition *is* diagnosed, learn as much as possible about it and the medicines used to treat it. Your knowledge is a weapon against any condition you face. Use it to make medicines an ally in treatment and to protect you or a loved one from possible harmful effects from the medicine itself.

As noted in each previous edition, no claim is made that *all* known actions, uses, side effects, adverse effects, precautions, interactions, etc., for a drug are included in the information provided in the sections that constitute this book. Although diligent care has been taken to ensure the accuracy of the information provided during the preparation of this revision, the continued accuracy and currentness are ever subject to change relative to the dissemination of new information derived from drug research, development, and general usage.

James Joseph Rybacki, Pharm. D.
August 1996

Points for Consideration by the Patient

Studies of medication usage performed over the past 15 years have shown that more than half of patients take their prescription drugs incorrectly. A study by Dr. Lucian L. Leape of Harvard found 334 drug errors in six months at two major teaching hospitals in the United States. Fourteen of these errors were life-threatening. A U.S. and Canadian study placed the financial cost at more than **9 billion dollars** in each country. The human cost cannot be calculated. There are a variety of reasons that contribute to this wasteful and sometimes hazardous practice. The following suggestions are offered to reduce confusion and misunderstanding and to increase the likelihood that you take the right drug for the right reason at the right time and in the right way.

If you are being treated for a recurrent or chronic disorder, such as asthma or diabetes, **learn as much as you can** about the nature and medical management of your condition. Dr. James Long's new book, *The Essential Guide to Chronic Disorders*, will be available in early 1997. Ask your physician and pharmacist for written information they may have available; visit your local libraries and bookstores for pertinent publications; consult local chapters of national organizations that provide educational materials for specific disorders. The more you know about your disorder and its treatment, the more you will be able to use your prescribed medications safely and effectively. Do not be afraid to ask your doctor or pharmacist questions—you help them when you help yourself. Any competent physician or pharmacist will welcome the chance to help you understand, regardless of how busy they may be.

Cooperate fully with your physician and pharmacist to ensure that the diagnosis of your disorder is as accurate as possible and that the treatment prescribed is the most appropriate for you. It is incumbent upon you to **share the responsibility** for obtaining safe and effective drug treatment. Be certain every prescriber and pharmacist who helps provide your health care knows **all** of the medicines you are taking, including prescription, nonprescription, and any herbal or nutritional support you take.

Try not to be unduly influenced by seductive advertising of prescription drug products through television commercials, magazine displays, celebrity endorsements, etc. Ask your physician and pharmacist for **printed information sheets** that provide unbiased, objective information regarding the drug's benefits and risks—and its appropriateness for you. Drug therapy **MUST** be individualized. **NEVER** take someone else's medicine because your symptoms sound just like theirs.

When Your Physician Prescribes a Drug for You

- Tell your doctor about any known drug allergies and of any prior drug-induced adverse effects.
- Inform your physician of **all other drugs** (prescription, nonprescription, herbal or nutritional) that you are taking currently. Some herbal extracts currently available may contain pharmacological doses of ingredients found in some prescription products. Make certain you include these in your medication history.
- Ask if there are any special precautions to observe: avoidance of certain foods, alcohol, exposure to sun, other drugs, or hazardous activities.
- Ask how long you should take the drug; if applicable, determine an approximate time for discontinuation.
- Ask your physician to include on the prescription label both the **name of the drug** and the **disorder** for which the drug is taken. For example: Capoten for hypertension.
- Ask your physician to give you a **written summary** of appropriate information about the drug prescribed. It is not surprising that you have difficulty remembering all of the information and instructions that you have been given verbally. A written summary will allow you to clarify and verify pertinent information as necessary.
- Ask your doctor if the medicine prescribed offers the best balance of price and outcomes for you. Ask if the dosing has been adjusted for any compromise in kidney or liver function which you may have.
- Be aware of the restrictions or limitations placed by your health care insurer which may impact on the physician's prescribing authority and the pharmacist's ability to fulfill your prescription.
- Tell your physician if new symptoms develop after you start taking the drug(s) prescribed.
- Be certain to keep follow-up appointments with your physician; the performance of many drugs must be monitored closely.
- If you go to a second physician, pharmacist, dentist, or other health

care provider, inform him or her of all medications you are taking currently—prescription and nonprescription. Remember any herbal remedies.

When You Obtain Your Prescription Drug(s) From Your Pharmacist

- Read your prescription carefully before submitting it to be filled. Verify that both the **name of the drug** and the **disorder** are specified. If these are not present, ask your pharmacist to contact your physician for permission to add them.
- If your prescription is a refill, verify that the drug issued is identical to the drug in your original supply. If it is not the same, ask your pharmacist to explain the difference. (Generic drug products from different manufacturers often vary in size, shape, color, etc.)
- Be aware that there are over 1,000 drug names that "look alike" in print or "sound alike" in speech. Examples: acetazolamide–acetohexamide, Acutrim–Accutane, Aralen–Arlidin, cyclosporine–cycloserine, Orinase–Ornade, Prilosec–Prozac, Xanax–Zantac. Mistaking one drug for the other can lead to serious dispensing errors. "Sound-alike" drugs are easily confused when a prescription is given by telephone. Since each drug of the pair is used to treat a distinctly different condition, the statement of the **disorder** within the prescription will alert the pharmacist and the patient to the mistake. Many of the most-often prescribed drugs are pictured in the Color Chart insert in this book.
- Ask the pharmacist to give you **printed information sheets** that provide specific information about the drug(s) prescribed for you. A variety of such sources of information geared specifically for the patient are now available to physicians and pharmacists for their patients' use. The information provided is similar to that presented in the Drug Profiles found in Section Two of this book, but usually is less comprehensive and less detailed.
- Read each warning label that the pharmacist attaches to the container—in addition to the main prescription label. These are important reminders regarding the proper use of the drug. They serve to distinguish between eyedrops and eardrops; they identify dosage forms that should not be altered (opened, crushed, or chewed), such as many sustained-release formulations; they provide numerous precautions that improve the effectiveness of your medication.
- If your pharmacist utilizes a computer system that records and analyzes each patient's drug history, take advantage of this excellent tool to prevent serious allergic reactions and significant drug interactions. Inform your pharmacist of all drugs (remember to include herbal remedies, megavitamins, alcohol, and nonprescription agents) you are currently taking.

Your Responsibilities—to Yourself—as a Patient

- Know both the generic and brand name of all drugs prescribed for you.
- If you are taking more than one drug, be sure that the label of each container includes the **name of the drug** and the **condition it treats**.
- Remember that foods can react with medicines. Something as simple as grapefruit juice is now known to interact with some high blood pressure medicines. The best liquid to take with most medicines is water, but not for all. Be aware.
- If you do not clearly understand the directions for using a drug, ask your physician or pharmacist before taking it.
- Remember that many nonprescription medicines were once available only with a prescription. Talk with your pharmacist or physician **BEFORE** combining any nonprescription or prescription medicines.
- Follow all dosing instructions carefully and completely. Comply fully to obtain the maximal benefit the drug can provide. For example, **DO NOT** stop taking an antibiotic 7 days into a 10-day prescription because you feel better. This can lead to serious treatment failure and resistant bacteria. If you have trouble remembering to take your medications on schedule, ask your pharmacist for a dosing calendar or a weekly medication box.
- If you are taking medications prescribed by more than one physician, check the **generic names** of all prescriptions to ensure that you are not taking duplicate drugs with different brand names. This could cause serious overdosage.
- Be certain all drugs you take are "in date"—have not expired according to the dating on the label.
- Consider the effective and timely control of pain a basic right to which you are entitled when you are in the hospital. The Agency for Health Care Policy and Research has released *Clinical Practice Guidelines* which clearly outline the management of cancer pain, but also broadly apply to the management of pain in general. It is reasonable to expect that your pain is responded to with as much care and attention as a high fever from an infection or a dangerously elevated blood pressure.

Suggestions for Containing the Costs of Drug Therapy

- Cooperate fully with your physician to ensure accurate diagnosis so that the initial selection of drugs will be as safe and effective as possible.
- Ask your physician to prescribe the drug that is most appropriate for you, selecting the product which offers the best balance of price and outcomes for you. If there appear to be several options to treat the condition which you are facing, ask your doctor what the expected

outcomes of the various treatments will be. For example, if you are challenged by several chronic diseases at the same time, what appears to be a more expensive therapy may have a better outcome for you than a less costly one. In a patient facing a single infection, unchallenged by other chronic diseases, a less costly, very specific antibiotic may offer an equal outcome and decreased expense.

- Ask your physician if the drug prescribed is available as an acceptable generic product that is less expensive than the brand-name product.
- Ask your doctor if there are any vitamins or minerals (such as folic acid for heart attacks or calcium for osteoporosis) that you should be taking to **PREVENT** a disease or condition for which your physician thinks you may be at risk.
- Comply fully with your physician's instructions regarding how to take the drugs prescribed.

Points for Consideration by the Pharmacist

The pharmacist is in a unique position to enhance and reinforce communication between the patient and the physician relative to the optimal use of drugs. Many pharmacists are being paid for their expertise in medicines (cognitive services) and in Veterans Administration hospitals are even prescribing medicines via guidelines. Many states have given pharmacists the opportunity to provide vaccinations, and large numbers of you are starting to offer them. In a setting where the pressure of time is somewhat less restrictive, the pharmacist is able to focus more on the identification, selection, and utilization of prescription drugs.

Today's pharmacist endorses the FDA initiative to define his or her role and responsibility as counselor to consumers regarding the proper use of medicinal drugs. The FDA's position is that the patient has a right to demand and receive essential drug information, and that the pharmacist should voluntarily initiate the appropriate dialogue to accomplish this. The FDA recommends that **printed information** be dispensed with the prescribed drug to reinforce verbal consultation by the pharmacist. Studies have established that the combined use of verbal consultation and printed information is the most effective means of patient education in drug use.

A study by Cavuto et al. from Georgetown of 50 pharmacies in the Washington, D.C., area must serve as a wake-up call regarding drug interactions. The study presented two prescriptions containing clear and potentially life-threatening drug interactions, yet nearly one-third of the pharmacies filled the prescriptions without comment. In community pharmacies and outpatient hospital or clinic sites, **you** are the final check before the patient gets the medicine. **Guard and value this role** above any distraction or volume of prescriptions which must be filled.

The outcomes of available therapeutic options will be the hallmark of the use of medicines for the future. Pharmacists need to understand the concepts of outcomes research; the FDA will be applying them to patient-directed advertising, physicians will be facing questions about who gets better on what medicine, and you will have a role in retrospective and potentially concurrent drug use review. Disease management and pharmacoeconomical principles will be widely applied.

Some pharmacists have made great inroads in clinical service by helping manage medicines for asthmatics, providing vaccines (where state law allows), offering smoking cessation groups, and helping those requiring anticoagulation. Contact your state board of pharmacy for more information. Many pharmacists are now accepting appointments and charging a fee for cognitive services.

Pharmacists should have a copy of the *Agency for Health Care Policy and Research Clinical Practice Guidelines Number 9* on the management of cancer pain, as well as copies of the patient guide on cancer pain. The Agency for Health Care Policy and Research is advocating effective and timely control of pain as a basic human right. This is a clear opportunity for you to help in offering effective therapeutic options and superb pharmaceutical care. Call 1–800–422–6237 for more information.

When You Fill a Prescription

- Clarify with the prescriber any prescription information that is illegible, uncertain, or a potential source for erroneous interpretation—by you or the patient.
- Be alert to the inherent hazard of "look-alike" and "sound-alike" drug names. This is an ongoing problem that increases with the proliferation of brand names; it is a significant cause of dispensing error. In accepting prescriptions by telephone, ask the caller to spell the name of the drug, as appropriate.
- As the situation warrants (multiple drugs taken concurrently, the older patient, etc.), include both the **name of the drug** and the respective **disorder** on the label. (Examples: Micronase for diabetes; Zantac for ulcer.) If required by jurisdictional regulation, consult the prescribing physician. The inclusion of the **disorder** on the label will serve to (1) reduce potential dispensing error caused by "look-alike" and "sound-alike" drug names; and (2) prevent the confusion that often occurs during the concurrent use of multiple drugs: mistaken identity of drug and purpose, mistakenly altered dosing schedules, etc.
- When needed, use all of the appropriate instructional add-on labels designed to enhance compliance and drug performance. Even

though people seem to understand while you are counseling them, they may forget once they return home.
- Check the stock bottle for accurate identification and appropriate dating. Be certain the appearance of the drug is uniform. If a technician fills the prescription, be certain you open the dispensing container as well as the completed prescription and check the drug personally.

When You Counsel the Patient as You Dispense the Filled Prescription

- If it seems advisable, ask the patient to read all of the labeling on the container. Clarify any points of confusion or misunderstanding.
- Verify that the patient recognizes the **name of the drug** and the **disorder being treated**. Explain what the drug is supposed to do.
- Review with the patient the details of dosing instructions: how much to take, when to take it, and for how long.
- Discuss the possibility of side effects and adverse effects that may occur while taking the drug(s) dispensed. Advise the patient about what to do if any of these occur.
- As appropriate, inform the patient of any precautions to observe while taking the drug. This includes the possibility of interactions with foods, beverages, and other drugs the patient may be taking. Specify any activities that should be avoided or modified.
- Provide **written information** about the drug(s) dispensed and the patient's **disorder** (if available).
- Be certain the patient knows how to store the medication properly. This not only includes refrigeration, but avoiding the humidity of the medicine chest. If any patient requests a non-childproof lid, remind him or her to keep the drug out of reach whenever children are visiting.
- Encourage the patient to call his or her physician if new symptoms develop while taking the medication.
- Remind the patient that nonprescription (over-the-counter) drugs can alter the effects of prescription drugs. Be certain to ask about any herbal remedies or megavitamins the patient may take. Encourage the patient to call your pharmacy or his/her physician whenever guidance is needed in this regard.
- Offer medication calendars or daily/weekly dose holders if you feel that compliance may be a problem. Reinforce the importance of taking medications exactly as directed.
- If your pharmacy utilizes a computerized information system that includes patient profiles (drug histories), invite the patient to participate in this program. Explain the service it provides in detecting possible contraindications and adverse drug effects, notably allergic re-

actions and drug interactions. Some systems provide a "reminder" service to alert patients that they are due for a refill of certain drugs being used for long-term therapy.
- Encourage the patient to ask questions—at the time of dispensing and later—whenever the need arises.

Suggestions for Containing the Costs of Drug Therapy

- As judgment dictates, fill the prescription with the most reasonably priced drug available—within legally possible and appropriate guidelines. Consult with the prescribing physician regarding generic substitution when feasible.
- If the patient is taking other drugs (prescribed by other physicians), explore the possibility of drug duplication—taking the same generic drug under more than one brand name.
- In conjunction with verbal counseling, provide written information designed to enhance patient compliance with dosing instructions.

Points for Consideration by the Physician

Critical paths, outcomes tracking and management, and closed formulary considerations have significantly changed the thinking and basic approach to many therapeutic decisions. I believe that a renewed focus on outcomes simply creates an atmosphere of continuous improvement and is just good medicine. One of the best colleagues to have in attaining the best outcomes from any medicine is a fully informed patient. Michael Weintraub, M.D., recognized this in 1991, when in his introduction to the *Yearbook of Drug Therapy* he stated, "In looking for trends in the medical literature, it is apparent that the need for the physician to be an educator of patients and their families is becoming greater and greater." In addition, citing an increased need for patient education, he summarized with the following opinion: "Treatment principles correctly applied by patients educated about their condition and involved in its management seem to be the wave of the future."

More than ever before, the volume and characteristics of the drugs in use today require deliberate individualization of treatment. The overall effectiveness of any drug therapy depends on how carefully the drug is selected, dispensed, and administered. Responsible communication between physician, pharmacist, nurse, and patient must be achieved to the greatest extent possible. This process begins with the physician.

When You Evaluate a Patient for Drug Therapy

- Review the patient's drug history for known drug allergies and prior drug-induced adverse reactions.
- Determine if the patient is currently under treatment by other health care providers.

- Ask about all drugs used currently—prescription and over-the-counter.
- Many over-the-counter agents were once prescription medicines. This may be a key fact for many of your patients. Make certain that you do not gloss over this aspect of the medicines they can take without ever obtaining your guidance.
- Remember the prevalence of herbal remedy and nutriceutical use. Include these substances in your questions.
- Considering a patient's history and lifestyle, think about diseases or conditions for which the patient is at risk and vitamins (such as folic acid for heart disease and calcium to prevent osteoporosis) or minerals that may be used to prevent the process. Rybacki's first recommendation: It is always better to prevent a disease or condition than to have to treat it once it occurs.
- Make certain that you are absolutely current. Many daily fax services are available which can be individualized to your practice and can easily be read after your morning rounds.
- Establish the nature and severity of the disorder under consideration for drug treatment.
- Elicit significant coexisting disorders—possible absolute contraindications for certain drugs.
- Evaluate any suspected or obvious organ dysfunction—possible relative contraindications for certain drugs. When creatinine values are available, take the time to calculate creatinine clearance. Many drugs have break points for adjustment of dosage at various levels of renal impairment. Even though an older patient's creatinine is within the "normal limits," their clearance will not be. For example, a 72-year-old, 70 kg man with a 1.4 creatinine will have a creatinine clearance of about 48.6 ml/min. This is **below the level where doses or intervals of renally eliminated medicines must be adjusted.** Hepatic disease will also impact doses or intervals for many drugs, particularly those which are highly protein-bound or heavily metabolized.
- Assess the patient's potential for compliance or noncompliance with drug therapy. Remember the expense that a given prescription asks your patient to face. The most brilliant prescription choice is totally ineffective if financial considerations prevent compliance. Once-a-day dosing is much easier for patients to remember, and combined with a dosing calendar gets excellent results.

When Selecting Drugs for Therapy

- Try to match the drug's power to the patient's problem. Avoid overprescribing—medicinal "overkill." For example: Mild to moderate stress reactions (situational anxiety—tension states) respond well to antianxiety drugs; they do not require antipsychotic medication. An uncomplicated urinary tract infection with a broadly sensitive single organism does not require a broad spectrum anti-infective drug.

- Obtain a copy of the *Agency for Health Care Policy and Research Clinical Practice Guidelines Number 9*. The AHCPR is advocating effective and timely pain control as a basic human right. Increase your awareness of the World Health Organization pain ladder and the use of the agents which are primary analgesics and adjuvants. AHCPR publications are great tools to help your patients understand their medicine and their disease.
- Always check for drug–drug, drug–food, and drug–disease interactions. Remember to take a "new" drug history periodically.
- Many new oral anti-infectives are effective against pathogens which historically required intravenous therapy. Although this allows you to avoid hospitalization, it makes the patient's compliance more critical.
- Consider the desired onset of drug action (immediate versus delayed) and the consequences or benefits of that effect.
- Choose the drug with the most favorable benefit/risk ratio: the best clinical effects with the least adverse reactions.
- When you prescribe narrow-therapeutic-window drugs that require periodic blood level determinations, be certain that blood sampling is done after the drug has reached its steady state (usually 5 half-lives). Understand which level is preferable to measure: "peak" level (as for theophylline), "trough" level (as for digoxin), and "peak and trough" for aminoglycosides (such as tobramycin). Many clinical pharmacists (the author included) will willingly calculate the best dose and interval for you, and make a consultative recommendation.
- Give due consideration to the patient's prior experience with other drugs similar to the one you are considering and prescribe accordingly. Prescribing a second drug from the same drug class from which a patient already had an allergic or adverse drug effect that required discontinuation of therapy is not prudent.
- Remember individual patient factors such as age, education, and cultural factors (including genetic effects on medication elimination).
- Think about the desired extent of effect (systemic or local).
- If drug treatment fails after a reasonable trial with good compliance, change to a drug of another chemical class if one is available for the specific disorder, or consider combination therapy with two medicines with different mechanisms of action. For example: if viral load decreases for a time, then increases in an AIDS patient, one of the newer nucleoside analogs and a protease inhibitor are indicated.
- Select the drugs you prescribe critically—utilizing independent, objective reviews of available information. The "most frequently prescribed" drug is not necessarily the best drug within its class. The large volume of a drug's use is frequently a reflection of its maker's marketing strategies and techniques and not an endorsement of any therapeutic advantage. Slick, glossy detail pieces should always be confirmed by primary literature.

- Even "drugs of choice" in objective reviews can be poor choices when you consider the characteristics of individual patients. A renally compromised patient may better tolerate an "alternate drug" with dual elimination (hepatic and renal) than a "drug of choice" that is limited to renal elimination.
- Remember the pharmacokinetic and pharmacodynamic changes that occur in those over 65 can lead to accumulation and excessive responses to "normal" doses and dosing intervals.
- Be objective and discerning as you review the claims made for a newly released drug within a sizable class of drugs already available. Only 20% of newly approved drugs each year are classified by FDA as truly innovative or more advantageous than similar drugs in current use. The remaining 80% are largely "me too" drugs with a limited history of use and a potential for "surprises" after a period of general use. It is advisable to select drugs with established records that show them to be the best within their respective classes.

When You Issue Prescriptions in Writing or by Telephone

- When prescribing for outpatient use, consider the value and advantage of including both the **name of the drug** and the **therapeutic indication** (the patient's disorder) on the prescription label. For example: Cafergot for migraine; Isordil for angina; Sinemet CR for Parkinson's. The inclusion of the disorder on the label will serve to (1) reduce potential dispensing error caused by "look-alike" and "sound-alike" drug names, and (2) prevent the confusion that so often occurs during the concurrent use of multiple drugs, especially among the elderly: mistaken identity of drug and purpose, mistakenly altered dosing schedules, etc.
- Respect your patients' wishes as to whether or not they *want* the name of the disorder written on the prescription label. If they prefer you not include it, recommend that they write it on the label themselves *after* the prescription is filled.
- Keep dosing instructions and schedules as simple as possible. When applicable, once-a-day dosing will do much to improve compliance.
- Alert the pharmacist to "look-alike" and "sound-alike" drug names. Print the drug name on written prescriptions. Spell the drug name when prescribing by telephone.

When Counseling Patients About Drug Therapy

- Briefly explain the nature of the patient's disorder and its treatment. Avoid the use of medical jargon; use language that is readily understood by the average person.
- Provide written information or references for educational material about the disorder. If the disorder is chronic in nature (diabetes, hy-

pertension), explain the need to continue drug therapy indefinitely, possibly for life.

- Briefly explain the name and nature of the drugs you are prescribing. Stress the importance of strict compliance with the instructions given for each medication. It is wise to alert the patient—in advance—to any potential adverse effects that may be characteristic of the drugs you are prescribing. The patient who experiences such effects is more likely to be understanding and forgiving if they do not come as a surprise to them.

- To supplement your discussion, **provide a printed document** that summarizes the essential information the patient needs to use the drug(s) safely and effectively. This is comforting to the patient and will save you an amazing number of telephone calls. Be certain the patient knows what to do if a dose is missed. Explore the feasibility of using an available computerized drug information program that prints out relevant information for your patients to take home. Such services can provide detailed descriptions of drugs, general guidelines for drug use, and personalized instructions.

- Explain the need for follow-up visits to monitor the effects of drug treatment and the course of the disorder.

- Explain that quite often drugs do not work in practice exactly as expected. Inform the patient to be alert to the possibility that a new symptom or sign *may* be drug-related. If one of your patients does experience a novel adverse drug reaction, it is critical that you (or your designate) call the FDA MedWatch at 1–800-332–1088. This fulfills your obligation to Phase Four reporting and makes medication use safer for everyone. Encourage the patient to call as needed regarding any aspect of drug treatment. Recognize the need to adjust drug selection and/or dosage regimens to accommodate individual variability. When altering medication schedules, be certain you adjust the size of the dose and/or the intervals of administration, as appropriate.

- As appropriate, give special attention to the older patient on drug therapy. Because the elderly (1) generally use multiple drugs concurrently, and (2) are more prone to experience adverse drug effects, it is advisable to conduct routine reviews of all drugs being taken each time a new drug is prescribed.

- If you refer any of your patients to a specialist, be certain to take a repeat medication history when they are returned to your care. Check for duplications in medicines by cross-referencing brand or generic names.

- Every six months, ask your patients to bring in all the prescription, nonprescription, and herbal medicines that they routinely take. This kind of "brown bag" session can help you best understand all of the potential or actual interactions of therapies your patient is or will be taking.

Remember: An informed patient can be your greatest ally in optimal therapeutics!

Suggestions for Containing the Costs of Drug Therapy

1. When you have selected the most appropriate drug, consider its cost. Which product of that drug is the most reasonably priced? If the patient requests an available generic product, direct the pharmacist to dispense one with certified bioequivalence. Because of generic product variability, caution the patient to have the prescription refilled with the identical generic (same manufacturer) each time.

2. Avoid polypharmacy whenever possible. Limit the number of drugs that the patient is taking concurrently to the fewest required. Do not let the cure become the disease. Medicate serious, significant disorders; discourage the use of drugs for minor, transient complaints.

3. Consider carefully any requests from patients for a prescription drug they have learned about through direct-to-consumer advertising, especially those with added inducements. Explain to your patients the profit motive of the producer and assure them that you will prescribe the drug that, in your judgment, is the most appropriate for them.

4 When circumstances permit, utilize home intravenous drug therapy in preference to hospitalization.

5. The move toward managed care and other health care reform initiatives brings increased scrutiny to the outcomes of your therapeutic and clinical decisions. Become more familiar with the expense of various medicinal options, as well as the specific patient populations where the benefit-to-risk and cost-to-outcome ratios make the most sense. Pharmacoeconomical and disease management approaches will bring the best balance of cost and outcome.

1

HOW TO USE THIS BOOK

2

GUIDELINES FOR SAFE AND EFFECTIVE DRUG USE

3

TRUE BREAKTHROUGHS IN MEDICINES

1

How to Use This Book

Your physician has advised you to take a drug (or drugs), or you have been directed to give a drug (or drugs) to someone in your care. The kind and amount of information you have been given about how to use these drugs, and what to expect from them, may vary tremendously. In many instances it will not be practical or possible for the physician to provide you with *all* the information that could be considered appropriate and useful, or it will be difficult for you to remember it. The aim of this book is to give you the kind of information you may need to supplement the direction and guidance you receive from your doctor.

The book consists of six sections. The first section will help you to better understand the complexities of modern drug therapy and help you to make the best use of the information contained in Sections Two through Six. An addition to this section is called "True Breakthroughs in Medicines" and will help identify completely new medicines, such as some of those from a prior edition's "The Leading Edge" section which have gained FDA approval. These medicines offer a novel drug molecule or completely new drug package or are the first new agents in many years for an existing disease or condition. These will be followed by full drug profiles in subsequent editions as more information becomes available.

Section Two has detailed Drug Profiles covering more than 300 generic prescription drugs and more than 2,000 brand names used widely in the United States and Canada. The selection of each drug is based upon three considerations: the extent of its use, the urgency of the conditions for which it is prescribed, and the volume and complexity of the information essential to its proper use. Profiles are arranged alphabetically by generic name. Read carefully to be sure you have the correct generic name.

Each Profile is presented in the same way. When you become familiar with the format, you will be able to quickly find specific items of information on any drug, without having to read the entire Profile. Each Drug Profile contains at least 45 categories of information, including:

Year Introduced

This tells you how long the drug has been in general use. The older the drug, the more likely its full spectrum of actions is known and the less likely its continued use will produce new surprises. The date given is the year the drug was introduced for human use anywhere in the world.

Drug Class

This identifies the principal therapeutic class(es) to which the drug belongs. When appropriate, the chemical and/or pharmacological class names are also given. The class is important because many actions, reactions, and interactions with other drugs are often shared by drugs of the same class. Throughout this book you will find reference to drugs by their class designation. (Section Four provides alphabetically arranged listings of the classes of drugs referred to in this guide.)

Prescription Required

This indicates whether a drug is a prescription or a nonprescription (over-the-counter) purchase. This designation can vary by country, hence the designation for each country is given when appropriate.

Controlled Drug

Drugs subject to regulation under the Controlled Substances Act of 1970 (those with abuse potential) are assigned to a specific schedule that governs their dispensing in the United States. A Canadian schedule is also given when applicable. A description of the schedules of controlled drugs is found at the back of this guide.

Available for Purchase by Generic Name

Increasing interest in generic drugs has been prompted by two issues of major significance. The first is concerned with the cost of prescription drugs. In general, costs can be greatly reduced by buying a generic equivalent of a brand-name product. The second issue relates to "bioavailability and bioequivalence"—the comparative composition, quality, and effectiveness of the generic versus the brand-name drug product. Further discussion of bioavailability and bioequivalence will be found in the Glossary, Section Five.

Brand Names

These names confirm that you are looking at the correct Drug Profile. They may also help you recognize a brand name that caused problems for you in the past. Brand names are listed for the United States and for Canada (✦). A combination drug (one with more than one active ingredient) is identified by [CD] following the brand name.

In some cases a name used in both the United States and Canada will represent entirely different generic drugs (in a single drug product), or a significantly different mixture of generic medicines in a combination drug product. The generic composition of such brand-name products is identified by country in the index. If you travel between the two countries, verify that the drug contains the same generic medicine(s).

Benefits versus Risks

This section summarizes the "pros" and "cons" for each drug. The Profiles use capital letters to emphasize the drug's principal benefits and risks, while lowercase letters are used for less critical benefits and risks. One look reveals the "comparative weights" of the two columns and gives an initial impression as to how a drug's benefits relate to its potential risks.

This presentation is not intended to be the principal basis for decision on whether or not to use the drug. Its purpose is to help you become more circumspect and discriminating in your use of drugs. The failure to give adequate attention to the individualization of drug selection and dosage is probably the greatest weakness seen in current drug therapy.

Principal Uses

A drug may be available as a single drug product or in combination with other drugs. In this section under the designation "As a Single Drug Product" are the primary use(s) of the drug when used alone. Under the designation "As a Combination Drug Product [CD]" are the primary use(s) when combined with other active drugs within the same tablet, capsule, etc. The uses stated are those determined by consensus within the medical community and substantiated by current scientific study. Combination drugs have been developed because some conditions have more than one cause, are characterized by a variety of symptoms, or may be treated in more than one way. Where appropriate, the logic for combining certain drugs to enhance their therapeutic value is explained. When you find the designation for combination drugs [CD] in the "Brand Names" list at the beginning of the Drug Profile, look under the "Principal Uses" section to learn more about the drug's role in combination products.

How This Drug Works

This simplified explanation is limited to how the drug acts to produce its principal (intended) therapeutic effect(s). If a specific method of action has not been established, the currently held theory is given.

Available Dosage Forms and Strengths

This represents a composite of available manufacturers' dosage forms (tablets, capsules, elixirs, etc.) and strengths, without company identification. Included are those dosage forms appropriate for use by outpatients and in extended care facilities and nursing homes. Dosage forms limited to hospital use are not included. Refer to Dosage Forms and Strengths in the Glossary for an explanation of those few abbreviations used to designate the strengths of each dosage form.

Usual Adult Dosage Range

The dosage information given represents a carefully derived consensus by appropriate authorities and is the currently recommended standard. It is provided as a guide that indicates the amount of the drug that is reasonably expected to be both effective and safe when properly used for its intended purpose. Under certain circumstances, your physician may elect to modify this "standard" dosage scheme. Adhere strictly to his or her prescribed dosages and schedules.

Conditions Requiring Dosing Adjustments

This section provides you with the latest information on conditions which require adjustments in the medicine dose or dosing. Problems in eliminating medicines from the body are surprisingly common causes of adverse drug effects. This is also a waste of money and may result in serious injury and hospitalization. If you have any compromise in kidney or liver function it is critical to ask your doctor if the medicine dose has been adjusted for it.

Dosing Instructions

Specific guidance is given here regarding the timing of oral medication with regard to food intake. In addition, there are occasions when an individual finds it difficult or impossible to swallow a tablet or a capsule, and the drug to be taken is not available in a liquid dosage form. On those occasions when the patient's condition urgently requires the medication, one may wish to crush the tablet or open the capsule and mix the contents with a palatable food or beverage for administration. Many of today's drugs are available in a bewildering array of solid dosage forms, some of which should *not* be altered to accommodate administration. This information category identifies those dosage forms of each drug that may be and those that should not be altered for administration. In addition, your pharmacist can provide appropriate guidance if you should need it.

Usual Duration of Use

Many factors influence the period of time required for any drug to exert beneficial effects: the nature and severity of the symptoms being treated, the formulation and strength of the drug, the presence or absence of food in the stomach, the ability of the patient to respond, and the concurrent use of other drugs, among others. The focus here is to prevent premature termination of medication in treatment situations where improvement may seem to you to be unreasonably slow. Where appropriate, limitations in the duration of use are given.

This Drug Should Not Be Taken If

These are the *absolute* contraindications to the use of the drug (see Contraindications in Glossary). It is most important that you alert your physician or dentist if any information in this category applies to you.

Inform Your Physician Before Taking This Drug If

This category lists the *relative* contraindications to the use of the drug. Here again, it is important that you communicate all relevant information to your physician or dentist.

Possible Side Effects

This category describes the natural, expected, and usually unavoidable actions of the drug—the normal and anticipated consequences of taking it. It is important to maintain a realistic perspective that balances the occurrence of side effects and the goals of treatment. Consult your physician for guidance whenever side effects are troublesome or distressing, so that appropriate adjustments of your treatment program can be made.

Possible Adverse Effects

This category includes those unusual, unexpected, and infrequent drug effects that are commonly referred to as adverse drug reactions. For the sake of evaluation, adverse effects are classified as mild or serious in nature. It is always wise to inform your physician as soon as you have reason to suspect you may be experiencing an adverse drug effect. Serious adverse reactions usually announce their development initially in the form of mild, unthreatening symptoms. It is important that you remain alert to significant changes in your well-being when you are taking a drug that is known to be capable of producing a serious adverse effect. It is also possible to experience an adverse reaction that has not yet been reported. Do not discount the possibility of an adverse effect just because it is not listed in this category. Following standard practice, some adverse reactions (and interactions) of certain drugs are listed as a precaution, because these reactions are associated with the use of a particular class of drugs. Although the literature may not document such reactions in connection with the use of an individual drug within that class, the possibility of their occurrence must be considered.

A word of caution is appropriate here. You have consulted your physician for medical evaluation and management. He or she has advised you to take a drug (or administer it to someone else). It is important that you recognize and understand that *in the vast majority of instances a properly selected drug has a comparatively small chance of producing serious harm.* Most of the drugs included in this book rarely produce serious adverse effects. Knowledge that a drug is capable of causing a serious adverse reaction should not deter you from using it when it has been properly selected and its use will be carefully supervised.

Possible Effects on Sexual Function

The growing interest and concern of the medical community and the general public regarding the potential effects of many drugs on sexual function justify this designated category for the provision of relevant information. This aspect of drug performance has not received the professional scrutiny or public disclosure commensurate with its importance. Currently available information (often inadequate and vague) from all reliable sources is presented for consideration. In the interest of compliance and effective management, both physician and patient are well advised to discuss frankly the full significance of any potential effect that proposed drug therapy could have on all aspects of sexual expression.

Adverse Effects That May Appear Similar to Natural Diseases or Disorders

The failure to recognize that a given symptom or disorder is actually drug-induced occurs with surprising frequency. Quite often this inadvertent error is compounded by the administration of yet another drug to relieve the "symptoms" (unrecognized manifestations) of a drug being taken on a regular basis. For milder symptoms (e.g., the nasal congestion and diarrhea caused by reserpine), the oversight may not be too serious. But in the case of Parkinson-like effects of some drugs, the mistake can be devastating. This category can alert you to this common flaw in the management of drug therapy.

Natural Diseases or Disorders That May Be Activated by This Drug

Similar to the situation described in the previous category, many drugs in common use are capable of "activating" latent disorders that may not be recognized as drug-induced. The development of a new and seemingly unrelated disorder during the course of any treatment program should arouse suspicion that it may be drug-related.

Possible Effects on Laboratory Tests

Most of the drugs in current use have multiple and significant effects on body chemistry and organ system functions. Some of these effects are intended and beneficial (therapeutic); others are unintended, unavoidable, and potentially harmful. Many of these effects can be detected and evaluated by a variety of specific laboratory tests. The timely use of appropriate tests enables the physician to monitor the performance of a drug and the course of the condition being treated. The tests included in this category are limited to those of practical importance for effective physician-patient communication and cooperation in managing the use of certain drugs. Knowledge of selected test results can greatly enhance the patient's understanding and skill in the proper use of medications.

Caution

This category provides information on certain aspects of drug action and/or drug use that require special emphasis. Occasionally these warnings may relate to information provided in other categories. When included here, such entries are of sufficient importance to warrant repetition.

Precautions for Use by Infants and Children

In addition to mandatory adjustments of drug dosage for infants and children under twelve years of age, some drugs and/or treatment situations call for special precautions. This category provides such information for selected drugs. When administering *any* prescription or over-the-counter drug, it is advisable to ask the attending physician about precautions to observe or procedures to follow.

Precautions for Use by Those Over 60 Years of Age

Changes in body composition and function occur naturally as part of normal aging. As would be expected, there is enormous individual variation in the speed with which such changes occur and the degree of these changes. With regard to medical management—and to drug therapy in particular—the assessment of one's "age" must be based upon the individual's mental and physical condition and never upon years alone. In general, however, it should be recognized that changes that accompany aging may affect the actions of the body on the drug, as well as the actions of the drug on the body. Appropriate precautions are outlined in this category.

Advisability of Use During Pregnancy: Pregnancy Category

Information regarding the safe use of a particular drug during pregnancy was one of the most forceful concerns that led to the formal petitioning of the Food and Drug Administration in 1975 for the provision of such guidance to the public. The FDA definitions of the five pregnancy categories are listed at the back of this book. It should be noted that the FDA does not make the initial category assignment; this is the responsibility of the manufacturer that markets the drug. The initial designation is then subject to review and modification by the FDA as deemed appropriate. The "Pregnancy Category" designations presented in each Profile were determined by the author after thorough review of pertinent literature and consultation with appropriate authorities. They are offered at this time for initial guidance only. They are in no sense "official" and do not have the endorsement of either the manufacturer or the FDA.

Advisability of Use If Breast-Feeding

Information presented here includes what could be ascertained regarding the effects of the drug on milk production, the presence of the drug in human milk, and the possible effects of the drug on the nursing infant. Prudent recommendations are given where appropriate.

Suggested Periodic Examinations While Taking This Drug

This category lists those examinations your physician may recommend you undergo while taking the drug(s) he or she has prescribed, in order to monitor your reaction to them and the course of your condition. You should remember that the advisability of performing such examinations varies greatly from one situation to another, and is best left to the judgment of your physician. The selection and timing of examinations are based on many variables, including your past and present medical history, the nature of the condition under treatment, the dosage and anticipated duration of drug use, and your physician's observations of your response to treatment. There may be many occasions when he or she will feel no examinations are necessary.

To assure optimal results from drug treatment, it is important that you keep your physician informed of all developments you think may be drug-related. If you are concerned you won't accurately remember everything at your next scheduled visit, continually make notes and review your notes with your doctor during your appointment.

While Taking This Drug, Observe the Following: Marijuana Smoking

The widespread "social" use of marijuana by virtually all age groups has led to inquiries regarding the possibility of interactions between the pharmacologically active chemicals in marijuana smoke and medicinal drugs in common use. Currently available literature on the health aspects of marijuana use contains very little practical information concerning the potential for drug interactions. The limited information presented in this category of selected Drug Profiles represents those *possible interactions* that are considered likely to occur in view of the known pharmacological effects of the principal components of marijuana and of the medicinal drug reviewed in the Profile. In most instances, the interaction statements are not based on documented evidence since very little is available. However, the conclusions stated—derived by logical inductive reasoning—represent the concurrence of authorities with expertise in this field.

While Taking This Drug, Observe the Following: Other Drugs

For clarification of this confusing and often controversial area of drug information, this category is divided into five subcategories of possible interactions between drugs. Observe carefully the wording of each sub-category heading (see also Interaction in Glossary). Some of the drugs listed as possible interactants do not have a representative Profile. If you are using one of these drugs, consult your physician or pharmacist for guidance regarding potential interactions. A brand name (or names) that follows the generic name of an interacting drug is given for purposes of illustration only. It is not intended to mean that the particular brand(s) named have interactions that are different from other brands of the same generic drug. If you are taking the generic drug, *all* brand names under which it is marketed are to be considered as possible interactants.

Driving, Hazardous Activities

In addition to driving motor vehicles, the information in this category applies to any activity of a dangerous nature, such as operating machinery, working on ladders, using power tools, and handling weapons.

Aviation Note

Until the publication of Dr. Stanley Mohler's *Medication and Flying: A Pilot's Drug Guide* in 1982, there was no authoritative source of current drug information written specifically to serve the needs of civil aviation. Military pilots enjoy the expert guidance and surveillance provided by the flight surgeon, but no tightly structured control system exists for their civilian counterparts. However, the need for practical information regarding the possible effects of medicinal drugs on flight performance is the same for pilots in all settings. This category is designed to inform the civilian pilot how a particular drug may affect his or her eligibility to fly and when it is advisable or necessary to consult a designated Aviation Medical Examiner or an FAA medical officer.

Occurrence of Unrelated Illness

This relates to those drugs that require careful regulation of daily doses to maintain a constant drug effect within critical limits, such as anticoagulants, antidiabetic medication, and digitalis. Emphasis is given to those interim illnesses, separate from the condition for which the drug has been prescribed, that might affect the established schedule of drug use.

Discontinuation

This aspect of drug use is often overlooked when a plan of drug therapy is first discussed. However, for some drugs it is mandatory that the patient be fully informed on *when* to discontinue, when *not* to discontinue, and precisely *how* to discontinue use of the drug.

Another consideration in discontinuation is the need to adjust the dosage schedules of other drugs being taken concurrently. The physician who is primarily responsible for your overall management must be kept informed of *all* the drugs you are taking at a given time.

The remaining information categories in the Drug Profile are self-explanatory.

Section Three is a new section which offers what are in the author's opinion those medicines that show great promise and are just over the horizon from FDA approval. Some of these medicines may not actually attain approval, but they give significant hope that they are worth consideration. The information may actually allow patients facing serious diseases to request to be included in scientific studies and obtain the medicine prior to actual approval.

Section Four is a presentation of Drug Classes arranged alphabetically according to their chemical or therapeutic class designation. The drugs within each class are listed alphabetically by their generic names. Because of their chemical composition and biological activities some drugs appear in two or more classes. For example, the drug product with the brand name Diuril will be represented by its generic name, chlorothiazide, in three drug classes: the Thiazide Diuretics (a chemical classification), the Diuretics (a drug action classification) and the Antihypertensives (a disease-oriented classification).

Frequently in the Drug Profiles in Section Two you are advised to "see (a particular) Drug Class." This alerts you to a possible contraindication for drug use, or to possible interactions with certain foods, alcohol, or other drugs. In each case, you can determine the more readily recognized brand names for each drug listed generically within a drug class by consulting the appropriate Drug Profile. Timely use of these references will enable you to avoid many possible hazards of medication.

Section Five is a glossary of drug-related terms used throughout the book. The preferred use of each term is explained. Frequent references to the Glossary are made in the Drug Profiles. Use of the Glossary will increase your understanding of how to recognize and interpret significant drug effects.

Section Six consists of tables of drug information. The title and introductory material explain the content and purpose of each table. The information in the tables is drawn from certain information categories in the Profiles and is rearranged to emphasize pertinent aspects of drug behavior. The tables are intended to provide another source of ready reference.

The index of brand and generic names in the back of the book is a single alphabetical listing that provides page references to the appropriate Drug Profile(s) for all drugs found in this book. Its usefulness will be enhanced if you first read the introductory explanation of the special features of this combined index.

2

Guidelines for Safe
and Effective Drug Use

DO NOT

- pressure your doctor to prescribe drugs that, in his or her judgment, you do not need. A pill is not always the answer.
- assume that all doctors automatically know all the drugs you take. Ask your doctor about nonprescription drugs you intend to take at the same time that you are taking drugs he or she prescribed.
- take prescription drugs on your own or on the advice of friends and neighbors because your symptoms are "just like theirs." Drug therapy must be individualized—based on liver and/or kidney function, medicines you currently take, and many other important factors.
- offer drugs prescribed for you to anyone else without a physician's guidance.
- change the dose or timing of any drug without the advice of your physician (except when the drug appears to be causing adverse effects).
- continue to take a drug that you feel is causing adverse effects, until you are able to reach your physician for clarification.
- store your medicines in a bathroom medicine cabinet. This is often an area of high humidity which can (even though the bottle is closed) enter the medicine and degrade the active drug. Select a kitchen cabinet out of reach of children for medication storage.
- take *any* drug (prescription or nonprescription) while pregnant or nursing an infant until you are assured by your physician that no harmful effects will occur to either mother or child. Remember that many herbal combinations may have active ingredients similar to those found in prescription medicines.
- take any more medicines than are absolutely necessary. (The greater

11

the number of drugs taken simultaneously, the greater the likelihood of adverse effects.)
- withhold from your physician important information about previous prescription or nonprescription drug experiences. He or she will want to know both beneficial and undesirable drug effects you have had.
- take any drug in the dark. Identify every dose of medicine carefully in adequate light to be certain you are taking the drug intended.
- keep drugs on a bedside table. Drugs for emergency use, such as nitroglycerin, are an exception. It is advisable to have only one such drug at the bedside for use during the night.

DO

- know the name (and correct spelling) of the drug(s) you are taking. It is best to know both the brand name and the generic name.
- read the package labels of all nonprescription drugs to become familiar with the contents of the product.
- follow the prescribed dosing schedules as closely as possible. Notify your doctor if it becomes necessary to make major changes in your treatment routine.
- thoroughly shake all liquid suspensions of drugs to ensure uniform distribution of ingredients.
- use a standardized measuring device for giving liquid medications by mouth. The household "teaspoon" varies greatly in size.
- follow your doctor's guidance on dietary and other measures designed to augment the actions of the drugs prescribed such as decreasing or eliminating salt from the diet when taking drug treatment for high blood pressure. This may help achieve desired drug effects with smaller doses.
- tell your anesthesiologist, surgeon, and dentist of *all* drugs you are taking, before any surgery.
- inform your doctor if you become pregnant while you are taking any drugs from any source.
- keep a written record of *all* drugs (prescription and nonprescription), vaccines, and herbal remedies you take during your entire pregnancy— name, dose, dates taken, and reasons for use.
- keep a written record of *all* drugs (and vaccines) to which you become allergic or experience an adverse reaction. This should be done for each member of the family, especially the elderly and infirm.
- keep a written record of *all* drugs (and vaccines) to which *your children* become allergic or experience an adverse reaction.
- fill out "Your Personal Drug Profile" (Table 14). Get the number of your Poison Control Center **today** and post it by your telephone. The worst time to try to find an emergency number is while there is a dire need for it.
- tell your doctor of all known or suspected allergies, especially allergies

to drugs. Be sure that allergies are a part of your medical record because people with allergies are four times more prone to drug reactions.

- call your doctor immediately if you think you are having an overdose, side effect, or an adverse effect from a drug.
- ask if it is safe to drive a car, operate machinery, or engage in other hazardous activities while taking the drug(s) prescribed.
- ask if it is safe to drink alcoholic beverages while taking the drug(s) prescribed. We often forget that alcohol is a drug with its own pharmacology and drug–drug interactions.
- determine if any particular foods, beverages, or other prescription or nonprescription medicines should be avoided while taking the drug(s) prescribed.
- keep all appointments for follow-up examinations or laboratory tests.
- ask for help to understand any point that confuses you. If you are concerned about remembering information or instructions for use, ask for written materials.
- throw away all outdated drugs.
- store all drugs to be retained for intermittent use out of the reach of children to prevent accidental poisoning. This is critical for those of you with grandchildren who visit infrequently.

PREVENTING ADVERSE DRUG REACTIONS

For the most part, we cannot identify with certainty the person who is at greater risk of experiencing a true adverse effect. Available tests for the early detection of toxicity are of definite value, but they do not provide as full a measure of protection as we could wish.

As our understanding of drug actions and reactions has expanded, we learned that many adverse effects are, to some extent, predictable and preventable. Several contributing factors are now well recognized, and specific recommendations exist to guide both physician and patient. These fall into 11 categories of consideration.

Previous Adverse Reaction to a Drug

Patients who have experienced an adverse drug reaction in the past are more likely to have adverse reactions to other drugs, even though the drugs are unrelated. This suggests that some people may have a genetic (inborn) predisposition to unusual or abnormal drug responses. *The patient should tell the physician of any history of prior adverse drug experiences*.

Allergies

Some people are allergic by nature (have hay fever, asthma, eczema, hives) and are more likely to develop allergies to drugs than are nonallergic individuals. The allergic patient must be watched very closely for the earliest indication of a developing hypersensitivity to any drug. Known drug allergies must be noted in the medical record. The patient must inform every health care provider that he or she is allergic by nature and is allergic to specific drugs by name. *The patient should provide this information without waiting to be asked*. Your doctor will then be able to avoid prescribing those drugs that could provoke an allergic reaction, as well as related drugs to which the patient may have developed a cross-sensitivity.

Contraindications

Both patient and physician must strictly observe all known contraindications to any drug under consideration. *Absolute contraindications* include those conditions and situations that prohibit the use of the drug for any reason. *Relative contraindications* are those conditions that, in the judgment of the physician, do not preclude the use of the drug altogether, but make it essential that special care be given to its use to prevent the intensification of preexisting disease or the development of new disease. Often, dosing adjustments, additional supportive measures, and close supervision are needed.

Precautions in Use

Patients should know any special precautions needed while taking a drug. This includes advisability of use during pregnancy or while nursing; precautions on sun exposure (or ultraviolet lamps); avoidance of extreme heat or cold, heavy physical exertion, etc.

Dosage

It is important to take the medicine exactly as prescribed. *This is most important with those drugs that have narrow margins of safety.* Even once-a-day medications should be taken at the same time of day or night to ensure the most constant blood drug levels. Call your doctor if circumstances (nausea, vomiting, diarrhea) interfere with taking the drug as prescribed.

Interactions

Some drugs can interact unfavorably with certain foods (including vitamins and some herbal remedies), alcohol, and other drugs (prescription and nonprescription) to produce serious adverse effects. *The patient must be told about all likely interactants* that could alter the action of the drug he or she is using. If, during the course of treatment, the patient has reason to feel he or she has discovered a new interaction of importance, tell your doctor so that its full significance can be determined.

Warning Symptoms

Many drugs will produce symptoms that are early indications of a developing adverse effect: for example, appearance of severe headaches and visual disturbances *before* the occurrence of a stroke in a woman taking oral contraceptives. *It is imperative that the patient be familiar with those symptoms and signs that could be early indicators of impending adverse reactions*. The patient is then empowered to act in his or her own behalf by calling their doctor **before** taking another dose of their medicine.

Examinations to Monitor Drug Effects

Many drugs in common use can damage vital body tissues (such as bone marrow, liver, kidney, eye structures, etc.)—especially when these drugs are used for a long time or are taken in high doses. Sometimes these adverse effects are not discovered until a newly approved drug has been in wide use for a long time. As our knowledge of such effects accumulates, we learn which kinds of drugs (by chemical structures) are most likely to produce such tissue reactions. We then know which drugs should be monitored closely to detect any tissue damage as early as possible. This damage may be reversible if found quickly. *The patient should cooperate fully with their doctor when he or she asks for periodic exams to check for adverse drug effects*.

Advanced Age and Debility

When we age or as some disease processes progress, decreasing functional capacity of vital organs can greatly influence the body's response to drugs. These patients often poorly tolerate drugs with inherent toxic potential and frequently need smaller doses at longer intervals. *The effects of drugs on the elderly and severely ill are often unpredictable*. Great care must be taken to prevent or minimize adverse effects.

Appropriate Drug Choice

The use of any medicine is always a benefit-to-risk decision. The medication used should offer the patient the best balance of overall cost (including lab tests) and outcomes (including quality of life). Many adverse reactions can be prevented if both physician and patient exercise good judgment and restraint.

Polypharmacy

Unfortunately, the cure can become the disease. Patients who are cared for by several physicians may end up with several drugs prescribed separately by more than one physician for different disorders—often without appropriate communication between patient and prescriber. This frequent practice can lead to serious drug–drug interactions. *The patient should routinely talk to* **each** *health care provider about all the drugs—prescription and nonprescription—that he or she may be taking at the time.* It is **mandatory** that each prescriber has this information before prescribing additional drugs.

DRUGS AND THE ELDERLY

Advancing age brings changes in structure and function that can significantly change the action of drugs. An impaired digestive system may interfere with drug absorption. Declines in liver and kidney ability to metabolize and eliminate drugs may result in toxic drug levels. We slowly lose the ability to maintain a "steady state" (homeostasis), and face increased sensitivity of many tissues to the actions of drugs, and altered responsiveness of the nervous and circulatory systems to typical drug doses. If aging causes deterioration of understanding, memory, vision, or physical coordination, people with such impairments may not always use drugs safely and effectively.

Adverse reactions to drugs occur three times more frequently in the older population. An unwanted drug response can change a functioning and independent older person with marginal health and reserves into a confused, incompetent, or helpless patient. For these reasons, drug treatment in the elderly must **always** be accompanied by the most careful consideration of the individual's health and tolerances. Once-daily dosing may be the only viable option.

Guidelines for the Use of Drugs by the Elderly

- Be certain that drug treatment is necessary. Many health problems of the elderly can be managed without the use of drugs.
- Avoid (if possible) the use of many drugs at one time.
- Dosing schedules should be as simple as possible. Once a medicine is selected, ask your doctor if a once- or twice-a-day formulation is available and appropriate.
- Treatment with most drugs is usually best begun by using smaller than standard doses. Maintenance doses should also be individualized. A maintenance dose is often smaller for persons over 60 years of age than for younger persons.
- Avoid large tablets and capsules if other dosage forms are available. Liquid preparations are easier for the elderly or debilitated to swallow.
- Have all drug containers labeled with the drug name and directions for use in large, easy-to-read letters.
- Ask the pharmacist to package drugs in easy-to-open containers. Avoid "child-proof" caps and stoppers.
- Do not take any drug in the dark. Identify each dose of medicine carefully in adequate light to be certain you are taking the drug intended.
- To avoid taking the wrong drug or an extra dose, do not keep drugs on

a bedside table. Drugs for emergency use, such as nitroglycerin, are an exception. It is advisable to have only one such drug at the bedside for use during the night.

• Drug use by older persons may require supervision. Observe drug effects continuously to ensure safe and effective use.

• Remember the adage: "Start low, go slow, and (when appropriate) learn to say no."

Drugs Best Avoided by the Elderly Because of Increased Possibility of Adverse Reactions

antacids (high sodium)*
barbiturates*
benzodiazepines
 (long-acting)
cyclophosphamide

diethylstilbestrol
estrogens
indomethacin
monoamine oxidase
 (MAO) inhibitors*

oxyphenbutazone
phenacetin
phenylbutazone
tetracyclines*

Drugs That Should Be Used by the Elderly in Reduced Dosages Until Full Effect Has Been Determined

anticoagulants (oral)*
antidepressants*
antidiabetic drugs*
antihistamines*
antihypertensives*
anti-inflammatory drugs*
barbiturates*
beta-blockers*
colchicine

cortisonelike drugs*
digitalis preparations*
diuretics* (all types)
ephedrine
epinephrine
haloperidol
isoetharine
nalidixic acid

narcotic drugs
prazosin
pseudoephedrine
quinidine
sleep inducers
 (hypnotics)*
terbutaline
thyroid preparations

Drugs That May Cause Confusion and Behavioral Disturbances in the Elderly

acyclovir
albuterol
amantadine
anticholinergics*
antidepressants*
antidiabetic drugs*
antihistamines*
anti-inflammatory drugs*
asparaginase
atropine* (and drugs
 containing belladonna)
barbiturates*
benzodiazepines*
beta-blockers*

bromocriptine
carbamazepine
cimetidine
digitalis preparations*
diuretics*
ergoloid mesylates
famotidine
haloperidol
levodopa
meprobamate
methocarbamol
methyldopa
narcotic drugs

nizatidine
pentazocine
phenytoin
primidone
quinidine
reserpine
ranitidine
sedatives
sleep inducers
 (hypnotics)*
thiothixene
tranquilizers (mild)*
trihexyphenidyl

Drugs That May Cause Orthostatic Hypotension in the Elderly

antidepressants*	neuroleptics*	selegiline
antihypertensives*	phenothiazines*	tranquilizers (mild)*
diuretics* (all types)	sedatives	vasodilators*

Drugs That May Cause Sluggishness, Unsteadiness, and Falling in the Elderly

barbiturates*	diazepam	methyldopa
beta-blockers*	diphenhydramine	prazepam
chlordiazepoxide	flurazepam	sleep inducers
clorazepate	halazepam	(hypnotics)*

Drugs That May Cause Constipation and/or Retention of Urine in the Elderly

acebutolol	calcium	ketorolac
amantadine	cholestyramine	metoclopramide
amiodarone	epinephrine	narcotic drugs
androgens	ergoloid mesylates	phenothiazines*
anticholinergics*	famotidine	ranitidine
antidepressants*	iron (some forms)	sucralfate
antiparkinsonism drugs*	isoetharine	terbutaline
atropinelike drugs*		

Drugs That May Cause Loss of Bladder Control (Urinary Incontinence) in the Elderly

diuretics* (all types)	(hypnotics)*	tranquilizers (mild)*
sedatives	tacrine	
sleep inducers	thioridazine	

THERAPEUTIC DRUG MONITORING
(Measuring Drug Levels in Blood)

The routine use of measuring drug levels in blood as an aid in managing drug therapy has evolved gradually since the early 1970s. Because individuals vary greatly in the nature and degree of their responses to drugs, it became apparent that greater precision in determining the best dose for each individual was needed. For many drugs, the clinical response seen by the physician clearly show that the drug is working as intended and that the dosage scheme is satisfactory. However, for some drugs—especially those with narrow safety margins—toxic reactions may closely resemble the symptoms of the disorder being treated. In many instances the pa-

*See Drug Class, Section Four.

tient's expected response is not in keeping with his or her clinical condition or program of drug therapy. By measuring the blood levels of certain drugs at appropriate times, the physician or clinical pharmacist can adjust dosing schedules more accurately, predict drug response more precisely, reduce the risk of toxicity, and achieve the best outcomes. Some medications require both a peak and trough level to ensure best results. The timing of the blood samples is critical. Sampling should be avoided during the two hours following oral administration; during this absorption period, blood levels do not represent tissue levels of the drug, and the tissue is where antibiotics actually work. The peak, or highest, level of the drug can measure several things: how effectively bacteria are killed or toxic levels within the body, for instance. The trough, or lowest, level tells how effectively the antibiotic is cleared from the body between doses. This can be important because if too much remains toxicity can result; if too little remains the bacteria may not be killed.

The following drugs are those most suitable for therapeutic drug monitoring. If you are using any of these on a regular basis, ask your doctor about the need for periodic measurement of drug levels in your blood. These numbers are ranges where effects are *usually* seen, but people react differently. The therapeutic ranges listed are not absolute fixed levels where lack of effect or toxicity definitely occur. Some have a therapeutic response at a level lower than the low end of the range. Generally in this case, the level should be followed closely and left alone. Correspondingly, a blood level higher than the high end of the range is not always toxic—but, as it means a level higher than desirable, dosing changes should be made. Fortunately most physicians "treat the patient, not the level."

Generic Name/Brand Name	Blood Level Range
acetaminophen/Tylenol, etc.	10–20 mcg/ml
amikacin/Amikin	12–25 mcg/ml (peak)
	5–10 mcg/ml (trough)
amitriptyline/Elavil, etc.	120–250 ng/ml
(combined with nortriptyline)	
amoxapine/Asendin	200–500 ng/ml
aspirin (other salicylates)	100–250 mcg/ml
carbamazepine/Tegretol	5–10 mcg/ml
chloramphenicol/Chloromycetin	10–25 mcg/ml
chlorpromazine/Thorazine	50–300 ng/ml
ciprofloxacin/Cipro	0.94–3.4 mcg/ml
clonazepam/Klonopin	10–50 ng/ml
cyclosporine/Sandimmune	100–150 ng/ml
desipramine/Norpramin, Pertofrane	150–300 ng/ml
digitoxin/Crystodigin	15–30 ng/ml
digoxin/Lanoxin	0.5–2.0 ng/ml
diltiazem/Cardizem	100–200 ng/ml
disopyramide/Norpace	2.0–4.5 mcg/ml
doxepin/Adapin, Sinequan	100–275 ng/ml

Generic Name/Brand Name	Blood Level Range
ethosuximide/Zarontin	40–100 mcg/ml
flecainide/Tambocor	0.2–1.0 mcg/ml
flucytosine/Ancobon	50–100 mcg/ml
gentamicin/Garamycin	4.0–10 mcg/ml (peak)
	less than 2 mcg/ml (trough)
gold salts/Auranofin, etc.	1.0–2.0 mcg/ml
imipramine/Janimine, Tofranil, etc.	150–300 ng/ml
kanamycin/Kantrex	25–35 mcg/ml
lidocaine/Xylocaine, etc.	2.0–5.0 mcg/ml
lithium/Lithobid, Lithotabs, etc.	0.3–1.3 mEq/L
mephobarbital/Mebaral	1–7 mcg/ml
methotrexate/Mexate	up to 0.1 mcmol/L
methsuximide/Celontin	up to 1.0 mcg/ml
metoprolol/Lopressor	20–200 ng/ml
mexiletine/Mexitil	0.75–2.0 mcg/ml
nifedipine/Procardia	25–100 ng/ml
nortriptyline/Aventyl, Pamelor	50–150 ng/ml
combined with amitriptyline	125–250 ng/ml
phenobarbital/Luminal, etc.	10–25 mcg/ml
phenytoin/Dilantin	10–20 mcg/ml
primidone/Mysoline	6–12 mcg/ml
procainamide/Pronestyl	4–10 mcg/ml
(NAPA metabolite)	4–10 mcg/ml
propranolol/Inderal	50–100 ng/ml
protriptyline/Vivactil	70–250 ng/ml
quinidine/Quinaglute, etc.	1.0–4.0 mcg/ml
(specific to quinidine test method)	
sulfadiazine/Microsulfon	100–120 mcg/ml
sulfamethoxazole/Gantanol	90–100 mcg/ml
theophylline/Aminophylline, etc.	10–20 mcg/ml
thioridazine/Mellaril	50–300 ng/ml
tobramycin/Nebcin	4.0–10 mcg/ml (peak)
	less than 2 mcg/ml (trough)
tocainide/Tonocard	5–12 mcg/ml
trimethadione/Tridione	10–30 mcg/ml
trimethoprim/Proloprim	1–3 mcg/ml
valproic acid/Depakene	50–100 mcg/ml
vancomycin/Vancocin	30–40 mcg/ml (peak)
	5–10 mcg/ml (trough)
verapamil/Calan	50–200 ng/ml

3

True Breakthroughs in Medicines

One of the continuing wonders of science, and of the many talented people who labor in its laboratories, are the constant advances being made in available medications. This section is offered to help you find out about some of them. Medicines which have recently been FDA-approved or offer novel approaches to treatment, or truly new uses of existing medicine are covered. I want to distinguish here between the "me too" products, which may be simply minor structural changes to an existing medicine made by a manufacturer in order to broaden a product line, from forward-looking advances that help make certain you are getting the latest treatment.

PROTEASE INHIBITORS

This new class of medicines used in the treatment of AIDS interferes with the ability of the virus to be made, resulting in noninfectious virus being released. The first study to look at combination treatment using indinavir (Crixivan), zidovudine, and lamivudine revealed a *huge decrease in viral load* and a *significant increase in protective CD4 cells*. More recent data also support the idea that this combination provides these benefits for a sustained period. The other currently available protease inhibitors are saquinavir (Invirase) and ritonavir (Norvir). Saquinavir in combination with zalcitabine showed a significant decrease in death from AIDS when compared to either agent used alone.

NALTREXONE

Naltrexone (ReVia) is an example of a new use for an older medicine and represents a totally new approach to treatment for people who have difficulty controlling their drinking. Exactly how naltrexone does this is uncertain, but it appears to decrease the craving for alcohol. Previously, a combination of counseling and aversive therapy (including other drugs that caused vomiting) were the available options. Naltrexone offers a level of control and more appealing treatment than was previously available.

ALENDRONATE

This new bisphosphonate was featured in last year's "Leading Edge" section, and has since gained FDA approval. Under the brand name Fosamax, this medicine is the first to show a significant increase in the amount of bone as well as a significant decrease in risk of fracture in patients who have gone through menopause. The medicine does not yet have FDA approval for prevention of osteoporosis, but the extension of alendronate for this purpose appears logical.

ACARBOSE

Acarbose (under the brand name Precose) is the first novel approach to gain approval in many years for managing diabetes in patients who do not require insulin. This drug is an alpha-glucosidase inhibitor, and as such works in a way unlike other currently available medicines. It appears to work by delaying the digestion of dietary sugar as well as the absorption of sugar or glucose from the diet. Acarbose can also be used in combination with existing sulfonylurea-type (see Drug Classes) oral blood-sugar-lowering medicines in order to achieve the best possible control of blood sugar.

ASPIRIN

While it may strike readers as odd to include this very old medicine, recent data from a large study over an extended period of time has shown some very valuable new uses: it may help prevent colon cancer in women, for one. Other studies have shown that aspirin helps prevent strokes. Aspirin is also FDA-approved for use in preventing heart attacks in people who have a specific kind of heart problem called unstable angina. If you've been diagnosed with heart problems, talk to your doctor to see if an aspirin every other day makes sense for you. Recent news reports of patients who, thinking they are having a heart attack, take an aspirin immediately and then go to the hospital, suggest that aspirin may have a clot-dissolving benefit, and could limit the severity of—and perhaps even prevent death from—a heart attack. Once started, the aspirin should be continued for at least 30 days after a heart attack. The FDA's response that new labeling for aspirin can be introduced immediately is promising. Patients at risk for heart attack, stroke, or bowel cancer should discuss regular aspirin use with their doctor before starting it. At your next office visit also discuss what to do if you experience symptoms of a heart attack. No drugs are without some drug and disease interactions. The same is true for aspirin, so it is important to talk with your doctor and find out if ongoing aspirin use can be of benefit to you.

LOSARTAN

This new treatment for high blood pressure, losartan (under the brand name Cozaar), is an angiotensin II inhibitor. It works in a way never previously used to fight high blood pressure. The benefit here is that people with high blood pressure, especially if it is resistant to older treatments, can achieve a new way to lower their blood pressure.

VACCINES

Many vaccines have been there to help us for many years, yet still I find that some fear exists regarding if and how they should be given. Prevention of disease is always the smartest option. I taught an advanced pharmacology course, and often said that my first recommendation was that it is *always* better to prevent a disease or condition than to have to treat it. Vaccines have prevented many deaths. Recently, vaccines have been FDA-approved that can prevent hepatitis A and chicken pox. The vaccine that prevents hepatitis B and the chicken pox vaccine have been recommended for routine use in all children. And finally, the flu vaccine is reformulated every year. I believe the benefits of this vaccine far outweigh the risks for most people. Talk with your doctor or pharmacist and make sure you and your family get all of the vaccine protection that is appropriate for them. In some states, pharmacists have been approved to give vaccinations. If this service is available where you live, discuss your options with your pharmacist.

LIPOSOMALLY ENCAPSULATED MEDICINES

Last year I first spoke of medicines being enclosed in liposomes. In those early days a medicine called amphotericin B[10] and one anticancer drug were being considered for FDA approval in either lipid-associated or liposomally encapsulated forms. Two of those products for treating serious fungal infections have been FDA-approved, while others are pending approval. The prime benefit is that much higher doses of these medicines can be used, in many cases with fewer side effects. This can also mean cure rates in patients with very resistant disease. The anticancer medicines have not yet received FDA approval in liposomally encapsulated forms.

THE FDA'S ACCELERATED APPROVAL PROCESS

This program, a brave departure from entrenched practice, was introduced by the FDA in order to make medicines used to treat AIDS available more rapidly. In a speech, President Clinton spoke about expanding this process to other life-threatening diseases, such as cancer. The accelerated approval process has not been without controversy; some scientists labeled it as cavalier and providing false hopes. I cannot agree, not only because of the willingness of the FDA to assume some controversy, but more importantly because of the courage of the patients who participate in new treatments knowing there are benefits and risks, some unrevealed as of yet.

POLYMER IMPLANT

Researchers at Johns Hopkins have formulated the first narcotic drug implant intended as a medication delivery system for use in treating pain in cancer patients. Dr. Stuart Grossman has lead the team that developed the polymer, and further envisions the polymer as being useful in meeting the needs of patients with serious pain as well as helping manage drug addiction. Medicine that is incorporated into the polymer is released in a steady amount over one to three months after it is implanted. Human clinical trials are expected to begin sometime in 1997.

DRUG PROFILES

Drugs Reviewed in This Section

Here you'll find detailed Drug Profiles of more than 300 drugs of major importance. Drug selection was governed by consideration of the following criteria:

1. The drug is used to treat or prevent a relatively serious or significant disease or disorder.

2. The drug is recognized by experts to be among the "best choices" within its class.

3. The drug has a current benefit-to-risk ratio that compares favorably with those available in its class.

4. The safe and effective use of the drug requires special information and guidance for both the health care practitioner (physician, dentist, pharmacist, nurse) and the health care consumer (patient and family).

5. The drug is suitable (safe and practical) for use in an outpatient setting (home, work site, school, etc.). It can be self-administered, or may require administration by trained medical personnel (as with home intravenous therapy, free-standing cancer, emergency or pain centers).

ACARBOSE (a KAR boz)

Introduced: 1996   **Prescription:** USA: Yes   **Available as Generic:**
No   **Class:** Antidiabetes agent, oral; alpha glucosidase inhibitor   **Con-**
trolled Drug: USA: No

Brand Name: Precose

BENEFITS versus RISKS

Possible Benefits	*Possible Risks*
EFFECTIVE LOWERING OF BLOOD SUGAR	Gas and abdominal pain (often decreases over time)
DECREASED RISK OF HIGH BLOOD PRESSURE, HEART DISEASE, AND OTHER LONG-TERM EFFECTS OF ELEVATED BLOOD SUGAR (WITH TIGHTER SUGAR CONTROL)	Mild possible decreases in hematocrit
COMBINED TREATMENT WITH A SULFONYLUREA FOR BETTER SUGAR CONTROL	

▷ **Principal Uses**

As a Single Drug Product: Uses currently included in FDA approved labeling: (1) Used as an additional (adjunct) agent to diet in patients with diabetes who do not require insulin injections, yet do not have sufficient blood sugar control with diet alone; (2) Used in combination with a sulfonylurea (see Drug Classes) if diet plus acarbose or diet and sulfonylurea do not acceptably control the blood sugar.

Other (unlabeled) generally accepted uses: None at present.

How This Drug Works: By blocking the enzymes intestinal alpha glucosidase and pancreatic alpha amylase, this medicine inhibits the digestion of sugar, and actually keeps sugar low after meals.

Available Dosage Forms and Strengths

Tablets — 50 mg, 100 mg

▷ **Recommended Dosage Ranges:** (Actual dosage and administration schedule must be determined by the physician or clinical pharmacist for each patient individually.)

Infants and Children: Safety and effectiveness have not been established in those less than 18 years old.

18 to 65 Years of Age: Initially 25 mg three times daily, taken at the start of each meal. The dose may then be increased as needed or tolerated to 50 mg three times daily taken at the start of each meal. Any needed dose increases are made at 4 to 8 week intervals in order to best identify the needed blood sugar response and minimize gastrointestinal side effects. If the response still is not acceptable, patients weighing more than 132 pounds (60 kg) may be given doses up to 100 mg three times daily. Those weighing less than 60 kg should NOT be given be given more than 50 mg three times daily. If a given dose increase does not result in better sugar control, consideration should be given to decreasing the dose.

Over 65 Years of Age: No specific recommendations at present.

Conditions Requiring Dosing Adjustments

Liver function: The GI tract, not the liver is involved in eliminating this medicine by metabolism. Specific dosing changes do not appear to be needed.

Kidney function: Increases in blood levels occur and further increase as kidney damage increases. Dose decreases may be needed, but specific guidelines are not available. Only about 2% of a given oral dose is usually absorbed.

▷ **Dosing Instructions:** This medicine should be taken after starting breakfast, lunch and dinner—after the first bite of a meal has been eaten. Gas (flatulence) or diarrhea are common side effects. These problems can be decreased by limiting sucrose in the diet. In general, diarrhea and gas decrease over time. Dosing changes are usually made at 4 to 8 week intervals. This helps find the best dose and blood sugar response, while minimizing the potential gas (flatulence) or diarrhea. Usually, the blood sugar is checked one hour after a meal (1 h post-prandial) and the dose adjusted to obtain the best balance of blood sugar and side effects.

Usual Duration of Use: The dose of this medicine must be individualized, and dose changes are made at 4 to 8 week intervals as needed and tolerated. Regular use is needed to see this drug's best effect in maintaining tighter blood glucose control. Since non-insulin dependent diabetes is a chronic condition, use of acarbose will be ongoing. Periodic hemoglobin A1C (glycosylated hemoglobin) tests and physician follow up are needed.

Possible Advantages of This Drug

May be used in combination with sulfonylurea oral hypoglycemics (see Drug Classes) to obtain the best control of blood sugar.

Works using a different (novel) mechanism than other oral hypoglycemic agents.

▷ **This Drug Should Not Be Taken If**
- you have had an allergic reaction to it previously.
- you are in diabetic ketoacidosis.
- you have a tendency to develop intestinal obstruction or have a partial obstruction of the intestine.
- you have inflammatory bowel disease or ulceration of the colon.
- your serum creatinine is greater than 2 mg per dl (talk with your doctor).
- you have cirrhosis of the liver.
- you have an intestinal condition that may worsen (such as a megacolon or bowel obstruction) if there is increased gas (flatus) formation in the intestine.
- you have a long standing (chronic) intestinal disease which alters digestion or your ability to absorb materials via the intestine.
- you are pregnant or are breast feeding your infant (no data exists on use in pregnancy or breast feeding).

▷ **Inform Your Physician Before Taking This Drug If**
- you do not know what the symptoms of hypoglycemia are.
- you have a history of kidney or liver disease.
- you plan to have surgery under general anesthesia in the near future.

- you take other prescription or nonprescription medications which were not discussed when acarbose was prescribed for you.
- you are unsure of how much to take or how often to take acarbose.

Possible Side Effects (natural, expected, and unavoidable drug actions)

Gas (flatulence) or diarrhea results from bacterial action on sugars in the intestine, and tends to decrease over time.

▷ **Possible Adverse Effects** (unusual, unexpected, and infrequent reactions)

If any of the following develop, consult your physician promptly for guidance.

Mild Adverse Effects

Allergic Reactions: Skin rash, itching.

Sleepiness, headache, dizziness (of questionable causation).

Pain or swelling of the belly (abdomen).

Very rare increased liver enzymes (associated in clinical trials with doses greater than 100 mg three times a day).

Serious Adverse Effects

May make other allergic reactions less responsive to treatment and more severe.

Low blood sugar if combined with sulfonylureas.

Anemia (rare and occurred in some studies and not in others).

▷ **Possible Effects on Sexual Function:**   None reported.

Possible Effects on Laboratory Tests

Hemoglobin A1C: trending more toward normal.

Blood sugar one hour after eating (post prandial): decreased.

Serum lipids: variable effect.

CAUTION

1. This medicine itself does not cause hypoglycemia, however; if it is combined with insulin or sulfonylureas, hypoglycemia may result.
2. If you develop an infection, loss of control of your diabetes may occur. Temporary use of insulin may be needed.
3. This medicine is only one part of the total program for managing your diabetes. A properly prescribed (and followed) diet and regular exercise are also still required for the best control of blood sugar.
4. If you develop kidney failure while taking this medicine, and see a specialist, be certain to inform your regular doctor. This medicine should not be used if your serum creatinine is greater than 2 mg per dl.

Precautions for Use

By Infants and Children: Safety and effectiveness for use by those under 18 years of age have not been established.

By Those over 60 Years of Age: Specific recommendations are not made at this time.

▷ **Advisability of Use During Pregnancy**

Pregnancy Category: B. See Pregnancy Risk Categories at the back of this book.

Animal studies: No significant increase in birth defects in rats or rabbits.

Human studies: Adequate studies of pregnant women are not available.

Use of this drug during pregnancy should occur only if clearly needed. Most clinicians use insulin as the drug of first choice for controlling blood sugar in pregnancy. Ask your doctor for help.

Advisability of Use if Breast-Feeding

Presence of this drug in breast milk: Yes, in rats. No human data available. Avoid drug or refrain from nursing.

Habit-Forming Potential: None.

Effects of Overdosage: Temporary increase in gas (flatus), abdominal discomfort and diarrhea.

Possible Effects of Long-Term Use: None reported.

Suggested Periodic Examinations While Taking This Drug (at physician's discretion)

Periodic blood sugar tests one hour after eating. Measurement of hemoglobin A1C levels are helpful. Tests of serum transaminases (a measure of liver function) should be obtained every 3 months during the first year of treatment and periodically thereafter.

▷ **While Taking This Drug, Observe the Following**

Foods: Follow the diet your doctor has prescribed for you closely. Tight blood sugar control will help you avoid or delay long term effects of your diabetes.

Beverages: No restrictions. May be taken with milk.

▷   *Alcohol:* An interaction is not expected with acarbose, however, if you are also taking a sulfonylurea (see Drug Classes), alcohol may exaggerate that drug's ability to lower the blood sugar, and can cause a disulfiramlike (see glossary) reaction with some sulfonylureas.

Tobacco Smoking: No interactions expected, however there are no studies that show smoking is good for you. Discuss ways to help you stop smoking with your doctor or pharmacist.

▷   *Other Drugs*

Acarbose may *increase* the effects of

- sulfonylureas (see Drug Classes) and result in excessive lowering of blood sugar. This is not an effect of acarbose on the sulfonylurea, but a result of its beneficial effect on blood sugar after meals. This may be used for therapeutic benefit.

Acarbose *taken concurrently* with

- clofibrate (Atromid-S) may result in hypoglycemia.
- digestive enzyme products that contain amylase or lipase may result in loss of blood sugar control.
- disopyramide (Norpace) may result in hypoglycemia.
- high dose aspirin or other salicylates and some NSAIDs (see Drug Classes) may result in hypoglycemia.
- insulin (see Drug Classes) poses an increased risk of hypoglycemia.
- sulfonamide antibiotics (see Drug Classes) may pose an increased risk for hypoglycemia.

The following drugs may *decrease* the effects of acarbose

- beta blockers (see Drug Classes).
- corticosteroids (see Drug Classes).
- calcium channel blockers (see Drug Classes).
- furosemide (Lasix) and bumetanide (Bumex)(see Drug Classes).
- isoniazid (INH).
- nicotinic acid.
- phenytoin (Dilantin).
- rifampin (Rifadin, others).

- thiazide diuretics (see Drug Classes).
- theophylline (Theodur, others).
- thyroid hormones (see Drug Classes).

▷ *Driving, Hazardous Activities:* Use caution until you see how drowsy and lethargic you may become.

Aviation Note: Diabetes *is a disqualification* for piloting. Consult a designated Aviation Medical Examiner.

Exposure to Sun: No restrictions.

Heavy Exercise or Exertion: Because this drug can lower the peak in blood sugar seen after meals, caution is advised regarding heavy exercise as the amount of blood sugar needed to sustain this kind of activity may not be present. Discuss dosing changes with your doctor.

Occurrence of Unrelated Illness: Illness can change blood sugar control, and temporary use of insulin may be required.

Discontinuation: Talk with your doctor before stopping acarbose if you are considering stopping this medicine.

ACEBUTOLOL (a se BYU toh lohl)

Introduced: 1973   **Prescription:** USA: Yes   **Available as Generic:** Yes   **Class:** Antihypertensive, heart rhythm regulator, beta-adrenergic blocker **Controlled Drug:** USA: No

Brand Name: Sectral, ✦Monitan, ✦Rhotral

BENEFITS versus RISKS	
Possible Benefits	*Possible Risks*
EFFECTIVE ANTIHYPERTENSIVE in mild to moderate high blood pressure MAY DECREASE the number of deaths which occur after a heart attack	CONGESTIVE HEART FAILURE in advanced heart disease Worsening of angina in coronary heart disease (abrupt withdrawal) Masking of low blood sugar (hypoglycemia) in drug-treated diabetes Rare lupus erythematosus syndrome

▷ **Principal Uses**

As a Single Drug Product: Uses currently included in FDA approved labeling: (1) Treatment of mild to moderate high blood pressure. Used alone or combined with other drugs. Also used to prevent premature ventricular heartbeats.

Other (unlabeled) generally accepted uses: Treatment of stable angina pectoris, use after a heart attack to help prolong life, may have a role in easing the symptoms of panic attacks.

How This Drug Works: By blocking part of the sympathetic nervous system, this drug slows the rate and contraction force of the heart. This reduces the extent of blood vessel contraction, expanding the walls and lowering the blood pressure. It also slows the speed of nerve impulses through the heart, which helps ease some heart rhythm disorders.

Available Dosage Forms and Strengths
> Capsules — 100 mg (in Canada), 200 mg, 400 mg

▷ **Recommended Dosage Ranges: (Actual dosage and administration schedule must be determined by the physician or clinical pharmacist for each patient individually.)**
> *Infants and Children:* Not indicated.
> *18 to 65 Years of Age:* Initially 400 mg daily, either as a single dose in the morning or as 200 mg taken morning and evening (12 hours apart). The usual maintenance dose is 400 to 800 mg/24 hours. The total dose should not exceed 1200 mg/24 hours, given as 600 mg twice daily.
> *Over 65 Years of Age:* Bioavailability (amount taken into your body) doubles. Lower maintenance doses are needed. **Maximum** daily dose is 800 mg per day.

Conditions Requiring Dosing Adjustments
> *Liver function:* Extensively metabolized in the liver. Used with caution in compromised liver function.
> *Kidney function:* Dose must be decreased by up to 75% in kidney failure.

▷ **Dosing Instructions:**   May be taken without regard to eating. Capsule may be opened when taken. Do not stop this drug abruptly.

Usual Duration of Use: Use on a regular schedule for 5 to 11 days is needed to see this drug's peak effect in lowering blood pressure or stopping premature heartbeats. Long-term use is determined by sustained benefit and patient response to a combined program (weight reduction, salt restriction, smoking cessation, etc.). See your doctor regularly.

Possible Advantages of This Drug
> Slows the heart less than most other beta blocker drugs, and less likely to cause asthma (in susceptible patients) when used in low doses.

▷ **This Drug Should Not Be Taken If**
> • you have had an allergic reaction to it previously.
> • you have congestive heart failure.
> • you have an abnormally slow heart rate or a serious form of heart block.
> • you are taking, or took within the past 14 days, any monoamine oxidase (MAO) type A inhibitor drug (see Drug Class, Section Four).

▷ **Inform Your Physician Before Taking This Drug If**
> • you have had an adverse reaction to any beta blocker (see Drug Class, Section Four).
> • you have serious heart disease, or episodes of heart failure.
> • you have hay fever (allergic rhinitis), asthma, chronic bronchitis or emphysema. Some drugs in this class should not be taken if you have asthma.
> • you have an overactive thyroid function (hyperthyroidism).
> • you have problems with circulation to your arms and legs (peripheral vascular disease).
> • you have a history of low blood sugar (hypoglycemia).
> • you have impaired liver or kidney function.
> • you have diabetes or myasthenia gravis.
> • you currently take any form of digitalis, quinidine or reserpine, or any calcium blocker drug (see Drug Class, Section Four).
> • you plan to have surgery under general anesthesia in the near future.

- you take other prescription or nonprescription medications which were not discussed when acebutolol was prescribed for you.
- you are unsure of how much to take or how often to take acebutolol.
- you have not asked if the dose prescribed was adjusted for your age.

Possible Side Effects (natural, expected, and unavoidable drug actions)

Lethargy and fatigability, cold extremities (rare), slow heart rate, light-headedness in upright position (see Orthostatic Hypotension in Glossary).

▷ **Possible Adverse Effects** (unusual, unexpected and infrequent reactions)

If any of the following develop, consult your physician promptly for guidance.

Mild Adverse Effects

Allergic Reactions: Skin rash, itching.

Headache, dizziness, insomnia, fatigue, or abnormal dreams.

Indigestion, nausea, constipation, diarrhea.

Decreased tearing with long term use.

Increased frequency and painful or nighttime urination.

Joint and muscle discomfort, fluid retention (edema).

Serious Adverse Effects

May make other allergic reactions less responsive to treatment and more severe.

Mental depression (rare), anxiety, low blood sugar.

Rare liver toxicity.

Chest pain, shortness of breath, precipitation of congestive heart failure.

Induction of bronchial asthma (in people with asthma).

Positive ANA and lupus erythematosus (up to 33%).

▷ **Possible Effects on Sexual Function:** Impotence (rare), decreased libido, Peyronie's disease (see Glossary).

Possible Effects on Laboratory Tests

Antinuclear Antibodies (ANA) and LE cells: often positive after 3 to 6 months. Free fatty acids (FFA): decreased.

Glucose tolerance test (GTT): decreased; abnormal tests at 60 and 120 minutes.

CAUTION

1. ***Do not stop this drug suddenly*** without the knowledge and help from your physician. Carry a note which says that you take this drug.
2. Call your physician or pharmacist before using nasal decongestants. These can cause sudden increases in blood pressure if taken with beta blockers.
3. Report the development of any tendency to emotional depression.

Precautions for Use

By Infants and Children: Safety and effectiveness for use by those under 12 years of age have not been established. If this drug is used, watch for fainting as a sign of low blood sugar (hypoglycemia) if a meal is skipped.

By Those over 60 Years of Age: All antihypertensive drugs should be used ***cautiously***. High blood pressure should be lowered slowly, avoiding the risks (such as stroke or heart attack) of excessively low blood pressure. Small doses and frequent blood pressure checks are indicated. Total daily dosage should not exceed 800 mg. Watch for dizziness, unsteadiness, tendency to fall, confusion, hallucinations, depression or urinary frequency.

▷ **Advisability of Use During Pregnancy**

Pregnancy Category: B. See Pregnancy Code at the back of this book.
Animal studies: No significant increase in birth defects in rats or rabbits.
Human studies: Adequate studies of pregnant women are not available.
Use this drug only if clearly needed. Ask your doctor for help.

Advisability of Use if Breast-Feeding

Presence of this drug in breast milk: Yes.
Avoid drug or refrain from nursing.

Habit-Forming Potential: None.

Effects of Overdosage: Weakness, slow pulse, low blood pressure, fainting, cold and sweaty skin, congestive heart failure, possible coma and convulsions.

Possible Effects of Long-Term Use: Decreased heart reserve and heart failure in some people with advanced heart disease.

Suggested Periodic Examinations While Taking This Drug (at physician's discretion)

Measurements of blood pressure, evaluation of heart function.

▷ **While Taking This Drug, Observe the Following**

Foods: No restrictions. Avoid excessive salt intake.

Beverages: No restrictions. May be taken with milk.

▷   *Alcohol:* Alcohol may exaggerate this drug's ability to lower the blood pressure and may increase its mild sedative effect.

Tobacco Smoking: Nicotine may reduce this drug's effectiveness in treating high blood pressure. May increase the closing of bronchial tubes seen in regular smokers.

▷   *Other Drugs*

Acebutolol may *increase* the effects of

• other antihypertensive drugs and excessively lower the blood pressure. Dosage adjustments may be necessary.
• reserpine (Ser-Ap-Es, etc.) and cause sedation, depression, slow heart rate and low blood pressure.

Acebutolol *taken concurrently* with

• amiodarone (Codarone) may result in severe slowing of the heart leading to sinus arrest. Use with great caution.
• clonidine (Catapres) may cause rebound high blood pressure if clonidine is withdrawn while acebutolol is still being taken.
• insulin may cause low blood sugar (hypoglycemia).
• nilvadipine (Escor) may pose a rare risk of heart failure (cardiac failure).
• NSAIDS (see Glossary) may result in decreased lowering of blood pressure.
• oral hypoglycemic agents (see Drug Classes) may result in slow recovery from low blood sugars.

The following drugs may *decrease* the effects of acebutolol

• indomethacin (Indocin), and some other "aspirin substitutes,"(NSAIDS) can blunt acebutolol's antihypertensive effect.

▷   *Driving, Hazardous Activities:* Use caution until you see how drowsy and lethargic you may become.

Aviation Note: The use of this drug *is a disqualification* for piloting. Consult a designated Aviation Medical Examiner.

Exposure to Sun: No restrictions.

Exposure to Heat: Hot environments can exaggerate the effects of this drug.

Exposure to Cold: The elderly must be careful in preventing hypothermia (see Glossary).

Heavy Exercise or Exertion: This drug can intensify the increased blood pressure (hypertensive) response to isometric exercise.

Avoid exertion causing dizziness, excessive fatigue or muscle cramps.

Occurrence of Unrelated Illness: Fevers can lower blood pressure and require decreased doses. Nausea or vomiting may interrupt the dosing schedule. Ask your doctor for help.

Discontinuation: Avoid stopping the drug suddenly. Slow reduction of dose over a period of 2 to 3 weeks is recommended. Ask your physician for guidance.

ACETAZOLAMIDE (a set a ZOHL a mide)

Introduced: 1953   **Prescription:** USA: Yes; Canada: Yes   **Available as Generic:** USA: Yes; Canada: No   **Class:** Anticonvulsant, antiglaucoma, diuretic, sulfonamides   **Controlled Drug:** USA: No; Canada: No

Brand Names: ✦Acetazolam, Ak-Zol, ✦Apo-Acetazolamide, Dazamide, Diamox, Diamox Sustained release, Diamox Sequles, Storzolamide

BENEFITS versus RISKS	
Possible Benefits	*Possible Risks*
REDUCTION OF INTERNAL EYE PRESSURE in selected cases of glaucoma	Rare bone marrow, liver, or kidney injury
CONTROL OF ABSENCE (PETIT MAL) SEIZURES	Acidosis with long-term use
	Increased risk of kidney stone
TREATMENT OF PERIODIC PARALYSIS	Tingling in the arms and legs (paresthesia)
REDUCTION OF FLUID IN CONGESTIVE HEART FAILURE OR DRUG-INDUCED EDEMA	Paralysis (rare)
	Bone weakening (with long-term use)
PREVENTION OR LESSENING OF SYMPTOMS OF ACUTE MOUNTAIN SICKNESS	

▷ **Principal Uses**

As a Single Drug Product: Uses currently included in FDA approved labeling: (1) Treatment of some kinds of glaucoma; (2) used with other drugs to manage petit mal epilepsy; (3) treats familial periodic paralysis and prevents altitude sickness.

Other (unlabeled) generally accepted uses: (1) Taken orally as a urine alkalinizing agent in patients who have had uric acid kidney stones; (2) given intravenously to increase elimination of some drugs in overdoses; (3) May be used in patients in intensive care units on ventilators to correct chemical imbalances; (3) may have a role in easing both kinetic and postural tremor in combination with other agents.

How This Drug Works: By blocking the effect of the enzyme carbonic anhydrase, it slows the formation of fluid (the aqueous humor) in the eye and increases the volume of urine. It causes fluid loss by lowering the hydrogen ion concentration in the kidney and increasing elimination of bicarbonate (a basic chemical), potassium, sodium and water.

Available Dosage Forms and Strengths

Capsules, prolonged-action (sustained release) — 500 mg

Injection — 500 mg per vial

Tablets — 125 mg, 250 mg

▷ **Recommended Dosage Ranges (Actual dosage and administration schedule must be determined by the physician or clinical pharmacist for each patient individually.)**

Infants and Children: Not indicated in infants.

Acute glaucoma in children: Give 5–10 mg/kg intramuscularly (IM) or intravenously (IV) every 6 hours.

Children with glaucoma: Give 8–30 mg/kg per day in three divided doses.

Epilepsy in children: Give 8–30 mg/kg per day in 1–4 divided doses. Lower doses used if drug is combined with other medications. (250 mg per day).

Diuretic in children: Give 5 mg/kg IV or orally once daily in the morning.

18 to 65 Years of Age: For glaucoma: 250 to 1000 mg/24 hours, in 2 or 3 doses. For epilepsy: 250 to 1000 mg/24 hours. As a diuretic: 250 to 375 mg/24 hours, in one morning dose for one or two days.

Over 65 Years of Age: Most of a given dose is eliminated via the kidneys. Use with caution in this age group, and start with the lower end of the dosage range.

Conditions Requiring Dosing Adjustments

Liver function: Used with extreme caution in patients with cirrhosis.

Kidney function: Used with extreme caution in kidney compromise, and the patient closely followed.

▷ **Dosing Instructions:** Best taken with food or milk to prevent stomach irritation. Tablet may be crushed. Diamox Sequels may be opened, but do not chew or crush contents.

Usual Duration of Use: Treatment of glaucoma and epilepsy require long-term use. If taken to control seizures, do not stop this drug abruptly. See your doctor regularly.

▷ **This Drug Should Not Be Taken If**

• you have had an allergic reaction to any form of it previously.
• you have serious liver or kidney disease.
• you have Addison's disease.
• your adrenal gland has failed.
• you have electrolyte problems (low sodium or potassium).
• you have some types of glaucoma.

▷ **Inform Your Physician Before Taking This Drug If**

• you have had an allergic reaction to any "sulfa" drug.
• you have gout or lupus erythematosus.
• you have emphysema or blockages of your lungs.
• you have a history of low blood platelets.

Possible Side Effects (natural, expected, and unavoidable drug actions)

Drowsiness, temporary nearsightedness.

▷ **Possible Adverse Effects** (unusual, unexpected, and infrequent reactions)
If any of the following develop, consult your physician promptly for guidance.

Mild Adverse Effects
Allergic Reactions: Skin rash, hives, drug fever.
Reduced appetite, indigestion, nausea.
Confusion, fatigue; weakness; dizziness; tingling of face, arms, or legs.
Tingling effect is a lowering of blood potassium, which often eases with time.
Excessive growth of hair in females.

Serious Adverse Effects
Allergic Reactions: Hemolytic anemia (see Glossary), spontaneous bruising (reduced blood platelet count, see Glossary).
Bone marrow depression (see Glossary)—fatigue, weakness, fever, sore throat, abnormal bleeding or bruising.
Hepatitis with jaundice (see Glossary)—yellow eyes and skin, dark-colored urine, light-colored stools.
Severe muscle weakness leading to paralysis (rare).
Weakness of the bones with long-term use (osteomalacia).

▷ **Possible Effects on Sexual Function:**   Decreased libido (male and female), impotence (both infrequent). Effects may begin after 2 weeks of use and subside when drug is stopped.

▷ **Adverse Effects That May Mimic Natural Diseases or Disorders**
Toxic liver reaction may suggest viral hepatitis.
Lupus erythematosuslike syndrome.

Natural Diseases or Disorders That May Be Activated by This Drug
Gout, acidosis caused by chronic obstructive lung disease—asthma, bronchitis, emphysema.

Possible Effects on Laboratory Tests
Complete blood counts: decreased red cells, hemoglobin, white cells and platelets.
Blood chloride level: increased.
Blood glucose level: increased in prediabetics and with use of oral antidiabetic drugs (see Drug Class, Section Four).
Blood lupus erythematosus (LE) cells: positive.
Blood theophylline tests: falsely increased.
Blood uric acid level: increased.

CAUTION
1. Watch for loss of diuretic (fluid) or seizure control effect.
2. Emotional depression can be an adverse effect of this drug.
3. May cause excessive loss of potassium. Ask your doctor about a high-potassium diet or potassium supplements.

Precautions for Use
By Infants and Children: Excess dose may cause drowsiness and numbness of the face and extremities. Not recommended for use as a diuretic in children.
By Those over 60 Years of Age: Do not exceed recommended doses. Increased dose may lead to weakness, confusion, numbness in the extremities and nausea. If taking a digitalis preparation (digitoxin, digoxin), you may need

a high-potassium diet or potassium supplements. Ask your doctor for advice.

▷ **Advisability of Use During Pregnancy**

Pregnancy Category: C. See Pregnancy Code at the back of this book.

Animal studies: Limb and skeletal defects reported in mice and rats.

Human studies: Adequate studies of pregnant women not available.

Avoid completely during the first 3 months and during labor and delivery.

Advisability of Use if Breast-Feeding

Presence of this drug in breast milk: Yes.

Diuretic effect may temporarily impair milk production. Watch nursing infant closely and stop drug or nursing if adverse effects develop.

Habit-Forming Potential: None.

Effects of Overdosage: Drowsiness, numbness and tingling, thirst, nausea, vomiting, confusion, excitement, convulsions, coma.

Possible Effects of Long-Term Use: The development of low blood potassium (first few weeks) and/or acidosis. Weakening of bones (osteomalacia).

Suggested Periodic Examinations While Taking This Drug (at physician's discretion)

Complete blood cell counts, measurements of blood sodium, potassium and uric acid levels, liver and kidney function tests.

▷ **While Taking This Drug, Observe the Following**

Foods: High-potassium diet may be advisable early in therapy. See Section Six for the Table of High Potassium Foods.

Beverages: No restrictions. May be taken with milk.

▷ *Alcohol:* Alcohol can blunt the anticonvulsant effect of this drug and reduce seizure control.

Tobacco Smoking: No interactions expected.

▷ *Other Drugs*

Acetazolamide may ***increase*** the effects of

• quinidine.

Acetazolamide may ***decrease*** the effects of

• lithium.

• oral hypoglycemic agents (see Drug Classes, section four).

Acetazolamide ***taken concurrently*** with

• aspirin may result in aspirin toxicity. Watch for ringing in the ears, confusion, rapid heart beat.

• amphetamines may result in amphetamine toxicity. Amphetamine dose must be decreased.

▷ *Driving, Hazardous Activities:* Usually no restrictions. Drowsiness or dizziness may occur.

Aviation Note: The use of this drug ***may be a disqualification*** for piloting. Consult a designated Aviation Medical Examiner.

Exposure to Sun: No restrictions.

ACETIC ACIDS
(Nonsteroidal Antiinflammatory Drugs)

Indomethacin (in doh METH a sin)   **Diclofenac** (di KLOH fen ak)   **Etodolac** (e TOE doh lak)   **Ketorolac** (KEY tor o lak)   **Nabumetone** (na BYU me tohn) **Sulindac** (sul IN dak)   **Tolmetin** TOHL met in)

Introduced: 1963, 1976, 1986, 1991, 1984, 1976, 1976, respectively   **Prescription:** USA: Yes; Canada: Yes   **Available as Generic:** USA: Yes: indomethacin, sulindac, tolmetin.; Canada: No   **Class:** NSAID, Mild analgesic   **Controlled Drug:** USA: No; Canada: No

Brand Names: Indomethacin: ✦Apo-Indomethacin, Indameth, ✦Indocid, ✦Indocid-SR, ✦Indocid PDA, Indocin, Indocin-SR, ✦Novomethacin, ✦Nu-Indo, Zendole, Diclofenac:, ✦Apo-Diclo, Cataflam, ✦Novo-Difenac, ✦Nu-Diclo, Voltaren, Voltaren SR, Voltaren Ophthalmic, Etodolac: Lodine, Ketorolac: Toradol, Acular (ketorolac ophthalmic), Nabumetone: Relafen, Sulindac: ✦Apo-Sulin, Clinoril, ✦Novo-Sundac, Tolmetin: Tolectin, Tolectin DS, Tolectin 600

BENEFITS versus RISKS	
Possible Benefits	*Possible Risks*
EFFECTIVE RELIEF OF MILD TO MODERATE PAIN AND INFLAMMATION	Gastrointestinal pain, ulceration, bleeding (rare)
Easy change from the IM or IV form to the oral form (ketorolac)	Liver or kidney damage (rare)
Decreased stomach (GI) problems (etodolac)	Fluid retention (rare)
	Rare bone marrow depression (rare)
	Mental depression, confusion
	Rare lung fibrosis (nabumetone)
	Rare pneumonitis (sulindac)
	Rare aseptic meningitis (diclofenac)
	Rare severe skin reaction (diclofenac, etodolac, ketorolac, and sulindac)

▷ **Principal Uses**

As a Single Drug Product: Uses currently included in FDA approved labeling: (1) All of the drugs in this class except ketorolac are approved to treat osteoarthritis; (2) all of the drugs in this class except ketorolac and etodolac are approved to relieve rheumatoid arthritis; (3) etodolac and ketorolac are used to treat mild to moderate pain; (4) diclofenac is useful in ankylosing spondylitis; (5) the sustained release form of indomethacin as well as the immediate release form of sulindac help symptoms of tendonitis, bursitis and acute painful shoulder; (6) tolmetin eases symptoms of juvenile rheumatoid arthritis; (7) sulindac therapy is useful in acute gout; (8) ophthalmic form of diclofenac is useful after cataract surgery.

Other (unlabeled) generally accepted uses: (1) Diclofenac used intramuscularly is effective in acute migraine headache and kidney colic; (2) indomethacin has recently proven to be useful in reducing systemic reactions in kidney transplants, and addressing low grade neonatal intraventricular hemorrhage; (3) ketorolac has been helpful in reducing swelling after cataract surgery and in treating reflex sympathetic dystrophy by injection; (4)

sulindac is effective in treating colon polyps (Gardner's syndrome) and easing diabetic neuropathic pain.

How These Drugs Work: It is thought that these drugs reduce tissue concentrations of prostaglandins (and related compounds), chemicals involved in the production of inflammation and pain.

Available Dosage Forms and Strengths

Indomethacin:

Capsules — 25 mg, 50 mg, 75 mg
Gelatin Capsule (Canada) — 25 mg, 50 mg
Capsules, SR (prolonged action) — 75 mg
Oral suspension — 25 mg/ 5 ml
Suppositories — 50 mg, 100 mg

Diclofenac sodium:

Suppositories — 50 mg, 100 mg (Canada)
Tablets — 25 mg, 50 mg
Prolonged action tablets — 50 mg, 75 mg, 100 mg (Canada)
Ophthalmic solution — 1 mg/ 1 ml

Etodolac:

Capsules — 200 mg, 300 mg

Ketorolac:

Tablets — 10 mg
Ophthalmic solution — 0.5%
Injection — 15 mg, 30 mg

Nabumetone:

Tablets — 500 mg, 750 mg

Sulindac:

Tablets — 150 mg, 200 mg

Tolmetin:

Capsules — 400 mg, 492 mg
Gelatin Capsule — 400 mg (Canada)
Tablets — 200 mg, 600 mg

▷ **Usual Adult Dosage Range:**   Indomethacin: For arthritis and related conditions: 25 to 50 mg 2 to 4 times daily. If needed and tolerated, dose may be increased by 25 or 50 mg/day at intervals of 1 week. For acute gout: 100 mg initially; then 50 mg 3 times/day until pain is relieved. Maximum daily dose is 200 mg.

Diclofenac potassium: Maximum daily dose is 200 mg.

Diclofenac sodium: 100 to 200 mg daily to start in 2 to 5 divided doses. Reduction to the minimum effective dose is advisable. Maximum daily dose is 225 mg.

Etodolac: For osteoarthritis: A starting dose of 800 to 1200 mg is given in divided doses. The lowest effective dose is advisable, and effective treatment has been accomplished with 200 to 400 mg daily. Maximum dose is 1200 mg daily.

Ketorolac: 10 mg is used every 4 to 6 hours for short-term treatment of pain. Maximum daily dose is 40 mg orally.

Nabumentone: 1000 mg daily as a single dose is given. Dosage is increased as needed and tolerated to 1500 mg daily. The lowest effective daily dose is advisable. Maximum daily dose is 2000 mg.

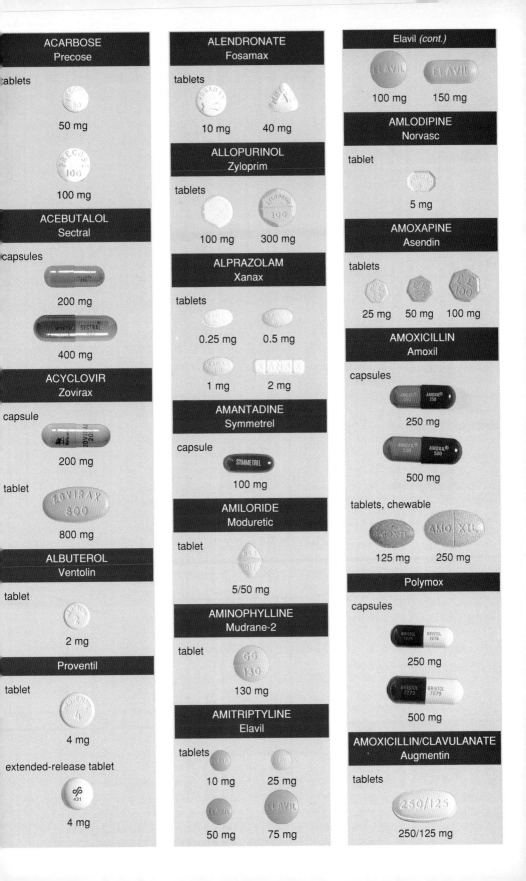

ACARBOSE
Precose

tablets

50 mg

100 mg

ACEBUTALOL
Sectral

capsules

200 mg

400 mg

ACYCLOVIR
Zovirax

capsule

200 mg

tablet

800 mg

ALBUTEROL
Ventolin

tablet

2 mg

Proventil

tablet

4 mg

extended-release tablet

4 mg

ALENDRONATE
Fosamax

tablets

10 mg   40 mg

ALLOPURINOL
Zyloprim

tablets

100 mg   300 mg

ALPRAZOLAM
Xanax

tablets

0.25 mg   0.5 mg

1 mg   2 mg

AMANTADINE
Symmetrel

capsule

100 mg

AMILORIDE
Moduretic

tablet

5/50 mg

AMINOPHYLLINE
Mudrane-2

tablet

130 mg

AMITRIPTYLINE
Elavil

tablets

10 mg   25 mg

50 mg   75 mg

Elavil (cont.)

100 mg   150 mg

AMLODIPINE
Norvasc

tablet

5 mg

AMOXAPINE
Asendin

tablets

25 mg   50 mg   100 mg

AMOXICILLIN
Amoxil

capsules

250 mg

500 mg

tablets, chewable

125 mg   250 mg

Polymox

capsules

250 mg

500 mg

AMOXICILLIN/CLAVULANATE
Augmentin

tablets

250/125 mg

AMOXICILLIN/CLAVULANATE
Augmentin

tablets (cont.)

500/125 mg

tablet, chewable

250/62.50 mg

AMPICILLIN
Omnipen

capsule

500 mg

Polycillin

capsules

250 mg

500 mg

Totacillin

capsule

250 mg

ASTEMIZOLE
Hismanal

tablet

10 mg

ATENOLOL
Tenormin

tablets

25 mg   50 mg   100 mg

AURANOFIN
Ridaura

capsule

3 mg

AZATHIOPRINE
Imuran

tablet

50 mg

AZITHROMYCIN
Zithromax

capsule

250 mg

BECLOMETHASONE
Beclovent

inhaler

Vanceril

inhaler

BENAZEPRIL
Lotensin

tablets

5 mg   10 mg   20 mg

BENZTROPINE
Cogentin

tablets

0.5 mg   1 mg   2 mg

BETAXOLOL
Kerlone

tablets

10 mg   20 mg

BITOLTEROL
Tornalate

inhaler

BROMOCRIPTINE
Parlodel

tablet

2.5 mg

BUMETANIDE
Bumex

tablets

0.5 mg   1 mg   2 mg

BUPROPION
Wellbutrin

tablets

75 mg   100 mg

BUSPIRONE
BuSpar

tablets

5 mg   10 mg

CAPTOPRIL
Capoten

tablets

12.5 mg   25 mg   50 mg

CARBAMAZEPINE
Tegretol

tablet

200 mg

tablet, chewable

100 mg

CARTEOLOL
Cartrol

tablet

2.5 mg

CEFACLOR
Ceclor

capsules

250 mg

500 mg

CEFADROXIL
Duricef

capsule

500 mg

tablet

1 gram

CEFIXIME
Suprax

tablet

400 mg

CEFPROZIL
Cefzil

tablets

250 mg   500 mg

CEFUROXIME
Ceftin

tablets

125 mg   250 mg

500 mg

CEPHALEXIN
Keflex

capsules

250 mg

500 mg

Keftab

tablet

500 mg

CHLORAMBUCIL
Leukeran

tablet

2 mg

CHLORAMPHENICOL
Chloromycetin

capsule

250 mg

CHLOROQUINE
Aralen

tablet

500 mg

CHLOROTHIAZIDE
Diuril

tablets

250 mg   500 mg

CHLORPROMAZINE
Thorazine

capsules, extended-release

75 mg   150 mg

tablets

100 mg   200 mg

CHLORPROPAMIDE
Diabinese

tablet

250 mg

CHLORTHALIDONE
Hygroton

tablets

25 mg   50 mg

CHOLESTYRAMINE

Questran Light

CHOLESTYRAMINE
(cont.)

Questran Powder

CIMETIDINE
Tagamet

tablets

200 mg   300 mg

400 mg   800 mg

CIPROFLOXACIN
Cipro

tablets

512   513

250 mg   500 mg

514

750 mg

CLARITHROMYCIN
Biaxin

tablets

250 mg   500 mg

CISAPRIDE
Prospulsid

tablets

10 mg   20 mg

CLOFAZIMINE
Lamprene

capsule

100 mg

CLOMIPRAMINE
Anafranil

capsules

25 mg   50 mg

75 mg

CLONAZEPAM
Klonopin

tablets

0.5 mg   1 mg

CLONIDINE
Catapres

tablets

0.1 mg   0.2 mg   0.3 mg

CLOTRIMAZOLE
Mycelex

troche

10 mg

CLOXACILLIN
Tegopen

capsules

250 mg   500 mg

CLOZAPINE
Clozaril

tablets

25 mg   100 mg

COLCHICINE
ColBENEMID

tablet

CROMOLYN
Intal

inhaler

CYCLOPHOSPHAMIDE
Cytoxan

tablets

25 mg   50 mg

CYCLOSPORINE
Sandimmune

capsule

25 mg

DESIPRAMINE
Norpramin

tablets

10 mg   25 mg

50 mg   75 mg

DEXAMETHASONE
Decadron (0.75mg) & Generic

tablets

0.5 mg   0.75 mg   4 mg

DEXFENFLURAMINE
Redux

tablet

15 mg

DIAZEPAM
Valium

tablets

2 mg   5 mg

Valrelease

capsule, extended-release

15 mg

DICLOFENAC
Voltaren

tablets

25 mg   75 mg

DIDANOSINE
Videx

tablet

25 mg

DIFLUNISAL
Dolobid

tablets

250 mg   500 mg

DIGOXIN
Lanoxicaps

capsules

0.1 mg   0.2 mg

Lanoxin

tablets

0.125 mg   0.25 mg   0.5 mg

DILTIAZEM
Cardizem

tablets

30 mg   60 mg

Cardizem *(cont.)*

90 mg

120 mg

Cardizem CD

capsules

180 mg

240 mg

300 mg

Cardizem SR

capsules

60 mg   90 mg

120 mg

DIPHENHYDRAMINE
Benadryl

capsules

25 mg   50 mg

DIPYRIDAMOLE
Persantine

tablets

50 mg   75 mg

DISOPYRAMIDE
Norpace

capsules

100 mg

Norpace *(cont.)*

150 mg

Norpace CR

capsules, extended-release

100 mg

150 mg

DISULFIRAM
Antabuse

tablets

250 mg   500 mg

DOXAZOSIN
Cardura

tablets

1 mg   2 mg

4 mg   8 mg

DOXEPIN
Sinequan

capsules

10 mg   25 mg

50 mg

DOXYCYCLINE
Zenith generic

tablet

100 mg

ENALAPRIL
Vasotec
tablet

2.5 mg

ERGOTAMINE
Ergostat
tablet

2 mg

ERYTHROMYCIN
Ery-Tab
tablet, delayed-release

333 mg

E-Mycin
tablets, delayed-release

250 mg   333 mg

Eryc
capsule, delayed-release

250 mg

Erythrocin
tablets

250 mg   500 mg

ESTROGENS
Estrace
tablets

1 mg   2 mg

Ogen
tablets

0.625 mg   1.5 mg

Premarin
tablets

0.3 mg   0.625 mg

0.9 mg   1.25 mg

2.5 mg

ETHAMBUTOL
Myambutol
tablet

400 mg

ETHOSUXIMIDE
Zarontin
capsule

250 mg

ETIDRONATE
Didronel
tablets

200 mg   400 mg

ETRETINATE
Tegison
capsules

10 mg   25 mg

FAMOTIDINE
Pepcid
tablets

20 mg   40 mg

FELODIPINE
Plendil
tablets

5 mg   10 mg

FENOPROFEN
Nalfon
capsule

200 mg

FINASTERIDE
Proscar
tablet

5 mg

FLUCONAZOLE
Diflucan
tablets

50 mg   100 mg

FLUCYTOSINE
Ancobon
capsule

500 mg

FLUOXETINE
Prozac
capsule

20 mg

FLUPHENAZINE
Prolixin

tablets

1 mg   5 mg

FLURAZEPAM
Dalmane

capsules

15 mg   30 mg

FLURBIPROFEN
Ansaid

tablets

ANSAID 50 mg   ANSAID 100 mg

50 mg   100 mg

FLUTAMIDE
Eulexin

capsule

SCHERING 525   SCHERING 525

125 mg

FOSINOPRIL
Monopril

tablets

10 mg   20 mg

FUROSEMIDE
Lasix

tablets

20 mg   40 mg

80 mg

GEMFIBROZIL
Lopid

tablet

Lopid

600 mg

GLIPIZIDE
Glucotrol

tablets

PFIZER 411   PFIZER 412

5 mg   10 mg

GLYBURIDE
DiaBeta

tablets

1.25 mg   2.5 mg   5 mg

Micronase

tablets

1.25 mg   2.5 mg   5 mg

GRISEOFULVIN
Fulvicin P/G

tablets

507   FULVICIN P/G

250 mg   330 mg

GUANFACINE
Tenex

tablets

1 mg   2 mg

HALOPERIDOL
Haldol

tablets

0.5 mg   1 mg   2 mg

Haldol (cont.)

HALDOL 5   HALDOL 10

5 mg   10 mg

HYDRALAZINE
Apresoline

tablet

101

100 mg

HYDROCHLOROTHIAZIDE
Esidrix

tablets

25 mg   50 mg

HYDROCODONE
(& acetaminophen)
Vicodin

tablet

VICODIN

5/500 mg

Vicodin ES

tablet

VICODIN ES

7.5/750 mg

HYDROXYCHLOROQUINE
Plaquenil

tablet

PLAQUENIL

200 mg

IBUPROFEN
Motrin

tablets

MOTRIN 400mg   MOTRIN 600mg

400 mg   600 mg

MOTRIN 800mg

800 mg

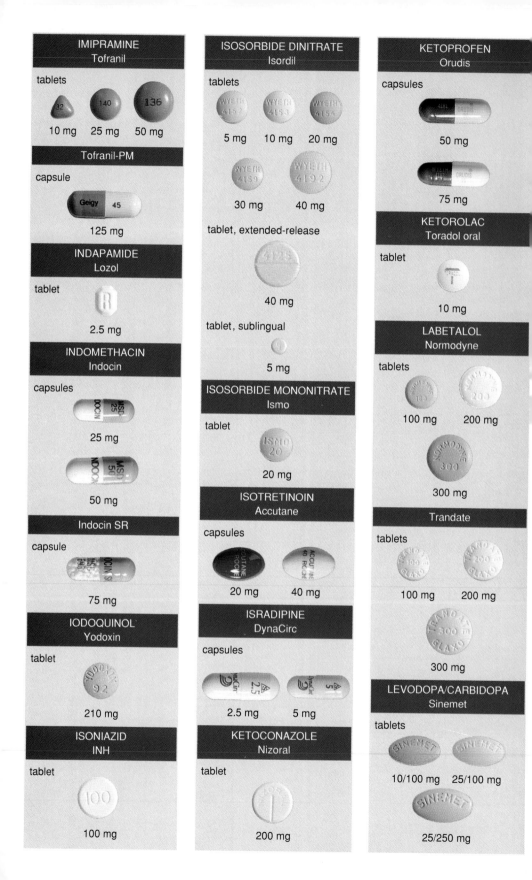

IMIPRAMINE
Tofranil

tablets

10 mg   25 mg   50 mg

Tofranil-PM

capsule

125 mg

INDAPAMIDE
Lozol

tablet

2.5 mg

INDOMETHACIN
Indocin

capsules

25 mg

50 mg

Indocin SR

capsule

75 mg

IODOQUINOL
Yodoxin

tablet

210 mg

ISONIAZID
INH

tablet

100 mg

ISOSORBIDE DINITRATE
Isordil

tablets

5 mg   10 mg   20 mg

30 mg   40 mg

tablet, extended-release

40 mg

tablet, sublingual

5 mg

ISOSORBIDE MONONITRATE
Ismo

tablet

20 mg

ISOTRETINOIN
Accutane

capsules

20 mg   40 mg

ISRADIPINE
DynaCirc

capsules

2.5 mg   5 mg

KETOCONAZOLE
Nizoral

tablet

200 mg

KETOPROFEN
Orudis

capsules

50 mg

75 mg

KETOROLAC
Toradol oral

tablet

10 mg

LABETALOL
Normodyne

tablets

100 mg   200 mg

300 mg

Trandate

tablets

100 mg   200 mg

300 mg

LEVODOPA/CARBIDOPA
Sinemet

tablets

10/100 mg   25/100 mg

25/250 mg

Sinemet CR

tablet, sustained-release

50/200 mg

LEVOTHYROXINE
Synthroid

tablets

0.025 mg 0.05 mg 0.075 mg

0.1 mg 0.112 mg 0.125 mg

0.15 mg 0.175 mg

LIOTHYRONINE
Cytomel

tablets

5 mcg 25 mcg

LISINOPRIL
Prinivil

tablets

5 mg 10 mg 20 mg

Zestril

tablets

5 mg 10 mg 20 mg

LITHIUM
Eskalith CR

tablet, controlled-release

450 mg

Lithobid

tablet

CIBA
65

300 mg

LOMEFLOXACIN
Maxaquin

tablet

MAXAQUIN
400

400 mg

LOPERAMIDE
Imodium

capsule

2 mg

LOVASTATIN
Mevacor

tablets

20 mg 40 mg

MAPROTILINE
Ludiomil

tablets

25 mg 50 mg

MECLOFENAMATE
Meclomen

capsule

100 mg

MEDROXYPROGESTERONE
Provera

tablets

2.5 mg 5 mg 10 mg

MEPERIDINE
Demerol

tablets

50 mg 100 mg

MERCAPTOPURINE
Purinethol

tablet

50 mg

MESALAMINE
Asacol

tablet

400 mg

METAPROTERENOL
Alupent

tablet

20 mg

METHADONE
Dolophine

tablet

5 mg

METHOTREXATE
Lederle generic

tablet

2.5 mg

METHYLPHENIDATE
Ritalin

tablets

5 mg 10 mg 20 mg

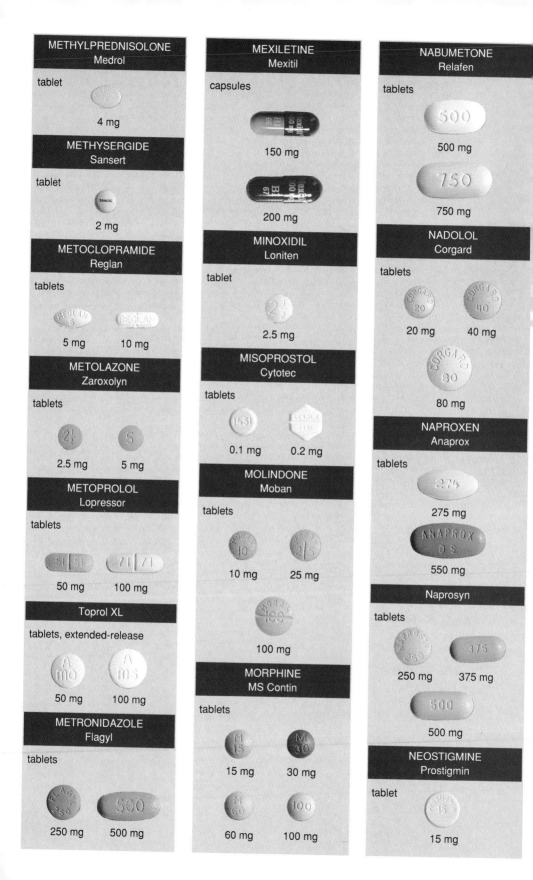

METHYLPREDNISOLONE
Medrol

tablet

4 mg

METHYSERGIDE
Sansert

tablet

2 mg

METOCLOPRAMIDE
Reglan

tablets

5 mg   10 mg

METOLAZONE
Zaroxolyn

tablets

2.5 mg   5 mg

METOPROLOL
Lopressor

tablets

50 mg   100 mg

Toprol XL

tablets, extended-release

50 mg   100 mg

METRONIDAZOLE
Flagyl

tablets

250 mg   500 mg

MEXILETINE
Mexitil

capsules

150 mg

200 mg

MINOXIDIL
Loniten

tablet

2.5 mg

MISOPROSTOL
Cytotec

tablets

0.1 mg   0.2 mg

MOLINDONE
Moban

tablets

10 mg   25 mg

100 mg

MORPHINE
MS Contin

tablets

15 mg   30 mg

60 mg   100 mg

NABUMETONE
Relafen

tablets

500 mg

750 mg

NADOLOL
Corgard

tablets

20 mg   40 mg

80 mg

NAPROXEN
Anaprox

tablets

275 mg

550 mg

Naprosyn

tablets

250 mg   375 mg

500 mg

NEOSTIGMINE
Prostigmin

tablet

15 mg

NIACIN
Nicobid
capsules, extended-release

250 mg

Slo-Niacin
tablets, extended-release

500 mg

NICARDIPINE
Cardene
capsules

20 mg

30 mg

NICOTINE
Nicorette chewing gum

2 mg

tablet

4 mg

NIFEDIPINE
Adalat
capsules

10 mg

20 mg

Procardia
capsules

10 mg

20 mg

Procardia XL
tablets, extended-release

30 mg   60 mg

90 mg

NITROFURANTOIN
Furadantin
tablets

50 mg

Macrodantin
capsules

50 mg   100 mg

NITROGLYCERIN
Nitrostat
tablets, sublingual

0.4 mg

NIZATIDINE
Axid
capsules

150 mg   300 mg

NORFLOXACIN
Noroxin
tablet

400 mg

NORTRIPTYLINE
Pamelor
capsules

10 mg   25 mg

50 mg   75 mg

OFLOXACIN
Floxin
tablets

200 mg   300 mg

400 mg

OLSALAZINE
Dipentum
capsule

250 mg

OMEPRAZOLE
Prilosec
capsule

20 mg

OXTRIPHYLLINE
Choledyl
tablet

200 mg

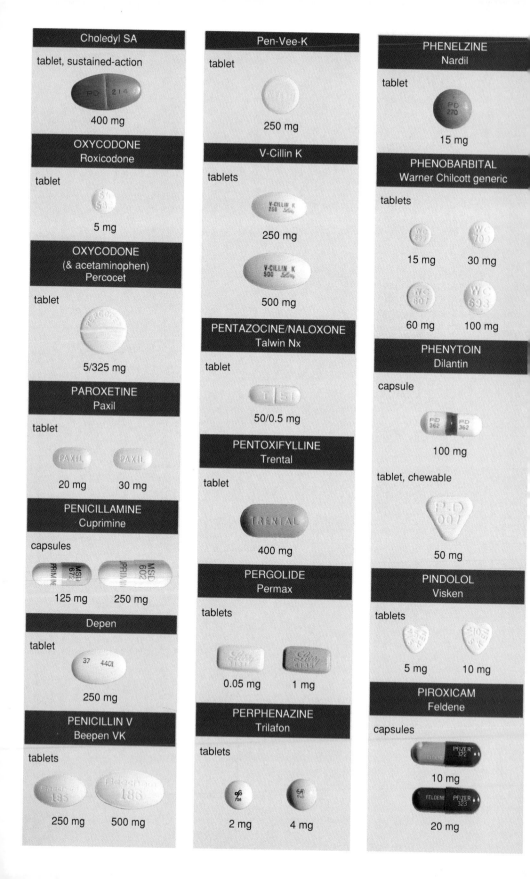

Choledyl SA
tablet, sustained-action

400 mg

OXYCODONE
Roxicodone

tablet

5 mg

OXYCODONE
(& acetaminophen)
Percocet

tablet

5/325 mg

PAROXETINE
Paxil

tablet

20 mg 30 mg

PENICILLAMINE
Cuprimine

capsules

125 mg 250 mg

Depen
tablet

250 mg

PENICILLIN V
Beepen VK

tablets

250 mg 500 mg

Pen-Vee-K
tablet

250 mg

V-Cillin K
tablets

250 mg

500 mg

PENTAZOCINE/NALOXONE
Talwin Nx

tablet

50/0.5 mg

PENTOXIFYLLINE
Trental

tablet

400 mg

PERGOLIDE
Permax

tablets

0.05 mg 1 mg

PERPHENAZINE
Trilafon

tablets

2 mg 4 mg

PHENELZINE
Nardil

tablet

15 mg

PHENOBARBITAL
Warner Chilcott generic

tablets

15 mg 30 mg

60 mg 100 mg

PHENYTOIN
Dilantin

capsule

100 mg

tablet, chewable

50 mg

PINDOLOL
Visken

tablets

5 mg 10 mg

PIROXICAM
Feldene

capsules

10 mg

20 mg

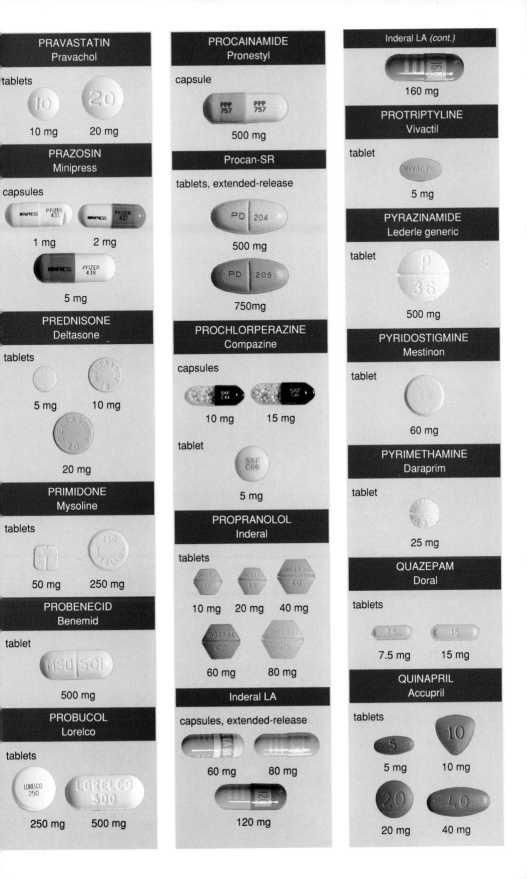

PRAVASTATIN
Pravachol

tablets

10 mg   20 mg

PRAZOSIN
Minipress

capsules

MINIPRESS PFIZER 431 — 1 mg   MINIPRESS PFIZER 437 — 2 mg

MINIPRESS PFIZER 438 — 5 mg

PREDNISONE
Deltasone

tablets

5 mg   10 mg

20 mg

PRIMIDONE
Mysoline

tablets

50 mg   250 mg

PROBENECID
Benemid

tablet

MSD 501 — 500 mg

PROBUCOL
Lorelco

tablets

LORELCO 250 — 250 mg   LORELCO 500 — 500 mg

PROCAINAMIDE
Pronestyl

capsule

PPP 757 PPP 757 — 500 mg

Procan-SR

tablets, extended-release

PD 204 — 500 mg

PD 205 — 750mg

PROCHLORPERAZINE
Compazine

capsules

SKF C44 — 10 mg   SKF C46 — 15 mg

tablet

SKF C66 — 5 mg

PROPRANOLOL
Inderal

tablets

INDERAL 10 — 10 mg   INDERAL 20 — 20 mg   INDERAL 40 — 40 mg

INDERAL 60 — 60 mg   INDERAL 80 — 80 mg

Inderal LA

capsules, extended-release

INDERAL LA 60 — 60 mg   80 mg

120 — 120 mg

Inderal LA *(cont.)*

160 mg

PROTRIPTYLINE
Vivactil

tablet

VIVACTIL — 5 mg

PYRAZINAMIDE
Lederle generic

tablet

p 36 — 500 mg

PYRIDOSTIGMINE
Mestinon

tablet

60 mg

PYRIMETHAMINE
Daraprim

tablet

43A — 25 mg

QUAZEPAM
Doral

tablets

7.5 — 7.5 mg   15 — 15 mg

QUINAPRIL
Accupril

tablets

5 — 5 mg   10 — 10 mg

20 — 20 mg   40 — 40 mg

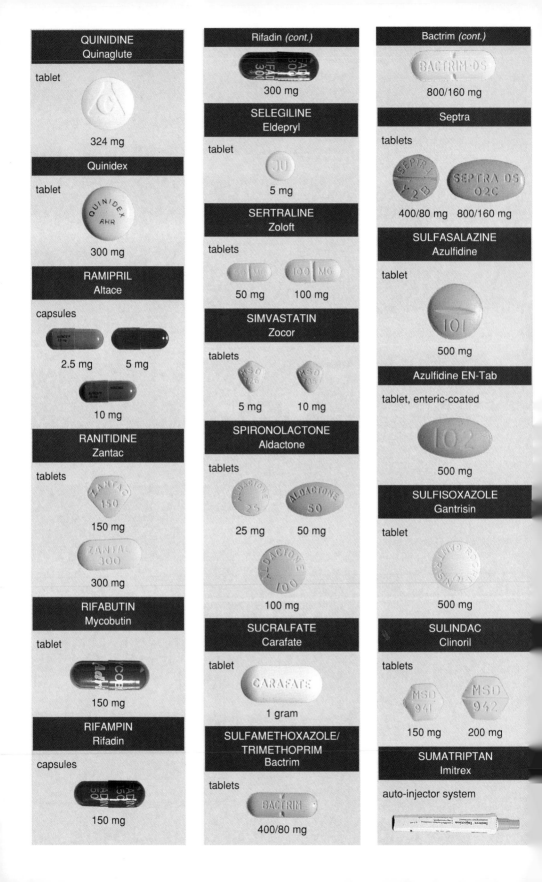

QUINIDINE
Quinaglute

tablet

324 mg

Quinidex

tablet

300 mg

RAMIPRIL
Altace

capsules

2.5 mg   5 mg

10 mg

RANITIDINE
Zantac

tablets

150 mg

300 mg

RIFABUTIN
Mycobutin

tablet

150 mg

RIFAMPIN
Rifadin

capsules

150 mg

Rifadin *(cont.)*

300 mg

SELEGILINE
Eldepryl

tablet

5 mg

SERTRALINE
Zoloft

tablets

50 mg   100 mg

SIMVASTATIN
Zocor

tablets

5 mg   10 mg

SPIRONOLACTONE
Aldactone

tablets

25 mg   50 mg

100 mg

SUCRALFATE
Carafate

tablet

1 gram

**SULFAMETHOXAZOLE/
TRIMETHOPRIM**
Bactrim

tablets

400/80 mg

Bactrim *(cont.)*

800/160 mg

Septra

tablets

400/80 mg   800/160 mg

SULFASALAZINE
Azulfidine

tablet

500 mg

Azulfidine EN-Tab

tablet, enteric-coated

500 mg

SULFISOXAZOLE
Gantrisin

tablet

500 mg

SULINDAC
Clinoril

tablets

150 mg   200 mg

SUMATRIPTAN
Imitrex

auto-injector system

TAMOXIFEN
Nolvadex

tablet

10 mg

TERAZOSIN
Hytrin

tablets

1 mg   2 mg

5 mg   10 mg

TERBUTALINE
Brethine

tablets

2.5 mg   5 mg

TERFENADINE
Seldane

tablet

60 mg

TETRACYCLINE
Achromycin V

capsule

250 mg

Sumycin

capsules

250 mg

500 mg

THEOPHYLLINE
Quibron-T/SR Dividose

tablet

300 mg

Slo-bid

capsules

50 mg   100 mg

200 mg

300 mg

Slo-Phyllin

capsules

125 mg

250 mg

tablet

200 mg

Theo-Dur

capsules

50 mg   75 mg

125 mg

200 mg

tablets

100 mg   200 mg

Theo-Dur *(cont.)*

300 mg   450 mg

Theo-24

capsule

300 mg

THIORIDAZINE
Mellaril

tablets

10 mg   25 mg

50 mg   100 mg

THIOTHIXENE
Navane

capsules

1 mg   2 mg

5 mg   10 mg

20 mg

TICLOPIDINE
Ticlid

tablet

250 mg

TIMOLOL
Blocadren

tablets

5 mg   10 mg

20 mg

TOLAZAMIDE
Tolinase
tablets

250 mg   500 mg

TOLBUTAMIDE
Orinase
tablet

500 mg

TOLMETIN
Tolectin
tablet

600 mg

Tolectin DS
capsule

400 mg

TRAZODONE
Desyrel
tablets

50 mg   100 mg

150 mg

TRIAMTERENE/
HYDROCHLOROTHIAZIDE
Dyazide
capsule

50/25 mg

Maxzide
tablets

37.5/25 mg   75/50 mg

TRIFLUOPERAZINE
Stelazine
tablets

1 mg   2 mg   5 mg

TRIMETHOPRIM
Trimpex
tablet

100 mg

VALACYCLOVIR
Valtrex
tablet

500 mg

VALPROIC ACID
Depakote Sprinkle
capsule

125 mg

Depakote
tablets

125 mg   250 mg

500 mg

VERAPAMIL
Calan
tablets

80 mg   120 mg

Calan SR
tablets, extended-release

120 mg   180 mg

240 mg

Verelan
capsules, extended-release

120 mg

180 mg

240 mg

WARFARIN
Coumadin
tablets

1 mg   2 mg   2.5 mg

5 mg   7.5 mg   10 mg

ZALCITABINE
Hivid
tablets

0.375 mg   0.750 mg

ZIDOVUDINE
Retrovir
capsule

100 mg

Sulindac: Therapy is started with 150 to 200 mg twice daily taken 12 hours apart. Maximum daily dose is 400 mg.

Tolmetin: 400 mg 3 times daily is started, with usual ongoing doses of 600 to 1600 mg as needed and tolerated. Total daily dose should not exceed 1600 mg for osteoarthritis or 2000 mg for rheumatoid arthritis.

Children two years of age or older may be given 20 mg per kg orally, divided into three or four doses daily. The dose may be increased as needed and tolerated to a maximum daily dose of 30 mg per kg.

Note: Actual dose and dosing schedule must be determined by the physician for each patient individually.

Conditions Requiring Dosing Adjustments

Liver function: These drugs are extensively metabolized in the liver. They should be used with caution in patients with liver compromise.

Kidney function: All nonsteroidal anti-inflammatory drugs may inhibit prostaglandins and alter kidney blood flow in patients with kidney (renal) compromise. Used with caution in patients with kidney compromise.

▷ **Dosing Instructions:**   Take with or following food to prevent stomach irritation. Take with a full glass of water and remain upright (do not lie down) for 30 minutes. Regular release tablets may be crushed, but not extended release forms. The regular capsules may be opened for administration, but not the prolonged-action capsules. Food actually increases absorption of nabumetone.

Usual Duration of Use: Continual use on a regular schedule for 1 to 2 weeks is usually necessary to determine drug benefit in relieving arthritic discomfort. The usual length of treatment for bursitis or tendonitis for indomethacin or sulindac is 7 to 14 days. Ketorolac is used for short-term pain treatment. Long-term use of the other agents in this class requires physician supervision and periodic evaluation.

▷ **These Drugs Should Not Be Taken If**
- you have had an allergic reaction to them previously.
- you are subject to asthma or nasal polyps caused by aspirin.
- you are pregnant (all NSAIDS during the last three months of pregnancy) or you are breast-feeding.
- you have active peptic ulcer disease or any form of gastrointestinal ulceration or bleeding.
- you have active liver disease.
- you have a bleeding disorder or a blood cell disorder.
- you have severe impairment of kidney function.
- you have porphyria (diclofenac, indomethacin).

▷ **Inform Your Physician Before Taking This Drug If**
- you are allergic to aspirin or to other aspirin substitutes.
- you have a history of peptic ulcer disease, Crohn's disease, ulcerative colitis or any type of bleeding disorder.
- you have a history of epilepsy, Parkinson's disease or mental illness (psychosis).
- you have impaired liver or kidney function.
- you have high blood pressure or a history of heart failure.
- you are taking: acetaminophen, aspirin or other aspirin substitutes or anticoagulants.

Possible Side Effects (natural, expected, and unavoidable drug actions)
Drowsiness, ringing in ears, fluid retention.

▷ **Possible Adverse Effects** (unusual, unexpected, and infrequent reactions)
If any of the following develop, consult your physician promptly for guidance.

Mild Adverse Effects
Allergic Reactions: Skin rash, hives, itching, localized swellings of face and/or extremities.
Headache, dizziness, feelings of detachment.
Mouth sores, indigestion, nausea, vomiting, diarrhea.
Ringing in the ears.
Temporary loss of hair (indomethacin).

Serious Adverse Effects
Allergic Reactions: Asthma, difficult breathing, mouth irritation.
Blurred vision, confusion, depression.
Active peptic ulcer, with or without bleeding.
Liver damage with jaundice (see Glossary).
Kidney damage with painful urination, bloody urine, reduced urine formation.
Rare bone marrow depression (see Glossary)—fatigue, weakness, fever, sore throat, abnormal bleeding or bruising.
Severe skin rash (Stevens-Johnson syndrome—diclofenac, ketorolac, etodolac, sulindac).
Peripheral neuritis (see Glossary)—numbness, pain, or weakness in extremities (indomethacin).
Rare lung fibrosis (nabumetone).
Rare pneumonitis (sulindac).
Rare aseptic meningitis (diclofenac).

▷ **Possible Effects on Sexual Function**
Enlargement and tenderness of both male and female breasts (indomethacin, sulindac).
Nonmenstrual vaginal bleeding (indomethacin).
Rare impotence (diclofenac, nabumetone).
Rare uterine bleeding (etodolac, sulindac).

Possible Delayed Adverse Effects: Mild anemia due to "silent" blood loss from the stomach.

▷ **Adverse Effects That May Mimic Natural Diseases or Disorders**
Liver reactions may suggest viral hepatitis.

Natural Diseases or Disorders That May Be Activated by These Drugs
Peptic ulcer disease, ulcerative colitis.

Possible Effects on Laboratory Tests
Complete blood cell counts: decreased red cells, hemoglobin, white cells and platelets.
Prothrombin time: increased.
Blood lithium level: increased.
Liver function tests: increased liver enzymes (ALT/GPT, AST/GOT and alkaline phosphatase), increased bilirubin.

Kidney function tests: increased blood creatinine and urea nitrogen (BUN) levels (kidney damage).

Fecal occult blood test: positive.

CAUTION

1. Dose should be limited to the smallest amount that produces reasonable improvement.
2. These drugs may mask early signs of infection. Tell your doctor if you think you are developing an infection of any kind.

Precautions for Use

By Infants and Children: Indomethacin: this drug frequently impairs kidney function in infants. Fatal liver reactions are possible in children between 6 and 12 years of age; avoid the use of this drug in this age group.

Diclofenac, etodolac, ketorolac, nabumetone, sulindac: Safety and efficacy for those under 12 years of age not established.

Tolmetin: Safety and efficacy for those under two years of age not established.

By Those over 60 Years of Age: Small doses are advisable until tolerance is determined. Watch for any signs of liver or kidney toxicity, fluid retention, dizziness, confusion, impaired memory, depression, peptic ulcer or diarrhea, often with rectal bleeding.

▷ Advisability of Use During Pregnancy

Pregnancy Category: Diclofenac, tolmetin: B. Ketorolac, nabumetone, sulindac and etodolac: C. Indomethacin, sulindac and tolmetin: (last three months): D. See Pregnancy Code at the back of this book.

Animal studies: Indomethacin: significant toxicity and birth defects reported in mice and rats.

Diclofenac: mouse, rat and rabbit studies reveal toxic effects on the embryo but no birth defects.

Ketorolac: rat and rabbit studies did not reveal teratogenicity, however, oral dosing after the 17th day of pregnancy caused increased pup mortality.

Nabumetone, tolmetin: rat and rabbit studies revealed no defects.

Human studies: Indomethacin: adequate studies of pregnant women are not available. However, birth defects have been attributed to the use of this drug during pregnancy.

The manufacturer recommends that indomethacin not be taken during pregnancy.

Diclofenac, nabumetone, sulindac, tolmetin: adequate studies of pregnant women are not available. Avoid this drug completely during the last 3 months of pregnancy. Use it during the first 6 months only if clearly needed. Ask your doctor for guidance.

Ketorolac: adequate studies of pregnant women are not available. Ask your doctor for guidance.

Etodolac: adequate studies of pregnant women not available. The manufacturer advises that this drug be avoided during pregnancy.

Advisability of Use if Breast-Feeding

Presence of this drug in breast milk: Yes: indomethacin, diclofenac, ketorolac.

Unknown: Etodolac, nabumetone, sulindac, tolmetin.

Avoid drug or refrain from nursing.

Habit-Forming Potential: None.

Effects of Overdosage: Drowsiness, agitation, confusion, nausea, vomiting, diarrhea, disorientation, seizures, coma.

Possible Effects of Long-Term Use: Indomethacin and tolmetin: eye changes: deposits in the cornea, alterations in the retina.

Suggested Periodic Examinations While Taking These Drugs (at physician's discretion)
Complete blood cell counts, liver and kidney function tests, complete eye examinations if vision is altered in any way.

▷ **While Taking These Drugs, Observe the Following**
Foods: No restrictions.
Nutritional Support: Indomethecin: take 50 mg of vitamin C (ascorbic acid) daily.
Beverages: No restrictions. May be taken with milk.

▷ *Alcohol:* Use with caution. Alcohol can irritate the stomach lining, and when this is added to irritation from these drugs, can increase the risk of stomach ulceration and/or bleeding.
Tobacco Smoking: No interactions expected.

▷ *Other Drugs*
Medications in this class may ***increase*** the effects of
• acetaminophen (Tylenol, etc.), and increase the risk of kidney damage; avoid prolonged use of this combination.
• anticoagulants such as warfarin (Coumadin, etc.), and increase the risk of bleeding; monitor prothrombin time, adjust dose accordingly.
• lithium, and cause lithium toxicity.
• cyclosporine (Sandimmune) and cause toxicity.
• methotrexate (Mexate, others) and cause toxic levels.
• thrombolytics such as streptokinase or TPA.
Medications in this class may ***decrease*** the effects of
• beta blocker drugs (see Drug Classes), and reduce their antihypertensive effectiveness.
• bumetanide (Bumex).
• captopril (Capoten).
• ethacrynic acid (Edecrin).
• furosemide (Lasix).
Medications in this class ***taken concurrently*** with the following drugs may increase the risk of bleeding; avoid these combinations:
• aspirin.
• diflunisal (Dolobid).
• dipyridamole (Persantine).
• sulfinpyrazone (Anturane).
• valproic acid (Depakene).

▷ *Driving, Hazardous Activities:* This drug may cause drowsiness, dizziness or impaired vision. Restrict activities as necessary.
Aviation Note: The use of this drug ***may be a disqualification*** for piloting. Consult a designated Aviation Medical Examiner.
Exposure to Sun: Use caution. Several of the medicines in this class have caused increased sensitivity (photosensitivity—see Glossary) to the sun.

ACYCLOVIR (ay SI kloh ver)

Other Name: Acycloguanosine

Introduced: 1979   **Prescription:** USA: Yes; Canada: Yes   **Available as**
Generic: No   **Class:** Antiviral   **Controlled Drug:** USA: No; Canada: No

Brand Name: Zovirax

> Author's note: This medication was rejected by the FDA for a change to non-prescription "over the counter" (OTC) status. This was based on fear of development of viral resistance—**not** safety issues.

<table>
<tr><td colspan="2" align="center">**BENEFITS versus RISKS**</td></tr>
<tr><td align="center">*Possible Benefits*</td><td align="center">*Possible Risks*</td></tr>
<tr><td>Faster recovery from initial episode of genital herpes
Prevention of recurrence of genital herpes
Lessens the severity of chicken pox in some children</td><td>Nausea, vomiting, diarrhea
Nervousness, depression
Joint and muscle pain
Seizures or coma with IV use (rare)</td></tr>
</table>

▷ **Principal Uses**

As a Single Drug Product: Uses currently included in FDA approved labeling: (1) Treats or helps prevent genital herpes; (2) used to lessen the severity of chicken pox in children using inhaled steroids or who have a lung disease or who are otherwise healthy; (3) treats shingles (Herpes zoster) which has recurred; (4) treats skin and mucous infections (mucocutaneous) caused by Herpes simplex in patients with immune problems; (5) used to treat brain infections caused by Herpes simplex; (6) used to prevent Herpes simplex virus infections in bone marrow transplant patients; (6) treats Varicella (chicken pox) in children over a year old who have a chronic pulmonary condition or have a chronic skin condition, children receiving short courses of corticosteroids via the lungs or children who are over 13 years old who are otherwise healthy.

Other (unlabeled) generally accepted uses: (1) Acyclovir helps treat Herpes simplex infections of the eye and rectum and pneumonia caused by the chicken pox (Varicella) virus; (2) some data to support its use in non-malignant skin growths in the throat (laryngeal papillomatosis); (3) it is a trial (in combination) AIDS treatment; (4) can prevent recurrent erythema multiforme that may occur with Herpes simplex infections.

How This Drug Works: By blocking genetic material formation of the herpes simplex virus, this drug stops viral multiplication and spread, reducing severity and duration of the herpes infection.

Available Dosage Forms and Strengths

Capsules — 200 mg
Intravenous — 500 mg, one gram
Oral suspension — 200 mg/ 5 ml
Tablets — 200 mg (Canada only), 400 mg and 800 mg
Ointment — 5%, 50 mg per gram (Canada)

▷ **Recommended Dosage Ranges (Actual dosage and administration schedule must be determined by the physician or clinical pharmacist for each patient individually.)**

Infants and Children: Safety and efficacy of oral use in children younger than 6 weeks of age has NOT been established.

Topical acyclovir use data in children less than 10 is lacking; however, the drug would be expected to follow the same patterns of side effects and risk benefit decisions as the oral formulation.

18 to 65 Years of Age: For initial episode of genital herpes—200 mg/ 4 hours for a total of 5 capsules daily for 10 consecutive days (total dose of 50 capsules). For intermittent recurrence—200 mg/4 hours for a total of 5 capsules daily for 5 consecutive days (total dose of 25 capsules). Start treatment at the earliest sign of recurrence. For prevention of frequent recurrence—400 mg taken 2 times daily for up to 12 months. For the ointment form—cover all infected areas every 3 hours for a total of 6 times daily for 7 consecutive days. Start treatment at the **earliest sign** of infection.

Treatment of chicken pox: 20 mg/kg (do not exceed 800 mg) orally, four times a day for 5 days. Start treatment at the first symptom or sign.

Over 65 Years of Age: The dose **must** be adjusted if the kidneys are impaired.

Conditions Requiring Dosing Adjustments

Liver function: Specific adjustment in liver dysfunction is not defined.

Kidney function: The dose MUST be adjusted in people with compromised kidney function.

Obesity: Dosing here (intravenous form) should be made on ideal body weight and given as 10 mg per kg. Maximum dose is 500 mg per square meter every eight hours.

▷ **Dosing Instructions:** May be taken without regard to food. Capsule may be opened to take it. Take the full course of the exact dose prescribed. Use a finger cot or rubber glove to apply the ointment.

Usual Duration of Use: Use on a regular schedule for 10 days is usually needed to see this drug's effect in reducing the severity and duration of the initial infection. Continual use for 6 months to 3 years may be needed to prevent frequent recurrence of herpes eruptions.

▷ **This Drug Should Not Be Taken If**
- you have had an allergic reaction to it previously.

▷ **Inform Your Physician Before Taking This Drug If**
- you have impaired liver or kidney function.
- you are taking any other drugs at this time.
- you think you are dehydrated.
- you are unsure of how much or how often to take acyclovir.

Possible Side Effects (natural, expected, and unavoidable drug actions)
With use of capsules—none.
With use of ointment—mild pain or stinging at site of application.

▷ **Possible Adverse Effects** (unusual, unexpected, and infrequent reactions)
If any of the following develop, consult your physician promptly for guidance.

Mild Adverse Effects
Allergic Reaction: Skin rash.

Headache, dizziness, nervousness, insomnia, depression, fatigue.

Nausea, vomiting, diarrhea.

Joint pains, muscle cramps.

Acne, hair loss.

Serious Adverse Effects

Superficial thrombophlebitis, enlarged lymph glands.

Seizures or coma with IV use (rare).

Kidney problems (rare).

Very rare colitis.

▷ **Possible Effects on Sexual Function:** Altered timing and pattern of menstruation.

Possible Effects on Laboratory Tests

Complete blood cell counts: decreased red cells and hemoglobin.

Blood urea nitrogen (BUN): increased.

Serum creatinine: increased.

CAUTION

1. This drug does **not** eliminate all herpes virus and is **not a cure**. Recurrence is possible. Resume treatment at the earliest sign of infection.
2. Avoid sexual intercourse if herpes blisters and swelling are present.
3. Do not exceed the prescribed dosage.
4. Tell your doctor if frequency or severity of infections don't improve.

Precautions for Use

By Infants and Children: Safety and effectiveness for use by those under 12 not established.

By Those over 60 Years of Age: Avoid dehydration. Drink 2 to 3 quarts of liquids daily.

▷ **Advisability of Use During Pregnancy**

Pregnancy Category: C. See Pregnancy Code at the back of this book.

The company has a pregnancy registry at 1–800–722–9292.

Animal studies: No birth defects found in mouse, rat or rabbit studies.

Human studies: The pregnancy registry has followed more than 400 cases to date. There was no consistent pattern of birth defects, and the number of patients (sample size) is still too small to detect small increases in risk. Avoid use if possible. Use only if clearly needed.

Advisability of Use if Breast-Feeding

Presence of this drug in breast milk: Yes.

Ask your physician for guidance.

Habit-Forming Potential: None.

Effects of Overdosage: Possible impairment of kidney function.

Possible Effects of Long-Term Use: Development of acyclovir-resistant strains of herpes virus. Treatment will fail if this occurs.

Suggested Periodic Examinations While Taking This Drug (at physician's discretion)

Kidney function tests.

▷ **While Taking This Drug, Observe the Following**

Foods: No restrictions.

Beverages: No restrictions. May be taken with milk. **Drink 2 to 3 quarts of liquids** (if not contraindicated for you) **daily.**

▷   *Alcohol:* Use caution; dizziness or fatigue may be accentuated.
    Tobacco Smoking: No interactions expected.
▷   *Other Drugs*
    The following drugs may ***increase*** the effects of acyclovir
- cyclosporine use may result in increased risk of kidney toxicity.
- probenecid (Benemid) may delay acyclovir elimination.

Acyclovir ***taken concurrently*** with
- meperidine may result in neurologic problems.
- varicella vaccine (Varivax) will blunt the vaccine effectiveness.
- zidovudine (AZT) may result in severe fatigue and lethargy.

▷   *Driving, Hazardous Activities:* Use caution if dizziness or fatigue occurs.
    Aviation Note: The use of this drug ***may be a disqualification*** for piloting. Consult a designated Aviation Medical Examiner.
    Exposure to Sun: No restrictions.

ALBUTEROL (al BYU ter ohl)

Other Name: Salbutamol

Introduced: 1968   **Prescription:** USA: Yes; Canada: Yes   **Available as Generic:** Yes   **Class:** Antiasthmatic, bronchodilator   **Controlled Drug:** USA: No; Canada: No

Brand Names: ✦Apo-Salvent, ✦Novo-Salmol, Proventil Inhaler, Proventil Repetabs, Proventil Tablets, ✦Salbutamol, ✦Ventodisk, Ventolin Inhaler, Ventolin Rotacaps, Ventolin syrup, Ventolin tablets, Volmax extended release tablets, ✦Volmax controlled release tablets

BENEFITS versus RISKS	
Possible Benefits	*Possible Risks*
VERY EFFECTIVE RELIEF OF BRONCHOSPASM	Increased blood pressure
	Fine hand tremor
	Irregular heart rhythm and fatalities (with excessive use)

▷ **Principal Uses**
    As a Single Drug Product: Uses currently included in FDA approved labeling: (1)Relieves acute bronchial asthma and reduces frequency and severity of chronic, recurrent asthmatic attacks. Helps prevent exercise induced bronchospasm in children ages 4 to 11.

How This Drug Works: By increasing cyclic AMP, this drug relaxes constricted bronchial muscles to relieve asthmatic wheezing.

Available Dosage Forms and Strengths
Aerosol — 90 mcg per actuation
Capsules for inhalation — 200 mcg
Nasal inhaler (Canada) — 100 mcg/dose
Solution for inhalation — 0.83 mg/ml and 5 mg/ml
Syrup — 2 mg/5 ml
Rotacaps — 200 mcg
Tablets — 2 mg, 4 mg
— 2.4 mg, 4.8 mg (Canada)

> Tablets, controlled release (Canada) — 4 mg, 8 mg
> Tablets, extended release — 4 mg, 8 mg, 9 mg
> Ventodisk (Canada) — 200 mcg and 400 mcg per disk

▷ **Recommended Dosage Ranges (Actual dosage and administration schedule must be determined by the physician or clinical pharmacist for each patient individually.)**
Inhaler—Adults and children 12 or older: Two inhalations repeated every 4 to 6 hours. For some patients, one inhalation every 4 hours may be enough. Taking a larger number of inhalations is **not** recommended. If the dose which has worked for you before does not provide relief, call your physician **immediately** as the status of your asthma must be examined. Tablets—2 to 4 mg 3 to 4 times daily, every 4 to 6 hours. **Do not exceed** 8 inhalations (720 mcg)/24 hours, or 32 mg (tablet form)/24 hours.

Conditions Requiring Dosing Adjustments
Liver function: Used with caution and in low doses in people with liver compromise.
Kidney function: No specific changes in dosing are available.
Coronary artery disease: A maximum starting dose should be 1 mg in order to avoid chest pain (angina).
Thyroid disease
People with low (hypoactive) thyroid may require increased doses.

▷ **Dosing Instructions:**   May be taken on empty stomach or with food or milk. Tablet may be crushed. For inhaler, follow the written instructions carefully. Do not use excessively.

Usual Duration of Use: Do not use beyond the time necessary to stop episodes of asthma.

▷ **This Drug Should Not Be Taken If**
• you have had an allergic reaction to any dosage form of it.
• you have an irregular heart rhythm.
• you are taking, or took within the past 2 weeks, any monoamine oxidase (MAO) type A inhibitor drug (see Drug Class, Section Four).

▷ **Inform Your Physician Before Taking This Drug If**
• you have a heart or circulatory disorder, especially high blood pressure or coronary heart disease.
• you have diabetes.
• you have an overactive thyroid (hyperthyroid).
• you are taking any form of digitalis or any stimulant drug.
• you take other prescription or nonprescription medications which were not discussed when albuterol was prescribed for you.
• you are unsure how much to take or how often to take albuterol.

Possible Side Effects (natural, expected, and unavoidable drug actions)
Aerosol—dryness or irritation of mouth or throat, altered taste.
Tablet—nervousness, palpitation.

▷ **Possible Adverse Effects** (unusual, unexpected, and infrequent reactions)
If any of the following develop, consult your physician promptly for guidance.
Mild Adverse Effects
Headache, dizziness (rare), restlessness, insomnia, fine hand tremor.

Nausea (rare), heartburn, vomiting.
Leg cramps, flushing of skin.
Difficulty urinating (rare).
Rapid heart rate.
Decreased platelets (after high doses).

Serious Adverse Effects

This drug may be dangerous if the medicine stops working and patients increase their dose and/or frequency, as it may result in rapid or irregular heart rhythm and fatalities.

Hallucinations or convulsions (with excessive dosing).
Decreased blood potassium (hypokalemia).
High blood sugar (hyperglycemia).

▷ **Possible Effects on Sexual Function:**   None reported.

Natural Diseases or Disorders That May Be Activated By This Drug

Latent coronary artery disease, diabetes or high blood pressure.

Possible Effects on Laboratory Tests

Blood aldosterone: increased.
Blood HDL cholesterol level: increased.
Blood glucose level: increased.
Blood potassium: decreased.

CAUTION

1. Use of this drug by inhalation with beclomethasone aerosol (Beclovent, Vanceril) may increase the risk of fluorocarbon propellant toxicity. Use albuterol aerosol 20 to 30 minutes *before* beclomethasone aerosol to reduce toxicity and enhance the penetration of beclomethasone.
2. Serious heart rhythm problems or cardiac arrest can result from excessive or prolonged inhalation.
3. Call your doctor if you begin to increase the number of times you use this drug on a daily basis.

Precautions for Use

By Infants and Children: Used to help prevent bronchospasm caused by exercise in children ages 4–11.

By Those over 60 Years of Age: Avoid excessive and continual use. If asthma is not relieved promptly, other drugs will have to be tried. Watch for nervousness, palpitations, irregular heart rhythm and muscle tremors.

▷ **Advisability of Use During Pregnancy**

Pregnancy Category: C. See Pregnancy Code at the back of this book.
Animal studies: Cleft palate reported in mice.
Human studies: Adequate studies of pregnant women are not available.
Avoid use during first 3 months if possible.

Advisability of Use if Breast-Feeding

Presence of this drug in breast milk: Unknown.
Avoid drug or refrain from nursing.

Habit-Forming Potential: A few cases of dependency and abuse have been described which may be used for the effect of the propellants or the drug itself.

Effects of Overdosage: Nervousness, palpitation, rapid heart rate, life-threatening arrhythmias, sweating, headache, tremor, vomiting, chest pain.

Possible Effects of Long-Term Use: Loss of effectiveness.

Suggested Periodic Examinations While Taking This Drug (at physician's discretion)
Blood pressure measurements, evaluation of heart status.

▷ **While Taking This Drug, Observe the Following**
Foods: No restrictions.
Beverages: Avoid excessive caffeine as found in coffee, tea, cola, chocolate.
▷ *Alcohol:* No interactions expected.
Tobacco Smoking: No interactions expected; however smoking may cause problems with other medications used to treat asthma. Ask your doctor for advice.
▷ *Other Drugs*
Albuterol *taken concurrently* with
- amphetamines may result in worsening of cardiovascular side effects.
- beta blockers such as propranolol results in loss of effect of both medications.
- monoamine oxidase (MAO) type A inhibitor drugs can cause very high blood pressure and undesirable heart stimulation.
- theophylline may result in rapid removal of theophylline and loss of therapeutic theophylline effect.
- tricyclic antidepressants (see Glossary) may cause a severe increase in blood pressure.
▷ *Driving, Hazardous Activities:* Use caution if excessive nervousness or dizziness occurs.
Aviation Note: The use of this drug *is a disqualification* for piloting. Consult a designated Aviation Medical Examiner.
Exposure to Sun: No restrictions.
Heavy Exercise or Exertion: Use caution. Excessive exercise can induce asthma in some asthmatics.

ALENDRONATE a LEN druh nate

Introduced: 1996 **Prescription:** USA: Yes **Available as Generic:**
No **Class:** Aminobisphosphonate **Controlled Drug:** USA: No
Brand Name: Fosamax

BENEFITS versus RISKS	
Possible Benefits	*Possible Risks*
EFFECTIVE TREATMENT OF OSTEOPOROSIS	Esophageal irritation (if not taken correctly)
INCREASE IN BONE MASS	Minor muscle pain
EXPECTED PREVENTION OF OSTEOPOROSIS	
DECREASED RISK OF BONE FRACTURES	
SYMPTOM RELIEF IN PAGET'S DISEASE	

▷ **Principal Uses**

> *As a Single Drug Product:* Uses currently included in FDA approved labeling: (1) Treatment of post-menopausal osteoporosis; (2) treatment of Paget's disease.

> Other (unlabeled) generally accepted uses: (1) Many clinicians are using this medicine in patients who do not want to take or who are not candidates for estrogen or progesterone therapy to prevent osteoporosis occurring after menopause; (2) may have a role in helping manage abnormally elevated blood calcium levels such as those seen with some cancers; (3) expected to work in the prevention and treatment of male osteoporosis.

How This Drug Works: This medicine works at the brush border of the osteoclast cell. This effectively prevents this cell from resorbing bone while letting the osteoblast or bone building cell continue to work. The net benefit is stronger bone and decreased risk of fractures.

Available Dosage Forms and Strengths

> Tablets — 10 mg and 40 mg

▷ **Recommended Dosage Ranges: (Actual dosage and administration schedule must be determined by the physician or clinical pharmacist for each patient individually.)**

> *Infants and Children:* Efficacy and safety are not established.

> *18 to 65 Years of Age:* In female post-menopausal osteoporosis: 10 mg taken once daily.

> Osteoporosis prevention: Expected to be 10 mg once daily.

> I strongly recommend an appropriate amount of dietary calcium and/or calcium supplementation to ensure adequate calcium intake *every day*. Discuss the need for vitamin D with your doctor. Calcium and vitamin D are critical in osteoporosis prevention and treatment.

> Paget's disease: 40 mg once daily for 6 months.

> *Over 65 Years of Age:* Same as in those 18 to 65 years old.

Conditions Requiring Dosing Adjustments

> *Liver function:* The liver is not involved in the elimination of this medicine. No changes needed.

> *Kidney function:* Lower doses are needed for patients with kidney compromise. Patients with creatinine clearances (see Glossary) of less than 35 ml per minute **should not** be given this medicine.

▷ **Dosing Instructions:**   TAKE THIS MEDICINE WITH 6 TO 8 OUNCES OF TAP WATER TO GET THE BEST RESULTS. DO NOT take this medicine with food or other medicines as the therapeutic benefit will be decreased. Take it at least half an hour before the first food or liquids (other than plain water) of the day. Waiting longer than 30 minutes to eat or drink will further improve the absorption of alendronate. In order to decrease the risk of irritation or ulceration of the esophagus DO NOT lie down for at least 30 minutes (preferably an hour) after taking this medication.

Usual Duration of Use: In Paget's disease, this medicine is used once daily for six months, with reassessment after that course of therapy. In treating osteoporosis in post-menopausal women, many physicians will obtain a bone mineral density test (DEXA is presently the most widely use) to help in the decision to start treatment, and then get a second measurement one to two years later in order to assess the outcome of therapy. Further study is needed to identify the best dosing strategies in long-term use of alendronate.

Possible Advantages of This Drug
This drug increases bone mass which decreases the risk of fractures.
This medicine also helps form bone of normal form (microarchitecture).
Better side effect profile than earlier bisphosphonates.
Greater maximum possible bone mass increase than other agents.

▷ This Drug Should Not Be Taken If
- you are allergic to the drug or any of the components of the tablets.
- you have a low blood calcium (hypocalcemia). Talk with your doctor.
- you have a significant kidney disease (this medicine should NOT be taken if creatinine clearance is less than 35 ml per minute).

▷ Inform Your Physician Before Taking This Drug If
- you have ulcers or inflammation of the duodenum.
- you have difficulty swallowing.
- you have esophageal disease.
- you have a vitamin D deficiency.
- you have a diet poor in calcium (low calcium diet).

Possible Side Effects (natural, expected, and unavoidable drug actions)
Irritation of the esophagus and potential ulceration (rare). This effect may be worsened if patients lie down soon after taking this medicine.

▷ Possible Adverse Effects (unusual, unexpected, and infrequent reactions)
If any of the following develop, consult your physician promptly for guidance.

Mild Adverse Effects
Allergic reactions: Rare skin rash or redness.
Headache.
Gas (flatulence), diarrhea.
Constipation.
Mild decrease in calcium (2% decrease in some patients taking 10 mg daily).
Mild decrease in phosphorous (up to 6%). Mild muscle pain (4.1% with the 10 mg dose).
Rare fever (drug fever) with intravenous use.

Serious Adverse Effects
Allergic reactions: None reported.
Esophageal ulceration (rare) may be worsened if you lie down immediately after taking this medicine. Best NOT to lie down for at least half an hour after taking this medicine.
One case report of a patient with a history of peptic ulcer disease who had stomach surgery and who was also taking aspirin developed an ulcer (anastomotic) and had mild hemorrhaging.

▷ Possible Effects on Sexual Function: None reported.

Possible Effects on Laboratory Tests
Serum calcium: lowered
Liver function tests: Rarely increased in patients given the intravenous form (asymptomatic and transient).

CAUTION

1. A "dear doctor" letter was sent out by the FDA warning of increased occurrence of esophageal ulceration. This may have been caused by patients taking the medicine with less water than directed. It is also advisable NOT TO LIE down for 30 minutes after taking this medicine.
2. Patients who take more than 10 mg of alendronate a day should avoid aspirin and aspirin-containing compounds because upper gastrointestinal adverse effects may be increased in this situation if the medicines are combined
3. Other causes of osteoporosis besides estrogen or aging (secondary osteoporosis) must be ruled out.

Precautions for Use

By Infants and Children: Safety and efficacy in this age group have not been established.

By Those over 60 Years of Age: The amount that goes into the body (bioavailability) and the places alendronate goes to (disposition) are similar as for those less than 60. No specific dosing changes are needed for those in this age group.

▷ **Advisability of Use During Pregnancy**

Pregnancy Category: C. See Pregnancy Risk Categories at the back of this book. Studies in rats have shown toxicity to the mother as well as neonatal death following dosing of alendronate during pregnancy. Adequate studies of pregnant women are not available. Avoid this medicine in pregnancy.

Advisability of Use if Breast-Feeding

Presence of this drug in breast milk: Unknown.

Avoid drug or refrain from nursing.

Habit-Forming Potential: None.

Effects of Overdosage: Nausea, vomiting, hypocalcemia and hypophosphatemia. Heartburn, ulceration of the upper gastrointestinal tract.

Possible Effects of Long-Term Use: Increased bone density and decreased fracture risk.

Suggested Periodic Examinations While Taking This Drug (at physician's discretion)

Measurement of bone mineral density.

Blood calcium.

Measurement of height.

▷ **While Taking This Drug, Observe the Following**

Foods: Intake of adequate elemental calcium is needed; however, calcium supplements (classified as a food) should be taken at least half an hour after taking alendronate.

Beverages: Any liquid other than water will decrease the amount of alendronate that gets into your body to help you. It is critical that this medicine only be taken with 6 to 8 ounces of water.

▷ *Alcohol:* Alcohol (especially in high doses) may act as a bone forming cell (osteoblast) poison and excessive use is a risk factor for osteoporosis.

Tobacco Smoking: Tobacco may act to increase the elimination of estrogen and is a risk factor for osteoporosis. Smoking is never advisable.

▷ *Other Drugs*
 Alendronate *taken concurrently* with
 • Antacids may decrease the total absorption of alendronate and decrease its therapeutic benefit.
 • Aspirin or aspirin-containing products may pose an increased risk of upper gastrointestinal adverse effects if more than 10 mg of alendronate is taken daily. Although other NSAIDs (see Drug Classes) were not presented as potential problems with alendronate doses greater than 10 mg, caution is advised.
 • estrogens (various) were taken by a small number of women in the clinical trials of this medicine without any adverse effects. The combination is not presently recommended because of lack of specific data.
 • foscavir (Foscarnet) may result in an additive decrease in calcium.
 • medicines in general should NOT be taken at the same time as alendronate. The most prudent approach is to separate any dose of alendronate and any other medicine by at least half an hour.
 The following drugs may *decrease* the effects of alendronate
 • Once again, because a small amount of alendronate gets into the body under the best conditions, it is prudent to only take alendronate with a full 6 to 8 ounces of water, and to take any other needed medicines at least half an hour after alendronate.
▷ *Driving, Hazardous Activities:* No specific limitations.
 Aviation Note: The use of this drug **is probably not a disqualification** for piloting. Consult a designated Aviation Medical Examiner.
 Exposure to Sun: No restrictions.
 Heavy Exercise or Exertion: If your bone density is low, heavy aerobic exercise may not be a good idea. Discuss this with your doctor. In general weight bearing exercise stimulates receptors (mechanoreceptors) to release factors that result in increased bone strength.
 Discontinuation: Talk with your doctor **before** stopping this medicine.

ALLOPURINOL (al oh PURE i nohl)

Introduced: 1963 **Prescription:** USA: Yes; Canada: Yes **Available as Generic:** USA: Yes; Canada: No **Class:** Antigout **Controlled Drug:** USA: No; Canada: No

Brand Names: ✦Alloprin, Lopurin, ✦Novopurol, ✦Purinol, Zurinol, Zyloprim

BENEFITS versus RISKS	
Possible Benefits	*Possible Risks*
EFFECTIVE CONTROL OF GOUT CONTROL OF HIGH BLOOD URIC ACID due to polycythemia, leukemia, cancer, and chemotherapy	Increased frequency of acute gout initially Peripheral neuritis Allergic reactions in skin, lung, blood vessels, and liver Bone marrow depression Kidney toxicity

▷ **Principal Uses**

As a Single Drug Product: Uses currently included in FDA approved labeling: (1) Used in long-term management of gout to *prevent* episodes of acute gout. (Does not relieve acute gout attacks.); (2) helps prevent excessive blood levels of uric acid in people who have recurrent uric acid kidney stones, those who are receiving chemotherapy or radiation therapy for cancer or people taking thiazide diuretics (see Drug Classes).

Other (unlabeled) generally accepted uses: (1) May be a great benefit in decreasing pain and occurrence of mouth sores in people receiving 5-fluorouracil chemotherapy.

How This Drug Works: By blocking the enzyme xanthine oxidase, it decreases uric acid formation.

Available Dosage Forms and Strengths

Tablets — 100 mg, 300 mg (and 200 mg in Canada)

▷ **Usual Adult Dosage Range:**   Initially 100 mg/24 hours. Increase by 100 mg/24 hours at intervals of 1 week until uric acid blood level is 6 mg/dl or less. Usual dose is 200 to 300 mg/24 hours for mild gout, and 400 to 600 mg/24 hours for moderate to severe gout. Daily doses of 300 mg or less may be taken as a single dose. Doses exceeding 300 mg daily should be divided into 2 or 3 equal portions; for the high uric acid levels associated with cancer, 600 to 800 mg/24 hours, divided into 3 equal portions. **Note: Actual dosage and administration schedule must be determined by the physician for each patient individually.**

Conditions Requiring Dosing Adjustments

Liver function: Need for dose adjustment in liver compromise is not documented.

Kidney function: Allopurinol dosing **must** be adjusted in renal compromise.

Malnutrition

Patients who are malnourished or who have been placed on low protein diets will not eliminate allopurinol normally and are at risk for toxicity. Doses **must** be decreased.

▷ **Dosing Instructions:**   Best taken with food or milk to reduce stomach irritation. Tablet may be crushed. Drink 2 to 3 quarts of liquids daily.

Usual Duration of Use: Blood uric acid levels often begin to decrease in 48 to 72 hours and may reach a normal range in 1 to 3 weeks. Regular use for several months may be needed to prevent attacks of acute gout. Continual use for many years may be needed for adequate control. See your doctor regularly.

▷ **This Drug Should Not Be Taken If**

• you have had an allergic reaction to it previously.
• you are experiencing an acute attack of gout at the present time.

▷ **Inform Your Physician Before Taking This Drug If**

• you have a personal or family history of hemochromatosis.
• you have a history of liver or kidney disease.
• you have had a blood cell or bone marrow disorder.
• you have any type of convulsive disorder (epilepsy).
• you take other prescription or nonprescription medications which were not discussed when allopurinol was prescribed for you.

- you are unsure of how much to take or how often to take allopurinol.
- you are on a low protein diet.

Possible Side Effects (natural, expected, and unavoidable drug actions)

Frequency and severity of episodes of acute gout may occur during the first several weeks of drug use. Ask your doctor about the need for other drugs during this period.

▷ **Possible Adverse Effects** (unusual, unexpected, and infrequent reactions)

If any of the following develop, consult your physician promptly for guidance.

Mild Adverse Effects

Allergic Reactions: Skin rash, hives, itching, drug fever.

Headache, dizziness, drowsiness.

Nausea, vomiting, diarrhea, stomach cramps.

Loss of scalp hair.

Serious Adverse Effects

Allergic Reactions: Severe skin reactions, high fever, chills, joint pains, swollen glands, kidney damage.

Hepatitis with or without jaundice (see Glossary)—yellow eyes and skin, dark-colored urine, light-colored stools.

Bone marrow depression (see Glossary).

Seizures, peripheral neuritis.

Bronchospasm (rare).

Eye damage (macular), cataract formation.

▷ **Possible Effects on Sexual Function:** Less than 1% and questionable cause: male infertility, male breast enlargement, impotence.

▷ **Adverse Effects That May Mimic Natural Diseases or Disorders**

Toxic liver reaction may suggest viral hepatitis.

Severe skin reactions may resemble the Stevens-Johnson syndrome (erythema multiforme).

Possible Effects on Laboratory Tests

Complete blood cell counts: decreased red cells, hemoglobin and platelets; increased eosinophils.

Liver function tests: increased ALT/GPT, AST/GOT, and alkaline phosphatase.

CAUTION

1. Early in treatment (first few weeks), the frequency of acute attacks of gout may increase. These subside with continuation of therapy.
2. This drug should not be started if acute gout symptoms are present as it will not help.
3. Vitamin C in doses of 2 grams or more daily can increase the risk of kidney stone formation during the use of allopurinol.
4. Allergic-type kidney damage can result if thiazide diuretics (see Drug Class, Section Four) are taken with allopurinol. Avoid this combination.
5. Patients on low protein diets will not eliminate allopurinol normally. Doses must be decreased.

Precautions for Use

By Infants and Children: Watch closely for allergic skin reactions and blood cell disorders. The toxicity of azathioprine (Imuran) or mercaptopurine (Purinethol) may be increased in children receiving chemotherapy.

By Those over 60 Years of Age: Smaller initial and maintenance doses of this drug must be used.

▷ **Advisability of Use During Pregnancy**
  Pregnancy Category: C. See Pregnancy Code at the back of this book.
    Animal studies: Results are conflicting and inconclusive.
    Human studies: Adequate studies of pregnant women are not available.
    Avoid use of drug during the first 3 months. Use during the last 6 months only if clearly needed.

Advisability of Use if Breast-Feeding
  Presence of this drug in breast milk: Yes.
  Avoid drug or refrain from nursing.

Habit-Forming Potential: None.

Effects of Overdosage: Nausea, vomiting or diarrhea. Hypersensitivity reactions, kidney and liver function decline.

Possible Effects of Long-Term Use: None identified.

Suggested Periodic Examinations While Taking This Drug (at physician's discretion)
  Blood uric acid levels, complete blood cell counts, liver and kidney function tests. If appropriate, eye examinations for possible cataract formation or macular damage. Complete blood counts.

▷ **While Taking This Drug, Observe the Following**
  Foods: Follow physician's advice regarding the need for a low-purine diet.
  Beverages: No restrictions. May be taken with milk.
▷ *Alcohol:* No interactions expected.
  Tobacco Smoking: No interactions expected.
▷ *Other Drugs*
    Allopurinol may *increase* the effects of
    • azathioprine (Imuran) and mercaptopurine (Purinethol), making dose decreases necessary.
    • oral anticoagulants (see Drug Classes) such as warfarin.
    • theophylline (aminophylline, Elixophyllin, Theo-Dur, etc.)
    Allopurinol *taken concurrently* with
    • ampicillin may increase the incidence of skin rash.
    • antacids containing aluminum will decrease the therapeutic effect of allopurinol.
    • captopril or other ACE inhibitors (see Drug Classes) can increase the likelihood of allergic reactions.
    • cyclophosphamide may result in cyclophosphamide toxicity.
    • cyclosporine can result in cyclosporine toxicity.
    • tamoxifen may result in increased allopurinol levels and increased risk of liver toxicity.
    • theophylline may increase theophylline to toxic levels.
    • vidarabine may increase risk of neurotoxicity.
▷ *Driving, Hazardous Activities:* Drowsiness may occur in some people. Use caution.
  Aviation Note: The use of this drug *may be a disqualification* for piloting. Consult a designated Aviation Medical Examiner.

Exposure to Sun: No restrictions.
Discontinuation: If you have a seizure disorder, this medicine dose should be
slowly decreased and then stopped.

ALPRAZOLAM (al PRAY zoh lam)

Introduced: 1973   **Prescription:** USA: Yes; Canada: Yes   **Available as**
Generic: Yes   **Class:** antianxiety drug, benzodiazepines   **Controlled**
Drug: USA: C-IV*; Canada: No

Brand Name: Xanax, Alprazolam Intensol, ✚Apo-Alpraz, Novo-Alprazol, ✚Nu-
Alpraz

Warning: The brand names Xanax and Zantac are similar and can lead to **serious** medication errors. These names represent very different drugs. Xanax
is the mild tranquilizer alprazolam. Zantac is ranitidine, used to treat peptic ulcer disease. Make sure your prescription was filled correctly.

BENEFITS versus RISKS

Possible Benefits	*Possible Risks*
RELIEF OF ANXIETY AND NERVOUS TENSION	Habit-forming potential with prolonged use
EFFECTIVE TREATMENT OF PANIC DISORDER	Minor impairment of mental functions with therapeutic doses
Wide margin of safety with therapeutic doses	Tachycardia and palpitations
May have some antidepressant activity	

▷ **Principal Uses**

As a Single Drug Product: Uses currently included in FDA approved labeling: (1)
Used for the short-term relief of mild to moderate anxiety and nervous tension; (2) helps relieve anxiety associated with neurosis; (3) eases irritable
bowel syndrome (see Glossary); (4) decreases the frequency and severity of
panic disorder.

Other (unlabeled) generally accepted uses: (1) May have a role in helping control extreme PMS symptoms; (2) can lessen a variety of types of cancer pain
when given with various narcotics; (3) eases agoraphobia; (4) can decrease
symptoms in essential tremor; (5) decreases the loudness of the sensation
of ear ringing in tinnitus.

How This Drug Works: Produces a calming effect by enhancing the action of
the nerve transmitter gamma-aminobutyric acid (GABA), which in turn
blocks higher brain centers.

Available Dosage Forms and Strengths

Tablets — 0.25 mg, 0.5 mg, 1 mg, 2 mg
Oral Solution — 0.25 mg, 0.5 mg, 1 mg/ 5 ml
— 0.25 mg/ 2.5 ml

*See Schedules of Controlled Drugs at the back of this book.

▷ **Usual Adult Dosage Range:**   For anxiety and nervous tension: 0.25 mg to 0.5 mg 3 times daily. Maximum dose is 4 mg/ 24 hours, taken in divided doses. For panic disorder: Initially 0.5 mg 3 times daily; increase dose by 1 mg every 3 to 4 days as needed and tolerated. Maximum daily dose is 10 mg.

Note: Actual dosage and administration schedule must be determined by the physician for each patient individually.

Conditions Requiring Dosing Adjustments

Liver function: Manufacturer recommends a starting dose of 0.25 mg in patients with advanced liver disease, with slow increase in dose only if needed.

Kidney function: Specific dosage reductions are not defined by the manufacturer.

Obesity

Takes a longer time to reach final concentrations in obese people. Doses should be calculated based on ideal rather than actual body weight.

Alcoholism

Because of some of the physiological and liver changes that can occur in alcoholism, the removal of this drug from the body may be delayed. Lower doses or longer times (intervals) between doses are needed.

▷ **Dosing Instructions:**   May be taken on empty stomach or with food or milk. Tablet may be crushed. Do not stop this drug abruptly if taken for more than 4 weeks.

Usual Duration of Use: Several days to several weeks. Avoid prolonged and uninterrupted use. Continual use should not exceed 8 weeks without evaluation by your doctor.

▷ **This Drug Should Not Be Taken If**
- you have had an allergic reaction to it previously.
- you are pregnant (first 3 months).
- you have acute narrow-angle glaucoma.
- you have myasthenia gravis.

▷ **Inform Your Physician Before Taking This Drug If**
- you have a history of palpitations and tachycardia (may be worsened).
- you are allergic to benzodiazepines (see Drug Class, Section Four).
- you are pregnant (last 6 months) or planning pregnancy.
- you are breast-feeding.
- you have a history of depression or serious mental illness (psychosis).
- you have a history of alcoholism or drug abuse.
- you have impaired liver or kidney function.
- you have open-angle glaucoma.
- you have a seizure disorder (epilepsy).
- you have severe chronic lung disease.
- you take other prescription or nonprescription medications which were not discussed when alprazolam was prescribed for you.
- you are unsure of how much alprazolam to take or how often to take it.

Possible Side Effects (natural, expected, and unavoidable drug actions)

Drowsiness, light-headedness.

▷ **Possible Adverse Effects** (unusual, unexpected, and infrequent reactions)

If any of the following develop, consult your physician promptly for guidance.

Mild Adverse Effects
> Allergic Reactions: Skin rash, hives.
> Headache, dizziness, drowsiness (most common effect—up to 50%), fatigue, blurred vision, dry mouth.
> Nausea, vomiting, constipation.

Serious Adverse Effects
> Confusion, hallucinations, depression, excitement, agitation (paradoxical reaction).
> Tachycardia and palpitations.
> Increased liver enzymes (rare).
> Low blood pressure (hypotension).

▷ **Possible Effects on Sexual Function:** Rare but documented: inhibited female orgasm (5 mg/day); impaired ejaculation (3.5 mg/day); decreased libido, impaired erection (4.5 mg/day); altered timing and pattern of menstruation (0.75 to 4 mg/day).

Possible Effects on Laboratory Tests
> Liver function tests: increased ALT/GPT, AST/GOT, rare and insignificant.
> Urine screening tests for drug abuse: may be **positive**. (Depends upon amount of drug taken and testing method.)

CAUTION
1. **Do not** stop taking this drug abruptly if it has been taken continually for more than 4 weeks.
2. Some nonprescription products have antihistamines (allergy and cold preparations, sleep aids) and can cause excessive sedation.

Precautions for Use
> *By Infants and Children:* Safety and effectiveness for use by those under 18 not established.
> *By Those over 60 Years of Age:* Starting dose should be 0.25 mg 2 or 3 times daily. Watch for excessive drowsiness, dizziness, unsteadiness and incoordination (possible low blood pressure).

▷ **Advisability of Use During Pregnancy**
> *Pregnancy Category:* D. See Pregnancy Code see at the back of this book.
> Animal studies: Diazepam (a closely related benzodiazepine) can cause cleft palate in mice and skeletal defects in rats. No data on alprazolam.
> Human studies: Some studies suggest an association between diazepam use and cleft lip and heart deformities. Adequate studies on the use of alprazolam by pregnant women are not available.
> Avoid use during entire pregnancy if possible.

Advisability of Use if Breast-Feeding
> Presence of this drug in breast milk: Yes.
> Avoid drug or refrain from nursing.

Habit-Forming Potential: This drug can cause psychological and/or physical dependence (see Glossary) if used in large doses for an extended period of time.

Effects of Overdosage: Marked drowsiness, weakness, feeling of drunkenness, staggering gait, tremor, stupor progressing to deep sleep or coma.

Possible Effects of Long-Term Use: Psychological and/or physical dependence.

Suggested Periodic Examinations While Taking This Drug (at physician's discretion)

None required for short-term use.

▷ **While Taking This Drug, Observe the Following**

Foods: No restrictions.

Beverages: Avoid excess intake of caffeine-containing beverages: coffee, tea, cola. This drug may be taken with milk.

▷ *Alcohol:* Use with extreme caution. Alcohol may increase the sedative effects of alprazolam. Alprazolam may increase the intoxicating effects of alcohol. Avoid alcohol completely—throughout the day and night—if you find it necessary to drive or to engage in *any* hazardous activity.

Tobacco Smoking: Heavy smoking may reduce the calming action of alprazolam.

Marijuana Smoking

Occasional (once or twice weekly): Mild increase in the sedative effect.

Daily: Marked increase in the sedative effect of this drug.

▷ *Other Drugs*

Alprazolam may ***increase*** the effects of
• digoxin (Lanoxin), and cause digoxin toxicity.

Alprazolam may ***decrease*** the effects of
• levodopa (Sinemet, etc.), and reduce its effect in treating Parkinson's disease.

The following drugs may ***increase*** the effects of alprazolam
• cimetidine (Tagamet).
• disulfiram (Antabuse).
• isoniazid (INH, Rifamate, etc.).
• omeprazole (Prilosec).
• oral contraceptives.
• fluoxetine (Prozac)
• valproic acid (Depakene).

The following drugs may ***decrease*** the effects of alprazolam
• carbamazepine (Tegretol).
• rifampin (Rimactane, etc.).
• theophylline (aminophylline, Theo-Dur, etc.).

Alprazolam ***taken concurrently*** with
• alcohol (ethanol) will worsen coordination and mental abilities.
• buspirone (Buspar) can result in additive CNS depression.
• benzodiazepines (see Drug Classes) can cause increased central nervous system (CNS) depression.
• narcotics (morphine, meperidine and others) will result in additive CNS depression.
• tricyclic antidepressants (see Drug Classes) results in additional (CNS) depression.

▷ *Driving, Hazardous Activities:* This drug can impair mental alertness, judgment, physical coordination and reaction time. Avoid hazardous activities accordingly.

Aviation Note: The use of this drug *is a disqualification* for piloting. Consult a designated Aviation Medical Examiner.

Exposure to Sun: Use caution, rare photosensitivity reports (see Glossary).

Discontinuation: If this drug has been taken for an extended period of time, do not stop it abruptly. Slowly reduce dose by 1 mg per week until a total daily dose of 4 mg is reached; by 0.5 mg per week until a total daily dose of 2 mg is reached; then by 0.25 mg per week thereafter. Ask your doctor for help.

AMANTADINE (a MAN ta deen)

Introduced: 1966   **Prescription:** USA: Yes; Canada: Yes   **Available as Generic:** USA: Yes; Canada: No   **Class:** Antiparkinsonism, antiviral
Controlled Drug: USA: No; Canada: No
Brand Names: Symadine, Symmetrel

BENEFITS versus RISKS	
Possible Benefits	*Possible Risks*
Partial relief of rigidity, tremor, and impaired motion in all forms of parkinsonism	Skin rashes, mild to severe
	Confusion, hallucinations
	Congestive heart failure
Prevention and treatment of respiratory infections caused by influenza type A viruses*	Increased prostatism (see Glossary)
	Abnormally low white blood cell counts

▷ **Principal Uses**

As a Single Drug Product: Uses currently included in FDA approved labeling: (1) Treats all forms of parkinsonism; (2) prevents or treats respiratory tract infections caused by influenza type A virus (although rimantidine is currently the drug of first choice because of amantidine's higher occurrence of CNS side effects); (3) treatment of drug-induced extrapyramidal symptoms (see Glossary).

Other (unlabeled) generally accepted uses: (1) May have a small role in helping manage behavioral problems which can happen after some brain injuries; (2) has had some success in reversing symptoms of mild dementia; (3) can ease some resistant myoclonic or absence seizures; (4) may help bed wetting (enuresis) in children; (5) eases fatigue in multiple sclerosis (MS) and may be of use in MS patients who experience fatigue that keeps them from living normally.

How This Drug Works: By increasing the nerve transmitter known as dopamine in some nerve centers, this drug reduces muscular rigidity, tremor and impaired movement associated with parkinsonism. By blocking penetration of infectious material from viruses into cells, this drug prevents development of influenza.

Available Dosage Forms and Strengths

Capsules — 100 mg
Syrup — 50 mg/ 5 ml

▷ **Usual Adult Dosage Range:** Antiparkinsonism: 100 mg once or twice daily. The total daily dose should not exceed 300 mg. Antiviral: 200 mg once daily; or 100 mg/12 hours. Children one to nine years old: For treatment of type A

*Does **NOT** prevent or treat viral infections other than those caused by influenza type A viruses.

flu: 4.4 to 8.8 mg per kg per day up to a maximum of 150 mg once daily. **Note: Actual dosage and administration schedule must be determined by the physician for each patient individually.**

Conditions Requiring Dosing Adjustments

Liver function: The liver is not known to be involved in the elimination of amantadine.

Kidney function: Must be carefully adjusted to blood levels in patients with kidney problems. Those with creatinine clearances of 30–50 ml per minute should receive 100 mg daily. Those with 15–29 clearance receive 100 mg every other day. Those with clearances less than 15 receive 200 mg once a week.

Epilepsy

Doses of 200 mg per day should be avoided as seizure risk may increase.

▷ **Dosing Instructions:** May be taken with or following meals. Can open the capsule to take it.

Usual Duration of Use: Use on a regular schedule for up to 2 weeks is usually needed to see this drug's effectiveness in relieving symptoms of parkinsonism. Long-term use (months to years) requires periodic check of response and dose changes. See your doctor on a regular basis.

Following exposure to influenza type A, peak protection requires continual daily dosage for at least 10 days. During influenza epidemics, this drug may be given for 6 to 8 weeks.

▷ **This Drug Should Not Be Taken If**
- you have had an allergic reaction to it previously.

▷ **Inform Your Physician Before Taking This Drug If**
- you have any type of seizure disorder.
- you have a history of serious emotional or mental disorder.
- you have a history of heart disease, especially previous heart failure.
- you have impaired liver or kidney function.
- you have a history of peptic ulcer disease.
- you have eczema or recurring eczemalike skin rashes.
- you are taking any drugs for emotional or mental disorders.
- you take other prescription or nonprescription medications which were not discussed when amantadine was prescribed for you.
- you have a history of low white blood cell counts.
- you are unsure of how much amantadine to take or how often to take it.

Possible Side Effects (natural, expected, and unavoidable drug actions)

Light-headedness, dizziness, weakness, feeling of impending faint in upright position (see Orthostatic Hypotension in Glossary). Dry mouth, constipation. Reddish-blue network pattern or patchy discoloration of the skin of the legs and feet (livedo reticularis); this is transient and unimportant.

▷ **Possible Adverse Effects** (unusual, unexpected, and infrequent reactions)
If any of the following develop, consult your physician promptly for guidance.

Mild Adverse Effects

Allergic Reaction: Skin rash.

Headache, nervousness, irritability, inability to concentrate, insomnia, nightmares.

Unsteadiness, visual disturbances, slurred speech.
Urine retention.
Loss of appetite, nausea, vomiting.
Serious Adverse Effects
Allergic Reaction: Severe eczemalike skin rashes.
Idiosyncratic Reactions: Confusion, depression, hallucinations.
Increased seizure activity in presence of epilepsy.
Swelling (fluid retention) of the arms, feet, or ankles.
Development of congestive heart failure (rare).
Aggravation of prostatism (see Glossary).
Difficulty breathing.
Elevated liver function tests.
Abnormally low white blood cell counts: fever, sore throat, infections.
Catatonia or seizures (if abruptly stopped).

▷ **Possible Effects on Sexual Function:**   None reported.

▷ **Adverse Effects That May Mimic Natural Diseases or Disorders**
Mood changes, confusion or hallucinations may suggest a psychotic disorder.
Swelling of the legs and feet may suggest (but not necessarily be indicative of) heart, liver or kidney disorder.

Natural Diseases or Disorders That May Be Activated by This Drug
Latent epilepsy, incipient congestive heart failure.

Possible Effects on Laboratory Tests
Liver function tests: increased liver enzymes (AST/GOT, alkaline phosphatase).
Kidney function tests: Transient increase in blood urea nitrogen (BUN).

CAUTION
1. NARROW margin of safety. Do not exceed a total dose of 400 mg/24 hours. Watch closely for adverse effects with doses over 200 mg/24 hours.
2. Initial benefit may only last 3 to 6 months in treatment of parkinsonism. If this occurs, ask your doctor if the dose should be adjusted or drug changed.
3. May increase susceptibility to German measles. Avoid exposure to anyone with active German measles.
4. Watch for early signs of congestive heart failure: shortness of breath on exertion or during the night while sleeping, mild cough, swelling of the feet and ankles. Report these developments promptly to your doctor.

Precautions for Use
By Infants and Children: Safety and effectiveness for use by those under 1 not established.
By Those over 60 Years of Age: Confusion, delirium, hallucinations and disorderly conduct may develop. Prostatism may be aggravated by this drug.

▷ **Advisability of Use During Pregnancy**
Pregnancy Category: C. See Pregnancy Code at the back of this book.
Animal studies: Birth defects reported in rat studies; no defects reported in rabbit studies.
Human studies: Adequate studies of pregnant women are not available. Avoid this drug during the first 3 months if possible. Ask your doctor for help.

Advisability of Use if Breast-Feeding
   Presence of this drug in breast milk: Yes.
   Nursing infant may develop skin rash, vomiting or retention of urine. Avoid drug or refrain from nursing.

Habit-Forming Potential: This drug has a potential for abuse because of its ability to cause euphoria, hallucinations and feelings of detachment.

Effects of Overdosage: Hyperactivity, disorientation, confusion, visual hallucinations, aggressive behavior, severe toxic psychosis, seizures, heart rhythm disturbances, drop in blood pressure.

Possible Effects of Long-Term Use: Livedo reticularis (see Possible Side Effects above). Congestive heart failure in predisposed individuals.

Suggested Periodic Examinations While Taking This Drug (at physician's discretion)
   White blood cell counts, liver and kidney function tests.
   Evaluation of heart function.

▷ **While Taking This Drug, Observe the Following**
   Foods: No restrictions.
   Beverages: No restrictions. May be taken with milk.
▷   *Alcohol:* This combination may impair mental function and lower blood pressure excessively.
   Tobacco Smoking: No interactions expected.
   Marijuana Smoking: No interactions expected.
▷   *Other Drugs*
      Amantadine may ***increase*** the effects of
      • atropinelike drugs that are used to treat parkinsonism, especially benztropine (Cogentin), orphenadrine (Disipal) and trihexyphenidyl (Artane). Amantadine can increase their therapeutic effectiveness, but if doses are too large, these drugs taken concurrently with amantadine may cause mental confusion, delirium, hallucinations and nightmares.
      • levodopa (Dopar, Larodopa, Sinemet, etc.), and enhance its therapeutic effectiveness. Combination may cause acute mental disturbances.
      The following drugs may ***increase*** the effects of amantadine
      • amphetamine and amphetaminelike stimulant drugs may cause excessive stimulation and adverse behavioral effects.
      • hydrochlorothiazide + triamterene may increase the blood level of amantadine and cause toxicity.
      Taken ***concurrently*** with
      • cotrimoxazole may increase risk of CNS stimulation or arrhythmias.
      • sulfamethoxazole may increase risk of CNS stimulation or arrhythmia.
      • trimethoprim may increase risk of CNS stimulation or arrhythmias.
▷   *Driving, Hazardous Activities:* This drug may cause drowsiness, dizziness, blurred vision or confusion. If these drug effects occur, avoid all hazardous activities.
   Aviation Note: The use of this drug ***may be a disqualification*** for piloting. Consult a designated Aviation Medical Examiner.
   Exposure to Sun: No restrictions.
   Exposure to Heat: No restrictions.
   Exposure to Cold: Use caution. Excessive chilling may enhance the development of livedo reticularis (see Possible Side Effects above).

Discontinuation: When used to treat parkinsonism, this drug should not be stopped abruptly. Sudden discontinuation may cause an acute parkinsonian crisis. When used to treat influenza A infections, this drug should be continued for 48 hours after the disappearance of all symptoms.

AMILORIDE (a MIL oh ride)

Introduced: 1967   **Prescription:** USA: Yes; Canada: Yes   **Available as**
Generic: Yes   **Class:** Diuretic   **Controlled Drug:** USA: No; Canada: No
Brand Names: ✦Apo-Amilzide, Midamor, ✦Moduret [CD], Moduretic [CD], ✦Nu-Amilzide [CD]

BENEFITS versus RISKS

Possible Benefits	*Possible Risks*
EFFECTIVE DIURETIC WITH DECREASED POTASSIUM LOSS	ABNORMALLY HIGH BLOOD POTASSIUM with excessive use
	Rare bone marrow depression
	Rare heart arrhythmias
	Rare kidney failure
	Rare liver toxicity

▷ **Principal Uses**

As a Single Drug Product: Uses currently included in FDA approved labeling: (1) Eliminates excessive fluid (edema) seen in congestive heart failure; (2) treats high blood pressure, especially good in those prone to low potassium; (3) treatment of thiazide-caused low blood potassium.

As a Combination Drug Product [CD]: Combined with other thiazide diuretics to prevent excess potassium loss.

Other (unlabeled) generally accepted uses: (1) May be able to help dissolve kidney stones in patients unable to tolerate surgery; (2) can help correct increased urination which occurs in patients taking lithium.

How This Drug Works: This drug promotes loss of sodium and water from the body and potassium retention by altering kidney enzymes that control urine formation.

Available Dosage Forms and Strengths

Tablets — 5 mg

▷ **Usual Adult Dosage Range:** One 5 mg dose a day, preferably in the morning. May increase up to 15 mg daily as needed and tolerated. Should not exceed 20 mg/24 hours. **Note: Actual dosage and administration schedule must be determined by the physician for each patient individually.**

Conditions Requiring Dosing Adjustments

Liver function: Used with extreme caution in patients with severe liver disease.
Kidney function: NOT used in patients who can't make urine or acute or chronic kidney failures.

▷ **Dosing Instructions:** Best taken when you wake up, with the stomach empty. Withhold food for 4 hours. May be taken with food if necessary to reduce stomach irritation. Tablet may be crushed for administration.

Usual Duration of Use: As needed to lose abnormal fluid or to normalize normal blood pressure. Intermittent or alternate-day use is recommended to minimize imbalance of sodium and potassium. See your doctor on a regular basis.

▷ **This Drug Should Not Be Taken If**
- you have had an allergic reaction to any form of it previously.
- your blood potassium level is above the normal range.
- you have nerve damage caused by diabetes (diabetic nephropathy).
- your kidneys are not producing urine.

▷ **Inform Your Physician Before Taking This Drug If**
- you are allergic to this drug or one similar to it.
- you have diabetes or glaucoma.
- you have a history of kidney disease or impaired kidney function.
- you take any other diuretic, blood pressure drug, any form of digitalis or lithium.
- you are unsure of how much amiloride to take or how often to take it.

Possible Side Effects (natural, expected, and unavoidable drug actions)
Abnormally high blood potassium level (10% of users), abnormally low blood sodium level, dehydration, constipation.

▷ **Possible Adverse Effects** (unusual, unexpected, and infrequent reactions)
If any of the following develop, consult your physician promptly for guidance.
Mild Adverse Effects
Allergic Reactions: Skin rash, itching.
Headache, dizziness, weakness, fatigue, numbness, and tingling.
Dry mouth, nausea, vomiting, stomach pains, diarrhea.
Loss of scalp hair.
Dizziness which occurs on standing (orthostatic hypotension).
Serious Adverse Effects
Idiosyncratic Reactions: Joint and muscle pains.
Abnormally high potassium level—marked fatigue and weakness, confusion, numbness and tingling of lips or extremities, slow and irregular heartbeats.
Rare liver or kidney toxicity.
Abnormally high sodium level.
Increased internal eye pressure (of concern in glaucoma).
Mental depression, visual disturbances, ringing in ears, tremors.
Aplastic anemia (see Glossary)—unusual fatigue or weakness, fever, sore throat, abnormal bleeding or bruising.
Palpitations and arrhythmias (rare).

▷ **Possible Effects on Sexual Function:**   More than 1%: decreased libido and impotence (5 to 10 mg/day).

▷ **Adverse Effects That May Mimic Natural Diseases or Disorders**
Nervousness, confusion or depression may mimic spontaneous mental disorder.

Natural Diseases or Disorders That May Be Activated by This Drug
Preexisting peptic ulcer, latent glaucoma.

Possible Effects on Laboratory Tests
Blood cholesterol level: decreased.

Blood creatinine level: increased with long-term use.

Blood potassium level: increased.

Blood uric acid level: increased with long-term use, especially if taken with thiazide diuretics.

Blood sodium level: decreased

CAUTION

1. Do **NOT** take potassium supplements, or eat more high-potassium foods.
2. More frequent potassium levels needed if you take digitalis compounds.
3. Do not stop this drug abruptly unless your doctor says you must.

Precautions for Use

By Infants and Children: Oral dosing with 0.625 mg per kg daily has been used to promote water loss (diuresis) in young patients weighing from 6 to 20 kg.

By Those over 60 Years of Age: Declines in kidney function may make it likely you will retain potassium. Limit use of this drug to periods of 2 to 3 weeks if possible. The dose MUST be reduced. This drug can cause excessive water loss, increased tendency of the blood to clot and increased risk of clots (thrombosis, heart attack, stroke).

▷ **Advisability of Use During Pregnancy**

Pregnancy Category: B. See Pregnancy Code at the back of this book.

Animal studies: No birth defects reported.

Human studies: Adequate studies of pregnant women are not available.

Use only if clearly needed.

Advisability of Use if Breast-Feeding

Presence of this drug in breast milk: Unknown, but probably present.

This drug may suppress milk production.

Avoid drug if possible. If use is necessary, watch nursing infant closely and stop drug or nursing if adverse effects develop.

Habit-Forming Potential: None.

Effects of Overdosage: Thirst, drowsiness, fatigue, weakness, nausea, vomiting, confusion, numbness and tingling of face and extremities, irregular heart rhythm, shortness of breath.

Suggested Periodic Examinations While Taking This Drug (at physician's discretion)

Complete blood counts; blood levels of sodium, potassium and chloride; kidney function tests; and check of water balance (state of hydration).

▷ **While Taking This Drug, Observe the Following**

Foods: Avoid excessive salt restriction and high-potassium foods.

Beverages: No restrictions. May be taken with milk.

▷ *Alcohol:* Use caution. Alcohol can exaggerate the blood-pressure-lowering effect of this drug and cause orthostatic hypotension (see Glossary).

Tobacco Smoking: No interactions expected.

▷ *Other Drugs*

Amiloride may ***increase*** the effects of

• other blood-pressure-lowering drugs. Dosage decreases may be needed.

Amiloride may ***decrease*** the effects of

• digoxin (Lanoxin, etc.), and reduce its effect in treating heart failure.

Amiloride *taken concurrently* with

- spironolactone (Aldactone, Aldactazide) or triamterene (Dyrenium, Dyazide) may cause dangerous blood potassium levels. Avoid combination.
- lithium may cause lithium accumulation to toxic levels.
- ACE inhibitors (see Drug Classes) such as benazopril may result in abnormally high blood potassium.
- NSAIDs (see Drug Classes) may decrease the lowering of blood pressure.
- potassium supplements may result in extremely elevated blood potassium levels.

▷ *Driving, Hazardous Activities:* May cause drowsiness, dizziness and orthostatic hypotension. If these drug effects occur, avoid hazardous activities.

Aviation Note: The use of this drug *may be a disqualification* for piloting. Consult a designated Aviation Medical Examiner.

Exposure to Sun: No restrictions.

Exposure to Heat: Caution advised. Excessive sweating can cause water, sodium and potassium imbalance. Hot environments can cause lowering of blood pressure.

Occurrence of Unrelated Illness: Call your doctor if you contract an illness causing vomiting or diarrhea.

Discontinuation: With high dosage or prolonged use, withdraw this drug gradually. Sudden withdrawal can cause excessive loss of potassium from the body.

AMINOPHYLLINE (am in OFF i lin)

Other Name: theophylline ethylenediamine

Introduced: 1910   **Prescription:** USA: Yes; Canada: Yes   **Available as Generic:** Yes   **Class:** Antiasthmatic, bronchodilator, xanthines   **Controlled Drug:** USA: No; Canada: No

Brand Names: Aminophyllin, Mudrane [CD], Mudrane GG [CD], ✦Palaron, Phyllocontin, Somophyllin, ✦Somophyllin-12, Truphylline

BENEFITS versus RISKS	
Possible Benefits	*Possible Risks*
EFFECTIVE PREVENTION AND RELIEF OF ACUTE BRONCHIAL ASTHMA	NARROW TREATMENT RANGE
	FREQUENT STOMACH DISTRESS
	Gastrointestinal bleeding
MODERATELY EFFECTIVE CONTROL OF CHRONIC, RECURRENT BRONCHIAL ASTHMA	Central nervous system toxicity, seizures
	Heart rhythm disturbances
Moderately effective symptomatic relief in chronic bronchitis and emphysema	

▷ **Principal Uses**

As a Single Drug Product: Uses currently included in FDA approved labeling: (1) Relieves shortness of breath and wheezing in acute bronchial asthma, helps prevent recurrence of asthmatic episodes; (2) Also useful in chronic obstructive pulmonary disease (COPD) typically used in combination with beta agonists and anticholinergics.

Other (unlabeled) generally accepted uses: None at present.

As a Combination Drug Product [CD]: Available in combination with several other drugs helpful in managing bronchial asthma and related conditions. Ephedrine enhances the bronchodilator effects; guaifenesin provides an expectorant effect that thins mucus secretions; mild sedatives such as phenobarbital are added to ease anxiety often seen in acute attacks of asthma.

How This Drug Works: This drug yields 79% theophylline, the active medicine. It inhibits the enzyme phosphodiesterase, and increases cyclic AMP. This causes relaxation of the muscles in the bronchial tubes and lung blood vessels, resulting in relief of bronchospasm, and improved lung circulation.

Available Dosage Forms and Strengths

Enema — 65.14 mg per ml
Injection — 25 mg per ml and 50 mg per ml (Canada)
Oral solution — 105 mg per 5-ml
Suppositories — 250 mg, 500 mg
Tablets — 100 mg, 200 mg
Tablets, enteric-coated — 100 mg, 200 mg
Tablets, extended release — 225 mg, 350 mg (Canada)

▷ **Recommended Dosage Ranges** (Actual dosage and administration schedule must be determined by the physician for each patient individually.)

Note: All doses of aminophylline are to be calculated as theophylline-equivalents; all dosages cited below are for theophylline.

Infants and Children: For acute attack of asthma (not currently taking theophylline)—loading dose of 5 to 6 mg/kg of body weight.

For acute attack if taking theophylline—a single dose of 2.5 mg/kg of body weight, if no signs of theophylline toxicity. Check blood levels.

For maintenance during acute attack—dosage is based on age:

Up to 6 months of age—0.07 for each week of age + 1.7 = the mg/kg of body weight, given every 8 hours.
6 months to 1 year of age—0.05 for each week of age + 1.25 = the mg/kg of body weight, given every 6 hours.
1 to 9 years of age—5 mg/kg of body weight, every 6 hours.
9 to 12 years of age—4 mg/kg of body weight, every 6 hours.
12 to 16 years of age—3 mg/kg of body weight, every 6 hours.

For chronic treatment to prevent recurrence of asthma—dosage is based on age:

Initially 16 mg/kg of body weight, in 3 or 4 divided doses at 6 to 8 hour intervals, up to a maximum of 400 mg daily. Increase dose as needed and tolerated by increments of 25% every 2 to 3 days. Limit total daily dosage as follows:

Up to 1 year of age—0.3 for each week of age + 8.0 = the mg/kg of body weight, per day.
1 to 9 years of age—22 mg/kg of body weight, per day.
9 to 12 years of age—20 mg/kg of body weight, per day.
12 to 16 years of age—18 mg/kg of body weight, per day.
16 years of age and over—13 mg/kg of body weight or 900 mg per day, whichever is less.

Note: Theophylline blood levels are needed periodically.

16 to 60 Years of Age: For acute attack of asthma (not currently taking theophylline)—loading dose of 5 to 6 mg/kg of body weight.

For acute attack while currently taking theophylline—a single dose of 2.5 mg/kg of body weight, if no signs of theophylline toxicity. Check blood levels of theophylline.

For maintenance during acute attack—for nonsmokers: 3 mg/kg of body weight, every 8 hours; for smokers: 4 mg/kg of body weight, every 6 hours.

For chronic treatment to prevent recurrence of asthma—initially 6 to 8 mg/kg of body weight, in 3 or 4 divided doses at 6 to 8 hour intervals, up to a maximum of 400 mg daily. Increase dose as needed and tolerated by increments of 25% every 2 to 3 days. The total daily dosage should not exceed 13 mg/kg of body weight or 900 mg, whichever is less.

Over 60 Years of Age: For acute attack—same as 16 to 60 years of age.

For maintenance during acute attack—2 mg/kg of body weight, every 8 hours.

Conditions Requiring Dosing Adjustments

Liver function: Dose **must** be decreased in liver compromise, and blood levels checked.

Kidney function: Lower doses will be needed and accumulation may occur. Check blood levels.

Obesity: This drug does not enter fatty tissue. Doses **must** be calculated on lean body weight.

Pulmonary edema: If fluid accumulates in the lungs, particularly acutely, the dose should be decreased to half the normal dose.

Fever: Extended periods of fever change the amount of space into which the drug distributes and also lowers the point at which seizures may occur. The dose of aminophylline may need to be decreased.

Congestive heart failure: Patients with this kind of heart failure should have doses decreased by 50% to avoid toxicity.

▷ **Dosing Instructions:** May be taken with or following food to reduce stomach irritation. Regular tablets may be crushed before taking. Enteric-coated and prolonged-action tablets should be swallowed whole and not altered. Shake the oral solution gently before measuring each dose. **Do not** refrigerate any liquid dosage forms of this drug.

▷ **Usual Duration of Use:** Use on a regular schedule for 48 to 72 hours is usually needed to see this drug's effectiveness in helping bronchial asthma and chronic lung disease. Long-term use (months to years) requires supervision and periodic evaluation by your physician. Consult your physician on a regular basis.

▷ **This Drug Should Not Be Taken If**
- you have had an allergic reaction to it, or to dyphylline, oxtriphylline or theophylline.
- you have active peptic ulcer disease.
- you have an uncontrolled seizure disorder.

▷ **Inform Your Physician Before Taking This Drug If**
- you have had an unfavorable reaction to any xanthine drug (see Drug Class, Section Four).
- you have a seizure disorder of any kind.
- you have a history of peptic ulcer disease.

- you have impaired liver or kidney function.
- you have had a temperature for a significant period of time.
- you have hypertension, heart disease or any heart rhythm disorder.
- you take other prescription or nonprescription medications which were not discussed when aminophylline was prescribed for you.
- you see a lung specialist for chronic pulmonary edema.
- you are unsure of how much aminophylline to take or how often to take it.

Possible Side Effects (natural, expected, and unavoidable drug actions)
Nervousness, insomnia, rapid heart rate, increased urine volume.

▷ **Possible Adverse Effects** (unusual, unexpected, and infrequent reactions)
If any of the following develop, consult your physician promptly for guidance.
Mild Adverse Effects
Allergic Reactions: Skin rash, hives.
Headache, dizziness, irritability, tremor, fatigue, weakness.
Appetite loss, nausea, vomiting, abdominal pain, diarrhea, excessive thirst.
Flushing of face.
Serious Adverse Effects
Idiosyncratic Reactions: Marked anxiety, confusion, behavioral disturbances.
Central nervous system toxicity: muscle twitching, seizures.
Heart rhythm abnormalities, rapid breathing, low blood pressure.
Gastrointestinal bleeding.
Worsening of migraines.
Increased fluid loss via the kidneys.

▷ **Possible Effects on Sexual Function:**   None reported.

Natural Diseases or Disorders That May Be Activated by This Drug
Latent peptic ulcer disease.

Possible Effects on Laboratory Tests
Blood uric acid level: increased.
Fecal occult blood test: positive (large doses may cause stomach bleeding).
Phenobarbital level: falsely decreased.

CAUTION
1. Do not combine this drug with other antiasthmatic drugs unless your doctor tells you to do so. Serious overdose could result.
2. Influenza vaccine may delay elimination and cause toxicity.

Precautions for Use
By Infants and Children: Do not exceed recommended doses. Watch for toxicity: irritability, agitation, tremors, lethargy, fever, vomiting, rapid heart rate and breathing, seizures. Check blood levels of drug during long-term use.
By Those over 60 Years of Age: Small starting doses are indicated. You may be more susceptible to stomach irritation, nausea, vomiting or diarrhea. This drug may cause a hyperactivity syndrome when used with coffee (caffeine) or nasal decongestants.

▷ **Advisability of Use During Pregnancy**
Pregnancy Category: C. See Pregnancy Code at the back of this book.
Animal studies: Significant birth defects due to this drug reported in mice.
Human studies: Adequate studies of pregnant women are not available. No increase in birth defects reported in 394 exposures to theophylline.

Avoid this drug during the first 3 months. Use it otherwise only if clearly needed. Ask your physician for guidance.

Advisability of Use if Breast-Feeding
Presence of this drug in breast milk: Yes.
Ask your doctor for help. It may be possible to take a typical dose **after** nursing and avoid the peak effect of the drug.

Habit-Forming Potential: None.

Effects of Overdosage: Nausea, vomiting, restlessness, irritability, confusion, delirium, seizures, high fever, weak pulse, coma.

Possible Effects of Long-Term Use: Gastrointestinal irritation.

Suggested Periodic Examinations While Taking This Drug (at physician's discretion)
MUST check blood theophylline levels. (See Therapeutic Drug Monitoring in Section One.)

▷ **While Taking This Drug, Observe the Following**
Foods: High carbohydrate meals may decrease absorption. High fat meals may decrease absorption.
Beverages: Avoid excess use of caffeine-containing beverages: coffee, tea, or cola.
▷ *Alcohol:* No interactions expected. May increase stomach irritation.
Tobacco Smoking: Can increase drug elimination and reduce effectiveness. Higher doses may be needed to maintain a therapeutic blood level.
▷ *Other Drugs*
Aminophylline may **decrease** the effects of
• adenosine (Adenocard).
• lithium (Lithane, Lithobid, etc.), and reduce its effectiveness.
• midazolam (Versed).
Aminophylline **taken concurrently** with
• amiodarone (Codarone) may cause a large increase in theophylline blood level.
• halothane (anesthesia) may cause heart rhythm abnormalities.
• imipenam-cilastatin (Primaxin) may result in large increases in theophylline levels and toxicity.
• phenytoin (Dilantin) may cause decreased effects of both drugs. Check blood levels and adjust dosages as appropriate.
The following drugs may **increase** the effects of aminophylline
• allopurinol (Lopurin, Zyloprim).
• azithromycin (Zithromax).
• caffeine (greater than 6 cups or IV form).
• cimetidine (Tagamet).
• ciprofloxacin (Cipro), and other quinolones (see Drug Classes) to various degrees.
• clarithromycin (Biaxin).
• disulfiram (Antabuse).
• erythromycin (E-Mycin, Erythrocin, etc.).
• ilsoniazid (INH).
• interferon alpha (Roferon).
• mexiletine (Mexitil).

- norfloxacin (Noroxin).
- oral contraceptives.
- pentoxyfylline (Trental).
- ranitidine (Zantac).
- tacrine (Cognex).
- thiabendazole (Mintezol)
- ticlopidine (Ticlid).
- troleandomycin (TAO).
- verapamil (Calan, Verelan, etc.)

The following drugs may *decrease* the effects of aminophylline

- albuterol.
- barbiturates (phenobarbital, etc.).
- beta blocker drugs (see Drug Classes).
- carbamazepine (Tegretol).
- primidone (Mysoline).
- rifampin (Rifadin, Rimactane, etc.).
- rifabutin (Mycobutin).
- tobacco smoke.

▷ *Driving, Hazardous Activities:* This drug may cause dizziness. Restrict activities as necessary.

Aviation Note: The use of this drug *may be a disqualification* for piloting. Consult a designated Aviation Medical Examiner.

Exposure to Sun: No restrictions.

Occurrence of Unrelated Illness: Acute viral respiratory infections can delay drug elimination. Watch closely for toxicity and the need to reduce dose or lengthen the dosing interval.

Discontinuation: Avoid prolonged and unnecessary use of this drug. When you have achieved an asthma-free state, slowly withdraw this drug over several days.

AMITRIPTYLINE (a mee TRIP ti leen)

Introduced: 1961   **Prescription:** USA: Yes; Canada: Yes   **Available as Generic:** Yes   **Class:** Antidepressant   **Controlled Drug:** USA: No; Canada: No

Brand Names: Amitril, ✦Apo-Amitriptyline, Elavil, ✦Elavil Plus [CD], Emitrip, Endep, Enovil, Etrafon [CD], Etrafon-A [CD], Etrafon-Forte [CD], ✦Levate, PMS-Levazine [CD], SK-amitriptyline, ✦Triavil [CD]

BENEFITS versus RISKS	
Possible Benefits	*Possible Risks*
EFFECTIVE RELIEF OF ENDOGENOUS DEPRESSION	ADVERSE BEHAVIORAL EFFECTS: Confusion, disorientation, hallucinations
Additive therapy in some pain syndromes	CONVERSION OF DEPRESSION TO MANIA in manic-depressive disorders
	Irregular heart rhythms
	Rare blood cell abnormalities

▷ **Principal Uses**

   As a Single Drug Product: Uses currently included in FDA approved labeling: (1) Relieves symptoms seen in spontaneous (endogenous) depression, and helps restore normal mood. This drug should be used only when a diagnosis of a true, primary depression of significant degree has been made; (2) has a role in relieving depression which is resistant (refractory) to single agent therapy.

   Other (unlabeled) generally accepted uses: (1) Additive (adjuvant) therapy in chronic pain and other pain syndromes; (2) helps ease agitation; (3) may have a role in diabetic neuropathic pain; (4) is an alternative in intractable hiccups; (5) used in combination with other medicines to ease the pain of postherpetic neuralgia; (6) may be of some benefit in easing the pain of chronic vulvar burning (vulvodynia); (7) used in fish (Ciguatera) poisoning.

   As a Combination Drug Product [CD]: Combined with chlordiazepoxide to relieve anxiety that may accompany depression. Also available in combination with perphenazine, a strong phenothiazine tranquilizer, to relieve severe agitation that may accompany depression.

How This Drug Works: Relieves depression by slowly restoring normal levels of norepinephrine and serotonin, chemicals that transmit nerve impulses.

Available Dosage Forms and Strengths

   Injection — 10mg/ ml
   Oral suspension — 10 mg/ 5 ml
   Tablets — 10 mg, 25 mg, 50 mg, 75 mg, 100 mg, 150 mg

▷ **Usual Adult Dosage Range:**   Intramuscular injection is given as 80 to 120 mg per day divided into four doses. Switch to the oral form is made as rapidly as possible. Oral dosing starts with 25 mg 2 to 4 times daily. Dose may be increased cautiously as needed and tolerated by 10 to 25 mg daily at intervals of 1 week. Usual maintenance dose is 50 to 100 mg/24 hours. Total dose should not exceed 150 mg/24 hours. When the best dose is found, it may be taken at bedtime as one dose. **Note: Actual dosage and administration schedule must be determined by the physician for each patient individually.**

Conditions Requiring Dosing Adjustments

   Liver function: Specific guidelines not available, however, low doses and a check of blood levels is prudent.

   Kidney function: Low doses and blood level checks are needed with kidney failure.

▷ **Dosing Instructions:**   May be taken without regard to meals. Tablet may be crushed to take it.

Usual Duration of Use: Some benefit may occur in 1 to 2 weeks, but adequate response may require continual use for 4 to 6 weeks or longer. Long-term use should not exceed 6 months without follow-up evaluation.

▷ **This Drug Should Not Be Taken If**

   • you are allergic to any of the brand names listed above.
   • you are taking or have taken within the past 14 days any monoamine oxidase (MAO) type A inhibitor drug (see Drug Class, Section Four).
   • you have heart induced chest pain (angina pectoris).

- you have a rapid heart rate which occurs spontaneously (paroxysmal tachycardia).
- you have heart (cardiovascular) disease or abnormal heart rhythms.
- you are recovering from a recent heart attack.
- you have narrow-angle glaucoma.
- you are pregnant.
- you have congestive heart failure.

▷ **Inform Your Physician Before Taking This Drug If**
- you are allergic to any tricyclic antidepressant (see Drug Class, Section Four).
- you have a history of: diabetes, epilepsy, glaucoma, heart disease, prostate gland enlargement or overactive thyroid function.
- you plan to have surgery under general anesthesia in the near future.
- you take other prescription or nonprescription medications which were not discussed when amitriptyline was prescribed for you.
- you are unsure of how much amitriptyline to take or how often to take it.
- you have a history of schizophrenia—this drug may worsen any paranoia.
- you have a history of prostate problems.
- you have a liver or kidney disorder.
- you have a blood cell disorder.
- you have a history of intestinal block (ileus).
- you have a history of sexual dysfunction.

Possible Side Effects (natural, expected, and unavoidable drug actions)
Drowsiness, blurred vision, dry mouth, constipation, impaired urination.

▷ **Possible Adverse Effects** (unusual, unexpected, and infrequent reactions)
If any of the following develop, consult your physician promptly for guidance.
Mild Adverse Effects
Allergic Reactions: Skin rash, hives, swelling of face or tongue, drug fever (see Glossary).
Headache, dizziness, weakness, fainting, unsteady gait, tremors.
Peculiar taste, irritation of tongue or mouth, nausea, indigestion.
Fluctuation of blood sugar levels.
Increased dental cavities (caries).
Restlessness and nightmares. Tingling of the extremities (paresthesias).
Change in the ability to perceive tones.
Serious Adverse Effects
Allergic Reactions: Hepatitis, with or without jaundice (see Glossary).
Idiosyncratic Reactions: Neuroleptic malignant syndrome (see Glossary).
Confusion and hallucinations.
Rare bowel obstruction (ileus).
Rare SIADH (see Glossary).
Excessively low blood pressure (hypotension).
Rare seizures.
Rare severe eye movement problems.
Heart palpitation and irregular rhythm.
Bone marrow depression (see Glossary)—fatigue, weakness, fever, sore throat, abnormal bleeding or bruising.

Peripheral neuritis (see Glossary)—numbness, tingling, pain, loss of arm or leg strength.

Parkinson-like disorders (see Glossary)—usually mild and infrequent; more likely to occur in the elderly.

Liver toxicity.

Worsening of paranoid psychosis in schizophrenic patients.

▷ **Possible Effects on Sexual Function:**   Decreased libido (rare), increased libido (antidepressant effect), impotence (rare), inhibited female orgasm, inhibited ejaculation, male and female breast enlargement, milk production, swelling of testicles. These effects usually disappear within 2 to 10 days after discontinuation of the drug.

▷ **Adverse Effects That May Mimic Natural Diseases or Disorders**

Liver toxicity may suggest viral hepatitis.

Natural Diseases or Disorders That May Be Activated by This Drug

Latent diabetes, epilepsy, glaucoma, impaired urination due to prostate.

Possible Effects on Laboratory Tests

Complete blood counts: decreased white cells and platelets; increased eosinophils.

Liver function tests: increased ALT/GPT, AST/GOT, alkaline phosphatase, increased bilirubin.

Blood glucose levels: increased and decreased (fluctuations).

CAUTION

1. Dosage must be individualized. Report for follow-up evaluation and laboratory tests as directed by your physician.
2. It is best to withhold this drug if electroconvulsive therapy (ECT, "shock" treatment) is to be used to treat your depression.

Precautions for Use

By Infants and Children: Safety and effectiveness for those under 12 years old not established.

By Those over 60 Years of Age: During the first 2 weeks of treatment watch for confusion, agitation, forgetfulness, disorientation, delusions and hallucinations. Decreased dose or discontinuation may be needed. Unsteadiness may predispose to falling and injury. May worsen impaired urination associated with prostate gland enlargement (prostatism).

▷ **Advisability of Use During Pregnancy**

Pregnancy Category: D. See Pregnancy Code at the back of this book.

Animal studies: Skull deformities reported in rabbits.

Human studies: No defects reported in 21 exposures. Adequate studies of pregnant women are not available.

Avoid use of drug during first 3 months. Use during last 6 months only if clearly needed.

Advisability of Use if Breast-Feeding

Presence of this drug in breast milk: Yes, in small amounts.

Watch nursing infant closely and stop drug or nursing if adverse effects start.

Habit-Forming Potential: Psychological or physical dependence is rare and unexpected.

Effects of Overdosage: Confusion, hallucinations, marked drowsiness, heart palpitations, dilated pupils, tremors, stupor, deep sleep, coma, convulsions.

Suggested Periodic Examinations While Taking This Drug (at physician's discretion)

Complete blood cell counts, liver function tests, serial blood pressure readings and electrocardiograms.

▷ **While Taking This Drug, Observe the Following**

Foods: Excessive vitamin C can result in an unexpected increase in decreased therapeutic benefit of amitriptyline. May also increase appetite and cause excessive weight gain.

Beverages: No restrictions. May be taken with milk.

▷ *Alcohol:* Avoid completely. Can markedly increase the intoxicating effects of alcohol and brain function depression.

Tobacco Smoking: May hasten the elimination of this drug. Higher doses may be necessary.

▷ *Other Drugs*

Amitriptyline may ***increase*** the effects of

- antihistamines (such as diphenhydramine-Benadryl, others) can increase the risk of urinary retention, chronic glaucoma and bowel obstruction (ileus). This is especially problematic in the elderly.
- atropinelike drugs (see Drug Classes).
- albuterol or other (amphetamines, epinephrine) direct sympathomimetic drugs.
- cimetidine (Tagamet)
- disulfiram (Antabuse) can worsen the disulfiram effect if alcohol is consumed.
- phenytoin.

Amitriptyline may ***decrease*** the effects of

- clonidine (Catapres).
- guanethidine (Ismelin).
- guanfacine (Hytrin).
- methyldopa can result in reduced amitriptyline and/or methyldopa benefits.

Amitriptyline ***taken concurrently*** with

- amphetamines can result in abnormally increased responses to amphetamines.
- anticoagulants such as warfarin may cause an increased risk of bleeding.
- carbamazepine (Tegretol) may decrease the blood level of amitriptyline.
- epinephrine may cause an increased risk of rapid heart rate and high blood pressure.
- estrogens (see Drug Classes) may result in abnormal body movements.
- ethanol (alcohol) may result in additive toxicity to the central nervous system.
- fluoxetine (Prozac) can result in very high levels of amitriptyline.
- fluvoxamine (Luvox) can result in very high levels of amitriptyline.
- monoamine oxidase (MAO) type A inhibitor drugs may cause high fever, delirium and convulsions (see Drug Classes).
- quinidine (Quinaglute, etc.) can result in increased antidepressant blood levels.
- thyroid preparations may impair heart rhythm and function. Ask your doctor for help with adjustment of thyroid dose.

▷ *Driving, Hazardous Activities:* This drug may impair mental alertness, judgment, physical coordination and reaction time. Avoid hazardous activities.

Aviation Note: The use of this drug **is a disqualification** for piloting. Consult a designated Aviation Medical Examiner.

Exposure to Sun: This drug may cause photosensitivity (see Glossary).

Exposure to Heat: This drug can inhibit sweating and impair the body's adaptation to hot environments, increasing the risk of heat stroke. Avoid saunas.

Exposure to Cold: Elderly should avoid conditions conducive to hypothermia (see Glossary).

Discontinuation: It is best to stop this drug gradually. Abrupt withdrawal after long-term use can cause headache, malaise and nausea.

AMLODIPINE (am LOH di peen)

Introduced: 1986   **Prescription:** USA: Yes   **Available as Generic:** No   **Class:** Antianginal, antihypertensive, calcium channel blocker   **Controlled Drug:** USA: No

Brand Name: Norvasc

Controversies In Medicine: Study data indicates that medicines in this class should NOT be used in some patients with extremely compromised hearts. There have also been several FDA hearings held on the calcium channel blocker class. **This medicine became the only calcium channel blocker to be FDA approved as safe for use in treating hypertension or angina in patients who also have congestive heart failure**. A recent FDA panel found medicines in this class to be safe and effective. A retrospective chart review yielded data that showed increased risks for nifedipine immediate release forms in those over 71, and cautioned physicians against using the immediate release form for indications other than angina. The immediate release form in question had never been approved for other uses. Most recently, a study of nearly 6,000 patients at Tel Aviv Medical Center found that there was no statistically significant increased risk of death in the patients who took calcium channel blockers versus those who did not.

BENEFITS versus RISKS	
Possible Benefits	*Possible Risks*
EFFECTIVE PREVENTION OF BOTH MAJOR TYPES OF ANGINA	DOSE-RELATED CHANGES IN HEART RHYTHM
EFFECTIVE TREATMENT OF HYPERTENSION	Peripheral edema (fluid retention in feet and ankles)
	Dose-related palpitations

▷ **Principal Uses**

As a Single Drug Product: Uses currently included in FDA approved labeling: Treatment of (1) angina pectoris due to coronary artery spasm (Prinzmetal's variant angina) that happens spontaneously and is not associated with exertion; (2) classical angina-of-effort (due to atherosclerotic disease of the coronary arteries) in people who have not responded to or can't tolerate nitrates or beta blocker drugs; (3) mild to moderate hypertension; (4)

treatment of hypertension or angina in patients who also have congestive heart failure.

Other (unlabeled) generally accepted uses: (1) Research has continued to accumulate which says medicines in this class can reverse or block the progression of fat build up and calcium depositing on the inside of blood vessels (atherosclerosis); (2) can help stop premature labor; (3) may help prevent migraine headaches.

How This Drug Works: By blocking the normal passage of calcium through cell walls, this drug inhibits the contraction of coronary arteries and peripheral arterioles. As a result of these combined effects, this drug

- prevents spontaneous spasm of the coronary arteries (Prinzmetal's type of angina).
- decreases rate and contraction force of the heart during exertion, reducing frequency of effort-induced angina.
- reduces contraction of peripheral arterial walls, resulting in lower blood pressure. This decreases the work of the heart during exertion and helps prevent angina.

Available Dosage Forms and Strengths

Tablets — 2.5 mg, 5 mg, 10 mg

▷ **Recommended Dosage Ranges** (Actual dosage and administration schedule must be determined by the physician for each patient individually.)

Infants and Children: Dosage not established.

12 to 60 Years of Age: 2.5 to 10 mg daily, in a single dose for high blood pressure. 5 to 10 mg daily in treating chronic angina.

Over 60 Years of Age: Same as 12 to 60 years of age.

Conditions Requiring Dosing Adjustments

Liver function: Patients with damaged livers should be started on a daily 2.5 mg dose for high blood pressure and 5 mg for angina, and have the medicine slowly increased as needed or tolerated.

Kidney function: No adjustment in dosing is needed.

Low protein or starvation

This drug is transported in the body by a protein called albumin. If protein is low as in liver failure or starvation, an increased effect may be seen with "normal" doses. Therapy should be started with low doses and increased only if needed or tolerated.

▷ **Dosing Instructions:** May be taken with or following food to reduce stomach irritation. The tablet may be crushed for administration.

Usual Duration of Use: Use on a regular schedule for 2 to 4 weeks is usually needed to see this drug's effectiveness in reducing the frequency and severity of angina and in controlling hypertension. For long-term use (months to years), determine the smallest effective dose. Periodic evaluation by your doctor is needed.

Possible Advantages of This Drug

Slow onset and prolonged effect, allowing effective once-a-day treatment for both angina and hypertension.

No adverse effects on heart function.

▷ **This Drug Should Not Be Taken If**

- you have had an allergic reaction to it previously.

- you have active liver disease.
- you have low blood pressure—systolic pressure below 90.
- you have atrioventricular block or sick sinus syndrome (talk to your doctor).
- you have a severe problem (dysfunction) in your left ventricle.
- you have a seriously contracted or narrowed (stenosed) aorta.

▷ **Inform Your Physician Before Taking This Drug If**
- you have had an unfavorable response to any calcium blocker drug.
- you are currently taking any form of digitalis or a beta blocker drug (see Drug Class, Section Four).
- you are taking any drugs that lower blood pressure.
- you have had congestive heart failure, heart attack or stroke.
- you are subject to disturbances of heart rhythm.
- you have a history of drug-induced liver damage.
- you are unsure of how much amlodipine to take or how often to take it.
- you have circulation problems in your hands.
- you have muscular dystrophy.

Possible Side Effects (natural, expected, and unavoidable drug actions)
Swelling of feet and ankles, flushing and sensation of warmth.

▷ **Possible Adverse Effects** (unusual, unexpected, and infrequent reactions)
If any of the following develop, consult your physician promptly for guidance.
Mild Adverse Effects
Allergic Reactions: Skin rash.
Headache (up to 12%), dizziness (3%), fatigue (4%).
Nausea (rare), constipation (rare).
Dose-related palpitations (rare at low dose, 4.5% at 10 mg doses).
Overgrowth of the gums (gingival hyperplasia) (up to 10% with drugs in the same class).
Increased urge to urinate at night.
Rare visual changes (eye pain, double vision).
Ringing in the ears (tinnitus) (rare).
Cough, muscle pain (rare).
Dose-related flushing (4.5% in women and 1.5% in men).
Elevated liver enzymes (may be a hypersensitivity—usually resolves).
Serious Adverse Effects
Allergic Reactions: None reported.
Idiosyncratic Reactions: Rare Parkinson-like symptoms.
Dose-dependent edema (up to 6.2 % in those over 65).
Rare exfoliative dermatitis or erythema multiforme.
Very rare agranulocytosis.
Rebound angina (if drug is abruptly stopped).
Difficulty breathing (dyspnea).
Dose-related abnormal heart rhythms (with higher doses).

▷ **Possible Effects on Sexual Function:**   Sexual dysfunction has been reported in both men and women as frequently as 1–2%.
Rare swelling and tenderness of male breast tissue (gynecomastia).

▷ **Adverse Effects That May Mimic Natural Diseases or Disorders**
An allergic rash and swelling of the legs may resemble erysipelas.

Possible Effects on Laboratory Tests

Liver function tests: transient increases in liver enzymes.

CAUTION

1. Tell all health care providers involved in your care that you are taking this drug. Note the use of this drug on your card of personal identification.
2. You may use nitroglycerin and other nitrate drugs as needed to relieve acute episodes of angina pain. If you notice that your angina attacks are becoming more frequent or intense, call your doctor promptly.

Precautions for Use

By Infants and Children: Safety and effectiveness for use by those under 12 not established.

By Those over 60 Years of Age: May be more susceptible to the development of weakness, dizziness, fainting and falling. Take necessary precautions to prevent injury. Starting doses should be lower in this age bracket.

▷ **Advisability of Use During Pregnancy**

Pregnancy Category: C. See Pregnancy Code at the back of this book.

Animal studies: No information available.

Human studies: Adequate studies of pregnant women are not available.

Avoid this drug during the first 3 months. Use during the last 6 months only if clearly needed. Ask physician for guidance.

Advisability of Use if Breast-Feeding

Presence of this drug in breast milk: Unknown.

Avoid drug or refrain from nursing.

Habit-Forming Potential: None.

Effects of Overdosage: Weakness, light-headedness, fainting, fast pulse, low blood pressure, slow heart beat, sinus arrest, heart attack, shortness of breath, flushed and warm skin, seizures, metabolic acidosis, low potassium and calcium.

Possible Effects of Long-Term Use: Overgrowth of the gums.

Suggested Periodic Examinations While Taking This Drug (at physician's discretion)

Evaluations of heart function, including electrocardiograms; measurements of blood pressure in supine, sitting and standing positions.

▷ **While Taking This Drug, Observe the Following**

Foods: No restrictions. Avoid excessive salt intake.

Beverages: No restrictions. May be taken with milk.

▷ *Alcohol:* Use caution. Alcohol may exaggerate the drop in blood pressure.

Tobacco Smoking: Nicotine may reduce the effectiveness of this drug. Ask your doctor to help.

Marijuana Smoking: Possible reduced effectiveness of this drug; mild to moderate increase in angina; possible changes in electrocardiogram, confusing interpretation.

▷ *Other Drugs*

Amlodipine *taken concurrently* with

- adenosine (Adenocard) may cause extended problems with slow heart rate.
- beta blocker drugs or digitalis preparations (see Drug Classes) may cause heart rate and rhythm problems.

- cyclosporine (Sandimmune) causes increased cyclosporine blood levels and increased risk of toxicity.
- rifampin (Rifater, others) may result in decreased therapeutic benefit of amlodipine.

The following drug may *increase* the effects of amlodipine

- cimetidine (Tagamet).

▷ *Driving, Hazardous Activities:* This drug may cause dizziness. Restrict activities as necessary.

Aviation Note: Coronary artery disease *is a disqualification* for piloting. Consult a designated Aviation Medical Examiner.

Exposure to Sun: No restrictions.

Exposure to Heat: Caution advised. Hot environments can exaggerate the blood-pressure-lowering effects of this drug. Observe for light-headedness or weakness.

Heavy Exercise or Exertion: This drug may improve your ability to be more active without resulting angina pain. Use caution.

Discontinuation: Do not stop this drug abruptly. Ask your doctor about gradual withdrawal. Observe for the possible development of rebound angina.

AMOXAPINE (a MOX a peen)

Introduced: 1970   **Prescription:** USA: Yes; Canada: Yes   **Available as Generic:** Yes   **Class:** Antidepressant   **Controlled Drug:** USA: No; Canada: No

Brand Name: Asendin

BENEFITS versus RISKS	
Possible Benefits	*Possible Risks*
EFFECTIVE RELIEF OF PRIMARY DEPRESSIONS: Endogenous, neurotic, reactive	ADVERSE BEHAVIORAL EFFECTS: Confusion, delusions, disorientation, hallucinations
	CONVERSION OF DEPRESSION TO MANIA in manic-depressive disorders
	Rare blood cell abnormalities
	Rare movement disorders
	Rare seizures
	Rare liver toxicity

▷ **Principal Uses**

As a Single Drug Product: Uses currently included in FDA approved labeling: (1) Provides symptomatic relief in all depressive neurosis, psychotic depression, psychotic depressive reaction and depression.

Other (unlabeled) generally accepted uses: (1) May be a second line agent in panic attacks; (2) can be of use in refractory atypical unipolar depression.

How This Drug Works: By increasing some nerve impulse transmitters (norepinephrine and serotonin) in brain tissue, this drug relieves symptoms of depression.

Available Dosage Forms and Strengths
Tablets — 25 mg, 50 mg, 100 mg, 150 mg

▷ **Usual Adult Dosage Range:**   Initially 50 mg 2 or 3 times daily. Dose may be increased cautiously on the fifth or sixth day as needed and tolerated to 100 mg 3 times daily. Usual maintenance dose is 120 to 300 mg/ 24 hours. Total dosage should not exceed 600 mg/24 hours. When individually determined, the best dose may be taken at bedtime as one dose, not to exceed 300 mg. If the dose is greater than 300 mg per day it should be separated into several smaller doses that are taken two or three times a day. With long-term use, reports of loss of benefit (tolerance) have been reported. Discuss this with your doctor if the drug seems to stop working for you. **Note: Actual dosage and administration schedule must be determined by the physician for each patient individually.**

Conditions Requiring Dosing Adjustments
Liver function: Lower doses, careful watch for adverse effects and blood levels are needed.
Kidney function: The steps taken for liver compromise are prudent with compromised kidneys.

▷ **Dosing Instructions:**   May be taken without regard to meals. May crush tablet to take it.

Usual Duration of Use: Benefit may be apparent within 4 to 7 days in some individuals, but continual use on a regular schedule for 2 to 3 weeks is usually needed to see the peak effect. Long-term use should not exceed 6 months without evaluation regarding the need for continuation. Ask your doctor.

▷ **This Drug Should Not Be Taken If**
- you have had an allergic reaction to it previously.
- you are taking or have taken within the past 14 days any monoamine oxidase (MAO) type B inhibitor drug (see Drug Class, Section Four).
- you are recovering from a recent heart attack.

▷ **Inform Your Physician Before Taking This Drug If**
- you are allergic or overly sensitive to other antidepressant drugs.
- you have a history of: diabetes, epilepsy, glaucoma, heart disease, paranoia, prostate gland enlargement, schizophrenia, urinary retention or overactive thyroid.
- you plan to have surgery under general anesthesia in the near future.
- you are unsure of how much amoxapine to take or how often to take it.
- you are pregnant or breast-feeding.
- you have asthma.
- you have liver or kidney disease.
- you have a history of a blood cell disorder.

Possible Side Effects (natural, expected, and unavoidable drug actions)
Drowsiness, blurred vision, dry mouth, constipation, impaired urination.

▷ **Possible Adverse Effects** (unusual, unexpected, and infrequent reactions)
If any of the following develop, consult your physician promptly for guidance.
Mild Adverse Effects
Allergic Reactions: Skin rash, hives, swellings, drug fever (see Glossary).

Insomnia, nervousness, palpitations, dizziness, unsteadiness, tremors, fainting.

Constipation, frequent urination.

Cavities (dental caries).

Blurred vision.

Peculiar taste, indigestion, nausea, vomiting.

Serious Adverse Effects

Idiosyncratic Reactions: Neuroleptic malignant syndrome (see Glossary), rare hepatitis.

Behavioral effects: Anxiety, confusion, excitement, disorientation, hallucinations, delusions.

Rapid heart rate (tachycardia).

Aggravation of paranoid psychosis and schizophrenia.

Aggravation of epilepsy (seizures).

Rare elevated blood glucose (hyperglycemia).

Seizures in those without a history of epilepsy.

Parkinson-like disorders (see Glossary).

Peripheral neuritis (see Glossary)—numbness, tingling, pain, loss of strength in arms and legs.

Reduced white blood cell count (agranulocytosis)—fever, sore throat.

Movement disorders (akathisia and extrapyramidal effects).

Hepatitis (rare).

▷ **Possible Effects on Sexual Function:** Decreased libido (150 mg/day), increased libido (antidepressant effect), inhibited ejaculation (75 to 150 mg/day), painful ejaculation (75 mg/day), inhibited female orgasm (100 mg/day), female breast enlargement/milk production (300 mg/day), altered menstrual timing and pattern (300 mg/day), swelling of testicles. These effects usually disappear within 2 to 10 days after discontinuation of the drug.

Natural Diseases or Disorders That May Be Activated by This Drug

Latent epilepsy, glaucoma, prostatism.

Possible Effects on Laboratory Tests

White blood cell counts: decreased.

Blood glucose: rarely increased.

Liver function tests: increased.

Alkaline phosphatase: increased.

CAUTION

1. Drug dose must be individualized. Blood levels may be needed.
2. Watch for toxicity: confusion, agitation, rapid heartbeat.
3. It is best to withhold this drug if electroconvulsive therapy (ECT, "shock" treatment) is to be used.

Precautions for Use

By Infants and Children: Safety and effectiveness for use by those under 16 not established.

By Those over 60 Years of Age: During the first 2 weeks of treatment, watch for confusion, restlessness, agitation, forgetfulness, disorientation, delusions and hallucinations. The dose may need to be reduced or the drug stopped. Unsteadiness may increase risk of falls or injury. This drug may worsen impaired urination seen in prostate gland enlargement (prostatism). Taking the total dose at bedtime can reduce the risk of postural hypotension (see Glossary).

▷ **Advisability of Use During Pregnancy**
  Pregnancy Category: C. See Pregnancy Code at the back of this book.
  Animal studies: Reveal toxic effects on the embryo in rats and rabbits but no birth defects in the newborn.
  Human studies: Adequate studies of pregnant women are not available.
  Avoid drug during first 3 months. Use during the last 6 months only if clearly needed.

Advisability of Use if Breast-Feeding
  Presence of this drug in breast milk: Yes, in small amounts.
  Watch infant closely and stop drug or nursing if adverse effects start.

Habit-Forming Potential: None.

Effects of Overdosage: Confusion, hallucinations, marked drowsiness, tremors, dilated pupils, cold skin, stupor, coma, convulsions, rapid heartbeat, high blood glucose, low blood pressure.

Suggested Periodic Examinations While Taking This Drug (at physician's discretion)
  Complete blood cell counts, serial blood pressure readings and electrocardiograms.

▷ **While Taking This Drug, Observe the Following**
  Foods: No restrictions. Drug may increase appetite and cause excessive weight gain.
  Beverages: No restrictions. May be taken with milk.
▷ *Alcohol:* Avoid completely. This drug can markedly increase the intoxicating effects of alcohol and accentuate its depressant action on brain function.
  Tobacco Smoking: May hasten the elimination of this drug. Higher doses may be necessary.
▷ *Other Drugs*
  Amoxapine may ***increase*** the effects of
  • amphetamines.
  • atropinelike drugs (see Drug Classes).
  • oral anticoagulants (warfarin, others). Increased INR testing is needed.
  Amoxapine may ***decrease*** the effects of
  • clonidine (Catapres).
  • guanethidine (Ismelin).
  • guanfacine (Tenex).
  Amoxapine ***taken concurrently*** with
  • acetazolamide can increase amoxapine blood levels.
  • antihistamines may increase urinary retention and dry mouth.
  • carbamazepine (Tegretol) may result in decreased antidepressant action.
  • cimetidine (Tagamet) may increase amoxapine levels and result in toxicity.
  • diphenhydramine (Benadryl) and other antihistamines can increase the risk of urine retention, chronic glaucoma or bowel obstruction (ileus).
  • monoamine oxidase (MAO) type A inhibitor drugs may cause high fever, delirium and convulsions (see Drug Classes).
  • phenytoin (Dilantin) may result in increased phenytoin levels.
  • quinidine (Quinaglute) may result in amoxapine toxicity.

- thyroid preparations may impair heart rhythm and function. Ask physician for guidance regarding adjustment of thyroid dose.

▷ *Driving, Hazardous Activities:* This drug may impair mental alertness, judgment, physical coordination and reaction time. Avoid hazardous activities.

Aviation Note: The use of this drug *is a disqualification* for piloting. Consult a designated Aviation Medical Examiner.

Exposure to Sun: Caution, this drug may cause photosensitivity (see Glossary).

Exposure to Heat: This drug can inhibit sweating and impair the body's adaptation to hot environments, increasing the risk of heat stroke. Avoid saunas.

Exposure to Cold: The elderly should use caution. Avoid conditions conducive to hypothermia (see Glossary).

Discontinuation: Slowly stop this drug. Abrupt withdrawal after long-term use can cause headache, malaise and nausea.

AMOXICILLIN (a mox i SIL in)

Introduced: 1969   **Prescription:** USA: Yes; Canada: Yes   **Available as Generic:** USA: Yes; Canada: No   **Class:** Anti-infective, penicillins   **Controlled Drug:** USA: No; Canada: No

Brand Names: Amoxil, ✦Apo-Amoxi, ✦Clavulin, Larotid, ✦Novamoxin, ✦Nu-Amoxi, Polymox, Trimox, Wymox

BENEFITS versus RISKS	
Possible Benefits	*Possible Risks*
EFFECTIVE TREATMENT OF INFECTIONS due to susceptible microorganisms	ALLERGIC REACTIONS, mild to severe Superinfections (yeast) Drug-induced colitis

▷ **Principal Uses**

As a Single Drug Product: Uses currently included in FDA approved labeling: Treatment of the following infections: (1) Some genitourinary tract infections; (2) acute uncomplicated gonorrhea, male and female; (3) a Drug of Choice for acute otitis media (middle ear infection); (4) some acute bacterial infections of the sinuses and throat; (5) some acute bacterial infections of the skin and soft tissues; (6) Haemophilus influenzae infections.

Other (unlabeled) generally accepted uses: Treatment of the following infections: (1) Bronchitis; (2) biliary tract infections; (3) Lyme disease; (4) typhoid fever; (5) gonorrheal infection of the urethra; (6) combination antibiotic treatment of duodenal ulcer caused by H. pylori; (7) prevention of bacterial endocarditis; (8) combination therapy of reactive lymphoid hyperplasia.

As a Combination Drug Product [CD]: See the following Drug Profile of Amoxicillin and Clavulanate.

How This Drug Works: This drug destroys susceptible infecting bacteria by interfering with their ability to produce new protective cell walls as they multiply and grow.

Available Dosage Forms and Strengths
        Capsules — 250 mg, 500 mg
Chewable tablets — 125 mg, 250 mg
        Oral liquid — 3 gram
Oral suspension — 50 mg per ml; 125 mg, 250 mg per 5 ml
Pediatric drops — 50 mg/ml

▷ **Recommended Dosage Ranges** (Actual dosage and administration schedule must be determined by the physician for each patient individually.)
Infants and Children: Up to 6 kg of body weight—25 to 50 mg every 8 hours.
6 to 8 kg of body weight—50 to 100 mg every 8 hours.
8 to 20 kg of body weight—6.7 to 13.3 mg/kg of body weight every 8 hours.
20 kg of body weight and over—same as 12 to 60 years of age.
12 to 60 Years of Age: Usual dose—250 to 500 mg every 8 hours. The total daily dose should not exceed 4.5 grams.
For gonorrhea—3 grams, together with 1 gram of probenecid, taken as a single dose.
For Lyme disease—250 to 500 mg, 3 or 4 times a day, for 10 to 30 days; dose and duration of treatment depends on severity of infection and response to treatment.
Over 60 Years of Age: Same as 12 to 60 years of age.

Conditions Requiring Dosing Adjustments
Liver function: Adjustments in dosing in liver compromise are not needed.
Kidney function: Dosing interval **must** be adjusted in renal compromise.

▷ **Dosing Instructions:**   May be taken on an empty stomach or with food, milk, fruit juice, ginger ale or other cold drinks. The capsule may be opened for administration. Shake the oral suspension well before measuring each dose. The tablets should be chewed or crushed.

Usual Duration of Use: For all streptococcal infections—not less than 10 consecutive days (without interruption) to reduce the possibility of rheumatic fever or glomerulonephritis. For all other infections—as long as needed to treat the infection.

▷ **This Drug Should Not Be Taken If**
   • you have had an allergic reaction to any dosage form of it previously.
   • you are certain you are allergic to *any* form of penicillin.

▷ **Inform Your Physician Before Taking This Drug If**
   • you suspect you are allergic to penicillin or have had a previous "reaction" to penicillin.
   • you are allergic to any cephalosporin drugs (Ancef, Ceporan, Ceporex, Kafocin, Keflex, Keflin, Kefzol, Loridine, others).
   • you are allergic by nature (hay fever, asthma, hives, eczema).
   • you are unsure of how much amoxicillin to take or how often to take it.
   • you have a history of liver or kidney disease.

Possible Side Effects (natural, expected, and unavoidable drug actions)
Superinfections (see Glossary), often due to yeast organisms.

▷ **Possible Adverse Effects** (unusual, unexpected, and infrequent reactions)
   If any of the following develop, consult your physician promptly for guidance.

Mild Adverse Effects
   Allergic Reactions: Skin rashes, hives, itching.
   Irritations of mouth and tongue, "black tongue," nausea, vomiting, mild diarrhea, dizziness (rare).
Serious Adverse Effects
   Allergic Reactions: Anaphylactic reaction (see Glossary), severe skin reactions, drug fever, swollen painful joints, sore throat, abnormal bleeding or bruising. Immune hemolytic anemia.
   Drug-induced pseudomembranous colitis: severe abdominal pain and cramping, marked diarrhea, bloody stools, fever.
   Rare liver or kidney toxicity.

▷ **Possible Effects on Sexual Function:**   None reported.

Possible Effects on Laboratory Tests
   White blood cell counts: decreased.

CAUTION
   1. Take the exact dose and the full course prescribed.
   2. Should not be used with antibiotics such as erythromycin or tetracycline.

Precautions for Use
   By Infants and Children: A rash occurs in approximately 90% of people who take this drug during an episode of infectious mononucleosis. The drug commonly causes diarrhea.
   By Those over 60 Years of Age: Natural changes in the skin may predispose to prolonged itching reactions in the genital and anal regions. Report such reactions promptly.

▷ **Advisability of Use During Pregnancy**
   Pregnancy Category: B. See Pregnancy Code at the back of this book.
      Animal studies: No information available.
      Human studies: Information from adequate studies of pregnant women indicates no increased risk of birth defects in 3546 pregnancies exposed to penicillin derivatives.
   Ask physician for guidance.

Advisability of Use if Breast-Feeding
   Presence of this drug in breast milk: Yes.
   The nursing infant may be sensitized to penicillin and may be at risk for developing diarrhea or yeast infections.
   Avoid drug if possible or refrain from nursing.

Habit-Forming Potential: None.

Effects of Overdosage: Possible nausea, vomiting and/or diarrhea.

Possible Effects of Long-Term Use: Superinfections, often due to yeast organisms.

Suggested Periodic Examinations While Taking This Drug (at physician's discretion)
   Complete blood cell counts.

▷ **While Taking This Drug, Observe the Following**
   Foods: No restrictions, minor decrease in absorption.
   Beverages: No restrictions. May be taken with milk, fruit juices or carbonated drinks.
▷ *Alcohol:* No interactions expected, but alcohol can blunt the immune response.

It is best NOT to drink while you have an infection severe enough to require antibiotics.

Tobacco Smoking: No interactions expected.

▷ *Other Drugs*

Amoxicillin may *decrease* the effects of
- oral contraceptives—*pregnancy* risk.

The following drugs may *decrease* the effects of amoxicillin
- antacids reduce the absorption of amoxicillin.
- chloramphenicol (Chloromycetin).
- erythromycin (Erythrocin, E-Mycin, etc.).
- tetracyclines (Achromycin, Declomycin, Minocin, etc.). (See Drug Class.)

Amoxicillin *taken concurrently* with
- H2 blockers (cimetidine, ranitidine, nizatidine or famotidine) may increase the absorption of amoxicillin.
- probenecid will increase the concentrations of amoxicillin in the body.

▷ *Driving, Hazardous Activities:* Be alert to the rare occurrence of dizziness and/or nausea, and restrict activities accordingly.

Aviation Note: The use of this drug *may be a disqualification* for piloting. Consult a designated Aviation Medical Examiner.

Exposure to Sun: No restrictions.

Special Storage Instructions: Oral suspension and pediatric drops should be refrigerated.

Observe the Following Expiration Times: Do not take the oral suspension or drops of this drug if older than 7 days when kept at room temperature or 14 days when kept refrigerated.

AMOXICILLIN/CLAVULANATE (a mox i SIL in/KLAV yu lan ayt)

Introduced: 1982   **Prescription:** USA: Yes; Canada: Yes   **Available as Generic:** USA: No; Canada: No   **Class:** Anti-infective, penicillins   **Controlled Drug:** USA: No; Canada: No

Brand Names: Augmentin, ✦Clavulin

BENEFITS versus RISKS	
Possible Benefits	*Possible Risks*
EFFECTIVE TREATMENT OF INFECTIONS due to susceptible microorganisms	ALLERGIC REACTIONS, mild to severe Superinfections (yeast) Drug-induced colitis Low white blood cells (rare)

▷ **Principal Uses**

As a Combination Drug Product [CD]: Uses currently included in FDA approved labeling: Treatment of the following infections: (1) Some genitourinary tract infections; (2) Some bacterial pneumonias; (3) Acute otitis media (middle ear infection) and sinusitis caused by certain bacteria; (4) Some acute bacterial infections of the skin and soft tissues.

Other (unlabeled) generally accepted uses: Treatment of the following infections: (1) bronchitis; (2) biliary tract infections; (3) chancroid; (4) cat bite infections.

How This Drug Works: Amoxicillin destroys susceptible infecting bacteria by interfering with their ability to produce new protective cell walls as they multiply and grow.

Clavulanate inhibits beta-lactamase enzymes produced by resistant bacteria. Clavulanate enhances the action of amoxicillin against resistant bacteria.

Available Dosage Forms and Strengths

Oral suspension — 125 mg (amoxicillin) and 31.25 mg (clavulanate) per 5 ml

— 250 mg (amoxicillin) and 62.5 mg (clavulanate) per 5 ml

Tablets — 250 mg (amoxicillin) and 125 mg (clavulanate)

— 500 mg (amoxicillin) and 125 mg (clavulanate)

Tablets, chewable — 125 mg (amoxicillin) and 31.25 mg (clavulanate)

— 250 mg (amoxicillin) and 62.5 mg (clavulanate)

▷ **Recommended Dosage Ranges** (Actual dosage and administration schedule must be determined by the physician for each patient individually.)

Infants and Children: Up to 40 kg of body weight—6.7 to 13.3 mg (amoxicillin)/kg of body weight every 8 hours.

40 kg of body weight and over—same as 12 to 60 years of age.

12 to 60 Years of Age: Usual dose—250 to 500 mg (amoxicillin) every 8 hours. The total daily dose (of amoxicillin) should not exceed 4.5 grams.

Over 60 Years of Age: Same as 12 to 60 years of age.

Note: The above doses refer to the amoxicillin component of this combination drug. The 250 mg regular tablet and the 250 mg chewable tablet contain different amounts of clavulanate and are not interchangeable. See **Dosage Forms** above.

Conditions Requiring Dosing Adjustments

Liver function: Specific guidelines do not exist regarding adjustment in liver failure.

Kidney function: Dose **must** be decreased in kidney compromise.

▷ **Dosing Instructions:**   May be taken on an empty stomach or with food, milk, fruit juice, ginger ale or other cold drinks. The oral suspension should be shaken well before measuring each dose. The regular tablets may be crushed for administration. The chewable tablets should be chewed or crushed.

Usual Duration of Use: For all streptococcal infections—not less than 10 consecutive days (without interruption) to reduce the possibility of developing rheumatic fever or glomerulonephritis. For all other infections—as long as necessary to eradicate the infection.

▷ **This Drug Should Not Be Taken If**
- you have had an allergic reaction to any dosage form of it previously.
- you are certain you are allergic to *any* form of penicillin.

▷ **Inform Your Physician Before Taking This Drug If**
- you suspect you are allergic to penicillin or have had a previous "reaction" to penicillin.
- you are allergic to cephalosporin drugs (Ancef, Ceporan, Ceporex, Kafocin, Keflex, Keflin, Kefzol, Loridine, others).

- you are allergic by nature (hay fever, asthma, hives, eczema).
- you are unsure of how much amoxicillin/clavulanate to take or how often to take it.
- you have a history of low blood counts.
- you have a history of liver or kidney disease.

Possible Side Effects (natural, expected, and unavoidable drug actions)
Superinfections (see Glossary), often due to yeast organisms.

▷ **Possible Adverse Effects** (unusual, unexpected, and infrequent reactions)
If any of the following develop, consult your physician promptly for guidance.
Mild Adverse Effects
Allergic Reactions: Skin rashes, hives, itching.
Irritations of mouth and tongue, "black tongue," nausea, vomiting, mild diarrhea, dizziness (rare).
Serious Adverse Effects
Allergic Reactions: Anaphylactic reaction (see Glossary), severe skin reactions, drug fever, swollen painful joints, sore throat, abnormal bleeding or bruising.
Drug-induced pseudomembranous colitis: severe abdominal pain and cramping, marked diarrhea, bloody stools, fever.
Low white blood cells (rare).
Hepatitis (rare).
Candidal vaginitis.

▷ **Possible Effects on Sexual Function:**   None reported.

Possible Effects on Laboratory Tests
White blood cell counts: decreased.

CAUTION
1. Take the exact dose and the full course prescribed.
2. Should not be used with erythromycin or tetracycline.

Precautions for Use
By Infants and Children: A generalized rash occurs in approximately 90% of individuals who take this drug during an episode of infectious mononucleosis. This drug may cause diarrhea, which sometimes necessitates discontinuation.
By Those over 60 Years of Age: Natural changes in the skin may predispose to prolonged itching reactions in the genital and anal regions. Report such reactions promptly.

▷ **Advisability of Use During Pregnancy**
Pregnancy Category: B. See Pregnancy Code at the back of this book.
Animal studies: No information available.
Human studies: Information from adequate studies of pregnant women indicates no increased risk of birth defects in 3546 pregnancies exposed to penicillin derivatives.
Ask physician for guidance.

Advisability of Use if Breast-Feeding
Presence of this drug in breast milk: Yes.

The nursing infant may be sensitized to penicillin and may be at risk for developing diarrhea or yeast infections.
Avoid drug if possible or refrain from nursing.

Habit-Forming Potential: None.

Effects of Overdosage: Possible nausea, vomiting and/or diarrhea.

Possible Effects of Long-Term Use: Superinfections, often due to yeast organisms.

Suggested Periodic Examinations While Taking This Drug (at physician's discretion)
Complete blood cell counts.

▷ **While Taking This Drug, Observe the Following**
Foods: No restrictions, may decrease absorption slightly so this is not of clinical importance.
Beverages: No restrictions. May be taken with milk, fruit juices or carbonated drinks.
▷ *Alcohol:* No interactions expected.
Tobacco Smoking: No interactions expected.
▷ *Other Drugs*
Amoxicillin/clavulanate may ***decrease*** the effects of
• oral contraceptives in some women, impair their effectiveness and result in pregnancy.
The following drugs may ***decrease*** the effects of amoxicillin/clavulanate
• antacids reduce the absorption of amoxicillin.
• chloramphenicol (Chloromycetin).
• erythromycin (Erythrocin, E-Mycin, etc.).
• tetracyclines (Achromycin, Declomycin, Minocin, etc.). (See Drug Class.)
Amoxicillin/clavulanate ***taken concurrently*** with
• H2 blockers (cimetidine, ranitidine, nizatidine or famotidine) may increase the absorption of amoxicillin.
• probenecid will increase the concentrations of amoxicillin in the body.
▷ *Driving, Hazardous Activities:* Be alert to the rare occurrence of dizziness and/or nausea, and restrict activities accordingly.
Aviation Note: The use of this drug ***may be a disqualification*** for piloting. Consult a designated Aviation Medical Examiner.
Exposure to Sun: No restrictions.
Special Storage Instructions: Oral suspension and pediatric drops should be refrigerated.
Observe the Following Expiration Times: Do not take the oral suspension or drops of this drug if older than 7 days when kept at room temperature or 14 days when kept refrigerated.

AMPICILLIN (am pi SIL in)

Introduced: 1961   **Prescription:** USA: Yes; Canada: Yes   **Available as Generic:** Yes   **Class:** Antibiotic, penicillins   **Controlled Drug:** USA: No; Canada: No

Brand Names: Amcill, ✦Ampicin, ✦Ampicin PRB [CD], ✦Ampilean, ✦Apo-Ampi, D-Amp, Faspak ampicillin, 500 Kit [CD], Nu-Ampi, ✦Novo-Ampicillin, Omnipen, Omnipen Pediatric Drops, Pardec capsules [CD], ✦Penbritin, Polycillin, Polycillin Pediatric Drops, Polycillin-PRB [CD], ✦Pondocillin, Principen, SK-Ampicillin, Totacillin

---

BENEFITS versus RISKS

Possible Benefits	*Possible Risks*
EFFECTIVE TREATMENT OF INFECTIONS due to susceptible microorganisms	ALLERGIC REACTIONS, mild to severe Superinfections (yeast) Drug-induced colitis Rare blood cell disorders Rare kidney problems

---

▷ **Principal Uses**

As a Single Drug Product: (1) Treats some infections of the skin and soft tissues, of the respiratory tract, of the gastrointestinal tract, and of the genitourinary tract (including some gonorrhea and vaginosis in females); (2) Also used to treat certain types of septicemia and meningitis.

As a Combination Drug Product [CD]: May be combined with probenecid (Benemid) to keep a therapeutic blood level.

How This Drug Works: This drug destroys susceptible infecting bacteria by interfering with their ability to produce new protective cell walls as they multiply and grow.

Available Dosage Forms and Strengths

Capsules — 250 mg, 500 mg
Oral suspension — 100 mg per ml, 125 mg, 250 mg, 500 mg per 5 ml
Pediatric drops — 100 mg per ml

▷ **Usual Adult Dosage Range:** 500 to 1000 mg every 6 hours or 50 to 100 mg per kg per day divided into four doses. The usual maximal dose is 6000 mg/24 hours. **Note: Actual dosage and administration schedule must be determined by the physician for each patient individually.**

Conditions Requiring Dosing Adjustments

Liver function: The liver is not significantly involved in the elimination of ampicillin.

Kidney function: Dose must be decreased in people with kidney damage.

▷ **Dosing Instructions:** Best taken on an empty stomach, 1 hour before or 2 hours after eating. Capsule may be opened for administration.

Usual Duration of Use: For all streptococcal infections—not less than 10 consecutive days (without interruption) to reduce the possibility of developing rheumatic fever or glomerulonephritis. For all other infections—as long as necessary to eradicate the infection or 48 to 72 hours after the patient is asymptomatic.

▷ **This Drug Should Not Be Taken If**

• you have had an allergic reaction to any dosage form of it previously.
• you are certain you are allergic to *any* form of penicillin.

▷ **Inform Your Physician Before Taking This Drug If**
  - you suspect you are allergic to penicillin or you have a previous "reaction" to penicillin.
  - you are allergic to cephalosporin antibiotics (Ancef, Ceporan, Ceporex, Kafocin, Keflex, Keflin, Kefzol, Loridine).
  - you are allergic by nature (hay fever, asthma, hives, eczema).
  - you are unsure of how much ampicillin to take or how often to take it.
  - you have mono (mononucleosis) as you are more likely to get a rash.
  - you have a history of blood disorders.
  - you have a history of kidney problems.

Possible Side Effects (natural, expected, and unavoidable drug actions)
  Superinfections (see Glossary), often due to yeast organisms.

▷ **Possible Adverse Effects** (unusual, unexpected, and infrequent reactions)
  If any of the following develop, consult your physician promptly for guidance.
  Mild Adverse Effects
  Allergic Reactions: Skin rashes, hives, itching.
  Irritations of mouth and tongue, "black tongue," nausea, vomiting, mild diarrhea, dizziness (rare).
  Muscle aches.
  Serious Adverse Effects
  Allergic Reactions: Anaphylactic reaction (see Glossary), severe skin reactions, drug fever, swollen painful joints.
  Idiosyncratic Reaction: Rare liver toxicity.
  Blood cell problems (agranulocytosis, thrombocytopenia, or hypoprothrombinemia): sore throat, abnormal bleeding or bruising.
  Rare kidney problems (interstitial nephritis).
  Rare seizures (high blood levels).
  Rare severe colon inflammation (pseudomembranous colitis).

▷ **Possible Effects on Sexual Function:**   May have a small effect in decreasing sperm counts in men.

Possible Effects on Laboratory Tests
  Complete blood cell counts: decreased red cells, white cells and platelets; increased eosinophils.
  Bleeding time: may be prolonged, related to dose of drug.
  Coombs' antiglobulin test: may be positive.
  Urine analysis: positive for red blood cells and casts.
  Urine sugar tests: using Tes-Tape—no drug effect; using Clinistix or Diastix— false low or negative; using Clinitest—
  false positive or negative.

CAUTION
  1. Take the exact dose and the full course prescribed.
  2. Should not be used with erythromycin or tetracycline.

Precautions for Use
  By Infants and Children: A generalized rash occurs in approximately 90% of individuals who take this drug during an episode of infectious mononucleo-

sis. This drug may cause diarrhea, which sometimes necessitates discontinuation.

By Those over 60 Years of Age: Natural changes in the skin may predispose to prolonged itching reactions in the genital and anal regions. Report such reactions promptly.

▷ **Advisability of Use During Pregnancy**
Pregnancy Category: B. See Pregnancy Code at the back of this book.
Animal studies: No birth defects due to this drug found in mice or rats.
Human studies: Information from adequate studies of pregnant women indicates no increased risk of birth defects in 3546 pregnancies exposed to penicillin derivatives.
Ask physician for guidance.

Advisability of Use if Breast-Feeding
Presence of this drug in breast milk: Yes, in small amounts.
The nursing infant may be sensitized to penicillin and may be at risk for developing diarrhea or yeast infections.
Avoid drug if possible or refrain from nursing.

Habit-Forming Potential: None.

Effects of Overdosage: Possible nausea, vomiting and/or diarrhea, seizures.

Possible Effects of Long-Term Use: Superinfections, often due to yeast organisms.

Suggested Periodic Examinations While Taking This Drug (at physician's discretion)
Complete blood cell counts.

▷ **While Taking This Drug, Observe the Following**
Foods: Will **decrease** the peak amount absorbed by 25–50%. Best to separate antibiotic doses and food by 1 to 2 hours.
Beverages: No restrictions. May be taken with milk.
▷ *Alcohol:* No interactions expected, however alcohol may blunt the immune response and lessen your ability to fight infection.
Tobacco Smoking: No interactions expected.
▷ *Other Drugs*
Ampicillin may *decrease* the effects of
• oral contraceptives (birth control pills) in some women, and impair their effectiveness in preventing pregnancy. Pregnancy may result unless an alternate method of birth control is used.
The following drugs may *decrease* the effects of ampicillin
• antacids reduce the absorption of ampicillin.
• chloramphenicol (Chloromycetin).
• erythromycin (Erythrocin, E-Mycin, etc.).
• tetracyclines (Achromycin, Declomycin, Minocin, etc.). (See Drug Class.)
Ampicillin *taken concurrently* with
• allopurinol may increase the risk of rashes.
• atenolol can blunt the therapeutic benefits of atenolol.
▷ *Driving, Hazardous Activities:* Be alert to the rare occurrence of dizziness and/or nausea, and restrict activities accordingly.

Aviation Note: The use of this drug *may be a disqualification* for piloting. Consult a designated Aviation Medical Examiner.

Exposure to Sun: No restrictions.

Special Storage Instructions: Oral suspension and pediatric drops should be refrigerated.

Observe the Following Expiration Times: Do not take the oral suspension or drops of this drug if older than 7 days when kept at room temperature or 14 days when kept refrigerated.

ASPIRIN* (AS pir in)

Other Names: ASA, acetylsalicylic acid

Introduced: 1899   **Prescription:** USA: No; Canada: No   **Available as Generic:** Yes   **Class:** analgesics, mild; antiplatelet, antipyretic, NSAID, salicylates   **Controlled Drug:** USA: No; Canada: No

Brand Names: Added Strength Analgesic Pain reliever, Alka-Seltzer Effervescent Pain Reliever & Antacid [CD], Alka-Seltzer Plus Cold, Alka-Seltzer Night Time [CD], Alka-Seltzer Plus [CD], Anacin [CD], Anacin Maximum Strength [CD], ✦Anacin w/Codeine [CD], ✦Ancasal, APC [CD], APC with codeine [CD], Arthritis Pain Formula [CD], Arthritis Strength Bufferin, A.S.A. Enseals, ✦Asasantine [CD], Ascriptin [CD], Ascriptin A/D [CD], Aspergum, ✦Aspirin*, Asprimox, ✦Astrin, Axotal [CD], Azdone [CD], Bayer Aspirin, Bayer Children's Chewable Aspirin, Bayer Enteric Aspirin, Bayer Plus, Buffaprin, Bufferin [CD], Bufferin Arthritis Strength [CD], Bufferin Extra Strength [CD], Bufferin w/Codeine [CD], Cama Arthritis Pain Reliever [CD], Carisoprodol Compound [CD], ✦C2 buffered [CD], Cope [CD], Coricidin [CD], ✦Coryphen, ✦Coryphen-Codeine [CD], Darvon Compound [CD], Direct Formulary Aspirin, ✦Dristan [CD], Easprin, Ecotrin, 8-Hour Bayer, Empirin, Empirin w/Codeine No. 2, 4 [CD], ✦Entrophen, Excedrin [CD], Excedrin Extra Strength Geltabs [CD], Fiorinal [CD], Fiorinal w/Codeine [CD], ✦Fiorinal-C 1/4, -C 1/2 [CD], Genprin, Halprin, Hepto [CD], Lortab ASA [CD], Low Dose Adult Chewable Aspirin, Marnal [CD], Maximum Bayer Aspirin, Measurin, Midol Caplets [CD], Momentum [CD], Norgesic [CD], Norgesic Forte [CD], Norwich Aspirin, ✦Novasen, Orphenadrine [CD], PAP with codeine [CD], Percodan [CD], Percodan-Demi [CD], ✦Phenaphen [CD], ✦Phenaphen No. 2, 3, 4 [CD], Propoxyphene compound [CD], ✦Riphen-10, Robaxisal [CD], ✦Robaxisal-C [CD], Roxiprin [CD], SK-65 Compound [CD], Soma Compound [CD], St. Joseph Children's Aspirin, ✦Supasa, Synalgos [CD], Synalgos-DC [CD], Talwin Compound [CD], Talwin Compound-50 [CD], ✦Tecnal tablet [CD], ✦Triaphen-10, ✦217 [CD], ✦217 Strong [CD], ✦292 [CD], ✦692 [CD], Vanquish [CD], Verin, Wesprin, Zorprin

   Author's note: Aspirin is featured in this edition's True Breakthroughs In Medicines section.

---

*In the United States *aspirin* is an official generic designation. In Canada *Aspirin* is the Registered Trade Mark of the Bayer Company Division of Sterling Drug Limited.

```
┌─────────────────────────────────────────────────────────────────┐
│                      BENEFITS versus RISKS                        │
│      Possible Benefits              Possible Risks                │
│  EFFECTIVE RELIEF OF MILD TO    Stomach irritation, bleeding, and/or │
│    MODERATE PAIN AND              ulceration                      │
│    INFLAMMATION                 Hearing loss                      │
│  REDUCTION OF FEVER             Decreased numbers of white blood  │
│  PREVENTION OF BLOOD CLOTS        cells and platelets             │
│  PREVENTION OF HEART ATTACK     Hemolytic anemia                  │
│  PREVENTION OF STROKE           Rare liver toxicity               │
│  PREVENTION OF COLON CANCER     Bronchospasm in asthmatics        │
│  MAY ACT TO LIMIT THE SIZE AND                                    │
│    SEVERITY OF A HEART ATTACK                                     │
│    ONCE IT HAS STARTED                                            │
└─────────────────────────────────────────────────────────────────┘
```

▷ **Principal Uses**

   As a Single Drug Product: Uses currently included in FDA approved labeling: (1) Relieves mild to moderate pain, and provides symptomatic relief in conditions causing inflammation or high fever. Treats musculoskeletal disorders, especially acute and chronic arthritis. Used selectively in low dosage to (2) reduce the risk of recurrent heart attack; (3) prevent platelet embolism to the brain (in men); (4) reduce the risk of clots (thromboembolism) in patients who have had a heart attack, in people with artificial heart valves and after hip surgery; (see Blood Platelets in Glossary.) (5) helps prevent recurrence of stroke in people who have suffered a stroke; (6) helps prevent stroke in patients who have had a transient ischemic attack (TIA).

   Other (unlabeled) generally accepted uses: (1) Can help prevent toxemia of pregnancy when used in low doses; (2) a very recent, well designed, large sample size study says that long-term use may decrease the risk of colon polyps or colon cancer in females. The data are large enough to be expected to apply to men as well; (3) another very recent study shows that aspirin may limit the size and severity of a heart attack when it is taken immediately after symptoms are recognized and is continued for at least 30 days after the heart attack.

   As a Combination Drug Product [CD]: Frequently combined with other mild or strong analgesic drugs to enhance pain relief. Also combined with antihistamines and decongestants in many cold preparations to relieve headache and general discomfort.

How This Drug Works: Reduces prostaglandins, chemicals involved in the production of inflammation and pain. By modifying the temperature-regulating center in the brain, dilating blood vessels, and increasing sweating, aspirin reduces fever. By preventing the production of thromboxane in blood platelets, aspirin inhibits formation of blood clots.

Available Dosage Forms and Strengths

                Capsules, enteric-coated — 500 mg
       Capsules, enteric-coated granules — 325 mg
                        Gum tablets — 227.5 mg
                       Suppositories — 60 mg, 120 mg, 125 mg, 130 mg, 195
                                       mg, 200 mg, 300 mg, 325 mg, 600 mg,
                                       650 mg, 1.2 grams

Tablets — 65 mg, 81 mg, 325 mg, 500 mg

Tablets, chewable — 81 mg

Tablets, enteric-coated — 81 mg, 165 mg, 325 mg, 500 mg, 650 mg, 975 mg

Tablets, prolonged-action — 650 mg, 800 mg

▷ **Usual Adult Dosage Range:**   For pain or fever—325 to 650 mg/4 hours as needed. For arthritis (and related conditions)—3600 to 5400 mg daily in divided doses. For the prevention of blood clots—80 to 150 mg daily or every other day. Low dose, long-term daily aspirin may also decrease risk of colon cancer. **Note: For long-term use, actual dosage and administration schedule must be determined by the physician for each patient individually.**

Conditions Requiring Dosing Adjustments

Liver function: This medication should be avoided in severe liver disease.

Kidney function: It should be avoided or used with caution in patients with kidney problems.

Glucose-6-Phosphate Dehydrogenase Deficiency

May cause destruction of red blood cells in patients with G-6-PD deficiency.

▷ **Dosing Instructions:**   Take with food, milk, or a full glass of water to reduce stomach upset. Regular tablets may be crushed and capsules opened for administration. Enteric-coated tablets, prolonged-action tablets, A.S.A. Enseals, Cama tablets and Ecotrin tablets should not be crushed.

Usual Duration of Use: Short-term use is recommended—3 to 5 days. Daily use should not exceed 10 days without physician supervision. Use on a regular schedule for 1 week is usually needed to determine this drug's effectiveness in relieving the symptoms of chronic arthritis. Must evaluate response and adjust dose in long-term use. Consult your physician on a regular basis.

▷ **This Drug Should Not Be Taken If**
- you have had an allergic reaction to any form of aspirin.
- you have any type of bleeding disorder (such as hemophilia).
- you have active peptic ulcer disease.
- you are in the last 3 months of pregnancy.
- it smells like vinegar. This indicates decomposition of aspirin.

▷ **Inform Your Physician Before Taking This Drug If**
- you are taking any anticoagulant drug.
- you are taking oral antidiabetic drugs.
- you have a history of peptic ulcer disease or gout.
- you have lupus erythematosus.
- you are pregnant or planning pregnancy.
- you have asthma, carditis or nasal polyps.
- you plan to have surgery of any kind in the near future.
- you take other prescription or nonprescription medications which were not discussed when aspirin was prescribed for you.
- you are unsure of how much aspirin to take or how often to take it.
- you have a history of liver or kidney problems.
- you have a deficiency of G-6-PD.
- you have a history of angina (may be worsened by this drug).

Possible Side Effects (natural, expected, and unavoidable drug actions)
Mild drowsiness in sensitive individuals.

▷ **Possible Adverse Effects** (unusual, unexpected, and infrequent reactions)
If any of the following develop, consult your physician promptly for guidance.

Mild Adverse Effects
Allergic Reactions: Skin rash, hives, nasal discharge (resembling hay fever), nasal polyps.
Stomach irritation, heartburn, nausea, vomiting, constipation.
Lowering of the blood sugar.

Serious Adverse Effects
Allergic Reactions: Acute anaphylactic reaction (see Glossary), allergic destruction of blood platelets (see Glossary) and bruising.
Idiosyncratic Reactions: Hemolytic anemia (see Glossary).
Erosion of stomach lining, with silent bleeding.
Activation of peptic ulcer, with or without hemorrhage.
Bone marrow depression (see Glossary)—fatigue, weakness, fever, sore throat, abnormal bleeding or bruising.
Hepatitis with jaundice (see Glossary)—yellow skin and eyes, dark-colored urine, light-colored stool (very rare).
Kidney damage, if used in large doses or for a prolonged period of time.
Bronchospasm when used in patients with nasal polyps, asthma.
May worsen angina attacks and increase their frequency.
Reye's syndrome if used during viral illness.

▷ **Possible Effects on Sexual Function:**   None reported.

▷ **Adverse Effects That May Mimic Natural Diseases or Disorders**
Liver damage may suggest viral hepatitis.

Possible Effects on Laboratory Tests
Complete blood counts: decreased red cells, hemoglobin, white cells and platelets.
Bleeding time: prolonged.
Prothrombin time: increased by large doses; decreased by small doses.
Blood glucose level: decreased in diabetics.
Blood uric acid level: increased by small doses; decreased by large doses.
Liver function tests: increased ALT/GPT, AST/GOT, alkaline phosphatase.
Kidney function tests: increased blood creatinine and urea nitrogen levels with long-term use; increased protein and kidney cells in urine.
Thyroid function tests: increased T_3 uptake, free T_3 and free T_4; decreased TSH, T_3, T_4, and free thyroxine index (FTI).
Urine sugar tests: false positive with Clinitest or Benedict's solution.
Fecal occult blood test: positive with large doses of aspirin.

CAUTION
1. Remember that aspirin is a drug. While it is one of our most useful drugs, we have an unrealistic sense of safety and its potential for adverse effects.
2. Make it a point to learn the contents of all drugs you take—those prescribed by your physician and over-the-counter (OTC) medicines.
3. Do NOT take more than 3 tablets (975 mg) at one time, allow at least 4 hours between doses and take no more than 10 tablets (3250 mg) in 24 hours without physician supervision.

4. Remember that aspirin can
   - cause new illnesses.
   - complicate existing illnesses.
   - complicate pregnancy.
   - complicate surgery.
   - interact unfavorably with other drugs.
5. When your physician asks "Are you taking any drugs?" the answer is **yes** if you are taking aspirin. This also applies to *any* nonprescription drug you may be taking. (See OTC Drugs in Glossary.)

Precautions for Use

By Infants and Children: Reye's syndrome (brain and liver damage in children, often fatal) can follow flu or chicken pox in children and teenagers. Some reports suggest that the use of aspirin by children with flu or chicken pox can increase the risk of developing this complication. Consult your physician before giving aspirin to a child or teenager with chicken pox, flu or similar infection.

Usual dosage schedule for children:

Up to 2 years of age—consult physician.
2 to 4 years of age—160 mg/4 hours, up to 5 doses/24 hours.
4 to 6 years of age—240 mg/4 hours, up to 5 doses/24 hours.
6 to 9 years of age—320 mg/4 hours, up to 5 doses/24 hours.
9 to 11 years of age—400 mg/4 hours, up to 5 doses/24 hours.
11 to 12 years of age—480 mg/4 hours, up to 5 doses/24 hours.

Do not exceed 5 days of continual use without consulting your physician.
Give all doses with food, milk or a full glass of water.

By Those over 60 Years of Age: Watch for signs of excessive dosage: nervous irritability, confusion, ringing in the ears, deafness, loss of appetite, nausea and stomach upset. Aspirin can cause serious bleeding from the stomach. This can occur as "silent" bleeding of small amounts over a long time, resulting in anemia. Sudden hemorrhage can occur, even without a history of stomach ulcer. Watch for gray to black colored stools—an indication of stomach bleeding.

▷ **Advisability of Use During Pregnancy**

Pregnancy Category: C. See Pregnancy Code at the back of this book.

Animal studies: Significant birth defects due to this drug have been reported.

Human studies: Information from studies of pregnant women indicates no increased risk of birth defects in 32,164 pregnancies exposed to aspirin. However, studies show that the regular use of aspirin during pregnancy is often detrimental to the health of the mother and to the welfare of the fetus. Anemia, hemorrhage before and after delivery and an increased incidence of stillbirths and newborn deaths have been reported. It is advisable to limit aspirin use during pregnancy to small doses and for brief periods of time. There are data which support use of aspirin in low doses to prevent toxemia of pregnancy in some women with a history of this problem. Ask your doctor for help. Avoid aspirin altogether during the last 3 months.

Advisability of Use if Breast-Feeding

Presence of this drug in breast milk: Yes.
Avoid drug or refrain from nursing.

Habit-Forming Potential: Extended high dose use may cause a psychological dependence (see Glossary).

Effects of Overdosage: Stomach distress, nausea, vomiting, ringing in the ears, dizziness, impaired hearing, blood chemistry imbalance, sweating, stupor, fever, deep and rapid breathing, muscular twitching, delirium, shock, hallucinations, convulsions.

Possible Effects of Long-Term Use

A form of psychological dependence (see Glossary).
Anemia due to chronic blood loss from erosion of stomach lining.
The development of stomach ulcer.
The development of "aspirin allergy"—nasal discharge, nasal polyps, asthma.
Kidney damage.
Prolonged bleeding time, critical in the event of injury or surgery.

Suggested Periodic Examinations While Taking This Drug (at physician's discretion)

Complete blood cell counts.
Kidney function tests and urine analyses.
Liver function tests.

▷ **While Taking This Drug, Observe the Following**

Foods: May decrease the total amount of aspirin per dose which is absorbed.
Nutritional Support: Do not take large doses of vitamin C while taking aspirin regularly.
Beverages: No restrictions. May be taken with milk.

▷ *Alcohol:* Concurrent use of alcohol and aspirin may significantly increase the risk of stomach damage and may prolong bleeding time.
Tobacco Smoking: No interactions expected.

▷ *Other Drugs*

Aspirin may *increase* the effects of
- oral anticoagulants (see Drug Classes), and cause abnormal bleeding.
- insulin and require dosage adjustment.
- oral antidiabetic drugs and insulin, and cause hypoglycemia (see Drug Classes). Dosage decrease is often necessary.
- heparin, and cause abnormal bleeding.
- methotrexate, and increase its toxic effects.
- valproic acid (Depakene).

Aspirin may *decrease* the effects of
- beta-adrenergic-blocking drugs (see Drug Classes).
- captopril (Capoten).
- furosemide (Lasix).
- spironolactone.
- other NSAIDS (see Drug Classes).
- probenecid (Benemid), and reduce its effectiveness in the treatment of gout—with aspirin doses of less than 2 grams/24 hours.
- spironolactone (Aldactone), and reduce its diuretic effect.
- sulfinpyrazone (Anturane), and reduce its effectiveness in the treatment of gout—with aspirin doses of less than 2 grams/24 hours.

Aspirin *taken concurrently* with
- diltiazem (Cardizem) may result in increased risk of bleeding.
- intrauterine devices (IUDs) may result in decreased IUD effectiveness.

- methotrexate (Mexate) and cause toxicity.
- valproic acid and cause toxic blood levels.
- high blood pressure (antihypertensive) medicines may blunt their therapeutic benefit, especially those which are diuretics such as furosemide (Lasix) or spironolactone.
- varicella vaccine (Varivax) may result in Reye's syndrome. **Avoid aspirin and other salicylates for 6 weeks following Varivax inoculation.**
- verapamil and cause increased bleeding risk.

The following drugs may *increase* the effects of aspirin
- acetazolamide (Diamox).
- para-aminobenzoic acid (Pabalate).
- cimetidine (Tagamet)

The following drugs may *decrease* the effects of aspirin
- antacids, in regular continual use.
- cortisonelike drugs (see Drug Classes).
- urinary alkalinizers (sodium bicarbonate, sodium citrate).

▷ *Driving, Hazardous Activities:* No restrictions or precautions.
Aviation Note: It is advisable to watch for mild drowsiness and restrict activities accordingly.
Exposure to Sun: Use caution, may cause photosensitivity.
Discontinuation: Aspirin should be stopped at least 1 week before surgery of any kind.

ASTEMIZOLE (a STEM i zohl)

Introduced: 1982   **Prescription:** USA: Yes; Canada: No   **Available as Generic:** No   **Class:** Antihistamines   **Controlled Drug:** USA: No; Canada: No
Brand Name: Hismanal

BENEFITS versus RISKS	
Possible Benefits	*Possible Risks*
EFFECTIVE, LONG-LASTING RELIEF OF ALLERGIC RHINITIS AND ALLERGIC SKIN DISORDERS MINIMAL DROWSINESS MINOR ANTICHOLINERGIC SIDE EFFECTS	RARE HEART RHYTHM DISTURBANCES Mild fatigue (infrequent)

▷ **Principal Uses**

As a Single Drug Product: Uses currently included in FDA approved labeling: (1) Provides symptomatic relief in allergic and related disorders: seasonal and perennial allergic rhinitis (hay fever), allergic conjunctivitis and vasomotor rhinitis; and hives or localized allergic swellings (angioedema); (2) helps relieve vertigo; (3) of use in chronic urticaria.

Other (unlabeled) generally accepted uses: (1) May have a role in relieving Lichen nitidus lesions; (2) may help ease some of the symptoms of asthma; (3) can help control chronic vertigo.

How This Drug Works: Antihistamines block the action of histamine, and the development of swelling and itch in the eyes, nose and skin.

Available Dosage Forms and Strengths
  Suspension — 2 mg per ml (Canada)
  Tablets — 10 mg

▷ **Usual Adult Dosage Range:** 10 mg once daily. The total daily dosage **MUST NOT** exceed 10 mg. Serious heart problems and death may result. **Note: Actual dosage and administration schedule must be determined by the physician for each patient individually.**

Conditions Requiring Dosing Adjustments
  Liver function: This drug should be used with caution in hepatic disease.
  Kidney function: Routine adjustment in kidney problems is not expected to be needed.

▷ **Dosing Instructions:** Take on an empty stomach, 1 hour before eating or 2 hours after eating. The tablet may be crushed for administration.

Usual Duration of Use: Regular use for 3 days is usually needed to see this drug's effectiveness in helping symptoms of allergic rhinitis and dermatosis. Some people may need to take this drug during the entire pollen season. However, antihistamines should not be taken continually (without interruption). Limit use to relieve symptoms. Talk with your doctor regularly.

Possible Advantages of This Drug
  Effective relief with once-a-day dosage.
  No loss of effectiveness with continual use.
  Minimal drowsiness or decreased alertness characteristic of many other antihistamines.
  No or very slight atropinelike (anticholinergic) effects.

▷ **This Drug Should Not Be Taken If**
  • you have had an allergic reaction to any form of it.
  • you are currently undergoing allergy skin tests.
  • you take: erythromycin, azithromycin, clarithromycin, itraconazole, fluconazole, fluvoxamine or ketoconazole.

▷ **Inform Your Physician Before Taking This Drug If**
  • you have had allergic reactions to antihistamines.
  • you have a history of heart rhythm disorders.
  • you have impaired liver or kidney function.
  • you take other prescription or nonprescription medications which were not discussed when astemizole was prescribed for you.
  • you are unsure of how much astemizole to take or how often to take it.

Possible Side Effects (natural, expected, and unavoidable drug actions)
  Dry nose, mouth, or throat.

▷ **Possible Adverse Effects** (unusual, unexpected, and infrequent reactions)
  If any of the following develop, consult your physician promptly for guidance.
  Mild Adverse Effects
  Allergic Reactions: Skin rash, itching.
  Headache, nervousness, fatigue.
  Increased appetite and weight, dry mouth, indigestion, nausea, diarrhea.
  Rare muscle aches.

Serious Adverse Effects
    Significant heart rhythm disorders (from excess dose or drug interactions).
    Rare paresthesias.
    Rare convulsions.
    Rare bronchospasm.

▷ **Possible Effects on Sexual Function**
    None reported.

Possible Effects on Laboratory Tests
    None reported.

CAUTION
    1. **NEVER** take more than prescribed; excess levels may cause serious heart rhythm disturbances.
    2. Do not take this drug with any form of erythromycin, azithromycin, clarithromycin, itraconazole, fluconazole, ketoconazole or sotolol.
    3. Report faintness, dizziness, heart palpitation or chest pain promptly.
    4. Stop this drug 4 days before diagnostic skin test. This drug can hide true allergy to the substances being skin tested (false negative).
    5. Do not use this drug if you have active bronchitis or pneumonia. It can thicken mucus, making it more difficult to remove.

Precautions for Use
    By Infants and Children: Safety and effectiveness for those under 12 years of age not established.
    By Those over 60 Years of Age: Increased risk of headache or fatigue. Use smaller doses at longer intervals.

▷ **Advisability of Use During Pregnancy**
    Pregnancy Category: C. See Pregnancy Code at the back of this book.
    Animal studies: No birth defects due to this drug reported.
    Human studies: Adequate studies of pregnant women are not available.
    Use this drug only if clearly needed. Ask your physician for guidance.

Advisability of Use if Breast-Feeding
    Presence of this drug in breast milk: Unknown.
    Avoid drug or refrain from nursing.

Habit-Forming Potential: None.

Effects of Overdosage: Serious heart rhythm abnormalities leading to death.

Possible Effects of Long-Term Use: None reported.

Suggested Periodic Examinations While Taking This Drug (at physician's discretion)
    Electrocardiograms for those with heart disorders.

▷ **While Taking This Drug, Observe the Following**
    Foods: No restrictions.
    Beverages: No restrictions. May be taken with milk.
▷   *Alcohol:* No interactions expected.
    Tobacco Smoking: No interactions expected.
▷   *Other Drugs:* Astemizole **taken concurrently** with the following drugs may cause increased blood levels of astemizole and resulting heart rhythm disturbances
        • azithromycin (Zithromax)

- clarithromycin (Biaxin)
- erythromycin
- fluconazole (Diflucan)
- fluvoxamine (Luvox)
- itraconazole (Sporonox)
- ketoconazole
- quinine (doses of 430 mg or higher)
- sotolol can cause heart arrhythmias by prolonging the QTC interval additively with astemizole.
- troleandomycin

Hazardous Activities: While this drug has minimal side effects compared to other antihistamines, use caution when first starting this medicine until you are certain of the effect the medicine has on you.

Aviation Note: The use of this drug **is probably not a disqualification** for piloting. Consult a designated Aviation Medical Examiner.

Exposure to Sun: Rare cases of photosensitivity have been reported (see Glossary).

ATENOLOL (a TEN oh lohl)

Introduced: 1973   **Prescription:** USA: Yes; Canada: Yes   **Available as Generic:** Yes   **Class:** Antianginal, antihypertensive, beta-adrenergic blocker
Controlled Drug: USA: No; Canada: No

Brand Names: ✦Apo-Atenolol, ✦Novo-Atenolol, ✦Nu-Atenolol, Tenoretic [CD], Tenormin

BENEFITS versus RISKS	
Possible Benefits	*Possible Risks*
EFFECTIVE ANTIANGINAL DRUG in the management of effort-induced angina EFFECTIVE, WELL-TOLERATED ANTIHYPERTENSIVE in mild to moderate high blood pressure	CONGESTIVE HEART FAILURE in advanced heart disease Worsening of angina in coronary heart disease (abrupt withdrawal) Masking of low blood sugar (hypoglycemia) in drug-treated diabetes Provocation of bronchial asthma (with high doses)

▷ **Principal Uses**

As a Single Drug Product: Uses currently included in FDA approved labeling: (1) Treats classical, effort-induced angina pectoris; (2) mild to moderately severe high blood pressure. May be used alone or in combination with other antihypertensive drugs, such as diuretics; (3) used following heart attacks to **help decrease risk of a second heart attack**, decrease the size of the heart attack and reduce risk of abnormal heart beats.

Other (unlabeled) generally accepted uses: (1) Can help people with stage fright; (2) may have a role in preventing migraine headaches; (3) can have an adjunctive role in alcohol withdrawal.

As a Combination Drug Product [CD]:

Used in combination with a thiazide diuretic to combine the benefits of a beta blocker with the excess fluid losing properties of a thiazide. This attacks high blood pressure using two different mechanisms.

How This Drug Works: By blocking certain actions of the sympathetic nervous system, this drug

- reduces the rate and contraction force of the heart, reducing the oxygen requirement for the heart as it works.
- reduces blood vessel wall contraction, resulting in their relaxation and expansion and consequent lowering of blood pressure.

Available Dosage Forms and Strengths

Tablets — 25 mg, 50 mg, 100 mg

▷ **Usual Adult Dosage Range:**   Initially 50 mg once daily. Dose may be increased gradually at intervals of 7 to 10 days as needed and tolerated up to 100 mg/24 hours. The usual maintenance dose is 50 to 100 mg/24 hours. The total dose should not exceed 100 mg/24 hours. After a heart attack (post MI): Within 12 hours after the attack, 5 mg of this drug is given intravenously. This is followed by a second 5 mg intravenous dose 10 minutes later. Twelve hours after the second intravenous dose, 50 mg is given orally, followed by a second 50 mg 12 hours later. Oral dosing is continued at 100 mg orally for the next 10 days. **Note: Actual dosage and administration schedule must be determined by the physician for each patient individually.**

Conditions Requiring Dosing Adjustments

Liver function: No decreases needed as the liver has a small role in eliminating atenolol.

Kidney function: The dose must be decreased with 25 mg a day as a maximum dose in some people.

▷ **Dosing Instructions:**   May be taken without regard to eating. Tablet may be crushed to take it. **DO NOT** stop this drug abruptly.

Usual Duration of Use: Use on a regular schedule for 3 to 7 days is usually needed to see this drug's effectiveness in lowering blood pressure. Long-term use of this drug will be decided by how much your blood pressure decreases over time in response to an overall treatment program (weight reduction, salt restriction, smoking cessation, etc.). See your physician on a regular basis.

Possible Advantages of This Drug: Least likely of all beta blocker drugs to cause central nervous system adverse effects: confusion, hallucinations, nervousness, nightmares.

▷ **This Drug Should Not Be Taken If**

- you have had an allergic reaction to it previously.
- you have congestive heart failure.
- you have an abnormally slow heart rate or a serious form of heart block.
- you are taking, or have taken within the past 14 days, any monoamine oxidase (MAO) type A inhibitor drug (see Drug Class, Section Four).
- you are in cardiogenic shock.

▷ **Inform Your Physician Before Taking This Drug If**
  • you have had an adverse reaction to any beta blocker drug (see Drug Class, Section Four).
  • you have a history of serious heart disease, with or without episodes of heart failure.
  • you have a history of hay fever (allergic rhinitis), asthma, chronic bronchitis, COPD or emphysema.
  • you have been taking clonidine.
  • you have a history of overactive thyroid function (hyperthyroidism).
  • you have a history of low blood sugar (hypoglycemia)—this drug may hide some of the symptoms occurring with hypoglycemia.
  • you have impaired liver or kidney function.
  • you have diabetes or myasthenia gravis.
  • you currently take any form of digitalis, quinidine or reserpine, or any calcium blocker drug (see Drug Class, Section Four).
  • you plan to have surgery under general anesthesia in the near future.
  • you take other prescription or nonprescription medications which were not discussed when atenolol was prescribed for you.
  • you are unsure of how much atenolol to take or how often to take it.

Possible Side Effects (natural, expected, and unavoidable drug actions)
  Lethargy, fatigability, cold extremities, slow heart rate, light-headedness in upright position (see Orthostatic Hypotension in Glossary).

▷ **Possible Adverse Effects** (unusual, unexpected, and infrequent reactions)
  If any of the following develop, consult your physician promptly for guidance.
  Mild Adverse Effects
  Allergic Reactions: Skin rash, itching.
  Headache, dizziness, drowsiness, abnormal dreams.
  Indigestion, nausea, diarrhea.
  Joint and muscle discomfort, fluid retention (edema).
  Serious Adverse Effects
  Mental depression, anxiety.
  Chest pain, shortness of breath, can lead to congestive heart failure.
  Induction of bronchial asthma (in asthmatic individuals).
  Angina or rebound hypertension (if abruptly stopped).
  Difficulty walking (intermittent claudication) (controversial).
  Psychosis (very rare).
  Systemic lupus erythematosus (rare).

▷ **Possible Effects on Sexual Function:**   Decreased libido and impaired potency (50 to 100 mg/day). This drug is less likely to cause reduced erectile capacity than most drugs of its class.

Possible Effects on Laboratory Tests
  Blood cholesterol levels: no effect with doses of 50 mg/day; increased with doses of 100 mg/day.
  Blood HDL cholesterol levels: no effect with doses of 50 mg/day; decreased with doses of 100 mg/day.
  Blood LDL cholesterol levels: no effect with doses of 50 mg/day; increased with doses of 100 mg/day.

Blood VLDL cholesterol levels: no effect with doses of 50 mg/day; increased with doses of 100 mg/day.

Blood triglyceride levels: no effect with doses of 50 mg/day; increased with doses of 100 mg/day.

CAUTION

1. **DO NOT stop this drug suddenly** without the knowledge and guidance of your physician. Always carry a note that says you take this drug.
2. Consult your physician or pharmacist before using nasal decongestants. These can cause sudden increases in blood pressure when combined with beta blocker drugs.
3. Report the development of any tendency to emotional depression.

Precautions for Use

By Infants and Children: Safety and effectiveness by those under 12 years of age not established. However, if this drug is used, watch for development of low blood sugar (hypoglycemia) especially if meals are skipped.

By Those over 60 Years of Age: Proceed **cautiously** with all antihypertensive drugs. High blood pressure should be reduced slowly, avoiding excessively low blood pressure. Small doses, and frequent blood pressure checks are needed. Sudden and excessive decrease in blood pressure can predispose to stroke or heart attack. Maximum daily dosage is 100 mg. Watch for dizziness, unsteadiness, tendency to fall, confusion, hallucinations, depression or urinary frequency.

▷ **Advisability of Use During Pregnancy**

Pregnancy Category: D. See Pregnancy Code at the back of this book.

Animal studies: Increased resorptions of embryo and fetus reported in rats, but no birth defects.

Human studies: Adequate studies of pregnant women are not available, but the drug has caused fetal harm.

This drug has been used during the last three months of pregnancy, however fetal growth may be slowed and the child may be born with low blood pressure and temperature. Ask your doctor for guidance.

Advisability of Use if Breast-Feeding

Presence of this drug in breast milk: Yes.

Avoid drug if possible. If drug is necessary, observe nursing infant for slow heart rate and indications of low blood sugar.

Habit-Forming Potential: None.

Effects of Overdosage: Weakness, slow pulse, low blood pressure, fainting, cold and sweaty skin, congestive heart failure, possible coma and convulsions.

Possible Effects of Long-Term Use: Reduced heart reserve and eventual heart failure in some people with advanced heart disease.

Suggested Periodic Examinations While Taking This Drug (at physician's discretion)

Measurements of blood pressure, evaluation of heart function.

▷ **While Taking This Drug, Observe the Following**

Foods: Can decrease total atenolol absorption by 20%. It is also best to avoid excessive salt intake.

Beverages: No restrictions. May be taken with milk.

▷ *Alcohol:* Use caution. Alcohol may exaggerate this drug's ability to lower blood pressure and may increase its mild sedative effect.

Tobacco Smoking: Nicotine may reduce this drug's effectiveness in treating high blood pressure. High doses may worsen bronchial tightening caused by regular smoking.

▷ *Other Drugs*

Atenolol may *increase* the effects of

- other antihypertensive drugs and cause excessive lowering of blood pressure. Dosage adjustments may be necessary.
- reserpine (Ser-Ap-Es, etc.) and cause sedation, depression, slowing of heart rate and lowering of blood pressure.

Atenolol *taken concurrently* with

- amiodarone (Codarone) may result in cardiac arrest.
- ampicillin may result in greater exercise induced tachycardia.
- calcium carbonate may result in large decreases in atenolol blood levels.
- clonidine (Catapres) requires close monitoring for rebound high blood pressure if clonidine is stopped while atenolol is still being taken.
- insulin requires close monitoring to avoid undetected hypoglycemia (see Glossary).
- oral hypoglycemics (see Drug Classes) may result in prolonged low blood sugar.
- phenothiazines (see Drug Classes) may increase the effects of both agents and result in phenothiazine toxicity or excessively low blood pressure.
- quinidine (Quinaglute) may cause additive lowering of the blood pressure.
- verapamil can result in undesirable slowing of the heart rate and excessively low blood pressure.

The following drugs may *decrease* the effects of atenolol

- indomethacin (Indocin), and possibly other "aspirin substitutes," or NSAIDs may impair atenolol's antihypertensive effect.

▷ *Driving, Hazardous Activities:* Use caution until the full extent of drowsiness, lethargy, and blood pressure change has been determined.

Aviation Note: The use of this drug *is a disqualification* for piloting. Consult a designated Aviation Medical Examiner.

Exposure to Sun: No restrictions.

Exposure to Heat: Caution advised. Hot environments can lower blood pressure and exaggerate the effects of this drug.

Exposure to Cold: Caution advised. Can enhance the circulatory deficiency that may occur with this drug. Elderly should be careful to prevent hypothermia (see Glossary).

Heavy Exercise or Exertion: Avoid exertion that causes light-headedness, excessive fatigue, or muscle cramping. This drug may worsen the blood pressure response to isometric exercise.

Occurrence of Unrelated Illness: Fever can lower blood pressure and require decreased dose. Nausea or vomiting may interrupt the dosing schedule. Ask your physician for help.

Discontinuation: Avoid stopping this drug suddenly. If possible, gradual reduction of dose over a period of 2 to 3 weeks is recommended. Ask your physician for help.

AURANOFIN (aw RAY noh fin)

Introduced: 1976   **Prescription:** USA: Yes; Canada: Yes   **Available as Generic:** No   **Class:** Antiarthritic   **Controlled Drug:** USA: No; Canada: No

Brand Name: Ridaura

BENEFITS versus RISKS	
Possible Benefits	*Possible Risks*
REDUCTION OF JOINT PAIN, TENDERNESS, AND SWELLING in active, severe RHEUMATOID ARTHRITIS	SIGNIFICANTLY REDUCED LEVELS OF RED AND WHITE BLOOD CELLS AND BLOOD PLATELETS (rare)
Medication effective when taken by mouth	LIVER DAMAGE WITH JAUNDICE (rare)
	Diarrhea
	Ulcerative colitis (rare)
	Skin rash
	Mouth sores
	Kidney toxicity (protein in the urine)
	Lung damage (rare)

▷ **Principal Uses**

As a Single Drug Product: Uses currently included in FDA approved labeling: Used *only* for severe rheumatoid arthritis in adults who have had an inadequate response to aspirin, aspirin substitutes or other antiarthritic drugs and treatment programs. Usually added to a well-established program of antiarthritic drugs of the aspirin-substitute (NSAID) class.

Other (unlabeled) generally accepted uses: (1) May have a role in helping decrease the need for steroid use in people with asthma; (2) can ease the symptoms of nodular vasculitis.

How This Drug Works: Unknown. It suppresses but does not cure arthritis and associated synovitis. It has an effect on specific cells (macrophages) and stops them from engulfing cell debris and also inhibits lysosomes.

Available Dosage Forms and Strengths

Capsules — 3 mg

▷ **Usual Adult Dosage Range:** 6 mg daily, taken either as one dose every 24 hours or as two doses of 3 mg each every 12 hours. If response is inadequate after 6 months of regular continual use does not produce an adequate response, the dose may be increased to 9 mg daily, taken as 3 doses of 3 mg each. If response remains inadequate after 3 months of 9 mg daily, this drug should be stopped. **Note: Actual dosage and administration schedule must be determined by the physician for each patient individually.**

Conditions Requiring Dosing Adjustments

Liver function: The liver is not involved in auranofin elimination. No dose decreases needed.

Kidney function: Blood levels are recommended, and decreased doses may be needed.

▷ **Dosing Instructions:** Take with or following food to reduce stomach irritation. Take the capsule whole with milk or a full glass of water.

Usual Duration of Use: Use on a regular schedule for 3 to 4 months is usually needed to see this drug's effectiveness in reducing joint pain, tenderness and swelling associated with rheumatoid arthritis. Long-term use will depend on how much benefit or the pattern of adverse effects experienced. Consult your physician on a regular basis.

▷ **This Drug Should Not Be Taken If**
  • you have had an allergic reaction from previous use of gold.
  • you have active ulcerative colitis.
  • you have a current blood cell or bone marrow disorder.
  • you have active liver or kidney disease.
  • you are pregnant or breast-feeding.
  • you have exfoliative dermatitis (ask your doctor).
  • you are taking penicillamine or antimalarial drugs for arthritis.
  • you have fibrous replacement of lung tissue (pulmonary fibrosis).

▷ **Inform Your Physician Before Taking This Drug If**
  • you have a history of allergic reactions to drugs.
  • you have diabetes.
  • you have a history of heart disease, high blood pressure, circulatory disorders, liver or kidney disease, or ulcerative colitis.
  • you are taking any other drugs at this time.
  • you are planning pregnancy in the near future.
  • you take other prescription or nonprescription medications which were not discussed when auranofin was prescribed for you.
  • you are unsure of how much auranofin to take or how often to take it.

Possible Side Effects (natural, expected, and unavoidable drug actions)
  Metallic taste.

▷ **Possible Adverse Effects** (unusual, unexpected, and infrequent reactions)
  If any of the following develop, consult your physician promptly for guidance.
  Mild Adverse Effects
  Allergic Reactions: Itching, skin rash.
  Sores in mouth (stomatitis) and throat and on tongue (glossitis), loss of appetite, nausea, vomiting, stomach cramps, diarrhea.
  Taste problems.
  Headache, partial or complete hair loss.
  Conjunctivitis.
  Serious Adverse Effects
  Allergic Reactions: Severe skin reactions, exfoliative dermatitis, pancreatitis.
  Fever, cough, shortness of breath, drug-induced pneumonia and lung damage.
  Liver damage with jaundice, ulcerative colitis.
  Kidney damage (nephrotoxicity).
  Blood cell and bone marrow toxicity—fatigue, weakness, sore throat, abnormal bleeding or bruising.
  Rare peripheral neuritis—pain, numbness, weakness of arms and legs.
  Pancreatitis (rare).

▷ **Possible Effects on Sexual Function:** Breast tenderness and swelling of male breast tissue (gynecomastia).

Possible Delayed Adverse Effects: Adverse effects may occur many months after treatment is stopped. This is due to accumulation of gold in body tissues and its slow elimination. Report any signs of toxicity to your physician promptly.

▷ **Adverse Effects That May Mimic Natural Diseases or Disorders**

Fever, cough and chest discomfort may suggest respiratory tract infections such as bronchitis or pneumonia.

Liver damage may suggest viral hepatitis.

Possible Effects on Laboratory Tests

Complete blood counts: decreased red cells, hemoglobin and white cells; increased eosinophils and platelets; these occur in about 13% of users.

CAUTION

1. Periodic examinations (blood and urine tests) are mandatory. Keep all appointments as directed by your physician.
2. Promptly tell your doctor if any signs of toxic reactions occur. If there is a delay in reaching your doctor, stop this drug until you obtain medical guidance.

Precautions for Use

By Infants and Children: Safety and effectiveness for those under 12 years of age not established.

By Those over 60 Years of Age: Use small doses initially and watch closely for indications of adverse effects.

▷ **Advisability of Use During Pregnancy**

Pregnancy Category: C. See Pregnancy Code at the back of this book.

Animal studies: Rabbit studies revealed an increase in resorptions, abortions and birth defects.

Human studies: Adequate studies of pregnant women are not available.

The manufacturer does not recommend the use of this drug during pregnancy.

Advisability of Use if Breast-Feeding

Presence of this drug in breast milk: Yes.

Avoid drug or refrain from nursing.

Habit-Forming Potential: None.

Effects of Overdosage: Nausea, vomiting, diarrhea, confusion, low blood platelets, kidney dysfunction, delirium, peripheral neuritis, lung damage, encephalopathy, necrosis of the liver.

Suggested Periodic Examinations While Taking This Drug (at physician's discretion)

Complete blood cell counts, urine analyses, liver and kidney function tests.

▷ **While Taking This Drug, Observe the Following**

Foods: No restrictions.

Beverages: No restrictions. May be taken with milk.

▷ *Alcohol:* Use caution. Alcohol may intensify the irritant effect of this drug on the stomach and intestines (gastrointestinal tract).

Tobacco Smoking: No interactions expected.

▷ *Other Drugs*
Auranofin may ***increase*** the effects of
- phenytoin (Dilantin), by increasing its blood level. Watch for indications of phenytoin toxicity.

Auranofin ***taken concurrently*** with
- Penicillamine may result in increased bone marrow depression.

▷ *Driving, Hazardous Activities:* Usually no restrictions.
Aviation Note: The use of this drug ***may be a disqualification*** for piloting. Consult a designated Aviation Medical Examiner.
Exposure to Sun: This drug may cause photosensitivity (see Glossary). Avoid sun and sun lamps.

AZATHIOPRINE (ay za THI oh preen)

Introduced: 1965   **Prescription:** USA: Yes; Canada: Yes   **Available as**
Generic: Yes   **Class:** Antiarthritic, immunosuppressive   **Controlled**
Drug: USA: No; Canada: No
Brand Name: Imuran

BENEFITS versus RISKS

Possible Benefits	*Possible Risks*
REDUCTION OF JOINT PAIN, TENDERNESS, AND SWELLING in active, severe RHEUMATOID ARTHRITIS	UNACCEPTABLE ADVERSE EFFECTS IN 15% OF USERS
PREVENTION OF REJECTION IN ORGAN TRANSPLANTATION	REDUCED LEVELS OF WHITE BLOOD CELLS
	REDUCED LEVELS OF RED BLOOD CELLS AND PLATELETS
	LIVER DAMAGE WITH JAUNDICE (rare)
	POSSIBLE INCREASED RISK OF MALIGNANCY (rare)

▷ **Principal Uses**
As a Single Drug Product: Uses currently included in FDA approved labeling: (1) Used to prevent rejection of transplanted organs (mainly kidney transplants); (2) also used in active, severe rheumatoid arthritis (in adults) that has failed conventional treatment.
Other (unlabeled) generally accepted uses: (1) Used to treat lupus erythematosus, ulcerative colitis, chronic active hepatitis and other "autoimmune" disorders; (2) decreases rejection rates as part of combination therapy in preventing heart transplant failures.

How This Drug Works: It is thought that by impairing purine metabolism, DNA and RNA, and inhibiting cell multiplication, this drug decreases the immune reaction that is responsible for rheumatoid arthritis, lupus erythematosus, etc.

Available Dosage Forms and Strengths
Injection — 100 mg per 20-ml vial
Tablets — 50 mg

▷ **Usual Adult Dosage Range:** As immunosuppressant—3 to 5 mg/kg of body weight daily, 1 to 3 days before transplantation surgery; for postoperative maintenance—1 to 2 mg/kg of body weight daily. In rheumatoid arthritis—1 mg/kg of body weight daily for 6 to 8 weeks; increase dose by 0.5 mg/kg of body weight every 4 weeks as needed and tolerated. Maximal daily dose is 2.5 mg/kg of body weight. Total dose may be taken once daily or divided into 2 equal doses taken 12 hours apart. **Note: Actual dosage and administration schedule must be determined by the physician for each patient individually.**

Conditions requiring dosing adjustments
Liver function: No specific dosing guidelines are available, however, the drug may need to be stopped if jaundice occurs. Liver function must be closely watched.
Kidney function: The dose must be decreased by up to 50% in kidney failure.

▷ **Dosing Instructions:** Take with or following food to reduce stomach upset. Tablet may be crushed.

Usual Duration of Use: Use on a regular schedule for 12 weeks is usually needed to determine this drug's effectiveness in helping rheumatoid arthritis. Successful use for up to 11 years has been reported. See your physician regularly.

▷ **This Drug Should Not Be Taken If**
- you have had an allergic reaction to it previously.
- you are pregnant, and this drug is prescribed to treat rheumatoid arthritis.
- you have an active blood cell or bone marrow disorder.
- you are taking, or have recently taken, any form of chlorambucil (Leukeran), cyclophosphamide (Cytoxan) or melphalan (Alkeran).

▷ **Inform Your Physician Before Taking This Drug If**
- you have any kind of active infection.
- you have any form of cancer.
- you have gout or are taking allopurinol (Zyloprim).
- you have a history of blood cell or bone marrow disorders.
- you have impaired liver or kidney function.
- you are taking a drug in the ACE inhibitor (see Drug Classes) class. Combination use of azathioprine with these medicines has severely lowered white blood cell counts.
- you are taking any form of gold, penicillamine or an antimalarial drug for arthritis.
- you plan pregnancy in the near future.
- you take other prescription or nonprescription medications which were not discussed when azathioprine was prescribed for you.
- you are unsure of how much azathioprine to take or how often to take it.

Possible Side Effects (natural, expected, and unavoidable drug actions)
Development of infection.

▷ **Possible Adverse Effects** (unusual, unexpected, and infrequent reactions)
If any of the following develop, consult your physician promptly for guidance.
Mild Adverse Effects
Allergic Reaction: Skin rash (rare).

Loss of appetite, nausea, vomiting, diarrhea (rare).
Sores on lips and in mouth.
Muscle aches.
Serious Adverse Effects
Allergic Reactions: Drug fever (see Glossary), joint and muscle pain.
Pancreatitis—severe stomach pain with nausea and vomiting (rare).
Bone marrow depression (see Glossary)—fatigue, weakness, fever, sore throat, abnormal bleeding or bruising.
Liver damage—yellow eyes and skin, dark-colored urine, light-colored stools (rare). (See Hepatitis and Jaundice in Glossary.)
Rare liver (hepatic) veno-occlusive disease.
Drug-induced pneumonia—cough, shortness of breath.
Development of cancer—skin cancer, reticulum-cell sarcoma, lymphoma, leukemia.

▷ **Possible Effects on Sexual Function:**   Reversal of male infertility due to sperm antibodies; this drug suppresses autoantibodies and permits the normal accumulation of sperm.

Possible Delayed Adverse Effects: Bone marrow depression may occur many weeks after stopping this drug.

▷ **Adverse Effects That May Mimic Natural Diseases or Disorders**
Liver damage may suggest viral hepatitis.

Possible Effects on Laboratory Tests
Complete blood cell counts: decreased red cells, hemoglobin, white cells and platelets.
Blood amylase and lipase levels: increased—possible pancreatitis.
Blood uric acid levels: increased with rapid tissue destruction; decreased in patients with gout.
Liver function tests: increased liver enzymes (ALT/GPT, AST/GOT and alkaline phosphatase); increased bilirubin.
Sperm counts: decreased.

CAUTION
1. Promptly report any indications of a developing infection—fever, chills, lip or mouth sores, etc.
2. Inform your physician promptly if you become pregnant.
3. Periodic blood counts are mandatory for the safe use of this drug.

Precautions for Use
By Infants and Children: Safety and effectiveness in those under 12 years of age not established.
By Those over 60 Years of Age: The smallest effective dose should be used as this reduces the risk of toxic reactions.

▷ **Advisability of Use During Pregnancy**
Pregnancy Category: D. See Pregnancy Code at the back of this book.
Animal studies: Birth defects reported in rodent studies.
Human studies: This drug exhibits teratogenic effects and also poses a risk of suppression of the immune system of the newborn. Adequate studies of pregnant women are not available.
Avoid completely during entire pregnancy if possible.

Advisability of Use if Breast-Feeding
Presence of this drug in breast milk: Yes.
Avoid drug or refrain from nursing.

Habit-Forming Potential: None.

Effects of Overdosage: Immediate—nausea, vomiting, diarrhea. Delayed—lowered white blood cell and platelet counts, liver and kidney toxicity.

Possible Effects of Long-Term Use: Susceptibility to infection, bone marrow depression, development of malignancies.

Suggested Periodic Examinations While Taking This Drug (at physician's discretion)
Complete blood cell counts, liver function tests.

▷ **While Taking This Drug, Observe the Following**
Foods: No restrictions.
Beverages: No restrictions. May be taken with milk.
▷ *Alcohol:* No interactions expected.
Tobacco Smoking: No interactions expected.
▷ *Other Drugs*
Azathioprine may *decrease* the effects of
• oral anticoagulants (warfarin, etc.), and require increased doses.
• certain muscle relaxants (gallamine, pancuronium, tubocurarine), and make it necessary to increase their dosage.
The following drugs may *increase* the effects of azathioprine
• allopurinol (Zyloprim) may increase its activity and toxicity and make it necessary to reduce its dosage.
Azathioprine *taken concurrently* with
• ACE inhibitors (see Drug Classes) such as captopril or enalapril may cause severe white blood cell count lowering or anemia.
• cotrimoxazole (Bactrim, others) can cause severe lowering of white blood cell counts.
• prednisolone will result in lower prednisolone blood levels and risk of decreased therapeutic benefit.
• warfarin (Coumadin) may result in decreased anticoagulant effectiveness.
▷ *Driving, Hazardous Activities:* No restrictions.
Aviation Note: The use of this drug *may be a disqualification* for piloting. Consult a designated Aviation Medical Examiner.
Exposure to Sun: No restrictions.
Discontinuation: A gradual reduction in dosage is preferable. Consult your physician for a withdrawal schedule.

AZITHROMYCIN (a zith roh MY sin)

Introduced: 1991   **Prescription:** USA: Yes   **Available as Generic:**
USA: No   **Class:** Anti-infective, macrolides   **Controlled Drug:** USA: No
Brand Name: Zithromax

```
┌─────────────────────────────────────────────────────────────────────┐
│                      BENEFITS versus RISKS                            │
│       Possible Benefits              Possible Risks                   │
│   Effective treatment of upper and   Mild gastrointestinal symptoms   │
│     lower respiratory tract infections   Drug-induced colitis (rare)  │
│     due to susceptible microorganisms   Superinfections (rare)        │
│   Effective treatment of skin infections                              │
│     due to susceptible microorganisms                                 │
│   Effective treatment of urethral and                                 │
│     cervical infections due to chlamydia                              │
│     trachomatis                                                       │
└─────────────────────────────────────────────────────────────────────┘
```

▷ **Principal Uses**

As a Single Drug Product: Uses currently included in FDA approved labeling: (1) Treatment of some upper respiratory tract infections—streptococcal pharyngitis and tonsillitis; (2) treatment of certain lower respiratory tract infections—acute bronchitis and pneumonia; (3) treatment of some skin (and skin structure) infections; (4) treatment of nongonococcal urethritis and cervicitis due to chlamydia trachomatis. Cultures and sensitivity testing needed; (5) treatment of AIDS related Mycobacterium avium complex.

Other (unlabeled) generally accepted uses: (1) May have a role in toxoplasmosis AIDS patients.

How This Drug Works: This drug prevents the growth of susceptible organisms by blocking the formation of life-sustaining proteins.

Available Dosage Forms and Strengths

Capsules — 250 mg
Oral suspension — 1 gram of powder

▷ **Recommended Dosage Ranges** (Actual dosage and administration schedule must be determined by the physician for each patient individually.)

Infants and Children: Dosage not established.

16 to 60 Years of Age: For pharyngitis/tonsillitis, bronchitis, pneumonia, and skin infections—500 mg as a single dose on the first day; then 250 mg once daily on days 2 through 4 for a total dose of 1.5 grams.

For nongonococcal urethritis and cervicitis—a single 1 gram (1,000 mg) dose.

Over 60 Years of Age: Same as 16 to 60 years of age. If liver or kidney function is limited, the dose must be reduced.

Conditions Requiring Dosing Adjustments

Liver function: Caution must be used in patients with impaired livers or bile tract disease (50% removal in the bile).

Kidney function: Less than 10% (4.6–6%) of this medicine is removed by the kidneys. No dosing changes in renal (kidney) compromise are expected to be needed.

▷ **Dosing Instructions:**   Do not take with food. Take at least 1 hour before eating or 2 hours after eating. Do not take antacids containing aluminum or magnesium with this drug. The capsule may be opened for administration.

Usual Duration of Use: Use on a regular schedule for 3 to 5 days is usually needed to see this drug's effectiveness in controlling infections. For streptococcal throat infections: the drug must be taken for at least 5 consecutive days (without interruption) to reduce the risk of rheumatic fever or glomerulonephritis.

Possible Advantages of This Drug

Broader spectrum of infectious microorganism coverage; equivalent to erythromycin, some penicillins and some cephalosporins. Effective with only 1 dose daily (easy to remember). Very well tolerated; infrequent and minor adverse effects.

▷ **This Drug Should Not Be Taken If**
- you have had an allergic reaction to it previously.
- you are taking astemizole.

▷ **Inform Your Physician Before Taking This Drug If**
- you are allergic to related drugs: clarithromycin, erythromycin, or troleandomycin.
- you have impaired liver function.
- you have a history of drug-induced colitis.
- you take other prescription or nonprescription medications which were not discussed when azithromycin was prescribed for you.
- you are unsure of how much azithromycin to take or how often to take it.

Possible Side Effects (natural, expected, and unavoidable drug actions)

Superinfections (see Glossary), usually due to yeast.

▷ **Possible Adverse Effects** (unusual, unexpected, and infrequent reactions)

If any of the following develop, consult your physician promptly for guidance.

Mild Adverse Effects

Allergic Reactions: Skin rash (rare).

Headache, dizziness, drowsiness, fatigue (all rare).

Palpitation, chest pain (rare).

Nausea, stomach pain, indigestion, diarrhea.

Serious Adverse Effects

Allergic Reactions: Rare angioedema (swelling of soft tissues).

Rare drug-induced jaundice (see Glossary).

Rare kidney problems (interstitial nephritis).

Rare drug-induced colitis.

Rare hearing loss.

▷ **Possible Effects on Sexual Function:**　None reported.

Possible Effects on Laboratory Tests

Complete blood cell counts: decreased white cells and platelets (1%).

Liver function tests: increased enzymes (ALT/GPT, AST/GOT and alkaline phosphatase); increased bilirubin (all 1–2%).

Kidney function tests: increased blood urea nitrogen (1%).

CAUTION

1. If diarrhea starts and continues for more than 24 hours, call your doctor promptly. This could be drug-induced colitis.
2. Take the full dosage and amount prescribed to prevent bacterial resistance.

Precautions for Use

By Infants and Children: Safety and effectiveness for use by those under 16 years of age have not been established.

By Those over 60 Years of Age: Consider dosage adjustment if liver or kidney function is severely impaired.

▷ **Advisability of Use During Pregnancy**

Pregnancy Category: B. See Pregnancy Code at the back of this book.

Animal studies: No drug-induced birth defects reported.

Human studies: Adequate studies of pregnant women are not available.

Use this drug only if clearly needed. Ask your physician for guidance.

Advisability of Use if Breast-Feeding

Presence of this drug in breast milk: Yes, in small amounts.

Watch nursing infant closely and stop drug or nursing if adverse effects develop.

Habit-Forming Potential: None.

Effects of Overdosage: Possible nausea, vomiting, abdominal discomfort and diarrhea.

Possible Effects of Long-Term Use: Superinfections, drug-induced colitis.

Suggested Periodic Examinations While Taking This Drug (at physician's discretion)

None.

▷ **While Taking This Drug, Observe the Following**

Foods: No restrictions.

Beverages: No restrictions.

▷ *Alcohol:* No interactions expected; however, alcohol can blunt the immune system and its use while having an infection is questionable.

Tobacco Smoking: No interactions expected.

▷ *Other Drugs*

Azithromycin may *increase* the effects of

- carbamazepine (Tegretol) may result in increased levels.
- cyclosporine (Sandimmune) may result in increased cyclosporine levels and toxicity.
- digoxin may result in increased blood levels of digoxin.
- ergotamine or other ergot derivatives. This effect has not been specifically reported for azithromycin (an azolide), but has been reported for other macrolide antibiotics. Increased watchfullness for adverse effects is warranted.
- phenytoin (Dilantin) may result in increased phenytoin levels.
- terfenadine may result in heart (cardiac) toxicity.
- theophylline (Theo-Dur, Theolair, etc.); monitor blood levels of theophylline if appropriate.
- warfarin (Coumadin); monitor INRs more frequently.

The following drugs may *decrease* the effects of azithromycin

- antacids containing aluminum or magnesium.

Azithromycin *taken concurrently* with

- astemizole (and perhaps other nonsedating antihistamines) may lead to severe adverse heart (cardiac) effects.

▷ *Driving, Hazardous Activities:* May cause dizziness, nausea and/or diarrhea. Restrict activities as needed.

Aviation Note: The use of this drug *may be a disqualification* for piloting. Consult a designated Aviation Medical Examiner.

Exposure to Sun: Use caution. This drug can cause photosensitivity (see Glossary).

BACAMPICILLIN (bak am pi SIL in)

Introduced: 1979   **Prescription:** USA: Yes; Canada: Yes   **Available as Generic:** No   **Class:** Antibiotic, penicillins   **Controlled Drug:** USA: No; Canada: No

Brand Names: ✦Penglobe, Spectrobid

BENEFITS versus RISKS	
Possible Benefits	*Possible Risks*
EFFECTIVE TREATMENT OF INFECTIONS due to susceptible microorganisms	ALLERGIC REACTIONS, mild to severe Superinfections (yeast) Drug-induced colitis

▷ **Principal Uses**

As a Single Drug Product: To treat some infections of the skin and skin structures, the upper and lower respiratory tract, and the genitourinary tract, including gonorrhea.

How This Drug Works: When it is absorbed from the gastrointestinal tract, bacampicillin is changed to ampicillin. When given in equivalent doses, bacampicillin provides peak blood levels that are 3 times higher than provided by ampicillin. This lets bacampicillin be effective when given every 12 hours, while ampicillin requires a dosing every 6 hours. (See ampicillin Drug Profile.)

Available Dosage Forms and Strengths

Oral suspension — 125 mg per 5 ml

Tablets — 400 mg and 800 mg (800 mg in Canada only)

▷ **Usual Adult Dosage Range:** 200 to 800 mg/12 hours. **Note: Actual dosage and administration schedule must be determined by the physician for each patient individually.**

Conditions Requiring Dosing Adjustments

Liver function: Caution is advised with use in moderate to severe liver compromise.

Kidney function: The dose must be decreased to 400 mg per day in moderate kidney failure. In severe kidney failure a dose of 400 mg every 36 hours is used.

▷ **Dosing Instructions:** Best taken on an empty stomach, 1 hour before or 2 hours after eating. The tablet may be crushed to take it.

Usual Duration of Use: Use on a regular schedule for 5 to 7 days is usually needed to see the effectiveness in eliminating the infection. Therapy is usually continued for 2 to 3 days after all indications of infection are gone. All streptococcal infections should be treated for at least 10 consecutive days (without interruption) to reduce risk of rheumatic fever or glomerulonephritis.

▷ **While Taking This Drug, Observe the Following**

▷ *Other Drugs*

Bacampicillin *taken concurrently* with

- allopurinol (Zyloprim) substantially increases skin rash occurrence.
- atenolol may result in increased exercise tachycardia.
- birth control pills (oral contraceptives) may result in loss of contraceptive effectiveness and pregnancy.
- disulfiram (Antabuse) can cause a disulfiramlike reaction (see Glossary). Avoid the combination of these 2 drugs.

The following drugs may *decrease* the effects of bacampicillin

- chloramphenicol (Chloromycetin).
- erythromycins (E-Mycin, Erythrocin, etc.).
- sulfonamides ("Sulfa" drugs, see Drug Classes).
- tetracyclines (see Drug Classes).

Note: The information categories provided in this Profile are appropriate for bacampicillin. For specific information that is normally found in those categories that have been omitted from this Profile, see the Drug Profile of ampicillin.

BECLOMETHASONE (be kloh METH a sohn)

Introduced: 1976   **Prescription:** USA: Yes; Canada: Yes   **Available as Controlled**
Generic: No   **Class:** antiasthmatic, cortisonelike drugs
Drug: USA: No; Canada: No

Brand Names: ✦Beclodisk, ✦Becloforte, Beclovent, ✦Beclovent Rotacaps, ✦Beclovent Rotahaler, Beconase AQ Nasal Spray, Beconase Nasal Inhaler, ✦Propaderm, ✦Propaderm-C, Vancenase AQ Nasal Spray, Vancenase Nasal Inhaler, Vanceril

BENEFITS versus RISKS	
Possible Benefits	*Possible Risks*
EFFECTIVE RELIEF OF ALLERGIC RHINITIS	FUNGUS INFECTIONS OF THE MOUTH AND THROAT
EFFECTIVE CONTROL OF SEVERE, CHRONIC ASTHMA	Localized areas of "allergic" pneumonia
	Changes in nasal mucosa

▷ **Principal Uses**

As a Single Drug Product: Uses currently included in FDA approved labeling: (1) Treats bronchial asthma in people who do not respond to bronchodilators and who need cortisonelike drugs for asthma control. This inhalation dosage form is much more advantageous than cortisone taken by mouth (swallowed) or by injection in that it works directly on the respiratory tract and does not require absorption and systemic distribution. This prevents the more serious adverse effects of long-term systemic cortisone use; (2) prevention of nasal polyps once they have been surgically removed; (3)

treats seasonal and perennial rhinitis in children and adults (Vancenase AQ nasal form).

Other (unlabeled) generally accepted uses: (1) Has a role in lung disease (bronchopulmonary dysplasia) in helping decrease the required daily dose of prednisone.

How This Drug Works: By increasing the amount of cyclic AMP, this drug may increase epinephrine, which opens the bronchial tubes and fights asthma. The drug can also reduce local inflammation in the lining of the respiratory tract.

Available Dosage Forms and Strengths
Nasal inhaler — 16.8 grams (200 doses of 42 mcg each)
Nasal spray — 0.042%
Oral inhaler — 16.8 grams (200 doses of 42 mcg each)

▷ **Usual Adult Dosage Range:**   Nasal inhaler—1 inhalation (42 mcg) 2 to 4 times daily. Oral inhaler—2 inhalations (84 mcg) 3 or 4 times daily. For severe asthma—12 to 16 inhalations daily. The maximal daily dose should not exceed 20 inhalations.

Children 6–12 years old may receive: Nasal inhaler—1 inhalation (42 mcg) in each nostril 3 times a day. Oral inhalation—maximum is 10 inhalations (420 mcg).

Note: Actual dosage and administration schedule must be determined by the physician for each patient individually.

Conditions Requiring Dosing Adjustments
Liver function: Use with caution in patients with liver compromise.
Kidney function: No adjustments in dosing expected to be needed.

▷ **Dosing Instructions:**   May be used without regard to eating. Rinse the mouth and throat (gargle) with water thoroughly after each inhalation.

Usual Duration of Use: Use on a regular schedule for 1 to 4 weeks is usually needed to see this drug's effectiveness in relieving severe, chronic allergic rhinitis and in controlling severe, chronic asthma. Long-term use must be physician supervised. See your doctor on a regular basis.

▷ **This Drug Should Not Be Taken If**
• you have had an allergic reaction to any of the brand names listed above.
• you are experiencing severe acute asthma or status asthmaticus that requires more intense treatment for prompt relief.
• your asthma can be controlled by other antiasthmatic drugs that are not related to cortisone.
• your asthma requires cortisonelike drugs infrequently for control.
• you have a form of nonallergic bronchitis with asthmatic features.

▷ **Inform Your Physician Before Taking This Drug If**
• you are now taking or have recently taken any cortisone-related drug (including ACTH by injection) for any reason (see Drug Class, Section Four).
• you have a history of tuberculosis of the lungs.
• you have chronic bronchitis or bronchiectasis.
• you think you have an active infection of any kind, especially a respiratory infection.
• you have recently been exposed to chicken pox.
• you are prone to nosebleeds (epistaxis).
• you are unsure of how much or how often to take beclomethasone.

Possible Side Effects (natural, expected, and unavoidable drug actions)
  Fungus infections (thrush) of the mouth and throat.

▷ **Possible Adverse Effects** (unusual, unexpected, and infrequent reactions)
  If any of the following develop, consult your physician promptly for guidance.
  Mild Adverse Effects
  Allergic Reaction: Skin rash (rare).
  Dryness of mouth, hoarseness, sore throat, cough.
  Nosebleeds (epistaxis).
  Serious Adverse Effects
  Allergic Reaction: Localized areas of "allergic" pneumonitis (lung inflammation).
  Bronchospasm, asthmatic wheezing (rare).
  Shrinking of the nasal tissues (nasal atrophy).
  Yeast infections (up to 41%).

▷ **Possible Effects on Sexual Function:**   None reported.

Natural Diseases or Disorders That May Be Activated by This Drug
  Cortisone-related drugs having systemic effects impair immunity and lead to reactivation of "healed" or dormant tuberculosis. People with a history of tuberculosis must be watched closely while using this drug.

Possible Effects on Laboratory Tests
  Blood cortisol levels: decreased.

CAUTION
  1. This drug should not be relied upon for immediate relief of acute asthma.
  2. If you were using cortisone-related drugs for your asthma *before* starting this inhaler, it may be necessary to resume the former cortisone-related drug if you experience injury or infection of any kind, or if you require surgery. Tell your doctor of your prior use of cortisone-related drugs taken either by mouth or by injection.
  3. If severe asthma returns while using this drug, notify your doctor immediately so that supportive treatment with cortisone-related drugs by mouth or injection can be provided as needed.
  4. Carry a personal identification card with a notation (if applicable) that you have used cortisone-related drugs within the past year. During periods of stress it may be necessary to resume cortisone treatment.
  5. Wait 5 to 10 minutes after using a bronchodilator inhaler like epinephrine, isoetharine, or isoproterenol (which should be used first) and inhalation of this drug. This will permit greater penetration of beclomethasone into the bronchial tubes. The delay between inhalations will also reduce the possibility of adverse propellant effects.
  6. This drug does NOT replace systemic steroids.

Precautions for Use
  By Infants and Children: Safety and effectiveness for use of the nasal inhaler by those under 6 years of age have not been established. Safety and effectiveness for use of the oral inhaler by those under 6 years of age have not been established. The maximal daily dose in children 6 to 12 years of age should not exceed 10 inhalations.
  By Those over 60 Years of Age: People with bronchiectasis should be watched closely for the development of lung infections.

▷ **Advisability of Use During Pregnancy**
   Pregnancy Category: C. See Pregnancy Code at the back of this book.
   Animal studies: Mouse, rat and rabbit studies reveal significant birth defects due to this drug.
   Human studies: Adequate studies of pregnant women are not available.
   Avoid drug during the first 3 months. Use infrequently and only as clearly needed during the last 6 months.

Advisability of Use if Breast-Feeding
   Presence of this drug in breast milk: Probably yes.
   Avoid drug or refrain from nursing.

Habit-Forming Potential: With recommended dosage, a state of functional dependence (see Glossary) is not likely to develop. There have been a small number of cases reported where the aerosol was abused for the effects of the fluorocarbon propellants.

Effects of Overdosage: Indications of cortisone excess (due to systemic absorption)—fluid retention, flushing of the face, stomach irritation, nervousness.

Suggested Periodic Examinations While Taking This Drug (at physician's discretion)
   Inspection of nose, mouth and throat for evidence of fungus infection. Inspection of the nose tissues for nasal atrophy. Assessment of adrenal function status in people who have used cortisone-related drugs over an extended period of time prior to using this drug.
   Lung X-ray of people with a prior history of tuberculosis.

▷ **While Taking This Drug, Observe the Following**
   Foods: No specific restrictions beyond those advised by your physician.
   Beverages: No specific restrictions.
▷ *Alcohol:* No interactions expected.
   Tobacco Smoking: No interactions expected. However, smoking can reduce the effectiveness of this drug. Follow your physician's advice.
▷ *Other Drugs*
   The following drugs may *increase* the effects of beclomethasone
   • inhalant bronchodilators—epinephrine, isoetharine, isoproterenol.
   • oral bronchodilators—aminophylline, ephedrine, terbutaline, theophylline, etc.
▷ *Driving, Hazardous Activities:* No restrictions.
   Aviation Note: The use of this drug and the disorder for which this drug is prescribed *may be disqualifications* for piloting. Consult a designated Aviation Medical Examiner.
   Exposure to Sun: No restrictions.
   Occurrence of Unrelated Illness: Acute infections, serious injuries, and surgical procedures can create an urgent need for additional supportive cortisone-related drugs given by mouth and/or injection. Notify your physician immediately in the event of new illness or injury of any kind.
   Discontinuation: If the regular use of this drug has made it possible to reduce or discontinue maintenance doses of cortisonelike drugs by mouth, *do not* stop this drug abruptly. If you must stop this drug, call your doctor. It may be necessary to resume cortisone preparations and to institute other measures for satisfactory management.

Special Storage Instructions

Store at room temperature. Avoid exposure to temperatures above 120 degrees F (49 degrees C). Do not store or use this inhaler near heat or open flame. Protect from light.

BENAZEPRIL (ben AY ze pril)

Introduced: 1985   **Prescription:** USA: Yes   **Available as Generic:**
No   **Class:** Antihypertensive, ACE inhibitor   **Controlled Drug:** USA: No
Brand Name: Lotensin, Lotensin HCT

BENEFITS versus RISKS	
Possible Benefits	*Possible Risks*
EFFECTIVE CONTROL OF MILD TO MODERATE HIGH BLOOD PRESSURE	Headache, dizziness, fatigue, low blood pressure (rare)
	Allergic swelling of face, tongue, throat, vocal cords (rare)
	Rare decreased hemoglobin

▷ **Principal Uses**

As a Single Drug Product: Uses currently included in FDA approved labeling: Treatment of mild to moderate high blood pressure, alone or in combination with a thiazide diuretic.

Other (unlabeled) generally accepted uses: (1) Helps relieve symptoms of congestive heart failure.

As a Combination Drug Product [CD]: Used to treat high blood pressure which has not responded to single agent treatment. The combination product has hydrochlorothiazide, a diuretic.

How This Drug Works: It is thought that by blocking certain enzyme systems (angiotensin-converting enzyme, ACE) that effect arteries, benazepril helps relax arterial walls throughout the body and lowers the blood pressure. This, in turn, reduces the workload of the heart and improves its performance.

Available Dosage Forms and Strengths

Lotensin Tablets — 5 mg, 10 mg, 20 mg, 40 mg

▷ **Recommended Dosage Ranges** (Actual dosage and administration schedule must be determined by the physician for each patient individually.)

Infants and Children: Dosage not established.

12 to 60 Years of Age: Initially 10 mg once daily for those not taking a diuretic; 5 mg once daily for those taking a diuretic. Usual maintenance dose is 20 to 40 mg/day taken in a single dose. If once-a-day dosing does not give stable control of blood pressure over a 24 hour period, divide the dose equally into morning and evening doses. The total daily dosage should not exceed 80 mg.

Over 60 Years of Age: Same as 12 to 60 years of age, if kidney function is normal. If kidney function is significantly impaired, reduce dose by 50%. The total daily dose should not exceed 40 mg.

Conditions Requiring Dosing Adjustments

Liver function: Dosage adjustment in cirrhosis is not currently considered necessary.

Kidney function: Some of this medicine is removed by the kidneys. For people with creatinine clearances of less than 30 ml/min., or serum creatinine concentrations of greater than 3 mg/dl, the initial dose should be 5 mg once daily.

▷ **Dosing Instructions:**   Take on an empty stomach or with food, at same time each day. The tablet may be crushed for administration.

Usual Duration of Use: Use on a regular schedule for 2 to 3 weeks is usually needed to see this drug's peak effect in controlling high blood pressure. Therapy may be long-term. See your physician on a regular basis.

Possible Advantages of This Drug

Usually controls blood pressure effectively with one daily dose.

Relatively low incidence of adverse effects.

No adverse influence on asthma, cholesterol blood levels or diabetes.

Sudden withdrawal does not result in a rapid increase in blood pressure.

▷ **This Drug Should Not Be Taken If**
- you have had an allergic reaction to it previously.
- you are pregnant (last 6 months).
- you currently have a blood cell or bone marrow disorder.
- you have an abnormally high level of blood potassium.

▷ **Inform Your Physician Before Taking This Drug If**
- you have had an allergic reaction to other ACE inhibitor drugs (see Drug Class, Section Four).
- you are planning pregnancy.
- you have a history of kidney disease or impaired kidney function.
- you have scleroderma or systemic lupus erythematosus or other autoimmune disease.
- you have cerebral artery disease.
- you have any form of heart disease.
- you are taking: other antihypertensives, diuretics, nitrates or potassium supplements.
- you plan to have surgery under general anesthesia in the near future.
- you are unsure of how much benazepril to take or how often to take it.
- you have renal artery stenosis (ask your doctor).
- you have liver disease.
- your face or tongue becomes swollen after you started taking this drug.
- you are taking an immunosuppressant drug.
- you think you are dehydrated.

Possible Side Effects (natural, expected, and unavoidable drug actions)

Dizziness, orthostatic hypotension (rare) (see Glossary), fainting (rare), increased blood potassium level (rare).

▷ **Possible Adverse Effects** (unusual, unexpected, and infrequent reactions)

If any of the following develop, consult your physician promptly for guidance.

Mild Adverse Effects

Allergic Reactions: Skin rash, itching (rare).

Headache, fatigue, drowsiness (rare), numbness and tingling (rare), weakness (rare).

Cough (up to 39%), chest pain, palpitation (rare).
Indigestion, nausea (rare), vomiting, constipation (rare).
Back pain (rare).
Serious Adverse Effects
Allergic Reactions: Swelling (angioedema) of face, tongue and/or vocal chords (rare); can be life-threatening.
Impairment of kidney function (rare).
Rare decreased hemoglobin.
Rare decreased white blood cell counts.
Angina and palpitations.
First dose low blood pressure.
Elevated blood potassium.
Psoriasis (rare).

▷ **Possible Effects on Sexual Function:**   Decreased libido, impotence (less than 1%). Rare enlargement and tenderness of male breast tissue.

Possible Effects on Laboratory Tests
Blood potassium level: increased.
Kidney function tests: blood urea nitrogen (BUN) and creatinine increased.
Blood glucose: rare increases.
Uric acid: rare increases.
Blood cholesterol: decreased (7.6–13.1%).

CAUTION
1. Ask your doctor if you should stop other antihypertensive drugs (especially diuretics) for 1 week before starting this drug.
2. **Inform your physician immediately if you become pregnant.** This drug should not be taken beyond the first 3 months of pregnancy.
3. **Report promptly** any signs of infection (fever, sore throat), and any weight gain, puffiness, swollen feet or ankles.
4. Do not use a salt substitute without your physician's knowledge and approval. (Many salt substitutes contain potassium.)
5. It is advisable to obtain blood cell counts and urine analyses **before** starting this drug.

Precautions for Use
By Infants and Children: Safety and effectiveness for use by those in this age group not established.
By Those over 60 Years of Age: Small starting doses are advisable. Sudden or excessive lowering of blood pressure can cause stroke or heart attack in people with impaired brain circulation or coronary artery heart disease.

▷ **Advisability of Use During Pregnancy**
Pregnancy Category: C during the first 3 months of pregnancy. D during the second or third trimester. See Pregnancy Code at the back of this book.
Animal studies: No birth defects found in mouse, rat or rabbit studies.
Human studies: The use of ACE inhibitor drugs during the last 6 months of pregnancy is known to possibly cause very serious injury and possible death to the fetus; skull and limb malformations, lung defects, and kidney failure have been reported in over 50 cases worldwide.
Avoid this drug completely during the last 6 months. During the first 3 months of pregnancy, use this drug only if clearly needed. Ask your physician for guidance.

Advisability of Use if Breast-Feeding
Presence of this drug in breast milk: Yes, in small amounts.
Ask your doctor for guidance.

Habit-Forming Potential: None.

Effects of Overdosage: Excessive drop in blood pressure, light-headedness, dizziness, fainting.

Possible Effects of Long-Term Use: Gradual increase in blood potassium level.

Suggested Periodic Examinations While Taking This Drug (at physician's discretion)
Before starting drug: Complete blood cell counts; urine analysis with measurement of protein content; blood potassium level.
During use of drug: Blood cell counts; measurements of blood potassium.

▷ **While Taking This Drug, Observe the Following**
Foods: Consult physician regarding salt intake. Ask about the benefits of weight loss if you are above your ideal body weight.
Nutritional Support: **Do not take** potassium supplements unless directed by your physician.
Beverages: No restrictions. May be taken with milk.
▷   *Alcohol:* Use caution. Alcohol may enhance the blood-pressure-lowering effect of this drug.
Tobacco Smoking: No interactions expected.
▷   *Other Drugs*
Benazepril **taken concurrently** with
• aspirin may decrease the benefit of benazepril on heart function.
• bumetanide (Bumex) or furosemide (Lasix) may cause severe lowering of blood pressure if patients suddenly stand.
• chlorpromazine (Thorazine) may cause excessive lowering of blood pressure.
• cyclosporine (Sandimune) may cause increased kidney toxicity.
• ketorolac (Toradol) can increase the risk of kidney (renal) toxicity.
• lithium may triple blood levels of lithium and result in lithium toxicity.
• phenothiazines (see Drug Classes) may cause sudden lowering of the blood pressure to undesirable levels.
• potassium preparations (K-Lyte, Slow-K, etc.) may cause increased blood levels of potassium with risk of serious heart rhythm disturbances.
• potassium-sparing diuretics: amiloride (Moduretic), spironolactone (Aldactazide), triamterene (Dyazide) may cause increased blood levels of potassium with risk of serious heart rhythm disturbances.
▷   *Driving, Hazardous Activities:* Be aware of possible drops in blood pressure with resultant dizziness or faintness.
Aviation Note: The use of this drug **may be a disqualification** for piloting. Consult a designated Aviation Medical Examiner.
Exposure to Sun: Caution advised. A similar drug of this class can cause photosensitivity.
Exposure to Heat: Caution advised. Excessive perspiring with resultant loss of body water may drop blood pressure.
Occurrence of Unrelated Illness: Promptly report vomiting or diarrhea. Fluid and chemical imbalances must be corrected as soon as possible.
Discontinuation: Talk to your doctor about withdrawal of this drug for any reason.

BENZTROPINE (BENZ troh peen)

Introduced: 1954   **Prescription:** USA: Yes; Canada: No   **Available as**
Generic: USA: Yes; Canada: Yes   **Class:** Antiparkinsonism, atropinelike
drugs   **Controlled Drug:** USA: No; Canada: No
Brand Names: ✦Apo-Benztropine, ✦Bensylate, Cogentin, ✦PMS Benztropine

---

BENEFITS versus RISKS

Possible Benefits	*Possible Risks*
PARTIAL RELIEF OF SYMPTOMS OF PARKINSON'S DISEASE RELIEF OF DRUG-INDUCED EXTRAPYRAMIDAL REACTIONS	Atropinelike side effects: blurred vision, dry mouth, constipation, impaired urination Toxic psychosis (rare) Tardive dyskinesia (rare)

▷ **Principal Uses**

As a Single Drug Product: Uses currently included in FDA approved labeling: (1) Used in combination with other therapy in of all types of parkinsonism to relieve the characteristic rigidity, tremor and sluggish movement. If relief is inadequate, it may be supplemented with more potent drugs such as levodopa and bromocriptine; (2) also used to control parkinsonian reactions that can result from some antipsychotic drugs, such as phenothiazines and related medicines; (3) used to help parkinsonian symptoms which can occur after encephalitis.

Other (unlabeled) generally accepted uses: (1) Combined with psychotherapy, this drug can help excessively sweaty palms; (2) can help drooling in developmentally disabled patients; (3) can relieve painful erections (priapism).

How This Drug Works: It decreases the symptoms of parkinsonism by restoring a more normal balance of chemicals responsible for nerve impulses in the brain (basal ganglia).

Available Dosage Forms and Strengths

Injection — 1 mg per ml

Tablets — 0.5 mg, 1 mg, 2 mg

▷ **Usual Adult Dosage Range:** For Parkinson's disease—0.5 to 2 mg daily, taken in a single dose at bedtime. For drug-induced parkinsonian reactions—1 to 4 mg daily, either in a single dose or in 2 to 3 divided doses. The total daily dose should not exceed 6 mg. For Parkinson's symptoms which occur after encephalitis: starting doses of 2 mg per day are used. The dose can then be increased as needed or tolerated to 4 to 6 mg per day. **Note: Actual dosage and administration schedule must be determined by the physician for each patient individually.**

Conditions Requiring Dosing Adjustments

Liver function: Use with caution in patients with impaired liver function.

Kidney function: Caution. Decreased kidney function may lead to an increased blood level and an increased risk of adverse effects.

▷ **Dosing Instructions:** May be taken with or following food to reduce stomach irritation. Tablet may be crushed for administration.

Usual Duration of Use: Use on a regular schedule for 2 to 4 weeks is usually necessary to see this drug's peak benefit in relieving symptoms of parkinsonism and to determine the best dosage schedule. Long-term use (months to years) requires physician supervision. See your doctor regularly.

▷ **This Drug Should Not Be Taken If**
- you have had an allergic reaction to any dosage form of it previously.
- it is prescribed for a child under 3 years of age.
- you have tardive dyskinesia.
- you have narrow angle glaucoma.

▷ **Inform Your Physician Before Taking This Drug If**
- you have had an unfavorable reaction to atropine or atropine-like drugs.
- you have glaucoma or myasthenia gravis.
- you have heart disease or high blood pressure.
- you have a history of liver or kidney disease.
- you have difficulty emptying the urinary bladder, especially if due to an enlarged prostate gland.
- you are taking, or have taken within the past 2 weeks, any monoamine oxidase (MAO) type A inhibitor drug (see Drug Class, Section Four).
- you take other prescription or nonprescription medications which were not discussed when benztropine was prescribed for you.
- you are unsure of how much benztropine to take or how often to take it.
- you will be exposed to extreme heat for extended periods such as some iron smelters or travelers to tropical climates.
- you have a history of bowel obstructions.

Possible Side Effects (natural, expected, and unavoidable drug actions)
Nervousness, blurring of vision, dryness of mouth, constipation, impaired urination. (These often subside as drug use continues.)

▷ **Possible Adverse Effects** (unusual, unexpected, and infrequent reactions)
If any of the following develop, consult your physician promptly for guidance.
Mild Adverse Effects
Allergic Reaction: Skin rashes.
Headache, dizziness, drowsiness, muscle cramps.
Indigestion, nausea, vomiting.
Memory problems.
Serious Adverse Effects
Idiosyncratic Reactions: Abnormal behavior, confusion, delusions, hallucinations, agitation.
Tardive dyskinesia (rare).
Dystonia (rare).
Bowel obstruction (rare).
Abnormal elevations of temperature (hyperthermia).

▷ **Possible Effects on Sexual Function**
Reversal of male impotence due to the use of fluphenazine (a phenothiazine antipsychotic drug).
Male infertility (0.5 to 6 mg/day).
May help treat priapism.

Natural Diseases or Disorders That May Be Activated by This Drug
Latent glaucoma, latent myasthenia gravis.

Possible Effects on Laboratory Tests
    None reported.

CAUTION
    1. Many over-the-counter (OTC) medications for allergies, colds and coughs contain drugs that should NOT be combined with benztropine. Ask your physician or pharmacist for help.
    2. This drug may aggravate tardive dyskinesia (see Glossary). Ask physician for guidance.

Precautions for Use
    By Infants and Children: Safety and effectiveness for those under 3 years of age not established. Children are especially susceptible to the atropinelike effects.
    By Those over 60 Years of Age: Small starting doses are advisable. Increased susceptibility to impaired thinking, confusion, nightmares, hallucinations, increased internal eye pressure (glaucoma) and impaired urination associated with prostate gland enlargement (prostatism).

▷ **Advisability of Use During Pregnancy**
    Pregnancy Category: C. See Pregnancy Code at the back of this book.
    Animal studies: No data available.
    Human studies: Adequate studies of pregnant women are not available.
    Avoid use if possible, especially close to delivery. This drug can impair the infant's intestinal tract following birth.

Advisability of Use if Breast-Feeding
    Presence of this drug in breast milk: Unknown.
    Ask your doctor for guidance.

Habit-Forming Potential: None with recommended doses. At higher doses it may cause euphoria and hallucinations, creating a potential for abuse.

Effects of Overdosage: Weakness; drowsiness; stupor; impaired vision; rapid pulse; excitement; confusion; hallucinations; dry, hot skin; skin rash; dilated pupils.

Possible Effects of Long-Term Use: Increased internal eye pressure—possible glaucoma, especially in the elderly.

Suggested Periodic Examinations While Taking This Drug (at physician's discretion)
    Measurement of internal eye pressure at regular intervals.

▷ **While Taking This Drug, Observe the Following**
    Foods: No restrictions.
    Beverages: No restrictions.
▷ *Alcohol:* Use caution. Alcohol may increase the sedative effects of this drug.
    Tobacco Smoking: No interactions expected.
▷ *Other Drugs*
        Benztropine may *decrease* the effects of
        • haloperidol (Haldol), and reduce its effectiveness.
        • phenothiazines (Thorazine, etc.), and reduce their effectiveness.
        The following drugs may *increase* the effects of benztropine
        • antihistamines may add to the dryness of mouth and throat.
        • tricyclic antidepressants (Elavil, etc.) may add to eye effects and further increase internal eye pressure (dangerous in glaucoma).

- monoamine oxidase (MAO) type A inhibitor drugs may intensify all effects of this drug (see Drug Class, Section Four).

Benztropine *taken concurrently* with

- amantadine (Symmetrel) may cause increased confusion and possible hallucinations.
- clozapine (Clozaril) can cause increased risk of elevated temperatures, neurologic adverse effects and bowel obstruction (ileus).

▷ *Driving, Hazardous Activities:* Drowsiness and dizziness may occur in sensitive individuals. Avoid hazardous activities until full effects and tolerance have been determined.

Aviation Note: The use of this drug *is a disqualification* for piloting. Consult a designated Aviation Medical Examiner.

Exposure to Sun: No restrictions.

Exposure to Heat: Use caution. This drug may reduce sweating, cause an increase in body temperature, and increase risk of heat stroke.

Heavy Exercise or Exertion: Use caution. Avoid in hot environments.

Discontinuation: Do not stop this drug abruptly. Ask your doctor how to reduce the dose gradually.

BETAXOLOL (be TAX oh lohl)

Introduced: 1983   **Prescription:** USA: Yes   **Available as Generic:** No   **Class:** Antihypertensive, beta-adrenergic blocker   **Controlled Drug:** USA: No

Brand Names: Betoptic, Betoptic-S, Kerlone

BENEFITS versus RISKS	
Possible Benefits	*Possible Risks*
EFFECTIVE, WELL-TOLERATED ANTIHYPERTENSIVE in mild to moderate high blood pressure	CONGESTIVE HEART FAILURE in advanced heart disease
EFFECTIVE TREATMENT OF CHRONIC, OPEN-ANGLE GLAUCOMA	Worsening of angina in coronary heart disease (abrupt withdrawal)
Treatment of ocular hypertension	Masking of low blood sugar (hypoglycemia) in drug-treated diabetes
	Provocation of bronchial asthma (with high doses)
	Rare anemia and low blood platelets

▷ **Principal Uses**

As a Single Drug Product: Uses currently included in FDA approved labeling: Used to treat: (1) mild to moderate high blood pressure; (2) chronic open-angle glaucoma (eye drops). May be used alone or combined with other antihypertensive drugs, such as diuretics; (3) ocular hypertension.

Other (unlabeled) generally accepted uses: (1) The oral form may help decrease mortality by reducing damage from a heart attack and making abnormal heart beats less likely; (2) helps decrease the occurrence and severity of chest pain (angina); (3) can be of help in easing aggressive behavior in selected psychiatric patients; (4) may help panic attacks; (5) can treat selected cases of stuttering.

How This Drug Works: By blocking certain actions of the sympathetic nervous system, this drug

- reduces the rate and contraction force of the heart, lowering blood ejection pressure and reducing the oxygen needed by the heart to work.
- relaxes contracted blood vessel walls, resulting in expansion and consequent lowering of blood pressure.
- reduces the internal pressure of the eye.

Available Dosage Forms and Strengths

Eye drops — 2.8 mg/ ml
        — 5.6 mg/ ml
Tablets — 10 mg, 20 mg

▷ **Usual Adult Dosage Range:**   Initially 10 mg once daily. Dose may be increased gradually at intervals of 7 to 14 days as needed and tolerated up to 20 mg/24 hours. The usual maintenance dose is 10 to 15 mg/24 hours. The total dose should not exceed 20 mg/24 hours.

For use in glaucoma: One or two drops of the 2.8 mg/ml solution or one drop of the 5.6 mg/ml. **Note: Actual dosage and administration schedule must be determined by the physician for each patient individually.**

Conditions Requiring Dosing Adjustments

Liver function: Use with caution; this drug is metabolized in the liver. Dose decreased are not; however, routinely needed.

Kidney function: Up to 12% of a dose is removed by the kidney. Starting dose is 5 mg in this case, and the dose is only increased as needed and tolerated by 5 mg every two weeks for a maximum of 20 mg daily.

▷ **Dosing Instructions:**   May be taken without regard to eating. The tablet may be crushed for administration. Do not stop this drug abruptly.

Usual Duration of Use: Use on a regular schedule for 10 to 14 days is usually needed to see this drug's effectiveness in lowering blood pressure. Long-term use will be determined by the success in lowering your blood pressure over time and your response to an overall treatment program of weight reduction, salt restriction, smoking cessation, etc. See your doctor regularly.

Possible Advantages of This Drug: Usually effective and well tolerated with a single dose daily.

▷ **This Drug Should Not Be Taken If**
- you have had an allergic reaction to it previously.
- you have congestive heart failure.
- you have an abnormally slow heart rate or a serious heart block.
- you are taking, or have taken within the past 14 days, any monoamine oxidase (MAO) type A inhibitor drug (see Drug Class, Section Four).

▷ **Inform Your Physician Before Taking This Drug If**
- you have had an adverse reaction to any beta blocker drug (see Drug Class, Section Four).
- you have a history of serious heart disease or episodes of heart failure.
- you have a history of hay fever (allergic rhinitis), asthma, chronic bronchi-

tis or emphysema. Some drugs in this class are contraindicated in asthmatics.

- you have a history of overactive thyroid function (hyperthyroidism).
- you have a history of low blood sugar (hypoglycemia).
- you have impaired liver or kidney function.
- you have narrowing of the vessels in your legs or arms (peripheral vascular disease). Discuss this with your doctor.
- you have diabetes or myasthenia gravis.
- you currently take: digitalis, quinidine or reserpine, or any calcium blocker drug (see Drug Class, Section Four).
- you plan to have surgery under general anesthesia in the near future.
- you take other prescription or nonprescription medications which were not discussed when betaxolol was prescribed for you.
- you are unsure of how much betaxolol to take or how often to take it.

Possible Side Effects (natural, expected, and unavoidable drug actions)

Lethargy, fatigue (up to 10%), cold extremities (rare), slow heart rate, lightheadedness in upright position (see Orthostatic Hypotension in Glossary).

▷ **Possible Adverse Effects** (unusual, unexpected, and infrequent reactions)

If any of the following develop, consult your physician promptly for guidance.

Mild Adverse Effects

Allergic Reactions: Skin rash (rare), itching.

Hair loss (rare).

Headache (up to 15%), dizziness, drowsiness, insomnia (rare), abnormal dreams (rare).

Indigestion, nausea (rare), diarrhea (rare).

Joint and muscle discomfort, fluid retention (edema) (rare).

Difficulty breathing (rare).

Serious Adverse Effects

Mental depression (rare), anxiety (rare).

Increased blood sugar (hyperglycemia) in non-insulin-dependent diabetics.

Chest pain, shortness of breath, congestive heart failure.

Induction of bronchial asthma (in asthmatic individuals).

Low blood platelets and anemia (rare).

Congestive heart failure (rare).

Difficulty breathing.

Angina (if drug abruptly stopped).

Intermittent problems walking (intermittent claudication) (rare).

Very rare myocardial infarction.

▷ **Possible Effects on Sexual Function:**   Decreased libido, impotence (1.2%).

Altered menstrual patterns.

▷ **Adverse Effects That May Mimic Natural Diseases or Disorders**

Reduced blood flow to extremities may mimic Raynaud's disease (see Glossary).

Possible Effects on Laboratory Tests

Glaucoma-screening test (measurement of internal eye pressure): pressure is decreased (false low or normal value).

Antinuclear antibodies (ANA) test: positive in 5.3% of users.

Blood potassium: slightly increased.

Blood platelet counts and hemoglobin: decreased (rarely).

Blood glucose: increased in non-insulin dependent diabetics.

CAUTION
1. ***Do not stop this drug suddenly*** without the knowledge of your doctor. Always carry a note with you that says you are taking this drug.
2. Ask your physician or pharmacist before using nasal decongestants. These can cause sudden increases in blood pressure when combined with beta blocker drugs.
3. Report the development of any tendency to emotional depression.

Precautions for Use

By Infants and Children: Safety and effectiveness for those under 12 years of age not established. However, if this drug is used, watch for the development of low blood sugar (hypoglycemia), especially if a meal is missed.

By Those over 60 Years of Age: **Caution**. High blood pressure should be slowly reduced, avoiding risks associated with excessively low blood pressure. Treatment should be started with 5 mg daily and blood pressure checked often. Sudden, rapid and excessive reduction of blood pressure can cause stroke or heart attack. Total daily dosage should not exceed 10 to 15 mg. Watch for dizziness, unsteadiness, tendency to fall, confusion, hallucinations, depression or urinary frequency. This age group is more prone to develop excessively slow heart rates and hypothermia.

▷ **Advisability of Use During Pregnancy**

Pregnancy Category: C. See Pregnancy Code at the back of this book.

Animal studies: Rat studies reveal increased resorptions of embryo and fetus, retarded growth and development of newborn and mild skeletal defects.

Human studies: Adequate studies of pregnant women are not available.

Avoid use of drug during the first 3 months if possible. Avoid use during labor and delivery because of the possible effects on the newborn infant.

Advisability of Use if Breast-Feeding

Presence of this drug in breast milk: Yes.

Avoid drug if possible. If drug is necessary, observe nursing infant for slow heart rate and indications of low blood sugar.

Habit-Forming Potential: None.

Effects of Overdosage: Weakness, slow pulse, low blood pressure, fainting, cold and sweaty skin, congestive heart failure, possible coma and convulsions.

Possible Effects of Long-Term Use: Reduced heart reserve and eventual heart failure in susceptible individuals with advanced heart disease.

Suggested Periodic Examinations While Taking This Drug (at physician's discretion)

Measurements of blood pressure, evaluation of heart function.

▷ **While Taking This Drug, Observe the Following**

Foods: No restrictions. Avoid excessive salt intake.

Beverages: No restrictions. May be taken with milk.

▷ *Alcohol:* Use with caution. Alcohol may exaggerate this drug's ability to lower blood pressure and may increase its mild sedative effect.

Tobacco Smoking: Nicotine may reduce this drug's effectiveness in treating high blood pressure. In addition, high drug doses worsen the constriction of bronchial tubes caused by regular smoking.

▷ *Other Drugs*

Betaxolol may ***increase*** the effects of
- other antihypertensive drugs and cause excessive lowering of blood pressure. Dosage decreases may be necessary.
- reserpine (Ser-Ap-Es, etc.) and cause sedation, depression, slowing of heart rate and lowering of blood pressure (light-headedness, fainting).
- verapamil and cause additive risk of congestive heart failure and slow heart rate (bradycardia).

Betaxolol ***taken concurrently*** with
- amiodarone (Codarone) may result in extremely slow heart rate and arrest.
- calcium channel blockers may cause severe lowering of blood pressure.
- clonidine (Catapres) requires close monitoring for rebound high blood pressure if clonidine is stopped while betaxolol is still taken.
- fluvoxamine (Luvox) may cause excessive slowing of the heart and very low blood pressure.
- insulin requires close following to avoid hypoglycemia (see Glossary).
- oral hypoglycemic drugs (see Drug Classes) may prolong recovery from low blood sugars.
- phenothiazines (see Drug Classes) may result in additive blood pressure lowering effects.

The following drugs may ***decrease*** the effects of betaxolol
- indomethacin (Indocin), and possibly other "aspirin substitutes," or NSAIDs may impair betaxolol's antihypertensive effect.

▷ *Driving, Hazardous Activities:* Use caution until the full extent of drowsiness, lethargy, and blood pressure change has been determined.

Aviation Note: The use of this drug ***is a disqualification*** for piloting. Consult a designated Aviation Medical Examiner.

Exposure to Sun: No restrictions.

Exposure to Heat: Caution advised. Hot environments can lower blood pressure and exaggerate the effects of this drug.

Exposure to Cold: Caution advised. Cold environments can enhance the circulatory deficiency in the extremities that may occur with this drug. The elderly should be careful to prevent hypothermia (see Glossary).

Heavy Exercise or Exertion: It is advisable to avoid exertion that produces light-headedness, excessive fatigue, or muscle cramping. The use of this drug may intensify the hypertensive response to isometric exercise.

Occurrence of Unrelated Illness: Fever can lower blood pressure and require adjustment of dosage. Nausea or vomiting may interrupt the dosing schedule. Ask your physician for help.

Discontinuation: Avoid sudden discontinuation of this drug in all situations. If possible, gradual reduction of dose over a period of 2 to 3 weeks is recommended. Ask your physician for specific guidance.

BITOLTEROL (bi TOHL ter ohl)

Introduced: 1985   **Prescription:** Yes   **Available as Generic:** No
Class: Antiasthmatic, bronchodilator   **Controlled Drug:** No
Brand Name: Tornalate

BENEFITS versus RISKS	
Possible Benefits	*Possible Risks*
EFFECTIVE PREVENTION AND RELIEF OF ASTHMA for 5 to 8 hours	Fine hand tremor
Nervousness
Throat irritation
Irregular heart rhythm (with excessive use)

▷ **Principal Uses**

As a Single Drug Product: Uses currently included in FDA approved labeling: (1) To relieve acute bronchial asthma and to reduce the frequency and severity of chronic, recurrent asthmatic attacks; (2) used to help those asthmatics dependent on steroids.

Other (unlabeled) generally accepted uses: (1) May be more useful than other agents in helping open the bronchi in patients with chronic obstructive pulmonary disease (COPD); (2) may have a role in preventing exercise-induced asthma.

How This Drug Works: By increasing cyclic AMP, this drug relaxes bronchial muscles and relieves asthmatic wheezing.

Available Dosage Forms and Strengths

Aerosol inhaler — 15 ml (300 inhalations of 0.37 mg each)

▷ **Usual Adult Dosage Range:** For acute bronchospasm—2 inhalations at intervals of 1 to 3 minutes, followed by a third inhalation in 3 to 4 minutes if needed. For prevention of bronchospasm—2 inhalations/8 hours. Maximum inhalation dose is 2 inhalations every 4 hours. For children over 12: same as adult bronchospasm dose. **Note: Actual dosage and administration schedule must be determined by the physician for each patient individually.**

Conditions Requiring Dosing Adjustments

Liver function: Use with caution in severe liver compromise.
Kidney function: Significant kidney removal; however, specific dosage guidelines are unavailable.

▷ **Dosing Instructions:** May be used without regard to eating. Follow the written directions for use carefully. Do not overuse.

Usual Duration of Use: Do not use beyond the time needed to stop episodes of acute asthma. Ask physician for help regarding use in preventing asthma attacks.

▷ **This Drug Should Not Be Taken If**

- you have had an allergic reaction to it previously.
- you currently have an irregular heart rhythm.
- you are taking, or have taken within the past 2 weeks, any monoamine oxidase (MAO) type A inhibitor drug (see Drug Class, Section Four).

▷ **Inform Your Physician Before Taking This Drug If**
- you have any type of heart or circulatory disorder, especially high blood pressure or coronary heart disease.
- you have diabetes, epilepsy or an overactive thyroid gland.
- you are taking any form of digitalis or any stimulant drug.
- you are unsure of how much bitolterol to take or how often to take it.
- you are pregnant and are nearing the time of delivery of your baby (may complicate labor and delivery).

Possible Side Effects (natural, expected, and unavoidable drug actions)
Dryness or irritation of mouth or throat.

▷ **Possible Adverse Effects** (unusual, unexpected, and infrequent reactions)
If any of the following develop, consult your physician promptly for guidance.
Mild Adverse Effects
Headache, dizziness, nervousness, insomnia (rare), fine tremor of hands (14%).
Nausea, indigestion.
Coughing.
Serious Adverse Effects
Excessive use can cause irregular heart rate or rhythm or increased blood pressure.
Paradoxical bronchospasm (rare).

▷ **Possible Effects on Sexual Function:**   None reported.

Natural Diseases or Disorders That May Be Activated by This Drug
Latent coronary artery disease, diabetes or high blood pressure.

Possible Effects on Laboratory Tests
None reported.

CAUTION
1. Combination use of this drug by inhalation with beclomethasone aerosol (Beclovent, Vanceril) may increase the risk of toxicity due to fluorocarbon propellants. Use bitolterol aerosol 20 to 30 minutes *before* beclomethasone aerosol. This will reduce toxicity risk and enhances penetration of beclomethasone.
2. Excessive or prolonged use of this drug by inhalation can reduce effectiveness and cause serious heart rhythm disturbances.

Precautions for Use
By Infants and Children: Safety and effectiveness for children under 12 years of age not established.
By Those over 60 Years of Age: Avoid excessive and continual use. If acute asthma is not relieved promptly, other drugs will be needed. Watch for development of nervousness, palpitations, irregular heart rhythm and muscle tremors.

▷ **Advisability of Use During Pregnancy**
Pregnancy Category: C. See Pregnancy Code at the back of this book.
Animal studies: Cleft palate reported in mice.
Human studies: Adequate studies of pregnant women are not available.
Avoid use during first 3 months if possible.

Advisability of Use if Breast-Feeding
Presence of this drug in breast milk: Unknown.
Avoid drug or refrain from nursing.

Habit-Forming Potential: None.

Effects of Overdosage: Nervousness, palpitation, rapid heart rate, sweating, headache, tremor, vomiting, abnormal heart rhythms, chest pain.

Possible Effects of Long-Term Use: Loss of effectiveness.

Suggested Periodic Examinations While Taking This Drug (at physician's discretion)
Blood pressure measurements, evaluation of heart status.

▷ **While Taking This Drug, Observe the Following**
Foods: No restrictions.
Beverages: Avoid excessive caffeine—coffee, tea, cola, chocolate.
▷ *Alcohol:* No interactions expected.
Tobacco Smoking: No interactions expected.
▷ *Other Drugs*
Bitolterol *taken concurrently* with
- monoamine oxidase (MAO) type A inhibitor drugs (see Drug Class, Section Four) may cause large increases in blood pressure and undesirable heart stimulation.

▷ *Driving, Hazardous Activities:* Use caution if excessive nervousness or dizziness occurs.
Aviation Note: The use of this drug *is a disqualification* for piloting. Consult a designated Aviation Medical Examiner.
Exposure to Sun: No restrictions.
Heavy Exercise or Exertion: Use caution. Excessive exercise can induce asthma in some people.

BROMOCRIPTINE (broh moh KRIP teen)

Introduced: 1975 **Prescription:** USA: Yes; Canada: Yes **Available as Generic:** No **Class:** Antiparkinsonism, ergot derivative **Controlled Drug:** USA: No; Canada: No
Brand Name: Parlodel, Normatine

BENEFITS versus RISKS	
Possible Benefits	*Possible Risks*
PARTIAL RELIEF OF SYMPTOMS OF PARKINSON'S DISEASE	ABNORMAL INVOLUNTARY MOVEMENTS AND ALTERED
CORRECTION OF INFERTILITY AND ABSENT MENSTRUATION in women with high prolactin levels	BEHAVIOR in users taking high doses
	Raynaud's phenomenon (see Glossary) in users taking high doses
	Low blood pressure

▷ **Principal Uses**
As a Single Drug Product: Uses currently included in FDA approved labeling: (1) Can be used to treat early-stage symptoms of Parkinson's disease. Often it is

used in conjunction with levodopa when levodopa starts to lose its effectiveness, or the patient cannot tolerate the adverse effects of levodopa and dosage adjustment or withdrawal is necessary; (2) treats disorders due to excessive production of prolactin by the pituitary gland: absence of menstruation, infertility, and inappropriate production of milk; (3) helps as an adjunct to surgery in acromegaly; (4) eases breast engorgement and galactorrhea in stress-induced hyperprolactinemia; (5) can help in functional infertility in females; (6) reduces the size of pituitary tumors.

Other (unlabeled) generally accepted uses: (1) Can help in patients who have had a stroke and have problems in speaking; (2) may have a small role in helping cocaine withdrawal; (3) may help return growth to normal in children experiencing abnormal skeletal growth.

Author's note: Bromocriptine is no longer FDA approved for the treatment of physiological lactation. This indication was withdrawn because the risks of the use of the drug outweigh the benefits for this indication.

How This Drug Works: By stimulating receptor sites (dopamine) in the brain (corpus striatum), this drug helps increase dopamine and relieve rigidity, tremor, and sluggish movement characteristic of Parkinson's disease. By inhibiting the production of the hormone prolactin by the anterior pituitary gland, this drug

- reduces the amount of prolactin in the blood and blocks breast milk production.
- reduces abnormally high levels of prolactin in the blood, restoring it to normal levels that permit menstrual regularity and fertility.

Available Dosage Forms and Strengths

Capsules — 5 mg
Tablets — 2.5 mg
Elixir — 4 mg/ 5 ml

▷ **Usual Adult Dosage Range:**   For Parkinson's disease—initially 1.25 to 2.5 mg once daily; for maintenance, 2.5 to 100 mg daily in divided doses. Increase dose by no more than 2.5 to 5 mg on alternate days. The usual dosage range is 10 to 40 mg daily. Do not exceed 100 mg daily. The lowest possible dose should be used. For absent menstruation and infertility—initially 2.5 mg one to 3 times daily with meals. Total dose can be increased by 2.5 mg every 3 to 7 days. Effective response may be seen at 2.5 to 15 mg per day. **Note: Actual dosage and administration schedule must be determined by the physician for each patient individually.**

Conditions Requiring Dosing Adjustments

Liver function: The dose should be decreased or the dosing interval lengthened; however, specific guidelines are not available.

Kidney function: Used with caution in severe renal failure only.

▷ **Dosing Instructions:**   Take with food or milk to reduce stomach irritation. Capsule may be opened and tablet may be crushed for administration.

Usual Duration of Use: Use on a regular schedule for 3 to 4 months is usually needed to determine this drug's effectiveness in controlling the symptoms of Parkinson's disease. Treatment for 4 to 12 weeks restores fertility and normal menstruation in most women; however, treatment may be necessary for 6 to 12 months. Long-term use (up to 3 years or more) must be under physician supervision and guidance. See your doctor regularly.

▷ **This Drug Should Not Be Taken If**
- you have had an allergic reaction to it previously.
- you have had a serious adverse effect from any ergot preparation.
- you have severe coronary artery disease or peripheral vascular disease.
- you are pregnant.

▷ **Inform Your Physician Before Taking This Drug If**
- you have constitutionally low blood pressure.
- you are taking any antihypertensive drugs or phenothiazines (see Drug Classes).
- you have coronary artery disease, especially with a history of heart attack (myocardial infarction).
- you have a history of heart rhythm abnormalities.
- you have impaired liver function.
- you have a seizure disorder (epilepsy).
- you take other prescription or nonprescription medications which were not discussed when bromocriptine was prescribed for you.
- you have an ulcer.
- you have a history of mental illness.
- you take other medicines that can lower blood pressure.
- you are unsure of how much bromocriptine to take or how often to take it.

Possible Side Effects (natural, expected, and unavoidable drug actions)
Fatigue, lethargy, light-headedness in upright position (see Orthostatic Hypotension in Glossary).

▷ **Possible Adverse Effects** (unusual, unexpected, and infrequent reactions)
If any of the following develop, consult your physician promptly for guidance.
Mild Adverse Effects
Allergic Reaction: Skin rash.
Headache, drowsiness, dizziness, fainting, nervousness, nightmares.
Nasal congestion, dry mouth, loss of appetite, nausea, vomiting, stomach cramps, constipation, diarrhea.
Serious Adverse Effects
Abnormal involuntary movements, confusion, hallucinations, incoordination, visual disturbances, depression, seizures.
Swelling of feet and ankles (edema).
Loss of urinary bladder control, inability to empty bladder.
Indications of "ergotism": numbness and tingling of fingers, cold hands and feet, muscle cramps of legs and feet.
Vomiting blood, bloody or black stools (gastrointestinal bleeding).
Retroperitoneal fibrosis.
May worsen existing ulcers.
Excessive lowering of blood pressure.
Worsening of mania in manic patients.
Vasospasms and potential for heart attack (very rare).
Lung changes (pulmonary fibrosis) with long-term use.

▷ **Possible Effects on Sexual Function:**   Rare occurrence of impotence. However, this drug can correct impotence and reduced libido when the problem is due to high blood levels of prolactin (a pituitary hormone).

▷ **Adverse Effects That May Mimic Natural Diseases or Disorders**
Effects on mental function and behavior may resemble psychotic disorders.

Natural Diseases or Disorders That May Be Activated by This Drug
Coronary artery disease with anginal syndrome, Raynaud's syndrome.

Possible Effects on Laboratory Tests
Blood alkaline phosphatase level: increased.

CAUTION
1. During treatment of parkinsonism, avoid excessive and hurried activity as improvement occurs; this will reduce the risk of falls and injury.
2. The neurological and psychiatric disturbances due to this drug may last for 2 to 6 weeks after stopping it.
3. During treatment to reduce the blood level of prolactin and restore normal menstruation and fertility, it is mandatory that you use a barrier method of contraception to prevent pregnancy. Oral contraceptives should not be used while taking bromocriptine.
4. If pregnancy occurs, notify your physician **immediately**.

Precautions for Use
By Infants and Children: Safety and effectiveness for those under 15 years of age not established.
By Those over 60 Years of Age: Your initial test dose should be 1.25 mg. Watch closely for light-headedness or faintness on attempting to stand after this first dose. You may be more susceptible to the development of impaired thinking, confusion, agitation, nightmares, hallucinations, nausea or vomiting. Close monitoring and careful dosage adjustments are mandatory.

▷ **Advisability of Use During Pregnancy**
Pregnancy Category: C. See Pregnancy Code at the back of this book.
Animal studies: Rabbit studies reveal an increase in cleft lip.
Human studies: Serious birth defects have been reported in infants whose mothers took this drug during early pregnancy. Because the incidence of these defects does not exceed that reported for the general population, a cause-and-effect relationship is uncertain. Information from adequate studies of pregnant women is not available.
Ask your doctor for advice on stopping therapy.

Advisability of Use if Breast-Feeding
This drug prevents the production of milk and makes nursing impossible.

Habit-Forming Potential: Use to treat cocaine craving may result in a chemical dependence on bromocriptine.

Effects of Overdosage: Weakness, low blood pressure, nausea, vomiting, diarrhea, confusion, agitation, hallucinations, loss of consciousness.

Possible Effects of Long-Term Use: Changes in lung tissue, thickening of the pleura and pleural effusion (fluid formation within the chest cage). These changes appear reversible after stopping the drug. Fibrosis (scar tissue formation) in the back wall of the abdominal cavity and contractures of the extremities have been reported.

Suggested Periodic Examinations While Taking This Drug (at physician's discretion)

Blood pressure measurements; CAT scan of the pituitary gland for enlargement due to tumor; pregnancy test; blood tests for anemia; evaluation of heart, lung and liver functions.

▷ **While Taking This Drug, Observe the Following**

Foods: No restrictions.

Beverages: No restrictions. May be taken with milk.

▷ *Alcohol:* Caution—alcohol can exaggerate the blood-pressure-lowering effects and sedative effects of this drug and also worsen nausea and abdominal side effects.

▷ *Other Drugs*

Bromocriptine *taken concurrently* with

- antihypertensive drugs (and other drugs that can lower blood pressure) requires careful monitoring for excessive drops in pressure. Dosage adjustments may be necessary.
- erythromycins (see Drug Classes) may result in increased bromocriptine levels and toxicity.
- phenylpropanolamine can result in bromocriptine toxicity.

The following drugs may *decrease* the effects of bromocriptine

- phenothiazines (see Drug Classes). It is probably best to avoid the concurrent use of these drugs until the results of further studies are available.

▷ *Driving, Hazardous Activities:* Be alert to the possible occurrence of orthostatic hypotension, dizziness, drowsiness or impaired coordination.

Aviation Note: Parkinsonism *is a disqualification* for piloting. The use of this drug otherwise *may be a disqualification* for piloting. Consult a designated Aviation Medical Examiner.

Exposure to Sun: No restrictions.

Discontinuation

Once this medicine is stopped, pituitary tumor regrowth and symptoms of hyperprolactinemia may occur again.

BUMETANIDE (byu MET a nide)

Introduced: 1983   **Prescription:** USA: Yes   **Available as Generic:** No   **Class:** Diuretic   **Controlled Drug:** USA: No   **Brand Name:** Bumex

BENEFITS versus RISKS	
Possible Benefits	*Possible Risks*
POTENT, EFFECTIVE DIURETIC BY MOUTH OR INJECTION	ABNORMALLY LOW BLOOD POTASSIUM with excessive use
	Decreased magnesium with chronic therapy
	Blood disorders (rare)

▷ **Principal Uses**

As a Single Drug Product: Uses currently included in FDA approved labeling: (1) Relieves retained fluid associated with congestive heart failure, liver disease or kidney disease; (2) helps edema in patients who don't respond or can't tolerate furosemide.

Other (unlabeled) generally accepted uses: (1) Used as an adjunct to other therapy in high blood pressure (hypertension); (2) can help older people decrease the number of times they must get up at night to urinate (nocturia); (3) eases the amount of fluid which can build up in the lungs (pulmonary edema).

How This Drug Works: Increases removal of salt and water from the body (through increased urine production), and reduces sodium and the volume of fluid in the blood.

Available Dosage Forms and Strengths

Injection — 0.25 mg per ml (2-ml ampules)

Tablets — 0.5 mg, 1 mg, 2 mg

▷ **Usual Adult Dosage Range:** 0.5 to 2 mg daily, usually taken in the morning as a single dose. If needed, an additional second or third dose may be taken later in the day at 4- to 5-hour intervals. The total daily dose should not exceed 10 mg. Alternate-day dosage (taken every other day) may be adequate for some individuals. **Note: Actual dosage and administration schedule must be determined by the physician for each patient individually.**

Conditions Requiring Dosing Adjustments

Liver function: Rapid body fluid removal can cause a coma in liver failure patients. Use of medicines in this class is only done under close medical supervision as in a hospital or outpatient care center.

Kidney function: **NOT** recommended for use in progressive renal failure.

▷ **Dosing Instructions:** May be crushed when taken and given with or following food to reduce stomach irritation.

Usual Duration of Use: Two to three days of use on a regular schedule is often needed to see peak effect in relieving fluid buildup (edema). Once peak benefit is realized, intermittent use reduces risk of sodium, potassium, magnesium and water imbalance. Long-term use requires physician supervision.

Possible Advantages of This Drug

Diuretic effect is usually complete in 4 hours; diuretic effect of furosemide usually lasts from 6 to 8 hours.

▷ **This Drug Should Not Be Taken If**

- you have had an allergic reaction to either dosage form previously.
- coma caused by liver failure is present.
- your kidneys are unable to produce urine.
- you have developed a marked increase in creatinine or BUN while taking this drug.
- severe electrolyte or fluid imbalance.

▷ **Inform Your Physician Before Taking This Drug If**

- you are allergic to any form of "sulfa" drug.
- you are pregnant or planning pregnancy.
- you have a blood disorder.
- you have impaired liver or kidney function.
- you have diabetes, a diabetic tendency or a history of gout.
- you have impaired hearing, or develop hearing loss during therapy.

- you are taking: cortisone, digitalis, oral antidiabetic drugs, insulin, probenecid (Benemid), indomethacin (Indocin), lithium or drugs for high blood pressure.
- you plan to have surgery under general anesthesia in the near future.
- you are unsure of how much to take or how often to take bumetanide.

Possible Side Effects (natural, expected, and unavoidable drug actions)

Light-headedness on arising from sitting or lying position (see Orthostatic Hypotension in Glossary).

Increase in level of blood sugar, affecting control of diabetes.

Increase in level of blood uric acid, affecting control of gout.

Decreased blood potassium and sodium with muscle weakness and cramping.

▷ **Possible Adverse Effects** (unusual, unexpected, and infrequent reactions)

If any of the following develop, consult your physician promptly for guidance.

Mild Adverse Effects

Allergic Reactions: Skin rashes, hives, itching.

Headache, dizziness, vertigo, fatigue, weakness, sweating, earache.

Nausea, vomiting, stomach pain, diarrhea.

Breast nipple tenderness, joint and muscle pains or cramps.

Serious Adverse Effects

Impaired hearing, development of liver coma (in preexisting liver disease).

Abnormally low magnesium, potassium, and sodium (electrolytes).

Rare low white blood cells and platelets (leukopenia and thrombocytopenia).

Kidney failure (rare).

Pancreatitis (rare).

Eye defects (rare).

Elevated blood glucose.

Lung fibrosis (rare).

Hearing toxicity (ototoxicity) (rare).

▷ **Possible Effects on Sexual Function:** Difficulty maintaining an erection; premature ejaculation (0.5 to 2 mg/day) (0.1 %).

Male breast enlargement and tenderness (gynecomastia) (rare).

Natural Diseases or Disorders That May Be Activated by This Drug

Latent diabetes, gout.

Possible Effects on Laboratory Tests

White blood cell counts: increased (usual); decreased (rare).

Blood platelets: decreased.

Blood sugar (glucose): increased.

Blood lithium levels: increased.

Blood uric acid levels: increased.

CAUTION

1. High doses can cause excessive excretion of water, sodium and potassium, with loss of appetite, nausea, weakness, confusion and profound drop in blood pressure (circulatory collapse).
2. May cause digitalis toxicity by depleting potassium. If you are taking a digitalis preparation (digitoxin, digoxin), ensure an adequate intake of high-potassium foods.

3. People with cirrhosis of the liver must never increase their dose unless told to do so by their doctor. Excess dosing can cause liver coma.
4. People who take lithium may experience lithium toxicity.

Precautions for Use

By Infants and Children: Safety and effectiveness for those under 18 years of age not established.

By Those over 60 Years of Age: Small starting doses are advisable. You may be more susceptible to the development of impaired thinking, orthostatic hypotension, potassium loss and elevation of blood sugar. Overdosage and prolonged use can cause excessive loss of body water, thickening of the blood, and an increased risk of blood clots, stroke, heart attack or thrombophlebitis.

▷ **Advisability of Use During Pregnancy**

Pregnancy Category: C. See Pregnancy Code at the back of this book.

Animal studies: Ten times the maximum therapeutic human dose caused bone defects in rabbits.

Human studies: Adequate studies of pregnant women are not available.

Only used in pregnancy if a very serious complication of pregnancy occurs for which this drug is significantly beneficial.

Advisability of Use if Breast-Feeding

Presence of this drug in breast milk: Unknown.

Avoid drug or refrain from nursing.

Habit-Forming Potential: None.

Effects of Overdosage: Weakness, lethargy, dizziness, confusion, nausea, vomiting, muscle cramps, thirst, electrolyte disturbances, drowsiness progressing to deep sleep or coma, weak and rapid pulse.

Possible Effects of Long-Term Use: Impaired balance of water, salt, and potassium in blood and body tissues. Dehydration with resultant increase in blood viscosity and potential for abnormal clotting. Development of diabetes in some patients.

Suggested Periodic Examinations While Taking This Drug (at physician's discretion)

Complete blood counts; blood levels of sodium, potassium, chloride, sugar, uric acid; liver and kidney function tests.

▷ **While Taking This Drug, Observe the Following**

Foods: Salt restriction and a high-potassium diet may be needed. Ask your doctor. See Section Six for the Table of High Potassium Foods.

Beverages: No restrictions unless directed by your doctor. May be taken with milk.

▷ *Alcohol:* Alcohol can exaggerate the blood-pressure-lowering effect of this drug and cause orthostatic hypotension (see Glossary).

Tobacco Smoking: No interactions expected. Follow your physician's advice regarding smoking.

▷ *Other Drugs*

Bumetanide may ***increase*** the effects of
• antihypertensive drugs. Careful decreases in dose are needed to prevent excessive lowering of the blood pressure.

Bumetanide *taken concurrently* with
- ACE inhibitors (see Drug Classes) may result in severe lowering of blood pressure on standing (postural or orthostatic hypotension).
- aminoglycoside antibiotics (amikacin, gentamicin, kanamycin, neomycin, streptomycin, tobramycin, viomycin) increase the risk of hearing loss.
- cortisone-related drugs may cause excessive potassium loss.
- digitalis-related drugs require very careful monitoring and dose adjustments to prevent serious disturbances of heart rhythm.
- aminoglycoside antibiotics (gentamycin, tobramicin, others) may result in increased risk of ear toxicity.
- lithium may increase the risk of lithium toxicity.

The following drugs may *decrease* the effects of bumetanide
- indomethacin (Indocin) or other NSAIDs (see Drug Classes) may reduce its diuretic effect.

▷ *Driving, Hazardous Activities:* **Caution.** Varying degrees of dizziness, weakness or orthostatic hypotension (see Glossary) may occur.

Aviation Note: The use of this drug *may be a disqualification* for piloting. Consult a designated Aviation Medical Examiner.

Exposure to Sun: No restrictions.

Occurrence of Unrelated Illness: Report vomiting or diarrhea promptly to your doctor.

Discontinuation: It may be advisable to stop this drug 5 to 7 days before major surgery. Consult your physician, surgeon, or anesthesiologist for help.

BUPROPION (byu PROH pee on)

Other Name: Amfebutamone

Introduced: 1986   **Prescription:** USA: Yes   **Available as Generic:** USA: No   **Class:** Antidepressant   **Controlled Drug:** USA: No

Brand Name: Wellbutrin

BENEFITS versus RISKS	
Possible Benefits	*Possible Risks*
EFFECTIVE TREATMENT OF MAJOR DEPRESSIVE DISORDERS	DRUG-INDUCED SEIZURES (rare)
Offers a different class than tricyclic, MAO, or SSRI antidepressants	Excessive mental stimulation: excitement, anxiety, confusion, hallucinations, insomnia
	Conversion of depression to mania in manic-depressive disorders

▷ **Principal Uses**

As a Single Drug Product: Uses currently included in FDA approved labeling: Treatment of major depressive disorders.

Other (unlabeled) generally accepted uses: (1) Chronic fatigue syndrome symptoms may be relieved by this medicine; (2) can significantly reduce cocaine craving when combined with psychotherapy; (3) is the agent of choice in patients who have had significant weight gain while taking tricyclic antidepressants; (4) has been helpful in a limited number of cases of low back pain which did not respond to other agents.

How This Drug Works: Bupropion increases the levels of two nerve transmitters (norepinephrine and dopamine). Animal studies demonstrate that this drug is primarily a brain stimulant.

Available Dosage Forms and Strengths

Tablets — 75 mg, 100 mg

▷ **Recommended Dosage Ranges** (Actual dosage and administration schedule must be determined by the physician for each patient individually.)

Infants and Children: Dosage not established for those under 18 years of age.

18 to 60 Years of Age: Initially (first 3 days), 100 mg in the morning, 100 mg in the evening; total daily dose of 200 mg.

On the fourth day, if needed and tolerated, increase dose to 100 mg in the morning, at noon, and in the evening; total daily dose of 300 mg. This schedule of 100 mg, 3 times daily, 6 hours apart, is now continued for 3 to 4 weeks.

If tolerated and improvement continues, the dose may be slowly increased if needed up to a maximum of 450 mg daily. Increases should not exceed 100 mg per day within a period of 3 days. No single dose should exceed 150 mg. If a daily dose of 450 mg is reached, take 150 mg in the morning, then 100 mg every 4 hours for 3 more doses.

The lowest dose that maintains remission of depression should be used. This drug should be stopped if significant improvement is not seen after an adequate trial of 450 mg daily. Doses higher than 450 mg daily appear to only increase the risk of seizures.

Over 60 Years of Age: Same as 18 to 60 years of age.

Conditions Requiring Dosing Adjustments

Liver function: In liver cirrhosis, lower dosages and caution in monitoring should be used.

Kidney function: The dose **must** be decreased in patients with compromised kidneys or who develop kidney compromise while taking this medicine.

▷ **Dosing Instructions:**   May be taken with food to reduce stomach upset. Best to swallow the tablet whole, not chewing or crushing it; this drug has a bitter taste and a local numbing effect on the lining of the mouth.

Usual Duration of Use: Use on a regular schedule for 4 to 6 weeks is usually needed to realize this drug's effectiveness in decreasing the symptoms of depression. Long-term use (months to years) requires periodic evaluation of response and dosage adjustment. See your doctor regularly.

Possible Advantages of This Drug

Causes less atropinelike side effects: Blurred vision, dry mouth, constipation, impaired urination.

Does not cause sedation or orthostatic hypotension (see Glossary).

▷ **This Drug Should Not Be Taken If**

- you have had an allergic reaction to it previously.
- you have a history of anorexia nervosa or bulimia.
- you have a seizure disorder of any kind.
- you are taking, or have taken within the past 14 days, any monoamine oxidase (MAO) type A inhibitor drug (see Drug Class, Section Four).

▷ **Inform Your Physician Before Taking This Drug If**

- you have had any adverse effects from antidepressant drugs.
- you are pregnant or planning pregnancy.

- you are breast-feeding currently.
- you have a history of mental illness, head injury, or brain tumor.
- you have a history of alcoholism or drug abuse.
- you have any kind of heart disease, especially a recent heart attack.
- you have impaired liver or kidney function.
- you take other prescription or nonprescription medications which were not discussed when bupropion was prescribed for you.
- you are unsure of how much to take or how often to take bupropion.

Possible Side Effects (natural, expected, and unavoidable drug actions)
Nervousness, anxiety, confusion, insomnia.
Weight loss of more than 5 pounds.

▷ **Possible Adverse Effects** (unusual, unexpected, and infrequent reactions)
If any of the following develop, consult your physician promptly for guidance.
Mild Adverse Effects
Allergic Reactions: Skin rash, itching (rare).
Headache, dizziness, tremor, agitation, or blurred vision.
Indigestion, nausea and vomiting, constipation.
Dry mouth.
Excessive sweating (diaphoresis).
Serious Adverse Effects
Drug-induced seizures (rare), more common with high doses.
Change of depression to mania in manic-depressive (bipolar) disorders.
Psychosis in patients with psychotic predisposition.
Decreased white blood cell counts.
Liver toxicity (rare).
Ringing in the ears (tinnitus).

▷ **Possible Effects on Sexual Function:**   Impotence (3%); however, one study reported a decrease in sexual dysfunction when patients were switched from fluoxetine (Prozac) to bupropion; altered menstruation (4%).

Possible Delayed Adverse Effects: None reported.

Natural Diseases or Disorders That May Be Activated by This Drug
Latent epilepsy, latent psychosis, manic phase of bipolar affective disorder.

Possible Effects on Laboratory Tests
White blood cell count: decreased.

CAUTION
1. Take exactly the amount prescribed; rapid dose increases can cause seizures. Watch closely for excessive stimulation.
2. Ask your physician or pharmacist before taking any other prescription or over-the-counter drug while taking this drug.
3. Do not take any monoamine oxidase (MAO) type A inhibitor drug while taking this drug (see Drug Class, Section Four). If you have taken a MAO inhibitor, then stopped it, wait 2 weeks before starting bupropion.

Precautions for Use
By Infants and Children: Safety and effectiveness for those under 18 years of age not established.
By Those over 60 Years of Age: Age-related liver or kidney function decline may require dose decreases.

▷ **Advisability of Use During Pregnancy**
  Pregnancy Category: B. See Pregnancy Code at the back of this book.
    Animal studies: Rat and rabbit studies reveal no significant birth defects.
    Human studies: Adequate studies of pregnant women are not available.
    Use this drug only if clearly needed. Ask your physician for guidance.

Advisability of Use if Breast-Feeding
  Presence of this drug in breast milk: Yes.
  Avoid drug or refrain from nursing.

Habit-Forming Potential: Remote with use of recommended doses. Slight potential for abuse by those who abuse stimulant drugs.

Effects of Overdosage: Headache, agitation, confusion, hallucinations, seizures, loss of consciousness.

Possible Effects of Long-Term Use: Electrocardiographic (ECG) changes: Premature beats, nonspecific ST-T wave changes.

Suggested Periodic Examinations While Taking This Drug (at physician's discretion)
  Liver and/or kidney function tests as appropriate.

▷ **While Taking This Drug, Observe the Following**
  Foods: No restrictions.
  Beverages: No restrictions. May be taken with milk.
▷ *Alcohol:* Avoid completely. Alcohol may predispose to the development of seizures.
  Tobacco Smoking: No interactions expected.
  Marijuana Smoking: Avoid completely; it may induce psychotic behavior.
▷ *Other Drugs*
    The following drugs *taken concurrently* with bupropion may increase the risk of major seizures
    • antidepressants (tricyclic).
    • clozapine (Clozaril).
    • fluoxetine (Prozac).
    • haloperidol (Haldol).
    • lithium.
    • loxapine.
    • maprotiline.
    • molindone.
    • phenothiazines.
    • thioxanthenes.
    • trazodone.
    Bupropion *taken concurrently* with
    • carbamazepine (Tegretol) may result in lowered carbamazepine levels.
    • levodopa results in increased nausea, restlessness and tremor.
    • phenobarbital may result in decreased levels.
    • phenytoin (Dilantin) may result in decreased phenytoin levels.
▷ *Driving, Hazardous Activities:* This drug may cause dizziness, drowsiness or seizures. Restrict activities as necessary.
  Aviation Note: The use of this drug *is a disqualification* for piloting. Consult a designated Aviation Medical Examiner.
  Exposure to Sun: No restrictions.
  Discontinuation: Do not stop this drug abruptly. Ask your physician for help.

BUSPIRONE (byu SPI rohn)

Introduced: 1979   **Prescription:** USA: Yes   **Available as Generic:**
No   **Class:** Antianxiety drug   **Controlled Drug:** USA: No
Brand Name: Buspar

BENEFITS versus RISKS	
Possible Benefits	*Possible Risks*
EFFECTIVE RELIEF OF MILD TO MODERATE ANXIETY	Mild dizziness, faintness, or headache (uncommon)
DECREASED RISK OF SEDATION OR DEPENDENCE THAN OTHER AGENTS	Tachycardia (rare)
	Rare restlessness, depression, tremor or rigidity (with high doses)

▷ **Principal Uses**

As a Single Drug Product: Uses currently included in FDA approved labeling: (1) Relieves mild to moderate anxiety and nervous tension. Particularly useful in the elderly, alcoholics and addiction-prone people because of its lack of significant sedative effects or abuse potential; (2) beneficial in decreasing self-injurious behaviors or aggression in developmentally disabled adults.

Other (unlabeled) generally accepted uses: (1) May have a benefit in reducing alcohol craving in alcoholics; (2) can help aggression or hyperactivity in autistics; (3) may decrease symptoms in obsessive-compulsive disorder; (4) can be of help in sexual dysfunction in people with generalized anxiety disorder; (4) may help decrease the urge to smoke in those addicted to nicotine.

How This Drug Works: This drug is thought to be a "mid-brain modulator" which causes changes in brain chemicals (dopamine, norepinephrine and serotonin) resulting in a calming effect. It is also a partial agonist at serotonin reuptake sites.

Available Dosage Forms and Strengths

Tablets — 5 mg, 10 mg

▷ **Usual Adult Dosage Range:**   Initially, 5 mg three times/day; if needed, increase dose by 5 mg/day every 2 to 3 days, with individual doses every 6 to 8 hours. The total daily dose should not exceed 60 mg. **Note: Actual dosage and administration schedule must be determined by the physician for each patient individually.**

Conditions Requiring Dosing Adjustments

Liver function: Used with caution in severe liver failure. Doses must be decreased.

Kidney function: Used with caution in severe kidney problems. Dose should be decreased to 25–50% of normal dose.

▷ **Dosing Instructions:**   The tablet may be crushed to take it and given without regard to food.

Usual Duration of Use: Use on a regular schedule for 7 to 10 days is usually needed to see this drug's benefit in relieving anxiety and nervous tension. Avoid uninterrupted use. Use intermittently and only as needed.

Possible Advantages of This Drug

Relieves anxiety or tension without severe sedation or impaired thinking. Does not cause withdrawal when it is stopped.

▷ **This Drug Should Not Be Taken If**
  • you have had an allergic reaction to it previously.
  • you take or have taken in the last two weeks, one of the MAO inhibitor drugs (see Drug Classes Section). May increase blood pressure.

▷ **Inform Your Physician Before Taking This Drug If**
  • you take other drugs that affect the brain or nervous system: Tranquilizers, sedatives, hypnotics, analgesics, narcotics, antidepressants, antipsychotic drugs, anticonvulsants or antiparkinsonians.
  • you have impaired liver or kidney function.
  • you take fluoxetine (Prozac) for depression.

Possible Side Effects (natural, expected, and unavoidable drug actions)
Mild drowsiness (less than with benzodiazepines), lethargy, fatigue.

▷ **Possible Adverse Effects** (unusual, unexpected, and infrequent reactions)
If any of the following develop, consult your physician promptly for guidance.
Mild Adverse Effects
Headache, dizziness, fatigue, faintness, excitement, nausea.
Insomnia and dream disturbances.
Serious Adverse Effects
Depression.
Tachycardia (rare).
With high doses: dysphoria, restlessness, rigidity, tremors.
Movement disorders (rare).

▷ **Possible Effects on Sexual Function:**   Increased or decreased libido, difficult or absent orgasm, inhibited ejaculation, impotence, breast milk production, altered timing or pattern of menstruation (10 to 40 mg/day).
May increase prolactin; however no reports of male breast tenderness or enlargement have been reported.

Possible Effects on Laboratory Tests
Growth hormone: Conflicting increases or lack of effect on growth hormone levels.
Blood prolactin levels: dose related increase.

CAUTION
This drug is reported to have very mild sedative effects and no abuse potential, however, it should be used with caution and only when clearly needed. Most use has been short-term. Some unexpected side effects or adverse effects may still be reported. Actual dysphoria has been reported with higher doses and may preclude its recreational use.

Precautions for Use
By Infants and Children: Safety and effectiveness by those under 18 years of age not established.
By Those over 60 Years of Age: Expected to be tolerated much better than benzodiazepines and barbiturates. Watch for increased dizziness or weakness and avoid falls.

▷ **Advisability of Use During Pregnancy**
Pregnancy Category: B. See Pregnancy Code at the back of this book.
Animal studies: No birth defects found in rat and rabbit studies.

Human studies: Adequate studies of pregnant women are not available.
Use this drug during pregnancy only when clearly needed. Advisable to avoid this drug during the first 3 months of pregnancy.

Advisability of Use if Breast-Feeding
Presence of this drug in breast milk: Excreted in rat milk; probably also in humans.
Avoid drug or refrain from nursing.

Habit-Forming Potential: Does not appear to cause addiction, however, more studies are needed. Higher doses result in a dysphoric reaction which may keep it from becoming a drug involved in recreational use.

Effects of Overdosage: Drowsiness, fatigue, nausea, dysphoria, tingling sensations (paresthesias), and a rare chance of seizures.

Possible Effects of Long-Term Use: None reported.

Suggested Periodic Examinations While Taking This Drug (at physician's discretion)
Periodic check of heart rate.

▷ **While Taking This Drug, Observe the Following**
Foods: No restrictions, taking with food may result in a clinically insignificant increase in absorption of this drug..
Beverages: No restrictions.
▷ *Alcohol:* Milder problems than diazepam (Valium), however, avoid the combination.
Tobacco Smoking: No interactions expected.
Marijuana Smoking: Additive increase in drowsiness.
▷ *Other Drugs:* Buspirone **taken concurrently** with
• MAO inhibitors (see Drug Classes) such as phenylzine (Parnate) may result in large blood pressure increases. Do not combine.
• fluoxetine (Prozac) may increase underlying anxiety or mental disorder such as obsessive compulsive disorder. Do not combine.
• fluvoxamine (Luvox) may result in serious slowing of the heart (bradycardia). Doses must be decreased.
• narcotics such as oxycodone (Percodan) may result in additive sedation and potential decreases in breathing (respiratory depression).
▷ *Driving, Hazardous Activities:* This drug may cause dizziness, faintness or fatigue. Restrict activities as necessary.
Aviation Note: The use of this drug **may be a disqualification** for piloting. Consult a designated Aviation Medical Examiner.
Exposure to Sun: No restrictions.

CALCITONIN (kal si TOH nin)

Other Names: Salcatonin, thyrocalcitonin

Introduced: 1977, Nasal spray form 1995   **Prescription:** USA: Yes; Canada: Yes   **Available as Generic:** USA: No; Canada: No   **Class:** antiosteoporotic, hormones   **Controlled Drug:** USA: No; Canada: No

Brand Names: Calcimar, Cibacalcin, Miacalcin Nasal Spray, Miacalcin Injection

---

BENEFITS versus RISKS

Possible Benefits	*Possible Risks*
PARTIAL RELIEF OF SYMPTOMS OF PAGET'S DISEASE OF BONE	Nausea (with or without vomiting)
NASAL FORM CAN INCREASE BONE MASS	Allergic reactions
Effective adjunctive treatment of postmenopausal osteoporosis	
Effective adjunctive treatment of abnormally high blood calcium levels (associated with malignant disease)	

▷ **Principal Uses**

As a Single Drug Product: Uses currently included in FDA approved labeling: (1) Treatment of symptomatic Paget's disease of bone (excessive bone growth of skull, spine and long bones); (2) combination treatment of post-menopausal osteoporosis, taken with calcium and vitamin D (also has a reasonably good effect on the pain of osteoporosis); (3) NASAL form approved for treatment of postmenopausal osteoporosis in women with low bone mass who had menopause 5 years previously; (4) adjunctive treatment of high blood calcium levels seen in bone cancer; (4) relieves symptoms of neurologic compression in Paget's disease.

Other (unlabeled) generally accepted uses: (1) Combination treatment of osteoporosis due to medicinal drugs, hormonal disorders, or immobilization taken with calcium and vitamin D; (2) may help aneurysmal bone cysts when directly injected into the cyst; (3) preliminary study indicates that this drug may be of benefit in preventing migraine headaches and reduce or eliminate the need for prophylactic medicines; (4) useful adjunct in cancer pain; (5) very beneficial in treating pain which occurs when an arm or leg has been amputated (phantom limb); (6) Early data gathered from several studies says this drug may also decrease risk of bone fractures in those with osteoporosis.

How This Drug Works: This hormone slows abnormally accelerated "bone turnover" that occurs in Paget's disease. Excessive replacement of bone loss is gradually reduced and a more normal balance is restored. In cancer of the bone, this drug slows bone destruction and decreases the transfer of calcium from bone to blood stream. In osteoporosis, this drug acts primarily on bone by blocking resorption (inhibiting osteoclasts) and allowing bone building cells to act. There are also effects on the intestine (calcium absorption) and the kidney (decreased calcium elimination) which are not fully defined.

Available Dosage Forms and Strengths

Calcitonin-Human

Injection — 500 mcg (0.5 mg)

Calcitonin-Salmon

Injection — 200 IU per ml

Nasal Spray — 200 IU per spray

▷ **Recommended Dosage Ranges** (Actual dosage and administration schedule must be determined by the physician for each patient individually.)

Skin Testing: Skin testing is accomplished by diluting 10 IU to one ml with 0.9% sodium chloride. One tenth ml of this dilution is injected onto the inner forearm (about one IU). A positive reaction occurs if more than mild skin reddening or weal is seen within 15 minutes. The drug should NOT be used if this positive reaction is seen.

Infants and Children: Dosage not established.

12 to 60 Years of Age: Calcitonin-Human

For Paget's disease—Initially 500 mcg (0.5 mg) daily, injected subcutaneously; after adequate response, dose may be decreased to 250 mcg (0.25 mg) daily, or 500 mcg (0.5 mg) 2 or 3 times per week. Severe cases may require 1 mg per day.

Calcitonin-Salmon

For Paget's disease—50 to 100 IU daily or every other day, injected subcutaneouly or intramuscularly; after adequate response, dose may be decreased to 50 IU daily, every other day, or 3 times per week.

For postmenopausal osteoporosis—100 IU daily, every other day, or 3 times per week, injected under the skin. If adverse effects are marked, reduce dose to 50 IU daily; then increase dose gradually over a period of 2 weeks.

NASAL Spray: 200 IU (one spray) daily. Nostrils should be alternated daily to help avoid nasal irritation. Calcium and vitamin D replacement is strongly recommended—such replacement can help keep you from drawing on your 'bone bank" (your bones) to maintain adequate calcium. For high blood calcium levels—Initially 4 IU/kg of body weight every 12 hours, injected subcutaneously or intramuscularly; as needed and tolerated, increase dose to 8 IU/kg of body weight every 12 hours; if necessary, the dose may be increased to a maximum of 8 IU/kg of body weight every 6 hours.

For adjunctive pain treatment: 100 to 200 IU daily, given intramuscularly or subcutaneously. Some clinicians have started using the nasal spray form (200 IU daily) for adjunctive pain therapy.

Over 60 Years of Age: Same as 12 to 60 years of age.

Conditions Requiring Dosing Adjustments

Liver function: No changes indicated.

Kidney function: Should be used with caution in blocked kidneys, as the attempt to lose water via the kidney (diuresis) will put added pressure on an overloaded system.

▷ **Dosing Instructions:**   The NASAL SPRAY form should be activated (as in package instructions), then the head placed upright, and then the spray tip placed firmly into the chosen nostril (remember to use a different nostril every day) and the pump depressed toward the bottle. Call your doctor if your nose becomes ulcerated. **Subcutaneous (under the skin)** injection is preferred for self-administration of the injectable form. Your doctor will teach you about proper injection technique. The daily dose may be given at bedtime with the stomach empty if you become nauseated.

Usual Duration of Use: Peak effect in treating Paget's disease is usually seen after 1–3 months of use on a regular schedule. If effective, the usual treatment is 6 months; and if response continues, the dose may be reduced during the next 6 months. Peak response may require treatment for up to 24 months. Long-term use (months to years) requires periodic physician eval-_ uation. Bone mineral density testing is strongly recommended Osteoporosis benefits should be followed by bone mineral density testing to decide the ongoing success of therapy or the need to change to another medicine.

Possible Advantages of This Drug
Calcitonin-human is less likely to induce allergic reactions than calcitonin-salmon, permitting treatment for longer periods of time.

▷ **This Drug Should Not Be Taken If**
  • you have had an allergic reaction to it previously.
  • you recently fractured a bone that has not healed completely.

▷ **Inform Your Physician Before Taking This Drug If**
  • you are allergic by nature (history of eczema, hives, hay fever, asthma).
  • you have known allergies to foreign proteins.
  • you are unsure of how much to take or how often to take it.
  • you develop sores in the nose following repeated intranasal use.
  • you will be unable to have follow-up laboratory testing of blood calcium.

Possible Side Effects (natural, expected, and unavoidable drug actions)
Salty or metallic taste in mouth.

▷ **Possible Adverse Effects** (unusual, unexpected, and infrequent reactions)
  If any of the following develop, consult your physician promptly for guidance.
  Mild Adverse Effects
  Allergic Reactions: Skin rash, hives, itching.
  Headache, dizziness, weakness.
  Loss of appetite, nausea, vomiting, stomach pain, diarrhea.
  Increased frequency of urination.
  Abnormal fluid accumulation (pedal edema).
  Shivering.
  Flushing of the face.
  Urination at night (nocturia).
  Serious Adverse Effects
  Allergic Reactions: Flushing, redness, tingling of face or extremities.
  Sugar (glucose) intolerance.
  Increased urination.
  Excessive lowering of calcium and rigidity (tetany) of muscles due to lack of calcium.
  Anaphylactic reactions.
  Severe ulceration of the nose (with nasal spray use).

▷ **Possible Effects on Sexual Function:**   None reported.

Possible Effects on Laboratory Tests
Blood alkaline phosphatase levels: decreased.
Blood calcium levels: decreased.
Urine hydroxyproline values: decreased.
Blood glucose: lack of diabetic control, glucose intolerance.

CAUTION
  1. It is best that your doctor perform a skin test before beginning treatment with calcitonin-salmon.

2. Eat a well-balanced diet with adequate calcium and vitamin D.
3. Tell your doctor if bone pain persists while taking this drug.

Precautions for Use

By Infants and Children: No specific information.

By Those over 60 Years of Age: Watch fluid balance closely if this drug is given to lower blood calcium.

▷ **Advisability of Use During Pregnancy**

Pregnancy Category: C. See Pregnancy Code at the back of this book.

Animal studies: No drug-induced birth defects reported.

Human studies: Adequate studies of pregnant women are not available.

Use this drug only if clearly needed. Ask your physician for help.

Advisability of Use if Breast-Feeding

Presence of this drug in breast milk: Yes.

Calcitonin taken in with breast milk is typically destroyed by infant stomach acids before it has any effect. Ask your doctor for guidance.

Habit-Forming Potential: None.

Effects of Overdosage: Nausea, vomiting.

Possible Effects of Long-Term Use: Antibodies may cause resistance and loss of effect. This occurs in approximately 50% of people after 2 to 18 months of treatment.

Suggested Periodic Examinations While Taking This Drug (at physician's discretion)

Measurements of blood calcium, phosphate, and alkaline phosphatase levels.

Measurement of urine hydroxyproline content.

Measurement of bone mineral density (BMD) by DEXA densitometry scanning.

▷ **While Taking This Drug, Observe the Following**

Foods: No restrictions.

Nutritional Support: Ensure adequate intake of calcium and vitamin D.

Beverages: No restrictions.

▷ *Alcohol:* No interactions expected, but alcohol (in higher doses) acts as a bone forming cell (osteoblast) poison and is a risk factor for osteoporosis.

Tobacco Smoking: No interactions expected, but smoking is a risk factor for osteoporosis.

▷ *Other Drugs:*

Calcitonin *taken concurrently* with

- ketoprofen may inhibit the calcium and uric acid distribution in the urine by calcitonin of pig origin. Changes with other calcitonins are not defined.
- Plicamycin will cause additive loss of calcium.

▷ *Driving, Hazardous Activities:* No restrictions.

Aviation Note: The use of this drug *may be a disqualification* for piloting. Consult a designated Aviation Medical Examiner.

Exposure to Sun: No restrictions.

Heavy Exercise or Exertion: As defined by your doctor. Remember, weight bearing exercise (if not contraindicated for you) actually helps osteoporosis by stimulating receptors (mechanoreceptors) to release factors that help structure healthy (normal architecture) bone.

Discontinuation: Your doctor should decide when to stop this drug.

Special Storage Instructions:
  Calcitonin-human—Store at a temperature below 25 degrees C (77 degrees F). Do not refrigerate. Protect from light.
  Calcitonin-salmon—Store in refrigerator, between 2 and 8 degrees C (36 and 46 degrees F). Do not freeze.
  Calcitonin-salmon Nasal Spray—store unopened in the refrigerator. Once it has been opened, the bottle can be kept at room temperature for two weeks.

CAPTOPRIL (KAP toh pril)

Introduced: 1979   **Prescription:** USA: Yes; Canada: Yes   **Available as**
Generic: Yes, recently approved.   **Class:** Antihypertensive, ACE inhibitor
Controlled Drug: USA: No; Canada: No

Brand Names: ♣Apo-Capto, Capoten, Capozide [CD], ♣Novo-Captopril, ♣Nu-Capto, ♣Syn-Captopril

BENEFITS versus RISKS	
Possible Benefits	*Possible Risks*
EFFECTIVE CONTROL OF MILD TO SEVERE HIGH BLOOD PRESSURE	Impaired white blood cell production (rare)
USEFUL ADJUNCTIVE TREATMENT FOR CONGESTIVE HEART FAILURE	Bone marrow depression (rare) Kidney damage (rare) Liver damage (rare)
MAY DECREASE RISK OF KIDNEY PROBLEMS IN DIABETICS TAKING INSULIN	
MAY REDUCE RISK OF DEATH AFTER A HEART ATTACK	

▷ **Principal Uses**
  As a Single Drug Product: Uses currently included in FDA approved labeling: (1) Treats all degrees of high blood pressure; (2) may help prevent death after heart attacks; (3) used in advanced heart failure; (4) used in type one insulin-dependent diabetics who have kidney problems and damage to the retina of the eye.
  Other (unlabeled) generally accepted uses: (1) Helps relieve symptoms of cystinuria; (2) may have some role in easing rheumatoid arthritis symptoms; (3) can help Raynaud's phenomenon symptoms.
How This Drug Works: It is thought that by blocking an enzyme system, this drug relaxes arterial walls and lowers the blood pressure. This, in turn, decreases the heart's work load and improves its performance. Use after heart attack appears to result from captopril blunting of response to catecholamines, free radical scavenging, as well as increased prostacyclin or bradykinin.

Available Dosage Forms and Strengths
  Tablets — 12.5 mg, 25 mg, 50 mg, 100 mg

▷ **Usual Adult Dosage Range:**   Initially 12.5 to 25 mg 2 or 3 times daily for 2 weeks. If necessary, dose may be increased to 50 mg 3 times daily. Usual maintenance dose is 50 to 100 mg 3 times daily. Total daily dose should not exceed 450 mg. After a heart attack: A test dose of 6.25 mg is given to see if excessive lowering of the blood pressure occurs. If the test is tolerated, 12.5 mg is given three times a day. This dose is then increased toward a goal of 50 mg three times a day. Diabetic kidney problems (nephropathy) and eye problems (retinopathy): Success has been achieved with 50 mg twice daily in two large studies. The manufacturer suggests a starting dose of 25 mg three times a day. Children (1.5 to 18 years old) with severe high blood pressure caused by the kidneys (renal hypertension) have been successfully treated using 1.3 mg per kg per day progressing to 2.2 mg per kg per day. **Note: Actual dosage and administration schedule must be determined by the physician for each patient individually.**

Conditions Requiring Dosing Adjustments
Liver function: Must used with extreme caution, and started at a lower dose in liver failure.
Kidney function: Increased blood level and risk of adverse effects (low blood counts and protein in the urine) if used in kidney failure. **Must** decrease dose according to decreases in creatinine clearance. The lowest effective dose must be used.

▷ **Dosing Instructions:**   Take on empty stomach, 1 hour before meals, at same time each day. Tablet may be crushed for administration.

Usual Duration of Use: Several weeks of use on a regular schedule is usually needed to see high blood pressure control. Use may be continued for life.

▷ **This Drug Should Not Be Taken If**
  • you have had an allergic reaction to it previously.
  • you are pregnant (last 6 months).
  • you currently have a blood cell or bone marrow disorder.
  • you have an abnormally high level of blood potassium.

▷ **Inform Your Physician Before Taking This Drug If**
  • you are allergic to ACE inhibitors (see Drug Classes).
  • you are planning pregnancy.
  • you have a history of kidney disease or impaired kidney function.
  • you have scleroderma or systemic lupus erythematosus.
  • you have any form of heart or liver disease.
  • you have diabetes.
  • you develop swelling of the tongue, face or throat while taking this drug.
  • you have an elevated potassium level.
  • you have a blood cell disorder.
  • you take: Other antihypertensives, diuretics, nitrates, allopurinol (Zyloprim), Indocin or potassium supplements.
  • you plan to have surgery under general anesthesia in the near future.
  • you have renal artery stenosis (ask your doctor).
  • you are taking medicines which suppress the immune system.
  • you are unsure of how much to take or how often to take captopril.

Possible Side Effects (natural, expected, and unavoidable drug actions)
Dizziness, light-headedness, fainting (excessive drop in blood pressure).

▷ **Possible Adverse Effects** (unusual, unexpected, and infrequent reactions)
If any of the following develop, consult your physician promptly for guidance.

Mild Adverse Effects

Allergic Reactions: Skin rash, swelling of face, hands, or feet; fever.

Lost or altered (metallic or salty) taste, mouth or tongue sores.

Nightmares, joint pain.

Cough.

Rare increased temperature (hyperthermia).

Rapid heart rate, palpitation.

Serious Adverse Effects

Bone marrow depression (neutropenia, anemia or aplastic anemia)—weakness, fever, sore throat, bleeding or bruising.

(This adverse effect is increased in those with collagen vascular disease and kidney impairment.)

Kidney damage—water retention (edema).

Elevated blood potassium (hyperkalemia).

Rare accumulation of fluid around the heart (pericarditis).

Rare hallucinations.

Rare Stevens-Johnson syndrome, lupus erythematosus, or other serious skin conditions.

Rare pancreatitis.

Liver damage—with or without jaundice.

▷ **Possible Effects on Sexual Function:** Decreased male libido (20% to 30%) with recommended dosage. Impotence. Rare swelling and tenderness of male breast tissue (gynecomastia).

Possible Effects on Laboratory Tests

Complete blood counts: decreased red cells, hemoglobin, white cells and platelets; increased eosinophils.

Blood antinuclear antibodies (ANA): increased.

Blood cholesterol and triglycerides: no effects.

Blood sodium level: decreased.

Blood urea nitrogen level (BUN): increased.

Liver function tests: increased liver enzymes (alkaline phosphatase, AST/GOT, LDH), increased bilirubin.

Urine ketone tests: false positive results with Keto-diastix and Chemstrip-6.

CAUTION

1. If possible, advisable to stop all other antihypertensive drugs (especially diuretics) for 1 week before starting captopril.
2. **Inform your physician immediately if you become pregnant.** This drug should not be taken beyond the first 3 months of pregnancy.
3. **Report promptly** any signs of infection (fever, sore throat), and any indications of water retention (weight gain, swollen feet or ankles).
4. Many salt substitutes contain potassium; ask your doctor before using.
5. Blood counts and urine analyses are needed **before** taking captopril.

Precautions for Use

By Infants and Children: Safety and effectiveness have not been established.

By Those over 60 Years of Age: Small starting doses are advisable. Sudden and excessive lowering of blood pressure can cause stroke or heart attack.

▷ **Advisability of Use During Pregnancy**

Pregnancy Category: C during the first three months. **D during the last six months** (last two trimesters). See Pregnancy Code at the back of this book.

Animal studies: No birth defects found in rat, rabbit or hamster studies. However, this drug was found to be toxic to the embryo and newborn.

Human studies: The use of ACE inhibitor drugs during the last 6 months of pregnancy is known to possibly cause very serious injury and possible death to the fetus; skull and limb malformations, lung defects, and kidney failure have been reported in over 50 cases worldwide.

Avoid this drug completely during the last 6 months. During the first 3 months of pregnancy, use this drug only if clearly needed. Ask your physician for guidance.

Advisability of Use if Breast-Feeding

Presence of this drug in breast milk: Yes, in small amounts.

Monitor nursing infant closely and discontinue drug or nursing if adverse effects develop.

Habit-Forming Potential: None.

Effects of Overdosage: Excessive drop in blood pressure—light-headedness, dizziness, fainting.

Possible Effects of Long-Term Use: Gradual increase in blood potassium level.

Suggested Periodic Examinations While Taking This Drug (at physician's discretion)

Complete blood cell count, urine analysis and blood potassium level before drug started. Once started: Blood counts every 2 weeks during the first 3 months, then periodically for duration of use. Urine protein every month for the first 9 months of treatment, then periodically for duration of use. Periodic measurements of blood potassium.

▷ **While Taking This Drug, Observe the Following**

Foods: Consult physician regarding salt intake.

Nutritional Support: **Do not take** potassium supplements unless directed by your physician.

Beverages: No restrictions. May be taken with milk.

▷ *Alcohol:* Alcohol can further lower blood pressure. Use with caution.

Tobacco Smoking: No interactions expected.

▷ *Other Drugs*

Captopril *taken concurrently* with

- allopurinol (Zyloprim) may increase risk of serious skin reactions.
- azathioprine may result in severe anemia.
- cyclosporine (Sandimune) may result in kidney failure that takes awhile to appear (delayed acute renal dysfunction).
- lithium may result in three times the expected lithium levels and **toxicity**.
- loop diuretics (such as Lasix or Bumex) (see Drug Classes) may result in excessively low blood pressure on standing (postural hypotension).
- phenothiazines (see Drug Classes) may result in postural hypotension.
- potassium preparations (K-Lyte, Slow-K, etc.) will increase blood potassium with risk of serious heart rhythm disturbances.
- potassium-sparing diuretics: amiloride (Moduretic), spironolactone (Aldactazide), triamterene (Dyazide) may increase blood levels of potassium with risk of serious heart rhythm disturbances.

The following drugs may *decrease* the effects of captopril
- antacids by decreasing captopril absorption. Separate doses by two hours.
- indomethacin (Indocin) or other NSAIDS (see Drug Classes).
- naloxone (Narcan).
- salicylates (aspirin, etc.).

▷ *Driving, Hazardous Activities:* Usually no restrictions. Be aware of possible drops in blood pressure with resultant dizziness or faintness.

Aviation Note: The use of this drug *may be a disqualification* for piloting. Consult a designated Aviation Medical Examiner.

Exposure to Sun: Caution advised. This drug can cause photosensitivity.

Exposure to Heat: Caution advised. Excessive perspiring may drop blood pressure.

Occurrence of Unrelated Illness: Report promptly any disorder that causes nausea, vomiting or diarrhea. Fluid and chemical imbalances must be corrected as soon as possible.

CARBAMAZEPINE (kar ba MAZ e peen)

Introduced: 1962   **Prescription:** USA: Yes; Canada: Yes   **Available as Generic:** Yes   **Class:** Anticonvulsant, antineuralgic, pain syndrome modifier **Controlled Drug:**   USA: No; Canada: No

Brand Names: ✦Apo-Carbamazepine, Epitol, ✦Mazepine, ✦Novo-Carbamaz, ✦PMS Carbamazepine, Tegretol, Tegretol Chewable tablet

BENEFITS versus RISKS	
Possible Benefits	*Possible Risks*
RELIEF OF PAIN IN TRIGEMINAL NEURALGIA	RARE BONE MARROW DEPRESSION (reduced formation of all blood cells)
EFFECTIVE CONTROL OF CERTAIN TYPES OF EPILEPTIC SEIZURES	Liver damage with jaundice
Relief of pain in some rare forms of nerve pain (neuralgia)	

▷ **Principal Uses**

As a Single Drug Product: Uses currently included in FDA approved labeling: (1) for relief of pain in true trigeminal neuralgia (tic douloureux) and glossopharyngeal neuralgia; (2) for control of several types of epilepsy, namely grand mal, tonic-clonic, psychomotor or temporal lobe, complex partial and mixed seizure patterns. Precise diagnosis and careful management are mandatory for its proper use.

Other (unlabeled) generally accepted uses: (1) Beneficial in bipolar affective disorders; (2) schizoaffective disorders; (3) resistant schizophrenia; (4) post traumatic stress disorder; (5) tabes dorsalis; (6) diabetic neuropathy; (7) hemifacial spasm; (8) cocaine withdrawal; (9) helps aggression in some Alzheimer's patients; (10) hiccups and belching associated with flutter of the diaphragm; (11) treats nerve problems resulting from thiamine deficiency; (12) may have a role in treating pain that occurs when an arm or leg is amputated (phantom limb pain); (13) may be of great benefit in a form of perceived repetitive ear noise called clicking tinnitus.

How This Drug Works: By reducing impulses at certain nerve terminals, this drug relieves or reduces pain (of trigeminal neuralgia) and also reduces the excitability of nerve fibers in the brain, decreasing the likelihood of seizures or reducing their frequency and severity.

Available Dosage Forms and Strengths
Oral suspension — 100 mg per 5 ml
            Tablets — 200 mg (400 mg in Canada)
Tablets, chewable — 100 mg

▷ **Usual Adult Dosage Range:**   Initially 200 mg/12 hours. Dose may be increased at weekly intervals by 200 mg/24 hours as needed and tolerated. Total daily dosage should not exceed 1200 mg. **Note: Actual dosage and administration schedule must be determined by the physician for each patient individually. Carbamazepine dosing should be guided by blood levels.**

Conditions Requiring Dosing Adjustments
Liver function: Used with extreme caution, in lower doses and watched closely in liver compromise patients. This medicine may have to be stopped in active liver disease.
Kidney function: Capable of being toxic to the kidneys. Used with extreme caution and in decreased dose in patients with kidneys that already do not work well.
Heart attack: Changes in blood distribution (perfusion) and protein binding may result in much higher than expected blood levels. Blood levels should be obtained more frequently to guide dose decreases and avoid toxicity.

▷ **Dosing Instructions:**   Take at same time each day, with or following food to reduce stomach irritation. Tablet may be crushed for administration.

Usual Duration of Use: Use on a regular schedule for 3 months is usually needed to see this drug's effect in relieving the pain of trigeminal neuralgia. Longer periods, with dosage adjustment, may be required to determine its ability to control epileptic seizures. Careful evaluation of individual tolerance and response should be made every 3 months during long-term treatment.

▷ **This Drug Should Not Be Taken If**
• you have had an allergic reaction to it previously.
• you have active liver disease.
• you currently have a blood cell or bone marrow disorder.
• you currently take, or have taken within the past 14 days, a monoamine oxidase (MAO) type A inhibitor (see Drug Class, Section Four).

▷ **Inform Your Physician Before Taking This Drug If**
• you have had an allergic reaction to any tricyclic antidepressant drug (see Drug Classes).
• you have taken this drug in the past.
• you have had any blood or bone marrow disorder, especially drug induced.
• you have a history of liver or kidney disease.
• you have had serious mental depression or other mental disorder.
• you have had thrombophlebitis.
• you have high blood pressure, heart disease or glaucoma.
• you take more than 2 alcoholic drinks a day.

- you take other prescription or nonprescription medications which were not discussed when carbamazepine was prescribed for you.
- you are unsure of how much to take or how often to take carbamazepine.
- you are pregnant.
- you are breast feeding your baby.

Possible Side Effects (natural, expected, and unavoidable drug actions)
Dry mouth and throat, constipation, impaired urination.

▷ **Possible Adverse Effects** (unusual, unexpected, and infrequent reactions)
If any of the following develop, consult your physician promptly for guidance.

Mild Adverse Effects
Allergic Reactions: Skin rash, hives, itching, drug fever.
Headache, dizziness, drowsiness, unsteadiness, fatigue, blurred vision, confusion.
Exaggerated hearing, ringing in ears.
Loss of appetite, nausea, vomiting, indigestion, diarrhea.
Water retention (edema), frequent urination.
Changes in skin pigmentation, hair loss.
Aching of muscles and joints, leg cramps.

Serious Adverse Effects
Allergic Reactions: Severe dermatitis with peeling of skin, irritation of mouth and tongue, swelling of lymph glands.
Idiosyncratic Reactions: Lung inflammation (pneumonitis): cough, shortness of breath.
Abnormal heartbeats (bradyarrhythmias).
Bone marrow depression (agranulocytosis, leukopenia, hemolytic or aplastic anemia) or thrombocytopenia (see Glossary)—fatigue, weakness, fever, sore throat, abnormal bleeding or bruising.
Liver damage with jaundice (see Glossary)—yellow eyes and skin, dark-colored urine, light-colored stools.
Kidney damage—reduced urine volume, uremic poisoning.
Mental depression and agitation/psychosis.
Paradoxical increase in seizures.
Drug induced meningitis (aseptic meningitis).
Low thyroid hormones.
Abnormally elevated urine output (SIADH).
Neuroleptic malignant syndrome (rare).
Rare abnormal movement and muscle contractions.
Rare pancreatitis.
Rare systemic lupus erythematosus.
Rare pseudolymphoma.
Rare aseptic meningitis.
Double vision, retinopathy, visual hallucinations, speech disturbances, peripheral neuritis (see Glossary).
Thrombophlebitis.
Rare porphyria.
Vitamin D deficiency (especially if other risk factors are present). This may lead to osteoporosis.

▷ **Possible Effects on Sexual Function**

Decreased libido and/or impotence (13%), male infertility. This drug is used to control hypersexuality (exaggerated sexual behavior) that can result from injury to the temporal lobe of the brain.

▷ **Adverse Effects That May Mimic Natural Diseases or Disorders**

Liver reactions may suggest viral hepatitis.

Rare lung reactions may suggest interstitial pneumonitis.

Natural Diseases or Disorders That May Be Activated by This Drug

Latent psychosis, systemic lupus erythematosus.

Possible Effects on Laboratory Tests

Complete blood cell: decreased red cells, hemoglobin, white cells and platelets; increased eosinophils, increased white cells.

Blood calcium level: decreased.

Blood prothrombin time: decreased.

Thyroid hormones: falsely decreased blood levels.

Blood urea nitrogen level (BUN): increased.

Liver function tests: increased liver enzymes (ALT/GPT, AST/GOT and alkaline phosphatase), increased bilirubin.

Urine pregnancy tests: false negative or inconclusive results with Prepurex, Predictor, Gonavislide, Pregnosticon.

CAUTION

1. Should be used only after less toxic drugs have failed.
2. *Before* the first dose is taken, blood cell counts, liver function tests and kidney function tests should be obtained.
3. Careful periodic testing for blood cell or bone marrow toxicity is *mandatory.*
4. *Should not be used* to prevent recurrence of trigeminal neuralgia when it is in remission.
5. *Do not stop this drug suddenly* if it is being used to control seizures.
6. If exposed to humidity, the tablet form hardens; this results in poor absorption from the gastrointestinal tract and erratic control of seizures. Store this drug in a cool, dry place; avoid bathrooms or other humid areas.

Precautions for Use

By Infants and Children: Safety and effectiveness by those under 6 years of age not established. Careful testing of blood production, liver and kidney function must be performed regularly. This drug can reduce the effectiveness of other anticonvulsant drugs. Blood levels of all anticonvulsant drugs should be checked if this drug is added to the treatment program.

By Those over 60 Years of Age: Can cause confusion and agitation. Watch for aggravation of glaucoma, coronary artery disease (angina) or prostatism (see Glossary).

▷ **Advisability of Use During Pregnancy**

Pregnancy Category: C. See Pregnancy Code at the back of this book.

Animal studies: Rat studies reveal significant birth defects.

Human studies: Adequate studies of pregnant women are not available.

Avoid completely during the first 3 months. Use during the last 6 months only if clearly needed.

Advisability of Use if Breast-Feeding
Presence of this drug in breast milk: Yes.
Avoid drug or refrain from nursing.

Habit-Forming Potential: None.

Effects of Overdosage: Dizziness, drowsiness, disorientation, tremor, involuntary movements, nausea, vomiting, flushed skin, dilated pupils, stupor progressing to coma.

Possible Effects of Long-Term Use: Water retention (edema), impaired liver function, possible jaundice.

Suggested Periodic Examinations While Taking This Drug (at physician's discretion)
Complete blood counts weekly during the first 3 months of treatment, and then monthly until the drug is stopped. Liver and kidney function tests. Complete eye examinations.

▷ **While Taking This Drug, Observe the Following**
Foods: No restrictions. There may be a minor increase in absorption if taken with food.
Beverages: No restrictions. May be taken with milk.
▷ *Alcohol:* Avoid alcohol use, unless your doctor approves alcohol use.
Tobacco Smoking: No interactions expected.
▷ *Other Drugs*
Carbamazepine may ***increase*** the effects of
• sedatives, tranquilizers, hypnotics, narcotics, and enhance their sedative effects.
Carbamazepine may ***decrease*** the effects of
• antidepressants (see Drug Classes).
• corticosteroids (see Drug Classes).
• cyclosporine (Sandimmune).
• doxycycline (Doxy-II, Vibramycin, etc.).
• felodipine (Plendil).
• haloperidol (Haldol) or other phenothiazines.
• isradipine (Dynacirc).
• itraconazole (Sporanox).
• birth control pills (oral contraceptives) and result in pregnancy.
• tetracyclines (see Drug Classes).
• valproic acid (Depakene, etc.).
• warfarin (Coumadin). Increased frequency of INR testing is indicated.
Carbamazepine ***taken concurrently*** with
• clozapine (Clozaril) may result in serious bone marrow suppression.
• felbamate (Felbatol) may result in decreased carbamazepine levels and seizures.
• lithium may cause serious neurological problems: Confusion, drowsiness, weakness, unsteadiness, tremors, and twitching.
• monoamine oxidase (MAO) type A inhibitor drugs (see Drug Classes) may cause severe toxic reactions.
• phenytoin (Dilantin, etc.) may cause unpredictable fluctuations of blood levels of both drugs and impair seizure control.
• terfenadine (Seldane) may result in carbamazepine toxicity.
• theophylline (Theo-Dur, etc.) may reduce the effects of both drugs.

The following drugs may *increase* the effects of carbamazepine
- cimetidine (Tagamet).
- danazol (Danocrine).
- diltiazem (Cardizem)—and perhaps other calcium channel blockers.
- fluvoxamine (Luvox) and result in toxicity.
- isoniazid (INH).
- macrolide antibiotics—erythromycins and clarithromycin.
- nicotinamide (nicotinic acid amide).
- propoxyphene (Darvon, Darvocet, etc.).
- rifampin and result in toxicity.
- troleandomycin (Tao).
- verapamil (Calan, Isoptin).

▷ *Driving, Hazardous Activities:* Can cause dizziness, drowsiness or blurred vision. Adjust activities.

Aviation Note: The use of this drug *is a disqualification* for piloting. Consult a designated Aviation Medical Examiner.

Exposure to Sun: This drug can cause photosensitivity (see Glossary). Use caution until sensitivity to sun is known.

Heavy Exercise or Exertion: Use caution if you have coronary artery disease. Can intensify angina and reduce tolerance for physical activity.

Occurrence of Unrelated Illness: Because of potential for serious adverse effects, you MUST tell each physician and dentist you see that you take carbamazepine.

Discontinuation: If treating trigeminal neuralgia, every 3 months attempts to reduce the maintenance dose or to stop this drug are needed. If used to control epilepsy, this drug *must not be stopped abruptly.*

Special Storage Instructions

Store the tablet form of this drug in a cool, dry place. Protect it from exposure to humid conditions (**do NOT store in a bathroom medicine cabinet**) as the tablets may lose potency.

CARTEOLOL (KAR tee oh lohl)

Introduced: 1983   **Prescription:** USA: Yes   **Available as Generic:** No   **Class:** Antihypertensive, beta-adrenergic blocker   **Controlled Drug:** USA: No

Brand Name: Cartrol, Ocupress, Optipress

BENEFITS versus RISKS	
Possible Benefits	*Possible Risks*
EFFECTIVE, WELL-TOLERATED ANTIHYPERTENSIVE	CONGESTIVE HEART FAILURE in advanced heart disease
EFFECTIVE GLAUCOMA TREATMENT	Worsening of angina in coronary heart disease (abrupt withdrawal)
	Masking of low blood sugar (hypoglycemia) in drug-treated diabetics
	Provocation of asthma in asthmatics

▷ **Principal Uses**

As a Single Drug Product: Uses currently included in FDA approved labeling: (1) Treatment of mild to moderate high blood pressure. May be used alone or in combination with other drugs, such as diuretics; (2) helps lower eye (intraocular) pressure in people with glaucoma.

Other (unlabeled) generally accepted uses: (1) Effective in helping increase the amount of exercise which can be performed before angina occurs; (2) can have a role in helping decrease aggressive behavior; (3) decreases the occurrence of abnormal heart rhythms; (3) other beta blockers have shown benefits in treating patients after heart attacks; however, studies using carteolol have not been performed; (4) may help lessen panic attacks.

How This Drug Works: By blocking certain actions of the sympathetic nervous system, this drug

- reduces the rate and contraction force of the heart, lowering the ejection pressure of blood leaving the heart.
- reduces the extent of blood vessel wall contraction, resulting in relaxation and expansion and lowering of blood pressure.
- reduces elevated eye pressure (intraocular) and relieves glaucoma symptoms.

Available Dosage Forms and Strengths

Tablets — 2.5 mg, 5 mg

Ophthalmic solution — 1 %

▷ **Usual Adult Dosage Range:**   For high blood pressure (hypertension): Initially 2.5 mg once daily. The dose may be increased gradually by 2.5 mg/day at intervals of 2 weeks as needed and tolerated up to 10 mg/day. For maintenance, 2.5 to 7.5 mg once daily is usually adequate. The total daily dose should not exceed 10 mg.

For glaucoma: One drop in the affected eye or eyes two times a day. **Note: Actual dosage and administration schedule must be determined by the physician for each patient individually.**

Conditions Requiring Dosing Adjustments

Liver function: Decreased doses needed in severe liver failure.

Kidney function: The kidney is the main route of elimination for this drug. Dosing interval **MUST** be decreased in kidney failure. In severe compromise, the drug is given every 48 to 72 hours.

▷ **Dosing Instructions:**   Tablet may be crushed and taken without regard to eating. Do not stop this drug abruptly.

Usual Duration of Use: Use on a regular schedule for up to 3 weeks may be needed to see this drug's effectiveness in lowering blood pressure. Long-term use of this drug (months to years) will be determined by the benefit in lowering your blood pressure over time and your response to a treatment program of weight reduction, salt restriction, smoking cessation, etc. See your doctor on a regular basis.

Possible Advantages of This Drug

Adequate control of blood pressure with a single daily dose.

Causes less slowing of the heart rate than most other beta blocker drugs.

▷ **This Drug Should Not Be Taken If**

- you have bronchial asthma
- you have had an allergic reaction to it previously.

- you have congestive heart failure.
- you have an abnormally slow heart rate or a serious heart block.
- you have a dissecting aortic aneurysm (ask your doctor).

▷ **Inform Your Physician Before Taking This Drug If**
- you have had an adverse reaction to any beta blocker (see Drug Classes).
- you have serious heart disease or episodes of heart failure.
- you have had hay fever (allergic rhinitis), asthma, chronic bronchitis or emphysema.
- you have a history of overactive thyroid function (hyperthyroidism).
- you have a history of low blood sugar (hypoglycemia).
- you have a history of diabetes.
- you have impaired liver or kidney function.
- you have diabetes or myasthenia gravis.
- you have a circulation problem (Raynaud's disorder, claudication pains in legs).
- you take any form of digitalis, quinidine or reserpine, or any calcium blocker drug (see Drug Classes).
- you plan to have surgery under general anesthesia in the near future.

Possible Side Effects (natural, expected, and unavoidable drug actions)
Lethargy and fatigability, cold extremities, slow heart rate, light-headedness in upright position (see Orthostatic Hypotension in Glossary).

▷ **Possible Adverse Effects** (unusual, unexpected, and infrequent reactions)
If any of the following develop, consult your physician promptly for guidance.
Mild Adverse Effects
Allergic Reactions: Skin rash (rare).
Dizziness, nervousness, drowsiness, insomnia, abnormal dreams.
Indigestion, nausea, vomiting, constipation, diarrhea.
Slight increase in blood potassium.
Cough, wheezing, or sinusitis (rare).
Joint and muscle discomfort, numbness of fingers or toes.
Episodic difficulty walking (intermittent claudication).
Tearing and irritation with use in the eye.
Serious Adverse Effects
Mental depression, anxiety.
Chest pain, irregular heartbeat, shortness of breath, can cause congestive heart failure.
Induction of bronchial asthma (in asthmatic patients).
Aggravation of myasthenia gravis.
May hide symptoms of low blood sugar.

▷ **Possible Effects on Sexual Function:**   Decreased libido, impotence.

▷ **Adverse Effects That May Mimic Natural Diseases or Disorders**
Decreased extremity blood flow may mimic Raynaud's phenomenon (see Glossary).

Natural Diseases or Disorders That May Be Activated by This Drug
Raynaud's disease, intermittent claudication, myasthenia gravis.

Possible Effects on Laboratory Tests
Blood creatine kinase level: increased.
Blood potassium: slight increase.

CAUTION
1. **Do not stop this drug suddenly** without the knowledge of your doctor. Carry a note that says you are taking this drug.
2. Ask your physician or pharmacist before using nasal decongestants. These can cause sudden increases in blood pressure when combined with beta blocker drugs.
3. Report any new tendency to emotional depression.

Precautions for Use
By Infants and Children: Safety and effectiveness by those under 12 years of age not established. However, if this drug is used, watch for the development of low blood sugar (hypoglycemia) especially if meals are skipped.
By Those over 60 Years of Age: **Caution.** Unacceptably high blood pressure should be reduced without creating excessively low blood pressure. Treatment should begin with small doses, and blood pressure should be checked often. Sudden and excessive reduction of blood pressure can lead to stroke or heart attack. Watch for dizziness, tendency to fall, confusion, hallucinations, depression or urinary frequency.

▷ **Advisability of Use During Pregnancy**
Pregnancy Category: C. See Pregnancy Code at the back of this book.
Animal studies: No birth defects due to this drug found in rat or rabbit studies.
Human studies: Adequate studies of pregnant women are not available.
Use this drug only if clearly needed. Ask physician for guidance.

Advisability of Use if Breast-Feeding
Presence of this drug in breast milk: Unknown in humans, yes in animals.
Avoid drug or refrain from nursing.

Habit-Forming Potential: None.

Effects of Overdosage: Weakness, slow pulse, low blood pressure, fainting, cold and sweaty skin, congestive heart failure, possible coma and convulsions.

Possible Effects of Long-Term Use: Reduced heart reserve and eventual heart failure in susceptible individuals with advanced heart disease.

Suggested Periodic Examinations While Taking This Drug (at physician's discretion)
Measurements of blood pressure, evaluation of heart function.

▷ **While Taking This Drug, Observe the Following**
Foods: No restrictions. Avoid excessive salt intake.
Beverages: No restrictions. May be taken with milk.
▷ *Alcohol:* Use caution. Alcohol may exaggerate this drug's ability to lower the blood pressure and may increase its mild sedative effect.
Tobacco Smoking: Nicotine may reduce this drug's effectiveness in treating high blood pressure. In addition, high doses may worsen constriction of the bronchial tubes caused by regular smoking.
▷ *Other Drugs*
Carteolol may **increase** the effects of
• other antihypertensive drugs, and cause excessive lowering of the blood pressure. Dosage adjustments may be necessary.

- reserpine (Ser-Ap-Es, etc.), and cause sedation, depression, slowing of the heart rate and low blood pressure. This combination is best avoided.
- theophyllines (aminophylline, dyphylline, oxtriphylline, etc.).
- verapamil (Calan, Isoptin), and cause excessive depression of heart function; monitor this combination closely.

Carteolol *taken concurrently* with

- amiodarone (Codarone) may cause severe slowing of the heart and sinus arrest. Do not combine these agents.
- clonidine (Catapres) requires close monitoring for rebound high blood pressure if clonidine is stopped while carteolol is still being taken. Severe rebound hypertension may occur.
- diltiazem (Cardizem) (like verapamil) may be very helpful in patients with normal heart function, but may result in
AV conduction problems.
- epinephrine (Adrenalin, etc.) may cause sudden rise in blood pressure followed by slowing of the heart rate. Avoid the combination.
- ergot preparations (ergotamine, methysergide, etc.) may enhance serious ergot-induced constriction of peripheral circulation.
- fluvoxamine (Luvox) may result in dangerous slowing of the heart or dangerously low blood pressure.
- insulin requires close monitoring to avoid hypoglycemia (see Glossary).
- nifedipine (dihydroperidine) may result in excessive lowering of the blood pressure.
- oral hypoglycemic agents (see Drug Classes) may cause prolonged recovery from hypoglycemia should it occur.
- phenothiazines (see Drug Classes) can cause increased effects of both drugs.

The following drugs may *decrease* the effects of carteolol

- indomethacin (Indocin), and possibly other "aspirin substitutes," or NSAIDs may impair carteolol's antihypertensive effect.

▷ *Driving, Hazardous Activities:* Use caution until the full extent of fatigue, dizziness and blood pressure change have been determined.

Aviation Note: The use of this drug *is a disqualification* for piloting. Consult a designated Aviation Medical Examiner.

Exposure to Sun: No restrictions.

Exposure to Heat: Caution advised. Hot environments can lower the blood pressure and exaggerate the effects of this drug.

Exposure to Cold: Caution advised. The elderly should take precautions to prevent hypothermia (see Glossary).

Heavy Exercise or Exertion: Avoid exertion that produces light-headedness, excessive fatigue or muscle cramping. The use of this drug can cause dangerously increased blood pressure with isometric exercise.

Occurrence of Unrelated Illness: Fever can lower the blood pressure and require decreased doses. Illnesses that cause nausea or vomiting may interrupt the regular dosage schedule. Ask your physician for guidance.

Discontinuation: **DO NOT STOP this drug suddenly**. If possible, gradual reduction of dose over a period of 2 to 3 weeks is recommended. Ask your physician for help.

CEFACLOR (SEF a klor)

Introduced: 1979   **Prescription:** USA: Yes; Canada: Yes   **Available as Generic:** Yes   **Class:** Antibiotic, cephalosporin   **Controlled Drug:** USA: No; Canada: No
Brand Name: Ceclor

BENEFITS versus RISKS	
Possible Benefits	*Possible Risks*
EFFECTIVE TREATMENT OF INFECTIONS due to susceptible microorganisms	ALLERGIC REACTIONS, mild to severe (may also be seen in those allergic to penicillin) Drug-induced colitis (rare) Superinfections (see Glossary)

▷ **Principal Uses**

As a Single Drug Product: Uses currently included in FDA approved labeling: (1) To treat certain infections of the skin and skin structures, the upper and lower respiratory tract (including middle ear infections and "strep" throat), some urinary tract and postoperative wound infections.

Other unlabeled, generally accepted uses: (1) may have an alternative role in helping prevent rheumatic fever if the bacteria are resistant to erythromycin.

How This Drug Works: This drug destroys susceptible infecting bacteria by interfering with their ability to produce new protective cell walls as they multiply and grow.

Available Dosage Forms and Strengths

Capsules — 250 mg, 500 mg

Oral suspension — 125 mg, 187 mg, 250 mg, 375 mg per 5-ml

▷ **Usual Adult Dosage Range:** 250 to 500 mg/8 hours. Total daily dose should not exceed 4 grams (4,000 mg).

In children: 20 to 40 mg per kg of body weight per day is given in divided doses every 8 hours. Maximum dose is 1 gram (1,000 mg) daily. **Note: Actual dosage and administration schedule must be determined by the physician for each patient individually.**

Conditions Requiring Dosing Adjustments

Liver function: Elimination by the liver has not been identified as yet.

Kidney function: Cefaclor is 40–80% eliminated by the kidney. For creatinine clearances (CrCl) of 10–50 ml/min., 50–100% of the usual dose at the normal interval is used. For CrCl of less than 10 ml/min., 50% of the usual dose at the usual time is given.

▷ **Dosing Instructions:** May be taken on an empty stomach or with food if stomach irritation occurs. Capsule may be opened for administration. Shake suspension well before measuring (use a measured dose cup or other calibrated dose measure) dose. Take the full course prescribed.

Usual Duration of Use: Continual use on a regular schedule for 3 to 5 days is usually necessary to determine this drug's effectiveness in controlling the infection under treatment. Response varies with the nature of the infection. Total treatment time will vary from 1 to 4 weeks. Some infections **require**

10 consecutive days of treatment to prevent the development of rheumatic fever. Follow your doctor's instructions about how long to take this medicine

▷ **This Drug Should Not Be Taken If**
- you are allergic to any cephalosporin antibiotic (see Drug Classes).

▷ **Inform Your Physician Before Taking This Drug If**
- you have a history of allergy to any penicillin (see Drug Classes).
- you have a history of regional enteritis or ulcerative colitis.
- you have impaired kidney function.

Possible Side Effects (natural, expected, and unavoidable drug actions)
Superinfections (see Glossary).

▷ **Possible Adverse Effects** (unusual, unexpected, and infrequent reactions)
If any of the following develop, consult your physician promptly for guidance.

Mild Adverse Effects
Allergic Reactions: Skin rash, itching, hives.
Nausea and vomiting or mild diarrhea (most common adverse effects).
Sore mouth or tongue.
Mild and reversible decrease in white blood cells (neutrophils).
Confusion, nervousness, insomnia, dizziness (rare).

Serious Adverse Effects
Allergic Reactions: Drug fever (see Glossary), anaphylactic reaction (see Glossary), Stevens-Johnson syndrome.
Idiosyncratic Reactions: Minor and temporary changes in white blood cell counts and liver function tests (infrequent).
Genital itching (may represent a fungus superinfection).
Serum sickness (itching, joint pain, and irritated swellings).
Increased BUN or serum creatinine (very rare).
Severe diarrhea, possibly indicating a drug-induced form of colitis (rare).
Increases in liver enzymes and jaundice (cholestatic) (rare).

▷ **Possible Effects on Sexual Function:**   None reported.

▷ **Adverse Effects That May Mimic Natural Diseases or Disorders**
Skin rash and fever may resemble measles.

Possible Effects on Laboratory Tests
Blood platelet counts: decreased (rare).
Liver enzymes: increased.
BUN and creatinine: increased.

CAUTION
This drug can cause a false positive test result for urine sugar when using Clinitest tablets, Benedict's solution or Fehling's solution, but not with Tes-Tape.

Precautions for Use
By Infants and Children: Not recommended for use in infants less than 1 month old. The maximal dose in children should not exceed 1 gram/24 hours.
By Those over 60 Years of Age: Dosage must be carefully individualized and based upon evaluation of kidney function. Natural changes in the skin may predispose to severe and prolonged itching reactions in the genital and anal regions. Such reactions should be reported promptly. The natural decline

in kidney function often requires a decrease in dose and achieves the same effect as a larger dose.

▷ **Advisability of Use During Pregnancy**
Pregnancy Category: B. See Pregnancy Code at the back of this book.
Animal studies: No birth defects reported.
Human studies: Information from adequate studies of pregnant women is not available.
Generally considered to be safe. Ask physician for guidance.

Advisability of Use if Breast-Feeding
Presence of this drug in breast milk: Yes, in small amounts.
Ask your doctor for advice.

Habit-Forming Potential: None.

Effects of Overdosage: Nausea, vomiting, stomach cramps and/or diarrhea.

Possible Effects of Long-Term Use: Superinfections (see Glossary).

Suggested Periodic Examinations While Taking This Drug (at physician's discretion)
Complete blood cell counts.
Liver enzymes.
BUN and creatinine with long-term therapy.

▷ **While Taking This Drug, Observe the Following**
Foods: Delays the absorption of this drug and may result in decreased antibiotic effect.
Beverages: No restrictions. May be taken with milk.
▷ *Alcohol:* No interactions expected.
Tobacco Smoking: No interactions expected.
▷ *Other Drugs*
Cefaclor *taken concurrently* with
• use of this drug with any aminoglycoside antibiotic (see Drug Classes) may result in increased kidney (renal) toxicity.
• birth control pills (oral contraceptives) may result in **decreased effectiveness** in preventing conception and pregnancy.
• loop diuretics such as ethacrynic acid may result in increased risk of kidney (renal) toxicity.
• probenecid (Benemid) will slow the elimination of cefaclor, resulting in higher blood levels and prolonged effect.
▷ *Driving, Hazardous Activities:* Usually no restrictions.
Aviation Note: The use of this drug *may be a disqualification* for piloting. Consult a designated Aviation Medical Examiner.
Exposure to Sun: No restrictions.
Special Storage Instructions: Oral suspension should be refrigerated.
Observe the Following Expiration Times: Do not take the oral suspension of this drug if it is older than 14 days.

CEFADROXIL (sef a DROX il)

Introduced: 1977   **Prescription:** USA: Yes; Canada: Yes   **Available as Generic:** Yes   **Class:** Antibiotic, cephalosporin   **Controlled Drug:** USA: No; Canada: No
Brand Names: Duricef, Ultracef

BENEFITS versus RISKS	
Possible Benefits	*Possible Risks*
EFFECTIVE TREATMENT OF INFECTIONS due to susceptible microorganisms	ALLERGIC REACTIONS, mild to severe
	Drug-induced colitis (rare)
	Superinfections (see Glossary)

▷ **Principal Uses**
   As a Single Drug Product: Uses currently included in FDA approved labeling: (1) To treat some infections of the skin and skin structures, the upper respiratory tract (including tonsillitis and "strep" throat) and certain infections of the urinary tract.
   Other (unlabeled) generally accepted uses: None.

How This Drug Works: This drug destroys susceptible infecting bacteria by interfering with their ability to produce new protective cell walls as they multiply and grow.

Available Dosage Forms and Strengths
            Capsules — 500 mg, 1000 mg
   Gelatin capsules (Canada) — 500 mg
            Oral suspension — 125 mg, 250 mg, 500 mg per 5-ml
            Tablets — 1000 mg (1 gram)

▷ **Usual Adult Dosage Range:** Skin infections—500 mg/12 hours, or 1 gram daily. "Strep" throat—500 mg/12 hours for 10 days. Urinary tract infections—500 mg to 1 gram/12 hours, or 1 to 2 grams daily. Total daily dosage should not exceed 6 grams.
   For children: 30 mg per kg per day, given in divided doses every 12 hours.
   Note: Actual dosage and administration schedule must be determined by the physician for each patient individually.

Conditions Requiring Dosing Adjustments
   Liver function: The liver is involved to a minimal degree, and no dosing changes are anticipated in liver compromise.
   Kidney function: With creatinine clearances of 10–50 ml/min., use the usual doses every 12 to 24 hours. For creatinine clearances less than 10 ml/min., usual doses are given every 24–48 hours.

▷ **Dosing Instructions:** May be taken on an empty stomach or with food if stomach irritation occurs. Capsule may be opened for administration. Shake suspension well before measuring dose. Take the full course prescribed.

Usual Duration of Use: Continual use on a regular schedule for 3 to 5 days is usually necessary to determine this drug's effectiveness in controlling the infection under treatment. Response varies with the nature of the infection. Total treatment time will vary from 1 to 4 weeks. Certain infections require that this drug be taken for 10 consecutive days to prevent the development of rheumatic fever. Follow your physician's instructions about how long to take this medicine.

▷ **This Drug Should Not Be Taken If**
  • you are allergic to any cephalosporin antibiotic (see Drug Classes).

▷ **Inform Your Physician Before Taking This Drug If**
  • you have a history of allergy to any form of penicillin (see Drug Classes).
  • you have a history of regional enteritis or ulcerative colitis.
  • you have impaired kidney function.

Possible Side Effects (natural, expected, and unavoidable drug actions)
  Superinfections (see Glossary).

▷ **Possible Adverse Effects** (unusual, unexpected, and infrequent reactions)
  If any of the following develop, consult your physician promptly for guidance.

Mild Adverse Effects
  Allergic Reactions: Skin rash, itching, hives, localized swellings.
  Headache, drowsiness, dizziness.
  Indigestion, stomach cramping, nausea, vomiting, mild diarrhea, sore mouth or tongue.

Serious Adverse Effects
  Allergic Reactions: Drug fever (see Glossary), joint aches and pains, anaphylactic reaction (see Glossary).
  Idiosyncratic Reactions: Minor and temporary changes in white blood cell counts and liver function tests (infrequent).
  Genital itching (may represent a fungus superinfection).
  Severe diarrhea, possibly indicating a drug-induced form of colitis (rare).

▷ **Possible Effects on Sexual Function:**   None reported.

▷ **Adverse Effects That May Mimic Natural Diseases or Disorders**
  Skin rash and fever may resemble measles.

Possible Effects on Laboratory Tests
  No significant effects reported.

CAUTION
  In the management of diabetes it should be noted that this drug can cause a false positive test result for urine sugar when using Clinitest tablets, Benedict's solution or Fehling's solution, but not with Tes-Tape.

Precautions for Use
  By Infants and Children: Dosage is based upon weight, and must be determined by the physician for each individual. Follow your physician's instructions exactly.
  By Those over 60 Years of Age: Dosage must be carefully individualized and based upon evaluation of kidney function. Natural changes in the skin may predispose to severe and prolonged itching reactions in the genital and anal regions. Such reactions should be reported promptly.

▷ **Advisability of Use During Pregnancy**
  Pregnancy Category: B. See Pregnancy Code at the back of this book.
    Animal studies: No birth defects reported.
    Human studies: Information from adequate studies of pregnant women is not available.
    Generally considered to be safe. Ask physician for guidance.

Advisability of Use if Breast-Feeding
>Presence of this drug in breast milk: Yes, in small amounts.
>Ask your doctor for guidance.

Habit-Forming Potential: None.

Effects of Overdosage: Nausea, vomiting, stomach cramps and/or diarrhea.

Possible Effects of Long-Term Use: Superinfections (see Glossary).

Suggested Periodic Examinations While Taking This Drug (at physician's discretion)
>Complete blood cell counts. Liver and kidney function tests.

▷ **While Taking This Drug, Observe the Following**
>*Foods:* No restrictions.
>*Beverages:* No restrictions. May be taken with milk.

▷ *Alcohol:* No interactions expected.
>*Tobacco Smoking:* No interactions expected.

▷ *Other Drugs*
>Cefadroxil *taken concurrently* with
>• aminoglycoside antibiotics (see Drug Classes) may cause an increased risk of kidney toxicity.
>• birth control pills (oral contraceptives) may result in **loss of contraceptive effect and pregnancy**.
>• probenecid (Benemid) will slow the elimination of cefadroxil, resulting in higher blood levels and prolonged effect.

▷ *Driving, Hazardous Activities:* Usually no restrictions. If drowsiness or dizziness occurs, restrict activities accordingly.
>*Aviation Note:* The use of this drug *may be a disqualification* for piloting. Consult a designated Aviation Medical Examiner.
>*Exposure to Sun:* No restrictions.
>*Special Storage Instructions:* Oral suspension should be refrigerated.
>*Observe the Following Expiration Times:* Do not take the oral suspension of this drug if it is older than 14 days.

CEFIXIME (sef IX eem)

Introduced: 1986   **Prescription:** USA: Yes   **Available as Generic:** No   **Class:** Antibiotic, cephalosporin   **Controlled Drug:** USA: No
Brand Name: Suprax

BENEFITS versus RISKS	
Possible Benefits	*Possible Risks*
EFFECTIVE TREATMENT OF INFECTIONS due to susceptible microorganisms	ALLERGIC REACTIONS Drug-induced colitis (rare) Superinfections (see Glossary) Low white blood cells (rare) Low blood platelets (rare)

▷ **Principal Uses**
>*As a Single Drug Product:* Uses currently included in FDA approved labeling: (1) Treats some infections of the middle ear, tonsils, throat, bronchial tubes and urinary tract.

Other (unlabeled) generally accepted uses: (1) Effective in uncomplicated cervical or urethral gonorrhea; (2) may have a role in treating resistant Salmonella infections; (3) helps Whipple's disease as part of combination therapy.

How This Drug Works: Destroys susceptible infecting bacteria by interfering with their ability to produce new protective cell walls as they multiply and grow.

Available Dosage Forms and Strengths

Oral suspension — 100 mg per 5 ml
Tablets — 200 mg, 400 mg

▷ **Usual Adult Dosage Range:**   400 mg daily, taken as a single dose or as 200 mg every 12 hours.

For children over 6 months of age: 8 mg per kg/day, all in one dose or divided into 2 doses.

For treatment of multi-drug resistant Salmonella: 20 mg per kg per day in divided doses every 12 hours for at least 12 days. For treatment of uncomplicated gonorrhea: 400 to 800 mg as a single dose. **Note: Actual dosage and administration schedule must be determined by the physician for each patient individually.**

Conditions Requiring Dosing Adjustments

Liver function: Dose changes not needed.

Kidney function: Dose **must be decreased** in mild to moderate kidney problems. In severe failure, a single dose every 48 hours is needed.

▷ **Dosing Instructions:**   May take on an empty stomach or with food if stomach irritation occurs. The tablet may be crushed and mixed with food (such as applesauce or ice cream) to help swallowing. Take the full course prescribed.

Usual Duration of Use: Continual use on a regular schedule for 3 to 5 days is needed to see this drug's effectiveness in controlling infections. Some infections require that the drug be taken for 10 consecutive days to prevent rheumatic fever. Follow your physician's instructions regarding duration of use. Call your doctor if your original symptoms and fever persist for more than 48 hours or worsen once you start taking this medicine. This may be a sign of bacteria which are not killed by the antibiotic (antimicrobial resistance).

▷ **This Drug Should Not Be Taken If**

- you are allergic to cephalosporin antibiotics (see Drug Classes).
- you have active colitis of any type.

▷ **Inform Your Physician Before Taking This Drug If**

- you are allergic to penicillin (see Drug Classes).
- you have a history of regional enteritis or ulcerative colitis.
- you have impaired kidney function.
- you have a history of low platelets or white blood cells.

Possible Side Effects (natural, expected, and unavoidable drug actions)

Superinfections (see Glossary): vaginitis (yeast infection).

▷ **Possible Adverse Effects** (unusual, unexpected, and infrequent reactions)

If any of the following develop, consult your physician promptly for guidance.

Mild Adverse Effects
Allergic Reactions: Skin rash, hives, itching, drug fever (see Glossary).
Nausea, indigestion, loose stools, diarrhea, abdominal pain.
Headache, dizziness.
Serious Adverse Effects
Allergic Reactions: Anaphylactoid reactions.
Severe diarrhea, possibly indicating a drug-induced form of colitis (rare). This can occur during use of the drug or months after it was stopped.
Low blood platelets (rare).
Low white blood cells (rare).
Kidney toxicity (rare).
Superinfections (see Glossary).
Other second- and third-generation cephalosporin have contributed to extended blood clotting times in debilitated patients. Caution should be given to long-term use of this drug in those with existing blood clotting disorders or in debilitated patients. Baseline INR testing may be needed.

▷ **Possible Effects on Sexual Function:** None reported.

▷ **Adverse Effects That May Mimic Natural Diseases or Disorders**
Skin rash may resemble measles.

Possible Effects on Laboratory Tests
Complete blood cell counts: transient decreases in white blood cells and platelets; no serious consequences reported.
INR: may be increased.

CAUTION
1. Otitis media (middle ear infection) should be treated with the oral suspension. Tablets should not be substituted for the suspension.
2. This drug can cause a false positive test result for urine sugar with using Clinitest tablets, Benedict's solution or Fehling's solution. Also causes a false positive reaction for urine ketones (nitroprusside tests).

Precautions for Use
By Infants and Children: Safety and effectiveness for use by those under 6 months of age have not been established.
By Those over 60 Years of Age: Must be individualized based on kidney function. Natural skin changes may make severe and prolonged itching reactions in genitals and anus likely. Such reactions should be reported promptly.

▷ **Advisability of Use During Pregnancy**
Pregnancy Category: B. See Pregnancy Code at the back of this book.
Animal studies: No birth defects reported in mouse and rat studies.
Human studies: Adequate studies of pregnant women are not available.
Generally considered to be safe. Ask physician for guidance.

Advisability of Use if Breast-Feeding
Presence of this drug in breast milk: Unknown.
Ask your doctor for help.

Habit-Forming Potential: None.

Effects of Overdosage: Nausea, vomiting, stomach cramps and/or diarrhea.

Possible Effects of Long-Term Use: Superinfections (see Glossary).

Suggested Periodic Examinations While Taking This Drug (at physician's discretion)
Complete blood cell counts.

▷ **While Taking This Drug, Observe the Following**
Foods: No restrictions.
Beverages: No restrictions. May be taken with milk.
▷ *Alcohol:* No interactions expected.
Tobacco Smoking: No interactions expected.
▷ *Other Drugs*
Cefixime *taken concurrently* with
- aminoglycoside antibiotics (see Drug Classes) may pose an increased risk of kidney toxicity.
▷ *Driving, Hazardous Activities:* Usually no restrictions. Observe for the rare occurrence of dizziness.
Aviation Note: The use of this drug *may be a disqualification* for piloting. Consult a designated Aviation Medical Examiner.
Exposure to Sun: No restrictions.
Special Storage Instructions: Keep oral suspension at room temperature. Do not refrigerate. Shake well before measuring dose.
Observe the Following Expiration Time: Do not take the oral suspension of this drug if older than 14 days.

CEFPROZIL (SEF pro zil)

Introduced: 1991   **Prescription:** USA: Yes   **Available as Generic:** No   **Class:** Anti-infective, cephalosporin   **Controlled Drug:** USA: No
Brand Name: Cefzil

BENEFITS versus RISKS	
Possible Benefits	*Possible Risks*
EFFECTIVE TREATMENT OF INFECTIONS due to susceptible microorganisms	ALLERGIC REACTIONS, mild to severe
	Drug-induced colitis (rare)
	Superinfections (see Glossary)

▷ **Principal Uses**
As a Single Drug Product: Uses currently included in FDA approved labeling (when caused by susceptible organisms): (1) Treatment of upper respiratory tract infections: Pharyngitis, tonsillitis, otitis media; (2) treatment of lower respiratory tract infections: Acute bronchitis and worsening (exacerbation) of chronic bronchitis, bacterial pneumonia; (3) treatment of skin and skin structure infections.
Other (unlabeled) generally accepted uses: None.

How This Drug Works: This drug destroys susceptible infecting bacteria by interfering with their ability to produce new protective cell walls as they multiply and grow.

Available Dosage Forms and Strengths
Oral suspension — 125 mg, 250 mg per 5 ml
Tablets — 250 mg, 500 mg

▷ **Recommended Dosage Ranges** (Actual dosage and administration schedule must be determined by the physician for each patient individually.)

Infants and Children: For otitis media (6 months to 12 years of age)—15 mg/kg of body weight every 12 hours, for 10 days.

13 to 60 Years of Age: Pharyngitis or tonsillitis—500 mg every 24 hours (once daily), for 10 days.

Acute or chronic bronchitis—500 mg every 12 hours, for 10 days.

Bacterial pneumonia—250 mg three times a day for 14 days.

Skin or skin structure infections—250 to 500 mg every 12 to 24 hours, for 10 days.

Over 60 Years of Age: Same as 13 to 60 years of age. Decreased dose in kidney failure.

Conditions Requiring Dosing Adjustments
Liver function: The liver is not known to be involved in elimination of this drug.

Kidney function: With severe kidney failure, **half** the dose can be given at the usual time.

Phenylketonuria (PKU): The suspension has 28 mg of phenylalanine in every 5 ml. This may preclude use of the drug in these patients.

▷ **Dosing Instructions:** Can take on an empty stomach or with food if stomach irritation occurs. The tablet may be crushed and mixed with food (such as applesauce or ice cream) if needed to help swallowing. Shake the oral suspension well before measuring each dose. Take the full course prescribed.

Usual Duration of Use: Continual use on a regular schedule for 3 to 5 days is needed to see how effective treatment will be. Some infections require 10 consecutive days to prevent the development of rheumatic fever. Follow your physician's instructions regarding how long it should be taken.

▷ **This Drug Should Not Be Taken If**
• you are allergic to cephalosporins (see Drug Classes).

▷ **Inform Your Physician Before Taking This Drug If**
• you are allergic to penicillin (see Drug Classes).
• you have a history of regional enteritis or ulcerative colitis.
• you have impaired kidney function.
• you have been taking this medicine as directed for 48 hours and your fever and other symptoms have worsened.
• you have a history of blood clotting disorders.
• you have a history of low white blood cell count.

Possible Side Effects (natural, expected, and unavoidable drug actions)
Superinfections (see Glossary) (rare); vaginitis (rare).

▷ **Possible Adverse Effects** (unusual, unexpected, and infrequent reactions)
If any of the following develop, consult your physician promptly for guidance.

Mild Adverse Effects
Allergic Reactions: Skin rash (rare), hives (rare).
Nausea, vomiting (rare), mild diarrhea.

Headache or hyperactivity (rare), dizziness or confusion (rare).
Increased liver enzymes.
Serious Adverse Effects
Low white blood cell count (rare).
Increased time for clotting to occur.
▷ **Possible Effects on Sexual Function:**   None reported.
▷ **Adverse Effects That May Mimic Natural Diseases or Disorders**
Skin rash may resemble measles.
Possible Effects on Laboratory Tests
White blood cell counts: decreased (very rare).
BUN: increased (0.1%).
Liver function tests: increased liver enzymes (ALT/GPT, AST/GOT).
Extended PTT tests.
Direct Coomb's test: positive.
CAUTION
This drug may cause a false positive test result for urine sugar when using Clinitest tablets, Benedict's solution or Fehling's solution.
Precautions for Use
By Infants and Children: Safety and effectiveness for those under 6 months of age not established.
By Those over 60 Years of Age: Dose must be individualized based on kidney function. Natural changes in the skin may predispose to severe and prolonged itching in the genital and anal regions. Such reactions should be reported promptly.
▷ **Advisability of Use During Pregnancy**
Pregnancy Category: B. See Pregnancy Code at the back of this book.
Animal studies: No birth defects reported in mouse, rat and rabbit studies.
Human studies: Adequate studies of pregnant women are not available.
Generally considered to be safe. Ask physician for guidance.
Advisability of Use if Breast-Feeding
Presence of this drug in breast milk: Unknown.
Ask your doctor for guidance.
Habit-Forming Potential: None.
Effects of Overdosage: Nausea, vomiting, stomach cramps and/or diarrhea.
Possible Effects of Long-Term Use: Superinfections (see Glossary).
Suggested Periodic Examinations While Taking This Drug (at physician's discretion)
Complete blood counts.
▷ **While Taking This Drug, Observe the Following**
Foods: No restrictions.
Beverages: No restrictions. May be taken with milk.
▷ *Alcohol:* No interactions expected. Excessive alcohol intake may blunt the immune response.
Tobacco Smoking: No interactions expected.
▷ *Other Drugs*
Cefprozil *taken concurrently* with
• aminoglycosides (see Drug Classes) may result in increased kidney toxicity.
• probenecid (Benemid) may cause higher blood levels and prolonged effect.

▷ *Driving, Hazardous Activities:* Usually no restrictions. Observe for the rare occurrence of dizziness.

Aviation Note: The use of this drug *may be a disqualification* for piloting. Consult a designated Aviation Medical Examiner.

Exposure to Sun: No restrictions.

Special Storage Instructions: Oral suspensions should be refrigerated.

Observe the Following Expiration Times: Discard unused portion after 14 days.

CEFTRIAXONE (SEF try ax own)

Introduced: 1984   **Prescription:** USA: Yes; Canada: Yes   **Available as Generic:** USA: No; Canada: No   **Class:** Antibiotic, cephalosporin   **Controlled Drug:** USA: No; Canada: No

Brand Name: Rocephin

BENEFITS versus RISKS	
Possible Benefits	*Possible Risks*
HOME IV TREATMENT OF ADVANCED LYME DISEASE (STAGE TWO OR THREE) AFTER HOSPITAL INDUCTION (initiation of intravenous therapy in the hospital). HOME IV TREATMENT OF OSTEOMYELITIS (BONE INFECTIONS) AFTER HOSPITAL INDUCTION. Home IV treatment of other serious infections	PALPITATIONS Hematological effects: Thrombocytosis, leukopenia, and anemia Pseudomembranous colitis (a serious colon inflammation)

▷ **Principal Uses**

As a Single Drug Product: Uses currently included in FDA approved labeling: (1) Treatment of: Lower respiratory infections, skin and skin structure infections, urinary tract infections, uncomplicated gonorrhea, pelvic inflammatory disease, bacterial septicemia, bone and joint infections, intra-abdominal infections, diabetic foot infections, gonorrhea, prosthetic joint infections, meningitis and surgical prophylaxis.

Other (unlabeled) generally accepted uses: (1) Intravenous treatment of late (stage two or three) Lyme disease; (2) treatment of chancroid; (3) initial treatment of epididymitis; (4) Shigella infection; (5) sexual assault cases.

How This Drug Works: Ceftriaxone inhibits the ability of bacteria to make protective cell walls. Ceftriaxone usually causes the death of the bacteria.

Available Dosage Forms and Strengths

250 mg of Rocephin—Boxes of one or ten vial(s)

500 mg of Rocephin—Boxes of one or ten vial(s)

1 gm of Rocephin—Boxes of one or ten vial(s) or piggyback bottles of ten

2 gm of Rocephin—Boxes of ten vials, or piggyback bottles of ten

10 gm of Rocephin—Box of one

1 gm or 2 gm ADD-Vantage packaging

How To Store

Following reconstitution with 0.9% sodium chloride, 5% dextrose or sterile water for injection—ceftriaxone solutions having 100 mg per ml are stable for three (3) days at room temperature or ten (10) days in the refrigerator. Consult guidelines and outdates from your provider regarding frozen ceftriaxone.

▷ **Recommended Dosage Ranges (Actual dosage and administration schedule must be determined by the physician for each patient individually.)**

Infants and Children: For neonates and children less than 12 for treatment of serious infections caused by susceptible organisms (other than CNS infections such as meningitis) is 50 to 75 mg per kg (mg/kg) per day given in two equally divided doses twelve hours apart (not to exceed 2 grams daily). Some doctors suggest that neonates one week old or younger be given 50 mg/kg per day, and that neonates older than one week and weighing 2 kg or less also receive 50 mg/kg per day, and 50–75 mg/kg per day be given to neonates older than one week and weighing more than 2 kg.

For meningitis (caused by susceptible organisms) the dose for neonates and children 12 or younger is 100 mg/kg daily, divided into two equal doses given every 12 hours. The American Academy of Pediatrics suggests 80–100 mg/kg be given once daily or in two equally divided doses every 12 hours for children older than one month. Because the once daily regimen is relatively new, I suggest that the 12 hour regimen be used.

12 to 60 Years of Age: The dosing of ceftriaxone for treatment of most infections (caused by susceptible organisms) is: 1–2 grams daily or in equally divided doses two times a day depending on the type and severity of the infection. Children older than 12 can be given the adult dose. Some physicians recommend that CNS infections in adults may require 4 grams daily. This is the maximum adult dosage recommended by the manufacturer.

Uncomplicated gonorrhea caused by penicillinase producing strains of Neisseria gonorrhea (PPNG) or nonpenicillinase producing strains may be treated by a single IM 250 mg dose of ceftriaxone. Disseminated gonococcal infection should be treated by 1 (one) gram of ceftriaxone IV or IM once a day for seven days. Acute sexually transmitted epididymitis in adults may be treated with a single 250 mg IM dose of ceftriaxone followed by seven days of oral tetracycline or erythromycin. For treatment of acute pelvic inflammatory disease (PID), a single 250 mg IM dose of ceftriaxone should be given and then followed by 100 mg of oral doxycycline two times a day for 10–14 days.

Treatment of serious arthritis, cardiac or neurologic complications of early or late (stage two or three) Lyme disease:

Arthritis—Ceftriaxone at a dose of 2 grams IV daily for adults. Children should be given 75–100 mg/kg/day IV.

Serious CNS Disease—Ceftriaxone at a dose of 2 grams IV daily for 21 days in adults. Children can be treated with 75–100 mg/kg IV daily for 21 days.

Cardiac Disease—Ceftriaxone 2 grams IV per day for 21 days in adults. Children can be given 75–100 mg/kg/day IV.

Surgical prophylaxis—Although ceftriaxone is FDA approved for surgical prophylaxis, we do not recommend its routine use. Other readily available agents are equally as effective, and much less expensive. Ceftriaxone use for surgical prophylaxis also increases the potential for resistance to this drug, and could decrease its usefulness in treating later infections.

Over 60 Years of Age: Same as 12 to 60 years of age.

Conditions Requiring Dosing Adjustments

Liver function: Patients with both liver and kidney problems should have drug levels checked, and a maximum total daily dose of 2 grams.

Kidney function: Compromise of the kidneys alone (see above) is cause for careful monitoring.

▷ **Dosing Instructions:** Bring refrigerated IV solutions to room temperature before using them. Do not use any IV solutions which contain particles or precipitates (are cloudy). Do not use outdated solutions—they will not treat your infection as effectively as IVs that have not expired.

Usual Duration of Use: In general, therapy should be continued (except gonorrhea) for at least 48 hours after the infection is gone and you are asymptomatic. For invasive infections, antibiotic therapy is usually continued for 5–7 days after negative bacteriologic cultures are obtained.

Gram negative bacillary meningitis should be treated for at least 21 days.

Osteomyelitis (bone infection) may require six weeks (42 days) of intravenous therapy with reassessment when the course of antibiotics is completed.

Continual use on a regular schedule for three weeks is usually needed to see this drug's effectiveness in Lyme disease. Lyme tests may remain positive for a significant amount of time even though the infection has been cured.

Possible Advantages of This Drug

Once or twice a day dosing is especially convenient for home IV therapy. Can be used with other antibiotics for a synergistic (much larger effect than either drug alone) effect against bacteria.

Currently a "Drug of Choice"

For second and third stage Lyme disease, for treatment of chancroid, for treatment of meningitis and epiglotitis caused by Hemophilus influenzae, meningitis caused by Neisseria meningitidis, Neisseria gonorrhea, and Salmonella typhi.

▷ **This Drug Should Not Be Taken If**
- you have had an allergic reaction to any dosage form of it previously or to any other cephalosporin (see Drug Classes).
- you have active colitis of any type.

▷ **Inform Your Physician Before Taking This Drug If**
- you have a hematologic (blood) disorder such as anemia.
- you have liver or kidney problems.
- you have a history of regional enteritis or ulcerative colitis.
- you have an allergy to any prescription or nonprescription medicines.
- you have an allergy to penicillin.
- you have a history of gallbladder disease.
- you have a clotting disorder of the blood.
- you are pregnant or plan to become pregnant.
- you take other prescription or nonprescription medicines which were not discussed with your doctor when this medicine was prescribed.

Possible Side Effects (natural, expected, and unavoidable drug actions)

Superinfections (see glossary) such as vaginitis (a vaginal yeast infection), oral yeast infections, and overgrowth of organisms with long-term use.

▷ **Possible Adverse Effects** (unusual, unexpected, and infrequent reactions)
If any of the following develop, consult your physician promptly for guidance.

Mild Adverse Effects

Allergic Reactions: Skin rash (erythematous and urticarial) (rare), pruritus (itching), fever and chills (rare).

Headache, flushing, dizziness, and sweating (rare); palpitations (very rare).

Transient diarrhea (42–44%) of children and (28%) of adults; asymptomatic gall bladder concretions (43%) in children receiving 60–100 mg/kg/day in one study; diarrhea, nausea, and vomiting (very rare).

Pain and induration at the injection site (intramuscular use) (rare).

Increased liver enzymes (SGOT and SGPT); increased BUN and the occurrence of urinary casts (rare); hematuria and glycosuria (blood and sugar in the urine) (very rare).

Epistaxis (nosebleeds) (very rare).

Serious Adverse Effects

Allergic Reactions: Bronchospasm, anaphylaxis, and serum sickness.

Palpitations (rare).

Leukopenia (rare), jaundice (very rare), hypoprothrombinemia (very rare), neutropenia, anemia, lymphopenia, and thrombocytopenia (rare); leukocytosis, lymphocytosis, monocytosis, and basophilia (very rare).

Rare gallbladder concretions, rare pseudomembranous colitis, rare reversible symptomatic biliary symptoms.

Very rare urolithiasis (kidney stone) with renal colic, decreased kidney function, and cholelithiasis.

▷ **Possible Effects on Sexual Function:**   None reported.

Possible Delayed Adverse Effects: Gallbladder (biliary) symptoms can be more likely with longer term high-dose therapy.

▷ **Adverse Effects That May Mimic Natural Diseases or Disorders**

Has been associated with the formation of biliary sludge in the gallbladder which mimics cholecystitis (gallbladder inflammation).

May result in jaundice as seen in hepatitis.

Markedly alters bacterial flora in the colon and may lead to hypoprothrombinemia as seen in malnutrition and chronic liver disease.

Natural Diseases or Disorders That May Be Activated by This Drug

Additive hypoprothrombinemia in malnutrition or chronic liver disease.

Possible Effects on Laboratory Tests

Complete blood cell counts: Eosinophilia, basophilia, monocytosis, leukocytosis, thrombocytosis, leukopenia, neutropenia, lymphopenias and thrombocytopenia have all occurred.

Prolongation of prothrombin times and hypoprothrombinemia has been reported.

Increased SGOT, SGPT, alkaline phosphatase and bilirubin.

Increased BUN, serum creatinine, urinary casts, glycosuria and hematuria.

Interferes with cupric sulfate (a specific chemical indicator) based tests for urine sugar such as Clinitest.

Manual tests for creatinine may be falsely elevated by ceftriaxone.

CAUTION

1. Ceftriaxone should be used with caution in people who are allergic to penicillin, whatever the symptoms were.
2. Jaundiced neonates are at risk of bilirubin encephalopathy.
3. Ceftriaxone made with bacteriostatic water containing benzyl alcohol should not be used for IM (intramuscular) use in neonates.

Precautions for Use

By Infants and Children: Specific dosing schedules have been developed for children less than 12.

By Those over 60 Years of Age: No changes indicated.

▷ **Advisability of Use During Pregnancy**

Pregnancy Category: B. See Pregnancy Code at the back of this book.

Animal studies: High dose studies in primates have not revealed teratogenicity or embryotoxicity. Mouse and rat studies using up to twenty times the usual human dose have not shown any toxicity to the embryo or fetus.

Human studies: Adequate studies of pregnant women are not available.

Ask your physician for guidance.

Advisability of Use if Breast-Feeding

Presence of this drug in breast milk: Ceftriaxone is distributed into the milk of nursing mothers.

This drug should be used with caution in nursing mothers.

Habit-Forming Potential: None.

Effects of Overdosage: This drug is safe over a wide dosage range, however, severe overdoses may increase the likelihood of listed adverse effects.

Possible Effects of Long-Term Use: Symptoms consistent with cholelithiasis (gall stones), Clostridium difficile mediated colitis, overgrowth of nonsusceptible organisms, prolongation of the prothrombin time.

Suggested Periodic Examinations While Taking This Drug (at physician's discretion)

Prothrombin time, CBC (complete blood count), SGOT and SGPT, BUN, creatinine and routine urinalysis.

▷ **While Taking This Drug, Observe the Following**

Foods: No restrictions as this is an intramuscular (IM) or intravenous (IV) medication.

Nutritional Support: Some studies have been performed with nutritional support compatibility—I recommend calling the manufacturer's scientific services division for TPN formulation combinations and percent decomposition over time.

Beverages: No restrictions.

▷ *Alcohol:* Severe nausea and vomiting reported rarely. Alcohol also blunts the immune response. Avoid alcohol while taking this drug.

Tobacco Smoking: No interactions expected.

Marijuana Smoking: No interactions expected.

▷   *Other Drugs*
     Ceftriaxone may *increase* the effects of
     • anticoagulants such as coumadin or heparin.
     Ceftriaxone *taken concurrently* with
     • alcohol may cause severe nausea and vomiting.
     • aminoglycosides may increase the effectiveness of both drugs against cer-
       tain bacteria. Can be a great therapeutic benefit.
     • aminoglycosides may increase the likelihood of kidney damage.
     • colistimethate may increase the renal toxicity of colistin.
     • cyclosporine may increase the cyclosporine level and toxicity risk.
     • ethacrynic acid may increase the risk of kidney damage.
     • furosemide may increase renal toxicity.
     • methotrexate may decrease the antibiotic effect.
     The following drugs may *decrease* the effects of ceftriaxone
     • methotrexate.
     • probenecid in high dose (1–2 grams).
▷   *Driving, Hazardous Activities:* Rarely cause of dizziness. Restrict activities as
       necessary.
     Aviation Note: The use of this drug *may be a disqualification* for piloting. Con-
       sult a designated Aviation Medical Examiner.
     Exposure to Sun: No restrictions.
     Special Storage Instructions: Refrigeration is preferred once the medicine is
       reconstituted as the time until expiration is greatly prolonged. Storage at
       room temperature is possible, but the medicine does not keep as long.
     Observe the Following Expiration Times: Because of the complexity of the situa-
       tion, contact the home IV service or hospital who provided the IV solutions
       to you.

CEFUROXIME (sef yur OX eem)

Introduced: 1976   **Prescription:** USA: Yes   **Available as Generic:**
Yes   **Class:** Antibiotic, cephalosporin   **Controlled Drug:** USA: No
Brand Name: Ceftin, Kefurox, Zinacef

BENEFITS versus RISKS	
Possible Benefits	*Possible Risks*
EFFECTIVE TREATMENT OF INFECTIONS due to susceptible microorganisms	ALLERGIC REACTIONS, mild to severe
	Drug-induced colitis (rare)
	Superinfections (see Glossary)

▷ **Principal Uses**
     As a Single Drug Product: Uses currently included in FDA approved labeling: (1)
       Used to treat some infections of the middle ear, bone, joints, wounds, ton-
       sils, throat, bronchial tubes, urinary tract and skin, open fractures and gon-
       orrhea.
     Other (unlabeled) generally accepted uses: (1) Transition to an agent taken by
       mouth (oral) from the intravenous form (step-down or antibiotic streamlin-

ing). This can give superb outcomes and also can decrease length of stay in the hospital.

How This Drug Works: This drug destroys susceptible infecting bacteria by interfering with their ability to produce new protective cell walls as they multiply and grow.

Available Dosage Forms and Strengths

Tablets — 125 mg, 250 mg, 500 mg

Intravenous — 750 mg/10 ml
— 750 mg/50 ml
— 750 mg/100 ml
— 1.5 g/100 ml
— 1.5 g/50 ml
— 1.5 g/20 ml
— 7.5 g/127 ml

Oral suspension — 125 mg/ 5 ml

▷ **Usual Adult Dosage Range:** Oral: 250 to 500 mg/12 hrs. Total daily dosage should not exceed 4 grams.

Intravenous: 750 mg to 1.5 grams every 8 hours.

For children:

Oral: 125 mg twice a day, 250 mg twice daily for treatment of otitis media.

Intravenous: Those over 3 months should be given 50 to 100 mg/kg per day divided every 6 to 8 hours. Maximum dose is 4 grams. **Note: Actual dosage and administration schedule must be determined by the physician for each patient individually.**

Conditions Requiring Dosing Adjustments

Liver function: Changes in dose or dosing interval are not needed.

Kidney function: Dosage changes needed in severe kidney compromise with a dose of 750 mg once daily in the most compromised kidneys. Dose must be repeated after dialysis as the drug is dialyzable.

▷ **Dosing Instructions:** May be taken on an empty stomach or with food if stomach irritation occurs. The tablet may be crushed and mixed with food (such as applesauce or ice cream) if necessary to facilitate swallowing. (Note: The crushed tablet has a persistent, bitter taste.) Take the full course prescribed.

Usual Duration of Use: Continual use on a regular schedule for 3 to 5 days is needed to see this drug's effectiveness in controlling infections. Response varies with the nature of the infection. Some infections require 10 consecutive days to prevent the development of rheumatic fever. Follow your doctor's advice.

▷ **This Drug Should Not Be Taken If**
- you are allergic to cephalosporins (see Drug Classes).

▷ **Inform Your Physician Before Taking This Drug If**
- you are allergic to penicillins (see Drug Classes).
- you have a history of regional enteritis or ulcerative colitis.
- you have a history of low white blood cell counts.
- you have impaired kidney function.

Possible Side Effects (natural, expected, and unavoidable drug actions)

Superinfections (see Glossary): vaginitis (rare).

▷ **Possible Adverse Effects** (unusual, unexpected, and infrequent reactions)
   If any of the following develop, consult your physician promptly for guidance.
   Mild Adverse Effects
      Allergic Reactions: Skin rash, hives, itching (all very rare).
      Nausea, vomiting (rare), loose stools (rare), mild diarrhea.
      Headache (very rare), dizziness (very rare).
   Serious Adverse Effects
      Severe diarrhea, possibly a sign of colitis caused by the drug (rare).
      Low white blood cell counts.
      Thrombophlebitis with the intravenous form (rare).

▷ **Possible Effects on Sexual Function:**   None reported.

▷ **Adverse Effects That May Mimic Natural Diseases or Disorders**
   Skin rash may resemble measles.

Possible Effects on Laboratory Tests
   White blood cell counts: decreased (very rare).
   Eosinophils: increased (14%).
   BUN: increased (rare).
   Liver function tests: increased liver enzymes (ALT/GPT, AST/GOT) in people
      with impaired liver function.

CAUTION
   This drug can cause a false positive test result for urine sugar when using
      Clinitest tablets, Benedict's solution or Fehling's solution.

Precautions for Use
   By Infants and Children: The usual dose is 125 mg/ 12 hours. For middle ear
      infection, the recommended dose for those under 2 years of age is 125 mg/
      12 hours, and 250 mg/ 12 hours for those over 2 years of age.
   By Those over 60 Years of Age: Must be individualized based on kidney function.
      Skin changes may predispose to severe and prolonged itching in the genital
      and anal regions. Such reactions should be reported promptly.

▷ **Advisability of Use During Pregnancy**
   Pregnancy Category: B. See Pregnancy Code at the back of this book.
      Animal studies: No birth defects reported in mouse and rat studies.
      Human studies: Adequate studies of pregnant women are not available.
      Generally considered to be safe. Ask physician for guidance.

Advisability of Use if Breast-Feeding
   Presence of this drug in breast milk: Yes, in small amounts.
   Ask your doctor for help.

Habit-Forming Potential: None.

Effects of Overdosage: Nausea, vomiting, stomach cramps and/or diarrhea.

Possible Effects of Long-Term Use: Superinfections (see Glossary).

Suggested Periodic Examinations While Taking This Drug (at physician's discretion)
   None.

▷ **While Taking This Drug, Observe the Following**
   Foods: No restrictions. Food enhances the absorption of this drug.
   Beverages: No restrictions. May be taken with milk.

▷ *Alcohol:* No interactions expected. Excessive alcohol intake may blunt the immune response.
    Tobacco Smoking: No interactions expected.
▷ *Other Drugs*
      Cefuroxime *taken concurrently* with
      • aminoglycoside antibiotics (see Drug Classes) may result in increased risk of kidney toxicity.
      • birth control pills (oral contraceptives) may result in loss of contraception and pregnancy.
      • probenecid (Benemid) will cause higher blood levels and prolonged effect.
▷ *Driving, Hazardous Activities:* Usually no restrictions. Observe for the rare occurrence of dizziness.
    Aviation Note: The use of this drug *may be a disqualification* for piloting. Consult a designated Aviation Medical Examiner.
    Exposure to Sun: No restrictions.

CEPHALEXIN (sef a LEX in)

Introduced: 1969   **Prescription:** USA: Yes; Canada: Yes   **Available as Generic:** Yes   **Class:** Antibiotic, cephalosporin   **Controlled Drug:** USA: No; Canada: No

Brand Names: ✦Apo-Cephalex, Cefanex, ✦Ceporex, Keflet, Keflex, Keftab, ✦Novo-lexin, ✦Nu-Cephalex

BENEFITS versus RISKS	
Possible Benefits	*Possible Risks*
EFFECTIVE TREATMENT OF INFECTIONS due to susceptible microorganisms	ALLERGIC REACTIONS, mild to severe
	Drug-induced colitis (rare)
	Hemolytic anemia (rare)
	Superinfections (see Glossary)

▷ **Principal Uses**
    As a Single Drug Product: Uses currently included in FDA approved labeling: (1) To treat certain infections of the skin and skin structures, the upper respiratory tract (including middle ear infections and "strep" throat), the genitourinary tract, prostate infections and certain infections involving bones and joints.
    Other (unlabeled) generally accepted uses: (1) Can have a role in treating streptococcal infections in patients who are penicillin allergic.
How This Drug Works: This drug destroys susceptible infecting bacteria by interfering with their ability to produce new protective cell walls as they multiply and grow.
Available Dosage Forms and Strengths
      Capsules — 250 mg, 500 mg
      Oral suspension — 125 mg, 250 mg per 5-ml Pediatric oral suspension
                — 100 mg per ml
      Tablets — 250 mg, 500 mg, 1000 mg (1 gram)

▷ **Usual Adult Dosage Range:**   250 to 500 mg/ 6 hours. Total daily dose should not exceed 4 grams.
   Use in children: 25 to 50 mg/kg per day in 2 to 4 divided doses. Maximum dose is 4 grams (4,000 mg).
   For otitis media: 75–100 mg/ kg per day in 4 divided doses. **Note: Actual dosage and administration schedule must be determined by the physician for each patient individually.**

Conditions Requiring Dosing Adjustments
   Liver function: No dosing changes needed. The liver is not significantly involved in the elimination of this drug.
   Kidney function: For creatinine clearances (CrCl) of 10–50 ml/min., give the usual dose every 6 hours. For CrCl less than 10 ml/min., give the usual dose every 8–12 hours.

▷ **Dosing Instructions:**   May be taken on an empty stomach or with food if stomach irritation occurs. Capsule may be opened and tablet may be crushed for administration. Shake suspension well before measuring dose. Take the full course prescribed.

Usual Duration of Use: Continual use on a regular schedule for 3 to 5 days is usually necessary to determine this drug's effectiveness in controlling the infection under treatment. Response varies with the nature of the infection. Total treatment time will vary from 1 to 4 weeks. Certain infections require that this drug be taken for 10 consecutive days to prevent the development of rheumatic fever. Follow your physician's instructions regarding duration of use.

▷ **This Drug Should Not Be Taken If**
   • you are allergic to any cephalosporin antibiotic (see Drug Classes).

▷ **Inform Your Physician Before Taking This Drug If**
   • you have a history of allergy to any form of penicillin (see Drug Classes).
   • you have a history of regional enteritis or ulcerative colitis.
   • you have impaired kidney function.
   • you have a history of a blood cell disorder, especially hemolytic anemia.
   • you have a seizure disorder.
   • you have a hearing disorder.

Possible Side Effects (natural, expected, and unavoidable drug actions)
   Superinfections (see Glossary).

▷ **Possible Adverse Effects** (unusual, unexpected, and infrequent reactions)
   If any of the following develop, consult your physician promptly for guidance.
   Mild Adverse Effects
   Allergic Reactions: Skin rash (very rare), itching, hives (very rare).
   Headache, drowsiness, dizziness.
   Irritation of mouth or tongue, stomach cramping, nausea, vomiting (rare), diarrhea (rare).
   Serious Adverse Effects
   Allergic Reactions: Drug fever (see Glossary), joint aches and pains, anaphylactic reaction (see Glossary).
   Idiosyncratic Reactions: Minor and temporary changes in white blood cell counts and liver function tests (infrequent).

Genital itching (may represent a fungus superinfection).
Severe diarrhea, possibly indicating a drug-induced form of colitis (rare).
Low white blood cells.
Hemolytic anemia (rare).

▷ **Possible Effects on Sexual Function:**   None reported.

▷ **Adverse Effects That May Mimic Natural Diseases or Disorders**
Skin rash and fever may resemble measles.

Possible Effects on Laboratory Tests
Complete blood cell counts: decreased white blood cells, increased eosinophils.
Urine sugar tests: false positive results with Benedict's solution, Fehling's solution and Clinitest.

CAUTION
1. This drug can cause a false positive test result for urine sugar when using Clinitest tablets, Benedict's solution or Fehling's solution, but not with Tes-Tape.
2. Do not use this drug concurrently with other antibiotics such as erythromycin or tetracyclines.

Precautions for Use
By Infants and Children: Not recommended for use in infants less than 1 year old. Monitor allergic children closely for evidence of developing allergy to this drug.
By Those over 60 Years of Age: Dosage must be carefully individualized and based upon evaluation of kidney function. Natural changes in the skin may predispose to severe and prolonged itching reactions in the genital and anal regions. Such reactions should be reported promptly.

▷ **Advisability of Use During Pregnancy**
Pregnancy Category: B. See Pregnancy Code at the back of this book.
Animal studies: No birth defects reported.
Human studies: Information from adequate studies of pregnant women is not available.
Generally considered to be safe. Ask physician for guidance.

Advisability of Use if Breast-Feeding
Presence of this drug in breast milk: Yes, in small amounts.
Ask your doctor for guidance.

Habit-Forming Potential: None.

Effects of Overdosage: Nausea, vomiting, stomach cramps and/or diarrhea, seizures.

Possible Effects of Long-Term Use: Superinfections (see Glossary).

Suggested Periodic Examinations While Taking This Drug (at physician's discretion)
Complete blood cell counts. Liver and kidney function tests.

▷ **While Taking This Drug, Observe the Following**
Foods: No restrictions.
Beverages: No restrictions. May be taken with milk.
▷ *Alcohol:* No interactions expected. Excessive alcohol intake may blunt the immune system.

Tobacco Smoking: No interactions expected.
▷ *Other Drugs*
Cephalexin ***taken concurrently*** with
- aminoglycoside antibiotics (see Drug Classes) as there is an increased risk of kidney toxicity.
- birth control pills (oral contraceptives) may cause loss of contraception and pregnancy.
- cholestyramine as it will result in decreased cephalexin absorption and lower benefit as an antibiotic.
- probenecid (Benemid) will slow the elimination of cephalexin, resulting in higher blood levels and prolonged effect.

▷ *Driving, Hazardous Activities:* Usually no restrictions. Use caution if drowsiness or dizziness occurs.
Aviation Note: The use of this drug ***may be a disqualification*** for piloting. Consult a designated Aviation Medical Examiner.
Exposure to Sun: No restrictions.
Special Storage Instructions: Oral suspension should be refrigerated.
Observe the Following Expiration Times: Do not take the oral suspension of this drug if it is older than 14 days.

CHLORAMBUCIL (klor AM byu sil)

Introduced: 1974   **Prescription:** USA: Yes; Canada: Yes   **Available as Generic:** USA: No; Canada: No   **Class:** Anticancer, immunosuppressant
Controlled Drug: USA: No; Canada: No

Brand Name: Leukeran

BENEFITS versus RISKS	
Possible Benefits	*Possible Risks*
EFFECTIVE PALLIATIVE TREATMENT FOR CHRONIC LYMPHOCYTIC LEUKEMIA	BONE MARROW DEPRESSION (see Glossary)
EFFECTIVE PALLIATIVE TREATMENT FOR HODGKIN'S DISEASE AND OTHER LYMPHOMAS	INCREASED SUSCEPTIBILITY TO INFECTIONS
	CENTRAL NERVOUS SYSTEM TOXICITY
Immunosuppression of nephrotic syndrome	Male and female sterility
	Drug-induced liver damage
Immunosuppression of rheumatoid arthritis	Drug-induced lung damage
	Development of secondary cancers

▷ **Principal Uses**
As a Single Drug Product: Uses currently included in FDA approved labeling: Treats (1) chronic lymphocytic leukemia; (2) Hodgkin's lymphoma and other malignant lymphomas.
Other (unlabeled) generally accepted uses: (1) Hairy cell leukemia; (2) multiple myeloma; (3) Letterer-Siwe disease; (4) nephrotic syndrome; (5) ova-

rian cancer; (6) may have a role in rheumatoid arthritis; (7) can have a short-term role in treating systemic lupus erythematosus.

How This Drug Works: This drug blocks genetic activity (impairs DNA and RNA), and inhibits production of essential proteins. This kills cancerous cells.

Available Dosage Forms and Strengths

Tablets — 2 mg

▷ **Usual Adult Dosage Range:** For leukemia and lymphoma: Initially (induction phase of 3–6 weeks) 0.1 to 0.2 mg per kilogram of body weight daily, or 3 to 6 mg per square meter of body surface daily (usually 4 to 10 mg daily) as a single dose or in divided doses. Maintenance dose: 2–4 mg per day or a maximum of 0.1 mg/kg daily.

For immunosuppression: 0.1 to 0.2 mg per kilogram of body weight daily, in a single dose, for 8 to 12 weeks.

Note: Actual dosage and administration schedule must be determined by the physician for each patient individually.

Conditions Requiring Dosing Adjustments

Liver function: Can cause liver damage. Used with extreme caution in liver compromise. Extensively metabolized.

Kidney function: Can cause bladder inflammation; caution advised in compromised urine outflow.

▷ **Dosing Instructions:** Tablet may be crushed, however, food may decrease absorption by up to 20%. Avoid this combination. See your doctor if vomiting prevents you from taking chlorambucil.

Usual Duration of Use: Use on a regular schedule for 3 to 4 weeks is usually required to see this drug's effectiveness in controlling leukemia or lymphoma; several months are needed to assess immunosuppression. Long-term use requires periodic evaluation of response and dose changes.

▷ **This Drug Should Not Be Taken If**
- you have had an allergic reaction to it previously.
- you have a significant degree of bone marrow depression.
- you currently have an uncontrolled infection.

▷ **Inform Your Physician Before Taking This Drug If**
- you are allergic to melphalan (Alkeran).
- you are pregnant, planning pregnancy, or breast-feeding.
- you have a history of bone marrow depression or a blood cell disorder.
- you have a history of gout or urate kidney stones.
- you have a seizure disorder of any kind.
- you have a history of porphyria.
- you have impaired liver or kidney function.
- you have had cancer chemotherapy or radiation therapy previously.
- you are taking drugs than can impair your immunity.
- you have recently had or been exposed to chicken pox or herpes zoster.

Possible Side Effects (natural, expected, and unavoidable drug actions)

Decreased white blood cell and platelet counts.

Decreased immunity; susceptibility to infections.

Increased blood levels of uric acid, formation of kidney stones.

▷ **Possible Adverse Effects** (unusual, unexpected, and infrequent
 reactions)
 **If any of the following develop, consult your physician promptly for
 guidance.**
 Mild Adverse Effects
 Allergic Reactions: Skin rash, itching, drug fever (see Glossary).
 Mouth and lip sores, nausea, vomiting.
 Serious Adverse Effects
 Allergic Reactions: Drug-induced hepatitis with jaundice.
 Cataract formation with high-dose usage.
 Central nervous system toxicity: agitation, confusion, hallucinations, sei-
 zures, tremors, paralysis.
 Peripheral neuritis (see Glossary).
 Lung damage: Cough, shortness of breath.
 Bone marrow damage, aplastic anemia (see Glossary).
 Leukemia (may depend on dose and length of treatment).
 Liver damage (hepatotoxicity and jaundice).
 Severe skin damage (toxic epidermal necrolysis).

▷ **Possible Effects on Sexual Function:**   Can inhibit reproduction: Stops sperm
 production (male sterility); altered menstrual patterns, blocks ovulation
 and menstruation (female sterility).

 Possible Delayed Adverse Effects: Severe bone marrow depression can hap-
 pen after the drug has been stopped.
 Secondary cancers (especially leukemia) have been reported.
 Lung damage (pulmonary fibrosis).

▷ **Adverse Effects That May Mimic Natural Diseases or Disorders**
 Drug-induced seizures may suggest epilepsy.
 Drug-induced jaundice may suggest viral hepatitis.

 Natural Diseases or Disorders That May Be Activated by This Drug
 Gout, urate kidney stones, porphyria, latent epilepsy.

 Possible Effects on Laboratory Tests
 Complete blood counts: decreased red cells, hemoglobin, white cells and
 platelets.
 Blood uric acid level: increased.
 Liver function tests: increased liver enzymes (ALT/GPT, AST/GOT), increased
 bilirubin, increased icterus index.
 Sperm counts: decreased or absent.

 CAUTION
   1. Long-term use of this drug in noncancerous conditions requires extreme
      caution. Risks include permanent sterility, lung damage, and the devel-
      opment of secondary cancers. It should only be used where less toxic
      medicines have failed.
   2. It is advisable to have any needed dental work done prior to using this
      drug. The bone marrow depression could lead to gum infection, excessive
      bleeding and delayed healing.
   3. If gout develops, allopurinol is the drug of choice for chlorambucil-
      caused gout symptoms.
   4. This drug impairs the body's ability to produce protective antibodies.

Both killed virus vaccines and live virus vaccines will not work. There is an increased risk that live virus vaccines may actually cause infection.

Three months to 1 year is needed for the immune system to recover after stopping this and similar drugs. Family members or people in close contact with chlorambucil patients should not receive the oral poliovirus vaccine. This eliminates risk of accidental exposure.

5. Immediately report: Onset of infection, unusual bruising or bleeding, excessive fatigue, tremors or muscle twitching, difficulty walking, loss of appetite with nausea or vomiting.

6. It is advisable to avoid pregnancy while taking this drug. A nonhormonal method of contraception is recommended. Call your doctor promptly if you think pregnancy has occurred.

Precautions for Use

By Infants and Children: Dosage schedules and treatment monitoring should be supervised by a qualified pediatrician.

Children with nephrotic syndrome can be more prone to drug-induced seizures.

By Those over 60 Years of Age: Watch closely for central nervous system toxicity.

▷ **Advisability of Use During Pregnancy**

Pregnancy Category: D. See Pregnancy Code at the back of this book.

Animal studies: Rat studies reveal drug associated defects of the nervous system, palate, skeleton and urogenital system.

Human studies: Adequate studies of pregnant women are not available. There are two known cases of an infant born with an absent kidney and ureter following exposure to this drug during early pregnancy.

If possible, this drug should be avoided during pregnancy, especially the first 3 months.

A nonhormonal contraceptive is generally advisable during treatment with this and similar drugs.

Advisability of Use if Breast-Feeding

Presence of this drug in breast milk: Unknown.

Avoid drug or refrain from nursing.

Habit-Forming Potential: None.

Effects of Overdosage: Fatigue, weakness, fever, sore throat, bruising, agitation, unstable gait, bone marrow depression, seizures.

Possible Effects of Long-Term Use: Permanent sterility; secondary cancers (leukemia); lung damage (pulmonary fibrosis).

Suggested Periodic Examinations While Taking This Drug (at physician's discretion)

Before drug treatment and *periodically* during drug use: Complete blood counts, uric acid levels, liver function tests, sperm counts.

▷ **While Taking This Drug, Observe the Following**

Foods: No restrictions.

Beverages: No restrictions. May be taken with milk. It is advisable to drink 2 to 3 quarts of liquids daily to reduce the risk of kidney stone formation.

▷ *Alcohol:* Use with caution. Avoid if platelet counts are low and there is a risk of stomach bleeding.

Tobacco Smoking: No interactions expected.

Marijuana Smoking: Best avoided. This could increase the risk of central nervous system toxicity.

▷ *Other Drugs*

Chlorambucil *taken concurrently* with

- aspirin may increase the risk of bruising or bleeding; the platelet-reduction effects of chlorambucil and the antiplatelet action of aspirin are additive; avoid aspirin while taking chlorambucil.
- antidepressant or antipsychotic (neuroleptic) drugs require careful monitoring; these drugs lower the seizure threshold and increase the risk of chlorambucil-induced seizures.
- other immunosuppressant drugs can increase the risk of infection and the development of secondary cancers.

▷ *Driving, Hazardous Activities:*

This drug may cause nervous agitation, confusion, hallucinations or seizures. Restrict activities as necessary.

Aviation Note:

The use of this drug *may be a disqualification* for piloting. Consult a designated Aviation Medical Examiner.

Exposure to Sun: No restrictions.

Discontinuation: Whether used as an anticancer drug or as an immunosuppressant, many factors will determine when and how this drug should be stopped. In order to get the greatest benefit, follow your doctor's advice.

CHLORAMPHENICOL (klor am FEN i kohl)

Introduced: 1947   **Prescription:** USA: Yes; Canada: Yes   **Available as Generic:** USA: Yes; Canada: No   **Class:** Antibiotic   **Controlled Drug:** USA: No; Canada: No

Brand Names: Ak-Chlor, Chloracol, Chlorofair, Chloromycetin, Chloroptic, Chloroptic SOP, Econochlor, ✤Elase-Chloromycetin, I-Chlor, ✤Isopto Fenicol, ✤Minims, ✤Nova-Phenicol, ✤Novochlorocap, ✤Ocu-Chlor, Ophthochlor, ✤Ophtho-Chloram, Ophthocort, ✤PMS-Chloramphenicol, ✤Sopamycetin, ✤Sopamycetin/HC

BENEFITS versus RISKS	
Possible Benefits	*Possible Risks*
VERY EFFECTIVE TREATMENT OF INFECTIONS due to susceptible microorganisms	BONE MARROW DEPRESSION APLASTIC ANEMIA (see Glossary) Peripheral neuritis (see Glossary) Liver damage, jaundice

▷ **Principal Uses**

As a Single Drug Product: Uses currently included in FDA approved labeling: (1) Very effective in a broad spectrum of serious infections. However, because of serious toxicity (fatal aplastic anemia), it is now reserved for life-threatening (such as meningitis) infections caused by resistant organisms, and for infections in people who cannot tolerate other appropriate anti-infective drugs; (2) used in eye (intraocular) infections.

Other (unlabeled) generally accepted uses: (1) May have a role in prevention of plague; (2) can help when applied topically to pressure sores; (3) can be used topically to treat acne.

How This Drug Works: This drug prevents the growth and multiplication of susceptible microorganisms by interfering with their formation of essential proteins.

Available Dosage Forms and Strengths
Previously available capsules and oral suspensions are no longer made

Cream — 1%
Eye/ear solutions — 0.5%
Eye ointment — 1%
Injection — 100 mg per ml
Ophthalmic/otic suspension — 2 mg per ml

▷ **Usual Adult Dosage Range:**   Ophthalmic: Chloramphenicol plus hydrocortisone suspension or solution is given as two drops to the affected eye every three hours day and night for 48 hours. After this, the time between doses is usually lengthened and therapy continued until 48 hours after the eye appears normal. Intravenous: Total daily dose is 50 to 100 mg per kg divided into four doses, 6 hours apart. **Note: Actual dosage and administration schedule must be determined by the physician for each patient individually.**

Conditions Requiring Dosing Adjustments
Liver function: Must be adjusted in liver failure based on blood levels.
Kidney function: Adjustments in dose or dosing interval are suggested based on blood levels.

▷ **Dosing Instructions:**   Shake ophthalmic or otic suspension well before dosing.

Usual Duration of Use: Use of the ophthalmic or otic preparations every 3 hours for 48 hours is needed to assess the benefit in fighting the infection. Use of the intravenous form on a regular schedule for 3 to 5 days is needed to see this drug's effectiveness in controlling the infection. Limit use to the time required to treat the infection. Repeated intravenous courses should be avoided if possible.

▷ **This Drug Should Not Be Taken If**
  • you have had an allergic reaction to it previously.
  • you have an active blood cell or bone marrow disorder (intravenous form).
  • for mild or trivial infections such as a sore throat (intravenous form).
  • you are pregnant.
  • the ophthalmic suspension has been prescribed in a patient with a viral disease of the cornea such as Herpes simplex or mycobacterial or fungal eye disease.
  • prescribed for a premature or newborn infant (under 2 weeks of age).

▷ **Inform Your Physician Before Taking This Drug If**
  • you have a history of a blood cell or bone marrow disorder.
  • you have impaired liver or kidney function.
  • you are taking anticoagulants.
  • you have a G-6-PD deficiency (ask your doctor).
  • you are planning pregnancy.

Possible Side Effects (natural, expected, and unavoidable drug actions)
Superinfections (see Glossary).

▷ **Possible Adverse Effects** (unusual, unexpected, and infrequent reactions)
  If any of the following develop, consult your physician promptly for guidance.
  Mild Adverse Effects
    Allergic Reactions: Skin rashes, hives, swelling of face or extremities, fever.
    Headache, confusion, peripheral neuritis (see Glossary)—numbness, pain, weakness in hands and/or feet.
    Sore mouth or tongue, "black tongue," nausea, vomiting, diarrhea.
  Serious Adverse Effects
    Allergic Reactions: Anaphylactic reaction (see Glossary), liver damage with jaundice (rare).
    Bone marrow depression (see Glossary)—fatigue, weakness, fever, sore throat, abnormal bleeding or bruising.
    Gray baby syndrome—heart and lung failure (cardiovascular–respiratory collapse) (intravenous form).
    Peripheral neuritis (with prolonged therapy).
    Porphyria (rare).
    Acidosis (metabolic).
    Pseudomembranous colitis (rare).
    Liver toxicity (rare).
    Severe skin syndrome (Stevens-Johnson).
    Optic neuritis (often dose-related).

▷ **Possible Effects on Sexual Function:**   None reported.

▷ **Adverse Effects That May Mimic Natural Diseases or Disorders**
  Liver reaction with jaundice may suggest viral hepatitis.

Possible Effects on Laboratory Tests
  Complete blood counts: decreased red cells, hemoglobin, white cells and platelets; increased white cells; increased eosinophils.
  Prothrombin time: increased.
  Blood glucose level: decreased.
  Liver function tests: increased liver enzymes (ALT/GPT, AST/GOT, alkaline phosphatase), increased bilirubin.
  Fecal occult blood: positive (intestinal bleeding or drug-induced colitis).

CAUTION
  1. This drug can cause serious bone marrow depression and aplastic anemia (see Glossary). Must not be used to treat trivial infections or as a preventive medication. Restricted to serious or life-threatening infections not responding to other anti-infective drugs.
  2. Troublesome and persistent diarrhea can develop. If diarrhea persists for more than 24 hours, stop this drug and call your doctor.

Precautions for Use
  By Infants and Children: Follow prescribed dosage exactly. Blood cell counts should be checked twice a week. Long-term use of this drug can cause optic neuritis; however, this may be prevented by taking vitamin B complex. Idiosyncratic aplastic anemia is rare (1 in 40,000 users), but may occur long after (weeks or months) this drug is stopped.
  By Those over 60 Years of Age: The natural decline in kidney function after 60 may require decreased doses. Skin changes after 60 may predispose to se-

vere itching reactions in the genital and anal regions. Report such reactions promptly.

▷ **Advisability of Use During Pregnancy**
> *Pregnancy Category:* C. See Pregnancy Code at the back of this book.
> Animal studies: Results are inconclusive.
> Human studies: Adequate studies of pregnant women are not available. Limited data (348 exposures) indicate that this drug does not cause birth defects. However, it has been shown to be potentially toxic for the fetus and newborn. Ask your physician for help.

Advisability of Use if Breast-Feeding
> Presence of this drug in breast milk: Yes.
> Avoid drug or refrain from nursing.

Habit-Forming Potential: None.

Effects of Overdosage: Possible nausea, vomiting, diarrhea.

Possible Effects of Long-Term Use: Superinfections, impaired vision, peripheral neuritis and bone marrow depression.

Suggested Periodic Examinations While Taking This Drug (at physician's discretion)
> Complete blood counts—before treatment is started and every 2 to 3 days during administration of drug.
> Liver and kidney function tests.

▷ **While Taking This Drug, Observe the Following**
> *Foods:* No restrictions.
> *Nutritional Support:* Supplemental vitamins B-2, B-6 and B-12 are recommended.
> *Beverages:* No restrictions. May be taken with milk.
▷ > *Alcohol:* Avoid completely if you have liver disease. Use caution: Some people may develop a disulfiramlike reaction (see Glossary).
> *Tobacco Smoking:* No interactions expected.
▷ > *Other Drugs*
> Chloramphenicol may *increase* the effects of
> • oral anticoagulants (Coumadin, dicumarol, etc.), and increase the risk of bleeding.
> • barbiturates (phenobarbital, etc.), and cause excessive sedation.
> • phenytoin (Dilantin), and cause phenytoin toxicity.
> • sulfonylureas (Diabinese, Dymelor, Orinase, Tolinase), and other oral hypoglycemic agents, and cause hypoglycemia (see Glossary).
> Chloramphenicol may *decrease* the effects of
> • some cephalosporins, especially ceftazidime.
> • cyclophosphamide.
> • iron preparations, used to treat anemia.
> • penicillins.
> • vitamin B-12.
> The following drugs may *decrease* the effects of chloramphenicol
> • barbiturates (phenobarbital, etc.).
> • rifabutin (Mycobutin).
> • rifampin (Rifadin, Rimactane, etc.).

▷ *Driving, Hazardous Activities:* Usually no restrictions. Watch for rare occurrence of confusion, and restrict activities accordingly.

Aviation Note: The use of this drug **may be a disqualification** for piloting. Consult a designated Aviation Medical Examiner.

Exposure to Sun: No restrictions.

CHLOROQUINE (KLOR oh kwin)

Introduced: 1964   **Prescription:** USA: Yes; Canada: Yes   **Available as Generic:** USA: Yes; Canada: No   **Class:** Amebecide, antimalarial   **Controlled Drug:** USA: No; Canada: No

Brand Name: Aralen, Kronofed-A-JR

Warning:

The brand names Aralen and Arlidin are similar and can be mistaken for each other; this can lead to serious medication errors. These names represent very different drugs. Verify that you are taking the correct drug.

BENEFITS versus RISKS	
Possible Benefits	*Possible Risks*
EFFECTIVE PREVENTION AND TREATMENT OF CERTAIN FORMS OF MALARIA	INFREQUENT BUT SERIOUS DAMAGE OF CORNEAL AND RETINAL EYE TISSUES
EFFECTIVE COMBINATION TREATMENT OF SOME FORMS OF AMEBIC INFECTION	RARE BUT SERIOUS BONE MARROW DEPRESSION; aplastic anemia, deficient white blood cells
Possibly effective in palindromic rheumatism	and platelets
Possibly effective in short-term treatment of systemic lupus erythematosus	Heart muscle damage (rare)
	Ear damage; hearing loss, ringing in ears (rare)
	Eye damage (rare)

▷ **Principal Uses**

As a Single Drug Product: Uses currently included in FDA approved labeling: (1) Treatment of acute attacks of certain types of malarial infection; (2) treatment for certain forms of amebic infection.

Other (unlabeled) generally accepted uses: (1) Reduce disease activity in refractory rheumatoid and juvenile arthritis; (2) suppress disease activity in certain types of lupus erythematosus (patients are switched to hydroxychloroquine as soon as possible); (3) treatment of sarcoidosis, polymorphous light eruption and porphyria; (4) may give dramatic results in palindromic rheumatism; (5) second line agent for people traveling in areas where there is risk of malaria.

How This Drug Works: In treating malaria and amebiasis, this drug impairs the function of DNA in the protozoa that cause these diseases.

As an antiarthritic and antilupus drug, it acts as a mild immunosuppressant. It accumulates in white blood cells and blocks many enzymes involved in tissue destruction.

Available Dosage Forms and Strengths
Injection — 50 mg per ml
Tablets — 250 mg, 500 mg

▷ **Usual Adult Dosage Range:**   For malaria suppression: 500 mg once every 7 days.

For malaria treatment: Initially 1 gram, followed by 500 mg in 6 to 8 hours; then 500 mg once a day on the second and third days.

For amebiasis (other than intestinal): Initially 250 mg 4 times daily for 2 days; then 250 mg 2 times daily for 2 to 3 weeks.

For rheumatoid arthritis: Up to 4 mg per kilogram of lean body weight daily.

For lupus erythematosus: Up to 4 mg per kilogram of lean body weight daily.

Note: Actual dosage and administration schedule must be determined by the physician for each patient individually.

Conditions Requiring Dosing Adjustments
Liver function: Blood levels are needed, and the dose should be adjusted (decreased) appropriately.

Kidney function: In severe kidney failure 50% of the normal dose should be used. If therapy is extended, 50 to 100 mg of chloroquine base should be given daily.

▷ **Dosing Instructions:**   Tablet may be crushed and taken with food or milk to reduce stomach irritation. Take full course of treatment as prescribed.

Note: For malaria prevention, begin medication 2 weeks before entering malarious area; continue medication while in the area and for 4 weeks after leaving the area.

For treating arthritis and lupus, take medication on a regular schedule daily; use for 6 months may be needed to see peak effect.

Usual Duration of Use: Use on a regular schedule for 2 weeks before exposure, during period of exposure, and 4 weeks after exposure is needed to realize effectiveness in preventing malaria. Use on a regular schedule for up to 6 months may be required to evaluate benefits in treating rheumatoid arthritis and lupus erythematosus. The drug is changed to hydroxychloroquine because it is less toxic. Long-term use (months to years) requires periodic physician evaluation of response and dose adjustments.

Possible Advantages of This Drug
May be more effective than hydroxychloroquine in some cases of lupus erythematosus.

▷ **This Drug Should Not Be Taken If**
- you have an allergy to chloroquine or hydroxychloroquine.
- you have an active bone marrow or blood cell disorder.
- you have significant pathology of the heart muscle (cardiomyopathy).
- you have existing visual field or retinal changes.

▷ **Inform Your Physician Before Taking This Drug If**
- you are pregnant or planning pregnancy.
- you have bone marrow depression or a blood cell disorder.
- you have a deficiency of glucose-6-phosphate dehydrogenase.
- you have any eye disorder, especially disease of the cornea or retina, or visual field changes.
- you have a history of movement disorders.

- you have a history of mental illness.
- you have impaired hearing or ringing in the ears.
- you have a seizure disorder.
- you have a history of peripheral neuritis.
- you have low blood pressure or a heart rhythm disorder.
- you have a history of peptic ulcer disease, Crohn's disease or ulcerative colitis.
- you have impaired liver or kidney function or porphyria.
- you have any form of psoriasis.
- you are taking antacids, cimetidine or penicillamine.

Possible Side Effects (natural, expected, and unavoidable drug actions)
Light-headedness (low blood pressure); blue-black discoloration of skin, fingernails, or mouth lining with long-term use.

▷ **Possible Adverse Effects** (unusual, unexpected, and infrequent reactions)
If any of the following develop, consult your physician promptly for guidance.
Mild Adverse Effects
Allergic Reactions: Skin rash, itching (more common in African-Americans).
Loss of hair color, loss of hair.
Headache, blurring of near vision (reading), ringing in ears.
Loss of appetite, nausea, vomiting, stomach cramps, diarrhea.
Serious Adverse Effects
Allergic Reactions: Severe skin rash (erythema multiforme).
Idiosyncratic Reactions: Hemolytic anemia in those with glucose-6-phosphate dehydrogenase deficiency in red blood cells.
Emotional or psychotic mental changes; seizures.
Movement disorders (ataxia, dyskinesias).
Loss of hearing.
Low blood sugar (hypoglycemia).
Amnesia (rare).
Excessive muscle weakness.
Eye damage (cornea and retina), with significant impairment of vision.
Heart rhythm abnormalities.
Aplastic anemia (see Glossary): abnormally low red cells (fatigue and weakness), low white blood cell counts (fever, sore throat, infections), abnormally low platelets (abnormal bruising or bleeding).

▷ **Possible Effects on Sexual Function:**   None reported.

Possible Delayed Adverse Effects: Retinal damage (reports of development 7 years after stopping) is more likely to occur following high-dose and/or long-term use.

▷ **Adverse Effects That May Mimic Natural Diseases or Disorders**
Central nervous system toxicity mimics unrelated neuropsychiatric disorder.
Seizures may suggest the onset of epilepsy.

Natural Diseases or Disorders That May Be Activated by This Drug
Porphyria, psoriasis.

Possible Effects on Laboratory Tests
Complete blood counts: decreased red cells, hemoglobin, white cells and platelets.
Liver function tests: increased liver enzymes (AST/GOT) and bilirubin.

Urine tests for drug abuse: *initial* test result may be falsely **positive**; *confirmatory* test will be **negative**. (Test results depend upon amount of drug taken and testing method used.)

Blood sugar (glucose): decreased.

Electrocardiogram: conduction abnormalities, prolonged QRS interval, T wave changes, heart block.

CAUTION

1. Will not prevent relapses in certain types of malaria. Ask your doctor for advice.
2. Not effective in treating acute amebic dysentery (intestinal infection) or asymptomatic carriers.
3. High-dose and/or long-term use of this drug may cause irreversible retinal damage; such use may also cause hearing loss due to nerve damage. Promptly report any vision or hearing changes.

Precautions for Use

By Infants and Children: This age group is very sensitive to the effects of this drug. Dosages should be chosen and therapy monitored by a qualified pediatrician.

By Those over 60 Years of Age: Reduced tolerance for high-dose and/or long-term use. Watch for behavioral changes, low blood pressure, heart rhythm disturbances, muscle weakness and changes in vision or hearing.

▷ **Advisability of Use During Pregnancy**

Pregnancy Category: C. See Pregnancy Code at the back of this book.

Animal studies: 47% of rat fetuses revealed undeveloped or partially developed eyes.

Human studies: Adequate studies of pregnant women are not available. A 1964 report includes drug-induced congenital deafness, retinal damage, gait instability and asymmetric body growth. A 1991 study of use in systemic lupus erythematosus concluded that the benefit outweighed the fetal risk.

Avoid use during pregnancy except for the suppression or treatment of malaria or amebic infection of the liver. Seek your doctor's advice.

Advisability of Use if Breast-Feeding

Presence of this drug in breast milk: Yes.

Avoid drug or refrain from nursing.

Habit-Forming Potential: None.

Effects of Overdosage: Drowsiness, headache, blurred vision, excitability, low blood pressure, seizures, coma.

Possible Effects of Long-Term Use: Irreversible eye damage (cornea and retina), hearing loss, myocarditis, muscle weakness, aplastic anemia.

Suggested Periodic Examinations While Taking This Drug (at physician's discretion)

Complete blood counts; liver and kidney function tests.

Serial blood pressure readings and electrocardiograms.

Neurological examinations for significant muscle weakness.

Complete eye examinations before starting high-dose or long-term treatment, then every 3 to 6 months during drug use.

Hearing tests as indicated.

▷ **While Taking This Drug, Observe the Following**
  Foods: No restrictions.
  Beverages: No restrictions. May be taken with milk.
▷ *Alcohol:* Use sparingly to minimize stomach irritation.
  Tobacco Smoking: No interactions expected.
▷ *Other Drugs*
    Chloroquine may *increase* the effects of
    • cyclosporine and increase risk of kidney toxicity.
    • penicillamine (Cuprimine, Depen), and increase its toxic potential.
    Chloroquine may *decrease* the effects of
    • ampicillin.
    • methotrexate
    • Rabies vaccine.
    The following drug may *increase* the effects of chloroquine
    • cimetidine (Tagamet).
    The following drugs may *decrease* the effects of chloroquine
    • magnesium salts and antacids.
▷ *Driving, Hazardous Activities:*
    This drug may cause light-headedness, blurred vision or impaired hearing.
      Restrict activities as necessary.
  Aviation Note:
    The use of this drug *may be a disqualification* for piloting. Consult a desig-
      nated Aviation Medical Examiner.
  Exposure to Sun: This drug may cause photosensitivity (see Glossary).
  Discontinuation: This drug should be stopped and prompt evaluation made if
      any changes in vision or hearing, seizures, unusual muscle weakness, infec-
      tion (fever, sore throat, etc.), abnormal bruising or bleeding occurs.

CHLOROTHIAZIDE (klor oh THI a zide)

Introduced: 1957   **Prescription:** USA: Yes   **Available as Generic:**
USA: Yes   **Class:** Antihypertensive, diuretic, thiazides   **Controlled Drug:**
USA: No

Brand Names: Aldoclor [CD], Diachlor, Diupres [CD], Diurigen, Diuril, SK-
  Chlorothiazide, ✤Supres [CD]

BENEFITS versus RISKS	
Possible Benefits	*Possible Risks*
EFFECTIVE, WELL-TOLERATED DIURETIC	Loss of body potassium
	Increased blood sugar
POSSIBLY EFFECTIVE IN MILD HYPERTENSION	Increased blood uric acid
	Increased blood calcium
ENHANCES EFFECTIVENESS OF OTHER ANTIHYPERTENSIVES	Blood cell disorders (rare)
Beneficial in treatment of diabetes insipidus	

Please see the thiazide diuretic profile for further information.

CHLORPROMAZINE (klor PROH ma zeen)

Introduced: 1952   **Prescription:** USA: Yes; Canada: Yes   **Available as**
Generic: Yes   **Class:** Antipsychotic, strong tranquilizer, phenothiazines
Controlled Drug: USA: No; Canada: No

Brand Names: ✦Chlorpromanyl, ✦Largactil, ✦Novochlorpromazine, Orma-
zine, Thora-Dex, Thorazine, Thorazine SR

BENEFITS versus RISKS

Possible Benefits	*Possible Risks*
EFFECTIVE CONTROL OF ACUTE MENTAL DISORDERS	SERIOUS TOXIC EFFECTS ON BRAIN with long-term use
Beneficial effects on thinking, mood, and behavior	Liver damage with jaundice (rare)
Moderately effective control of nausea and vomiting	Rare blood disorders: hemolytic anemia, abnormally low white blood count
	Eye toxicity

▷ **Principal Uses**

As a Single Drug Product: Uses currently included in FDA-approved labeling: (1) Treats acute and chronic psychotic disorders such as agitated depression, schizophrenia and mania; (2) it can be used for presurgical anxiety; (3) helps reduce symptoms in porphyrias and tetanus; (4) is used to stop pro-longed hiccups; (5) lessens or stops vomiting caused by toxic chemotherapy or a potent drug used to treat fungal infections (amphotericin B).

Other (unlabeled) generally accepted uses: (1) Can be of help in complicated drug withdrawal cases; (2) lessens the symptoms of Tourette's syndrome; (3) may be of help in combination therapy of tuberculosis; (4) can be used intravenously after some heart surgery.

How This Drug Works: By inhibiting the action of dopamine, this drug acts to correct an imbalance of nerve impulses found in some mental disorders.

Available Dosage Forms and Strengths

Capsules, prolonged-action — 30 mg, 75 mg, 150 mg, 200 mg, 300 mg
Concentrate — 30 mg per ml and 100 mg per ml
Oral drops — 40 mg per ml
Injection — 25 mg per ml
Suppositories — 25 mg, 100 mg
Syrup — 10 mg per 5-ml
Tablets — 10 mg, 25 mg, 50 mg, 100 mg, 200 mg

▷ **Usual Adult Dosage Range:** Initially 10 to 25 mg 3 or 4 times daily. Dose may be increased by 20 to 50 mg at 3- to 4-day intervals as needed and tolerated. Usual dosage range is 300 to 800 mg daily. Extreme range is 25 to 2000 mg daily. Total daily dosage should not exceed 2000 mg. **Note: Actual dosage and administration schedule must be determined by the physician for each patient individually.**

Conditions Requiring Dosing Adjustments

Liver function: Used with caution and in decreased dose in patients with com-promised livers. Can also be a cause of a specific kind of (cholestatic) jaun-dice.

Kidney function: Blood levels are recommended if used in severe kidney compromise.

▷ **Dosing Instructions:**   Tablets may be crushed and taken with or after meals to reduce stomach irritation. Prolonged-action capsules may be opened, but not crushed or chewed.

Usual Duration of Use: Use on a regular schedule for several weeks is usually needed to see this drug's effectiveness in controlling psychotic disorders. If benefits are not seen in 6 weeks, it should be stopped. Long-term use (months to years) requires periodic physician evaluation.

▷ **This Drug Should Not Be Taken If**
   • you are allergic to any form of this drug.
   • you have active liver disease.
   • you have taken a large amount of alcohol or narcotics.
   • you have cancer of the breast.
   • you have a current blood cell or bone marrow disorder.

▷ **Inform Your Physician Before Taking This Drug If**
   • you are allergic or very sensitive to any phenothiazine drug (see Drug Classes).
   • you have impaired liver or kidney function.
   • you have any type of seizure disorder.
   • you have diabetes, glaucoma or heart disease.
   • you have a history of lupus erythematosus.
   • you work in extreme heat or are typically exposed to organophosphorous insecticides.
   • you are taking any drug with sedative effects.
   • you plan to have surgery with anesthesia (general or spinal) soon.

Possible Side Effects (natural, expected, and unavoidable drug actions)
   Drowsiness (usually during the first 2 weeks), orthostatic hypotension (see Glossary), blurred vision, dry mouth, nasal congestion, constipation, impaired urination.
   Pink or purple coloration of urine, of no clinical significance.

▷ **Possible Adverse Effects** (unusual, unexpected, and infrequent reactions)
   If any of the following develop, consult your physician promptly for guidance.
   Mild Adverse Effects
   Allergic Reactions: Skin rash, hives, low-grade fever.
   Lowering of body temperature, especially in the elderly.
   Increased appetite and weight gain.
   Weakness, agitation, insomnia, impaired day and night vision.
   Chronic constipation, fecal impaction.
   Serious Adverse Effects
   Allergic Reactions: Hepatitis with jaundice (see Glossary), usually between second and fourth week; high fever; asthma; anaphylactic reaction (see Glossary).
   Idiosyncratic Reactions: Neuroleptic malignant syndrome (see Glossary).
   Depression, disorientation, seizures.
   Disturbances of heart rhythm, rapid heart rate.
   Hemolytic or aplastic anemia (see Glossary).

Low blood platelets (rare).

Low white blood cells—fever, sore throat, infections.

Parkinson-like disorders (see Glossary); muscle spasms of face, jaw, neck, back, extremities.

Prolonged drop in blood pressure with weakness, perspiration, and fainting.

Drop in blood pressure on standing (orthostatic hypotension).

▷ **Possible Effects on Sexual Function**

Decreased libido and impotence (1200 mg/day); inhibited ejaculation (400 mg/day); priapism (see Glossary) (250 mg/day); male infertility (30 to 800 mg/day); enlargement of male breasts, enlargement of female breasts with milk production, cessation of menstruation (30 to 800 mg/day).

▷ **Adverse Effects That May Mimic Natural Diseases or Disorders**

Nervous system reactions may suggest Parkinson's disease.

Liver reactions may suggest viral hepatitis.

Reactions resembling systemic lupus erythematosus can occur.

Natural Diseases or Disorders That May Be Activated by This Drug

Latent epilepsy, glaucoma, diabetes mellitus (25%), prostatism (see Glossary).

Possible Effects on Laboratory Tests

Complete blood counts: decreased red cells, hemoglobin, white cells and platelets; increased eosinophils (often warns of jaundice).

Antinuclear antibodies (ANA): positive in 63% of long-term users.

Blood cholesterol level: increased (with liver damage).

Blood glucose level: increased with long-term use.

Glucose tolerance test (GTT): decreased; 40% abnormal with chronic use.

Partial thromboplastin time: increased.

Blood uric acid level: decreased.

Liver function tests: increased liver enzymes (ALT/GPT, AST/GOT and alkaline phosphatase); increased bilirubin.

Urine pregnancy tests: false positive results with frog, rabbit and immunological tests.

CAUTION

1. Many over-the-counter medications (see OTC Drugs in Glossary) for allergies, colds and coughs should not be combined with this drug. Ask your physician or pharmacist for help.
2. Antacids that contain aluminum and/or magnesium can lower absorption of this drug and reduce its effect.
3. Obtain prompt evaluation of any change or disturbance of vision.
4. This drug can cause false positive pregnancy tests.

Precautions for Use

By Infants and Children: This drug has been used in neonates. Younger children may require more frequent dosing. Do not use in children of any age with symptoms suggestive of Reye syndrome (see Glossary). Watch carefully for blood cell changes.

By Those over 60 Years of Age: You may be more susceptible to the development of drowsiness, lethargy, constipation, lowering of body temperature (hypothermia) and orthostatic hypotension (see Glossary). Can worsen existing prostatism (see Glossary). Parkinson-like reactions and/or tardive dyskinesia (see discussion of these terms in Glossary) are more likely. Symptoms must be recognized early since they may become irreversible.

▷ **Advisability of Use During Pregnancy**

Pregnancy Category: C. See Pregnancy Code at the back of this book.

Animal studies: No birth defects reported in rodent studies. However, rodent studies suggest possible permanent neurological damage to the fetus.

Human studies: No increase in birth defects reported in 284 exposures. Adequate studies of pregnant women are not available.

Limit use to small and infrequent doses only when clearly needed. Avoid drug during the last month of pregnancy.

Advisability of Use if Breast-Feeding

Presence of this drug in breast milk: Yes, in small amounts.

Ask your doctor for advice.

Habit-Forming Potential: None.

Effects of Overdosage: Marked drowsiness, weakness, tremor, agitation, unsteadiness, deep sleep, coma, convulsions.

Possible Effects of Long-Term Use: Tardive dyskinesia in 10% to 20% (see Glossary); eye changes—cataracts and pigmentation of retina; gray to violet pigmentation of skin in exposed areas, more common in women; severe ulcerative colitis.

Suggested Periodic Examinations While Taking This Drug (at physician's discretion)

Complete blood counts, especially between four to ten weeks of treatment.

Liver function tests, electrocardiograms.

Complete eye examinations—eye structures and vision.

Careful tongue inspection for fine, involuntary, wavelike movements that could be the beginning of tardive dyskinesia.

▷ **While Taking This Drug, Observe the Following**

Foods: No restrictions.

Nutritional Support: A riboflavin (vitamin B-2) supplement should be taken with long-term use.

Beverages: Caffeine may lessen calming effect of drug. May be taken with milk.

▷ *Alcohol:* Avoid completely. Increases phenothiazine sedative action and accentuates their depressant effects on brain function and blood pressure. Phenothiazines can increase the intoxicating effects of alcohol.

Tobacco Smoking: Possible reduction of drowsiness from drug.

Marijuana Smoking: Moderate increase in drowsiness; worsened orthostatic hypotension; increased risk of precipitating latent psychoses.

▷ *Other Drugs*

Chlorpromazine may *increase* the effects of

• all sedatives or narcotics, especially meperidine (Demerol).

• all atropinelike drugs, and cause nervous system toxicity.

• zolpidem (Ambien).

Chlorpromazine may *decrease* the effects of

• guanethidine (Ismelin, Esimil), and reduce its effectiveness in lowering blood pressure.

• oral hypoglycemic agents (see Drug Classes).

Chlorpromazine *taken concurrently* with
- amphetamine will cause decreased effect of both drugs.
- ACE inhibitors (see Drug Classes) cause excessive lowering of blood pressure.
- beta blockers (see Drug Classes) can intensify the effects of both drugs.
- lithium may result in a decrease in lithium or chlorpromazine effectiveness.
- propranolol (Inderal) may cause increased effects of both drugs; watch drug effects closely—doses may have to be decreased.
- valproic acid can result in elevated valproic acid blood levels and toxicity.

The following drugs may *decrease* the effects of chlorpromazine
- antacids containing aluminum and/or magnesium.
- benztropine (Cogentin).
- trihexyphenidyl (Artane).

▷ *Driving, Hazardous Activities:* This drug can impair mental alertness, judgment and physical coordination. Avoid hazardous activities.

Aviation Note: The use of this drug *is a disqualification* for piloting. Consult a designated Aviation Medical Examiner.

Exposure to Sun: Use caution. Some phenothiazines cause photosensitivity (see Glossary).

Exposure to Heat: Use caution and avoid excessive heat. This drug can impair body temperature regulation and increase the risk of heat stroke.

Exposure to Cold: Use caution and dress warmly. Increased risk of hypothermia in the elderly.

Discontinuation: After long-term use, do not stop this drug suddenly. Gradual withdrawal over 2 to 3 weeks. Do not stop this drug without your physician's knowledge and approval. Schizophrenia relapse rate after discontinuation is 50% to 60%.

CHLORPROPAMIDE (klor PROH pa mide)

Introduced: 1958 **Prescription:** USA: Yes; Canada: Yes **Available as Generic:** Yes **Class:** Antidiabetic, sulfonylureas **Controlled Drug:** USA: No; Canada: No

Brand Names: ✦Apo-Chlorpropamide, ✦Chloronase, Diabinese, Glucamide

---

BENEFITS versus RISKS

Possible Benefits	*Possible Risks*
Help in regulating blood sugar in noninsulin-dependent diabetes (adjunctive to appropriate diet and weight control)	HYPOGLYCEMIA, severe and prolonged Allergic skin reactions (some severe) Water retention Liver damage Blood cell and bone marrow disorders (rare)

▷ **Principal Uses**

As a Single Drug Product: Uses currently included in FDA approved labeling: Helps control mild to moderate type II diabetes mellitus (adult, maturity-onset) that does not require insulin, but is not adequately controlled by diet alone.

Other (unlabeled) generally accepted uses: (1) May be of help in easing abnormal urine output (SIADH); (2) can be used as a test to define some genetic characteristics of diabetes (CPAF test); (3) can be of benefit in some people who have an excessive reaction to sugar (reactive hypoglycemia).

How This Drug Works: This drug (1) stimulates the secretion of insulin if the pancreas is capable of responding to stimulation, and (2) enhances the utilization of insulin by appropriate tissues.

Available Dosage Forms and Strengths

Tablets — 100 mg, 250 mg

▷ **Usual Adult Dosage Range:** Initially 250 mg daily with breakfast. After 5 to 7 days, dose may be increased to 500 mg daily if needed and tolerated. Total daily dosage should not exceed 750 mg. A "loading" or priming dose is not necessary and should not be given. **Note: Actual dosage and administration schedule must be determined by the physician for each patient individually.**

Conditions Requiring Dosing Adjustments

Liver function: The dose **must** be decreased in patients with liver compromise.
Kidney function: Prudent to change to a drug such as tolbutamide in kidney failure.

▷ **Dosing Instructions:** Tablet may be crushed when taken. Taking with food reduces stomach irritation.

Usual Duration of Use: Use on a regular schedule for 1 to 2 weeks is usually needed to see peak effect in controlling diabetes. Failure to respond to maximum doses in 1 month is a primary failure. Up to 15% of those who respond initially may develop secondary failure of the drug within a year. Periodic measurement of blood sugar is needed. See your physician on a regular basis.

▷ **This Drug Should Not Be Taken If**

• you have had an allergic reaction to it previously.
• you have severe impairment of liver or kidney function.
• you are pregnant.
• you make ketone bodies (ketosis). Ask your doctor.
• you are a brittle, juvenile or unstable diabetic.

▷ **Inform Your Physician Before Taking This Drug If**

• you are allergic to other sulfonylurea drugs or to "sulfa" drugs.
• your diabetes has been unstable or "brittle" in the past.
• you have a history of blood disorders.
• you do not know how to recognize or treat hypoglycemia (see Glossary).
• you have a history of congestive heart failure, kidney disease, peptic ulcer disease, cirrhosis of the liver, hypothyroidism or porphyria.
• you have G6PD deficiency (ask your doctor).

Possible Side Effects (natural, expected, and unavoidable drug actions)

If drug dose is excessive or food intake is delayed or inadequate, low blood sugar (hypoglycemia) will occur as a drug effect.

▷ **Possible Adverse Effects** (unusual, unexpected, and infrequent reactions)

If any of the following develop, consult your physician promptly for guidance.

Mild Adverse Effects
  Allergic Reactions: Skin rash, hives, itching, drug fever.
  Headache, ringing in ears, weakness, numbness and tingling.
  Indigestion, nausea, vomiting, diarrhea (may be severe).
Serious Adverse Effects
  Allergic Reactions: Hepatitis with jaundice (see Glossary), severe skin reactions.
  Idiosyncratic Reaction: Hemolytic anemia (see Glossary).
  Disulfiramlike reaction with concurrent use of alcohol (see Glossary).
  Water retention (edema), weight gain.
  SIADH (talk to your doctor).
  Lowered thyroid function (hypothyroidism).
  Bone marrow depression (see Glossary)—fatigue, weakness, fever, sore throat, abnormal bleeding or bruising.
  Abnormal heartbeats (very rare).
  Persistent diarrhea (pseudomembranous colitis) (rare).
  Severe skin reactions (Stevens-Johnson syndrome) (rare).

▷ **Possible Effects on Sexual Function:**   None reported.

▷ **Adverse Effects That May Mimic Natural Diseases or Disorders**
  Liver reactions may suggest viral hepatitis.

Natural Diseases or Disorders That May Be Activated by This Drug
  Acute intermittent porphyria, congestive heart failure (in predisposed individuals), peptic ulcer disease.

Possible Effects on Laboratory Tests
  Complete blood cell counts: decreased red cells, hemoglobin, white cells and platelets; increased eosinophils (allergic reaction).
  Blood sodium: increased or decreased.
  Prothrombin time: increased (with liver damage).
  Blood thyroxine (T_4) level: decreased.
  Liver function tests: increased liver enzymes (ALT/GPT, AST/GOT and alkaline phosphatase), increased bilirubin.

CAUTION
  1. Must be only one part of a total diabetes management program. It is not a substitute for a prescribed diet and regular exercise.
  2. Over time (usually several months), this drug may lose its effectiveness in controlling blood sugar levels. Periodic follow-up examinations are necessary.
  3. This drug has a long duration of action (up to 60 hours). It can produce severe and prolonged hypoglycemia, especially in the elderly.

Precautions for Use
  By Infants and Children: This drug does not work in type I (juvenile, growth-onset) insulin-dependent diabetes.
  By Those over 60 Years of Age: Should be avoided in this age group. Because its effect lasts such a long time, it can accumulate and cause marked and prolonged hypoglycemia. Repeated hypoglycemia in the elderly can cause brain damage.

▷ **Advisability of Use During Pregnancy**
  Pregnancy Category: C by manufacturer, D by some researchers. See Pregnancy Code at the back of this book.

Animal studies: Specific studies have not been conducted in animals.
Human studies: Adequate studies of pregnant women are not available.
Ask your doctor for guidance. Insulin is clearly the drug of choice during
pregnancy to control glucose levels.

Advisability of Use if Breast-Feeding
Presence of this drug in breast milk: Yes.
Avoid drug or refrain from nursing.

Habit-Forming Potential: None.

Effects of Overdosage: Symptoms of mild to severe hypoglycemia: headache,
light-headedness, faintness, nervousness, confusion, tremor, sweating,
heart palpitation, weakness, hunger, nausea, vomiting, stupor progressing
to coma.

Possible Effects of Long-Term Use: Reduced function of the thyroid gland
(hypothyroidism). Reports of increased frequency and severity of heart and
blood vessel diseases associated with long-term use of this class of drugs
was based on study of tolbutamide, but may apply to any drug in this class.
A direct cause-and-effect relationship (see Glossary) is tenuous. Ask your
physician for guidance.

Suggested Periodic Examinations While Taking This Drug (at physician's discretion)
Complete blood cell counts, liver function tests, thyroid function tests, periodic evaluation of heart and circulatory system.

▷ **While Taking This Drug, Observe the Following**
Foods: Follow the diabetic diet prescribed by your physician.
Beverages: As directed in the diabetic diet. May be taken with milk.
▷   *Alcohol:* Avoid this combination. Alcohol can exaggerate this drug's hypoglycemic effect. This drug can also cause a disulfiramlike reaction (see Glossary): facial flushing, sweating, palpitation.
Tobacco Smoking: No interactions expected.
▷   *Other Drugs*
The following drugs may ***increase*** the effects of chlorpropamide
• ammonium chloride.
• aspirin, aspirin-containing combination drugs (see Aspirin profile), and
other salicylates.
• beta blockers (see Drug Classes) and cause slowed recovery from any low
blood sugars which may occur.
• calcium channel blockers (see Drug Classes).
• chloramphenicol (Chloromycetin).
• clofibrate (Atromid S).
• dicumarol.
• fenfluramine (Pondimin).
• monoamine oxidase (MAO) type A inhibitor drugs (see Drug Classes).
• NSAIDs (see Drug Classes).
• some "sulfa" drugs: sulfamethoxazole (Gantanol), sulfisoxazole (Gantrisin), Septra, Bactrim.
The following drugs may ***decrease*** the effects of chlorpropamide
• diazoxide (Proglycem).
• phenothiazines (see Drug Classes).

- rifampin (Rifadin, Rimactane).
- sodium bicarbonate.
- thiazide diuretics (see Drug Classes).

▷ *Driving, Hazardous Activities:* Dosing, eating schedule and physical activities must be carefully regulated to prevent hypoglycemia. Know the early symptoms of hypoglycemia so you can avoid hazardous activities and take corrective measures.

Aviation Note: Diabetes *is a disqualification* for piloting. Consult a designated Aviation Medical Examiner.

Exposure to Sun: Use caution. Drugs of this class can cause photosensitivity (see Glossary).

Occurrence of Unrelated Illness: Acute infections, illnesses causing vomiting or diarrhea, serious injuries and surgical procedures can change diabetic control and may require insulin use. Consult your physician promptly.

Discontinuation: Only about 12% of patients remain well controlled by this drug for more than 6 to 7 years. It is advisable to evaluate the continued benefit of this drug every 6 months.

CHLORTHALIDONE (klor THAL i dohn)

Introduced: 1960   **Prescription:** USA: Yes; Canada: Yes   **Available as Generic:** USA: Yes; Canada: Yes   **Class:** Antihypertensive, diuretic   **Controlled Drug:** USA: No; Canada: No

Brand Names: ✢Apo-Chlorthalidone, Combipres [CD], Demi-Regroton [CD], Hygroton, ✢Hygroton-Reserpine [CD], Hylidone, ✢Novothalidone, Regroton [CD], Tenoretic [CD], Thalitone, ✢Uridon

BENEFITS versus RISKS	
Possible Benefits	*Possible Risks*
EFFECTIVE, WELL-TOLERATED DIURETIC	Loss of body potassium
POSSIBLY EFFECTIVE IN MILD HYPERTENSION	Increased blood sugar, uric acid, and calcium
ENHANCES EFFECTIVENESS OF OTHER ANTIHYPERTENSIVES	Rare blood cell disorders
Beneficial in treatment of diabetes insipidus	

Please see the thiazide diuretic profile for further information.

CHOLESTYRAMINE (koh LES tir a meen)

Introduced: 1959   **Prescription:** USA: Yes; Canada: No   **Available as Generic:** USA: No; Canada: No   **Class:** Anticholesterol   **Controlled Drug:** USA: No; Canada: No

Brand Names: Questran, Questran Light

```
┌─────────────────────────────────────────────────────────────────┐
│                    BENEFITS versus RISKS                          │
│      Possible Benefits                   Possible Risks           │
│  EFFECTIVE REDUCTION OF TOTAL   Constipation (may be severe)      │
│    CHOLESTEROL AND              Reduced absorption of fat, fat-soluble │
│    LOW-DENSITY CHOLESTEROL        vitamins (A, D, E, and K) and folic │
│    IN TYPE IIa CHOLESTEROL        acid                            │
│    DISORDERS (15% to 25%        Reduced formation of prothrombin  │
│    reduction of total cholesterol, 25%   with resultant bleeding  │
│    to 35% reduction of LDL                                        │
│    cholesterol)                                                   │
│  EFFECTIVE RELIEF OF ITCHING                                      │
│    associated with biliary obstruction                            │
│  Effective binding of medicines in drug                           │
│    overdoses                                                      │
└─────────────────────────────────────────────────────────────────┘
```

▷ **Principal Uses**

As a Single Drug Product: Uses currently included in FDA approved labeling: Used to (1) treat a new condition called arteriohepatic dysplasia which results in liver and heart problems; (2) reduces abnormally high blood levels of total cholesterol and low density (LDL) cholesterol in Type IIa cholesterol disorders; (3) relieves itching due to the deposit of bile acids in the skin associated with partial biliary obstruction; (4) reduces risk of heart disease in men with type II hyperlipoproteinemia.

Other (unlabeled) generally accepted uses: (1) May be of help in biliary fistulas and skin irritations seen in colostomy; (2) can help lower thyroid hormone levels if too much thyroid hormone has been given in error; (3) may help treat cholesterol ester storage disease (CESD); (4) helps relapses of resistant diarrhea (pseudomembranous colitis).

How This Drug Works: It combines with bile acids and bile salts in the intestinal tract, and forms insoluble complexes that are excreted in the feces. This process stimulates conversion of cholesterol to bile acids to replace the loss; and reduces cholesterol levels. By reducing the blood levels of bile acids, this drug reduces bile acids deposited in the skin and relieves itching.

Available Dosage Forms and Strengths

Cans — 378 grams

Packets — 4 grams and 9 grams

▷ **Usual Adult Dosage Range:**   9 grams of powder (equivalent to 4 grams of cholestyramine) 1 to 6 times daily. Dose may be increased slowly as needed and tolerated. The total daily dosage should not exceed 72 grams of powder (32 grams of cholestyramine). **Note: Actual dosage and administration schedule must be determined by the physician for each patient individually.**

Conditions Requiring Dosing Adjustments

Liver function: Cholestyramine is eliminated via the feces—no liver involvement.

Kidney function: This medication is **not** absorbed, and the kidney is not involved.

▷ **Dosing Instructions:** Always take just before or with a meal; this drug is ineffective when taken without food. Mix the powder thoroughly in 4 to 6 ounces of water, fruit juice, milk, thin soup or a soft food like applesauce; do not use carbonated beverages. **Do not take it in its dry form.**

Usual Duration of Use: Use on a regular schedule for up to 3 weeks may be needed to see this drug's benefit in lowering excessively high cholesterol. Duration of use should not exceed 3 months if an adequate response does not occur. Long-term use (months to years) requires periodic evaluation of response.

▷ **This Drug Should Not Be Taken If**
- you have had an allergic reaction to it previously.
- you have complete biliary obstruction.
- you have type three, four, or five hyperlipoproteinemia, as this drug does not work in these conditions. Ask your doctor.

▷ **Inform Your Physician Before Taking This Drug If**
- you are prone to constipation.
- you have peptic ulcer disease.
- you have a bleeding disorder of any kind.
- you have impaired kidney function.
- you have phenylketonuria (PKU).
- you have a bleeding disorder.

Possible Side Effects (natural, expected, and unavoidable drug actions)
Constipation; interference with normal fat digestion and absorption; reduced absorption of vitamins A, D, E, and K and folic acid.

▷ **Possible Adverse Effects** (unusual, unexpected, and infrequent reactions)
If any of the following develop, consult your physician promptly for guidance.
Mild Adverse Effects
Allergic Reactions: Skin rash, hives, tongue irritation, anal itching.
Loss of appetite, heartburn, abdominal discomfort, excessive gas, nausea, vomiting, diarrhea.
Serious Adverse Effects
Allergic Reaction: Asthmalike wheezing.
Vitamin K deficiency and increased bleeding tendency.
Impaired absorption of calcium; predisposition to osteoporosis.
Gallbladder colic.
Disruption of acid–base balance (acidosis).

▷ **Possible Effects on Sexual Function:** Increased libido (questionable).

Natural Diseases or Disorders That May Be Activated by This Drug
Peptic ulcer disease; steatorrhea (excessive fat in stools) with large doses.

Possible Effects on Laboratory Tests
Blood cholesterol and triglyceride levels: decreased (therapeutic effect).
Blood hemoglobin and iron levels: decreased (drug impairs absorption of iron).
Prothrombin time: increased (drug impairs absorption of vitamin K).
Liver function tests: increased liver enzymes (ALT/GPT, AST/GOT) in a few cases; not thought to be liver damage.

Urine calcium: increased (drug impairs absorption of calcium from intestine).

CAUTION

1. The powder should never be taken in its dry form; always mix it thoroughly with a suitable liquid before swallowing.
2. Use stool softeners and laxatives as needed if constipation develops.
3. This drug may bind other drugs and impair their absorption. It is advisable to take *all other drugs* 1 to 2 hours before or 4 to 6 hours after taking this drug.

Precautions for Use

By Infants and Children: Safety and effectiveness for those under 6 years of age not established. Watch carefully for development of acidosis and vitamin A or folic acid deficiency. (Ask your doctor for help.)

By Those over 60 Years of Age: Increased risk of developing severe constipation. Impaired kidney function may predispose to the development of acidosis.

▷ **Advisability of Use During Pregnancy**

Pregnancy Category: C. See Pregnancy Code at the back of this book.
Animal studies: No information available.
Human studies: Adequate studies of pregnant women are not available.
Use this drug only if clearly needed. Ensure adequate intake of vitamins and minerals. Ask physician for guidance.

Advisability of Use if Breast-Feeding

Presence of this drug in breast milk: No.
Breast-feeding is permitted.

Habit-Forming Potential: None.

Effects of Overdosage: Progressive constipation.

Possible Effects of Long-Term Use

Deficiencies of vitamins A, D, E and K and folic acid.
Calcium deficiency, osteoporosis. Bone mineral density testing is recommended.
Acidosis due to excessive retention of chloride.

Suggested Periodic Examinations While Taking This Drug (at physician's discretion)

Measurements of blood levels of total cholesterol, low density (LDL) cholesterol and high density (HDL) cholesterol.
Hemoglobin and red blood cell studies for possible anemia.

▷ **While Taking This Drug, Observe the Following**

Foods: Avoid foods that tend to constipate (cheeses, etc.).
Nutritional Support: Ask your doctor about the need for supplements of vitamins A, D, E and K, folic acid and calcium.
Beverages: Avoid carbonated beverages. Ensure adequate liquid intake (up to 2 quarts daily). This drug may be taken with milk.

▷ *Alcohol:* No interactions expected.
Tobacco Smoking: No interactions expected.

▷ *Other Drugs*

Cholestyramine may ***decrease*** the effects of
• acetaminophen; give 2 hours before cholestyramine.
• digitoxin and digoxin; give 2 hours before.

- fluvastatin (Lescol).
- furosemide (lasix).
- iron preparations; give 2 to 3 hours before.
- methotrexate; give 3 hours before cholestyramine.
- metronidazole (Flagyl).
- NSAIDS (some acidic ones such as piroxicam and sulindac).
- oral hypoglycemic agents (see Drug Classes).
- penicillin G.
- phenobarbital; give 2 hours before.
- thiazide diuretics (see Drug Classes); give 2 hours before.
- thyroxin; give 5 hours before.
- warfarin; give 6 hours after.

Cholestyramine *taken concurrently* with

- amiodarone (Codarone) can result in lowered amiodarone blood levels and decreased effectiveness.

▷ *Driving, Hazardous Activities:* No restrictions.

Aviation Note: The use of this drug *is usually not a disqualification* for piloting. Consult a designated Aviation Medical Examiner.

Exposure to Sun: No restrictions.

Discontinuation: The dose of any potentially toxic drug taken concurrently must be reduced appropriately when this drug is discontinued.

CIMETIDINE (si MET i deen)

Introduced: 1976, OTC version 1996   **Prescription:**   USA: Yes in one form. An OTC form is now available; Canada: Yes

Author's note: This drug received FDA approval as Tagamet HB, a nonprescription form for heartburn.

Please see histamine (H-2) blocking drug for further information.

CIPROFLOXACIN (sip roh FLOX a sin)

Introduced: 1984   **Prescription:**   USA: Yes   **Available as Generic:** USA: No   **Class:**   Anti-infective, fluoroquinolone   **Controlled Drug:**   USA: No

Brand Name: Ciloxan, Cipro

Warning: **Reports are being made for some drugs in this class which find tendon rupture as a rare adverse effect. Ask your doctor about limits on strenuous exercise while you are taking this medicine. A rare idiosyncratic reaction has also been reported which presents as mental confusion and disorientation. Use of this medicine after head trauma may be a risk factor. If you have suffered a fall, ask your doctor if a medicine in a different antibiotic class should be substituted. If you are taking this drug and notice a change in your thinking, call your doctor.**

BENEFITS versus RISKS	
Possible Benefits	*Possible Risks*
HIGHLY EFFECTIVE TREATMENT FOR INFECTIONS OF THE LOWER RESPIRATORY TRACT, URINARY TRACT, BONES, JOINTS, AND SKIN TISSUES due to susceptible organisms Effective treatment for some forms of bacterial gastroenteritis (diarrhea)	Very rare drug-induced colitis Very rare hallucination or seizure Tendon rupture (rare)

▷ **Principal Uses**

As a Single Drug Product: Uses currently included in FDA approved labeling: Treats responsive infections (in adults) of: (1) the lower respiratory tract (lungs and bronchial tubes); (2) the urinary tract (kidneys, bladder, urethra (including uncomplicated gonorrhea) and prostate gland); (3) the digestive tract (small intestine and colon); (4) bones and joints; (5) skin and related tissues; (6) used in an ophthalmic preparation to treat bacterial conjunctivitis caused by Strep pneumoniae and Staph organisms; (7) ophthalmic preparation used to treat eye (corneal) ulcers caused by Pseudomonas Serratia and Staph.

Other (unlabeled) generally accepted uses: (1) Can have a role in treating cholera where the organisms are resistant to doxycycline; (2) lessens symptoms or prevents traveler's diarrhea; (3) can be of use in treating some unusual organisms such as aeromonas, cat scratch fever or chancroid.

How This Drug Works: It blocks the bacterial enzyme DNA gyrase (required for DNA synthesis and cell reproduction), and arrests bacterial growth (in low concentrations) and kills bacteria (in high concentrations).

Available Dosage Forms and Strengths

Tablets — 250 mg, 500 mg, 750 mg
Ophthalmic solution — 0.3%

▷ **Usual Adult Dosage Range:**   250 mg to 750 mg/12 hours, depending upon the nature and severity of the infection. The total daily dosage should not exceed 1500 mg.

Ophthalmic: 1 or 2 drops instilled in the eye every 2 hours while awake for 2 days, then 1 or 2 drops for 5 more days which is given every 4 hours while awake. **Note: Actual dosage and administration schedule must be determined by the physician for each patient individually.**

Conditions Requiring Dosing Adjustments

Liver function: Used with caution in severe liver failure.

Kidney function: Dose **must** be decreased (or interval lengthened) in kidney compromise.

Cystic Fibrosis

A loading dose as well as ongoing doses of 750 mg every 8 hours is given in cystic fibrosis patients. This dosing gives blood levels which are more aggressive versus the bacteria which usually cause infections in these patients.

▷ **Dosing Instructions:** May be taken with or without food and may be crushed. Best taken 2 hours after eating. Drink large amounts of fluids during treatment. Avoid aluminum or magnesium antacids, iron, zinc or calcium for 2 hours before and after taking this medicine.

Usual Duration of Use: Use on a regular schedule for 7 to 14 days is needed to see this drug's effectiveness in eradicating infection. The drug should be continued for at least 2 days after all indications of infection have disappeared. Bone and joint infections may be treated for 6 weeks or longer. Long-term use requires periodic evaluation of response.

Possible Advantages of This Drug

Very broad spectrums of antibacterial activity of all currently available oral antimicrobial drugs.

Among the most potent anti-infective actions of quinolones.

Highly effective in treating numerous types of infection caused by a wide spectrum of bacteria.

Provides effective drug levels in the prostate gland (a difficult place to penetrate).

▷ **This Drug Should Not Be Taken If**
- you have had an allergic reaction to it or any quinolone drug previously.
- you are pregnant or breast-feeding.
- you have a seizure disorder that is not adequately controlled.
- it is prescribed for a person under 18 years of age.

▷ **Inform Your Physician Before Taking This Drug If**
- you are allergic to cinoxacin (Cinobac), nalidixic acid (NegGram), norfloxacin (Noroxin), or other quinolone drugs.
- you have a seizure disorder or a circulatory disorder of the brain.
- you have impaired liver or kidney function.
- you have a history of mental disorders (psychosis).
- you are taking any form of probenecid or theophylline.

Possible Side Effects (natural, expected, and unavoidable drug actions)

Superinfections (see Glossary). Permanent greenish tooth discoloration if used in infants.

▷ **Possible Adverse Effects** (unusual, unexpected, and infrequent reactions)

If any of the following develop, consult your physician promptly for guidance.

Mild Adverse Effects

Allergic Reactions: Rash, itching, localized swelling (all rare).

Dizziness, headache, weakness, migraine, anxiety, abnormal vision (all rare).

Nausea, diarrhea, vomiting, indigestion (all rare).

Muscle aches.

Burning feeling in the eye when the ophthalmic solution is used.

Serious Adverse Effects

Allergic Reactions: Anaphylaxis.

Idiosyncratic Reactions: Mental confusion and incapacitation.

Central nervous system stimulation: restlessness, tremor, confusion, hallucinations, seizures (all very rare).

Kidney disease (interstitial nephritis) (rare).

Tendon rupture (rare).

Decreased vision (with ophthalmic use) (rare).
Rare abnormal heart beats or palpitations.
Liver toxicity (rare).

▷ **Possible Effects on Sexual Function:**   None reported.

▷ **Natural Diseases or Disorders That May Be Activated by This Drug**
Latent epilepsy, latent gout.

Possible Effects on Laboratory Tests
Kidney function: increased blood creatinine and urea nitrogen (BUN) (rare).
Liver function tests: increased as a sign of liver toxicity (rare).

CAUTION

1. With high doses or prolonged use, crystal formation in the kidney may occur. This can be prevented by drinking large amounts of water, up to 2 quarts/24 hours.
2. May decrease saliva formation; make dental cavities or gum disease more likely. Consult your dentist if dry mouth persists.
3. Strenuous exercise is NOT recommended while this medicine is being taken.
4. If a sudden change in mental status is noticed, call your doctor immediately.

Precautions for Use
By Infants and Children: Avoid the use of this drug completely. Impairs normal bone growth and development.
By Those over 60 Years of Age: Impaired kidney function may require dosage reduction.
If taking theophylline with this drug, the theophylline dose must be decreased.

▷ **Advisability of Use During Pregnancy**
Pregnancy Category: C. See Pregnancy Code at the back of this book.
Animal studies: No birth defects due to this drug found in mouse or rat studies. Rabbit studies showed maternal weight loss and increased abortions. This drug can impair normal bone development in immature dogs.
Human studies: Adequate studies of pregnant women are not available. However, the potential for adverse effects on fetal bone development contraindicates the use of this drug during entire pregnancy.

Advisability of Use if Breast-Feeding
Presence of this drug in breast milk: Probably yes.
Avoid drug or refrain from nursing.

Habit-Forming Potential: None.

Effects of Overdosage: Confusion, headache, abdominal pain, diarrhea, liver toxicity, seizures, kidney toxicity and hallucinations.

Possible Effects of Long-Term Use: Superinfections (see Glossary); crystal formation in kidneys.

Suggested Periodic Examinations While Taking This Drug (at physician's discretion)
Liver function tests, urine analysis.

▷ **While Taking This Drug, Observe the Following**

Foods: Caffeine will remain in your system longer than usual.

Dairy foods will decrease the effectiveness of ciprofloxacin by decreasing the amount absorbed.

Beverages: No restrictions. May be taken with milk.

▷ *Alcohol:* No interactions expected.

Tobacco Smoking: No interactions expected.

▷ *Other Drugs*

Ciprofloxacin may *increase* the effects of
- theophylline, and cause theophylline toxicity.

The following drug may *increase* the effects of ciprofloxacin
- probenecid (Benemid).

Ciprofloxacin *taken concurrently* with
- azlocillin may result in ciprofloxacin toxicity.
- caffeine will result in increased caffeine levels.
- cyclosporine (Sandimmune) may result in increased risk of kidney toxicity.
- foscarnet may result in an increased risk of seizures.
- phenytoin (Dilantin) may result in increased or decreased Dilantin levels.
- warfarin can result in increased risk of bleeding.

The following drugs may *decrease* the effects of ciprofloxacin
- antacids containing aluminum or magnesium can reduce the absorption of ciprofloxacin and lessen its effectiveness.
- calcium supplements.
- didanosine.
- iron salts.
- sucralfate.
- zinc salts.

▷ *Driving, Hazardous Activities:* May cause dizziness and impair vision. Restrict activities as necessary.

Aviation Note: The use of this drug *may be a disqualification* for piloting. Consult a designated Aviation Medical Examiner.

Exposure to Sun: May rarely cause photosensitivity (see Glossary). Sunglasses are advised if eyes are overly sensitive to bright light.

Heavy Exercise or Exertion: Several reports have surfaced regarding tendon rupture in patients on this medication. It is prudent to avoid heavy exercise or exertion while you are taking this medicine.

Discontinuation: If you experience no adverse effects from this drug, take the full course prescribed for best results. Ask your doctor when to stop treatment.

CISAPRIDE (SIS a pryde)

Introduced: 1993   **Prescription:** USA: Yes; Canada: Yes   **Available as Generic:** USA: No; Canada: No   **Class:** Gastrointestional drug   **Controlled Drug:** USA: No; Canada: No

Brand Names: Propulsid, ✦Prepulsid

BENEFITS versus RISKS

Possible Benefits	*Possible Risks*
EFFECTIVE TREATMENT OF NOCTURNAL HEARTBURN	Diarrhea, cramping
FEW CENTRAL NERVOUS SIDE EFFECTS	Joint pain
May have a role in helping diabetic gastroparesis	

▷ **Principal Uses**

As a Single Drug Product: Uses currently included in FDA approved labeling: (1) Used to relieve symptoms of reflux esophagitis; (2) helps decrease nocturnal heartburn caused by gastroesophageal reflux disease.

Other (unlabeled) generally accepted uses: (1) May have a role in helping improve delayed stomach emptying which may lead to anorexia nervosa; (2) can help children with chronic constipation; (3) helps relieve slow emptying of the stomach (diabetic gastroparesis) often seen in diabetes; (4) relieves slowed stomach emptying caused by morphine; (5) decreases pain and flatulence in irritable bowel syndrome; (6) helps the gallbladder work better in patients with myotonic muscular dystrophy; (7) can be of help in promoting defecation in patients with spinal cord injury.

How This Drug Works: Increases the movement of the esophagus (by activating a specific muscarinic receptor) and increases contractions in the stomach and helps it to empty.

Available Dosage Forms and Strengths

Tablets — 10 mg, 20 mg

Oral suspension — 1 mg per ml

▷ **Recommended Dosage Ranges (Actual dosage and administration schedule must be determined by the physician for each patient individually.)**

Infants and Children: Safety and efficacy not established in children or infants.

12 to 60 Years of Age: For relief of nocturnal heartburn: 10 to 20 mg four times a day given 15 minutes before meals and at bedtime.

For reflux esophagitis: 10 mg four times a day combined with cimetidine one gram a day.

For diabetic gastroparesis: 10 mg four times a day given 15 minutes before meals and at bedtime.

Over 60 Years of Age: Same as 12 to 60 years of age.

Conditions Requiring Dosing Adjustments

Liver function: Patients with liver failure should be given 50% of the usual dose. The dose may then be increased (titrated upward) as needed and tolerated.

Kidney function: Dose changes are not needed in kidney failure, but metabolites may accumulate.

▷ **Dosing Instructions:**   This medicine should be taken 15 minutes before meals and at bedtime for best effect.

Usual Duration of Use: Use on a regular schedule for 8 to 12 weeks may be needed to see the peak benefit in treating chronic functional constipation. Up to 12 weeks may be needed to realize the full therapeutic effect when used in therapy of reflux esophagitis. Long-term use (months to years) requires periodic physician evaluation of response and dosage adjustment.

Possible Advantages of This Drug
Significant decrease in central nervous side effects compared to metoclopramide.

Currently a "Drug of Choice"
for patients who are unable to tolerate metoclopramide and are using it for a condition which cisapride effectively treats.

▷ **This Drug Should Not Be Taken If**
- you have had an allergic reaction to any dosage form of it previously.
- you have gastrointestinal obstruction, hemorrhage or perforation.
- you are taking fluconazole, miconazole, itraconazole, ketoconazole or macrolide antibiotics such as clarithromycin, erythromycin or troleandomycin)

▷ **Inform Your Physician Before Taking This Drug If**
- you currently take a benzodiazepine drug (see Drug Classes Section).
- you have an abnormally fast heart beat.
- you take other prescription or nonprescription medicines which were not discussed with your doctor when cisapride was prescribed.

Possible Side Effects (natural, expected, and unavoidable drug actions)
Sleepiness and fatigue (rare).

▷ **Possible Adverse Effects** (unusual, unexpected, and infrequent reactions)
If any of the following develop, consult your physician promptly for guidance.
Mild Adverse Effects
Allergic Reactions: Skin rash and itching.
Depression (rare), somnolence and fatigue (rare), rare joint pain.
Abnormal vision (rare).
Occasional headache, dizziness, and sleep disturbances.
Rhinitis, sinusitis, or coughing (rare).
Diarrhea, abdominal pain, joint pain (infrequent).
Urinary incontinence (rare).
Serious Adverse Effects
Allergic Reactions: Anaphylactoid reaction (see Glossary).
Rare increases in heart rate, palpitations, or abnormal heartbeat.

▷ **Possible Effects on Sexual Function:**   None reported.

Possible Delayed Adverse Effects: None defined.

Possible Effects on Laboratory Tests
Liver function tests: increased liver enzymes (SGOT, SGPT and CPK).

CAUTION
1. May cause increased heart rate. Notify physician if this occurs.
2. Report promptly any increased tendency to depression.

Precautions for Use
By Infants and Children: Safety and effectiveness for children not established.
By Those over 60 Years of Age: Specific changes not required.

▷ **Advisability of Use During Pregnancy**
Pregnancy Category: C. See Pregnancy Code at the back of this book.
Animal studies: Has caused prolongation of breeding interval in female rats.
Embryotoxic and fetotoxic in high dose studies in rats.

Human studies: Adequate studies of pregnant women are not available. Used as a benefit to risk decision in pregnancy. Ask your doctor for help.

Advisability of Use if Breast-Feeding
Presence of this drug in breast milk: Yes.
Monitor nursing infant closely and discontinue drug or nursing if adverse effects develop.

Habit-Forming Potential: None.

Effects of Overdosage: Nausea, vomiting, flatulence, increased urination and diarrhea

Possible Effects of Long-Term Use: None defined.

Suggested Periodic Examinations While Taking This Drug (at physician's discretion)
Complete blood counts: Periodically.

▷ **While Taking This Drug, Observe the Following**
Foods: No restrictions, but food may actually increase the blood level obtained.
Beverages: No restrictions.
▷ *Alcohol:* Sedative effects of alcohol will be increased.
Tobacco Smoking: No interactions expected.
Marijuana Smoking: May cause additive drowsiness.
▷ *Other Drugs*
Cisapride may *decrease* the effects of .
• warfarin (Coumadin) and decrease benefits. More frequent prothrombin times are indicated, and dosing should be adjusted if needed.
Cisapride *taken concurrently* with
• cimetidine (Tagamet) results in increased cisapride levels and potential cisapride toxicity. Cisapride dose may need to be decreased.
• diazepam (Valium) can lead to up to a 17% increase in the peak drug level.
• itraconazole (Sporonox), ketoconazole (Nizoral), fluconazole (Diflucan) or miconazole (Monistat IV) can lead to cisapride toxicity and abnormal heart effects.
• macrolide antibiotics such as clarithromycin (Biaxin), erythromycin (E-mycin, others) or troleandomycin can lead to cisapride toxicity.
▷ *Driving, Hazardous Activities:* This drug may cause some drowsiness. Restrict activities as necessary.
Aviation Note: The use of this drug *may be a disqualification* for piloting. Consult a designated Aviation Medical Examiner.
Exposure to Sun: No restrictions.
Discontinuation: If this medication is stopped and you have been taking an anticoagulant, INR (prothrombin time) testing will be needed.

CLARITHROMYCIN (klar ith roh MY sin)

Introduced: 1991   **Prescription:**   USA: Yes   **Available as Generic:**
USA: No   **Class:**   Anti-infective, macrolide   **Controlled Drug:**   USA: No
Brand Name: Biaxin

BENEFITS versus RISKS	
Possible Benefits	*Possible Risks*
EFFECTIVE TREATMENT OF UPPER AND LOWER RESPIRATORY TRACT INFECTIONS due to susceptible microorganisms	Mild gastrointestinal symptoms Drug-induced colitis (rare) Superinfections (rare)
EFFECTIVE TREATMENT OF SKIN INFECTIONS due to susceptible microorganisms	

▷ **Principal Uses**

As a Single Drug Product: Uses currently included in FDA approved labeling: (1) Treatment of certain upper respiratory tract infections—maxillary sinusitis, pharyngitis, tonsillitis; (2) treatment of some lower respiratory tract infections—acute bronchitis and pneumonia; (3) treatment of certain skin (and skin structure) infections. As necessary, bacterial cultures and sensitivity testing should be performed; (4) treatment of mycobacterium avium complex (MAI) infections; (5) prevention of disseminated mycobacterium avium complex in advanced HIV.

Other (unlabeled) generally accepted uses: (1) Combination antibiotic treatment of duodenal ulcer disease caused by H. pylori; (2) can have a role in combination therapy of some toxoplasmosis infections.

How This Drug Works: This drug prevents the growth and multiplication of susceptible organisms by interfering with their formation of essential proteins.

Available Dosage Forms and Strengths

Tablets — 250 mg, 500 mg
Oral suspension granules — 125 and 250 mg

▷ **Recommended Dosage Ranges** (Actual dosage and administration schedule must be determined by the physician for each patient individually.)

Infants and Children: Used to treat otitis media (caused by H. influenza, M. catarrhalis or S. pneumoniae) in children: The dose here is 7.5 mg per kg twice daily up to a maximum of 500 mg twice a day for 10 days. For Mycobacterium avium complex infections in children: The dose is 7.5 mg per kg twice daily to a maximum of 500 mg twice a day. If this dose is successful, therapy is continued for life.

12 to 60 Years of Age: For pharyngitis/tonsillitis—250 mg/12 hours for 10 days. For maxillary sinusitis—500 mg/12 hours for 14 days. For acute bronchitis—250–500 mg/12 hours for 7 to 14 days. For pneumonia—250 mg/12 hours for 7 to 14 days. For skin infections—250 mg/12 hours for 7 to 14 days.

Over 60 Years of Age: Same as 12 to 60 years of age. Dose must be reduced in kidney compromise.

Conditions Requiring Dosing Adjustments

Liver function: If kidney function is normal, dose decrease not needed with liver problems.

Kidney function: The dose **must be decreased** or **the time between doses (dosing interval) prolonged** in patients with compromised kidneys.

▷ **Dosing Instructions:**   May be taken with or without food. The tablet may be crushed when taken.

Usual Duration of Use: Use on a regular schedule for 4 to 6 days is usually needed to see this drug's benefit in controlling responsive infections. For streptococcal throat infections; not less than 10 consecutive days (without interruption) will reduce the risk of rheumatic fever or glomerulonephritis. Use should stop when the infection is eliminated.

Possible Advantages of This Drug

Single drug effectiveness against a broader spectrum of bacteria; equivalent to erythromycin, some penicillins and some cephalosporins. Effective with only 2 doses daily. Can be taken without regard to eating.

Very well tolerated; infrequent and minor adverse effects.

▷ **This Drug Should Not Be Taken If**
- you have had an allergic reaction to it previously.

▷ **Inform Your Physician Before Taking This Drug If**
- you are allergic to: azithromycin, erythromycin, or troleandomycin.
- you have impaired liver or kidney function.
- you have a history of drug-induced colitis.
- you have a history of low blood platelets.
- you are pregnant or planning pregnancy.

Possible Side Effects (natural, expected, and unavoidable drug actions)

Superinfections (see Glossary).

▷ **Possible Adverse Effects** (unusual, unexpected, and infrequent reactions)

If any of the following develop, consult your physician promptly for guidance.

Mild Adverse Effects

Allergic Reactions: Pruritic rash.

Headache (rare).

Abnormal taste, nausea, stomach pain, indigestion, diarrhea.

Serious Adverse Effects

Allergic Reactions: Leukocytoclastic vasculitis.

Drug-induced colitis (rare).

Low blood platelets (rare).

Kidney toxicity (rare).

Acute psychosis (two recent case reports) (very rare).

▷ **Possible Effects on Sexual Function:**   None reported.

Possible Effects on Laboratory Tests

INR (prothrombin time): increased (1%).

Liver function tests: increased liver enzymes (ALT/GPT, AST/GOT and alkaline phosphatase), increased bilirubin (all less than 1%).

Kidney function tests: increased blood urea nitrogen (4%).

CAUTION

1. If diarrhea starts and continues for more than 24 hours, call your doctor promptly. This could be the onset of drug-induced colitis.
2. Take the full amount prescribed to help prevent resistant bacteria.

Precautions for Use

By Infants and Children: Safety and effectiveness for those under 12 years of age not established.

By Those over 60 Years of Age: Consider dosage adjustment if kidney function is severely impaired.

▷ **Advisability of Use During Pregnancy**
Pregnancy Category: C. See Pregnancy Code at the back of this book.
  Animal studies: Monkey, rabbit, rat and mouse studies have demonstrated adverse effects on fetal development and pregnancy outcome.
  Human studies: Adequate studies of pregnant women are not available.
  This drug should not be used during pregnancy except where no alternative treatment is appropriate. Ask your doctor for help.

Advisability of Use if Breast-Feeding
  Presence of this drug in breast milk: Probably yes.
  Watch nursing infant closely and stop the drug or nursing if adverse effects develop.

Habit-Forming Potential: None.

Effects of Overdosage: Possible nausea, vomiting, abdominal discomfort and diarrhea.

Possible Effects of Long-Term Use: Superinfections, drug-induced colitis.

Suggested Periodic Examinations While Taking This Drug (at physician's discretion)
  Repeat complete blood count (CBC)

▷ **While Taking This Drug, Observe the Following**
Foods: No restrictions.
Beverages: No restrictions. May be taken with milk.
▷ *Alcohol:* No interactions expected.
Tobacco Smoking: No interactions expected.
▷ *Other Drugs*
    Clarithromycin may *increase* the effects of
    • astemizole and cause life-threatening heart rhythms.
    • carbamazepine (Tegretol); check blood levels of carbamazepine.
    • digoxin (Lanoxin).
    • tacrolimus (Prograft).
    • terfenadine (Seldane) and cause life-threatening heart rhythms.
    • theophylline (Theo-Dur, Theolair, etc.); monitor blood levels of theophylline if appropriate.
    • warfarin and cause bleeding.
    Clarithromycin *taken concurrently* with
    • cyclosporine (Sandimune) may lead to cyclosporine toxicity.
    • dihydroergotamine can lead to increased levels and dihydroergotamine toxicity.
    • ergotamine can cause toxicity.
    • zidovudine may lead to decreased levels and lack of zidovudine effectiveness.
▷ *Driving, Hazardous Activities:* This drug may cause nausea and/or diarrhea. Restrict activities as necessary.
Aviation Note: The use of this drug *may be a disqualification* for piloting. Consult a designated Aviation Medical Examiner.
Exposure to Sun: No restrictions.

CLINDAMYCIN (klin da MY sin)

Introduced: 1973   **Prescription:** USA: Yes; Canada: Yes   **Available as Generic:** USA: Yes; Canada: No   **Class:** Antibiotic   **Controlled Drug:** USA: No; Canada: No

Brand Names: Cleocin, Cleocin T, ✣Dalacin C, ✣Dalacin T

BENEFITS versus RISKS

Possible Benefits	*Possible Risks*
EFFECTIVE TREATMENT FOR SERIOUS INFECTIONS OF THE LOWER RESPIRATORY TRACT, ABDOMINAL CAVITY, GENITAL TRACT IN WOMEN, BLOOD STREAM (SEPTICEMIA), SKIN AND RELATED TISSUES caused by susceptible organisms	SEVERE DRUG-INDUCED COLITIS (fatalities reported)
Combination treatment of Pneumocystis carinii pneumonia	Rare liver injury with jaundice
Effective for the local treatment of acne	Rare reduction in white blood cell and platelet counts

---

▷ **Principal Uses**

As a Single Drug Product

Uses currently included in FDA approved labeling: (1) Treats serious and unusual infections of the lungs and bronchial tubes, organs and tissues within the abdominal cavity, the genital tract and pelvic organs in women, the skin and soft tissue structures and generalized infections involving the bloodstream; (2) used in topical form to treat acne.

Other (unlabeled) generally accepted uses: (1) Treatment of resistant gum disease, and malaria; (2) prevention of infection of the heart; (3) combination treatment of pneumocystis carinii pneumonia, an infection associated with AIDS; (4) may have a role in combination therapy of Toxoplasmosis infections of the brain in AIDS patients.

How This Drug Works: By blocking the formation of critical growth and reproductive proteins, this drug (in low concentrations) stops multiplication of bacteria and (in high concentrations) kills bacteria.

Available Dosage Forms and Strengths

Capsules — 75 mg, 150 mg, 300 mg

Injection — 150 mg per ml

Oral solution — 75 mg per 5 ml

Topical gel — 10 mg per ml

Topical lotion — 1%

Topical solution — 10 mg per ml

Vaginal cream — 2%

▷ **Usual Adult Dosage Range:** For infections of average severity: 150 to 300 mg/6 hours; for more severe infections: 300 to 450 mg/6 hours. The total daily dosage should not exceed 1800 mg. In treating acne: The topical formulation is applied to the affected area twice daily. In PCP pneumonia in AIDS patients: Intravenous or oral therapy: 900 to 2700 mg daily given in divided doses every 6 hours in combination with primaquine (15 to 30 mg of base daily). **Note: Actual dosage and administration schedule must be determined by the physician for each patient individually.**

Conditions Requiring Dosing Adjustments
   Liver function: The dose must be decreased with liver compromise, and blood levels checked.
   Kidney function: Serum levels should be checked in patients with renal compromise, and the dose adjusted appropriately.

▷ **Dosing Instructions:**   Take the capsule with a full glass of water or with food to prevent irritation. The capsule may be opened and the contents mixed with food for administration. Shake the oral solution well before measuring the dose. Do not refrigerate the oral solution; chilling can cause it to thicken, making it difficult to take. The topical lotion should be shaken well before it is applied.

Usual Duration of Use: Use on a regular schedule for 3 to 5 days is usually needed to see this drug's effect in controlling infections.

Possible Advantages of This Drug: Bacterial sensitivity testing may show this drug to be more effective than other antibiotics in treating some severe infections.

▷ **This Drug Should Not Be Taken If**
   • you are allergic to either clindamycin or lincomycin.
   • it is prescribed for a mild or trivial infection.
   • you have a history of Crohn's disease or ulcerative colitis.

▷ **Inform Your Physician Before Taking This Drug If**
   • you have a history of allergy to any drug.
   • you have a history of drug-induced colitis.
   • you are allergic by nature: Hay fever, asthma, hives, eczema.
   • you have a history of previous yeast infections.
   • you have a blood disorder.
   • you have myasthenia gravis.
   • you have impaired liver or kidney function.
   • you plan to have surgery under general anesthesia in the near future.

Possible Side Effects (natural, expected, and unavoidable drug actions)
   Superinfections (see Glossary).

▷ **Possible Adverse Effects** (unusual, unexpected, and infrequent reactions)
   If any of the following develop, consult your physician promptly for guidance.
   Mild Adverse Effects
   Allergic Reactions: Skin rashes, hives.
   Nausea, vomiting, mild diarrhea, stomach pain.
   Multiple joint pains (rare).
   Serious Adverse Effects
   Allergic Reactions: Severe skin reactions: erythema multiforme (Stevens-Johnson syndrome).
   Toxic liver reaction with jaundice (see Glossary).
   Severe colitis with persistent diarrhea; stools may contain blood and/or mucus.

Rare reduction of white blood cell and platelet counts.
Neuromuscular blockade (dose-related) (rare).

▷ **Possible Effects on Sexual Function:**   None reported.

Possible Delayed Adverse Effects: Severe colitis with diarrhea (pseudomembranous colitis) may start several weeks after stopping this drug.

▷ **Adverse Effects That May Mimic Natural Diseases or Disorders**
Liver reactions may suggest viral hepatitis.
Multiple joint pains may suggest the onset of arthritis.

▷ **Natural Diseases or Disorders That May Be Activated by This Drug**
Crohn's disease, ulcerative colitis, myasthenia gravis.

Possible Effects on Laboratory Tests
Complete blood counts: decreased white cells and platelets; increased eosinophils (allergic reaction).
Liver function tests: uncommon, mild and transient increases in liver enzymes (ALT/GPT, AST/GOT, alkaline phosphatase).

CAUTION
1. Persistent diarrhea can develop in some patients. If diarrhea persists longer than 24 hours, stop the drug and call your doctor.
2. If surgery under general anesthesia is planned, the anesthetic must be carefully chosen to prevent clindamycin-induced excessive muscle relaxation (neuromuscular blockade) and breathing problems.

Precautions for Use
By Infants and Children: Safety and effectiveness for those under 1 month of age not established. Use with caution.
By Those over 60 Years of Age: Diarrhea will be more common in this age group. Watch for development of yeast infection of the skin in the genital and anal regions, a form of superinfection (see Glossary). Report such developments promptly to your physician.

▷ **Advisability of Use During Pregnancy**
Pregnancy Category: B. See Pregnancy Code at the back of this book.
Animal studies: No birth defects due to this drug found in mouse or rat studies.
Human studies: Adequate studies of pregnant women are not available. Use this drug only if clearly needed. Ask your physician for guidance.

Advisability of Use if Breast-Feeding
Presence of this drug in breast milk: Yes.
Avoid drug or refrain from nursing.

Habit-Forming Potential: None.

Effects of Overdosage: Nausea, vomiting, cramping, diarrhea.

Possible Effects of Long-Term Use
Superinfections, especially from yeast organisms.
Severe colitis with persistent diarrhea.

Suggested Periodic Examinations While Taking This Drug (at physician's discretion)
Complete blood cell counts, liver function tests.

▷ **While Taking This Drug, Observe the Following**
   Foods: No restrictions.
   Beverages: No restrictions. May be taken with milk.
▷ *Alcohol:* No interactions expected.
   Tobacco Smoking: No interactions expected.
▷ *Other Drugs*
   Clindamycin **taken concurrently** with
   • antidiarrheal drugs (diphenoxylate, loperamide, paregoric) may result in
     worsening of the underlying colitis. Avoid the combination.
   • antimyasthenic drugs (ambenonium, neostigmine, pyridostigmine) may
     reduce their benefit in relieving muscle weakness of myasthenia gravis.
   • dantrolene or other skeletal muscle relaxants may result in enhanced or
     protracted and potentially dangerous muscle relaxation.
   The following drugs may **decrease** the effects of clindamycin
   • chloramphenicol (Chloromycetin).
   • macrolide antibiotics such as erythromycin (E.E.S., E-Mycin, etc.), clari-
     thromycin or azithromycin.
▷ *Driving, Hazardous Activities:* This drug may cause nausea and diarrhea. Restrict activities as necessary.
   Aviation Note: The use of this drug **may be a disqualification** for piloting. Consult a designated Aviation Medical Examiner.
   Exposure to Sun: Use caution until sensitivity is determined.
   Discontinuation: If tolerated, take the full course prescribed. When used to treat
   infections that may predispose to rheumatic fever or nephritis, take continually in full dosage for no less than 10 days.
   Special Storage Instructions: Oral solution should be kept at room temperature;
   do not refrigerate.
   Observe the Following Expiration Times: Do not take the oral solution if it is
   older than 14 days.

CLOMIPRAMINE (kloh MI pra meen)

Introduced: 1970   **Prescription:** USA: Yes; Canada: Yes   **Available as
Generic:** USA: No; Canada: No   **Class:** Antidepressant   **Controlled Drug:**
USA: No; Canada: No

Brand Name: Anafranil

BENEFITS versus RISKS	
Possible Benefits	*Possible Risks*
EFFECTIVE TREATMENT OF SEVERE OBSESSIVE-COMPULSIVE NEUROSIS	DRUG-INDUCED SEIZURES (rare) ADVERSE BEHAVIORAL EFFECTS Conversion of depression to mania in manic-depressive (bipolar) disorders
Effective relief of symptoms of some types of endogenous depression	Aggravation of schizophrenia Rare liver toxicity Rare bone marrow depression and blood cell disorders

▷ **Principal Uses**

As a Single Drug Product: Uses currently included in FDA approved labeling: (1) Relieves manifestations of severe, disabling obsessive-compulsive disorder.

Other (unlabeled) generally accepted uses: (1) Relieves symptoms of panic attacks; (2) helps some phobias; (3) may help repetitive symptoms in autistics; (4) could have a role in diabetic neuropathy; (5) can help premature ejaculation; (6) may relieve severity of hair pulling syndromes, severe nail biting and arm burning in obsessive-compulsive patients; (7) can help relieve symptoms in severe premenstrual syndrome.

How This Drug Works: By increasing brain levels of some nerve transmitters, principally serotonin, this drug reduces the frequency and intensity of obsessive and compulsive behavior patterns.

Available Dosage Forms and Strengths

Capsules — 10 mg (Canada only), 25 mg, 50 mg, 75 mg

▷ **Usual Adult Dosage Range:**   Initially 25 mg daily, taken in the evening. Dose may be increased cautiously as needed and tolerated by 25 mg daily at intervals of 3 to 4 days until a dose of 100 mg daily is reached in 2 weeks. This larger dose should be divided and taken after meals. The usual maintenance dose is 50 mg to 150 mg/24 hours. The total daily dosage should not exceed 250 mg. (When determined, the optimal daily requirement may be given at bedtime as a single dose.) **Note: Actual dosage and administration schedule must be determined by the physician for each patient individually.**

Conditions Requiring Dosing Adjustments

Liver function: The dose should be decreased in patients with liver compromise.
Kidney function: Changes in dose are not usually needed.

▷ **Dosing Instructions:**   May be taken without regard to meals. If needed, the capsule may be opened and may be taken with or following food to reduce stomach upset.

Usual Duration of Use: Use on a regular schedule for 3 to 4 weeks is usually needed to see this drug's benefit in controlling obsessive-compulsive behavior; peak response may require 3 or more months of use. Long-term use (months to years) requires periodic evaluation.

▷ **This Drug Should Not Be Taken If**
- you have had an allergic reaction to it previously.
- you are taking, or have taken within the past 14 days, any monoamine oxidase (MAO) type A inhibitor drug (see Drug Classes).
- you have active bone marrow depression or a current blood cell disorder.
- you have had a recent heart attack (myocardial infarction).
- you have narrow-angle glaucoma.

▷ **Inform Your Physician Before Taking This Drug If**
- you have had an adverse reaction to an antidepressant drug, especially one of the tricyclic class.
- you have a history of bone marrow or blood cell disorder.
- you have any type of seizure disorder.
- you have increased internal eye pressure.
- you have any type of heart disease, especially coronary artery disease or a heart rhythm disorder.

- you are subject to bronchial asthma.
- you have impaired liver or kidney function.
- you have any type of thyroid disorder or are taking thyroid medication.
- you have a history of suicide attempts.
- you have an adrenalin-producing tumor.
- you have prostatism (see Glossary).
- you have a history of alcoholism.
- you plan to have surgery under general anesthesia in the near future.

Possible Side Effects (natural, expected, and unavoidable drug actions)
Drowsiness, increased sweating, light-headedness, blurred vision, dry mouth, constipation, impaired urination.

▷ **Possible Adverse Effects** (unusual, unexpected, and infrequent reactions)
If any of the following develop, consult your physician promptly for guidance.
Mild Adverse Effects
Allergic Reactions: Skin rash, itching, drug fever (see Glossary).
Headache, dizziness, nervousness, impaired memory, weakness, tremors, insomnia, muscle cramps, flushing.
Increased appetite, weight gain.
Altered taste, indigestion, nausea, vomiting, diarrhea.
Serious Adverse Effects
Allergic Reactions: Drug-induced hepatitis, with or without jaundice.
Idiosyncratic Reactions: Neuroleptic malignant syndrome (see Glossary).
Adverse behavioral effects: confusion, delirium, disorientation, delusions, hallucinations, paranoia.
Seizures; reduced control of epilepsy.
Aggravation of paranoid psychoses and schizophrenia.
Heart rhythm disturbances.
Bone marrow depression (see Glossary): fatigue, weakness, fever, sore throat, infections, abnormal bleeding or bruising.
SIADH and severe lowering of blood sodium.
Liver toxicity.
Serotonin syndrome.

▷ **Possible Effects on Sexual Function**
Altered libido, impaired (delayed) ejaculation, impotence, inhibited male orgasm, inhibited female orgasm, abnormal sperm formation, female breast enlargement with milk production.

▷ **Adverse Effects That May Mimic Natural Diseases or Disorders**
Liver toxicity may suggest viral hepatitis.

Natural Diseases or Disorders That May Be Activated by This Drug
Latent epilepsy, glaucoma, prostatism, schizophrenia.

Possible Effects on Laboratory Tests
Complete blood cell counts: decreased red cells, hemoglobin, white cells and platelets.
Liver function tests: increased liver enzymes (ALT/GPT, AST/GOT)—liver damage.
Thyroid function tests: decreased TT3 and FT3.
Blood sodium: severely lowered in cases of drug-induced SIADH.

CAUTION
1. Watch for toxicity: Confusion, agitation, rapid heart rate, heart irregularity. Blood levels will clarify the situation.
2. Use with caution in schizophrenia. Watch closely for deterioration of thinking or behavior.
3. Use with caution in epilepsy. Watch for any change in the frequency or severity of seizures.

Precautions for Use

By Infants and Children: Safety and effectiveness for those under 10 years of age not established. Dose and management should be supervised by a properly trained pediatrician. Total daily dosage should not exceed 200 mg.

By Those over 60 Years of Age: Start treatment with 10 mg at bedtime. Dose may be increased gradually as needed and tolerated to 75 mg daily in divided doses. During the first 2 weeks of treatment, watch for behavioral reactions: Restlessness, agitation, forgetfulness, disorientation, delusions or hallucinations. Also observe for unsteadiness and instability that may predispose to falling. This drug may aggravate prostatism.

▷ ## Advisability of Use During Pregnancy

Pregnancy Category: C. See Pregnancy Code at the back of this book.

Animal studies: No drug-induced birth defects reported in mouse or rat studies.

Human studies: Adequate studies of pregnant women are not available.

Use only if clearly needed. Avoid use during the last 3 months, if possible, to prevent withdrawal symptoms in the newborn infant: irritability, tremors, seizures.

Advisability of Use if Breast-Feeding

Presence of this drug in breast milk: Yes.

Avoid drug or refrain from nursing.

Habit-Forming Potential: Psychological or physical dependence is rare and unexpected. This drug is not liable to abuse.

Effects of Overdosage: Confusion, delirium, hallucinations, drowsiness, tremors, unsteadiness, heart irregularity, seizures, stupor, sweating, fever.

Possible Effects of Long-Term Use: Neuroleptic malignant syndrome (see Glossary): Fever, fast or irregular heartbeat, fast breathing, sweating, weakness, muscle stiffness, seizures, loss of bladder control.

Suggested Periodic Examinations While Taking This Drug (at physician's discretion)

Monitoring of blood drug levels as appropriate.

Complete blood cell counts; liver and kidney function tests.

Serial blood pressure readings and electrocardiograms.

Measurement of internal eye pressure.

▷ ## While Taking This Drug, Observe the Following

Foods: No specific restrictions. May need to limit food intake to avoid excessive weight gain.

Beverages: No restrictions. May be taken with milk.

▷ *Alcohol:* Avoid completely. This drug can markedly increase the intoxicating effects of alcohol; the combination can depress brain function significantly.

Tobacco Smoking: May delay the elimination of this drug and require dosage adjustment.

Marijuana Smoking: Increased drowsiness and mouth dryness; and reduced effectiveness.

▷ *Other Drugs*

Clomipramine may *increase* the effects of
- all drugs with sedative effects; observe for excessive sedation.
- all drugs with atropinelike effects (see Drug Classes).

Clomipramine may *decrease* the effects of
- clonidine (Catapres).
- guanadrel (Hylorel).
- guanethidine (Ismelin, Esimil).

Clomipramine *taken concurrently* with
- anticonvulsants requires careful monitoring for changes in seizure patterns and need to adjust anticonvulsant dosage.
- monoamine oxidase (MAO) type A inhibitor drugs (see Drug Classes) may cause high fever, seizures and excessive rise in blood pressure; avoid combining these drugs and provide periods of 14 days between administration of either.
- stimulant drugs (amphetamine, cocaine, epinephrine, phenylpropanolamine, etc.) may cause severe high blood pressure and/or high fever.
- thyroid preparations may increase the risk of heart rhythm disorders.
- warfarin may cause an increased warfarin effect and bleeding.

The following drugs may *increase* the effects of clomipramine
- ACE inhibitors (see Drug Classes).
- cimetidine (Tagamet).
- estrogens.
- fluoxetine (Prozac).
- fluvoxamine (Luvox).
- haloperidol (Haldol).
- methylphenidate (Ritalin).
- birth control pills (oral contraceptives).
- phenothiazines (see Drug Classes).
- quinidine.
- ranitidine (Zantac).
- sertraline (Zoloft).
- verapamil (Calan, others).

The following drugs may *decrease* the effects of clomipramine
- barbiturates (see Drug Classes).
- carbamazepine (Tegretol).
- chloral hydrate (Noctec, Somnos, etc.).
- lithium (Lithobid, Lithotab, etc.).
- reserpine (Serpasil, Ser-Ap-Es, etc.).

▷ *Driving, Hazardous Activities:*

This drug may cause seizures and impair alertness, judgment, physical coordination and reaction time. Restrict activities as necessary.

Aviation Note:

The use of this drug *is a disqualification* for piloting. Consult a designated Aviation Medical Examiner.

Exposure to Sun: No restrictions.

Exposure to Heat: Use caution. This drug may impair the body's adaptation to hot environments, increasing the risk of heat stroke. Avoid saunas.

Exposure to Environmental Chemicals: This drug may mask the symptoms of poisoning due to handling certain insecticides (organophosphorous types). Read their labels carefully.

Discontinuation: It is advisable to stop this drug gradually over a period of 3 to 4 weeks. Abrupt withdrawal after prolonged use may cause nausea, vomiting, diarrhea, headache, dizziness, malaise, disturbed sleep and irritability. Obsessive-compulsive behavior may worsen when this drug is stopped. It may be necessary to adjust the dosages of other drugs taken concurrently when this drug is discontinued.

CLONAZEPAM (kloh NA ze pam)

Introduced: 1977   **Prescription:** USA: Yes; Canada: Yes   **Available as Generic:** No   **Class:** Anticonvulsant, benzodiazepines   **Controlled Drug:** USA: C-IV*; Canada: No

Brand Names: Klonopin, ✦Rivotril

Warning: The brand name Klonopin and the generic name clonidine are similar and can be mistaken for each other; this can lead to serious medication errors. These names represent very different drugs. Verify that you are taking the correct drug.

BENEFITS versus RISKS	
Possible Benefits	*Possible Risks*
EFFECTIVE CONTROL OF SOME TYPES OF PETIT MAL, AKINETIC, AND MYOCLONIC SEIZURES	Paradoxical reactions: excitement, agitation, hallucinations
Possibly effective in the management of panic disorders	Minor impairment of mental functions
	Rare blood cell disorders: anemia, abnormally low white blood cell and platelet counts
	Increased salivation (of concern for those with chronic lung disease)

▷ **Principal Uses**

As a Single Drug Product: Uses currently included in FDA approved labeling: (1) Treats several types of epilepsy: petit mal variations, akinetic, myoclonic and absence seizure patterns

Other (unlabeled) generally accepted uses: (1) Helps control panic disorder; (2) eases symptoms of Tourette's syndrome; (3) relieves trigeminal neuralgia; (4) helps resistant depression; (5) can ease drug-induced mania.

How This Drug Works: This drug produces an anticonvulsant effect by increasing the action of a nerve transmitter (gamma-aminobutyric acid), which then blocks seizures.

*See Schedules of Controlled Drugs at the back of this book.

Available Dosage Forms and Strengths
   Tablets — 0.5 mg, 1 mg, 2 mg

▷ **Usual Adult Dosage Range:**   Initially 0.5 mg three times daily. The dose may be increased by 0.5 mg to 1.0 mg every three days, as needed and tolerated, until seizures are controlled. Total daily dose should not exceed 20 mg. **Note: Actual dosage and administration schedule must be determined by the physician for each patient individually.**

Conditions Requiring Dosing Adjustments
   Liver function: The dose **must** be decreased in liver compromise.
   Kidney function: Watch for signs and symptoms of accumulation (see overdosage).

▷ **Dosing Instructions:**   May be taken on empty stomach or with food or milk. The tablet may be crushed for administration. Do not stop this drug abruptly if taken for control of seizures, or if taken for more than 4 weeks to control panic attacks.

Usual Duration of Use: Use on a regular schedule for 2 to 3 weeks may be needed to see this drug's benefit in reducing the frequency and severity of seizures. Peak control will require careful dosage adjustments over a period of several months. Long-term use (months to years) requires ongoing supervision and periodic evaluation by your physician.

▷ **This Drug Should Not Be Taken If**
   • you have had an allergic reaction to it previously.
   • you have acute narrow-angle glaucoma.
   • you have active liver disease.

▷ **Inform Your Physician Before Taking This Drug If**
   • you are allergic to any benzodiazepine (see Drug Classes).
   • you have a history of alcoholism or drug abuse.
   • you are pregnant or planning pregnancy.
   • you have palpitations, as this drug may worsen palpitations.
   • you have impaired liver or kidney function.
   • you have a history of serious depression or mental disorder.
   • you have any of the following: asthma, emphysema, chronic bronchitis, myasthenia gravis.
   • you have acute intermittent porphyria.

Possible Side Effects (natural, expected, and unavoidable drug actions)
   Drowsiness, lethargy, unsteadiness, increased salivation.

▷ **Possible Adverse Effects** (unusual, unexpected, and infrequent reactions)
   If any of the following develop, consult your physician promptly for guidance.
   Mild Adverse Effects
   Allergic Reactions: Skin rash, hives, itching.
   Headache, dizziness, blurred vision, double vision, slurred speech, impaired memory, confusion, depression.
   Muscle weakness, ataxia, uncontrolled body movements.
   Palpitations (rare).
   Rare hair loss.
   Weight gain.
   Nausea, vomiting, constipation, diarrhea, impaired urination, incontinence in older patients.

Serious Adverse Effects

Idiosyncratic Reactions: Paradoxical responses of excitement, hyperactivity, agitation, anger, hostility.

Hallucinations, seizures.

Rare blood disorders: abnormally low red blood cell, white blood cell, and platelet counts.

Porphyria.

Abnormal eye movements.

Increased secretions and breathing problems, especially in those with chronic lung disease.

▷ **Possible Effects on Sexual Function:** Increased libido, enlargement of male breasts. May cause abnormally early (precocious) secondary sex characteristics in children.

Possible Effects on Laboratory Tests

Complete blood cell counts: decreased red cells, hemoglobin, white cells and platelets.

Urine screening tests for drug abuse; may be *positive*. (Test results depend upon amount of drug taken and testing method used.)

Liver function tests: increased.

CAUTION

1. This drug should not be stopped abruptly if used to control seizures.
2. Some over-the-counter drug products that contain antihistamines (allergy and cold preparations, sleep aids) can cause excessive sedation if combined with clonazepam.
3. Adverse behavioral reactions are more common in people with brain damage, mental retardation or psychiatric disorders.
4. A decreased response to this drug occurs in approximately 30% of users within 3 months after initiating treatment. Dosage adjustment may be necessary to restore seizure control.

Precautions for Use

By Infants and Children: This drug is used to treat infants and children of all ages. Careful dosage adjustment based on weight and age is mandatory. Abnormal behavioral responses are more common in children.

By Those over 60 Years of Age: Smaller doses and longer intervals are suggested. Watch for development of lethargy, indifference, fatigue, weakness, unsteadiness, disturbing dreams, nightmares and paradoxical reactions of excitement, agitation, anger, hostility and rage.

▷ **Advisability of Use During Pregnancy**

Pregnancy Category: C. See Pregnancy Code at the back of this book.

Animal studies: This drug causes cleft palates, open eyelids, fused rib structures and limb defects in rabbits.

Human studies: Adequate studies of pregnant women are not available.

It is advisable to avoid this drug during the first 3 months if possible. Frequent use in late pregnancy may cause the "floppy infant" syndrome in the newborn: weakness, lethargy, unresponsiveness, depressed breathing, low body temperature.

Advisability of Use if Breast-Feeding

Presence of this drug in breast milk: Yes.

Avoid drug or refrain from nursing.

Habit-Forming Potential: This drug can produce psychological and/or physical dependence (see Glossary) if used in large doses for an extended period of time.

Effects of Overdosage: Marked drowsiness, weakness, confusion, slurred speech, staggering gait, tremor, stupor progressing to deep sleep or coma.

Possible Effects of Long-Term Use: Benefits versus risks must be considered carefully during the extended use of this drug in children. Possible adverse effects on physical or mental development may not be apparent for many years.

Suggested Periodic Examinations While Taking This Drug (at physician's discretion)
During long-term use: Complete blood cell counts; liver function tests.

▷ **While Taking This Drug, Observe the Following**
Foods: No restrictions.
Beverages: No restrictions. May be taken with milk.
▷   *Alcohol:* Use with extreme caution. Alcohol may increase the depressant effects of this drug on the brain. It is advisable to avoid alcohol completely—throughout the day and night—if it is necessary to drive or to engage in any hazardous activity.
Tobacco Smoking: No interactions expected.
Marijuana Smoking: Increased sedation and significant impairment of intellectual and physical performance.
▷   *Other Drugs*
Clonazepam *taken concurrently* with
• amiodarone (Codarone) may decrease elimination of clonazepam and also worsen toxicity by causing low thyroid function.
• carbamazepine (Tegretol) may decrease blood levels and hence benefits of both medications.
• desipramine, imipramine and other tricyclic antidepressants (see Drug Classes) can decrease the tricyclic antidepressant blood level and lessen its therapeutic benefit.
• MAO inhibitors (see Drug Classes) may result in very low blood pressure and worsening of sedation and respiratory depression.
• valproic acid (Depakene, etc.) may cause continuous absence seizures.
The following drugs may *increase* the effects of clonazepam
• cimetidine (Tagamet).
• disulfiram (Antabuse).
• omeprazole (Prilosec).
• oral contraceptives (birth control pills).
The following drugs may *decrease* the effects of clonazepam
• theophylline (aminophylline, Theo-Dur, etc.).
▷   *Driving, Hazardous Activities:* This drug can impair mental alertness, judgment, physical coordination and reaction time. Avoid hazardous activities accordingly.
Aviation Note:
The use of this drug *is a disqualification* for piloting. Consult a designated Aviation Medical Examiner.
Exposure to Sun: No restrictions.

Discontinuation: Do not stop clonazepam suddenly if it is being used to control any type of seizure, or if it has been taken for more than 4 weeks to treat other conditions. Dosage should be tapered gradually to prevent a withdrawal syndrome that could include depression, confusion, hallucinations, tremor, seizures, muscle cramping, sweating and vomiting.

CLONIDINE (KLOH ni deen)

Introduced: 1969   **Prescription:** USA: Yes; Canada: Yes   **Available as**
Generic: USA: Yes; Canada: No   **Class:** Antihypertensive   **Controlled**
Drug: USA: No; Canada: No

Brand Names: ✣Apo-Clonidine, Catapres, Catapres-TTS, Combipres [CD], ♣Dixarit, ✣Nu-Clonidine

<table>
<tr><td colspan="2" align="center">BENEFITS versus RISKS</td></tr>
<tr><td align="center">Possible Benefits</td><td align="center">Possible Risks</td></tr>
<tr><td>EFFECTIVE ANTIHYPERTENSIVE in mild to moderate high blood pressure</td><td>ACUTE WITHDRAWAL SYNDROME (rebound hypertension) with abrupt discontinuation</td></tr>
<tr><td>Effective control of menopausal hot flashes (in selected cases)</td><td>Raynaud's phenomenon (cold fingers or toes)</td></tr>
<tr><td>Effective help in narcotic withdrawal</td><td></td></tr>
</table>

▷ **Principal Uses**

As a Single Drug Product: Uses currently included in FDA approved labeling: Used in combination with other medicines which are usually drugs of first choice in starting treatment of mild to moderate high blood pressure. Generally not used to start therapy. It may also be added as a "step 3 or 4" drug, replacing drugs that cause marked orthostatic hypotension (see Glossary).

Other (unlabeled) generally accepted uses: (1) Helps prevent migraine headache; (2) may help improve outcomes in patients with head injuries; (3) can aid menopausal hot flashes and treat severe menstrual cramps; (4) helps to lessen symptoms of alcohol or narcotic drug withdrawal; (4) has a role in some cases of abnormal heart rhythms (atrial fibrillation; (5) some data to suggest a role for intravenous use after a heart attack to limit the size of the heart damage (infarct); (6) early studies suggest a benefit in attention deficit disorder (ADHD).

As a Combination Drug Product [CD]: Available in combination with chlorthalidone, a diuretic product previously termed a "step 1" or drug of first choice in treating hypertension. The different ways in which these drugs work complement each other, making the combination a more effective antihypertensive.

How This Drug Works: By decreasing the activity of part of the brain (vasomotor center), this drug limits the ability of the sympathetic nervous system to constrict blood vessels and increase blood pressure.

Available Dosage Forms and Strengths

Patches — 2.5 mg, 5.0 mg, 7.5 mg
Tablets — 0.1 mg, 0.2 mg, 0.3 mg

▷ **Usual Adult Dosage Range:**   Tablets—initially 0.1 mg twice daily. Increased by 0.1 to 0.2 mg daily as needed and tolerated. Usual range is 0.2 to 0.8 mg daily, taken in 2 doses. Total daily dosage should not exceed 2.4 mg. Medicated patches are applied once a week. Hypertension in children has been treated with 5 to 10 micrograms per kilogram per day divided into two or three doses. **Note: Actual dosage and administration schedule must be determined by the physician for each patient individually.**

Conditions Requiring Dosing Adjustments
Liver function: This drug is changed into 6 active forms. The dose **must** be decreased in liver compromise.
Kidney function: Presently, dosing changes are not thought to be needed in mild to severe kidney failure. Some kidney patients may require higher maintenance doses to get the best blood pressure.

▷ **Dosing Instructions:**   Tablets may be taken without regard to eating. The tablet may be crushed for administration.

Usual Duration of Use: Use on a regular schedule for 2 to 3 weeks is usually needed to see this drug's benefit in lowering high blood pressure. Long-term use (months to years) requires physician supervision and guidance.

▷ **This Drug Should Not Be Taken If**
- you have had an allergic reaction to it previously.
- you have a problem in your heart that impacts the timing of the heartbeat or transmission of electrical impulses through the heart.

▷ **Inform Your Physician Before Taking This Drug If**
- you have a circulatory disorder of the brain.
- you have angina or coronary artery disease.
- you have or have had serious emotional depression.
- you have a very slow heart rate.
- you have Buerger's disease or Raynaud's phenomenon.
- you are taking a tricyclic antidepressant (see Drug Classes).
- you are taking any sedative or hypnotic drugs or an antidepressant.
- you plan to have surgery under general anesthesia in the near future.

Possible Side Effects (natural, expected, and unavoidable drug actions)
Drowsiness, dry nose and mouth, constipation (common), decreased heart rate, mild orthostatic hypotension (see Glossary).

▷ **Possible Adverse Effects** (unusual, unexpected, and infrequent reactions)
If any of the following develop, consult your physician promptly for guidance.
Mild Adverse Effects
Allergic Reactions: Skin rash, hives, localized swellings, itching.
Headache, dizziness, fatigue, anxiety, sleep disorders (nightmares or vivid dreaming), dry and burning eyes.
Painful parotid (salivary) gland, nausea, vomiting.
Weight gain, urinary retention.
Dry mouth.
Urination at night (rare).
Thinning of hair (rare).
Serious Adverse Effects
Idiosyncratic Reaction: Raynaud's phenomenon (see Glossary).

Aggravation of congestive heart failure, heart rhythm disorders.
Depression, hallucinations, or psychosis (rare).
Corneal ulcers (rare).
Liver toxicity (very rare).
Acute pancreatitis (rare).
Slow heart beat (bradycardia).

▷ **Possible Effects on Sexual Function:**   Decreased libido in 10% (0.2 to 0.8 mg/day); impotence in 8% to 24% (0.5 to 3.6 mg/day); impaired ejaculation (rare); enlargement of male breasts (gynecomastia) (0.2 to 0.8 mg/day). Precocious puberty in females.

Possible Effects on Laboratory Tests
Blood cholesterol or triglyceride levels: no consistent or significant effects.
Blood sodium level: increased.
Liver function: Rare increases of enzymes (ALT/GPT, AST/GOT, alkaline phosphatase).

CAUTION
1. ***Do not stop this drug suddenly.*** Sudden withdrawal can cause a severe and possibly fatal reaction.
2. Hot weather or fever can reduce blood pressure significantly. Dose adjustments may be necessary.
3. Report the development of any tendency to emotional depression.

Precautions for Use
By Infants and Children: Initial doses of 5–10 micrograms per kg per day divided into two or three doses have been used. A larger evening dose and smaller morning dose can help minimize sedation during school hours.
By Those over 60 Years of Age: ***Proceed cautiously*** with this drug. High blood pressure should be reduced slowly without the risks associated with excessively low blood pressure. Low initial doses and frequent blood pressure checks are needed. Watch for development of light-headedness, dizziness, unsteadiness, fainting and falling. Sedation and dry mouth occur in 50% of elderly users. Promptly report any changes in mood or behavior: Depression, delusions, hallucinations.

▷ **Advisability of Use During Pregnancy**
Pregnancy Category: C. See Pregnancy Code at the back of this book.
Animal studies: No birth defects reported. However, this drug is toxic to the embryo in low dosage.
Human studies: Adequate studies of pregnant women are not available.
The manufacturer recommends that this drug be avoided by women who are or who may become pregnant. Ask physician for guidance.

Advisability of Use if Breast-Feeding
Presence of this drug in breast milk: Yes.
This drug may impair milk production. Monitor nursing infant closely and discontinue drug or nursing if adverse effects begin.

Habit-Forming Potential: A small number of reports regarding abuse of this drug have surfaced. It may give extreme grogginess and lethargy when combined with diazepam (Valium).

Effects of Overdosage: Marked drowsiness, weakness, dry mouth, slow pulse, low blood pressure, vomiting, stupor progressing to coma.

Possible Effects of Long-Term Use: Development of tolerance (see Glossary) with loss of drug effect; weight gain due to salt and water retention; temporary sexual impotence.

Suggested Periodic Examinations While Taking This Drug (at physician's discretion)
Blood pressure measurements, monitoring of body weight.

▷ **While Taking This Drug, Observe the Following**
Foods: Avoid excessive salt. Ask physician for help with degree of salt restriction.
Beverages: No restrictions. May be taken with milk.
▷ *Alcohol:* Use with extreme caution. Combined effects can cause marked drowsiness and exaggerated reduction of blood pressure.
Tobacco Smoking: No expected interactions. Heed your doctor's advice about stopping tobacco use.
▷ *Other Drugs*
Clonidine may *decrease* the effects of
- levodopa (Larodopa, Sinemet, etc.), causing an increase in parkinsonism symptoms.

Clonidine *taken concurrently* with
- beta-adrenergic-blocking drugs (Inderal, Lopressor, etc.) may increase the risk of rebound hypertension if clonidine is stopped first. Best to stop the beta blocker first and then withdraw clonidine gradually.
- naloxone (Narcan, Talwin NX) may blunt the therapeutic effect of clonidine and result in a hypertensive response.
- niacin may decrease the facial flushing side effect of niacin.

The following drugs may *decrease* the effects of clonidine
- tricyclic antidepressants (Elavil, Sinequan, etc.) may reduce its effectiveness in lowering blood pressure.

▷ *Driving, Hazardous Activities:* Use caution. This drug can cause drowsiness and can impair mental alertness, judgment and coordination.
Aviation Note: Hypertension (high blood pressure) *is a disqualification* for piloting. Consult a designated Aviation Medical Examiner.
Exposure to Sun: No restrictions.
Exposure to Heat: Use caution. Hot environments may reduce the blood pressure; be alert to the possibility of orthostatic hypotension (see Glossary).
Exposure to Cold: Use caution. May cause painful blanching and numbness of the hands and feet on exposure to cold air or water (Raynaud's phenomenon).
Heavy Exercise or Exertion: Use caution. Isometric exercises—the "overload" technique for strengthening individual muscles—can raise blood pressure significantly. This drug may intensify the hypertensive response to isometric exercise. Ask physician for guidance.
Occurrence of Unrelated Illness: Fever may lower the blood pressure. Repeated vomiting may prevent the regular use of this drug and cause an acute withdrawal reaction. Consult your physician.
Discontinuation: **Do not stop this drug suddenly.** A severe withdrawal reaction can occur within 12 to 48 hours after the last dose. Best to gradually decrease the dose over 3 to 4 days, and check blood pressure often.

CLOTRIMAZOLE (kloh TRIM a zohl)

Introduced: 1976   **Prescription:** USA: Yes; Canada: Yes   **Available as Generic:** USA: Yes; Canada: No   **Class:** Antifungal   **Controlled Drug:** USA: No; Canada: No

Brand Names: ✦Canesten, Clotrimaderm, Clotrimazole, Gyne-Lotrimin, ✦Lotriderm, Lotrimin, Lotrimin AF, Lotrisone, Mycelex, Mycelex-7, Mycelex-G, ✦Myclo, ✦Neo-Zol

Warning: The brand names Mycelex and Myoflex are similar and can be mistaken for each other; this can lead to serious medication errors. These names represent very different drugs. Verify that you are using the correct drug.

BENEFITS versus RISKS

Possible Benefits	*Possible Risks*
EFFECTIVE TREATMENT AND PREVENTION OF CANDIDA (YEAST) INFECTIONS OF THE MOUTH AND THROAT (THRUSH)	Skin and mucous membrane irritation due to sensitization (drug-induced allergy)
EFFECTIVE TREATMENT OF CANDIDA (YEAST) INFECTIONS OF THE SKIN	Nausea, vomiting, stomach cramping, diarrhea (when swallowed)
EFFECTIVE TREATMENT OF CANDIDA (YEAST) INFECTIONS OF THE VULVA AND VAGINA	
EFFECTIVE TREATMENT OF TINEA (RINGWORM) INFECTIONS OF THE SKIN	

▷ **Principal Uses**

As a Single Drug Product: Uses currently included in FDA approved labeling: (1) Treatment of candida (yeast) infections of the skin, mouth, throat, vulva and vagina; (2) treatment of tinea and related infections: ringworm of the body, groin (jock itch), and feet (athlete's foot), due to susceptible fungal organisms.

Other (unlabeled) generally accepted uses: Prevention of candida (yeast) infections of the mouth and throat in the management of AIDS.

How This Drug Works: By damaging cell walls and blocking essential enzymes, this drug inhibits fungal cell growth and reproduction (with low drug concentrations) and kills fungus (with high drug concentrations).

Available Dosage Forms and Strengths

Cream — 1% (10 mg per gram)
Lotion — 1% (10 mg per gram)
Topical Solution — 1% (10 mg per ml)
Mouth lozenges — 10 mg
Vaginal Cream — 1% (10 mg per gram), 2%
Vaginal Tablets — 100 mg, 200 mg, 500 mg

▷ **Recommended Dosage Ranges** (Actual dosage and administration schedule must be determined by the physician for each patient individually.)

Infants and Children: Use of lozenges not recommended for children under 5 years of age; for 5 years and older—dissolve 1 lozenge slowly and completely in mouth 5 times a day for 14 days, longer if necessary.

12 to 60 Years of Age: For Candida infections of mouth and throat—Dissolve 1 lozenge slowly and completely in mouth 5 times a day for 14 days; extended treatment will be necessary for people with AIDS.

For candida and tinea infections of skin—apply cream, lotion or solution to infected areas twice a day, morning and evening.

For candida infections of vulva and vagina—1 applicatorful (5 grams) of cream intravaginally at bedtime for 7 to 14 consecutive days; or 1 100 mg tablet intravaginally at bedtime for 7 days, or 2 100 mg tablets intravaginally at bedtime for 3 days; one-dose treatment: 1 500 mg tablet intravaginally at bedtime, one time only.

Over 60 Years of Age: Same as 12 to 60 years of age.

Conditions Requiring Dosing Adjustments

Liver function: The drug goes out via the bile—dose decreased if bile duct is blocked.

Kidney function: Dosing changes are not needed.

▷ **Dosing Instructions:**   Dissolve lozenge in mouth completely, swallowing saliva as it accumulates. Do not chew the lozenge or swallow it whole. Take full course prescribed.

Usual Duration of Use: Use on a regular schedule for 1 to 2 weeks is usually needed to see this drug's benefit in controlling yeast or tinea infection. Long-term use (as in management of AIDS) requires periodic evaluation of response and dosage adjustment. Treatment failure may also be an indication to change to combination HIV therapy or to change agents.

Possible Advantages of This Drug

Reasonably effective with minimal toxicity.

More palatable than nystatin.

▷ **This Drug Should Not Be Taken If**

• you have had an allergic reaction to it previously.

▷ **Inform Your Physician Before Taking This Drug If**

• you are allergic to related antifungal drugs: fluconazole, itraconazole, ketoconazole, miconazole.

Possible Side Effects (natural, expected, and unavoidable drug actions)

None.

▷ **Possible Adverse Effects** (unusual, unexpected, and infrequent reactions)

If any of the following develop, consult your physician promptly for guidance.

Mild Adverse Effects

Allergic Reactions: Skin rash, hives, itching, burning, swelling, blistering (not present prior to treatment).

Nausea, vomiting, stomach cramping, diarrhea (when swallowed).

Serious Adverse Effects
Allergic Reactions: Sensitization of tissues (where applied locally) that will react allergically with future drug application.
Liver toxicity (with oral form) (rare).

▷ **Possible Effects on Sexual Function:** None.

Possible Delayed Adverse Effects: Local tissue sensitization to this drug.

Possible Effects on Laboratory Tests
Liver function tests: Increased liver enzyme AST/GOT in 15% of users.

CAUTION
1. Avoid contact of cream, lotion and solution with the eyes.
2. Do not cover applied cream or lotion with an occlusive dressing.

Precautions for Use
By Infants and Children: Use of lozenges by those under 5 years of age is not recommended.
By Those over 60 Years of Age: No problems reported.

▷ **Advisability of Use During Pregnancy**
Pregnancy Category: B. See Pregnancy Code at the back of this book.
Animal studies: No drug-induced birth defects were found in mouse, rat or rabbit studies.
Human studies: Adequate studies of pregnant women are not available.
Use this drug only if clearly needed. Ask your physician for guidance.

Advisability of Use if Breast-Feeding
Presence of this drug in breast milk: Unknown.
Watch infant closely and stop drug or nursing if adverse effects start.

Habit-Forming Potential: None.

Effects of Overdosage: Excessive use of lozenges may cause nausea, vomiting or diarrhea.

Possible Effects of Long-Term Use: None reported.

Suggested Periodic Examinations While Taking This Drug (at physician's discretion)
Chronic oral use: liver function tests.

▷ **While Taking This Drug, Observe the Following**
Foods: No restrictions.
Beverages: No restrictions.
▷ *Alcohol:* No interactions expected.
Tobacco Smoking: No interactions expected.
▷ *Other Drugs:* Clotrimazole *taken concurrently* with
• cyclosporine (Sandimmune) may result in cyclosporine toxicity.
• tacrolimus (Prograf) can result in kidney toxicity and increased potassium and glucose.
▷ *Driving, Hazardous Activities:* No restrictions.
Aviation Note: No restrictions.
Exposure to Sun: No restrictions.
Discontinuation: As directed by your physician.

CLOXACILLIN (klox a SIL in)

Introduced: 1962   **Prescription:** USA: Yes; Canada: Yes   **Available as**
Generic: USA: Yes; Canada: No   **Class:** Antibiotic, penicillin   **Controlled**
Drug: USA: No; Canada: No

Brand Names: ✦Apo-Cloxi, ✦Bactopen, Cloxapen, ✦Novo-Cloxin, ✦Nu-Cloxi,
✦Orbenin, Tegopen

BENEFITS versus RISKS	
Possible Benefits	*Possible Risks*
EFFECTIVE TREATMENT OF INFECTIONS due to susceptible microorganisms	ALLERGIC REACTIONS, mild to severe Superinfections (yeast) Drug-induced colitis Rare blood cell disorders

▷ **Principal Uses**

As a Single Drug Product: Uses currently included in FDA approved labeling: Used to (1) treat infections that are caused by bacteria (principally Staphylococcus). Treats infections of the skin and skin structures, the upper and lower respiratory tract (including "strep" throat) and infections that are widely scattered throughout the body.

Other (unlabeled) generally accepted uses: (1) May have a limited role in treatment of bone infections where intravenous medicines are not tolerated.

How This Drug Works: This drug destroys susceptible infecting bacteria by interfering with their ability to produce new protective cell walls as they multiply and grow.

Available Dosage Forms and Strengths

Capsules — 250 mg, 500 mg
Oral suspension — 125 mg per 5-ml
Oral liquid — 125 mg per 5-ml

▷ **Usual Adult Dosage Range:** Usually, 250 to 500 mg every 6 hours (4 doses/24 hours). The maximum dose is 6000 mg/24 hours. For children weighing less than 20 kilograms (44 pounds): 50–100 mg per kilogram per day divided into four doses. Children greater than 20 kg receive the adult dose. The intravenous route may be required for severe infections. **Note: Actual dosage and administration schedule must be determined by the physician for each patient individually.**

Conditions Requiring Dosing Adjustments

Liver function: Significantly metabolized to both active and inactive metabolites. This medication is also highly protein bound. The dose or dosing interval is decreased in liver disease.

Kidney function: This drug is eliminated through the bile and the urine. Monitor the patient closely if there is severe kidney compromise.

▷ **Dosing Instructions:** Take on empty stomach, 1 hour before or 2 hours after eating, at same times each day. Capsule may be opened for administration.

Usual Duration of Use: As long as necessary to eradicate the infection. For all streptococcal infections: not less than 10 consecutive days (without interruption) to reduce the possibility of developing rheumatic fever or glomerulonephritis.

▷ **This Drug Should Not Be Taken If**
  - you have had an allergic reaction to any dosage form of it previously.
  - you are certain you are allergic to *any* form of penicillin.

▷ **Inform Your Physician Before Taking This Drug If**
  - you suspect you may be allergic to penicillin or you have a history of a previous "reaction" to penicillin.
  - you are allergic to cephalosporin antibiotics (Ancef, Ceporan, Ceporex, Duricef, Kafocin, Keflex, Keflin, Kefzol, Loridine).
  - you are allergic by nature—hay fever, asthma, hives, eczema.
  - you have a history of kidney disease, regional enteritis or ulcerative colitis.
  - you have a history of liver or kidney failure.

Possible Side Effects (natural, expected, and unavoidable drug actions)
  Superinfections (see Glossary), often due to yeast organisms.

▷ **Possible Adverse Effects** (unusual, unexpected, and infrequent reactions)
  If any of the following develop, consult your physician promptly for guidance.
  Mild Adverse Effects
  Allergic Reactions: Skin rashes, hives, itching.
  Irritations of mouth and tongue, unpleasant taste, nausea, vomiting, mild diarrhea.
  Serious Adverse Effects
  Allergic Reactions: Anaphylactic reaction (see Glossary); severe skin reactions; drug fever; swollen, painful joints; sore throat.
  Agranulocytosis (decrease in certain infection-fighting white blood cells) (rare).
  Pseudomembranous colitis—severe diarrhea.
  Blood clotting problems (hypoprothrombinemia) (rare).
  Kidney problems (interstitial nephritis).
  Liver problems (cholestatic jaundice) (rare).

▷ **Possible Effects on Sexual Function:**   None reported.

Possible Effects on Laboratory Tests
  Complete blood cell counts: decreased white cells; increased eosinophils (allergic reaction).

CAUTION
  1. Take the exact dose and the full course prescribed.
  2. This drug should not be used at the same time as antibiotics like erythromycin or tetracycline.

Precautions for Use
  By Infants and Children: Dosage is based on age and weight. Talk to your doctor about the precise dosage schedule.
  By Those over 60 Years of Age: It is advisable to evaluate kidney function before and during use of this drug to determine the need for dosage adjustment. Natural changes in the skin may predispose to prolonged itching reactions in the genital and anal regions. Report such reactions promptly.

▷ **Advisability of Use During Pregnancy**

Pregnancy Category: B. See Pregnancy Code at the back of this book.

Animal studies: No birth defects reported in rabbit studies.

Human studies: Information from adequate studies of pregnant women indicates no increased risk of birth defects in 3546 pregnancies exposed to penicillin derivatives.

Use only if clearly needed. Ask physician for guidance.

Advisability of Use if Breast-Feeding

Presence of this drug in breast milk: Probably, yes.

The nursing infant may be sensitized to penicillin and may be at risk for diarrhea or yeast infections. Avoid drug if possible or refrain from nursing.

Habit-Forming Potential: None.

Effects of Overdosage: Possible nausea, vomiting and/or diarrhea.

Possible Effects of Long-Term Use: Superinfections, often due to yeast organisms.

Suggested Periodic Examinations While Taking This Drug (at physician's discretion)

Complete blood cell counts. Liver and kidney function tests with long-term use.

▷ **While Taking This Drug, Observe the Following**

Foods: No restrictions.

Beverages: No restrictions.

▷ *Alcohol:* No interactions expected. Excessive alcohol may blunt the immune response.

Tobacco Smoking: No interactions expected.

▷ *Other Drugs*

Cloxacillin may *decrease* the effects of

• Birth control pills (oral contraceptives) in some women, and impair their effectiveness in preventing pregnancy.

The following drugs may *decrease* the effects of cloxacillin

• antacids may reduce the absorption of cloxacillin.

• chloramphenicol (Chloromycetin).

• erythromycin (Erythrocin, E-Mycin, etc.).

• tetracyclines (Achromycin, Declomycin, Minocin, etc.). (see Drug Classes).

Cloxacillin *taken concurrently* with

• warfarin (Coumadin) may intensify the anticoagulant effect and increase risk of bleeding.

▷ *Driving, Hazardous Activities:* Usually no restrictions.

Aviation Note: The use of this drug *may be a disqualification* for piloting. Consult a designated Aviation Medical Examiner.

Exposure to Sun: No restrictions.

Special Storage Instructions: Keep capsules in a tightly closed container at room temperature. Keep oral solution in the refrigerator.

Observe the Following Expiration Times: Oral solution kept refrigerated is good for 14 days; when kept at room temperature, it is good for only 3 days.

CLOZAPINE (KLOH za peen)

Introduced: 1975   **Prescription:** USA: Yes   **Available as Generic:** USA: No   **Class:** Strong tranquilizer (Antipsychotic)   **Controlled Drug:** USA: No

Brand Name: Clozaril

Note: In the United States, this drug is available only by special arrangement through the Clozaril Patient Management System, which was administered by Caremark Homecare Corporation, and is now administered by HMI. The toll free number is: 800–648-1975. Ask your doctor for help.

BENEFITS versus RISKS

Possible Benefits	*Possible Risks*
EFFECTIVE CONTROL OF SEVERE SCHIZOPHRENIA that has failed to respond adequately to other appropriate drugs Improvement in 30% of refractory cases	SERIOUS BLOOD CELL DISORDERS: abnormally low white blood cell and platelet counts (rare) DRUG-INDUCED SEIZURES (depending upon size of dose)

▷ **Principal Uses**

As a Single Drug Product: Uses currently included in FDA approved labeling: Used in managing severe schizophrenia that has failed to respond to adequate trials of other standard antipsychotic medications (treatment resistant). Because of its potential for causing serious blood cell disorders and seizures, its use is reserved for the severely ill schizophrenic patient.

Other (unlabeled) generally accepted uses: (1) Severe and refractory bipolar disorder; (2) severe tardive dyskinesia (dystonic subtype)—a syndrome which can happen after some medicines are used to treat psychosis; (3) psychosis occurring after labor with lactation.

How This Drug Works: By blocking the place (receptor) where dopamine works in some parts of the brain, this drug helps correct an imbalance of nerve impulses that causes schizophrenic thought disorders.

Available Dosage Forms and Strengths

Tablets — 25 mg, 100 mg

▷ **Usual Adult Dosage Range:**   Initially 12.5 mg one or two times a day; the dose is gradually increased by 25 mg to 50 mg daily, as tolerated, to reach a dose of 300 mg to 450 mg daily (divided into three doses) by the end of two weeks. Later increases should be limited to 100 mg one or two times a week. Average dosage requirements are 600 mg daily. Total daily dosage should not exceed 900 mg. **Note: Actual dosage and administration schedule must be determined by the physician for each patient individually.**

Conditions Requiring Dosing Adjustments

Liver function: Eliminated in the liver, however no specific dosing guidelines are available.

Kidney function: Patients with kidney failure should be watched closely for adverse effects.

▷ **Dosing Instructions:**   May be taken without regard to meals or with food if necessary to reduce stomach irritation. The tablet may be crushed for administration.

Usual Duration of Use: This drug's benefits may be seen after 2 to 4 weeks of regular use. Peak effect usually requires three months. If no significant benefit is seen within 6 to 8 weeks, the drug should be stopped. Long-term use requires periodic evaluation of response and dosage adjustment.

Possible Advantages of This Drug
Rarely causes significant sexual dysfunction.
Low incidence of Parkinson-like reactions (see Glossary).
Does not cause tardive dyskinesia (see Glossary).

Currently a "Drug of Choice"
for treatment of severe schizophrenia in patients who have not responded to other standard antipsychotic drugs.

▷ **This Drug Should Not Be Taken If**
• you have had an allergic reaction to it previously.
• you have experienced severe bone marrow depression (impaired white blood cell production) with previous use of this drug.
• you presently have any type of bone marrow or blood cell disorder.
• you are currently taking any other drug that can cause bone marrow depression (see Glossary).

▷ **Inform Your Physician Before Taking This Drug If**
• you have a history of any type of seizure disorder.
• you have a history of narrow-angle glaucoma.
• you have any type of heart or circulatory disorder, especially heart rhythm abnormalities or hypertension.
• you have impaired liver or kidney function.
• you have prostatism (see Glossary).

Possible Side Effects (natural, expected, and unavoidable drug actions)
Drowsiness, dizziness, light-headedness, orthostatic hypotension (see Glossary).
Blurred vision, salivation, dry mouth, impaired urination (rare), constipation.

▷ **Possible Adverse Effects** (unusual, unexpected, and infrequent reactions)
If any of the following develop, consult your physician promptly for guidance.
Mild Adverse Effects
Allergic Reactions: Skin rash (rare); drug fever (see Glossary), which usually occurs within the first 3 weeks of treatment and is self-limiting.
Headache, tremor, fainting, sleep disorders, restlessness, confusion, depression (rare).
Weight gain.
Rapid heartbeat, hypertension, chest pain (rare).
Nausea, indigestion, vomiting, diarrhea (rare).
Serious Adverse Effects
Allergic Reactions: Asthmatic-type respiratory reaction (rare).
Bone marrow depression: specific impairment of white blood cell production with potential for serious infection.

Drug-induced seizures, dose-related.
Tardive dyskinesia (very rare).
Abnormally low blood pressure on standing (orthostatic hypotension).
Anticholinergic syndrome (rare).
Neuroleptic malignant syndrome (rare).

▷ **Possible Effects on Sexual Function**
Decreased libido and impotence (infrequent and dose related—over 150 mg), abnormal ejaculation (1%), priapism (see Glossary).

▷ **Adverse Effects That May Mimic Natural Diseases or Disorders**
Drug-induced fever may suggest systemic infection. Because of the risk of bone marrow depression and secondary infection, any occurrence of fever must be carefully evaluated.
Drug-induced seizures may suggest the possibility of epilepsy.

Natural Diseases or Disorders That May Be Activated by This Drug
Latent glaucoma, prostatism.

Possible Effects on Laboratory Tests
White blood cell counts: decreased.

CAUTION
1. Baseline white blood cell counts must be checked before clozapine treatment is started; follow-up counts must be made every week during the entire course of treatment and for 4 weeks after discontinuation of clozapine.
2. Promptly report any signs of infection: fever, sore throat, flulike symptoms, skin infections, painful urination, etc.
3. Report promptly light-headedness or dizziness on rising from a sitting or lying position; this could be orthostatic hypotension (see Glossary).
4. Call your doctor before taking any other medication. This includes all prescription and over-the-counter drugs.

Precautions for Use
By Infants and Children: An open label trial of 11 patients from 12 to 17 years old used 12.5 to 25 mg per day as a starting dose, and increased every 4 days by one or two times the starting dose. This dosing strategy was used to treat refractory childhood onset schizophrenia. Mean trial dose was 370 mg per day.
By Those over 60 Years of Age: Increased risk of orthostatic hypotension, confusion, blood problems and prostatism. Report related symptoms promptly.

▷ **Advisability of Use During Pregnancy**
Pregnancy Category: B. See Pregnancy Code at the back of this book.
Animal studies: No birth defects due to this drug reported.
Human studies: Adequate studies of pregnant women are not available.
Use this drug only if clearly needed.

Advisability of Use if Breast-Feeding
Presence of this drug in breast milk: Unknown.
Avoid drug or refrain from nursing.

Habit-Forming Potential: None.

Effects of Overdosage: Marked drowsiness, delirium, hallucinations, rapid and irregular heartbeat, irregular breathing, fainting.

Possible Effects of Long-Term Use: None reported to date.

Suggested Periodic Examinations While Taking This Drug (at physician's discretion)
>White blood and differential counts prior to starting therapy, every week during therapy and for 4 weeks after stopping therapy.
>Serial blood pressure measurements and electrocardiograms.

▷ **While Taking This Drug, Observe the Following**
Foods: No restrictions.
Beverages: No restrictions. May be taken with milk.
▷   *Alcohol:* Avoid completely. Alcohol increases sedation and accentuates its brain function and blood pressure depression. This drug can increase the intoxicating effects of alcohol.
Tobacco Smoking: May accelerate the elimination of this drug and require increased dosage.
Marijuana Smoking: Moderate increase in drowsiness; accentuation of orthostatic hypotension; increased risk of aggravating psychosis.
▷   *Other Drugs*
Clozapine may ***increase*** the effects of
• drugs with sedative actions; observe for excessive sedation.
• drugs with atropinelike actions (see Drug Classes).
• antihypertensive drugs; observe for excessive lowering of blood pressure.
Clozapine ***taken concurrently*** with
• other bone marrow depressant drugs such as carbamazepine (Tegretol) may increase the risk of impaired white blood cell production.
• cimetidine (Tagamet) can result in a toxic level of clozapine.
• erythromycin (E-Mycin, others) can result in increased clozapine concentrations and potential toxicity. This has been seen in a single case report, but caution is advised.
• fluvoxamine (Luvox) can result in clozapine toxicity.
• lithium (Lithobid, Lithotab, etc.) may increase the risk of confusional states, seizures and neuroleptic malignant syndrome (see Glossary).
• Monoamine Oxidase Inhibitors (MAO inhibitors—see Drug Class) may cause abnormally low blood pressure and exaggerated central nervous system response.
• phenytoin (Dilantin) can cause a decreased clozapine level and result in breakthrough schizophrenia.
• risperidone (Risperdal).
• warfarin (Coumadin) and cause an increased risk of bleeding.
▷   *Driving, Hazardous Activities:*
This drug may cause drowsiness, dizziness, blurred vision, confusion and seizures. Restrict activities as necessary.
Aviation Note:
The use of this drug ***is a disqualification*** for piloting. Consult a designated Aviation Medical Examiner.
Exposure to Sun: No restrictions.
Exposure to Heat: Use caution. This drug can cause fever and can impair the body's adaptation to heat.
Occurrence of Unrelated Illness: Infections must be vigorously treated. White blood cell response to infection must be followed closely.

Discontinuation: If possible, this drug should be discontinued gradually over a period of 1 to 2 weeks. If abrupt withdrawal is necessary, observe carefully for recurrence of psychotic symptoms.

CODEINE (KOH deen)

Introduced: 1886   **Prescription:** USA: Yes; Canada: Yes   **Available as Generic:** Yes   **Class:** Analgesic, narcotic, opioid   **Controlled Drug:** USA: C-II*; Canada: N

Brand Names: A.B.C. compound with codeine [CD], AC & C [CD], Accopain, Actagen-C [CD], Actifed w/Codeine [CD], Afed-C [CD], Alamine-C [CD], Alamine Expectorant [CD], Ambenyl Expectorant [CD], Ambenyl Syrup [CD], Anacin 3 with Codeine #2–4, Anacin w/Codeine [CD], APC with Codeine [CD], Atasol-8, -15, -30 [CD], Ban-Tuiss C [CD], Benylin Syrup w/Codeine [CD], Bromanyl Cough Syrup [CD], Bromotuss, Bromphen DC [CD], Bufferin w/Codeine [CD], Butalbital compound [CD], ✦C2 buffered, ✦C2 with codeine, Chemdal Expectorant [CD], Chem-Tuss NE [CD], Chlor-Trimeton Expectorant [CD], Coactifed [CD], Codehist Elixir, Codehist DH, ✦Coricidin with Codeine [CD], ✦Coryphen-Codeine [CD], Deproist [CD], Dimetane Cough Syrup-DC [CD], Dimetane Expectorant-C [CD], Dimetapp-C [CD], Dimetapp w/Codeine [CD], Empirin w/Codeine No. 2, 4 [CD], Empracet w/Codeine No. 3, 4 [CD], ✦Empracet-30, -60 [CD], ✦Emtec-30 [CD], ✦Exdol-8, -15, -30 [CD], ✦Extra Strength Acetaminophen, ✦Fiorinal-C 1/4, -C 1/2 [CD], Fiorinal w/Codeine No. 1, 2, 3 [CD], Gecil [CD], Glydeine, Isoclor Expectorant [CD], ✦Lenoltec w/Codeine No. 1, 2, 3, 4 [CD], ✦Mersyndol, Naldecon-CX [CD], Normatane [CD], Novadyne DH [CD], ✦Novahistex C [CD], ✦Novo-Gesic, Nucochem [CD], Nucofed [CD], ✦Omni-Tuss [CD], Oridol-C [CD], Panadol with codeine [CD], ✦Paveral, Pediacof [CD], Penntuss [CD], ✦Phenaphen No. 2, 3, 4 [CD], Phenaphen w/Codeine No. 2, 3, 4 [CD], Phenergan w/Codeine [CD], Poly-Histine [CD], Promethazine CS [CD], Pyra-Phed [CD], ✦Robaxacet-8, Robaxisal-C [CD], ✦Rounox w/Codeine [CD], SK-Apap [CD], Tamine Expectorant DC [CD], ✦Tecnal C [CD], Terpin Hydrate and Codeine [CD], Triafed with codeine [CD], Triaminic Expectorant w/Codeine [CD], ✦Triatec-8, 30 [CD], ✦Tussaminic C Forte [CD], ✦Tussaminic C Ped [CD], ✦Tussi-Organidin [CD], ✦Tylenol w/Codeine [CD], Tylenol w/Codeine No. 1, 2, 3, 4 [CD], Tylenol w/Codeine Elixir [CD], ✦222 [CD], ✦282 [CD], ✦292 [CD], ✦318 A.C. & C. [CD], ✦VC Expectorant with Codeine, ✦Veganin [CD]

BENEFITS versus RISKS	
Possible Benefits	*Possible Risks*
EFFECTIVE RELIEF OF MODERATE TO SEVERE PAIN	Low potential for habit formation (dependence)
VERY EFFECTIVE CONTROL OF COUGH	Mild allergic reactions (infrequent)
	Nausea, constipation

*See Schedules of Controlled Drugs at the back of this book.

▷ **Principal Uses**

As a Single Drug Product: Uses currently included in FDA approved labeling: (1) relieves moderate to severe pain; (2) controls cough. Its widest use is as an ingredient in analgesic preparations and cough remedies.

Other (unlabeled) generally accepted uses: None.

As a Combination Drug Product [CD]: Codeine is combined with other analgesics (aspirin and acetaminophen) on the World Health Organization Pain Ladder to increase overall pain control. It is also added to cough mixtures containing antihistamines, decongestants and expectorants.

How This Drug Works: By depressing some brain functions, this drug decreases pain perception, calms emotional responses to pain and reduces cough reflex sensitivity.

Available Dosage Forms and Strengths

Injection — 30 mg per ml and 60 mg per ml

Tablets — 15 mg, 30 mg, 60 mg

Tablets, soluble — 15 mg, 30 mg, 60 mg

▷ **Usual Adult Dosage Range:**   As analgesic—15 to 60 mg/3 to 6 hours. Current pain theory says that the drug should be scheduled, not taken in response to pain as in the past. For cough—10 to 20 mg/4 to 6 hours as needed. Total daily dosage should not exceed 200 mg for pain or 120 mg for cough. **Note: Actual dosage and administration schedule must be determined by the physician for each patient individually.**

Conditions Requiring Dosing Adjustments

Liver function: The dose must be decreased in liver compromise.

Kidney function: In moderate to severe kidney failure, the dose is decreased by up to 75%.

▷ **Dosing Instructions:**   Tablet may be crushed, then taken with or following food to reduce stomach irritation or nausea.

Usual Duration of Use: As required to control pain or cough. Continual use should not exceed 5 to 7 days without reassessment of need.

▷ **This Drug Should Not Be Taken If**

- you have had an allergic reaction to any dosage form of it previously.
- you are having an acute attack of asthma.
- your breathing is depressed (respiratory depression).

▷ **Inform Your Physician Before Taking This Drug If**

- you have a history of drug abuse or alcoholism.
- you have impaired liver or kidney function.
- you have gallbladder disease, a seizure disorder or an underactive thyroid gland.
- you have chronic lung disease (COPD)
- you have low blood calcium (increased sensitivity to this medicine).
- you have a history of porphyria.
- you tend to be constipated.
- you are taking any other drugs that have a sedative effect.
- you plan to have surgery under general anesthesia in the near future.

Possible Side Effects (natural, expected, and unavoidable drug actions)

Drowsiness, light-headedness, dry mouth, urinary retention, constipation.

▷ **Possible Adverse Effects** (unusual, unexpected, and infrequent reactions)
   If any of the following develop, consult your physician promptly for guidance.
   Mild Adverse Effects
   Allergic Reactions: Skin rash, hives, itching.
   Dizziness, impaired concentration, sensation of drunkenness, confusion, depression, blurred or double vision.
   Nausea, vomiting.
   Serious Adverse Effects
   Allergic Reactions: Anaphylaxis (rare), severe skin reactions.
   Idiosyncratic Reactions: Delirium, hallucinations, excitement, increased sensitivity to pain after the analgesic effect has worn off.
   Seizures (rare), impaired breathing.
   Porphyria (rare).
▷ **Possible Effects on Sexual Function:**   None reported.
▷ **Adverse Effects That May Mimic Natural Diseases or Disorders**
   Paradoxical behavioral disturbances may suggest psychotic disorder.

Possible Effects on Laboratory Tests
   Blood platelet counts: decreased.
   Blood amylase and lipase levels: increased (natural side effect).
   Urine screening tests for drug abuse: may be **positive**. (Test results depend upon amount of drug taken and testing method used.)

CAUTION
   1. If you have asthma, chronic bronchitis or emphysema, excessive use of this drug may cause respiratory difficulty, thickening of bronchial secretions and decrease of needed cough reflex.
   2. Combining this drug with atropinelike drugs can increase the risk of urinary retention and reduced intestinal function.
   3. Do not take this drug following acute head injury.

Precautions for Use
   By Infants and Children: Do not use this drug in children under 2 years of age because of their vulnerability to life-threatening respiratory depression. Children 2 to 6 years old: 1 mg per kilogram per day divided into four equal doses. Maximum dose is 30 mg per day. Children 6–12 years of age can receive 5 to 10 mg per dose every 4 to 6 hours to a maximum of 60 mg per 24 hours.
   By Those over 60 Years of Age: Small starting doses and short-term use is indicated. Expect increased risk of drowsiness, dizziness, unsteadiness, falling, urinary retention and constipation (often leading to fecal impaction).
▷ **Advisability of Use During Pregnancy**
   Pregnancy Category: C. D if used in high doses or for prolonged periods near the time the baby is about to be born. See Pregnancy Code at the back of this book.
   Animal studies: Skull defects reported in hamster studies.
   Human studies: Adequate studies of pregnant women are not available. Some studies suggest an increase in significant birth defects when this drug is taken during the first 6 months of pregnancy. Codeine taken during the last few weeks before delivery can cause withdrawal symptoms in the newborn.
   Use this drug only if clearly needed and in small, infrequent doses.

Advisability of Use if Breast-Feeding
Presence of this drug in breast milk: Yes, in small amounts.
Avoid drug or refrain from nursing.

Habit-Forming Potential: Psychological and/or physical dependence can develop with use of large doses for an extended period of time. However, true dependence is infrequent and unlikely with prudent use.

Effects of Overdosage: Drowsiness, restlessness, agitation, nausea, vomiting, dry mouth, vertigo, weakness, lethargy, stupor, coma, seizures.

Possible Effects of Long-Term Use: Psychological and physical dependence, chronic constipation.

Suggested Periodic Examinations While Taking This Drug (at physician's discretion)
None.

▷ **While Taking This Drug, Observe the Following**
Foods: No restrictions.
Beverages: No restrictions. May be taken with milk.
▷ *Alcohol:* Use extreme caution. Codeine intensifies the intoxicating effects of alcohol, and alcohol intensifies the depressant effects of codeine on brain function, breathing and circulation.
Tobacco Smoking: No interactions expected, but tobacco smoking may cause a decrease in pain tolerance and require an increased or more frequent dose of codeine.
Marijuana Smoking: Increased drowsiness and pain relief; mental and physical performance will be impaired.
▷ *Other Drugs*
Codeine may *increase* the effects of
• other drugs with sedative effects.
• atropinelike drugs, and increase the risk of constipation and urinary retention.
• monoamine oxidase inhibitors (MAO) and also increase central nervous symptoms and depression.
▷ *Driving, Hazardous Activities:* This drug can impair mental alertness, judgment, reaction time and physical coordination. Avoid hazardous activities accordingly.
Aviation Note: The use of this drug *is a disqualification* for piloting. Consult a designated Aviation Medical Examiner.
Exposure to Sun: No restrictions.
Discontinuation: Best to limit this drug to short-term use. If extended use occurs, discontinuation should be gradual to minimize possible effects of withdrawal (usually mild with codeine).

COLCHICINE (KOL chi seen)

Introduced: 1763   **Prescription:** USA: Yes; Canada: No   **Available as Generic:** Yes   **Class:** Antigout   **Controlled Drug:** USA: No; Canada: No
Brand Names: Col-probenecid [CD], Colbenemid [CD], Cosalide, Proben-C [CD]

BENEFITS versus RISKS	
Possible Benefits	*Possible Risks*
EFFECTIVE RELIEF OF ACUTE GOUT SYMPTOMS	Loss of hair
	Rare bone marrow depression (see Glossary)
Prevention of recurrent gout attacks	
Prevention of attacks of Mediterranean fever	Rare peripheral neuritis (see Glossary)
	Rare liver damage

▷ **Principal Uses**

As a Single Drug Product: Uses currently included in FDA approved labeling: (1) Reduces the pain, swelling and inflammation associated with acute attacks of gout (however; many rheumatologists prefer NSAIDS (see Drug Classes) as drugs of first choice in acute gout) ; (2) it is also used in smaller doses to prevent recurrent gout attacks.

Other (unlabeled) generally accepted uses: (1) Prevention and control of attacks of familial Mediterranean fever; (2) may have a role in easing symptoms of Behcet's disease; (3) limited use in cirrhosis of the liver; (4) damaged disk syndrome may be helped in some patients; (5) may have a role in recurrent pericarditis; (6) can be of help in pseudogout; (7) appears to be of benefit in some lung disease (idiopathic pulmonary fibrosis); (8) has a role in treatment of some cases of refractory immune thrombocytopenic purpura.

As a Combination Drug Product [CD]: Colchicine combined with probenecid enhances its ability to prevent recurrent attacks of gout. Colchicine is most effective in relieving acute gout; it has some effect in preventing recurrent and chronic discomfort. Probenecid increases removal of uric acid by the kidneys and reduces risk of acute gout. This dual action is more effective than either drug used alone in the long-term management of gout.

How This Drug Works: By decreasing joint tissue acid, this drug decreases painful deposit of uric acid crystals and acute inflammation and pain. (Colchicine does not lower uric acid in the blood or increase urine removal.)

Available Dosage Forms and Strengths

Injection — 1 mg per 2 ml

Tablets — 0.5 mg, 0.6 mg (also 1 mg in Canada)

▷ **Usual Adult Dosage Range:**   For acute attack—0.5 to 1.2 mg initially, followed by 0.5 to 0.65 mg/1 to 2 hours until pain is relieved or nausea, vomiting or diarrhea occurs. Maximum total dose is 10 mg. For prevention of recurrent attacks—0.5 to 0.65 mg, 1 to 3 times/day. **Note: Actual dosage and administration schedule must be determined by the physician for each patient individually.**

Conditions Requiring Dosing Adjustments

Liver function: Caution must be used, and the dose decreased if there is a bile obstruction.

This drug should NOT be used in people with both liver and kidney compromise.

Kidney function: For severe kidney failure, 50% of the usual dose should be given. Ongoing prophylactic use should be avoided in moderate (CCl less than 50) kidney problems.

▷ **Dosing Instructions:** The tablet may be crushed, then either taken on an empty stomach or with food to reduce nausea or stomach irritation. Start treatment at the first sign of an acute attack. Take the exact dose prescribed.

Usual Duration of Use: For acute attack—stop the drug when pain is relieved or when nausea, vomiting or diarrhea occurs; do not start this drug for 3 days without asking your doctor. For prevention—use the smallest dose that works; consult your doctor about dosage schedule and duration.

▷ **This Drug Should Not Be Taken If**
- you have had an allergic reaction to it previously.
- you have an active stomach or duodenal ulcer.
- you have active ulcerative colitis.
- you have a severe kidney or liver disorder.
- you have a serious heart disorder.
- you have a history of blood cell disorders.

▷ **Inform Your Physician Before Taking This Drug If**
- you have a history of peptic ulcer disease or ulcerative colitis.
- you develop diarrhea and vomiting while taking this drug.
- you have any type of heart disease.
- you have impaired liver or kidney function.
- you plan to have surgery in the near future.

Possible Side Effects (natural, expected, and unavoidable drug actions)
Nausea, vomiting, abdominal cramping, diarrhea.

▷ **Possible Adverse Effects** (unusual, unexpected, and infrequent reactions)
If any of the following develop, consult your physician promptly for guidance.
Mild Adverse Effects
Allergic Reactions: Skin rash, hives, fever.
Serious Adverse Effects
Allergic Reaction: Anaphylactic reaction (see Glossary).
Loss of hair.
Bone marrow depression (see Glossary)—fatigue, weakness, fever, sore throat, abnormal bleeding or bruising.
Peripheral neuritis (see Glossary)—numbness, tingling, pain, weakness in hands and/or feet.
Myopathy with nerve symptoms (facial palsy and weakness) (especially with long-term use).
Porphyria.
Drooping of the eyes (ptosis).
Inflammation of colon with bloody diarrhea.
Thrombophlebitis with intravenous use.
Liver damage.

▷ **Possible Effects on Sexual Function:** Reversible absence of sperm (azoospermia).

Possible Delayed Adverse Effects: Impaired production of sperm, possibly resulting in birth defects of child that was conceived while father was taking this drug.

Natural Diseases or Disorders That May Be Activated by This Drug
Peptic ulcer disease, ulcerative colitis.

Possible Effects on Laboratory Tests

Complete blood cell counts: decreased red cells, hemoglobin, white cells and platelets; increased white cells (follows initial decrease).

Prothrombin time: decreased (with concurrent use of warfarin).

Blood vitamin B_{12} level: decreased.

Liver function tests: increased liver enzymes (ALT/GPT, AST/GOT and alkaline phosphatase), increased bilirubin.

Fecal occult blood test: positive.

Sperm counts: decreased (may be marked).

CAUTION

1. If this drug causes vomiting and/or diarrhea before relief of joint pain, discontinue it and inform your physician.
2. Try to limit each course of treatment for acute gout to 4 to 8 mg. Do not exceed 3 mg/24 hours or a total of 10 mg/course.
3. Omit drug for 3 days between courses to avoid toxicity.
4. Carry this drug with you while traveling if you are subject to attacks of acute gout.
5. The stress of surgery can cause an acute attack of gout. Ask your doctor how much colchicine should be taken before and after surgery to prevent gout.

Precautions for Use

By Infants and Children: Use for preventing (prophylaxis) familial Mediterranean fever in children 6 to 13 years of age was given as 0.5 mg per day and increased by 0.5 mg per day to symptom control or a maximum of 2 mg per day. For other uses in children, dosage has not been established. Ask physician for guidance.

By Those over 60 Years of Age: Because the dosage needed to relieve acute gout often causes vomiting and/or diarrhea, extreme caution is advised if you have heart or circulatory disorders, reduced liver or kidney function, or general debility.

▷ Advisability of Use During Pregnancy

Pregnancy Category: C by one manufacturer, and D by another. See Pregnancy Code at the back of this book.

Animal studies: This drug causes significant birth defects in hamsters and rabbits.

Human studies: Adequate studies of pregnant women are not available. However, it is reported that colchicine can cause harm to the fetus.

Avoid during entire pregnancy if possible. Ask physician for guidance.

Advisability of Use if Breast-Feeding

Presence of this drug in breast milk: Yes.

Ask your doctor for help.

Habit-Forming Potential: None.

Effects of Overdosage: Nausea, vomiting, abdominal cramping, diarrhea (may be bloody), burning sensation in throat and skin, weak and rapid pulse, progressive paralysis, inability to breathe.

Possible Effects of Long-Term Use: Hair loss, aplastic anemia (see Glossary), peripheral neuritis (see Glossary).

Suggested Periodic Examinations While Taking This Drug (at physician's discretion)

Complete blood cell counts, uric acid blood levels to monitor status of gout, sperm analysis for quantity and condition, liver function tests.

▷ **While Taking This Drug, Observe the Following**

Foods: Follow physician's advice regarding the need for a low-purine diet.

Beverages: Drink at least 3 quarts of liquids/24 hours. This drug may be taken with milk. Some "herbal teas" (promoted as being beneficial for arthritis) contain phenylbutazone and other potentially toxic ingredients. Avoid herbal teas if you are not certain of their source, content and medicinal effects.

▷ *Alcohol:* No interactions expected. Combination may increase the risk of gastrointestinal irritation or bleeding and raise uric acid blood levels.

Tobacco Smoking: No interactions expected.

▷ *Other Drugs*

Colchicine *taken concurrently* with

• allopurinol (Zyloprim), probenecid (Benemid) or sulfinpyrazone (Anturane) can prevent attacks of acute gout that often occur when treatment with these drugs is first started.

• cyanocobalamin will decrease absorption of the vitamin B12.

• cyclosporine (Sandimmune) may increase cyclosporine levels and result in toxicity.

• erythromycins (EES, azithromycin, clarithromycin) and result in toxic colchicine blood levels.

▷ *Driving, Hazardous Activities:* Usually no restrictions when taken continually in small (preventive) doses. May cause nausea, vomiting and/or diarrhea when taken in larger (treatment) doses.

Aviation Note: The use of this drug *may be a disqualification* for piloting. Consult a designated Aviation Medical Examiner.

Exposure to Sun: No restrictions.

Exposure to Cold: This drug can lower body temperature. Use caution to prevent excessive lowering (hypothermia), especially in those over 60 years of age.

Occurrence of Unrelated Illness: Acute attacks of gout may result from injury or illness. Call your doctor for dosing adjustment if injury or new illness occurs.

COLESTIPOL (koh LES ti pohl)

Introduced: 1974   **Prescription:** USA: Yes; Canada: Yes   **Available as Generic:** USA: No; Canada: No   **Class:** Anticholesterol   **Controlled Drug:** USA: No; Canada: No

Brand Name: Colestid

BENEFITS versus RISKS	
Possible Benefits	*Possible Risks*
EFFECTIVE REDUCTION OF TOTAL CHOLESTEROL AND LOW-DENSITY CHOLESTEROL IN TYPE IIa CHOLESTEROL DISORDERS	Constipation (may be severe) Reduced absorption of fat, fat-soluble vitamins (A, D, E, and K) and folic acid
EFFECTIVE RELIEF OF ITCHING associated with biliary obstruction	Reduced formation of prothrombin with resultant bleeding

▷ **Principal Uses**

As a Single Drug Product: Uses currently included in FDA approved labeling: (1) Used in combination with diet changes to decrease blood cholesterol and low density (LDL) cholesterol in Type IIa cholesterol disorders; (2) eases itching due to the deposit of bile acids in the skin associated with partial biliary obstruction; (3) helps remove buildup on interior of blood vessels (atherosclerosis).

Other (unlabeled) generally accepted uses: (1) Data from one study showed that colestipol in combination with lovastatin actually caused regression of plaque buildup (atherosclerosis) inside blood vessels.

How This Drug Works: This drug combines with bile acids and salts and is excreted in the feces. This removal of bile acids stimulates conversion of cholesterol to bile acids to replace the loss; this in turn reduces the blood levels of cholesterol. By reducing the blood levels of bile acids, this drug hastens clearance of bile acids in the skin and relieves itching.

Available Dosage Forms and Strengths

Bottles — 250 grams and 500 grams
Packets — 5 grams
Flavored Colestid Granules — 5 grams per dose

▷ **Usual Adult Dosage Range:**   Initially 5 grams of powder 3 times daily. Dose may be increased slowly as needed and tolerated to 30 grams daily in 2 to 4 divided doses. **Note: Actual dosage and administration schedule must be determined by the physician for each patient individually.**

Conditions Requiring Dosing Adjustments

Liver function: This medication is eliminated via the feces, and the liver is not involved.

Kidney function: No changes are needed in renal compromise as the drug is not absorbed.

▷ **Dosing Instructions:**   Always take just before or with a meal; this drug is ineffective when taken without food. Mix the powder thoroughly in 4 to 6 ounces of water, fruit juice, tomato juice, milk, thin soup or a soft food like applesauce. **Do not take it in its dry form.**

Usual Duration of Use: Use on a regular schedule for 4 to 6 weeks is usually needed to see this drug's effectiveness in lowering high blood levels of cholesterol. The drug should be stopped if an acceptable response is not seen after 3 months. Long-term use (months to years) requires periodic physician evaluation of response and dosage adjustment.

▷ **This Drug Should Not Be Taken If**

- you have had an allergic reaction to it previously.
- you have complete biliary obstruction.

▷ **Inform Your Physician Before Taking This Drug If**

- you are prone to constipation.
- you have low thyroid function (hypothyroidism).
- you have peptic ulcer disease.
- you have a bleeding disorder of any kind.
- you have impaired kidney function.

Possible Side Effects (natural, expected, and unavoidable drug actions)
Constipation; interference with normal fat digestion and absorption; reduced absorption of vitamins A, D, E, and K and folic acid. Binds to vitamin B12—intrinsic factor complex.

▷ **Possible Adverse Effects** (unusual, unexpected, and infrequent reactions)
If any of the following develop, consult your physician promptly for guidance.

Mild Adverse Effects
Allergic Reactions: Skin rash (rare), hives, tongue irritation, anal itching.
Headache, dizziness, weakness, muscle and joint pains.
Constipation, loss of appetite, indigestion, heartburn, abdominal discomfort, excessive gas, nausea, vomiting, diarrhea.

Serious Adverse Effects
Vitamin K deficiency and increased bleeding tendency.
Impaired absorption of calcium; predisposition to osteoporosis.
Gallbladder colic (questionable).
Hypothyroidism.
Disruption of normal acid–base balance of the body (metabolic acidosis).

▷ **Possible Effects on Sexual Function:**   None reported.

Natural Diseases or Disorders That May Be Activated by This Drug
Peptic ulcer disease; steatorrhea (excessive fat in stools) with large doses.

Possible Effects on Laboratory Tests
Blood cholesterol and triglyceride levels: decreased (therapeutic effect).
Blood thyroxine (T_4) level: decreased when colestipol and niacin are taken concurrently (in presence of normal thyroid function).

CAUTION
1. Never take the powder in its dry form; always mix it thoroughly with a suitable liquid before swallowing.
2. Watch carefully for constipation; use stool softeners and laxatives as needed.
3. This drug may bind other drugs taken concurrently and impair their absorption. It is advisable to take **all other drugs** 1 to 2 hours before or 4 to 6 hours after taking this drug.

Precautions for Use
By Infants and Children: Safety and effectiveness for those under 12 years of age not established. Watch carefully for the possible development of acidosis and vitamin A or folic acid deficiency. (Ask your physician for guidance.)
By Those over 60 Years of Age: Increased risk of severe constipation. Impaired kidney function may predispose to the development of acidosis.

▷ **Advisability of Use During Pregnancy**
Pregnancy Category: C. See Pregnancy Code at the back of this book.
Animal studies: No information available.
Human studies: Adequate studies of pregnant women are not available.
Use this drug only if clearly needed. Ensure adequate intake of vitamins and minerals to satisfy needs of mother and fetus.

Advisability of Use if Breast-Feeding
Presence of this drug in breast milk: No.
Breast-feeding is permitted.

Habit-Forming Potential: None.

Effects of Overdosage: Progressive constipation.

Possible Effects of Long-Term Use: Deficiencies of vitamins A, D, E and K and folic acid. Calcium deficiency, osteoporosis. Acidosis due to excessive retention of chloride. Binding of the B-12 intrinsic factor complex may lead to blood cell problems.

Suggested Periodic Examinations While Taking This Drug (at physician's discretion)

Measurements of blood levels of total cholesterol, low density (LDL) cholesterol and high density (HDL) cholesterol.

Hemoglobin and red blood cell studies for possible anemia.

Thyroid function tests.

▷ **While Taking This Drug, Observe the Following**

Foods: Avoid foods that tend to constipate (cheeses, etc.).

Nutritional Support: Ask your doctor if you need supplements of vitamins A, D, E and K, folic acid and calcium.

Beverages: Ensure adequate liquid intake (up to 2 quarts daily). This drug may be taken with milk.

▷ *Alcohol:* No interactions expected.

Tobacco Smoking: No interactions expected.

▷ *Other Drugs*

Colestipol may *decrease* the effects of

- acetaminophen; give 2 hours before colestipol.
- aspirin; give 2 hours before.
- digitoxin and digoxin; give 2 hours before.
- furosemide; give 4 hours before.
- hydrocortisone; 2 hours before.
- iron preparations; give 2 to 3 hours before.
- penicillin G; give 2 hours before.
- phenobarbital; give 2 hours before.
- tetracycline; give 2 hours before.
- thiazide diuretics (see Drug Classes); give 2 hours before.
- thyroxine; give 5 hours before.
- vitamin B12.

▷ *Driving, Hazardous Activities:* No restrictions.

Aviation Note: The use of this drug *is usually not a disqualification* for piloting. Consult a designated Aviation Medical Examiner.

Exposure to Sun: No restrictions.

Discontinuation: The dose of any toxic drug combined with colestipol must be reduced when this drug is stopped. Once colestipol is stopped, cholesterol levels usually return to pretreatment levels in 1 month.

CROMOLYN (KROH moh lin)

Other Names: Cromolyn sodium, sodium cromoglycate

Introduced: 1968   **Prescription:** USA: Yes; Canada: Yes   **Available as Generic:** USA: No; Canada: No   **Class:** antiasthmatic drug, preventive

Controlled Drug: USA: No; Canada: No

Brand Names: Crolom, Gastrocrom, Intal, ✦Intal Spincaps, ✦Intal Syncroner, ✦Nalcrom, Nasalcrom, Opticrom, ✦Rynacrom

BENEFITS versus RISKS	
Possible Benefits	*Possible Risks*
LONG-TERM PREVENTION OF RECURRENT ASTHMA ATTACKS	Rare anaphylactic reaction (see Glossary)
Prevention of acute asthma due to allergens or exercise	Rare spasm of bronchial tubes, increased wheezing
Prevention and treatment of allergic rhinitis	Rare allergic pneumonitis (allergic reaction in lung tissue)
Prevention of bronchospasm	
Relief of allergic conjunctivitis	
Treatment of giant papillary conjunctivitis	

▷ **Principal Uses**

As a Single Drug Product: Uses currently included in FDA approved labeling: (1) *Prevents* allergic reactions in the nose (allergic rhinitis, hay fever) and the bronchial tubes (bronchial asthma). Does not help asthma once an attack starts. It is also used to treat allergic rhinitis (70% effective) and conjunctivitis; (2) helps prevent exercise- or environmentally-induced asthma; (3) treatment of mastocytosis and management of several allergy-related skin disorders.

Other (unlabeled) generally accepted uses: (1) Helps modify the reactions in food allergies; (2) may have a small place in the therapy of Bell's palsy.

How This Drug Works: It blocks the release of histamine (and other chemicals) that worsen allergic reactions. This drug prevents the sequence of events that lead to swelling and itching and to constriction of bronchial tubes (asthma).

Available Dosage Forms and Strengths

Capsules, oral — 100 mg
Eye drops — 2% and 4%
Inhalation aerosol — 0.8 mg per metered spray
Inhalation capsules (powder) — 20 mg
Inhalation solution — 20 mg per ampul
Nasal insufflation (powder) — 10 mg per cartridge
Nasal solution — 40 mg per ml

▷ **Usual Adult Dosage Range**

Eye drops: 1 to 2 drops 4 to 6 times daily at regular intervals.

Inhalation aerosol: 1.6 mg (2 inhalations) 4 times daily at regular intervals for prevention of asthma, or as a single dose 10 to 15 minutes before exposure to prevent acute allergen-induced or exercise-induced asthma.

Inhalation powder: 20 mg (1 capsule) 4 times daily at regular intervals for long-term prevention of asthma; 20 mg (1 capsule) as a single dose 10 to 15 minutes before exposure to prevent acute allergen-induced or exercise-induced asthma. Total daily maximum dosage is 160 mg (8 capsules).

Inhalation solution: Same as inhalation powder.

Nasal insufflation: Initially 10 mg in each nostril every 4 to 6 hours as needed; reduce to every 8 to 12 hours for maintenance.

Nasal solution: 2.6 mg to 5.2 mg in each nostril 3 to 6 times daily as needed.

Note: Actual dosage and administration schedule must be determined by the physician for each patient individually.

Conditions Requiring Dosing Adjustments
Liver function: If the bile duct is damaged by liver disease, the dose must be decreased.
Kidney function: The dose should be decreased in kidney failure.

▷ **Dosing Instructions:**   Follow instructions provided with all of the dosage forms, especially the inhalers. Do not swallow the capsules; the powder is intended for inhalation. (If the capsule is accidentally swallowed, the drug will cause no beneficial or adverse effects.)

Usual Duration of Use: Use on a regular schedule for 4 to 6 weeks is usually needed to see this drug's benefit in preventing asthma attacks or allergic rhinitis. Long-term use (months to years) requires periodic physician evaluation.

Possible Advantages of This Drug
May be quite effective in the young asthmatic.
Usually well tolerated.
Serious adverse effects are very rare.

▷ **This Drug Should Not Be Taken If**
• you have had an allergic reaction to any dosage form of it previously.

▷ **Inform Your Physician Before Taking This Drug If**
• you are allergic to milk, milk products or lactose. (The inhalation powder contains lactose.)
• you have impaired liver or kidney function.
• you have soft contact lenses (these should not be worn while using the eye drops).
• you have angina or a heart rhythm disorder. (The inhalation aerosol contains propellants that could be hazardous.)

Possible Side Effects (natural, expected, and unavoidable drug actions)
Unpleasant taste with use of inhalation aerosol.
Mild throat irritation, hoarseness, cough. (These can be minimized by a few swallows of water after each inhalation of powder.)

▷ **Possible Adverse Effects** (unusual, unexpected, and infrequent reactions)
If any of the following develop, consult your physician promptly for guidance.
Mild Adverse Effects
Allergic Reactions: Skin rash, hives, itching.
Headache, dizziness, drowsiness.
Nausea, vomiting, urinary urgency and pain (dysuria), joint and muscle pain.
Stinging or burning of the eyes with ophthalmic use.
Cough and bronchial irritation.
Nosebleed with nasal solution use.
Serious Adverse Effects
Allergic Reactions: Rare anaphylactic reaction (see Glossary). Allergic pneumonitis (allergic reaction in lung tissue).
Propellants in the metered dose inhaler may cause problems in patients with disease of the heart arteries or a history of abnormal heart rhythms.
Rare arteritis.

▷ **Possible Effects on Sexual Function:**   None reported.

Possible Effects on Laboratory Tests
None reported.

CAUTION
1. This drug only helps *prevent* bronchial asthma—used **before** the start of acute bronchial constriction (asthmatic wheezing).
2. *Do not* use this drug during an acute attack of asthma; it could worsen and prolong asthmatic wheezing.
3. This drug does *not* block the benefits of drugs which relieve acute asthma attacks after they start. Cromolyn is used *before and between* acute attacks to help keep them from starting; bronchodilators are used *during* acute attacks.
4. If you are using a bronchodilator drug by inhalation, it is best to take it about 5 minutes before inhaling cromolyn.
5. If this drug has allowed you to decrease or eliminate steroids, and you are unable to tolerate it, ask your doctor about the need to start steroids once again.

Precautions for Use
By Infants and Children: Safety and effectiveness for those under 5 years of age not established for the metered dose inhaler. Inhalation capsules: For children 2 years and older: 20 mg (contents of one capsule) inhaled four times a day. Young children may find a nebulized solution easier than the powder.
By Those over 60 Years of Age: This drug does not work in the management of chronic bronchitis or emphysema.

▷ **Advisability of Use During Pregnancy**
Pregnancy Category: B. See Pregnancy Code at the back of this book.
Animal studies: Mouse, rat and rabbit studies revealed no birth defects due to this drug.
Human studies: Adequate studies of pregnant women are not available.
Use this drug only if clearly needed.

Advisability of Use if Breast-Feeding
Presence of this drug in breast milk: Unknown.
Avoid drug or refrain from nursing.

Habit-Forming Potential: None.

Effects of Overdosage: No significant effects reported.

Possible Effects of Long-Term Use: Allergic reaction of lung tissue (allergic pneumonitis, very rare).

Suggested Periodic Examinations While Taking This Drug (at physician's discretion)
Sputum analysis and X-ray if symptoms suggest allergic pneumonitis.

▷ **While Taking This Drug, Observe the Following**
Foods: Follow physician prescribed diet. Avoid all foods to which you are allergic.
Beverages: Avoid all beverages to which you may be allergic.
▷   *Alcohol:* No interactions expected.
Tobacco Smoking: Follow your physician's advice regarding smoking.
▷   *Other Drugs:* Cromolyn may allow reduced dosage of cortisonelike drugs in the management of chronic asthma. Ask your doctor about dosage adjustment.

▷ *Driving, Hazardous Activities:* This drug may cause dizziness. Restrict activities as necessary.

Aviation Note: The use of this drug *may be a disqualification* for piloting. Consult a designated Aviation Medical Examiner.

Exposure to Sun: No restrictions.

Heavy Exercise or Exertion: This drug may prevent exercise-induced asthma if taken 10 to 15 minutes before exertion. It is most effective in young people.

Discontinuation: If cromolyn has made it possible to reduce or stop maintenance doses of cortisonelike drugs, and you find it necessary to discontinue cromolyn, watch closely for a sudden return of asthma. You may have to start a cortisonelike drug as well as other measures to control asthma.

Special Storage Instructions: Keep the powder cartridges in a dry, tightly closed container. Store in a cool place but not in the refrigerator. Do not handle the cartridges or the inhaler when hands are wet.

CYCLOPHOSPHAMIDE (si kloh FOSS fa mide)

Introduced: 1959   **Prescription:** USA: Yes; Canada: Yes   **Available as Generic:** No   **Class:** Anticancer, immunosuppressive   **Controlled Drug:** USA: No; Canada: No

Brand Names: Cytoxan, Neosar, ✦Procytox

BENEFITS versus RISKS	
Possible Benefits	*Possible Risks*
CURE OR CONTROL OF CERTAIN TYPES OF CANCER	REDUCED WHITE BLOOD CELL COUNT
PREVENTION OF REJECTION IN ORGAN TRANSPLANTATION	SECONDARY INFECTION
	URINARY BLADDER BLEEDING
Possibly beneficial in the treatment of rheumatoid arthritis and lupus erythematosus	HEART, LUNG, LIVER, OR KIDNEY DAMAGE
	Loss of hair
Possibly beneficial in selected cases of nephrotic syndrome in children	

▷ **Principal Uses**

As a Single Drug Product: Uses currently included in FDA approved labeling: (1) Treatment of various forms of cancer, notably malignant lymphomas, multiple myeloma, sarcomas, retinoblastomas, leukemias and cancers of the breast and ovary; (2) because this drug exerts a suppressant effect on the immune system, it is also used to prevent rejection in organ transplantation and to treat certain autoimmune disorders; (3) also used to treat some resistant forms of nephrotic syndrome.

Other (unlabeled) generally accepted uses: (1) Used to prepare patients for autologous bone marrow transplants; (2) part of several combination chemotherapy regimens; (3) helps overall survival in combination therapy of lung or fallopian tube cancer; (4) can be part of combination therapy for Ewing's sarcoma; (5) may be of help in patients with lupus erythematosus who have interstitial lung disease or nephritis; (6) secondary role in prostate cancer; (7) has a secondary role in treating the serious anemia (aplastic anemia) that can be seen in lupus erythematosus.

How This Drug Works: Because of its ability to kill cancer cells during all phases of their development and reproduction, this drug suppresses the primary growth and secondary spread (metastasis) of certain types of cancer.

Available Dosage Forms and Strengths
Injection — vials of 100 mg, 200 mg, 500 mg, 1 gram and 2 grams
Tablets — 25 mg, 50 mg

▷ **Usual Adult Dosage Range:**   Oral form: 60 to 120 mg per square meter of body surface area daily or 400 mg per square meter of body surface area on days 1 to 5 every 3 to 4 weeks. As therapy continues, the dose is adjusted according to how the tumor responds or unacceptable low white blood cell counts develop. Intravenous: 1000 to 1500 mg per square meter every 3 to 4 weeks, adjusted the same as the oral form. **Note: Actual dosage and administration schedule must be determined by the physician for each patient individually.**

Conditions Requiring Dosing Adjustments
Liver function: Dose changes are not required in liver compromise.
Kidney function: In moderate to severe kidney problems, the dose is decreased by 75–50%.

▷ **Dosing Instructions:**   Tablets may be crushed, and are best taken on an empty stomach. However, if nausea or indigestion occurs, this drug may be taken with or following food. Total liquid intake should be no less than 3 quarts/ 24 hours to reduce the risk of bladder irritation.

Usual Duration of Use: Use on a regular schedule is required to achieve and maintain a significant remission of the cancer. Duration of use depends on the response of the cancer and patient tolerance of the drug.

▷ **This Drug Should Not Be Taken If**
- you have had an allergic reaction to any dosage form of it previously.
- you have an active infection of any kind.
- you have bloody urine for any reason.
- you have kidney (renal) failure with creatinine clearance less than 30 ml per minute (talk with your doctor).
- you are pregnant.

▷ **Inform Your Physician Before Taking This Drug If**
- you have impaired liver or kidney function.
- you have a blood cell or bone marrow disorder.
- you have had previous chemotherapy or X-ray therapy for any type of cancer.
- you take, or have taken within the past year, any cortisonelike drug (adrenal corticosteroids).
- you have diabetes.
- you plan to have surgery under general anesthesia in the near future.

Possible Side Effects (natural, expected, and unavoidable drug actions)
Bone marrow depression (see Glossary)—low production of white blood cells and, to a lesser degree, red blood cells and blood platelets (see Glossary).

Possible effects include fever, chills, sore throat, fatigue, weakness, abnormal bleeding or bruising.

Leukemia has been reported following cyclophosphamide therapy.

Impairment of natural resistance (immunity) to infection.

Weakening of the heart muscle (cardiomyopathy).

Excessive urination (SIADH).

Cystitis or hemorrhagic cystitis.

Ninefold increase in bladder cancer risk.

▷ **Possible Adverse Effects** (unusual, unexpected, and infrequent reactions)

If any of the following develop, consult your physician promptly for guidance.

Mild Adverse Effects

Allergic Reaction: Skin rash (rare).

Headache, dizziness, blurred vision.

Loss of scalp hair (50% of users), darkening of skin and fingernails, transverse ridging of nails.

Loss of appetite, nausea, vomiting, ulceration of mouth, diarrhea (may be bloody).

Serious Adverse Effects

Idiosyncratic Reaction: Hemolytic anemia (see Glossary).

Liver damage with jaundice—yellow eyes and skin, dark-colored urine, light-colored stools.

Kidney damage—impaired kidney function, reduced urine volume, bloody urine.

Severe inflammation of bladder—painful urination, bloody urine.

Drug-induced damage of heart and lung tissue.

Severe lung damage (interstitial pneumonitis).

▷ **Possible Effects on Sexual Function**

Suppression of ovarian function—irregular menstrual pattern or cessation of menstruation (18% to 57% depending upon dose and duration of use).

Testicular suppression—reduced or no sperm production (100% of users).

Possible Delayed Adverse Effects

Development of other types of cancer (secondary malignancies).

Development of severe cystitis with bleeding from the bladder wall. (May occur many months after the last dose.)

Possible Effects on Laboratory Tests

Complete blood cell counts: decreased red cells, hemoglobin, white cells and platelets.

Prothrombin time: increased.

Liver function tests: increased liver enzymes (ALT/GPT, AST/GOT and alkaline phosphatase), increased bilirubin.

CAUTION

1. This drug may interfere with the normal healing of wounds.

2. This drug can cause significant changes in genetic material in both men and women (sperm and eggs or ova). Patients taking this drug **must** understand the potential for serious defects in children that are conceived during or following the course of medication.

3. This drug can suppress natural resistance (immunity) to infection, resulting in life-threatening illness.

4. Avoid live-virus vaccines while taking this drug (talk with your doctor about this).

Precautions for Use

By Infants and Children: This drug should not be given if the child is dehydrated. Adequate fluid intake to ensure a copious urine volume for 4 hours following each dose is needed. Prevent exposure of child to anyone with active chicken pox or shingles. This drug may cause ovarian or testicular sterility.

By Those over 60 Years of Age: Increased risk of serious bladder problems (chemical cystitis). Patients **MUST** drink large amounts of water in order to keep the bladder flushed. This may increase the risk of urinary retention in men with prostatism (see Glossary).

▷ **Advisability of Use During Pregnancy**

Pregnancy Category: D. See Pregnancy Code at the back of this book.

Animal studies: Significant birth defects reported in mice, rat and rabbit studies.

Human studies: Information from studies of pregnant women indicates that this drug can cause serious birth defects or fetal death.

Avoid completely during the first 3 months. Use of this drug during the last 6 months must be carefully individualized.

Advisability of Use if Breast-Feeding

Presence of this drug in breast milk: Yes.

Avoid drug or refrain from nursing.

Habit-Forming Potential: None.

Effects of Overdosage: Nausea, vomiting, diarrhea, bloody urine, water retention, weight gain, severe bone marrow depression, severe infections.

Possible Effects of Long-Term Use: Development of fibrous tissue in lungs; secondary malignancies.

Suggested Periodic Examinations While Taking This Drug (at physician's discretion)

Complete blood cell counts, every 2 to 4 days during initial treatment; then every 3 to 4 weeks during maintenance treatment.

Liver and kidney function tests.

Thyroid function tests (if symptoms warrant).

▷ **While Taking This Drug, Observe the Following**

Foods: No restrictions.

Beverages: No restrictions. May be taken with milk.

▷ *Alcohol:* No interactions expected.

Tobacco Smoking: No interactions expected.

▷ *Other Drugs*

Cyclophosphamide *taken concurrently* with

- allopurinol (Zyloprim) may increase the extent of bone marrow depression.
- chloramphenicol can decrease cyclophosphamide effectiveness.
- ciprofloxacin (Cipro) can result in lowered ciprofloxacin levels and the need for a larger than usual dose.
- digoxin may decrease digoxin absorption and impair digoxin effectiveness.
- hydrochlorothiazide and other thiazide diuretics (see Drug Classes) may worsen the lowering of white blood cells (myelosuppression) caused by cyclophosphamide.

- influenza vaccine (and perhaps other vaccines) may have decreased ability to confer immunity.
- pentostatin may cause fatal heart damage.
- succinylcholine can result in succinylcholine toxicity.

▷ *Driving, Hazardous Activities:* Use caution if dizziness occurs.

Aviation Note: The use of this drug *may be a disqualification* for piloting. Consult a designated Aviation Medical Examiner.

Exposure to Sun: No restrictions.

Occurrence of Unrelated Illness: Any signs of infection—fever, chills, sore throat, cough or flulike symptoms must be promptly reported. This drug may have to be stopped until the infection is controlled. Consult your physician.

CYCLOSPORINE (SI kloh spor een)

Other Names: Ciclosporin, cyclosporin A

Introduced: 1983   **Prescription:** USA: Yes; Canada: Yes   **Available as**
Generic: USA: No; Canada: No   **Class:** Immunosuppressant   **Controlled**
Drug: USA: No; Canada: No

Brand Name: Sandimmune, Neoral

BENEFITS versus RISKS	
Possible Benefits	*Possible Risks*
EFFECTIVE PREVENTION AND TREATMENT OF REJECTION IN ORGAN TRANSPLANTATION	MARKED KIDNEY TOXICITY DEVELOPMENT OF HYPERTENSION
Limited effectiveness in the treatment of Crohn's disease, myasthenia gravis, severe psoriasis, rheumatoid arthritis	Excessive hair growth
	Overgrowth of gums
	Liver toxicity
	Low white blood cell count
	Development of lymphoma

▷ **Principal Uses**

As a Single Drug Product: Uses included in FDA approved labeling: (1) Helps prevent (in conjunction with cortisonelike drugs) organ rejection in kidney, liver and heart transplantation; (2) helps treat rejection crisis.

Other (unlabeled) generally accepted uses: (1) Used in transplantation of the bone marrow; (2) used investigationally in a variety of diseases involving the immune system such as: Sjogren's, Crohn's and Grave's disease, psoriasis, myasthenia gravis, bullous pemphigoid, pulmonary fibrosis associated with rheumatoid arthritis, rheumatoid arthritis, Sweet's syndrome, insulin-dependent diabetes, and aplastic anemia; (3) may have a role in treating male pattern baldness; (4) can help canker sores (apthous stomatitis); (5) used to help severe, steroid-dependent asthma; (6) can have a role in treating severe skin reactions (toxic epidermal necrolysis) to phenytoin (Dilantin).

How This Drug Works: By inhibiting some lymphocytes (white blood cells) and their growth factors, this drug suppresses the rejection of transplanted organs.

Available Dosage Forms and Strengths
>Capsules, soft gelatin—25 mg, 100 mg
>Injection, intravenous—50 mg per ml
>Oral solution (note: a microemulsion (Neoral) is NOT the same as Sandimmune.)—100 mg per ml

▷ **Usual Adult Dosage Range:** Initially 15 mg/kg/day taken 4 to 12 hours prior to transplantation surgery. This dose is continued following surgery for 1 to 2 weeks; then the dose is gradually reduced by 5% per week to a maintenance dose of 5 to 10 mg/kg/day. A new dosing strategy NOT using weight (using only the lowest blood level) has been developed. Rectal dosing for ulcerative colitis has been given in a range of 250 to 350 mg per day. The microemulsion formulation offers more consistent pharmacokinetics. If Neoral is used: it should be given at the same time each day in two equally divided doses. If conversion is made from oral Sandimune to Neoral, the Neoral dose is usually started at the same daily dose as the Sandimmune. Cyclosporine trough levels should be measured twice a week when patients are converted to Neoral who were taking more than 10 milligrams per kilogram per day of Sandimmune. **Note: Actual dosage and administration schedule must be determined by the physician for each patient individually.**

Conditions Requiring Dosing Adjustments
Liver function: The dose must be adjusted (based on blood levels) in liver compromise. Much of the drug is eliminated in the bile.
Kidney function: This drug is capable of causing marked kidney toxicity. Caution is critical. Dosing usually does not change, but more frequent blood levels are indicated.
Diabetes: People who are diabetic and subsequently have kidney or pancreatic transplants will need larger than usual doses.
Hypercholesterolemia: If the blood cholesterol is 50% above normal, the dose must be decreased by 50% in order to avoid toxicity.
Obesity: Because of the way the drug is distributed in the body, the dosing of this medication **must** be based on ideal (a calculation which helps eliminate the weight which is fat) body weight.
Cystic fibrosis: It is very difficult to appropriately dose this medication in patients who have this disease. Some patients will require as much as two times the usual dose. The dose should be adjusted to drug levels.
Multiple organ transplants: Patients with multiple transplants (such as pancreas and kidney) often need an increased dose of cyclosporine in order to achieve the desired effect. The dose should be determined based on blood levels.

▷ **Dosing Instructions:** Preferably taken with or immediately following food to reduce stomach irritation. The capsule should be swallowed whole; do not open, crush or chew. The oral solution should be mixed with milk, chocolate milk or orange juice (at room temperature) in a glass or ceramic cup; do not use a wax-lined or plastic container. Stir well and drink immediately. It is advisable to take this drug at the same time each day to maintain steady blood levels.

Usual Duration of Use: Use on a regular schedule for several weeks is usually needed to see this drug's effectiveness in preventing organ rejection or stopping rejection that is already underway. Long-term use (months to years) requires periodic evaluation of response, blood tests and dosage adjustment.

▷ **This Drug Should Not Be Taken If**
- you have had an allergic reaction to it previously.
- you are taking any immunosuppressant drug other than cortisonelike preparations.
- you have an active lymphoma of any type.
- you have an active, uncontrolled infection, especially chicken pox or shingles.

▷ **Inform Your Physician Before Taking This Drug If**
- you are pregnant or breast-feeding.
- you have a history of liver or kidney disease, or impaired liver or kidney function.
- you have a history of hypertension or gout.
- you have a chronic gastrointestinal disorder.
- you are taking a potassium supplement or drugs that can raise the blood level of potassium.
- you have a seizure disorder.
- you have a history of a blood cell disorder.
- you are taking other medicines which may be toxic to the kidney.

Possible Side Effects (natural, expected, and unavoidable drug actions)
Predisposition to infections.

▷ **Possible Adverse Effects** (unusual, unexpected, and infrequent reactions)
If any of the following develop, consult your physician promptly for guidance.

Mild Adverse Effects
Allergic Reactions: Skin rash, itching.
Excessive hair growth, acne (rare).
Headache, confusion (rare), tremors (21 to 55%).
Mouth sores (rare), gum overgrowth (frequent in some reports), nausea/vomiting, diarrhea.
Changes in facial features (dysmorphosis).

Serious Adverse Effects
Allergic Reactions: Anaphylactoid reaction (see Glossary) to intravenous solution (rare).
Severe kidney injury.
Hypertension, mild to severe (up to half).
Seizures (up to ¼ of liver transplant patients).
Cortical blindness.
Liver injury.
Pancreatitis (rare).
Low white blood cell count (leukopenia).
Low blood platelets (rare).
High blood potassium levels.
High blood glucose.

High uric acid levels and gout.
Low blood magnesium.
Lymphoma (rare), possibly drug-induced.
Elevation of blood potassium.
Relapse of lupus erythematosus.
Increased risk of skin cancers (risk increased by sun or UV light exposure).

▷ **Possible Effects on Sexual Function**
Enlargement and tenderness of male breast (1 to 4%).

▷ **Adverse Effects That May Mimic Natural Diseases or Disorders**
Liver toxicity may suggest viral hepatitis.

Natural Diseases or Disorders That May Be Activated by This Drug
Latent infections, hypertension, gout.

Possible Effects on Laboratory Tests
Complete blood cell counts: decreased red cells, hemoglobin and white cells.
Blood potassium level: increased.
Blood uric acid level: increased.
Blood platelets, white cells, magnesium: decreased.
Liver function tests: increased liver enzymes (ALT/GPT, AST/GOT and alkaline phosphatase), increased bilirubin.
Kidney function tests: blood creatinine and urea nitrogen levels (BUN) increased; urine casts present.

CAUTION
1. Report promptly any indications of infection of any kind.
2. Promptly report swollen glands, sores or lumps in the skin, abnormal bleeding or bruising.
3. Inform your physician promptly if you become pregnant.
4. Periodic laboratory tests are mandatory.
5. Best to avoid immunizations and contact with people who have recently taken oral poliovirus vaccine.

Precautions for Use
By Infants and Children: This drug has been used successfully and safely in children of all ages.
By Those over 60 Years of Age: The dose must be adjusted to any decline in kidney function.

▷ **Advisability of Use During Pregnancy**
Pregnancy Category: C. See Pregnancy Code at the back of this book.
Animal studies: Rat and rabbit studies reveal that this drug is toxic to the embryo and fetus. No drug-induced birth defects were found.
Human studies: Adequate studies of pregnant women are not available.
Avoid this drug during entire pregnancy unless it is clearly needed.

Advisability of Use if Breast-Feeding
Presence of this drug in breast milk: Yes.
Avoid drug or refrain from nursing.

Habit-Forming Potential: None.

Effects of Overdosage: Headache, painful sensations in hands and feet, flushing of the face, gum soreness and bleeding, high blood pressure, atrial fibrillation, respiratory distress syndrome, seizures, coma, hallucinations, neurotoxicity, electrolyte disturbances, liver toxicity.

Possible Effects of Long-Term Use: Irreversible kidney damage, severe hypertension, abnormal growth of gums.

Suggested Periodic Examinations While Taking This Drug (at physician's discretion)
Measurement of cyclosporine blood levels.
Complete blood cell counts.
Liver and kidney function tests.
Measurement of magnesium, potassium and uric acid blood levels.
Serial blood pressure measurements.

▷ **While Taking This Drug, Observe the Following**
Foods: Avoid excessive intake of high-potassium foods. See Table section. Food may also increase the peak blood level of cyclosporine.
Beverages: Grapefruit juice increases blood levels. Milk may increase blood levels.
▷ *Alcohol:* Large amounts of alcohol may increase blood levels of cyclosporine.
Tobacco Smoking: This interaction has not been well studied, but since smoking changes the elimination of some other medications, smoking is not recommended while taking this drug.
▷ *Other Drugs*
Cyclosporine *taken concurrently* with
• ACE (see Drug Classes) inhibitors may increase the risk of kidney problems.
• amphotericin B can cause serious kidney toxicity.
• aspirin substitutes (nonsteroidal anti-inflammatory drugs or NSAIDs) may increase kidney toxicity.
• aminoglycoside antibiotics (see Drug Classes) may increase kidney toxicity.
• azathioprine may increase immunosuppression.
• calcium channel blockers (see Drug Classes) may result in cyclosporine toxicity.
• ciprofloxacin (and other fluoroquinolones—see Drug Class) may increase risk of kidney toxicity.
• cotrimoxazole may result in decreased cyclosporine effectiveness as well as kidney toxicity.
• cyclophosphamide may increase immunosuppression.
• digoxin may result in serious digoxin toxicity.
• furosemide may result in increased risk of gout.
• ganciclovir may result in increased kidney toxicity.
• histamine H2 inhibitors (see Drug Classes) and ketoconazole may experience decreased cyclosporine blood levels.
• imipenem/cilastatin may result in neurotoxicity.
• lovastatin may increase risk of muscle toxicity (moypathy) or kidney failure.
• methylprednisolone may cause seizures.
• metronidazole may result in increased cyclosporine levels and toxicity.

- nifedipine may worsen abnormal gum growth (gingival hyperplasia) and also cause nefedipine toxicity (low blood pressure and abnormal heart beats).
- pravastatin can cause myopathy.
- simvastatin may cause myopathy.
- sulfamethoxazole and/or trimethoprim may increase kidney toxicity.
- tacrolimus can cause kidney toxicity.
- verapamil may increase immunosuppression.
- vaccines may blunt the benefit of the vaccine.

The following drugs may *increase* the effects of cyclosporine

- acetazolamide.
- allopurinol.
- amiodarone.
- ceftriaxone.
- clarithromycin.
- colchicine.
- danazol or other anabolic steroids.
- diltiazem.
- econazole.
- erythromycin.
- fluconazole.
- itraconazole.
- ketoconazole.
- miconazole.
- methyltestosterone.
- metoclopramide.
- oral contraceptives (birth control pills).
- terconazole.

The following drugs may *decrease* the effects of cyclosporine

- carbamazepine.
- isoniazid.
- nafcillin.
- octreotide.
- phenobarbital.
- phenytoin.
- quinine.
- rifabutin.
- rifampin.
- sulfadimidine, sulfadiazine and/or trimethoprim.
- ticlopidine.

▷ *Driving, Hazardous Activities:*
This drug may cause confusion or seizures. Restrict activities as necessary.

Aviation Note: The use of this drug *may be a disqualification* for piloting. Consult a designated Aviation Medical Examiner.

Exposure to Sun: Exposure to sunlight or other ultraviolet (UV) radiation may increase the risk of skin cancer.

Discontinuation: Do not stop this drug without your physician's guidance.

Special Storage Instructions: Keep the gelatin capsules in the blister packets until ready for use. Store below 77 degrees F (25 degrees C).

Keep the oral solution in a tightly closed container. Store below 86 degrees F (30 degrees C). Do not refrigerate.

Observe the Following Expiration Times: The oral solution must be used within 2 months after opening.

DESIPRAMINE (des IP ra meen)

Introduced: 1964   **Prescription:** USA: Yes; Canada: Yes   **Available as**
Generic: USA: Yes; Canada: Yes   **Class:** Antidepressant   **Controlled**
Drug: USA: No; Canada: No
Brand Names: Norpramin, Pertofrane

BENEFITS versus RISKS	
Possible Benefits	*Possible Risks*
EFFECTIVE RELIEF OF ENDOGENOUS DEPRESSION Possibly beneficial in other depressive disorders	ADVERSE BEHAVIORAL EFFECTS: confusion, disorientation, delusions, hallucinations CONVERSION OF DEPRESSION TO MANIA in manic-depressive (bipolar) disorders Aggravation of paranoia and schizophrenia Drug-induced heart rhythm disorders Abnormally low white blood cell and platelet counts

▷ **Principal Uses**

As a Single Drug Product: Uses currently included in FDA approved labeling: (1) Relieves severe depression. This drug is more likely to work in primary (endogenous) depression than in secondary, reactive (exogenous) depression.
Other (unlabeled) generally accepted uses: (1) Chronic pain syndromes, including diabetic neuropathy; (2) treatment of attention deficit disorder in children over 6 years of age and in adolescents; (3) decreases the symptoms of panic disorder; (4) helps treat resistant malaria; (5) may help reduce binge eating in bulimia.

How This Drug Works: By increasing brain concentrations of some nerve impulse transmitters (norepinephrine and serotonin), this drug relieves the symptoms associated with depression.

Available Dosage Forms and Strengths
Capsules — 25 mg, 50 mg
Tablets — 10 mg, 25 mg, 50 mg, 75 mg, 100 mg, 150 mg

▷ **Usual Adult Dosage Range:** Initially 25 mg 2 to 4 times daily. Dose may be increased cautiously as needed and tolerated by 25 mg daily at intervals of 1 week. The usual maintenance dose is 100 mg to 200 mg/24 hours. The total daily dosage should not exceed 300 mg. (When determined, the optimal daily requirement may be given at bedtime as a single dose.) **Note: Actual dosage and administration schedule must be determined by the physician for each patient individually.**

Conditions Requiring Dosing Adjustments

Liver function: The dose should be decreased in patients with compromised livers.

Kidney function: Can cause urine retention—used with caution in kidney compromise with urine outflow problems.

▷ **Dosing Instructions:**   May be taken without regard to meals. The capsule may be opened and the tablet may be crushed for administration.

Usual Duration of Use: Use on a regular schedule for 3 to 4 weeks is usually needed to see this drug's effectiveness in relieving depression; peak response may require 3 months of use. Delusional patients may require seven weeks to benefit. Long-term use (months to years) requires periodic evaluation of response and dosage adjustment.

▷ **This Drug Should Not Be Taken If**
- you have had an allergic reaction to it previously.
- you are taking, or have taken within the past 14 days, any monoamine oxidase (MAO) type A inhibitor drug (see Drug Classes).
- you have had a recent heart attack (myocardial infarction).
- you have narrow-angle glaucoma.

▷ **Inform Your Physician Before Taking This Drug If**
- you have had an adverse reaction to any other antidepressant drug.
- you have any type of seizure disorder.
- you have increased internal eye pressure.
- you have any type of heart disease, especially a heart rhythm disorder.
- you have any type of thyroid disorder or are taking thyroid medication.
- you have thought about or attempted suicide.
- you have diabetes or sugar intolerance.
- you take levodopa (increased risk of heart rhythm problems with high desipramine doses).
- you have prostatism (see Glossary).
- you plan to have surgery under general anesthesia in the near future.

Possible Side Effects (natural, expected, and unavoidable drug actions)

Mild drowsiness, light-headedness (low blood pressure), blurred vision, dry mouth, constipation, impaired urination.

▷ **Possible Adverse Effects** (unusual, unexpected, and infrequent reactions)

If any of the following develop, consult your physician promptly for guidance.

Mild Adverse Effects

Allergic Reactions: Skin rash, hives, swelling of face or tongue, drug fever (see Glossary).

Headache, dizziness, weakness, unsteadiness, tremors, fainting.

Irritation of tongue or mouth, altered taste, difficulty talking (rare), indigestion, nausea.

Fluctuations of blood sugar.

Serious Adverse Effects

Allergic Reactions: Drug-induced hepatitis, with or without jaundice; anaphylactoid reaction (see terms in Glossary).

Adverse behavioral effects: confusion, disorientation, delusions, hallucinations.

Seizures; reduced control of epilepsy.

Aggravation of paranoid psychoses and schizophrenia.

Heart rhythm disturbances, myocarditis.

Parkinson-like disorders, peripheral neuritis (see both terms in Glossary).

Abnormally low white blood cell and platelet counts: fever, sore throat, infections, abnormal bleeding or bruising.

Neuroleptic malignant syndrome.

▷ **Possible Effects on Sexual Function:**   Decreased libido, increased libido (antidepressant effect), impotence, painful male orgasm, male breast enlargement, female breast enlargement with milk production, swelling of testicles, decreased sperm viability.

▷ **Adverse Effects That May Mimic Natural Diseases or Disorders**

Liver toxicity may suggest viral hepatitis.

Natural Diseases or Disorders That May Be Activated by This Drug

Latent diabetes, epilepsy, glaucoma, prostatism.

Possible Effects on Laboratory Tests

Complete blood cell counts: decreased red cells, hemoglobin, white cells and platelets; increased eosinophils (allergic reaction).

Blood glucose levels: unexplained fluctuations.

Liver function tests: increased liver enzymes (ALT/GPT, AST/GOT and alkaline phosphatase), increased bilirubin (all rare).

Thyroid function tests: decreased TSH and mean free thyroxin.

CAUTION

1. Should only be used when a true, primary, endogenous depression (not reactive) has been diagnosed.
2. Watch for indications of toxicity: confusion, agitation, rapid heart rate, heart irregularity. Blood levels will be needed.
3. It is advisable to withhold this drug if electroconvulsive therapy (ECT) is to be used to treat the depression.

Precautions for Use

By Infants and Children: Safety and effectiveness for those under 6 years of age not established. This drug is being used experimentally to treat children who have attention deficit syndrome, with or without hyperactivity. Dosage and management must be supervised by a properly trained pediatrician.

By Those over 60 Years of Age: Initiate treatment with 25 mg 1 or 2 times daily to evaluate tolerance. During the first 2 weeks of treatment, watch for confusion, restlessness, agitation, forgetfulness, disorientation, delusions or hallucinations. Also observe for unsteadiness and instability that may predispose to falling. This drug may aggravate prostatism.

▷ **Advisability of Use During Pregnancy**

Pregnancy Category: C. See Pregnancy Code at the back of this book.

Animal studies: Birth defects reported in rat and rabbit studies.

Human studies: Adequate studies of pregnant women are not available.

Use only if clearly needed. Avoid during the first 3 months if possible.

Advisability of Use if Breast-Feeding

Presence of this drug in breast milk: Yes, in small amounts.

Monitor nursing infant closely and discontinue drug or nursing if adverse effects develop.

Habit-Forming Potential: Psychological or physical dependence is rare and unexpected. Some patients may seek to abuse this medicine for its ability to create anticholinergic delirium.

Effects of Overdosage: Confusion, hallucinations, drowsiness, tremors, heart irregularity, seizures, stupor, hypothermia (see Glossary).

Possible Effects of Long-Term Use: None reported.

Suggested Periodic Examinations While Taking This Drug (at physician's discretion)
Complete blood cell counts, liver function tests.
Serial blood pressure readings and electrocardiograms.

▷ **While Taking This Drug, Observe the Following**
Foods: No specific restrictions. Limiting food intake may avoid excess weight gain.
Beverages: No restrictions. May be taken with milk.
▷ *Alcohol:* **Avoid completely.** This drug can markedly increase the intoxicating effects of alcohol; the combination can depress brain function.
Tobacco Smoking: May accelerate the elimination of this drug and require increased dosage.
Marijuana Smoking
Occasional (once or twice weekly): Transient increase in drowsiness and mouth dryness.
Daily: Persistent drowsiness and mouth dryness; possible reduced effectiveness of this drug.
▷ *Other Drugs*
Desipramine may *increase* the effects of
• all drugs with sedative effects; watch for excessive sedation.
• all drugs with atropinelike effects (see Drug Classes).
Desipramine may *decrease* the effects of
• clonidine (Catapres).
• guanfacine (Tenex).
• guanethidine (Ismelin, Esimil).
• levodopa by decreasing absorption of the levodopa.
Desipramine *taken concurrently* with
• albuterol may increase the effect of albuterol on the blood vessels.
• anticonvulsants requires careful monitoring for changes in seizure patterns and need to adjust anticonvulsant dosage (carbamazepine-Tegretol or phenytoin-Dilantin are examples).
• large doses (greater than 2 grams per day) of vitamin C may lead to increased removal of desipramine and the need to increase the dose.
• ethchlorvynol (Placidyl) may cause delirium; avoid concurrent use.
• monoamine oxidase (MAO) type A inhibitor drugs (see Drug Classes) may cause high fever, seizures and excessive rise in blood pressure; avoid concurrent use of these drugs and provide periods of 14 days between administration of either.
• quinidine may cause desipramine toxicity.
• stimulant drugs (amphetamine, cocaine, epinephrine, phenylpropanolamine, etc.) may cause severe high blood pressure and/or high fever.
• thyroid preparations may increase the risk of heart rhythm disorders.

- warfarin may cause an increased risk of bleeding. Increased testing of INR is indicated.

The following drugs may *increase* the effects of desipramine
- cimetidine (Tagamet).
- fluoxetine (Prozac).
- fluvoxamine (Luvox).
- methylphenidate (Ritalin).
- phenothiazines (see Drug Classes).

The following drugs may *decrease* the effects of desipramine
- barbiturates (see Drug Classes).
- chloral hydrate (Noctec, Somnos, etc.).
- clonazepam.
- estrogen (see Drug Profile for brand names).
- lithium (Lithobid, Lithotab, etc.).
- oral contraceptives (see Drug Profile for brand names) (birth control pills).
- reserpine (Serpasil, Ser-Ap-Es, etc.).

▷ *Driving, Hazardous Activities:* This drug may impair mental alertness, judgment, physical coordination and reaction time. Restrict activities as necessary.

Aviation Note: The use of this drug *is a disqualification* for piloting. Consult a designated Aviation Medical Examiner.

Exposure to Sun: Use caution. This drug may cause photosensitivity (see Glossary) and changes in iris and skin pigment color with sun exposure.

Exposure to Heat: Use caution. This drug can inhibit sweating and impair adaptation to hot environments, increasing the risk of heat stroke. Avoid saunas.

Exposure to Cold: The elderly should use caution and avoid conditions conducive to hypothermia (see Glossary).

Exposure to Environmental Chemicals: This drug may mask the symptoms of poisoning due to handling certain insecticides (organophosphorus types). Read labels carefully.

Discontinuation: It is advisable to stop this drug gradually. Abrupt withdrawal after prolonged use may cause headache, malaise and nausea. When this drug is stopped, it may be necessary to adjust the dosages of other drugs taken concurrently.

DEXAMETHASONE (dex a METH a sohn)

Introduced: 1958   **Prescription:** USA: Yes; Canada: Yes   **Available as Generic:** USA: Yes; Canada: Yes   **Class:** Cortisonelike drugs   **Controlled Drug:** USA: No; Canada: No

Brand Names: Acroseb-Dex, ♣Ak-Dex, Ak-Trol [CD], Baldex, Dalalone, Dalalone DP, Dalalone LA, Decaderm, Decadron, Decadron Nasal Spray, Decadron-LA, Decadron Phosphate Ophthalmic, Decadron Phosphate Respihaler, Decadron Phosphate Turbinaire, Decadron w/Xylocaine [CD], Decaject, Decaject LA, Decaspray, Deenar [CD], ♣Deronil, Dex-4, Dexacen-4, Dexacen LA-8, Dexameth, Dexasone, Dexasone-LA, Dexo-LA, Dexon, Dexone, Dexone-E, Dexone-LA, Hexadrol, Maxidex, Mymethasone,

✦Neodecadron Eye-Ear, Neodexair, Neomycin-Dex, Ocu-Trol [CD], ✦Ora-dexon, ✦PMS-Dexamethasone, ✦SK-Dexamethasone, ✦Sofracort, Solurex, Solurex-LA, ✦Spersadex, Tobradex

---

BENEFITS versus RISKS

Possible Benefits	*Possible Risks*
EFFECTIVE RELIEF OF SYMPTOMS IN A WIDE VARIETY OF INFLAMMATORY AND ALLERGIC DISORDERS EFFECTIVE IMMUNOSUPPRESSION in selected benign and malignant disorders	Long-term use (exceeding 2 weeks) is associated with many possible adverse effects: ALTERED MOOD AND PERSONALITY, CATARACTS, GLAUCOMA, HYPERTENSION, ARRHYTHMIAS, PEPTIC ULCERS, PANCREATITIS, OSTEOPOROSIS, ASEPTIC BONE NECROSIS, INCREASED SUSCEPTIBILITY TO INFECTIONS

▷ **Principal Uses**

As a Single Drug Product: Uses currently included in FDA approved labeling: (1) Used in the management of serious skin disorders, asthma, lymphoma, brain edema, shock, systemic lupus erythematosus and all types of major rheumatic disorders including bursitis, systemic lupus erythematosus, ten-donitis and most forms of arthritis; (2) topical cream is used to treat ec-zema, psoriasis, dermatitis and lichen planus.

Other (unlabeled) generally accepted uses: (1) Adrenal insufficiency; (2) acute airway obstruction; (3) mountain sickness; (4) vomiting caused by chemo-therapy; (5) cardiopulmonary bypass; (6) refractory depression; (7) relief of symptoms of cancer which has spread to the brain (metastasis); (8) used in combination regimens to control multiple myeloma; (9) may have a role in extreme cases of pneumocystis carinii pneumonia; (10) can help suppress male hormones (androgens) in women with acne, hirsutism or hair loss (androgenic alopecia) caused by androgens.

How This Drug Works: Inhibits defensive functions of certain white blood cells. It reduces the production of lymphocytes and some antibodies and acts as an immunosuppressant.

Available Dosage Forms and Strengths

Aerosol — 0.01% and 0.04%

Aerosol inhaler — 84 mcg per spray

Cream — 0.1%

Elixir — 0.5 mg per 5-ml

Eye ointment — 0.05%

Gel — 0.1%

Injection — 4 mg per ml, 8 mg per ml, 10 mg per ml, 16 mg per ml, 20 mg per ml and 24 mg per ml

Oral solution — 0.5 mg per 0.5 ml and 0.5 mg per 5 ml

Solution — 0.1%

Suspension — 0.1%

Tablets — 0.25 mg, 0.5 mg, 0.75 mg, 1 mg, 1.5 mg, 2 mg, 4 mg, 6 mg

▷ **Usual Adult Dosage Range:**   Oral: 0.75 to 9 mg daily divided into 2 to 4 doses. Oral dose for children: 0.03 to 0.15 mg per kg per day divided into equal doses given every 6 to 12 hours. **Note: Actual dosage and administration schedule must be determined by the physician for each patient individually.**

Conditions Requiring Dosing Adjustments

Liver function: This drug is eliminated via the liver, however, no specific guidelines for dosing adjustments are available.

Kidney function: Used with caution as it can cause alkalosis (a change toward a more basic condition in the body's chemistry).

Obesity: Dosing on a mg per kg per day basis is recommended. Best to measure free urinary cortisol as well.

▷ **Dosing Instructions:**   Tablet may be crushed and taken with or following food to prevent stomach irritation, preferably in the morning.

Usual Duration of Use: For acute disorders: 4 to 10 days. For chronic disorders: according to individual requirements. Length of therapy should not exceed the time needed to obtain adequate symptomatic relief in acute self-limiting conditions; or the time required to stabilize a chronic condition and permit gradual withdrawal. Because of its long duration of action, this drug is not appropriate for alternate day administration.

▷ **This Drug Should Not Be Taken If**
- you have had an allergic reaction to any dosage form of it previously.
- you have active peptic ulcer disease.
- you have an active herpes simplex infection of the eye.
- you have a systemic fungal infection (talk with your doctor).
- you have osteoporosis.
- your sputum consistently grows Candida albicans (a yeast which may grow very quickly if steroids suppress your immune system).
- you have a psychoneurosis or psychosis.
- you have active tuberculosis.

▷ **Inform Your Physician Before Taking This Drug If**
- you have had an unfavorable reaction to any cortisonelike drug.
- you have a history of peptic ulcer disease, thrombophlebitis or tuberculosis.
- you have: diabetes, glaucoma, high blood pressure, deficient thyroid function or myasthenia gravis.
- you start to have restricted motion, increased pain, fever or joint swelling These may be early signs of a septic arthritis.
- you plan to have surgery of any kind in the near future.

Possible Side Effects (natural, expected, and unavoidable drug actions)

Increased appetite, weight gain, retention of salt and water, excretion of potassium, increased susceptibility to infection.

▷ **Possible Adverse Effects** (unusual, unexpected, and infrequent reactions) **If any of the following develop, consult your physician promptly for guidance.**

Mild Adverse Effects

Allergic Reaction: Skin rash.

Headache, dizziness, insomnia.

Acid indigestion, abdominal distention.

Muscle cramping and weakness.

Vaginal itching.

Easy bruising (Echymosis).

Acne, excessive growth of facial hair.

Serious Adverse Effects

Mental and emotional disturbances of serious magnitude.

Reactivation of latent tuberculosis.

Development of peptic ulcer.

Inflammation of the pancreas.

Thrombophlebitis (inflammation of a vein with the formation of blood clot)—pain or tenderness in thigh or leg, or swelling of the foot, ankle, or leg.

Pulmonary embolism (movement of a blood clot to the lung)—sudden shortness of breath, pain in the chest, coughing, bloody sputum.

Low blood platelets.

Abnormal lipids (cholesterol, triglycerides, LDLs).

Abnormal heart rhythm.

Cushing's syndrome.

Suppression of the adrenal gland.

High blood pressure (may be lessened by alternate-day therapy).

High blood sugar.

Excessively low blood potassium.

Superinfections of the stomach.

Abnormally slow heartbeat in infants.

Increased pressure in the eye.

Cataracts or glaucoma.

Pneumocystis carinii pneumonia.

Precipitation of porphyria.

Rare excessive thyroid function (questionable causality).

Myopathy.

Bone death (aseptic necrosis or avascular necrosis).

Osteoporosis.

▷ **Possible Effects on Sexual Function:**   Altered timing and pattern of menstruation.

▷ **Adverse Effects That May Mimic Natural Diseases or Disorders**

Pattern of symptoms and signs resembling Cushing's syndrome.

Natural Diseases or Disorders That May Be Activated by This Drug

Latent diabetes, glaucoma, peptic ulcer disease, tuberculosis.

Possible Effects on Laboratory Tests

Blood amylase level: increased (possible pancreatitis).

Blood glucose level: increased.

Digoxin testing: may falsely increase digoxin results.

Glucose tolerance test (GTT): decreased.

Blood potassium level: decreased.

Thyroid function tests: decreased.

CAUTION

1. Best to carry a card noting that you are taking this drug, if your course of treatment is to exceed 1 week.

2. Do not stop this drug abruptly if it is used for long-term treatment.

3. If vaccination against measles, rabies, smallpox or yellow fever is required, stop this drug 72 hours before vaccination and do not resume it for at least 14 days after vaccination.

Precautions for Use

By Infants and Children: Avoid prolonged use if possible. During long-term use, watch for suppression of normal growth and the possibility of increased intracranial pressure. Following long-term use, the child may be at risk for adrenal gland deficiency during stress for as long as 18 months after cessation.

By Those over 60 Years of Age: Avoid prolonged use of this drug. Continual use (even in small doses) can increase the severity of diabetes, enhance fluid retention, raise blood pressure, weaken resistance to infection, induce stomach ulcer and accelerate the development of cataract and osteoporosis.

▷ **Advisability of Use During Pregnancy**

Pregnancy Category: C. See Pregnancy Code at the back of this book.

Animal studies: Birth defects reported in mice, rats and rabbits.

Human studies: Adequate studies of pregnant women are not available.

Avoid completely during the first 3 months. Limit use during the last 6 months as much as possible. If used, examine infant for possible deficiency of adrenal gland function.

Advisability of Use if Breast-Feeding

Presence of this drug in breast milk: Yes.

Avoid drug or refrain from nursing.

Habit-Forming Potential: Use to suppress symptoms over an extended period of time may produce a state of functional dependence (see Glossary). In treating asthma and rheumatoid arthritis, it is best to keep the dose as small as possible and to attempt drug withdrawal after periods of reasonable improvement. Such procedures may reduce the degree of "steroid rebound"— the return of symptoms as the drug is withdrawn.

Effects of Overdosage: Fatigue, muscle weakness, stomach irritation, acid indigestion, excessive sweating, facial flushing, fluid retention, swelling of extremities, increased blood pressure.

Possible Effects of Long-Term Use: Increased blood sugar (possible diabetes), increased fat deposits on the trunk of the body ("buffalo hump"), rounding of the face ("moon face"), thinning and fragility of skin, loss of texture and strength of bones (osteoporosis, aseptic necrosis), cataracts, glaucoma, retarded growth and development in children.

Suggested Periodic Examinations While Taking This Drug (at physician's discretion)

Measurements of blood pressure, blood sugar and potassium levels.

Complete eye examinations at regular intervals.

Chest X-ray if history of tuberculosis.

Determination of the rate of development of the growing child to detect retardation of normal growth.

▷ **While Taking This Drug, Observe the Following**

Foods: No interactions expected. Ask physician about salt restriction or need for potassium-rich foods. During long-term use of this drug, it is advisable to eat a high-protein diet.

Nutritional Support: During long-term use, take a vitamin D supplement. During wound repair, take a zinc supplement.

Beverages: No restrictions. Drink all forms of milk liberally.

▷ *Alcohol:* No interactions expected. Caution if you are prone to peptic ulcer disease.

Tobacco Smoking: Nicotine increases the blood levels of naturally produced cortisone and related hormones. Heavy smoking may add to the expected actions of this drug and requires close observation for excessive effects.

Marijuana Smoking: May cause additional impairment of immunity.

▷ *Other Drugs*

Dexamethasone may ***decrease*** the effects of
- isoniazid (INH, Niconyl, etc.).
- salicylates (aspirin, sodium salicylate, etc.).
- vaccines, by blunting the immune response to them.

Dexamethasone ***taken concurrently*** with
- carbamazepine (Tegretol) will reduce the effectiveness of dexamethasone.
- loop diuretics such as furosemide (Lasix) or bumetanide can result in additive potassium loss.
- oral anticoagulants may either increase or decrease their effectiveness; ask your doctor about prothrombin time testing and dosage adjustment.
- oral hypoglycemic agents (see Drug Classes) will decrease their effectiveness.

The following drugs may ***decrease*** the effects of dexamethasone
- antacids may reduce its absorption.
- barbiturates (Amytal, Butisol, phenobarbital, etc.).
- phenytoin (Dilantin, etc.).
- phenobarbital.
- primidone.
- rifabutin.
- rifampin (Rifadin, Rimactane, etc.).

▷ *Driving, Hazardous Activities:* Usually no restrictions. Be alert to the rare occurrence of dizziness.

Aviation Note: The use of this drug ***may be a disqualification*** for piloting. Consult a designated Aviation Medical Examiner.

Exposure to Sun: No restrictions.

Occurrence of Unrelated Illness: This drug may decrease natural resistance to infection. Call your doctor if you develop an infection of any kind. It may also reduce your body's ability to respond to the stress of acute illness, injury or surgery. Keep your physician fully informed of any significant health changes.

Discontinuation: Do not stop this drug abruptly after chronic use. Ask your doctor for help regarding gradual withdrawal. For a period of 2 years after discontinuing this drug, it is essential in the event of illness, injury or surgery that you inform attending medical personnel that you have used this drug in the past.

DEXFENFLURAMINE (dex FEN flur a MEEN)

Introduced: 1996   **Prescription:** USA: Yes; Canada: Yes   **Available as Generic:** USA: No   **Class:** Serotonin reuptake inhibitor, Weight loss agent **Controlled Drug:** USA: Yes,C-IV*

Brand Names: Redux

> **Warning:** A REVIEW OF EARLY DATA HAS FOUND THE RISK OF PRI-MARY PULMONARY HYPERTENSION TO BE SIGNIFICANTLY HIGHER THAN REPORTED EARLIER. The makers of dexfenfluramine caution that this product is not for use by those seeking cosmetic weight loss. Its use should be reserved for the seriously overweight—at least 30% over their desirable weight or 20% over their desirable weight when other risk factors are present.

BENEFITS versus RISKS	
Possible Benefits	*Possible Risks*
EFFECTIVE WEIGHT LOSS FOR UP TO ONE YEAR	RARE PULMONARY HYPERTENSION
	Drowsiness

▷ **Principal Uses**

As a Single Drug Product: Uses currently included in FDA approved labeling: (1) Used in the management of obesity, including weight loss and helping to maintain weight loss in people on a reduced calorie diet; (2) recommended for use in obese people with an initial body mass index (BMI, a calculation which takes the patient's weight in kg divided by their height in meters squared) greater than 30 kg per square meter or 27 kg per square meter in the presence of other risk factors (such as diabetes, hyperlipidemia or hypertension).

Other (unlabeled) generally accepted uses: None.

How This Drug Works: This medicine helps treat obesity by decreasing the desire to eat by increasing serotonin (a nerve transmitter) in brain synapses. It accomplishes this effect by both stimulating release of serotonin from synaptosomes and also inhibiting serotonin reuptake. Clinical trial data showed that dexfenfluramine resulted in decreased appetite and possible slowing of stomach (gastric) emptying. Patients also ate fewer carbohydrates and had decreased craving between meals for high carbohydrate snack foods.

Available Dosage Forms and Strengths

Capsules — 15 mg

▷ **Recommended Dosage Ranges (Actual dosage and administration schedule must be determined by the physician for each patient individually.)**

One capsule (15 mg) twice a day, with meals. Doses greater than 30 mg daily are not recommended.

Conditions Requiring Dosing Adjustments

Liver function: This drug is metabolized in the liver, however, no specific guidelines for dosing adjustments are available.

Kidney function: Fenfluramine and norfenfluramine (a liver metabolite) combined are up to 30% removed by the kidneys, however, no specific guidelines for dosing adjustments are available.

Obesity: No significant differences between final medicine levels (steady state drug concentrations) in non-obese or obese people.

▷ **Dosing Instructions:**   Capsule may be taken with or following food, twice daily.

Usual Duration of Use: Initial studies done in 1995 were three month placebo controlled, and were usually used in conjunction with a low-calorie diet or counseling. Longer term use should be discussed with your doctor. Safety and effectiveness for longer than one year have not been determined. Clinical trial data also showed that patients benefited from lower cholesterol and blood pressure while realizing weight loss as well. Patients who do not lose four pounds during the initial four weeks of therapy should be re-evaluated to make certain they are taking their medicine correctly. If dexfenfluramine has been taken correctly, and a four pound weight loss has not occurred during the initial four weeks of therapy, consideration should be given to stopping dexfenfluramine. Ongoing use requires periodic physician follow up.

▷ **This Drug Should Not Be Taken If**
- you have had an allergic reaction to any dosage form of it previously.
- you have pulmonary hypertension.
- you have glaucoma.
- you take or have taken a monoamine oxidase (MAO) inhibitor (see Drug Classes) within the last 14 days.

▷ **Inform Your Physician Before Taking This Drug If**
- you have cardiovascular disease or have had an unfavorable reaction to any serotonin reuptake inhibitor.
- you have a history of abnormal heart rhythms.
- you have a history of kidney or liver compromise.
- you have a history of psychiatric disorders or drug abuse.
- you have a history of porphyria.
- you have taken other weight loss medicines (anorexigens) in the last year.
- you develop unexplained difficulty in breathing, fainting, chest pain or swelling of the ankles. These may be early symptoms of pulmonary hypertension.

Possible Side Effects (natural, expected, and unavoidable drug actions)
None reported as yet.

▷ **Possible Adverse Effects** (unusual, unexpected, and infrequent reactions)
If any of the following develop, consult your physician promptly for guidance.
Mild Adverse Effects
Allergic Reaction: Skin rash.
Tiredness or drowsiness.
Headache, dizziness or reactive depression.
Sleep disturbances.
Diarrhea.
Lowering of the blood pressure (may be of therapeutic benefit).
Dry mouth.
Nausea, vomiting or constipation.
Increased urination (polyuria).
Serious Adverse Effects
Rare case reports of dysphoria or suicidal tendency.

Depression, serious enough to lead 5% of the patients in clinical trials to discontinue use.

Rare cases of primary pulmonary hypertension.

▷ **Possible Effects on Sexual Function:** Menstrual disorders (less than 2% in clinical trials). Infrequent impotence occurred in clinical trials.

Possible Effects on Laboratory Tests

Serum cholesterol: decreased.

Drug testing: may cause false-positive tests for amphetamines.

CAUTION

1. Best to carry a card noting that you are taking this drug, if your course of treatment is to exceed 1 week.
2. May increase insulin sensitivity in obese patients. If insulin is taken at the same time as this medicine, the dose may be able to be decreased.
3. This medicine may cause false-positive urine drug tests for amphetamines.
4. Other conditions (organic causes) leading to obesity (such as low activity of the thyroid gland—hypothyroidism) should be ruled out prior to starting this medicine.
5. Safety and efficacy of use of dexfenfluramine with other weight loss agents have NOT been established. Combination therapy is NOT recommended.

Precautions for Use

By Infants and Children: Safety and effectiveness have not been established in those less than 18 years old.

By Those over 60 Years of Age: The drug levels this medicine achieves and the places in the body where this medicine goes are no different for those over 60 than those under 60. Caution should be used (as with all medicines active in the central nervous system) in treating elderly patients with dexfenfluramine.

▷ **Advisability of Use During Pregnancy**

Pregnancy Category: C. See Pregnancy Code at the back of this book.

Animal studies: Decreased weight gain, reduced numbers of placental implantations and fewer live young (as well as delayed bone formation or ossification) was reported in rats. These rats were given 2.5–5 times the human dose of dexfenfluramine.

Human studies: Adequate studies of pregnant women are not available.

NOT recommended for pregnant women.

Advisability of Use if Breast-Feeding

Presence of this drug in breast milk: Yes in rats, unknown in humans.

Avoid drug or refrain from nursing.

Habit-Forming Potential: The possibility of physical dependence is low. Further study is needed to confirm an accurate probability of dependence risk. There was no evidence of addictive or drug seeking behavior in pre-marketing studies.

Effects of Overdosage: During post-marketing reports sent in over 10 years in Europe, 66 cases of overdoses show: Agitation, drowsiness, mydriasis, shivering, nausea and vomiting.

Possible Effects of Long-Term Use: Weight loss (the desired effect). Some reports of higher occurrence (although still rare) of pulmonary hypertension with long-term use have been made.

Suggested Periodic Examinations While Taking This Drug (at physician's discretion)
Periodic weights.

▷ **While Taking This Drug, Observe the Following**
Foods: No interactions expected.
Nutritional Support: Dietary counseling and physician or dietitian directed diets are suggested.
Beverages: No restrictions except as described in your dietary guidelines.
▷ *Alcohol:* Since dexfenfluramine may cause drowsiness and also has significant central nervous system (CNS) effects, caution is advised. Discuss this with your doctor before drinking alcohol.
Tobacco Smoking: No interactions are described in the current literature. There is no data showing that smoking is good for you. Please discuss ways to quit smoking with your doctor or pharmacist.
Marijuana Smoking: May cause additive drowsiness.
▷ *Other Drugs*
Dexfenfluramine *taken concurrently* with
- anti-migraine agents (such as sumatriptan or Imitrex) and dihydroergotamine may rarely result in a serotonin syndrome. This combination of agents is NOT advisable.
- central nervous system active medicines (see Drug Classes of benzodiazepines, opioids, phenothiazines and others) may have additive effects. Caution is advised.
- insulin (various brands) may increase the sensitivity of the body to insulin (in obese patients) and enable a decreased insulin dose to give a larger than expected effect. More frequent fingerstick glucose testing is recommended, with ongoing insulin doses adjusted to blood sugar levels.
- monoamine oxidase (MAO) inhibitors (see Drug Classes) may result in serious, even fatal reactions. Fourteen days should pass after stopping a MAO inhibitor and starting dexfenfluramine. Three weeks should pass after stopping dexfenfluramine and starting a MAO inhibitor.
- some oral hypoglycemic agents (see Drug Classes) may increase their effectiveness.
▷ *Driving, Hazardous Activities:* Use caution. In one large study which lasted a year, this medicine caused tiredness in more than a quarter of patients but drowsiness in only 5% of those who took this medicine.
Aviation Note: The use of this drug *may be a disqualification* for piloting. Consult a designated Aviation Medical Examiner.
Exposure to Sun: No restrictions at present.
Occurrence of Unrelated Illness: Since weight loss may modify the need for medicines used to control blood pressure, lipids, and dexfenfluramine itself may increase sensitivity to insulin; medicines used in these conditions may need to be adjusted.
Discontinuation: Ask your doctor for help if you are considering stopping this medicine.

DIAZEPAM (di AZ e pam)

Introduced: 1963   **Prescription:** USA: Yes; Canada: Yes   **Available as Generic:** Yes   **Class:** antianiexty drug, mild tranquilizer, benzodiazepines **Controlled Drug:** USA: C-IV*; Canada: No

Brand Names: ♣Apo-Diazepam, Diastat, ♣Diazemuls, Diazepam Intensol Oral Solution, ♣Meval, ♣Novodipam, ♣Rival, Valcaps, Valium, Valrelease, Vazepam, ♣Vivol, Zetran

---

BENEFITS versus RISKS

Possible Benefits	*Possible Risks*
RELIEF OF ANXIETY AND NERVOUS TENSION	Habit-forming potential with prolonged use
Wide margin of safety with therapeutic doses	Minor impairment of mental functions
	Respiratory depression
	Very rare jaundice
	Very rare blood cell disorders

▷ **Principal Uses**

As a Single Drug Product: Uses included in FDA approved labeling: (1) Provides short-term relief of mild to moderate anxiety; (2) relieves the symptoms of acute alcohol withdrawal: agitation, tremors, hallucinations, incipient delirium tremens; (3) eases skeletal muscle spasm; (4) provides short-term control of certain types of seizures (epilepsy, fever induced and status epilepticus); (5) short-term relief of insomnia; (6) adjunctive use in endoscopic procedures; (7) decreases anxiety prior to electrical defibrillation of the heart (cardioversion); (8) eases severe muscle spasms.

Other (unlabeled) generally accepted uses: (1) Helps prevent LSD flashbacks; (2) short-term treatment of sleep walking; (3) treatment of persistent hiccups; (4) adjunctive treatment of catatonia.

How This Drug Works: By enhancing the nerve transmitter gamma-aminobutyric acid (GABA), this drug helps block higher brain centers and causes calming.

Available Dosage Forms and Strengths

Capsules, prolonged-action (sustained release) — 15 mg

Concentrate — 5 mg per ml

Injection — 5 mg per ml

Oral solution — 5 mg per ml, 5 mg per 5-ml

Tablets — 2 mg, 5 mg, 10 mg

▷ **Usual Adult Dosage Range:** For anxiety: Given as 2 to 10 mg, 2 to 4 times daily. Dose may be increased cautiously as needed and tolerated. After 1 week of continual use, the total daily dose may be taken at bedtime. Total daily dose should not exceed 60 mg. The sustained release form can be given once daily if the total daily dose is decided to 15 mg given as 5 mg three times daily. **Note: Actual dosage and administration schedule must be determined by the physician for each patient individually.**

*See Schedules of Controlled Drugs at the back of this book.

Conditions Requiring Dosing Adjustments

Liver function: The dose **must** be decreased by 50% in patients with liver compromise.

Kidney function: Caution—if 15 mg or more is given daily, diazepam metabolites may accumulate.

Obesity: Obese patients may take longer than non-obese patients to accumulate this medicine. The time that it takes to remove diazepam (elimination half life) is prolonged in obese people. This means that obese people may take a much longer time to get the peak effect of diazepam and will also take a longer time to remove the drug from their body.

▷ **Dosing Instructions:**   The tablet may be crushed and taken on empty stomach or with food or milk. The prolonged-action capsule should not be opened. Do not stop this drug abruptly if taken for more than 4 weeks.

Usual Duration of Use: Use on a regular schedule for 3 to 5 days is usually needed to see this drug's effectiveness in relieving moderate anxiety. Limit continual use to 1 to 3 weeks. Avoid uninterrupted and prolonged use.

▷ **This Drug Should Not Be Taken If**
- you have had an allergic reaction to any dosage form of it previously.
- you have acute narrow-angle glaucoma.
- it is prescribed for a child under 6 months of age.

▷ **Inform Your Physician Before Taking This Drug If**
- you are allergic to any benzodiazepine (see Drug Classes).
- you have a history of alcoholism or drug abuse.
- you are pregnant or planning pregnancy.
- you have impaired liver or kidney function.
- you have a history of serious depression or mental disorder.
- you have: asthma, emphysema, epilepsy, or myasthenia gravis.

Possible Side Effects (natural, expected, and unavoidable drug actions)

Drowsiness, lethargy, unsteadiness (rare), "hangover" effects on the day following bedtime use.

▷ **Possible Adverse Effects** (unusual, unexpected, and infrequent reactions)

If any of the following develop, consult your physician promptly for guidance.

Mild Adverse Effects

Allergic Reactions: Rashes (rare), hives.

Dizziness, fainting, blurred or double vision, slurred speech, sweating, nausea.

Ringing in the ears.

Sedation, impaired motor skills.

Serious Adverse Effects

Allergic Reactions: Liver damage with jaundice (see Glossary), kidney damage, abnormally low blood platelet count, anaphylaxis.

Respiratory depression.

Bone marrow depression—low white blood cells, fever, sore throat.

Severe lowering of blood pressure, slow heart rate, and cardiac arrest has been reported after rapid intravenous dosing.

Amnesia.

Obsessive-compulsive disorder following extended use and abrupt with-drawal.

Paradoxical responses of excitement, agitation, anger, rage.

▷ **Possible Effects on Sexual Function**

Altered timing and pattern of menstruation.

Small doses (2 to 5 mg/day) may help the anxiety seen in many cases of impotence in men and inhibited sexual responsiveness in women.

Larger doses (10 mg/day or more) can decrease libido, impair potency in men and inhibit orgasm in women.

Swelling and tenderness of male breast tissue (gynecomastia). Abnormally prolonged erections (priapism).

▷ **Adverse Effects That May Mimic Natural Diseases or Disorders**

Liver reaction with jaundice may suggest viral hepatitis.

Possible Effects on Laboratory Tests

White blood cell counts: decreased.

Blood thyroxine (T_4) level: decreased.

Liver function tests: increased liver enzymes (ALT/GPT, AST/GOT and alkaline phosphatase), increased bilirubin (all rare).

Urine sugar tests: no drug effect with TesTape; low test results with Clinistix and Diastix.

Urine screening tests for drug abuse: may be **positive**. (Test results depend upon amount of drug taken and testing method used.)

CAUTION

1. This drug should not be stopped abruptly if it has been taken continually for more than 4 weeks.
2. Some nonprescription (over-the-counter or OTC) drug products that contain antihistamines (allergy and cold preparations, sleep aids) can cause excessive sedation if combined with diazepam.

Precautions for Use

By Infants and Children: This drug should not be used in hyperactive or psychotic children. Watch for excessive sedation and incoordination. Usual dose in children for muscle relaxation or sedation is 0.1 to 0.8 mg per kg per day divided into equal doses and given every 8 hours or as often as every 6 hours. The drug has been used intravenously to help seizures in neonates.

By Those over 60 Years of Age: Small doses are indicated. Observe for lethargy, indifference, fatigue, weakness, unsteadiness, disturbing dreams, nightmares and paradoxical reactions of excitement, agitation, anger, hostility and rage.

▷ **Advisability of Use During Pregnancy**

Pregnancy Category: D. See Pregnancy Code at the back of this book.

Animal studies: Cleft palate reported in mice; skeletal defects in rats.

Human studies: Available information is conflicting and inconclusive. Some findings of increased serious birth defects. Other studies have found no significant increase in birth defects.

Frequent use in late pregnancy can cause the "floppy infant" syndrome in the newborn: weakness, lethargy, unresponsiveness, depressed breathing, low body temperature.

Avoid use during entire pregnancy.

Advisability of Use if Breast-Feeding
Presence of this drug in breast milk: Yes.
Avoid drug or refrain from nursing.

Habit-Forming Potential: This drug can produce psychological and/or physical dependence (see Glossary), especially if used in large doses for an extended period of time.

Effects of Overdosage: Marked drowsiness, weakness, feeling of drunkenness, staggering gait, tremor, stupor progressing to deep sleep or coma.

Possible Effects of Long-Term Use: Psychological and/or physical dependence, rare blood cell disorders.

Suggested Periodic Examinations While Taking This Drug (at physician's discretion)
Complete blood cell counts during long-term use.

▷ **While Taking This Drug, Observe the Following**
Foods: No restrictions.
Beverages: Avoid excessive intake of caffeine-containing beverages: coffee, tea, cola. May be taken with milk.

▷ *Alcohol:* **Avoid this combination**. Alcohol increases the absorption of this drug and adds to its depressant effects on the brain. It is advisable to avoid alcohol completely—throughout the day and night—if it is necessary to drive or to engage in any hazardous activity.

Tobacco Smoking: Heavy smoking may reduce the calming action of this drug.
Marijuana Smoking: Increased sedation and impairment of intellectual and physical performance.

▷ *Other Drugs*
Diazepam may ***increase*** the effects of
• digoxin (Lanoxin), and cause digoxin toxicity.
• phenytoin (Dilantin), and cause phenytoin toxicity.
Diazepam may ***decrease*** the effects of
• levodopa (Sinemet, etc.), and reduce its effectiveness in treating Parkinson's disease.
Diazepam ***taken concurrently*** with
• fluvoxamine (Luvox) can result in serious accumulation of diazepam and toxicity.
• narcotics or other centrally active medicines may cause additive respiratory depression or decreased levels of consciousness.
The following drugs may ***increase*** the effects of diazepam
• cimetidine (Tagamet).
• disulfiram (Antabuse).
• isoniazid (INH, Rifamate, etc.).
• omeprazole (Prilosec).
• oral contraceptives.
• sertraline (Zoloft).
• valproic acid (Depakene).
The following drugs may ***decrease*** the effects of diazepam
• ranitidine (Zantac).
• rifampin (Rimactane, etc.).
• rifabutin.
• theophylline (aminophylline, Theo-Dur, etc.).

▷   *Driving, Hazardous Activities:* This drug can impair mental alertness, judgment, physical coordination and reaction time. Avoid hazardous activities accordingly.

Aviation Note: The use of this drug *is a disqualification* for piloting. Consult a designated Aviation Medical Examiner.

Exposure to Sun: No restrictions.

Exposure to Heat: Because of reduced urine volume, this drug may accumulate in the body and produce effects of overdosage.

Discontinuation: Avoid sudden discontinuation if this drug has been taken for over 4 weeks without interruption. Dosage should be tapered gradually to prevent a withdrawal syndrome that could include depression, confusion, hallucinations, tremor, seizures, muscle cramping, sweating and vomiting.

DICLOFENAC (di KLOH fen ak)

Introduced: 1976   **Prescription:** USA: Yes; Canada: Yes   **Available as Generic:** USA: No; Canada: No   **Class:** Mild analgesic, NSAID   **Controlled Drug:** USA: No; Canada: No

Brand Name: Apo-Diclo, Arthrotec, Cataflam, Novo-Difenac, Nu-Diclo, Voltaren, Voltaren Ophthalmic

Please see the acetic acid NSAIDs profile for further information.

DIDANOSINE (di DAN oh seen)

Other Names: Dideoxyinosine, DDI

Introduced: 1991   **Prescription:** USA: Yes; Canada: Yes   **Available as Generic:** USA: No; Canada: No   **Class:** Antiviral   **Controlled Drug:** USA: No; Canada: No

Brand Name: Videx

BENEFITS versus RISKS	
Possible Benefits	*Possible Risks*
DELAYED PROGRESSION OF DISEASE IN HIV-INFECTED INDIVIDUALS WITH AIDS OR AIDS-RELATED COMPLEX	DRUG-INDUCED PANCREATITIS DRUG-INDUCED PERIPHERAL NEURITIS Drug-induced seizures Rare liver damage

▷ **Principal Uses**

As a Single Drug Product: Uses currently included in FDA approved labeling: (1) Treatment of human immunodeficiency virus (HIV) infections in adults and children (6 months of age or older) with advanced disease who cannot tolerate zidovudine or who have shown significant deterioration during zidovudine therapy. This drug is not a cure for AIDS, and it does not reduce the risk of transmission of HIV infection to others through sexual contact or contamination of blood.

Other (unlabeled) generally accepted uses: (1) Used in combination with hydroxyurea (Hydrea) to treat AIDS.

How This Drug Works: By interfering with essential HIV enzyme systems, this drug prevents growth and reproduction of HIV particles in infected cells, limiting the severity and extent of HIV infection.

Available Dosage Forms and Strengths
> Powder for oral solution — 2 grams or 4 grams per bottle
> Powder for oral solution — packets of 100 mg, 167 mg, 250 mg, 375 mg
> Tablets, chewable/dispersible — 25 mg, 50 mg, 100 mg, 150 mg

Author's note: The company is actively investigating other formulations for this medicine.

▷ **Recommended Dosage Ranges** (Actual dosage and administration schedule must be determined by the physician for each patient individually.)

Infants and Children: For those 6 months of age or older, dosage is based on dosage form and body surface area:

Pediatric oral solution (reconstituted and admixed with buffers)—125 mg (12.5 ml)/12 hours for body surface area of 1.1–1.4 m^2, 94 mg (9.5 ml)/12 hours for body surface area of 0.8–1 m^2, 62 mg (6 ml)/12 hours for body surface area of 0.5–0.7 m^2, 31 mg (3 ml)/12 hours for body surface area of 0.4 m^2 or less.

Chewable/dispersible tablets—100 mg/12 hours for body surface area of 1.1–1.4 m^2, 75 mg/12 hours for body surface area of 0.8–1 m^2, 50 mg/12 hours for body surface area of 0.5–0.7 m^2, 25 mg/12 hours for body surface area of 0.4 m^2 or less. In children 1 year of age or older, each dose should be 2 tablets to ensure that adequate buffering is provided to prevent destruction (degradation) of the drug in stomach acid. In children younger than 1 year of age, 1 tablet will provide adequate buffering.

12 to 60 Years of Age: Dosing as follows:

Adult oral solution (buffered)—250 mg every 12 hours for those weighing more than 60 kg, 167 every 12 hours for those weighing less than 60 kg.

Chewable/dispersible tablets—200 mg every 12 hours for body weight of 60 kg or more, 125 mg every 12 hours for body weight of less than 60 kg.

Over 60 Years of Age: Same as 12 to 60 group. Dose reduced in impaired liver or kidney function.

Conditions Requiring Dosing Adjustments

Liver function: Up to 60% of a given dose is changed by the liver to other compounds. There is an increased risk of liver toxicity if used in people with compromised livers. Dose must be decreased if used in liver failure.

Kidney function: Dose **must** be decreased in mild to moderate kidney failure. There is also an increased risk of magnesium toxicity and drug-induced pancreatitis in patients with kidney problems.

▷ **Dosing Instructions:**   Best taken on an empty stomach, 2 hours before or 2 hours after eating.

The pediatric oral solution is first reconstituted with water and then combined with equal quantities of antacid (such as Mylanta or Maalox). This mixture must be shaken thoroughly before measuring each dose.

The adult oral solution is made by stirring 1 packet into 120 ml (4 ounces) of water until the powder is dissolved; this may take up to 3 minutes. The powder should not be mixed with fruit juice or other acidic liquid. The entire 4 ounce solution should be swallowed immediately.

The chewable/dispersible buffered tablets should be thoroughly chewed, crushed or dispersed in water before swallowing. To disperse the tablet(s), stir the prescribed number in at least 30 ml (1 ounce) of water until a uniform suspension is obtained. Swallow the entire preparation immediately.

Author's note: Current HIV therapy involves combination use of agents from different drug classes to attack the AIDS virus from different points and delay resistance. Many clinicians are using viral load or burden (see Glossary) as an indicator for success of treatment or to show a need for changes in therapy.

Usual Duration of Use:

Use on a regular schedule for several months is usually needed to see this drug's effectiveness in slowing AIDS progression. Long-term use (months to years) requires periodic physician evaluation.

Possible Advantages of This Drug

Does not cause serious bone marrow depression (production of blood cells). Less frequent liver toxicity.

▷ **This Drug Should Not Be Taken If**

- you have had an allergic reaction to it previously.
- you have active liver disease.
- you have had pancreatitis recently.

▷ **Inform Your Physician Before Taking This Drug If**

- you have had allergic reactions to any drugs in the past.
- you are taking any other drugs currently.
- you have a history of pancreatitis or peripheral neuritis.
- you have a history of gout or high blood uric acid level.
- you have a history of alcoholism.
- you have a history of diarrhea
- you have a history of phenylketonuria.
- you have a history of low blood platelets or blood disorder.
- you have a history of low blood potassium.
- you have a history of heart failure.
- you have a seizure disorder.
- you have impaired liver or kidney function.

Possible Side Effects (natural, expected, and unavoidable drug actions)

Mild decreases in red blood cell, white blood cell, and platelet counts in adults. Mild increases in blood uric acid levels.

▷ **Possible Adverse Effects** (unusual, unexpected, and infrequent reactions)

If any of the following develop, consult your physician promptly for guidance.

Mild Adverse Effects

Allergic Reactions: Skin rash and itching (occasional in adults and common in pediatric patients).

Headache, dizziness, insomnia, nervousness, confusion, rare visual disturbances.

Nausea, vomiting, stomach pain and diarrhea (¼ of adults and frequent in pediatric patients), dry mouth and altered taste, yeast infection of mouth (rare).

Lowered blood pressure.

Rare loss of color in the retina (retinal depigmentation).

Asthma, cough.

Loss of hair, muscle and joint pains.

Serious Adverse Effects

Drug-induced pancreatitis, usually seen in the first 6 months.

Drug-induced peripheral neuritis (see Glossary), usually occurring after 2 to 6 months of treatment. This effect also appears to be dose-related.

Electrolyte imbalance (low potassium magnesium or calcium).

High blood sugar.

Excessive lowering of blood pressure and passing out (syncope).

Serious skin rash (Stevens-Johnson syndrome).

Seizures (may be due to electrolyte problems).

Lowered white blood cell counts, lowered granulocyte (a specific white blood cell) counts, and lowered blood platelets (69%) in pediatric patients.

Optic neuritis and blindness (rare).

Rare liver damage.

Rare kidney damage.

▷ **Possible Effects On Sexual Function:** None reported.

▷ **Adverse Effects That May Mimic Natural Diseases or Disorders**

Drug-induced liver reaction (rare at less than 0.2%) may suggest viral hepatitis.

Possible Effects on Laboratory Tests

Complete blood cell counts: decreased red cells and white cells (3–5%); decreased platelets (1%).

Blood amylase level: increased (7–18%).

Blood uric acid level: increased (6%).

Blood electrolytes: low calcium, potassium and magnesium.

Liver function tests: increased liver enzymes (ALT/GPT, AST/GOT and alkaline phosphatase), increased bilirubin (1–9% of adults and higher in pediatric patients).

CAUTION

1. This drug **does not cure HIV infection** or reduce the risk of transmitting infection to others.
2. Report development of stomach pain with nausea and vomiting; this could indicate pancreatitis.
3. Report the development of pain, numbness, tingling or burning in the hands or feet; this could be peripheral neuritis. It may be necessary to stop this drug.

Precautions for Use

By Infants and Children: Safety and effectiveness for those under 6 months of age not established. Children are also at risk for developing pancreatitis and peripheral neuritis. It is recommended that detailed eye examinations be performed every 6 months and at any time that visual disturbance occurs.

By Those over 60 Years of Age: Reduced kidney function may require dosage reduction.

▷ **Advisability of Use During Pregnancy**

    Pregnancy Category: B. See Pregnancy Code at the back of this book.

    Animal studies: Rat and rabbit studies show no birth defects.

    Human studies: Adequate studies of pregnant women not available.

    Consult your physician for specific guidance.

Advisability of Use if Breast-Feeding

    Presence of this drug in breast milk: Unknown.

    Avoid drug or refrain from nursing.

    Note: HIV has been found in human breast milk. Breast-feeding may result in transmission of HIV infection to the nursing infant.

Habit-Forming Potential: None.

Effects of Overdosage: Nausea, vomiting, stomach pain, diarrhea, pain in hands and feet, irritability, confusion.

Possible Effects of Long-Term Use: Peripheral neuritis (see Glossary).

Suggested Periodic Examinations While Taking This Drug (at physician's discretion)

    Complete blood cell counts before starting treatment and weekly thereafter until tolerance is established.

    Electrolytes.

    Blood amylase levels, fractionated for salivary gland and pancreatic origin.

    Liver and kidney function tests.

    Viral load or viral burden in order to assess success of treatment.

    CD4 counts.

▷ **While Taking This Drug, Observe the Following**

    Foods: High fat foods can decrease didanosine absorption and lower therapeutic benefit.

    Beverages: No restrictions.

▷   *Alcohol:* No interactions expected.

    Tobacco Smoking: No interactions expected.

▷   *Other Drugs*

    Didanosine may ***increase*** the effects of

    • zidovudine (Retrovir), and enhance its antiviral effect against HIV.

    Didanosine may ***decrease*** the effects of

    • dapsone, and render it ineffective; avoid concurrent use.

    • ketoconazole, if taken at the same time; take ketoconazole at least 2 hours before taking didanosine.

    • ciprofloxacin (Cipro), if taken at the same time; take ciprofloxacin at least 2 hours before taking didanosine.

    • itraconazole. Separate dosing by at least two hours.

    • tetracyclines (see Drug Classes), if taken at the same time; take tetracyclines at least 2 hours before taking didanosine.

    Didanosine ***taken concurrently*** with

    • antacids will decrease didanosine absorption and lower its therapeutic benefit.

    • histamine (H-2) blocking drugs (see Drug Classes)—cimetidine, etc.,—may increase didanosine toxicity.

    • pentamidine or sulfamethoxazole may increase the risk of drug-induced pancreatitis; watch for significant symptoms.

- triazolam (Halcion), may cause confusion.
- zalcitabine (Hivid), will cause increased neurotoxicity.

▷ *Driving, Hazardous Activities:* This drug may cause dizziness and impaired vision. Restrict activities as necessary.

Aviation Note: The use of this drug *is a disqualification* for piloting. Consult a designated Aviation Medical Examiner.

Exposure to Sun: No restrictions.

Discontinuation: Do not stop this drug without your physician's knowledge and guidance.

DIFLUNISAL (di FLU ni sal)

Introduced: 1977   **Prescription:** USA: Yes; Canada: Yes   **Available as Generic:** No   **Class:** Mild analgesic   **Controlled Drug:** USA: No; Canada: No

Brand Name: Dolobid

Please see the new combined nonsteroidal (similar in composition to propionic acids) anti-inflammatory profile.

DIGITOXIN (di ji TOX in)

Introduced: 1942   **Prescription:** USA: Yes; Canada: Yes   **Available as Generic:** Yes   **Class:** Digitalis preparations   **Controlled Drug:** USA: No; Canada: No

Brand Names: Crystodigin, ✦Digitaline

Please see the digoxin profile for further information.

DIGOXIN (di JOX in)

Introduced: 1934   **Prescription:** USA: Yes; Canada: No   **Available as Generic:** Yes   **Class:** Digitalis preparations   **Controlled Drug:** USA: No; Canada: No

Brand Names: Lanoxicaps, Lanoxin, ✦Novodigoxin, Sk-Digoxin

BENEFITS versus RISKS	
Possible Benefits	*Possible Risks*
EFFECTIVE HEART STIMULANT IN CONGESTIVE HEART FAILURE EFFECTIVE PREVENTION AND TREATMENT OF CERTAIN HEART RHYTHM DISORDERS	NARROW TREATMENT RANGE Frequent and sometimes serious disturbances of heart rhythm

▷ **Principal Uses**

As a Single Drug Product: Uses in current FDA approved labeling: (1) Treatment of congestive heart failure; (2) restoration and maintenance of normal heart rate and rhythm in cases of atrial fibrillation, atrial flutter, PAT and atrial/supraventricular tachycardia.

Other (unlabeled) generally accepted uses: (1) post-operative arrhythmias; (2) helps to increase left ventricular function in patients with pacemakers; (3) may have a role in Wolff-Parkinson-White Syndrome.

How This Drug Works: Increases force of heart muscle contraction by increasing calcium. Slows the pacemaker and delays electrical transmission through the heart and helps restore normal rate and rhythm.

Available Dosage Forms and Strengths

　Elixir, pediatric — 0.05 mg per ml
　　　Capsules — 0.05 mg, 0.1 mg, 0.2 mg
　　　Injection — 0.1 mg per ml and 0.25 mg per ml
　　　Tablets — 0.0625 mg (Canada), 0.125 mg, 0.25 mg, 0.5 mg

Author's note: dosing and timing of doses is critical for this medication because the difference between toxic blood levels and therapeutic blood levels is small. Be CERTAIN you understand how and when to take this medicine.

▷ **Usual Adult Dosage Range:**   Loading dose: 10 micrograms per kilogram of lean body weight. 10–15 micrograms per kg may be needed if digoxin is being used to control abnormal heart rhythms (such as atrial fibrillation). This loading dose can be given orally or intravenously, and once calculated is often given as 50% in the first dose with the remainder divided into smaller doses and given at 6 to 8 hour intervals until the desired response is achieved. The usual maintenance dose (the ongoing dose used after loading is achieved) is 0.125 to 0.5 milligrams per day. In neonatal and pediatric patient, a similar loading and maintenance dose strategy is used, but the amount on a mg per kg basis is much different than that for adults. **Note: Actual dosage and administration schedule must be determined by the physician for each patient individually.**

Conditions Requiring Dosing Adjustments

　Liver function: Used with caution and blood levels should be obtained more frequently.

　Kidney function: Dose **must** be adjusted in kidney compromise. Smaller doses and some cases of dosing every other day may be needed.

▷ **Dosing Instructions:**   Tablet may be crushed, and best taken at the same time each day on an empty stomach. Can be taken with or following food if desired; milk and dairy products may delay absorption but do not reduce the amount of drug absorbed. The capsule should be swallowed whole.

Usual Duration of Use: Use on a regular schedule for 7 to 10 days is needed to see this drug's effectiveness in relieving heart failure or controlling heart rhythm disorders. Long-term use requires physician supervision and periodic assessment of continued need.

▷ **This Drug Should Not Be Taken If**
　• you have had an allergic reaction to any dosage form of it previously.
　• you are in ventricular fibrillation (a life-threatening heart rhythm).

▷ **Inform Your Physician Before Taking This Drug If**
　• you have had an unfavorable reaction to a digitalis preparation.
　• you have taken any digitalis preparation within the past 2 weeks.
　• you now take (or have recently taken) any diuretic (urine-producing) drug.

- you have a history of severe lung disease.
- you have abnormal heart rhythms or certain problems with the aorta.
- you have sustained damage to the heart muscle (myocardium).
- you have a history of low blood potassium or magnesium.
- you have impaired liver or kidney function.
- you have a history of thyroid function disorder.

Possible Side Effects (natural, expected, and unavoidable drug actions)
Slow heart rate, rare enlargement or sensitivity of the male breast.

▷ **Possible Adverse Effects** (unusual, unexpected, and infrequent reactions)
If any of the following develop, consult your physician promptly for guidance.
Mild Adverse Effects
Allergic Reactions: Skin rash, hives.
Headache, drowsiness, lethargy, confusion, changes in vision: "halo" effect, blurring, spots, double vision, yellow-green vision.
Changes in vaginal tissue (vaginal cornification).
Nightmares.
Loss of appetite, nausea, vomiting, diarrhea—early signs of adult toxicity.
Serious Adverse Effects
Idiosyncratic Reactions: Hallucinations, facial neuralgias, peripheral neuralgias, blindness (very rare).
Low blood platelets (rare and probably an immune reaction).
Rare psychosis and hallucinations (associated with toxic levels).
Rare serious skin rash (Stevens-Johnson syndrome).
Disorientation, most common in the elderly.
Heart rhythm disturbances.

▷ **Possible Effects on Sexual Function**
Decreased libido and impotence in 35% of male users.
Enlargement and tenderness of male breasts (gynecomastia).
Both effects are attributed to digoxin's estrogenlike action.

▷ **Adverse Effects That May Mimic Natural Diseases or Disorders**
Drug-induced mental changes may be mistaken for senile dementia or psychosis.

Possible Effects on Laboratory Tests
White blood cell counts: decreased.
Blood testosterone level: decreased 30% in men with long-term use.

CAUTION
1. Adhere strictly to prescribed dosage schedules. Do not raise or lower the dose without first consulting your doctor.
2. If you take calcium supplements, ask your physician for help. Avoid large doses.
3. Best to carry a card that says you are taking this drug.
4. Avoid taking over-the-counter antacids and cold, cough and allergy remedies without consulting your physician.

Precautions for Use
By Infants and Children: Observe carefully for indications of toxicity: slow heart rate (below 60 beats/minute), irregular heart rhythms.

By Those over 60 Years of Age: You may have reduced drug tolerance; smaller doses are advisable. Watch for early toxicity: headache, dizziness, fatigue, weakness, lethargy, depression, confusion, nervousness, agitation, delusions, difficulty with reading. Promptly call your doctor if these happen.

▷ **Advisability of Use During Pregnancy**

Pregnancy Category: C. See Pregnancy Code at the back of this book.

Animal studies: No birth defects reported.

Human studies: Adequate studies of pregnant women not available. However, no birth defects from the therapeutic use of this drug have been reported.

Use this drug only if clearly needed. Overdosage can be harmful to the fetus.

Advisability of Use if Breast-Feeding

Presence of this drug in breast milk: Yes.

Monitor nursing infant closely and discontinue drug or nursing if adverse effects develop.

Habit-Forming Potential: None.

Effects of Overdosage: Loss of appetite, excessive saliva, nausea, vomiting, diarrhea, serious disturbances of heart rate and rhythm, intestinal bleeding, drowsiness, headache, confusion, delirium, hallucinations, convulsions.

Possible Effects of Long-Term Use: None reported.

Suggested Periodic Examinations While Taking This Drug (at physician's discretion)

Measurements of blood levels of digoxin, calcium, magnesium and potassium; electrocardiograms.

Time to sample blood for digoxin level: 6–8 hours after last dose, or just before next dose.

Recommended therapeutic range: 0.5–2.0 ng/ml.

▷ **While Taking This Drug, Observe the Following**

Foods: Talk to your doctor about the advisability of eating high-potassium foods. The peak concentration and absorption rate will be decreased if digoxin is taken with food.

Beverages: Avoid excessive amounts of caffeine-containing beverages: coffee, tea, cola. May be taken with milk.

▷ *Alcohol:* No interactions expected.

Tobacco Smoking: Nicotine can cause heart muscle irritability and predispose to serious rhythm disturbances. Best to abstain from all forms of tobacco.

Marijuana Smoking: Possible accentuation of heart failure; reduced digoxin effect; possible changes in electrocardiogram, confusing interpretation.

▷ *Other Drugs*

Digoxin *taken concurrently* with

• calcium (intravenously) may cause a fatal interaction.

• digoxin immune FAB (Digibind) will result in decreased blood levels. This is used to therapeutic advantage in digoxin toxicity.

• diuretics (other than spironolactone and triamterene) can cause serious heart rhythm disturbances due to excessive loss of potassium.

• propranolol or other beta blocking medicines (see Drug Classes) may cause very slow heart rate.

- quinidine may result in decreased digoxin effectiveness and increased digoxin toxicity; careful dosage adjustments are necessary.
- succinylcholine.

The following drugs may ***increase*** the effects of digoxin
- alprazolam (Xanax).
- amiloride (Midamor).
- amiodarone (Codarone).
- amphotericin B (Abelcet, Fungizone).
- benzodiazepines (Librium, Valium, etc.; see Drug Class Section).
- captopril (Capoten, Capazide).
- cyclosporine (Sandimune).
- diltiazem (Cardizem) and other calcium channel blockers (see Drug Classes).
- disopyramide (Norpace).
- erythromycin (EES, Erythrocin, etc.). May also occur with clarithromycin and azithromycin.
- ethacrynic acid.
- flecainide (Tambocor).
- hydroxychloroquine.
- ibuprofen (Advil, Medipren, Motrin, Nuprin, etc.).
- indomethacin (Indocin).
- itraconazole.
- methimazole (Tapazole).
- nifedipine (Adalat, Procardia).
- phenytoin (Dilantin).
- propafanone (Rhythmol).
- propylthiouracil (Propacil).
- quinine.
- tetracyclines (see Drug Classes).
- tolbutamide (Orinase).
- trazodone (Desyrel).
- verapamil (Calan, Verelan, others).

The following drugs may ***decrease*** the effects of digoxin
- aluminum-containing antacids (Amphojel, Maalox, etc.).
- bleomycin (Blenoxane).
- carmustine (Bicnu).
- cholestyramine (Questran).
- colestipol (Colestid).
- cyclophosphamide (Cytoxan).
- cytarabine (Cytosar).
- doxorubicin (Adriamycin).
- fluvoxamine (Luvox).
- kaolin/pectin (Donagel, others).
- methotrexate (Mexate).
- metoclopramide (Reglan).
- neomycin.
- penicillamine (Cuprimine, Depen).
- procarbazine (Matulane).
- rifampin or rifabutin.

- sucralfate (Carafate).
- sulfa antibiotics or sulfasalazine.
- thyroid hormones.
- vincristine (Oncovin).

▷ *Driving, Hazardous Activities:* Usually no restrictions. However, this drug may cause drowsiness, vision changes and nausea. Restrict activities as necessary.

Aviation Note: Heart function disorders ***are a disqualification*** for piloting. Consult a designated Aviation Medical Examiner.

Exposure to Sun: No restrictions.

Occurrence of Unrelated Illness: Vomiting or diarrhea can seriously alter this drug's effectiveness. Notify your physician promptly.

Discontinuation: This drug may be continued indefinitely. Do not stop it without consulting your physician.

DILTIAZEM (dil TI a zem)

Introduced: 1977   **Prescription:** USA: Yes; Canada: Yes   **Available as Generic:** Yes   **Class:** Antianginal, antihypertensive, calcium channel blocker
Controlled Drug: USA: No; Canada: No
Brand Names: ✦Apo-Diltiaz, Cardizem, Cardizem CD, Cardizem SR, Dilacor XR, Diltiazem, ✦Novo-Diltiazem, ✦Nu-Diltiaz, ✦Syn-Diltiazem, Tiazac

Controversies In Medicine: Study data indicates that medicines in this class should NOT be used in some patients with extremely compromised hearts. There have also been several FDA hearings held on the calcium channel blocker class. Be certain to ask your doctor about your cardiac output and if the benefits of this medicine outweigh the risks of its use. A recent FDA panel found medicines in this class to be safe and effective. A retrospective chart review yielded data that showed increased risks for nifedipine immediate release forms in those over 71, and cautioned physicians against using the immediate release form for indications other than angina. The immediate release form in question had never been approved for other uses. Most recently, a study of nearly 6,000 patients at Tel Aviv Medical Center found that there was no statistically significant increased risk of death in the patients who took calcium channel blockers versus those who did not.

BENEFITS versus RISKS	
Possible Benefits	*Possible Risks*
EFFECTIVE PREVENTION OF BOTH MAJOR TYPES OF ANGINA	Depression, confusion
	Low blood pressure
EFFECTIVE CONTROL OF MILD TO MODERATE HYPERTENSION	Heart rhythm disturbance
	Fluid retention
	Liver damage (very rare)
	Rare muscle damage

▷ **Principal Uses**

As a Single Drug Product: Uses currently included in FDA approved labeling: Treats (1) angina pectoris due to coronary artery spasm (Prinzmetal's variant angina) that occurs spontaneously or is associated with exertion; (2)

classical angina-of-effort (due to atherosclerotic disease); (3) mild to moderate hypertension.

Other (unlabeled) generally accepted uses: (1) unstable angina; (2) congestive heart failure; (3) migraine prophylaxis; (4) prevention of abnormal protein excretion in the urine; (5) treatment of abnormal heart rhythms; (6) treatment of build up of abnormal plaques on the inside of blood vessels (atherosclerosis); (7) may help prevent abnormal growth of the left side of the heart (left ventricular hypertrophy) in patients who have suffered a heart attack; (8) can be of benefit in patients with esophageal disorders; (9) may have a role in helping ease the symptoms of an overactive thyroid gland (hyperthyroidism); (10) can ease symptoms of Raynaud's phenomena; (11) can have a role in preserving function in kidney and heart transplant patients; (12) may protect against heart attacks or variant or unstable angina which can occur after (post-operatively) coronary artery bypass grafting.

How This Drug Works: By blocking normal calcium movement through certain cell walls (needed for nerve and muscle tissue), this drug slows electrical activity in the conduction system of the heart and inhibits the contraction of coronary arteries and peripheral arterioles. As a result of these combined effects, this drug

- prevents spontaneous coronary artery spasm (Prinzmetal's angina).
- reduces the rate and contraction force of the heart during exertion, lowers the oxygen needs of heart muscle, and reduces the occurrence of effort-induced angina (classical angina pectoris).
- reduces contraction of peripheral arterial walls, resulting in relaxation and consequent lowering of blood pressure. This further reduces heart work load during exertion and helps prevent angina.

Available Dosage Forms and Strengths

Tablets (immediate release) — 30 mg, 60 mg, 90 mg, 120 mg

Capsules (extended release) — 120 mg, 180 mg, 240 mg, 300 mg

Capsules (sustained release) — 60 mg, 90 mg, 120 mg

▷ **Usual Adult Dosage Range:** Initially 30 mg, 3 or 4 times daily. Dose may be increased gradually at 1 to 2 day intervals as needed and tolerated. Total daily dosage should not exceed 360 mg. **Note: Actual dosage and administration schedule must be determined by the physician for each patient individually.**

Conditions Requiring Dosing Adjustments

Liver function: Maximum daily dose in patients with liver compromise should be 90 mg. Rarely causes hepatoxicity, and a benefit to risk decision must be made.

Kidney function: May be one of the best to use in kidney compromise since it has such a large percentage of liver metabolism and fecal excretion. Caution must still be used however, as the drug can be a rare cause of kidney compromise.

▷ **Dosing Instructions:** Tablet may be crushed and is best taken before meals and at bedtime.

Usual Duration of Use: Use on a regular schedule for 2 to 4 weeks is required to see this drug's effectiveness in decreasing frequency and severity of angina and in lowering elevated blood pressure. The smallest effective dose should be used in long-term therapy (months to years).

Possible Advantages of This Drug
Often effective as single drug therapy.
Does not reduce blood supply to kidneys.
Does not raise blood cholesterol levels.
Does not induce asthma in susceptible individuals.

▷ **This Drug Should Not Be Taken If**
- you have had an allergic reaction to it previously.
- you have "sick sinus" syndrome (and do not have an artificial pacemaker).
- you have second-degree or third-degree heart block.
- you have low blood pressure—systolic pressure below 90.
- you have heart failure (talk with our doctor).
- you have advanced stenosis of the aorta.

▷ **Inform Your Physician Before Taking This Drug If**
- you had an unfavorable response to any calcium blocker drug.
- you currently take any form of digitalis or a beta blocker (see Drug Classes).
- you have a history of congestive heart failure.
- you have atrial fibrillation (talk with your doctor).
- you have impaired liver or kidney function.
- you have a history of drug-induced liver damage.

Possible Side Effects (natural, expected, and unavoidable drug actions)
Fatigue (rare), light-headedness, heart rate and rhythm changes in some people (rare).

▷ **Possible Adverse Effects** (unusual, unexpected, and infrequent reactions)
If any of the following develop, consult your physician promptly for guidance.

Mild Adverse Effects

Allergic Reactions: Skin rash (rare), hives, itching.

Headache (may be self-limiting), drowsiness, dizziness (occasional and dose-related), nervousness, sleep problems, depression, confusion, hallucinations.

Very rare desire to be in constant motion (acathisia).

Overgrowth of the gums (gingival hyperplasia).

Increased urination (rare).

Flushing, palpitations, fainting, slow heart rate, low blood pressure.

Nausea (rare), indigestion, heartburn, vomiting, diarrhea, constipation.

Serious Adverse Effects

Serious disturbances of heart rate and/or rhythm, fluid retention (edema), congestive heart failure.

Drug-induced myopathy or liver damage (very rare).

Very rare lowering of a specific kind of white blood cell (granulocytes).

Very rare lowering of blood platelets.

▷ **Possible Effects on Sexual Function:**   Impotence is reported in less than 1% of users. Rare cases of swelling or tenderness of the male breast tissue (gynecomastia). One reported case of heavy vaginal bleeding.

Possible Effects on Laboratory Tests
Blood total cholesterol and triglyceride levels: no effects.
Blood HDL cholesterol level: increased.
Blood LDL and VLDL cholesterol levels: no effects.

CAUTION
1. Tell all physicians and dentists or other people who provide health care that you take this drug. Note the use of this drug on your card of personal identification.
2. You may use nitroglycerin and other nitrate drugs as needed to relieve acute angina pain. However, if your angina attacks become more frequent or intense, call your doctor promptly.

Precautions for Use
By Infants and Children: Safety and effectiveness for those under 12 years of age not established.
By Those over 60 Years of Age: May be more likely to have weakness, dizziness, fainting and falling. Take necessary precautions to prevent injury. Report promptly any changes in your pattern of thirst and urination.

▷ **Advisability of Use During Pregnancy**
Pregnancy Category: C. See Pregnancy Code at the back of this book.
Animal studies: Embryo and fetal deaths and skeletal birth defects reported in mice, rats and rabbits.
Human studies: Adequate studies of pregnant women not available.
Avoid this drug during the first 3 months.
Use during the last 6 months only if clearly needed. Ask physician for help.

Advisability of Use if Breast-Feeding
Presence of this drug in breast milk: Yes.
Avoid drug or refrain from nursing.

Habit-Forming Potential: None.

Effects of Overdosage: Weakness, light-headedness, fainting, slow pulse, low blood pressure, shortness of breath, congestive heart failure.

Possible Effects of Long-Term Use: None reported.

Suggested Periodic Examinations While Taking This Drug (at physician's discretion)
Evaluations of heart function, including electrocardiograms; liver and kidney function tests, with long-term use.

▷ **While Taking This Drug, Observe the Following**
Foods: May increase absorption and cause a 30% increase in blood levels. Avoid excessive salt intake.
Beverages: No restrictions. May be taken with milk.
▷ *Alcohol:* Use with caution. Alcohol may exaggerate the drop in blood pressure.
Tobacco Smoking: Nicotine may reduce the effectiveness of this drug. Follow your physician's advice regarding smoking.
Marijuana Smoking: Possible reduced effectiveness of this drug; mild to moderate increase in angina; possible changes in electrocardiogram, confusing interpretation.
▷ *Other Drugs*
Diltiazem *taken concurrently* with
• aspirin can result in prolonged bleeding time or hemorrhage.
• beta blocker drugs or digitalis preparations (see Drug Classes Section) may affect heart rate and rhythm. Careful physician monitoring is necessary if these drugs are combined.
• carbamazepine (Tegretol) may result in toxicity and seizures.

- cyclosporine (Sandimmune) may result in cyclosporine toxicity and kidney failure.
- digoxin can result in digoxin toxicity.
- lithium can result in psychosis and neurotoxicity.
- oral hypoglycemic agents (see Drug Classes) such as glipizide (Glucotrol) may result in greater than expected lowering of blood sugar and hypoglycemia.
- phenytoin decreases phenytoin metabolism and causes phenytoin toxicity.
- rifampin may result in decreased diltiazem effectiveness.
- rifabutin may decrease diltiazem blood levels.
- tacrolimus (Prograf) may result in tacrolimus accumulation and tacrolimus toxicity.

The following drugs may *increase* the effects of diltiazem
- cimetidine (Tagamet).
- fluvoxamine (Luvox).
- ranitidine (Zantac).

▷ *Driving, Hazardous Activities:* Usually no restrictions. This drug may cause drowsiness or dizziness. Limit activities as necessary.

Aviation Note: Coronary artery disease *is a disqualification* for piloting. Consult a designated Aviation Medical Examiner.

Exposure to Sun: This drug may cause photosensitivity (see Glossary).

Exposure to Heat: Caution advised. Hot environments can exaggerate the blood-pressure-lowering effects of this drug. Observe for light-headedness or weakness.

Heavy Exercise or Exertion: This drug may improve ability to be more active without angina pain. Use caution and avoid excessive exercise that could impair heart function in the absence of warning pain.

Discontinuation: Do not stop this drug abruptly. Ask your doctor about gradual withdrawal.

DIPHENHYDRAMINE (di fen HI dra meen)

Introduced: 1946   **Prescription:** USA: Varies; Canada: No   **Available as Generic:** Yes   **Class:** Hypnotic, antihistamines   **Controlled Drug:** USA: No*; Canada: No

Brand Names: Acetaminophen-PM, Allerdryl, Allergy capsules, Allergy formula, Allermax, ✦Ambenyl Expectorant [CD], Ambenyl Syrup [CD], Anacin P.M. Aspirin free, Banophen, Bayer Select, Beldin Syrup, Bena-D, Benahist, Benadryl, Benadryl 25, Benylin, ✦Benylin Decongestant [CD], ✦Benylin Pediatric Syrup, ✦Benylin Syrup w/Codeine [CD], ✦Caladryl [CD], Caldyphen lotion, Children's Complete Allergy, Complete Allergy Medication, Compoz, Dermarest, Di-Delamine, Dihydrex, Diphendryl, Diphenhist, Dormarex 2, ✦Ergodryl [CD], Excedrin P.M. [CD], Extra Strength Tylenol PM, Gecil, Genahist, Gen-D-Phen, Hydramine, ✦Insomnal, Kolex, ✦Mandrax [CD], Medi-Phedryl, Midol-PM, Nervine Nightime Sleep, Nidryl Elixir,

*Ambenyl Syrup is C-V. See Schedules of Controlled Drugs at the back of this book.

Nighttime Cold Medicine [CD], Nite-Time, Noradryl [CD], Noradryl 25, Nytol, Pain Relief PM [CD], Pathadryl, ✦PMS-Diphenhydramine, Sinutab Maximum Strength, Sk-Diphenhydramine, Sleep, Sleep-Eze 3, ✦Sleep-Eze D, Sominex, Sominex 2, Theraflu Cold Medicine, Nighttime Strength, Twilite, Tylenol PM Extra Strength, Unisom Sleepgels, Valdrene, Valu-dryl Allergy Medicine [CD], Wal-ben, Wal-dryl, Wehydryl

---

BENEFITS versus RISKS

Possible Benefits	*Possible Risks*
EFFECTIVE RELIEF OF ALLERGIC RHINITIS AND ALLERGIC SKIN DISORDERS	Marked sedation
	Atropinelike effects
	Accentuation of prostatism (see Glossary)
EFFECTIVE, NONADDICTIVE SEDATIVE AND HYPNOTIC	
Treatment of anaphylaxis	
Prevention and relief of motion sickness	
Partial relief of symptoms of Parkinson's disease	

▷ **Principal Uses**

As a Single Drug Product: Uses currently included in FDA approved labeling: (1) Prevention or treatment of motion sickness (control of dizziness, nausea and vomiting); (2) treatment of drug-induced parkinsonian reactions, especially in children or the elderly; (3) treatment of conditions caused by histamine release (such as allergic drug reactions); (4) used as a short-term sleep aid.

Other (unlabeled) generally accepted uses: (1) cough suppression; (2) eases the symptoms of the common cold; (3) can have a role in easing the discomfort of mucositis caused by radiation therapy.

As a Combination Drug Product [CD]: This drug may have a mild suppressant effect on coughing. It is combined with expectorants and codeine or dextromethorphan in some cough products.

How This Drug Works: This drug blocks the action of histamine after it has been released. Its natural side effects are used to advantage: sedative action is used to induce drowsiness and sleep; its atropinelike action is used in motion sickness and Parkinson-related disorders.

Available Dosage Forms and Strengths

Capsules — 25 mg, 50 mg
Cream — 1%
Elixir — 12.5 mg per 5-ml (14% alcohol)
Spray — 1%
Syrup — 12.5 mg, 13.3 mg per 5-ml
Tablets — 25 mg, 50 mg

▷ **Usual Adult Dosage Range:** 25 to 50 mg/4 to 6 hours. Total daily dosage should not exceed 300 mg. When used as a sleep aid (hypnotic) 50 mg at bedtime is often used. **Note: Actual dosage and administration schedule must be determined by the physician for each patient individually.**

Conditions Requiring Dosing Adjustments

Liver function: Caution—single doses are not expected to be a problem, however, the use of multiple doses in patients with liver compromise has not been studied.

Kidney function: In severe kidney failure, the dose is given every 12 to 18 hours.

▷ **Dosing Instructions:**   Tablet may be crushed and capsule may be opened, and best taken with or following food.

Usual Duration of Use: Use on a regular schedule for 2 to 3 days is needed to see effectiveness in relieving the symptoms of allergic rhinitis and dermatosis. If not effective after 5 days, this drug should be stopped. As a bedtime sedative (hypnotic), use only as needed. Avoid long-term use without interruption.

▷ **This Drug Should Not Be Taken If**
- you have had an allergic reaction to any dosage form of it previously.
- you are taking, or have taken during the past 2 weeks, any monoamine oxidase (MAO) type A inhibitor drug (see Drug Classes).
- you have chicken pox.

▷ **Inform Your Physician Before Taking This Drug If**
- you have had an unfavorable response to any antihistamine drug.
- you have narrow-angle glaucoma.
- you have peptic ulcer disease, with any degree of pyloric obstruction.
- you have prostatism (see Glossary).
- you are subject to bronchial asthma or seizures (epilepsy).
- you have difficulty urinating.
- you have G-6-PD deficiency.

Possible Side Effects (natural, expected, and unavoidable drug actions)
Drowsiness; weakness; dryness of nose, mouth, and throat; constipation.

▷ **Possible Adverse Effects** (unusual, unexpected, and infrequent reactions)
If any of the following develop, consult your physician promptly for guidance.

Mild Adverse Effects
Allergic Reactions: Skin rash, hives.
Headache, dizziness, inability to concentrate, nervousness, blurred or double vision, difficult urination.
Reduced tolerance for contact lenses.
Nausea, vomiting, diarrhea.

Serious Adverse Effects
Allergic Reaction: Anaphylactic reaction (see Glossary).
Idiosyncratic Reactions: Insomnia, excitement, confusion.
Hemolytic anemia (see Glossary).
Reduced white blood cell count—fever, sore throat, infections.
Blood platelet destruction (see Glossary)—abnormal bleeding or bruising.
Movement disorders (dyskinesias).
Porphyria.

▷ **Possible Effects on Sexual Function:**   Shortened menstrual cycle (early arrival of expected menstrual onset).

Natural Diseases or Disorders That May Be Activated by This Drug
Latent epilepsy, glaucoma, prostatism.

Possible Effects on Laboratory Tests
Red blood cell counts and hemoglobin: decreased.
Urine screening tests for drug abuse: *initial* test result may be falsely **positive**; *confirmatory* test result will be **negative**. (Test results depend upon amount of drug taken and testing method used.)

CAUTION
1. Stop this drug 5 days before diagnostic skin testing procedures in order to prevent false negative test results.
2. Do not use if you have active bronchial asthma, bronchitis or pneumonia.

Precautions for Use
By Infants and Children: This drug should not be used in premature or full-term newborn infants. Doses for children should be small, as the young child is especially sensitive to the effects of antihistamines on the brain and nervous system. For use to decrease coughing (antitussive)in children 6 to 12 years old is 12.5 mg every 4 to 6 hours The maximum daily dose here is 75 mg per day. Avoid the use of this drug in the child with chicken pox or a flulike infection—may adversely affect Reye syndrome if it develops.

By Those over 60 Years of Age: Increased risk of drowsiness, dizziness and unsteadiness, and impairment of thinking, judgment and memory. Can increase the degree of impaired urination associated with prostate enlargement (prostatism). Sedative effects may be misinterpreted as senility or emotional depression.

▷ **Advisability of Use During Pregnancy**
Pregnancy Category: B by the manufacturer. See Pregnancy Code at the back of this book.
Animal studies: No birth defects reported in rats or rabbits.
Human studies: Information from studies of pregnant women indicates no significant increase in birth defects in 2948 exposures to this drug. A withdrawal syndrome of tremor and diarrhea has been reported in a 5-day-old infant whose mother used this drug (150 mg daily) during pregnancy.
Avoid drug during the last 3 months. Use sparingly during the first 6 months only if clearly needed.

Advisability of Use if Breast-Feeding
Presence of this drug in breast milk: Yes.
Avoid drug or refrain from nursing.

Habit-Forming Potential: Combination use of pentazocine and diphenhydramine has become an abused intravenous drug combination. There have been rare reports of a withdrawal syndrome after use of high diphenhydramine doses.

Effects of Overdosage: Marked drowsiness, confusion, incoordination, unsteadiness, muscle tremors, stupor, coma, seizures, fever, flushed face, dilated pupils, weak pulse, shallow breathing.

Possible Effects of Long-Term Use:　The development of tolerance (see Glossary) and reduced effectiveness of drug.

Suggested Periodic Examinations While Taking This Drug (at physician's discretion)

Complete blood cell counts.

▷ **While Taking This Drug, Observe the Following**

Foods: No restrictions.

Beverages: No restrictions. May be taken with milk.

▷　*Alcohol:* Use extreme caution. The combination of alcohol and antihistamines can cause rapid and marked sedation.

Tobacco Smoking: No interactions expected.

Marijuana Smoking: Increased drowsiness and mouth dryness; accentuation of impaired thinking.

▷　*Other Drugs*

Diphenhydramine may *increase* the effects of

- amitriptyline and cause increased urinary retention.
- all drugs with a sedative effect such as benzodiazepines, tricyclic antidepressants, and narcotics (see Drug Classes), and cause oversedation.
- atropine and atropinelike drugs (see Drug Classes).

The following drugs may *increase* the effects of diphenhydramine

- monoamine oxidase (MAO) type A inhibitor drugs (see Drug Classes) delay elimination, exaggerating and prolonging its action.

Diphenhydramine *taken concurrently* with

- phenothiazines (see Drug Classes) may result in increased difficulty urinating, intestinal obstruction or glaucoma, especially in those over 70 years old.
- temazepam in pregnancy may result in increased death of the fetus.
- tricyclic antidepressants (see Drug Classes) may cause increased risk of urinary retention.

▷　*Driving, Hazardous Activities:* This drug may impair mental alertness, judgment, physical coordination and reaction time. Restrict activities as necessary.

Aviation Note: The use of this drug *is a disqualification* for piloting. Consult a designated Aviation Medical Examiner.

Exposure to Sun: Caution—this drug may cause photosensitivity (see Glossary).

Exposure to Environmental Chemicals: The insecticides Aldrin, Dieldrin and Chlordane may decrease the effectiveness of this drug. Sevin may increase the sedative effects of this drug.

DISOPYRAMIDE (di so PEER a mide)

Introduced: 1969　**Prescription:** USA: Yes; Canada: Yes　**Available as Generic:** USA: Yes; Canada: No　**Class:** Antiarrhythmic　**Controlled Drug:** USA: No; Canada: No

Brand Names: Napamide, Norpace, Norpace CR, Pisopyramide, ✤Rythmodan, ✤Rythmodan-LA

```
┌─────────────────────────────────────────────────────────────────┐
│                      BENEFITS versus RISKS                        │
│        Possible Benefits              Possible Risks              │
│   EFFECTIVE TREATMENT OF        NARROW TREATMENT RANGE            │
│     SELECTED HEART RHYTHM       LOW BLOOD PRESSURE               │
│     DISORDERS                   LOW BLOOD SUGAR                  │
│                                   (INFREQUENT)                    │
│                                 AGRANULOCYTOSIS (RARE)           │
│                                 Peripheral neuropathy            │
│                                 Liver toxicity                    │
│                                 Heart conduction and rhythm      │
│                                   abnormalities                   │
│                                 Frequent atropinelike side effects│
└─────────────────────────────────────────────────────────────────┘
```

▷ **Principal Uses**

As a Single Drug Product: Uses currently included in FDA approved labeling: (1) This drug is used to treat abnormal rhythms in the ventricles of the heart (ventricular arrhythmias). It is classified as a Type 1 antiarrhythmic agent, similar to procainamide and quinidine in its actions.

Other (unlabeled) generally accepted uses: (1) It is used to abolish and prevent the recurrence of premature beats arising in the atria (upper chambers) and the ventricles (lower chambers) of the heart; (2) also useful in the treatment and prevention of abnormally rapid heart rates (tachycardia) that originate in the atria or the ventricles; (3) eases arrhythmias and abnormal pressures in the heart arising from cardiomyopathy or subaortic stenosis.

How This Drug Works: By slowing the activity of the pacemaker and delaying the transmission of electrical impulses through the conduction system and muscle of the heart, this drug assists in restoring normal heart rate and rhythm.

Available Dosage Forms and Strengths

Capsules — 100 mg, 150 mg

Capsules, prolonged-action — 100 mg, 150 mg, 250 mg LA (in Canada)

Tablet, controlled release — 150 mg, 250 mg (Canada)

▷ **Usual Adult Dosage Range:**   For most adults, 600 mg per day is given. For the immediate release form: 150 mg every 6 hours. For the controlled release form: 300 mg every 12 hours. Should not exceed 1600 mg/24 hours—reserved for refractory cases. A loading dose has been used if there is a critical need for quick control: for patients weighing more than 50 kg, 300 mg of the immediate release form is used. For patients weighing less than 50 kg, 200 mg of the immediate release form is used. **Note: Actual dosage and administration schedule must be determined by the physician for each patient individually.**

Conditions Requiring Dosing Adjustments

Liver function: The dose should be decreased in patients with liver compromise by 25 to 50%.

Kidney function: The dose **must** be adjusted in kidney compromise. In moderate to severe kidney failure, the immediate release form usual dose is only given every 12 to 24 hours. This drug may cause urine retention and should be used with caution in patients with urinary outflow problems.

▷ **Dosing Instructions:** The regular capsules may be opened to take them, and are best taken on an empty stomach, 1 hour before or 2 hours after eating. However, it may be taken with or following food to reduce stomach irritation. The prolonged-action capsules should not be opened, chewed or crushed.

Usual Duration of Use: Use on a regular schedule for 2 to 4 days is needed to see this drug's effectiveness in correcting or preventing rhythm disorders. Long-term use requires physician supervision and periodic evaluation.

▷ **This Drug Should Not Be Taken If**
- you have had an allergic reaction to it previously.
- you have second-degree or third-degree heart block.
- you have sick sinus syndrome (talk with your doctor).

▷ **Inform Your Physician Before Taking This Drug If**
- you have had unfavorable reactions to other antiarrhythmic drugs.
- you have heart disease of any kind, especially "heart block."
- you have a history of atrial fibrillation.
- you have a history of low blood potassium.
- you have a history of low blood pressure.
- you have a history of low white blood cells.
- you have impaired liver or kidney function.
- you have glaucoma, a family history of glaucoma or myasthenia gravis.
- you have an enlarged prostate gland.
- you are prone to low blood sugars.
- you take any form of digitalis or any diuretic drug that can cause loss of body potassium (ask your doctor).

Possible Side Effects (natural, expected, and unavoidable drug actions)
Drop in blood pressure in susceptible individuals.
Dry mouth, constipation, blurred vision, impaired urination.

▷ **Possible Adverse Effects** (unusual, unexpected, and infrequent reactions)
If any of the following develop, consult your physician promptly for guidance.
Mild Adverse Effects
Allergic Reactions: Skin rash, itching.
Headache, nervousness, fatigue, muscular weakness, mild aches.
Blurred vision.
Loss of appetite, indigestion, nausea, vomiting, diarrhea.
Serious Adverse Effects
Idiosyncratic Reaction: Acute psychotic behavior (rare).
Severe drop in blood pressure, fainting.
Progressive heart weakness, predisposing to congestive heart failure.
Inability to empty urinary bladder, prostatism (see Glossary).
Abnormal heart rhythms.
Peripheral neuropathy.
Low blood sugar (glucose).
Jaundice (see Glossary).
Porphyria (rare).
Abnormally low white blood cell count (rare).

▷ **Possible Effects on Sexual Function:** Rare impotence (300 mg/day); enlargement and tenderness of male breasts.

▷ **Adverse Effects That May Mimic Natural Diseases or Disorders**
Reversible jaundice may suggest viral hepatitis.

Natural Diseases or Disorders That May Be Activated by This Drug
Glaucoma, myasthenia gravis.

Possible Effects on Laboratory Tests
White blood cell counts: decreased.
Liver function tests: increased liver enzymes (ALT/GPT, AST/GOT and alkaline phosphatase), increased bilirubin.

CAUTION
1. Thorough heart exam (including electrocardiograms) is critical prior to using this drug.
2. Periodic heart exams are needed to follow drug responses. Some people may have heart rhythm or function declines. Close monitoring of heart rate, rhythm and overall performance is essential.
3. Dosage must be individualized. Do not change your dosage without the knowledge and supervision of your physician.
4. Talk with your doctor about the signs and symptoms of low blood sugar.
5. Do not take any other antiarrhythmic drug while taking this drug unless directed to do so by your doctor.

Precautions for Use
By Infants and Children: In pediatric patients, disopyramide is given on a mg per kg basis. The dose is then divided into equal doses and given at times determined by the patient response. For example, some patients from one to four years old will receive 10 to 20 mg per kg per day divided into equal doses and given every 6 hours. Initial use of this drug requires hospitalization and supervision by a qualified pediatrician.
By Those over 60 Years of Age: Reduced kidney function may require dose reductions. This drug can aggravate existing prostatism (see Glossary) and promote constipation. Observe carefully for light-headedness, dizziness, unsteadiness and tendency to fall.

▷ **Advisability of Use During Pregnancy**
Pregnancy Category: C. See Pregnancy Code at the back of this book.
Animal studies: No birth defects reported in rats and rabbits.
Human studies: Adequate studies of pregnant women are not available. It has been reported that this drug can cause contractions of the pregnant uterus.
Use this drug only if clearly needed. Ask your physician for guidance.

Advisability of Use if Breast-Feeding
Presence of this drug in breast milk: Yes.
Avoid drug or refrain from nursing.

Habit-Forming Potential: None.

Effects of Overdosage: Dryness of eyes, nose, mouth and throat; impaired urination; constipation; marked drop in blood pressure; abnormal heart rhythms; congestive heart failure.

Possible Effects of Long-Term Use: None reported.

Suggested Periodic Examinations While Taking This Drug (at physician's discretion)
  Electrocardiograms, complete blood counts, potassium blood levels.

▷ **While Taking This Drug, Observe the Following**
  Foods: No restrictions. Ask physician regarding need for salt restriction and advisability of eating potassium-rich foods.
  Beverages: No restrictions. May be taken with milk.
▷ *Alcohol:* Use caution. Alcohol can increase the blood-pressure-lowering effects and the blood-sugar-lowering effects of this drug.
  Tobacco Smoking: Nicotine can cause irritability of the heart and reduce the effectiveness of this drug. Follow physician's advice regarding smoking.
▷ *Other Drugs*
  Disopyramide may ***increase*** the effects of
  • antihypertensive drugs, and cause excessive lowering of blood pressure.
  • atropinelike drugs (see Drug Classes).
  • warfarin (Coumadin, etc.); check prothrombin times, adjust dosing.
  Disopyramide may ***decrease*** the effects of
  • ambenonium (Mytelase).
  • neostigmine (Prostigmin).
  • pyridostigmine (Mestinon).
  Benefits of these three drugs in treating myasthenia gravis may be reduced.
  Disopyramide ***taken concurrently*** with
  • amiodarone may result in an abnormal heart effect (Torsades de Pointes).
  • beta blockers (see Drug Classes) may result in abnormally low heart rates.
  • digoxin can cause digoxin toxicity.
  • erythromycins (EES, others) can cause increased disopyramide blood concentrations and abnormal heart effects. Caution is advised in combining azithromycin or clarithromycin because they are structurally similar.
  • insulin or oral hypoglycemic (see Drug Classes) agents may result in abnormally low blood sugars.
  • phenobarbital may result in loss of disopyramide effectiveness.
  • phenytoin can result in decreased disopyramide effectiveness and accumulation of a metabolite of phenytoin which causes a severe increase in anticholinergic (see Glossary) effects.
  • potassium supplements may result in elevated potassium levels which can lead to disopyramide toxicity.
  • quinidine can cause increases in disopyramide blood levels and decrease in quinidine levels.
  • verapamil can precipitate or worsen congestive heart failure.
  • warfarin may cause increased risk of bleeding. INR should be checked more frequently if these medicines are combined.
  The following drugs may ***decrease*** the effects of disopyramide
  • all diuretics that promote potassium loss.
  • rifampin (Rimactane, Rifadin).
  • rifabutin.
▷ *Driving, Hazardous Activities:* May cause dizziness or blurred vision. Limit activities as needed.
  Aviation Note: The use of this drug ***may be a disqualification*** for piloting. Consult a designated Aviation Medical Examiner.

Exposure to Sun: Use caution. This drug causes photosensitization (see Glossary).

Exposure to Heat: Use caution. The use of this drug in hot environments may increase the risk of heat stroke.

Occurrence of Unrelated Illness: Vomiting, diarrhea or dehydration can affect this drug's action adversely. Report such developments promptly.

Discontinuation: This drug should not be stopped abruptly following long-term use. Ask your doctor for help regarding gradual dose reduction.

DISULFIRAM (di SULF i ram)

Introduced: 1948   **Prescription:** USA: Yes; Canada: Yes   **Available as**
Generic: USA: Yes; Canada: No   **Class:** Antialcoholism   **Controlled**
Drug: USA: No; Canada: No

Brand Name: Antabuse

BENEFITS versus RISKS	
Possible Benefits	*Possible Risks*
EFFECTIVE ADJUNCT IN THE TREATMENT OF CHRONIC ALCOHOLISM	DANGEROUS REACTIONS WITH ALCOHOL INGESTION
	Acute psychotic reactions (uncommon)
	Drug-induced liver damage (rare)
	Drug-induced optic and/or peripheral neuritis (rare)
	Low blood platelets (rare)

▷ **Principal Uses**

As a Single Drug Product: Uses currently included in FDA approved labeling: (1) Deter abusive drinking of alcoholic beverages. It does not abolish the craving or impulse to drink.

Other (unlabeled) generally accepted uses: (1) Limited use in helping skin problems (dermatitis) caused by nickel exposure; (2) some data increasing infection fighting cells (CD4) in AIDS.

How This Drug Works: After alcohol is taken, this drug blocks normal liver enzyme activity after the conversion of alcohol to acetaldehyde. This causes excessive accumulation of acetaldehyde, and produces the disulfiram (Antabuse) reaction (see Glossary).

Available Dosage Forms and Strengths

Tablets — 250 mg, 500 mg

▷ **Usual Adult Dosage Range:** Once all signs of alcoholic intoxication are gone and no less than 12 hours after the last alcohol containing drink, treatment is started with 500 mg/day for 1 to 2 weeks. This is followed by a maintenance dose of 250 mg/day. The range of the maintenance dose is 125 mg to 500 mg/day and is individually determined. Total daily dosage should not exceed 500 mg. **Note: Actual dosage and administration schedule must be determined by the physician for each patient individually.**

Conditions Requiring Dosing Adjustments

Liver function: This drug is a benefit to risk decision in mild liver compromise. Disulfiram is clearly contraindicated in portal hypertension and active hepatitis.

Kidney function: Dosing adjustments are not indicated.

Diabetes: People with diabetes who take disulfiram can be at increased risk for diabetic blood vessel (micro and macrovascular) problems. The risk is worsened by potential adverse drug effects such as increased cholesterol levels and peripheral neuropathy.

Lung disease: Accumulation of a metabolite may occur in severe lung problems. Drug levels or dose reduction will be needed.

▷ **Dosing Instructions:**   The tablet may be crushed and taken with or following food to decrease stomach irritation.

Usual Duration of Use: Use on a regular schedule for several months is needed to see this drug's effectiveness in deterring alcohol use. If tolerated well, use should continue until permanent self-control and sobriety is seen.

▷ **This Drug Should Not Be Taken If**
- you have had a severe allergic reaction to disulfiram. (Note: The interaction of disulfiram and alcohol is *not an allergic* reaction.)
- you have taken any form of alcohol within the past 12 hours.
- you are pregnant.
- you have a history of psychosis.
- you are taking paraldehyde.
- you have significant exposure to ethylene dibromide where you live or work. Disulfiram inhibits the removal of this chemical and enhances the ability of ethylene dibromide to cause cancer.
- you are taking (or have taken recently) metronidazole (Flagyl).
- you have coronary heart disease or a serious heart rhythm disorder.

▷ **Inform Your Physician Before Taking This Drug If**
- you have used disulfiram in the past.
- you do not intend to avoid alcohol completely while taking this drug.
- you do not understand what will happen if you drink alcohol while taking this drug.
- you are planning pregnancy in the near future.
- you have a history of diabetes, epilepsy, kidney or liver disease.
- you take oral anticoagulants, digitalis, isoniazid, paraldehyde or phenytoin (Dilantin).
- you have a history of low thyroid function (hypothyroidism).
- you have a history of lung disease.
- you plan to have surgery under general anesthesia while taking this drug.

Possible Side Effects (natural, expected, and unavoidable drug actions)

Drowsiness, lethargy during early use.

Offensive breath and body odor.

▷ **Possible Adverse Effects** (unusual, unexpected, and infrequent reactions)

If any of the following develop, consult your physician promptly for guidance.

Mild Adverse Effects

Allergic Reactions: Skin rash, hives.

Headache, dizziness, restlessness, tremor.

Metallic or garliclike taste, indigestion (usually subsides in 2 weeks).

Serious Adverse Effects

Allergic Reactions: Severe skin rashes, drug-induced hepatitis (rare).

Idiosyncratic Reaction: Acute toxic effect on brain including abnormal movements and psychotic behavior.

Optic or peripheral neuritis (see Glossary).

Seizures.

May increase risk for blood vessel problems in people with diabetes.

Low thyroid function.

Low blood platelets (extremely rare).

Decreased or increased blood pressure.

Carpal tunnel syndrome.

▷ **Possible Effects on Sexual Function:** Decreased libido and/or impaired erection in users taking recommended doses of 125 to 500 mg/day.

▷ **Adverse Effects That May Mimic Natural Diseases or Disorders**

Liver reaction may suggest viral hepatitis.

Brain toxicity may suggest spontaneous psychosis.

Possible Effects on Laboratory Tests

Blood cholesterol level: increased.

Prothrombin time: increased (taken concurrently with warfarin).

Liver function tests: liver enzymes increased (ALT/GPT, AST/GOT and alkaline phosphatase), increased bilirubin.

CAUTION

1. No one should take this drug while in a state of alcoholic intoxication.
2. The patient must be fully informed about the purpose and actions of this drug *before* treatment is started.
3. Long-term use requires exam for reduced thyroid function.
4. Carry a personal identification card noting you are taking this drug.

Precautions for Use

By Infants and Children: Safety and effectiveness for those under 12 years of age not established.

By Those over 60 Years of Age: Watch for excessive sedation when the drug is started. *Do not* perform an "alcohol trial" to see the effects of this drug.

▷ **Advisability of Use During Pregnancy**

Pregnancy Category: C. See Pregnancy Code at the back of this book.

Animal studies: No defects reported in rats and hamsters.

Human studies: Two reports indicate that 4 of 8 fetuses exposed had serious birth defects. Adequate studies of pregnant women are not available.

Avoid this drug completely if possible.

Advisability of Use if Breast-Feeding

Presence of this drug in breast milk: Unknown.

Talk with your doctor as this is a benefit of the drug versus the risk of adverse effects to the fetus question.

Habit-Forming Potential: None.

Effects of Overdosage: Marked lethargy, impaired memory, altered behavior, confusion, unsteadiness, weakness, stomach pain, nausea, vomiting, diarrhea.

Possible Effects of Long-Term Use: Decreased function of thyroid gland.

Suggested Periodic Examinations While Taking This Drug (at physician's discretion)
Visual acuity, liver function tests, thyroid function tests.

▷ **While Taking This Drug, Observe the Following**
Foods: Avoid all foods prepared with alcohol, including sauces, marinades, vinegars, desserts, etc. Ask when dining out about use of alcohol in cooking food.

Beverages: Avoid all punches, fruit drinks, etc., that may contain alcohol. This drug may be taken with milk.

▷ *Alcohol: **Avoid completely in all forms*** while taking this drug and for 14 days following the last dose. Combination of disulfiram and alcohol—even in small amounts—produces the disulfiram (Antabuse) reaction. This starts in 5 to 10 minutes after ingesting alcohol and consists of: intense flushing, severe headache, shortness of breath, chest pains, nausea, repeated vomiting, sweating and weakness. If large amounts of alcohol are taken, the reaction may progress to blurred vision, vertigo, confusion, marked drop in blood pressure and loss of consciousness. Severe reactions may lead to convulsions and death. The reaction may last from 30 minutes to several hours, depending upon the amount of alcohol and disulfiram in the body.

Tobacco Smoking: No interactions expected.
Marijuana Smoking: Possible increase in drowsiness and lethargy.

▷ *Other Drugs*
Disulfiram may ***increase*** the effects of
• oral anticoagulants (warfarin, etc.), and increase the risk of bleeding; dosage adjustments may be necessary.
• chlordiazepoxide (Librium) and diazepam (Valium), and cause oversedation. Other benzodiazepines such as alprazolam, clonazepam, clorazepate, flurazepam, halazepam, prazepam or triazolam may also be subject to this interaction.
• paraldehyde, and cause excessive depression of brain function.
• phenytoin (Dilantin), and cause toxicity; dosage must be decreased.
Disulfiram may ***decrease*** the effects of
• perphenazine (Tilafon, etc.).
Disulfiram ***taken concurrently*** with
• bacampicillin (Spectrobid) can theoretically cause a disulfiram reaction, but no cases have been reported.
• cisplatin (Platinol) can increase risk of toxicity of cisplatin.
• cyclosporine (Sandimune) may result in a disulfiram reaction as there is alcohol in the intravenous and oral forms of cyclosporine.
• isoniazid (INH, etc.) may cause acute mental problems and incoordination.
• metronidazole (Flagyl) may cause acute mental and behavioral disturbances, making it necessary to stop treatment.
• omeprazole (Prilosec) may result in increased disulfiram levels and toxicity.
• OTC cough syrups, tonics, etc., containing alcohol may cause a disulfiram (Antabuse) reaction; avoid concurrent use. (See OTC Drugs in Glossary.)

- paraldehyde may result in a disulfiram reaction.
- theophylline can lead to theophylline toxicity because the metabolism of theophylline is decreased.
- warfarin will result in an increased risk of bleeding. Increased INR testing is recommended.

The following drugs may *increase* the effects of disulfiram

- amitriptyline (Elavil), and perhaps other tricyclic antidepressants may enhance the disulfiram + alcohol interaction; avoid concurrent use of these drugs.

▷ *Driving, Hazardous Activities:* This drug may cause drowsiness or dizziness. Limit activities as necessary.

Aviation Note: Alcoholism *is a disqualification* for piloting. Consult a designated Aviation Medical Examiner.

Exposure to Sun: No restrictions.

Exposure to Environmental Chemicals: Thiram, a pesticide, and carbon disulfide, a pesticide and industrial solvent, can have additive toxic effects. Watch for toxic effects on the brain and nervous system.

Discontinuation: Drug treatment is only part of your total program. Do not stop it without the knowledge and guidance of your physician. If it must be stopped abruptly, there are no symptoms. However, no alcohol should be ingested for 14 days following discontinuation.

DORNASE ALPHA (DOOR nase AL fa)

Introduced: 1994   **Prescription:** USA: Yes; Canada: Yes   **Available as Generic:** USA: No; Canada: No   **Class:** anticystic fibrosis agent   **Controlled Drug:** USA: No; Canada: No

Brand Names: Pulmozyme

BENEFITS versus RISKS	
Possible Benefits	*Possible Risks*
DECREASED MUCOUS VISCOSITY	Hoarseness
IMPROVED LUNG FUNCTION	Antibodies to DNA
DECREASED OCCURRENCE OF	Facial swelling (edema)
RESPIRATORY INFECTIONS	
DECREASED NUMBER OF	
HOSPITALIZATIONS	

▷ **Principal Uses**

As a Single Drug Product: Uses currently included in FDA approved labeling: (1) Management of cystic fibrosis in conjunction with standard therapies.

Other (unlabeled) generally accepted uses: (1) may have a role in chronic bronchitis.

How This Drug Works: The sputum of people with cystic fibrosis contains large amounts of DNA and is much thicker than normal. Dornase breaks the DNA down, making the sputum easier to remove. Other undiscovered mechanisms may also account for its benefits.

Available Dosage Forms and Strengths
Solution — 2.5 ml ampules of 1.0 mg/ml dornase alpha (2.5 mg)

How To Store
This drug should be stored at 36–46 degrees Fahrenheit and should be protected from light. Unused ampules should be stored in their protective pouch in the refrigerator.

▷ **Recommended Dosage Ranges (Actual dosage and administration schedule must be determined by the physician for each patient individually.)**
Infants and Children: Safety and efficacy for those under 5 not established.
5 to 60 Years of Age: One 2.5 mg dose administered by one of the tested nebulizers each day. Some selected patients may benefit from twice daily dosing (older patients).
Over 60 Years of Age: Same as 12 to 60 years of age.

Conditions Requiring Dosing Adjustments
Liver function: Not defined.
Kidney function: Not defined.

▷ **Dosing Instructions:** The solution must be kept in the refrigerator and protected from strong light. The drug should not be used if it is cloudy or discolored. Do **not** mix dornase with other medications. Clinical trials have only been conducted with the Hudson T Up-draft ll, Marquest Acorn ll and Pulmo-Aide compressor. The reusable PARI LC Jet nebulizer and PARI PRONEB compressor were also tested. Do **not** use with other equipment.

Usual Duration of Use:
Use on a regular schedule for eight days usually determines effectiveness in cystic fibrosis. Long-term use (up to 12 months has been studied) requires periodic physician evaluation of response and dosage adjustment.

Possible Advantages of This Drug
Reduction in number of infections, use of antibiotics and hospitalizations with minimal side effects.

▷ **This Drug Should Not Be Taken If**
• you have had an allergic reaction to any dosage form of it previously.
• you have an allergy to Chinese hamster ovary cells.

▷ **Inform Your Physician Before Taking This Drug If**
• you had a rash after the last dose was taken.
• you are uncertain how to use the nebulizer or compressor.
• you are uncertain of how much dornase alpha to take or how often to take it.

Possible Side Effects (natural, expected, and unavoidable drug actions)
Hoarseness.

▷ **Possible Adverse Effects** (unusual, unexpected, and infrequent reactions)
If any of the following develop, consult your physician promptly for guidance.
Mild Adverse Effects
Allergic Reactions: Rash.
Mild pharyngitis or laryngitis.
Conjunctivitis.
Chest pain (has been reported). Facial swelling (rare).

Serious Adverse Effects
> Allergic Reactions: None defined at present.
> Antibodies to DNA (2–4%).

▷ **Possible Effects on Sexual Function:** None reported.

Possible Delayed Adverse Effects: None reported.

Possible Effects on Laboratory Tests
> Antibodies to DNA.

CAUTION
> 1. This drug should only be used with one of the studied nebulizers and compressors.
> 2. Do not use the drug if it is cloudy or discolored.

Precautions for Use
> *By Infants and Children:* Safety and effectiveness for those under 5 years of age not established.
> *By Those over 60 Years of Age:* No changes or precautions.

▷ **Advisability of Use During Pregnancy**
> *Pregnancy Category:* B. See Pregnancy Code at the back of this book.
> Animal studies: Studies in rats and rabbits at up to 600 times the usual human dose have not revealed any harm to the fetus.
> Human studies: Adequate studies of pregnant women are not available.
> Ask your doctor for guidance.

Advisability of Use if Breast-Feeding
> Presence of this drug in breast milk: Unknown.
> Avoid drug or refrain from nursing.

Habit-Forming Potential: None.

Effects of Overdosage: Single doses of up to 180 times the usual human dose in rats and monkeys have been well tolerated.

Possible Effects of Long-Term Use: Not defined.

Suggested Periodic Examinations While Taking This Drug (at physician's discretion)
> Periodic pulmonary function tests.

▷ **While Taking This Drug, Observe the Following**
> *Foods:* No restrictions.
> *Nutritional Support:* Continued enzyme and nutritional support is still needed.
> *Beverages:* No specific restrictions.
▷ *Alcohol:* Follow your doctor's advice relative to alcohol use.
> *Tobacco Smoking:* Follow your doctor's advice regarding smoking. There is no data that says smoking is good for you. Talk with your doctor or pharmacist regarding ways to help you stop smoking.
▷ *Other Drugs:* Clinical studies have revealed that dornase is compatible with medications typically used in management of cystic fibrosis. Specific adverse drug interactions are not documented at present.
▷ *Driving, Hazardous Activities:* Specific limitations because of drug effects are not defined at present.
> *Aviation Note:* The use of this drug *may be a disqualification* for piloting. Consult a designated Aviation Medical Examiner.

Exposure to Sun: No restrictions.

Discontinuation: This drug's benefits stop soon after its regular use is stopped. It must be continued indefinitely to continue to benefit.

Special Storage Instructions: This medicine should be stored in the refrigerator in its protective pouch.

DOXAZOSIN (dox AY zoh sin)

Introduced: 1986   **Prescription:** USA: Yes   **Available as Generic:** No   **Class:** Antihypertensive   **Controlled Drug:** USA: No

Brand Name: Cardura

BENEFITS versus RISKS

Possible Benefits	*Possible Risks*
EFFECTIVE TREATMENT OF MILD TO MODERATE HYPERTENSION when used alone or in combination with other antihypertensive drugs	"First dose" drop in blood pressure, but without fainting Dizziness Fluid retention Rapid heart rate (rare)

▷ **Principal Uses**

As a Single Drug Product: Uses currently included in FDA approved labeling: (1) Once daily treatment of mild to moderate hypertension.

Other (unlabeled) generally accepted uses: (1) Used in conjunction with other drugs to treat congestive heart failure; (2) used to treat pheochromocytoma; (3) useful in prostate problems (symptomatic benign prostatic hyperplasia).

How This Drug Works: By blocking certain actions of the sympathetic nervous system, this drug causes direct relaxation of blood vessel walls and lower blood pressure.

Decreases the peak pressure of the detrusor muscle, prevents alpha-1 receptor stimulation and, as such occurs, prevents smooth muscle contractions in the prostatic urethra and bladder neck and helps urine outflow.

Available Dosage Forms and Strengths

Tablets — 1 mg, 2 mg, 4 mg, 8 mg

▷ **Usual Adult Dosage Range:** Started with a "test dose" of 1 mg to check patient's response within the first 2 to 6 hours. If tolerated, dose is increased cautiously (as needed and tolerated) every 2 weeks and taken as a single dose at bedtime. Doses in excess of 4 mg may increase the occurrence of lightheadedness or dizziness, and should be avoided. Total daily dosage should not exceed 16 mg. For benign prostatic hyperplasia (BPH), a similar test dose is used and usual effective doses are from 4 to 12 milligrams. **Note: Actual dosage and administration schedule must be determined by the physician for each patient individually.**

Conditions Requiring Dosing Adjustments

Liver function: Extreme caution and lower doses **must** be used if the drug is used in patients with liver compromise.

Kidney function: Doses of 1–16 mg have been used. In one study of kidney compromise, one mg decreased the blood pressure for three days.

▷ **Dosing Instructions:**   The tablet may be crushed and is best taken at bedtime to avoid orthostatic hypotension (see Glossary). May be taken without regard to food.

Usual Duration of Use: Use on a regular schedule for 6 to 8 weeks is needed to see this drug's benefit in controlling hypertension. Long-term use (months to years) requires physician supervision and evaluation.

Possible Advantages of This Drug
May be used to initiate treatment.
Effective with once-a-day dosage.
Causes depression or impotence infrequently.
Lowers blood cholesterol and sugar levels.
Does not lose effectiveness with long-term use.

▷ **This Drug Should Not Be Taken If**
- you have had an allergic reaction to this drug or to prazosin (Minipress) or terazosin (Hytrin).
- you have active liver disease.

▷ **Inform Your Physician Before Taking This Drug If**
- you have had orthostatic hypotension (see Glossary) when using other antihypertensive drugs.
- you have a history of mental depression.
- you have impaired circulation to the brain, or a history of stroke.
- you have coronary artery disease.
- you are taking other medicine to help lower your blood pressure.
- you have had a stroke and have high blood pressure.
- you have a history of low white blood cells.
- you have active liver disease or impaired liver function.
- you have impaired kidney function.
- you have angina (active coronary artery disease) and you are not taking a beta-blocking drug. (Consult your physician.)
- you plan to have surgery under general anesthesia in the near future.

Possible Side Effects (natural, expected, and unavoidable drug actions)
Orthostatic hypotension, drowsiness, salt and water retention, dry mouth (rare), nasal congestion, constipation (rare).

▷ **Possible Adverse Effects** (unusual, unexpected, and infrequent reactions)
If any of the following develop, consult your physician promptly for guidance.
Mild Adverse Effects
Allergic Reaction: Skin rash (rare), itching (rare).
Headache, dizziness, fatigue, weakness (rare), nervousness (rare), numbness and tingling (rare), blurred vision (rare).
Palpitation (rare), rapid heart rate (rare), shortness of breath (rare).
Nausea, diarrhea (rare), indigestion (rare).
Increased urination (rare).
Serious Adverse Effects
Mental depression (rare).
Arrhythmias.

Decreased blood sugar (glucose).
Low white blood cell counts (has not caused symptoms in patients who had
follow-up visits).

▷ **Possible Effects on Sexual Function:**   Impotence (2%).

Natural Diseases or Disorders That May Be Activated by This Drug
Latent coronary artery insufficiency.

Possible Effects on Laboratory Tests
White blood cell counts: rare occurrence of mild decrease while taking drug.
Blood lipid tests: decreased total cholesterol, LDL-cholesterol and choles-
terol/HDL ratio; decreased triglycerides; increased HDL.
Blood sugar level: variable decreases.

CAUTION
1. Watch for "first dose" response of precipitous drop in blood pressure,
with or without fainting; this usually happens in the first 6 hours. Starting dose is 1 mg taken at bedtime for the first week; remain supine after
taking these trial doses.
2. Impaired liver function will increase drug level and require smaller than
usual doses.
3. Ask your doctor or pharmacist before you take over-the-counter remedies for allergic rhinitis or head colds; these preparations contain drugs
that may interact with doxazosin.

Precautions for Use
By Infants and Children: Safety and effectiveness for those under 12 years of age
not established.
By Those over 60 Years of Age: Therapy is started with no more than 1 mg/day for
the first week. Subsequent increases in dose must be very gradual. Orthostatic hypotension can cause unexpected falls and injury; sit or lie down
promptly if you feel light-headed or dizzy. Report dizziness or chest pain
promptly.

▷ **Advisability of Use During Pregnancy**
Pregnancy Category: B. See Pregnancy Code at the back of this book.
Animal studies: No birth defects found in rat or rabbit studies.
Human studies: Adequate studies of pregnant women are not available.
Use this drug only if clearly needed. Ask your physician for guidance.

Advisability of Use if Breast-Feeding
Presence of this drug in breast milk: Unknown.
Watch nursing infant closely and discontinue drug or nursing if adverse ef-
fects develop.

Habit-Forming Potential: None.

Effects of Overdosage: Orthostatic hypotension, headache, generalized flushing, rapid heart rate, extreme weakness, irregular heart rhythm, circulatory
collapse.

Possible Effects of Long-Term Use: None reported.

Suggested Periodic Examinations While Taking This Drug (at physician's dis-
cretion)
Measurements of blood pressure in lying, sitting and standing positions.
Measurements of body weight to check for fluid retention.

▷ **While Taking This Drug, Observe the Following**

    Foods: No restrictions. Avoid excessive salt intake.

    Beverages: No restrictions. May be taken with milk.

▷   *Alcohol:* Use with extreme caution. Alcohol can exaggerate the blood-pressure-lowering actions of this drug and cause excessive reduction.

    Tobacco Smoking: Nicotine can contribute to this drug's ability to intensify coronary insufficiency. All forms of tobacco should be avoided.

▷   *Other Drugs*

    The following drugs may *increase* the effects of doxazosin

- beta-adrenergic-blocking drugs (see Drug Classes); severity and duration of the "first dose" response may be increased.

    The following drugs may *decrease* the effects of doxazosin

- estrogens.
- indomethacin (Indocin) and other NSAIDs.

▷   *Driving, Hazardous Activities:* This drug may cause dizziness or drowsiness. Restrict activities as necessary.

    Aviation Note: The use of this drug *is a disqualification* for piloting. Consult a designated Aviation Medical Examiner.

    Exposure to Sun: No restrictions.

    Exposure to Cold: Use caution. Cold environments may increase coronary insufficiency (angina) and hypothermia (see Glossary).

    Heavy Exercise or Exertion: Excessive exertion can augment this drug's ability to induce angina.

    Discontinuation: If you are taking this drug for congestive heart failure, do not stop it abruptly. Ask your physician for guidance.

DOXEPIN (DOX e pin)

Introduced: 1969　**Prescription:** USA: Yes; Canada: Yes　**Available as Generic:** USA: Yes; Canada: No　**Class:** Antidepressant　**Controlled Drug:** USA: No; Canada: No

Brand Names: Adapin, Sinequan, ✦Triadapin, Zonalon

BENEFITS versus RISKS	
Possible Benefits	*Possible Risks*
EFFECTIVE RELIEF OF ENDOGENOUS DEPRESSION	ADVERSE BEHAVIORAL EFFECTS: Confusion, disorientation, hallucinations, delusions
EFFECTIVE RELIEF OF ANXIETY AND NERVOUS TENSION	CONVERSION OF DEPRESSION TO MANIA in manic-depressive (bipolar) disorders
Possibly beneficial in other depressive disorders	Aggravation of schizophrenia and paranoia
	Rare blood cell disorders
	Rare liver toxicity
	Low blood pressure on standing

▷ **Principal Uses**

    As a Single Drug Product: Uses currently included in FDA approved labeling: (1) To relieve the symptoms associated with spontaneous (endogenous) depression, refractory depression, neurotic depression, mixed depression anxiety and depression and anxiety in alcoholism; (2) helps treat sleep disturbances; (3) treats depression and anxiety associated with alcoholism.

Other (unlabeled) generally accepted uses: (1) Helps decrease the frequency of urination at night in patients with excessive activity of the detrusor muscle; (2) has a role in pain management in cancer patients; (3) can ease the extent of lowered blood glucose (postprandial hypoglycemia) which occurs after meals in some patients; (4) may help in the management of posttraumatic stress disorder; (5) helps people troubled by itching and swelling of unknown cause (idiopathic urticaria); (6) may help ease the craving which occurs when people try to stop smoking.

How This Drug Works: Relieves depression by slowly restoring to normal levels chemicals (norepinephrine and serotonin) that transmit nerve impulses.

Available Dosage Forms and Strengths
Capsules — 10 mg, 25 mg, 50 mg, 75 mg, 100 mg, 150 mg
Oral concentrate — 10 mg per ml
Topical Cream — 50 mg per gram

▷ **Usual Adult Dosage Range:**   Initially 25 mg 3 to 4 times daily. Dose may be increased cautiously as needed and tolerated by 10 to 25 mg daily at intervals of 1 week. Usual maintenance dose is 75 to 150 mg/24 hours. Usually, there is no greater benefit achieved by using more than 300 mg/24 hours. There have been rare uses of 500 mg per day. When the optimal requirement is determined, it may be taken at bedtime as one dose. **Note: Actual dosage and administration schedule must be determined by the physician for each patient individually.**

Conditions Requiring Dosing Adjustments
Liver function: Doxepin has rarely caused hepatitis. This drug should be used with caution and in reduced dose in patients with liver compromise.
Kidney function: Used with caution in patients with compromised kidneys and urine outflow problems.

▷ **Dosing Instructions:**   May be taken without regard to meals. Capsule may be opened for administration.

Usual Duration of Use: Some benefit may be apparent within to 2 weeks, but adequate response may require continual use for 3 weeks or longer. Long-term use should not exceed 6 months without evaluation regarding the need for continuation of the drug. Consult your physician on a regular basis.

▷ **This Drug Should Not Be Taken If**
• you have had an allergic reaction to it previously.
• you are taking or have taken within the past 14 days any monoamine oxidase (MAO) type A inhibitor drug (see Drug Classes).
• you are recovering from a recent heart attack.
• you have significant urine retention.
• you have narrow-angle glaucoma.

▷ **Inform Your Physician Before Taking This Drug If**
• you are allergic or sensitive to any other tricyclic antidepressant (see Drug Classes).
• you have a history of any of the following: Diabetes, epilepsy, glaucoma,

heart disease, liver compromise, prostate gland enlargement or overactive thyroid function.
- you are pregnant or are breast feeding.
- you plan to have surgery under general anesthesia in the near future.

Possible Side Effects (natural, expected, and unavoidable drug actions)
Drowsiness, blurred vision, dry mouth, constipation, impaired urination.

▷ **Possible Adverse Effects** (unusual, unexpected, and infrequent reactions)
If any of the following develop, consult your physician promptly for guidance.
Mild Adverse Effects
Allergic Reactions: Skin rash, hives, swelling of face or tongue, drug fever (see Glossary).
Blurred vision.
Ringing in the ears (rare).
Stinging or burning of the skin with application of doxepin cream.
Headache, dizziness, drowsiness, weakness, fainting, unsteady gait, tremors.
Increased appetite, craving for sweets, weight gain.
Peculiar taste, irritation of tongue or mouth, nausea, indigestion.
Fluctuation of blood sugar levels.
Serious Adverse Effects
Allergic Reactions: Hepatitis, with or without jaundice (see Glossary).
Confusion, hallucinations, agitation, restlessness, delusions.
Bone marrow depression (see Glossary)—fatigue, weakness, fever, sore throat, abnormal bleeding or bruising (reported for other drugs of this class).
Peripheral neuritis (see Glossary)—numbness, tingling, pain, loss of strength in arms and legs.
Rare elevations in temperature.
Seizures (rare).
Rare kidney damage.
Low blood pressure on standing.
Parkinson-like disorders (see Glossary)—usually mild and infrequent; more likely to occur in the elderly.
Abnormal heart rhythm or rate.

▷ **Possible Effects on Sexual Function:**   Female breast enlargement with milk production; swelling of testicles.
Enlargement and tenderness of male breast tissue (gynecomastia).
Ejaculation disorder.
Painful and persistent erection (priapism).

▷ **Adverse Effects That May Mimic Natural Diseases or Disorders**
Liver toxicity may suggest viral hepatitis.

Natural Diseases or Disorders That May Be Activated by This Drug
Latent diabetes, epilepsy, glaucoma, impaired urination due to prostate gland enlargement (prostatism, see Glossary).

Possible Effects on Laboratory Tests
White blood cell and platelet counts: may be decreased.
Liver function tests: increased.
Blood sugar (glucose): may be increased.

CAUTION
1. Dosage must be adjusted for each person individually. Report for follow-up evaluation and laboratory tests as directed by your physician.
2. It is advisable to withhold this drug if electroconvulsive therapy (ECT, "shock" treatment) is to be used to treat your depression.

Precautions for Use
By Infants and Children: Safety and effectiveness for those under 12 years of age not established.
By Those over 60 Years of Age: During the first 2 weeks of treatment, watch for development of confusion, agitation, forgetfulness, disorientation, delusions and hallucinations. Reduction of dosage or discontinuation may be necessary. Unsteadiness may predispose to falling and injury. This drug can increase the degree of impaired urination associated with prostate gland enlargement (prostatism).

▷ **Advisability of Use During Pregnancy**
Pregnancy Category: C. See Pregnancy Code at the back of this book.
Animal studies: No birth defects reported in rats, rabbits, dogs or monkeys.
Human studies: Adequate studies of pregnant women are not available.
Use this drug only if clearly needed. If possible, avoid use during the first 3 months and the last month. Ask physician for guidance.

Advisability of Use if Breast-Feeding
Presence of this drug in breast milk: Yes.
Monitor nursing infant very closely and discontinue drug or nursing if adverse effects develop.

Habit-Forming Potential: None.

Effects of Overdosage: Confusion, hallucinations, marked drowsiness, heart palpitations, dilated pupils, tremors, stupor, deep sleep, coma, convulsions.

Suggested Periodic Examinations While Taking This Drug (at physician's discretion)
Complete blood cell counts, liver function tests, serial blood pressure readings and electrocardiograms.

▷ **While Taking This Drug, Observe the Following**
Foods: No restrictions. This drug may increase the appetite and cause excessive weight gain.
Beverages: No restrictions. May be taken with milk.
▷ *Alcohol:* Avoid completely. This drug can markedly increase the intoxicating effects of alcohol and accentuate its depressant action on brain function.
Tobacco Smoking: May hasten the elimination of this drug. Higher doses may be necessary.
Marijuana Smoking: Possible increase in heart rate.
▷ *Other Drugs*
Doxepin may *increase* the effects of
• albuterol on blood vessels.
• atropinelike drugs (see Drug Classes).
• dicumarol, and increase the risk of bleeding; dosage adjustments may be necessary.
• other drugs with central nervous system effects (narcotics, benzodiazepines, etc.).

- phenytoin (Dilantin).
- thyroid hormones.

Doxepin may *decrease* the effects of
- clonidine (Catapres).
- guanethidine (Ismelin).

Doxepin *taken concurrently* with
- monoamine oxidase (MAO) type A inhibitor drugs may cause high fever, delirium and convulsions (see Drug Classes).
- carbamazepine (Tegretol) may decrease the effectiveness of doxepin.
- cimetidine (Tagamet) may result in doxepin toxicity (urine retention, dry mouth).
- diphenhydramine (Benadryl) or other drugs with anticholinergic actions may result in increased risk of urine retention or bowel obstruction.
- epinephrine will result in an exaggerated increase in blood pressure.
- estrogens may change the action of doxepin.
- fluoxetine (Prozac) can result in doxepin toxicity.
- meperidene (Demerol) may result in an increased risk of respiratory depression.
- methylphenidate (Ritalin) can result in doxepin toxicity.
- paroxetine (Paxil) can cause increased doxepin levels and toxicity.
- pseudoephedrine will result in abnormal increases in blood pressure and should not be combined in therapy.
- propoxyphene (Darvon) can result in doxepin toxicity.
- quinidine (Quinaglute) can result in doxepin toxicity.
- sertraline (Zoloft) can result in increased doxepin levels.
- verapamil (Calan, Verelan, others) may result in increased doxepin levels.
- warfarin will result in prolonged action of the anticoagulant. More frequent INR testing is needed.

▷ *Driving, Hazardous Activities:* This drug may impair mental alertness, judgment, physical coordination and reaction time. Avoid hazardous activities.

Aviation Note: The use of this drug *is a disqualification* for piloting. Consult a designated Aviation Medical Examiner.

Exposure to Sun: Use caution until sensitivity to sun has been determined. This drug may cause photosensitivity (see Glossary).

Exposure to Heat: This drug can inhibit sweating and impair the body's adaptation to hot environments, increasing the risk of heat stroke. Avoid saunas.

Exposure to Cold: The elderly should use caution and avoid conditions conducive to hypothermia (see Glossary).

Discontinuation: It is advisable to discontinue this drug gradually. Abrupt withdrawal after long-term use can cause headache, malaise and nausea.

DOXYCYCLINE (dox ee SI kleen)

Introduced: 1967   **Prescription:** USA: Yes; Canada: Yes   **Available as Generic:** USA: Yes; Canada: No   **Class:** Antibiotic, tetracyclines   **Controlled Drug:** USA: No; Canada: No

Brand Names: Apo-Doxy, Apo-Doxy-Tabs, ✦Doryx, Doryx, Doxy 100, 200, Doxy Caps, Doxychel, ✦Doxycin, Doxy-Lemmon, Novopharm, Vibramycin, Vibra-Tabs, ✦Vibra-Tabs C-Pak

```
┌─────────────────────────────────────────────────────────────────────┐
│                      BENEFITS versus RISKS                            │
│        Possible Benefits              Possible Risks                  │
│   EFFECTIVE TREATMENT OF          ALLERGIC REACTIONS, mild to         │
│   INFECTIONS due to susceptible     severe                            │
│   microorganisms                  Liver reaction with jaundice (rare) │
│                                   Kidney toxicity                     │
│                                   Fungal superinfections              │
│                                   Drug-induced colitis                │
│                                   Blood cell disorders                │
└─────────────────────────────────────────────────────────────────────┘
```

▷ **Principal Uses**

As a Single Drug Product: Uses currently included in FDA approved labeling: (1) Treats a broad range of infections caused by susceptible bacteria and protozoa; (2) treats and prevents "traveler's diarrhea"; (3) treats syphilis in people who are penicillin allergic; (4) helps prevent malaria in travelers.

Other (unlabeled) generally accepted uses: (1) treatment of early Lyme disease; (2) treatment of sexual assault victims; (3) treatment of prostatitis; (4) can help in some cases of PMS; (5) may be of benefit in some cases of male infertility of unexplained origin.

How This Drug Works: Prevents growth and multiplication of susceptible bacteria by interfering with formation of essential proteins and causing leaky cell walls.

Available Dosage Forms and Strengths

> Capsules — 50 mg, 100 mg
> Capsules, coated pellets — 100 mg
> Delayed release capsule — 100 mg
> Injection — 100 mg per vial and 200 mg per vial
> Oral suspension — 25 mg per 5-ml
> Syrup — 50 mg per 5-ml
> Tablets — 50 mg, 100 mg

▷ **Usual Adult Dosage Range:**   100 mg/12 hours the first day; then 100 mg once daily. Some severe infections may require ongoing therapy of 100 mg every 12 hours. Total daily dosage should not exceed 300 mg. **Note: Actual dosage and administration schedule must be determined by the physician for each patient individually.**

Conditions Requiring Dosing Adjustments

Liver function: Patients with both liver and kidney compromise should have the dose decreased. This drug can cause liver problems, and a benefit to risk decision should be made in patients with liver compromise.

Kidney function: Patients with moderate to severe kidney failure should be given the usual dose, but only every 12 to 24 hours.

Malnutrition: Lower than expected levels may occur in patients with malnutrition. If clinical progress is not as expected, the dose may need to be increased.

▷ **Dosing Instructions:**   The tablet may be crushed and the capsule opened, then best taken on an empty stomach, 1 hour before or 2 hours after eating. If stomach irritation occurs, it may be taken with food or milk. (Unlike other tetracyclines, the doxycycline absorption is not significantly changed by food or milk.) Take at same time each day, with a full glass of water or milk. Take the full course prescribed.

Usual Duration of Use: The time needed to control the infection and be free of fever and symptoms for 48 hours. This varies with the nature of the infection.

▷ **This Drug Should Not Be Taken If**
- you are allergic to any tetracycline drug (see Drug Classes).
- you are pregnant or breast-feeding.
- you have severe liver disease.

▷ **Inform Your Physician Before Taking This Drug If**
- you are taking a penicillin antibiotic (see Drug Classes).
- you have a history of any of the following: Liver or kidney disease, lupus erythematosus.
- it is prescribed for a child under 8 years old.
- you are taking any anticoagulant drug.
- you plan to have surgery under general anesthesia in the near future.

Possible Side Effects (natural, expected, and unavoidable drug actions)
Superinfections (see Glossary), often due to yeast organisms. These can occur in the mouth, intestinal tract, rectum, and/or vagina, resulting in rectal and vaginal itching.

▷ **Possible Adverse Effects** (unusual, unexpected, and infrequent reactions)
If any of the following develop, consult your physician promptly for guidance.
Mild Adverse Effects
Allergic Reactions: Skin rash, hives, itching of hands and feet, swelling of face or extremities.
Loss of appetite, nausea, vomiting, diarrhea.
Loss of smell (anosmia) (rare).
Irritation of mouth or tongue, "black tongue," sore throat, abdominal cramping or pain.
Increased eosinophils.
Distortion of smell (dysosmia), perception of foul odors.
Serious Adverse Effects
Allergic Reactions: Anaphylactic reaction (see Glossary), asthma, fever, swollen joints, abnormal bleeding or bruising, jaundice (see Glossary).
Permanent discoloration and/or malformation of teeth when taken by children under 8 years of age, including unborn child and infant.
Ulceration of the esophagus.
Liver toxicity.
Systemic lupus erythematosus (rare).
Blood cell disorders (hemolytic anemia, thrombocytopenia, neutropenia, or eosinophilia).
Kidney toxicity.
Serious skin reactions (erythema multiforme or Stevens-Johnson syndrome).

▷ **Possible Effects on Sexual Function:**   None reported.

Natural Diseases or Disorders That May Be Activated by This Drug
Systemic lupus erythematosus.

Possible Effects on Laboratory Tests

Complete blood cell counts: decreased red cells, hemoglobin, white cells and platelets; increased eosinophils (allergic reaction).

Prothrombin time: increased.

Kidney function tests: increased blood creatinine and urea nitrogen (BUN) levels; increased urine protein (kidney damage).

CAUTION

1. Antacids and preparations containing aluminum, bismuth, iron, magnesium or zinc can prevent adequate drug absorption.
2. Troublesome and persistent diarrhea can occur. If diarrhea persists for more than 24 hours, stop this drug and call your doctor.

Precautions for Use

By Infants and Children: If possible, tetracyclines should not be given to those under 8 years old because of the risk of permanent tooth discoloration and deformity. Rarely, infants may develop increased intracranial pressure within the first 4 days of receiving this drug. Tetracyclines may inhibit normal bone growth and development.

By Those over 60 Years of Age: Natural skin changes may predispose to severe and prolonged itching reactions in the genital and anal regions.

▷ ## Advisability of Use During Pregnancy

Pregnancy Category: D. See Pregnancy Code at the back of this book.

Animal studies: Tetracycline causes limb defects in rats, rabbits and chickens.

Human studies: Information from studies of pregnant women indicates that drugs of this class can cause impaired development and discoloration of teeth and other developmental defects.

It is advisable to avoid this drug completely during entire pregnancy.

Advisability of Use if Breast-Feeding

Presence of this drug in breast milk: Yes.

Avoid drug or refrain from nursing.

Habit-Forming Potential: None.

Effects of Overdosage: Nausea, vomiting, diarrhea, acute liver damage (rare).

Possible Effects of Long-Term Use: Superinfections (see Glossary), prolongation of prothrombin time.

Suggested Periodic Examinations While Taking This Drug (at physician's discretion)

Complete blood cell counts, liver and kidney function tests.

During extended use, sputum and stool examinations may detect early superinfection due to yeast organisms.

▷ ## While Taking This Drug, Observe the Following

Foods: Avoid meats and iron-fortified cereals and supplements for 2 hours before and after taking this drug. Avoid combination with dairy products or calcium supplements.

Beverages: No restrictions. May be taken with milk or carbonated beverages.

▷ *Alcohol:* Shortened half life and decreased antibiotic benefit. Best avoided if you have active liver disease.

Tobacco Smoking: No interactions expected.

▷ *Other Drugs*
Doxycycline may *increase* the effects of
  - oral anticoagulants such as warfarin, and make it necessary to reduce their dosage.
  - digoxin (Lanoxin), and cause digitalis toxicity.
  - lithium (Eskalith, Lithane, etc.), and increase the risk of lithium toxicity.
Doxycycline may *decrease* the effects of
  - birth control pills (oral contraceptives), and **impair their effectiveness, resulting in pregnancy.**
  - penicillins, and impair their effectiveness in treating infections.
The following drugs may *decrease* the effects of doxycycline
  - antacids (aluminum and magnesium preparations, sodium bicarbonate, etc.) may reduce drug absorption.
  - barbiturates (see Drug Classes).
  - bismuth preparations (Pepto-Bismol, etc.).
  - calcium supplements (various).
  - carbamazepine (Tegretol).
  - cimetidine (Tagamet).
  - phenobarbital.
  - phenytoin (Dilantin).
  - iron and mineral preparations (such as zinc salts) may reduce drug absorption.

▷ *Driving, Hazardous Activities:* Usually no restrictions. Watch for nausea or diarrhea.
Aviation Note: The use of this drug *may be a disqualification* for piloting. Consult a designated Aviation Medical Examiner.
Exposure to Sun: Use caution—tetracyclines can cause photosensitivity (see Glossary).

ENALAPRIL (e NAL a pril)

Introduced: 1981   **Prescription:** USA: Yes   **Available as Generic:** No   **Class:** Antihypertensive, ACE inhibitor   **Controlled Drug:** USA: No
Brand Names: ✤Vaseretic (also available in US) [CD], Vasotec

BENEFITS versus RISKS	
Possible Benefits	*Possible Risks*
EFFECTIVE CONTROL OF MILD TO SEVERE HIGH BLOOD PRESSURE	Headache, dizziness, fatigue, and low blood pressure (all infrequent)
Possibly beneficial as adjunctive treatment in selected cases of congestive heart failure	Bone marrow depression (rare)
	Allergic swelling of face, tongue, or vocal cords (very rare)
	Increased blood potassium (rare)

▷ **Principal Uses**
As a Single Drug Product
Uses currently included in FDA approved labeling: (1) treatment of all degrees of high blood pressure; (2) adjunctive treatment of symptomatic congestive heart failure.

Other (unlabeled) generally accepted uses: (1) angina therapy; (2) captopril induced protein in the urine; (3) kidney failure in diabetics; (4) pheochromocytoma (a rare tumor which increases blood pressure).

How This Drug Works: By blocking certain enzyme systems (angiotensin converting enzymes—ACE) that influence arterial function, this drug contributes to relaxation of arterial walls and lowers blood pressure. This reduces the workload of the heart and improves its performance.

Available Dosage Forms and Strengths
Injection — 1.25 mg per ml
Tablets — 2.5 mg, 5 mg, 10 mg, 20 mg

▷ **Usual Adult Dosage Range:** For high blood pressure: Initially 5 mg once daily for weeks. Usual maintenance dose is 10 to 40 mg/day in a single dose or divided into 2 equal doses. Total daily dose should not exceed 40 mg if kidney function is impaired.

For heart failure: 2.5 to 10 mg once or twice daily. Usually combined with other medications. Maximum is 40 mg daily. **Note: Actual dosage and administration schedule must be determined by the physician for each patient individually.**

Conditions Requiring Dosing Adjustments
Liver function: In patients with liver compromise, the dose may need to be **increased** because less of the drug is activated.
Kidney function: Patients with mild to moderate kidney failure can be given 5 mg per day. In severe kidney failure, maximum dose is 2.5 mg per day.
Diabetes: Patients with diabetes with decreased creatinine clearance and protein in the urine (proteinuria) should be given decreased doses.

▷ **Dosing Instructions:** Tablet may be crushed and taken on an empty stomach or with food, at same time each day.

Usual Duration of Use: Use on a regular schedule for several weeks is needed to see this drug's effectiveness in controlling high blood pressure. Treatment of high blood pressure usually requires the long-term therapy.

▷ **This Drug Should Not Be Taken If**
• you have had an allergic reaction to it previously.
• you have angioedema from other ace inhibitors (swelling of the tongue, face or glottis).
• you are pregnant (last 6 months).
• you have active liver disease.

▷ **Inform Your Physician Before Taking This Drug If**
• you have had an allergic reaction (or other adverse effect) from any other ACE inhibitor (see Drug Classes).
• you are planning pregnancy.
• you have severe liver disease.
• you take immunosuppressant medicines.
• you currently have a blood cell or bone marrow disorder.
• you have a history of kidney disease or impaired kidney function.
• you have scleroderma or systemic lupus erythematosus.
• you have an abnormally high level of blood potassium.
• you have any form of heart disease.

- you have renal artery stenosis (talk with your doctor).
- you have diabetes.
- you are taking other antihypertensives, diuretics, nitrates or potassium supplements.
- you have an autoimmune disease.
- you have swelling of the face or tongue. Call your doctor immediately if this occurs.
- you plan to have surgery under general anesthesia in the near future.

Possible Side Effects (natural, expected, and unavoidable drug actions)

Dizziness, light-headedness, fainting (excessive drop in blood pressure).

▷ **Possible Adverse Effects** (unusual, unexpected, and infrequent reactions)

If any of the following develop, consult your physician promptly for guidance.

Mild Adverse Effects

Allergic Reactions: Skin rash, itching.

Headache, fatigue, drowsiness, nervousness, numbness and tingling, insomnia.

Rapid heart rate, palpitation.

Indigestion, taste disorders, stomach pain, nausea, vomiting, diarrhea.

Vulvovaginal itching.

Excessive sweating, muscle cramps.

Cough.

Ringing in the ears.

Baldness (rare).

Dizziness.

Serious Adverse Effects

Allergic Reactions: Swelling (angioedema) of face, tongue, and/or vocal cords: Can be life-threatening.

Bone marrow depression—fatigue, weakness, fever, sore throat, abnormal bleeding or bruising (very rare).

Problems with blood clotting (reduced platelet aggregation).

Excessively low blood pressure.

Pancreatitis (rare).

Kidney toxicity.

Liver toxicity.

Rare peripheral neuropathy.

Laryngeal edema (rare).

Depression (rare).

Hallucinations (rare).

Elevated blood potassium (rare).

▷ **Possible Effects on Sexual Function:**   Rare report of impotence, rare swelling and tenderness of male breast tissue (gynecomastia). Rare itching of the vulva and vagina.

Possible Effects on Laboratory Tests

Blood eosinophil counts: increased (allergic reaction).

Blood creatinine level: increased.

Blood potassium level: increased.

Blood uric acid level: decreased.

CAUTION

1. Consult your physician regarding the advisability of discontinuing other antihypertensive drugs (especially diuretics) for 1 week before starting this drug.
2. **Tell your doctor immediately if you become pregnant.** This drug should not be taken beyond the first 3 months of pregnancy.
3. **Report promptly** any signs of infection (fever, sore throat), or water retention (weight gain, puffiness, swollen feet or ankles).
4. Do not use a salt substitute without your physician's knowledge and approval. (Many salt substitutes contain potassium.)
5. Blood counts and urine analyses are needed **before** starting this drug.

Precautions for Use

By Infants and Children: Safety and effectiveness for those in this age group not established.

By Those over 60 Years of Age: Small starting doses are advisable. Sudden or excessive lowering of blood pressure can predispose to stroke or heart attack.

▷ **Advisability of Use During Pregnancy**

Pregnancy Category: D during the last six months (second and third trimesters). C during the first three months. See Pregnancy Code at the back of this book.

Animal studies: No birth defects found in rat or rabbit studies.

Human studies: Use of ACE inhibitor drugs during the last 6 months of pregnancy is known to possibly cause very serious injury and death to the fetus; skull and limb malformations, lung defects, and kidney failure have been reported in over 50 cases worldwide.

Avoid this drug completely during the last 6 months of pregnancy. During the first 3 months, ask your physician for help.

Advisability of Use if Breast-Feeding

Presence of this drug in breast milk: Yes.

Watch nursing infant closely and discontinue drug or nursing if adverse effects develop.

Habit-Forming Potential: None.

Effects of Overdosage: Excessive drop in blood pressure—light-headedness, dizziness, fainting.

Possible Effects of Long-Term Use: Gradual increase in blood potassium level.

Suggested Periodic Examinations While Taking This Drug (at physician's discretion)

Before starting drug: Complete blood cell counts; urine analysis with measurement of protein content; blood potassium level.

During use of drug: Blood cell counts; measurements of blood potassium.

▷ **While Taking This Drug, Observe the Following**

Foods: Consult physician regarding salt intake.

Nutritional Support: **Do not take** potassium supplements unless directed by your physician.

Beverages: No restrictions. May be taken with milk.

▷ *Alcohol:* Use caution until combined effect has been determined. Alcohol may enhance the blood-pressure-lowering effect of this drug.

Tobacco Smoking: No interactions expected.

▷ *Other Drugs*

Enalapril *taken concurrently* with

- allopurinol can result in serious skin reactions.
- aspirin or other NSAIDs (see Drug Classes) can lessen therapeutic benefit of enalapril.
- azathioprine can cause severe impairment of blood formation (myelosuppression).
- cyclosporine (Sandimmune) can cause acute kidney failure.
- ethacrynic acid can cause excessive lowering of blood pressure.
- lithium can lead to lithium toxicity.
- loop diuretics (see Drug Classes) can cause severe lowering of blood pressure upon standing up from a sitting position.
- oral hypoglycemic agents (glyburide-Glynase, others) may result in decreased insulin resistance and the need to decrease the dose of the oral hypoglycemic agent.
- phenothiazines (see Drug Classes) can cause additive lowering of blood pressure.
- potassium preparations (K-Lyte, Slow-K, etc.) may cause increased blood levels of potassium with risk of serious heart rhythm disturbances.
- potassium-sparing diuretics: amiloride (Moduretic), spironolactone (Aldactazide), triamterene (Dyazide) may cause increased potassium with risk of serious heart rhythm disturbances.
- rifampin or rifabutin may cause decreased therapeutic benefit from enalapril.
- thiazide diuretics (hydrochlorothiazide, others) may result (especially in older people) in increased levels of enalaprilat (the active medicine) and increased reduction in blood pressure. Doses may need to be decreased if this combination is used.

▷ *Driving, Hazardous Activities:* Usually no restrictions. Be aware of possible drops in blood pressure with resultant dizziness or faintness.

Aviation Note: The use of this drug *may be a disqualification* for piloting. Consult a designated Aviation Medical Examiner.

Exposure to Sun: Caution advised. A similar drug from this class can cause photosensitivity.

Exposure to Heat: Caution advised. Avoid excessive perspiring with resultant loss of body water and drop in blood pressure.

Occurrence of Unrelated Illness: Promptly report any nausea, vomiting or diarrhea. Fluid and chemical imbalances must be corrected as soon as possible.

EPINEPHRINE (ep i NEF rin)

Other Name: Adrenaline

Introduced: 1900   **Prescription:** USA: Varies; Canada: No   **Available as Generic:** USA: Yes; Canada: No   **Class:** Antiasthmatic, antiglaucoma, decongestant   **Controlled Drug:** USA: No; Canada: No

Brand Names: Adrenalin, Adreno-Mist, Ana-Kit, Asthmahaler, Asthmanephrine, Bronkaid Mist, ✦Bronkaid Mistometer, ✦Citanest Forte, Duranest

[CD], ✦Dysne-Inhal, Epifrin, E-Pilo Preparations [CD], Epinal Ophthalmic, EpiPen, Epitrate, Marcaine, Medihaler-Epi Preparations, Micronephrine, Norocaine, Octocaine, P1E1, P2E1, P3E1, P4E1, P6E1, Primatene Mist, Propine Ophthalmic, Sensoricaine, Sus-Phrine, Thalfed [CD], Therex [CD], ✦Ultracaine, Vaponefrin, Xylocaine

---

BENEFITS versus RISKS

Possible Benefits	*Possible Risks*
EFFECTIVE RELIEF OF SEVERE ALLERGIC (ANAPHYLACTIC) REACTIONS	Significant increase in blood pressure (in sensitive people)
TEMPORARY RELIEF OF ACUTE BRONCHIAL ASTHMA	Idiosyncratic Reaction: pulmonary edema (fluid formation in lungs)
Reduction of internal eye pressure (treatment of glaucoma)	Heart rhythm disorders (in sensitive individuals)
Relief of allergic congestion of the nose and sinuses	

▷ **Principal Uses**

As a Single Drug Product: Uses currently included in FDA approved labeling: (1) Inhalation to relieve acute attacks of bronchial asthma; (2) as a decongestant for symptomatic relief of allergic nasal congestion and as eye drops in the management of glaucoma; (3) used in treatment of anaphylactic shock; (4) used in emergency situations to treat abnormal heart rhythms and in cardio-pulmonary resuscitation; (5) used as an aid to increase the beneficial effects of topical anesthetics.

Other (unlabeled) generally accepted uses: (1) septic shock; (2) wheezing in infants; (3) croup; (4) can have a role in easing painful erections (priapism).

How This Drug Works: By stimulating some nerve terminals (sympathetic), this drug acts to

- contract blood vessel walls and raise the blood pressure.
- inhibit release of histamine into skin and internal organs.
- dilate constricted bronchial tubes, increasing the size of the airways and improving the ability to breathe.
- decrease fluid formation in the eye, increase its outflow from the eye and reduce internal eye pressure.
- decrease the amount of blood in the nose, shrinking swelling (decongestion) and expanding the nasal airway.

Available Dosage Forms and Strengths

Aerosol — 0.2 mg, 0.27 mg, 0.3 mg per spray
Eye drops — 0.1%, 0.25%, 0.5%, 1% and 2%
Injection — 0.01 mg, 0.1 mg, 1 mg, 5 mg per ml
Nose drops — 0.1%
Solution for nebulizer — 1%, 1.25% and 2.25%

▷ **Usual Adult Dosage Range:** Aerosols: 1 inhalation, repeated in 1 to 2 minutes if needed; wait 4 hours before next inhalation. Eye drops: 1 drop/12 hours. Dosage may vary with product; follow printed instructions and label directions. **Note: Actual dosage and administration schedule must be determined by the physician for each patient individually.**

Conditions Requiring Dosing Adjustments
   Liver function: Dosage reduction is not needed in liver compromise.
   Kidney function: Dosage adjustment is not defined in kidney compromise.

▷ **Dosing Instructions:**   Aerosols and inhalation solutions: After first inhalation, wait 1 to 2 minutes to determine if a second inhalation is necessary. If relief does not occur within 20 minutes of use, and difficult breathing persists, stop this drug and seek medical attention **promptly. Avoid prolonged and excessive use**. Eye drops: During instillation of drops and for 2 minutes following, press finger against the tear sac (inner corner of eye) to prevent rapid absorption of drug into body circulation.

Usual Duration of Use: According to individual needs. Long-term use requires physician supervision.

▷ **This Drug Should Not Be Taken If**
   • you have had an allergic reaction to any dosage form of it previously.
   • you have narrow-angle glaucoma.
   • you are in shock.
   • you have organic brain damage.
   • you are in labor—as it may delay the second stage of labor.
   • you are to undergo general anesthesia with cyclopropane or halogenated hydrocarbons.
   • your heart is dilated and you have a coronary deficiency.
   • you have experienced a recent stroke or heart attack.

▷ **Inform Your Physician Before Taking This Drug If**
   • you have any degree of high blood pressure.
   • you have any form of heart disease, especially coronary heart disease (with or without angina), or a heart rhythm disorder.
   • you have diabetes or overactive thyroid function (hyperthyroidism).
   • you have a history of stroke.
   • you have a chronic lung disease
   • you take: monoamine oxidase (MAO) type A inhibitors, phenothiazines (see Drug Classes Section), digitalis preparations or quinidine.

Possible Side Effects (natural, expected, and unavoidable drug actions)
   In some people—restlessness, anxiety, headache, tremor, palpitation, cold hands and feet, dryness of mouth and throat (with use of aerosol).

▷ **Possible Adverse Effects** (unusual, unexpected, and infrequent reactions)
   If any of the following develop, consult your physician promptly for guidance.
   Mild Adverse Effects
   Allergic Reactions: Skin rash; eyedrops may cause redness, swelling, and itching of the eyelids.
   Weakness, dizziness, pallor.
   Serious Adverse Effects
   Idiosyncratic Reaction: Sudden development of excessive fluid in the lungs (pulmonary edema).
   In predisposed individuals—excessive rise in blood pressure with risk of stroke (cerebral hemorrhage).
   Rapid heart rate and arrhythmias.
   Seizures (rare).

Porphyria (rare).

Pulmonary edema.

Pigmentation of the eye.

Kidney toxicity (rare).

Porphyria (rare).

▷ **Possible Effects on Sexual Function:** May be of help in painful and abnormally prolonged erections (priapism).

Possible Effects on Laboratory Tests

Complete blood counts: red cells and white cells increased; eosinophils decreased.

Blood glucose level: increased.

Urine sugar tests: false low or negative results with Clinistix; true positive with Benedict's or Fehling's solution.

Acidosis.

Blood platelets: temporarily increased.

CAUTION

1. Medication failure can result from frequent repeat use at short intervals. If this develops, avoid use for 12 hours, and a normal response should return.

2. Excessive use of aerosol preparations in asthmatics has been associated with sudden death.

3. This drug can cause significant irritability of the nerve pathways (conduction system) and muscles of the heart, predisposing to serious heart rhythm disorders. Consult your doctor if you have a heart disorder.

4. This drug can increase blood sugar level. If you have diabetes, test for sugar often to detect significant changes.

5. If you become unresponsive to this drug and you substitute isoproterenol (Isuprel), allow an interval of 4 hours between drugs.

6. Promptly throw this drug away if a pink to red to brown or cloudiness (precipitation) occurs.

Precautions for Use

By Infants and Children: Use cautiously in small doses until tolerance is determined. Watch for any indications of weakness, light-headedness or inclination to faint.

By Those over 60 Years of Age: Small doses are indicated. Observe for: Nervousness, headache, tremor, rapid heart rate. If you have hardening of the arteries (arteriosclerosis), heart disease, high blood pressure, Parkinson's disease or prostatism (see Glossary), this drug may aggravate your disorder. Ask your doctor for help.

▷ **Advisability of Use During Pregnancy**

Pregnancy Category: C. See Pregnancy Code at the back of this book.

Animal studies: Birth defects reported in rats.

Human studies: Adequate studies of pregnant women are not available.

This drug can cause significant reduction of oxygen supply to the fetus. Use it only if clearly needed and in small, infrequent doses. Avoid during the first 3 months and during labor and delivery.

Advisability of Use if Breast-Feeding

Presence of this drug in breast milk: Yes.

Avoid drug or refrain from nursing.

Habit-Forming Potential: Tolerance to this drug can develop with frequent use (see Glossary), but dependence does not occur.

Effects of Overdosage: Nervousness, throbbing headache, dizziness, tremor, palpitation, disturbance of heart rhythm, difficult breathing, abdominal pain, vomiting of blood.

Possible Effects of Long-Term Use: "Epinephrine-fastness": loss of ability to respond to this drug's bronchodilator effect. With long-term treatment of glaucoma: Pigment deposits on eyeball and eyelids, possible damage to retina, impaired vision, blockage of tear ducts.

Suggested Periodic Examinations While Taking This Drug (at physician's discretion)

Blood pressure measurements; blood or urine sugar measurements in diabetics; vision testing and measurement of internal eye pressure in glaucoma.

▷ **While Taking This Drug, Observe the Following**

Foods: No restrictions, except those that cause you to have asthma.

Beverages: No restrictions.

▷ *Alcohol:* Alcoholic beverages can increase the urinary excretion of this drug.

Tobacco Smoking: No interactions expected. Follow physician's advice regarding smoking as it affects the condition under treatment.

▷ *Other Drugs*

Epinephrine *taken concurrently* with

- some beta blockers (carteolol, nadolol, propranolol) may cause increased blood pressure and decreased heart rate.
- chlorpromazine (Thorazine) or other phenothiazines (see Drug Classes) may cause decreased blood pressure and increased heart rate.
- furazolidone (Furoxone) may cause increased blood pressure.
- guanethidine (Esimil, Ismelin) may cause increased blood pressure.
- halothane may cause abnormal heartbeats.
- pilocarpine (Ocusert) may cause increased myopia.
- tricyclic antidepressants (amitriptyline, etc.) may cause increased blood pressure and heart rhythm disturbances.

▷ *Driving, Hazardous Activities:* This drug may cause dizziness or nervousness. Limit activities as necessary.

Aviation Note: The use of this drug *may be a disqualification* for piloting. Consult a designated Aviation Medical Examiner.

Exposure to Sun: No restrictions.

Heavy Exercise or Exertion: No interactions expected. However, exercise can induce asthma in sensitive individuals.

Occurrence of Unrelated Illness: Use caution in presence of severe burns. This drug can increase drainage from burned tissue and cause significant loss of tissue fluids and blood proteins.

Discontinuation: If this drug fails to provide relief after an adequate trial, stop it and call your doctor. It is dangerous to increase the dosage or frequency.

Special Storage Instructions: Protect drug from exposure to air, light and heat. Keep in a cool place, preferably in the refrigerator.

ERGOTAMINE (er GOT a meen)

Introduced: 1926   **Prescription:** USA: Yes; Canada: Yes   **Available as Generic:** No   **Class:** Antimigraine, ergot derivative   **Controlled Drug:** USA: No; Canada: No

Brand Names: ✦Bellergal [CD], Bellergal-S [CD], ✦Bellergal Spacetabs [CD], Cafergot [CD], Cafergot P-B [CD], Cafetrate [CD], Ercaf [CD], ✦Ergodryl [CD], Ergomar, Ergostat, Genergen, ✦Gravergol [CD], ✦Gynergen, Medihaler Ergotamine, ✦Megral [CD], Oxoids, Spastrin [CD], Wigraine [CD], Wigrettes

---

BENEFITS versus RISKS

Possible Benefits	*Possible Risks*
PREVENTION AND RELIEF OF VASCULAR HEADACHES: migraine, migrainelike and histamine headaches	GANGRENE OF THE FINGERS, TOES, OR INTESTINE AGGRAVATION OF CORONARY ARTERY DISEASE (ANGINA) INCREASED RISK OF ABORTION (if used during pregnancy)

▷ **Principal Uses**

As a Single Drug Product: Uses currently included in FDA approved labeling: (1) This drug is used to treat vascular headaches, especially migraine and "cluster" headaches. It is often effective in stopping the headache if taken within the first hour following the onset of pain. It may be used on a short-term basis in an attempt to prevent or abort "cluster" headaches during the period of their occurrence. The inhalation form provides rapid onset of action.

Other (unlabeled) generally accepted uses: (1) Helps to ease the symptoms of narcolepsy; (2) may have a role in patients who have a C5 quadriplegia in helping to treat excessive lowering of blood pressure which occurs on rising from a sitting position.

As a Combination Drug Product [CD]: This drug is combined with caffeine to take advantage of caffeine's ability to enhance its absorption. This makes a smaller dose of ergotamine effective, and reduces the risk of adverse effects with repeated use. This drug is also combined with belladonna (atropine) and one of the barbiturates to provide preparations that help premenstrual tension and the menopausal syndrome—nervousness, nausea, hot flushes and sweating.

How This Drug Works: By constricting the walls of blood vessels in the head, this drug prevents or relieves the excessive expansion (dilation) that causes the pain of migrainelike headaches.

Available Dosage Forms and Strengths

Aerosol — 9 mg per ml (0.36 mg/inhalation)
Nasal inhaler (Canada) — 9 mg/ml (360 mcg per dose)
Suppositories — 2 mg (in combination with 100 mg of caffeine)
Tablets, sublingual — 2 mg

▷ **Usual Adult Dosage Range:**   Inhalation: 1 spray (0.36 mg) at the onset of headache; repeat 1 spray after 30 to 60 minutes as needed for relief, up to a maximum of 6 sprays/24 hours. Do not exceed 15 sprays/week. Sublingual tablets: Dissolve 2 mg under tongue at the onset of headache; repeat 2 mg in 30 to 60 minutes as needed, up to a maximum of 6 mg/attack. Do not exceed 6 mg/24 hours or 10 mg/week. **Note: Actual dosage and administration schedule must be determined by the physician for each patient individually.**

Conditions Requiring Dosing Adjustments
Liver function: Should be used with caution in patients with liver compromise.
Kidney function: This drug is a rare cause of acute renal failure, and should be used with caution in patients with compromised kidneys.

▷ **Dosing Instructions:**   Follow written instructions and doses **carefully**. The regular tablets (combination drug) may be crushed for administration; the sustained-release tablets should be taken whole (not crushed). Sublingual tablets should be dissolved under the tongue, not swallowed.

Usual Duration of Use: Use on a regular schedule for several episodes of headache is often needed to see this drug's effectiveness in aborting or relieving the pain of vascular headache. Do not exceed recommended dosage schedules. If headaches are not controlled after several trials of maximal doses, ask your doctor about other treatments.

▷ **This Drug Should Not Be Taken If**
- you have had an allergic reaction to any dosage form.
- you are pregnant.
- you have a severe infection.
- you have any of the following conditions:
  angina pectoris (coronary artery disease)
  Buerger's disease
  hardening of the arteries (arteriosclerosis)
  high blood pressure (severe hypertension)
  ischemic heart disease
  peptic ulcer
  kidney disease or impaired kidney function
  liver disease or impaired liver function
  Raynaud's phenomenon
  thrombophlebitis
  severe itching

▷ **Inform Your Physician Before Taking This Drug If**
- you are allergic or overly sensitive to *any* ergot preparation.
- you are planning to have a face lift (rhytidectomy). This drug may cause serious skin flap problems.

Possible Side Effects (natural, expected, and unavoidable drug actions)
Usually infrequent and mild with recommended doses.
Some people may have cold hands and feet, with mild numbness and tingling.

▷ **Possible Adverse Effects** (unusual, unexpected, and infrequent reactions)
If any of the following develop, consult your physician promptly for guidance.

Mild Adverse Effects

Allergic Reactions: Localized swellings (angioedema), itching.

Headache, drowsiness, dizziness, confusion.

Chest pain, abdominal pain, numbness and tingling of fingers and toes, muscle pains in arms or legs.

Nausea, vomiting, diarrhea.

Serious Adverse Effects

Gangrene of the extremities—coldness; numbness; pain; dark discoloration; eventual loss of fingers, toes, or feet.

Gangrene of the intestine—severe abdominal pain and swelling; emergency surgery required.

Retroperitoneal fibrosis.

Fibrous changes in the lung (pleuropulmonary fibrosis).

Pain syndromes (reflex sympathetic dystrophy).

Insufficient blood flow to the heart (myocardial ischemia).

Arrhythmias.

Fibrous changes in the heart (myocardial fibrosis).

Porphyria.

Lesions of the rectum or anus (anorectal lesions).

Kidney failure.

▷ **Possible Effects on Sexual Function:**   None reported.

Natural Diseases or Disorders That May Be Activated by This Drug

Angina pectoris (coronary artery insufficiency), Buerger's disease, Raynaud's syndrome.

Possible Effects on Laboratory Tests

None reported.

CAUTION

1. Excessive use of this drug can provoke migraine headache and increase the frequency of its occurrence.
2. Do not exceed a total dose of 6 mg/24 hours or 10 mg/week of the oral form.
3. Individual drug sensitivity varies greatly. Some may have early toxic effects while taking recommended doses. Promptly report: Numbness in fingers or toes, muscle cramping, chest pain.

Precautions for Use

By Infants and Children: Safety and effectiveness for those under 12 years of age not established.

By Those over 60 Years of Age: Natural circulation changes may make you more susceptible to adverse effects of this drug. See the preceding list of disorders that are contraindications for the use of this drug.

▷ **Advisability of Use During Pregnancy**

Pregnancy Category: X. See Pregnancy Code at the back of this book.

Animal studies: Fetal deaths reported due to this drug.

Human studies: Information from studies of pregnant women indicates that this drug can cause abortion.

This drug should be avoided during the entire pregnancy.

Advisability of Use if Breast-Feeding

Presence of this drug in breast milk: Yes.

Avoid drug or refrain from nursing.

Habit-Forming Potential: None.

Effects of Overdosage: Manifestations of "ergotism": coldness of skin, severe muscle pains, tingling and burning pain in hands and feet, loss of blood supply to extremities resulting in tissue death (gangrene) in fingers and toes. Acute ergot poisoning: nausea, vomiting, diarrhea, cold skin, numbness of extremities, confusion, seizures, coma.

Possible Effects of Long-Term Use: A form of functional dependence (see Glossary) may develop, resulting in withdrawal headaches when the drug is discontinued.

Suggested Periodic Examinations While Taking This Drug (at physician's discretion)

Evaluation of circulation (blood flow) to the extremities.

▷ **While Taking This Drug, Observe the Following**

Foods: No interactions expected. Avoid all foods to which you are allergic; some migraine headaches are due to food allergies.

Beverages: No restrictions.

▷ *Alcohol:* Best avoided; alcohol can intensify vascular headache.

Tobacco Smoking: Best avoided; nicotine can further reduce the restricted blood flow produced by this drug.

Marijuana Smoking: Best avoided; additive effects can increase the coldness of hands and feet.

▷ *Other Drugs*

Ergotamine may *decrease* the effects of

• nitroglycerin, and reduce its effectiveness in preventing or relieving angina pain.

The following drugs may *increase* the effects of ergotamine

• beta blockers (see Drug Classes).
• dopamine.
• erythromycins: clarithromycin, E-Mycin, Eryc, etc. Azithromycin has not been reported to cause this effect.
• sumatriptan (Imitrex) can also result in extended vasospastic reactions.
• troleandomycin (TAO).

▷ *Driving, Hazardous Activities:* This drug may cause drowsiness or dizziness. Restrict activities as necessary.

Aviation Note: Vascular headache *is a disqualification* for piloting. Consult a designated Aviation Medical Examiner.

Exposure to Sun: No restrictions.

Exposure to Cold: Avoid as much as possible. Cold further reduces restricted blood flow to the extremities.

Discontinuation: Following long-term use, it may be necessary to withdraw this drug gradually to prevent withdrawal headache. Ask physician for guidance.

ERYTHROMYCIN (er ith roh MY sin)

Introduced: 1952　**Prescription:** USA: Yes; Canada: Yes　**Available as Generic:** Yes　**Class:** Antibiotic, macrolide　**Controlled Drug:** USA: No; Canada: No

Brand Names: AK-Mycin Ophthalmic, Akne-Mycin, ✦Apo-Erythro Base, ✦Apo-Erythro E-C, ✦Apo-Erythro-ES, ✦Apo-Erythro-S, A/T/S, Benzamycin [CD], C-Solve 2, EES, EES 200, EES 400, Emgel, E-Mycin, E-Mycin controlled release, E-Mycin E, E-Mycin 333, Eramycin, ✦Erybid, Eryc, Erycette, Eryderm, Erygel, Erymax, Erypar, EryPed, Ery-Tab, Erythrocin, ✦Erythromid, E-Solve 2, ETS-2%, Ilosone, Ilotycin, ✦Novorythro, PCE, Pediamycin, ✦Pediazole [CD], ✦PMS-Erythromycin, Robimycin, Sans-Acne, SK-Erythromycin, Staticin, ✦Stievamycin, T-Stat, Wyamycin E, Wyamycin S

BENEFITS versus RISKS	
Possible Benefits	*Possible Risks*
EFFECTIVE TREATMENT OF INFECTIONS due to susceptible microorganisms	Allergic reactions, mild and infrequent
	Liver reaction (most common with erythromycin estolate)
	Drug-induced colitis (rare)
	Superinfections (rare)

▷ **Principal Uses**

As a Single Drug Product: Uses currently included in FDA approved labeling: Treatment of (1) skin and skin structure infections (such as acne and Strep); (2) upper and lower respiratory tract infections, including "Strep" throat, diphtheria and several types of pneumonia; (3) gonorrhea and syphilis; (4) amebic dysentery; (5) Legionnaire's disease and (5) long-term prevention of recurrences of rheumatic fever. Effective use requires the precise identification of the causative organism and determination of its sensitivity to erythromycin; (6) treatment of mycoplasma pneumonia; (7) listeriosis; (8) neonatal conjunctivitis; (9) pertussis; (10) urethritis, (11) treatment of ear infections (otitis media).

Other (unlabeled) generally accepted uses: (1) Treatment of early Lyme disease; (2) treatment of Campylobacter jejuni infections; (3) used in chancroid; (4) helps sterilize the bowel before surgical procedures; (5) may help threatened preterm labor if the cause is ureaplasma organisms; (6) helps impetigo; (7) may have a role in Ogilvie's syndrome in restoring normal bowel function.

How This Drug Works: This drug prevents the growth and multiplication of susceptible organisms by interfering with their formation of essential proteins.

Available Dosage Forms and Strengths

Capsules — 125 mg, 250 mg
Capsules, enteric-coated — 125 mg, 250 mg
Drops — 100 mg per ml
Eye ointment — 5 mg per gram
Gel — 2%
Oral suspension — 125 mg, 250 mg per 5 ml
Skin ointment — 2%
Tablets — 250 mg, 500 mg
Tablets, chewable — 125 mg, 200 mg, 250 mg
Tablets, delayed release — 250 mg, 333 mg
Tablets, dispersible (Canada) — 500 mg

Tablets, enteric-coated — 250 mg, 333 mg, 500 mg
Tablets, film-coated — 250 mg, 500 mg
Topical solution — 1.5% and 2%

▷ **Usual Adult Dosage Range:**   250 to 500 mg/6 hours, according to nature and severity of infection. Total daily dosage should not exceed 4 grams. For endocarditis prophylaxis (stearate oral form): 1 gram 2 hours before procedure and 500 mg 6 hours later.
Pediatrics: oral erythromycin is usually given at a dose of 30 to 50 mg per kilogram per day and is divided into three or four doses. **Note: Actual dosage and administration schedule must be determined by the physician for each patient individually.**

Conditions Requiring Dosing Adjustments
Liver function: This drug is metabolized in the liver, and will accumulate in patients with liver compromise. Decreased doses may be needed. It should be used with caution in patients with biliary tract disease.
Kidney function: Patients with severe kidney failure can be given 50–75 % of the usual dose at the usual time. It is a rare cause of interstitial nephritis (inflammation of a specific part of the kidney).

▷ **Dosing Instructions:**   Nonenteric-coated preparations should be taken 1 hour before or 2 hours after eating. Enteric-coated preparations may be taken without regard to food. Regular uncoated capsules may be opened and tablets may be crushed for administration; coated and prolonged-action preparations should be swallowed whole. Ask pharmacist for guidance.

Usual Duration of Use: Use on a regular schedule for 3 to 5 days is necessary to determine this drug's effectiveness in controlling infections. For streptococcal infections: Not less than 10 consecutive days (without interruption) to reduce the possibility of developing rheumatic fever or glomerulonephritis. The duration of use should not exceed the time required to eliminate the infection.

▷ **This Drug Should Not Be Taken If**
• you have had an allergic reaction to any form of erythromycin previously.
• you have active liver disease (estolate form).
• you are allergic to para amino benzoic acid type anesthetics (of concern with intramuscular form of erythromycin).
• you are taking terfenadine or astemizole.

▷ **Inform Your Physician Before Taking This Drug If**
• you have a history of a previous "reaction" to erythromycin.
• you are allergic by nature: Hay fever, asthma, hives, eczema.
• you have a blood disorder.
• you have an abnormal heart rhythm.
• you have a history of porphyria.
• you have a history of kidney disorder.
• you have myasthenia gravis.
• you have a hearing disorder.
• you have taken the estolate form of erythromycin previously.

Possible Side Effects (natural, expected, and unavoidable drug actions)
Superinfections (see Glossary).

▷ **Possible Adverse Effects** (unusual, unexpected, and infrequent reactions)
If any of the following develop, consult your physician promptly for guidance.

Mild Adverse Effects
Allergic Reactions: Skin rash, hives, itching.
Nausea, vomiting, diarrhea, abdominal cramping.

Serious Adverse Effects
Allergic Reaction: Rare anaphylactic reaction (see Glossary).
Idiosyncratic Reactions: Liver reaction—nausea, vomiting, fever, jaundice (usually but not exclusively associated with erythromycin estolate).
Decreased white blood cells (rare).
Abnormal heart rhythm (rare).
Worsening of myasthenia gravis.
Low body temperature (hypothermia) (rare).
Pseudomembranous colitis (rare).
Pancreatitis (rare).
Kidney problems (interstitial nephritis).
Hearing loss (ototoxicity).

▷ **Possible Effects on Sexual Function:**   None reported.

▷ **Adverse Effects That May Mimic Natural Diseases or Disorders**
Liver toxicity may resemble acute gallbladder disease or viral hepatitis.

Possible Effects on Laboratory Tests
Complete blood cell counts: white cells may increase or decrease; eosinophils increased (allergic reaction); platelets decreased.
Prothrombin time: increased (drug taken concurrently with warfarin).
Liver function tests: liver enzymes increased (ALT/GPT, AST/GOT and alkaline phosphatase), increased bilirubin.

CAUTION
1. Take the **full dosage prescribed** to help prevent resistant bacteria.
2. If you have a history of liver disease or impaired liver function, avoid any form of erythromycin estolate.
3. If diarrhea develops and continues for more than 24 hours, consult your physician promptly.

Precautions for Use
By Infants and Children: Watch allergic children closely for indications of developing allergy to this drug. Observe also for evidence of gastrointestinal irritation.
By Those over 60 Years of Age: Watch for itching reactions in the genital and anal regions, often due to yeast superinfections. Observe also for evidence of hearing loss. Report such developments promptly.

▷ **Advisability of Use During Pregnancy**
Pregnancy Category: B. See Pregnancy Code at the back of this book.
Animal studies: Studies of rats are inconclusive.
Human studies: Information from adequate studies of pregnant women is not available.
Generally thought to be safe during entire pregnancy, *except for erythromycin estolate*; this form of erythromycin can cause toxic liver reactions during pregnancy and should be avoided.

Advisability of Use if Breast-Feeding
　Presence of this drug in breast milk: Yes.
　Watch nursing infant closely and discontinue drug or nursing if adverse effects develop.

Habit-Forming Potential: None.

Effects of Overdosage: Possible nausea, vomiting, diarrhea and abdominal discomfort.

Possible Effects of Long-Term Use: Superinfections (see Glossary).

Suggested Periodic Examinations While Taking This Drug (at physician's discretion)
　Liver function tests if the estolate form is used.

▷ **While Taking This Drug, Observe the Following**
　Foods: New formulation absorption is decreased by more than 70% (especially high fat meals) and effectiveness may be seriously compromised.
　Beverages: Avoid fruit juices and carbonated beverages for 1 hour after taking any nonenteric-coated preparation. May be taken with milk.
▷　*Alcohol:* Avoid if you have impaired liver function or are taking the estolate form.
　Tobacco Smoking: No interactions expected.
▷　*Other Drugs*
　　Erythromycin may ***increase*** the effects of
　　• carbamazepine (Tegretol), and cause toxicity.
　　• digoxin (Lanoxin), and cause toxicity.
　　• ergotamine (Cafergot, Ergostat, etc.), and cause impaired circulation to extremities.
　　• methylprednisolone (Medrol), and prednisone and cause excess steroid effects.
　　• theophylline (aminophylline, Theo-Dur, etc.), and cause toxicity.
　　• warfarin (Coumadin), and increase the risk of bleeding.
　　Erythromycin may ***decrease*** the effects of
　　• clindamycin.
　　• lincomycin.
　　• penicillins.
　　Erythromycin ***taken concurrently*** with
　　• astemizole may cause serious arrhythmias.
　　• birth control pills (oral contraceptives) can cause loss of effectiveness and result in pregnancy.
　　• cyclosporine (Sandimune) may result in cyclosporine toxicity.
　　• disopyramide may cause heart (cardiac) arrhythmias.
　　• loratadine (Claritin) may result in increased loratadine levels, but does not appear to cause the serious arrythmias of some of the other nonsedating antihistamines. Since loratadine levels may be increased, it may be prudent to decrease loratadine doses while taking erythromycin.
　　• lovastatin can cause rhabdomyolysis (serious muscle damage).
　　• midazolam may lead to excessive central nervous system depression.
　　• terfenadine can cause cardiac (heart) arrhythmias.
　　• triazolam may cause toxicity.
　　• trimexate decreases trimexate metabolism and leads to toxicity.
　　• valproic acid can lead to toxic blood levels.

▷ *Driving, Hazardous Activities:* This drug may cause nausea and/or diarrhea. Restrict activities as necessary.

Aviation Note: The use of this drug **may be a disqualification** for piloting. Consult a designated Aviation Medical Examiner.

Exposure to Sun: No restrictions.

Special Storage Instructions: Keep liquid forms refrigerated.

Observe the Following Expiration Times: Freshly mixed oral suspension—14 days. Premixed oral suspension—18 months. Ask pharmacist for help.

ESTROGENS (ES troh jenz)

Other Names: Chlorotrianisene, conjugated estrogens, esterified estrogens, estradiol, estriol, estrone, estropipate, quinestrol

Introduced: 1933 **Prescription:** USA: Yes; Canada: Yes **Available as Generic:** USA: Yes; Canada: No **Class:** Female sex hormones **Controlled Drug:** USA: No; Canada: No

Brand Names: ✤C.E.S., ✤Climestrone, ✤Congest, Delestrogen, DV, Estinyl, Estrace, Estraderm, Estraguard, Estratab, Estrovis, Feminone, ✤Femogen, ✤Femogex, Gynetone, Gynogen LA, Menest, Menotab, Menotab-M, Menrium [CD], Milprem [CD], ✤Minestrin, ✤Neo-Pause, ✤Oestrilin, Ogen, PMB [CD], PMS-Estradiol, Premarin, Prempro (a single tablet form with conjugated estrogens and medroxyprogesterone has been FDA approved), Progynon Pellet, TACE, Valergen-10, Vivelle (transdermal), White Premarin

BENEFITS versus RISKS	
Possible Benefits	*Possible Risks*
RELIEF OF MENOPAUSAL HOT FLASHES AND NIGHT SWEATS	INCREASED RISK OF CANCER OF THE UTERUS with 3 years of continual use
PREVENTION OR RELIEF OF ATROPHIC VAGINITIS, ATROPHY OF THE VULVA AND URETHRA	INCREASED RISK OF BREAST CANCER (EVEN IF COMBINED WITH A PROGESTERONE)
PREVENTION OF OSTEOPOROSIS	
Prevention of thinning of the skin	Increased frequency of gallstones
Mental tonic effect	Accelerated growth of preexisting fibroid tumors of the uterus
Prevention of postmenopausal cardiovascular disease	Fluid retention
	Postmenopausal bleeding
	Deep vein thrombophlebitis and thromboembolism (less likely with conjugated estrogens, more likely with synthetic unconjugated hormones)
	Increased blood pressure (rare)
	Decreased sugar tolerance (rare)

▷ **Principal Uses**

As a Single Drug Product: This widely used hormone is very effective when administered in proper dosage and carefully supervised. Its primary use is supplemental ("replacement" therapy) when used to treat the following conditions: (1) ovarian failure or removal in the young woman; (2) the menopausal syndrome; (3) postmenopausal atrophy of genital tissues; and (4) postmenopausal osteoporosis. It is also used in selected cases of breast cancer and prostate cancer.

As a Combination Drug Product [CD]: Estrogen is available in combination with chlordiazepoxide (Librium) and with meprobamate (Equanil, Miltown). These mild tranquilizers are added to provide a calming effect that makes the combination more effective in treating selected cases of the menopausal syndrome. See the Drug Profile of the Oral Contraceptives for a discussion of the combination of estrogens and progestins.

Estrogen is also available in new combination packaging to help patients remember to take their medicine.

How This Drug Works: When used to correct hormonal deficiency states, estrogens restore normal cellular activity by increasing nuclear material and protein synthesis. The frequency and intensity of menopausal symptoms are reduced when normal tissue levels of estrogen are restored.

Available Dosage Forms and Strengths

Capsules — 12 mg, 25 mg, 72 mg (TACE)
Tablets — 0.02 mg, 0.05 mg, 0.1 mg, 0.3 mg, 0.5 mg, 0.625 mg, 0.9 mg, 1.25 mg, 2.5 mg
Transdermal patch — 0.025 mg (2 mg), 0.05 mg (4 mg) and 0.1 mg (8 mg)
— 2 mg (only in Canada)
Vaginal cream — 0.1 mg, 0.625 mg, 1.5 mg per gram

▷ **Usual Adult Dosage Range:**   For conjugated and esterified estrogens: 0.3 to 1.25 mg daily for 21 days. Omit for 7 days. Repeat cyclically as needed. For other forms of estrogen: consult your physician. **Note: Actual dosage and administration schedule must be determined by the physician for each patient individually.**

Conditions Requiring Dosing Adjustments

Liver function: The dose should be decreased in mild liver disease. Estrogens should not be used in acute or severe liver compromise. This drug can be lithogenic (capable of causing stones) in the bile.

Kidney function: No expected dosing changes in kidney compromise.

▷ **Dosing Instructions:**   The tablets may be crushed and may be taken without regard to food. The capsules should be taken whole.

Usual Duration of Use: Use on a regular schedule for 10 to 20 days is needed to see this drug's effectiveness in menopausal symptoms. Long-term use requires supervision and periodic evaluation by your physician every 6 months.

▷ **This Drug Should Not Be Taken If**
- you have had an allergic reaction to any form of it previously.
- you have a history of thrombophlebitis, embolism, heart attack or stroke.
- you have seriously impaired liver function or recent onset liver disease.
- you have abnormal and unexplained vaginal bleeding.
- you have sickle cell disease.
- you have or are suspected to have breast cancer (may be used to treat some kinds of breast cancer).

- known or suspected estrogen dependent cancer (you doctor would determine this).
- you are pregnant.

▷ **Inform Your Physician Before Taking This Drug If**
- you have had an unfavorable reaction to estrogen therapy previously.
- you have a history of cancer of the breast or reproductive organs.
- you have: Fibrocystic breast changes, fibroid tumors of the uterus, endometriosis, migrainelike headaches, epilepsy, asthma, heart disease, high blood pressure, gallbladder disease, diabetes or porphyria.
- you smoke tobacco on a regular basis.
- you have a history of blood-clotting disorders.
- you plan to have surgery in the near future.

Possible Side Effects (natural, expected, and unavoidable drug actions)

Fluid retention, weight gain, "breakthrough" bleeding (spotting in middle of menstrual cycle), altered menstrual pattern, resumption of menstrual flow (bleeding from the uterus) after a period of natural cessation (postmenopausal bleeding), increased susceptibility to yeast infection of the genital tissues.

▷ **Possible Adverse Effects** (unusual, unexpected, and infrequent reactions)

If any of the following develop, consult your physician promptly for guidance.

Mild Adverse Effects

Allergic Reactions: Skin rash, hives, itching.

Headache, nervous tension, irritability, accentuation of migraine headaches.

Nausea, vomiting, bloating, diarrhea.

Tannish pigmentation of the face.

Serious Adverse Effects

Idiosyncratic Reaction: Cutaneous porphyria—fragility and scarring of the skin.

Emotional depression.

Can produce or worsen high blood pressure.

Gallbladder disease, benign liver tumors, jaundice, rise in blood sugar.

Erosion of uterine cervix, enlargement of uterine fibroid tumors.

Thrombophlebitis (inflammation of a vein with formation of blood clot)—pain or tenderness in thigh or leg, with or without swelling of foot or leg.

Pulmonary embolism (movement of blood clot to lung)—sudden shortness of breath, pain in chest, coughing, bloody sputum.

Benign liver tumors (adenomas).

Systemic lupus erythematosus (rare).

Stroke (blood clot in brain)—headaches, blackout, sudden weakness or paralysis of any part of the body, severe dizziness, altered vision, slurred speech, inability to speak.

Endometrial cancer (how long increased risk continues if the drug is stopped is not clear).

Porphyria (rare).

Retinal thrombosis (blood clot in eye vessels)—sudden impairment or loss of vision.

Heart attack (blood clot in coronary artery)—sudden pain in chest, neck, jaw, or arm; weakness; sweating; nausea. Has been associated with women taking higher doses and with men using estrogen to treat prostate cancer, however, this is not clearly decided as yet. Estrogen in lower doses appears to decrease overall risk of heart attack.

Increased risk of breast cancer (even if combined with a progesterone) (with long-term use—nine years).

Conjugated estrogens were not associated with increased overall relative risk of breast cancer in one large study.

▷ **Possible Effects on Sexual Function**

Swelling and tenderness of breasts, milk production.

Increased vaginal secretions.

Possible Delayed Adverse Effects: Estrogens taken during pregnancy can predispose the female child to the later development of cancer of the vagina or cervix following puberty.

▷ **Adverse Effects That May Mimic Natural Diseases or Disorders**

Liver reactions may suggest viral hepatitis.

Natural Diseases or Disorders That May Be Activated by This Drug

Latent hypertension, diabetes mellitus, acute intermittent porphyria.

Possible Effects on Laboratory Tests

Red blood cells, hemoglobin and platelets: decreased.

Blood calcium level: increased.

Blood total cholesterol level: decreased (treatment effect); increased in post menopausal women.

Blood LDL cholesterol level: decreased in post menopausal women.

Blood triglyceride level: no drug effect in post menopausal women.

Blood glucose level: increased.

Glucose tolerance test (GTT): decreased.

Blood thyroid hormone (T_3 and T_4) levels: increased.

Blood uric acid level: decreased.

Liver function tests: increased liver enzymes (ALT/GPT, AST/GOT and alkaline phosphatase), increased bilirubin.

CAUTION

1. To avoid prolonged (uninterrupted) stimulation of breast and uterine tissues, estrogen should be taken in cycles of 3 weeks on and 1 week off of medication.

2. The estrogen in estrogen vaginal creams is absorbed systemically. It may also be absorbed through the penis during sexual intercourse and can cause enlargement and tenderness of male breast tissue.

Precautions for Use

By Those over 60 Years of Age: Very limited usefulness after 60. Restricted to women who are at increased risk for osteoporosis. In this age group, it is advisable to attempt relief of hot flushes with nonestrogenic medications. During use, report promptly any indications of impaired circulation: speech disturbances, altered vision, sudden hearing loss, vertigo, sudden weakness or paralysis, angina, leg pains.

▷ **Advisability of Use During Pregnancy**

Pregnancy Category: X. See Pregnancy Code at the back of this book.

Animal studies: Genital defects reported in mice and guinea pigs; cleft palate reported in rodents.

Human studies: Information from studies of pregnant women indicates that estrogens can masculinize the female fetus. In addition, limb defects and heart malformations have been reported.

It is now known that estrogens taken during pregnancy can predispose the female child to the development of cancer of the vagina or cervix following puberty. *Avoid estrogens completely during entire pregnancy.*

Advisability of Use if Breast-Feeding

Presence of this drug in breast milk: Yes, in minute amounts.

Estrogens in large doses can suppress milk formation.

Breast-feeding is considered to be safe during the use of estrogens.

Malnourished mothers may have unacceptable decreases in protein and nitrogen in their breast milk if this drug is used while breast feeding.

Habit-Forming Potential: There has been some suggestion of estrogens having potential for pscyhological dependence and tolerance because of their mood elevating properties, but clinical reports have not been presented.

Effects of Overdosage: Headache, drowsiness, nausea, vomiting, fluid retention, abnormal vaginal bleeding, breast enlargement and discomfort.

Possible Effects of Long-Term Use: High blood pressure, gallbladder disease with gallstone formation, increased growth of benign fibroid tumors of the uterus. Several reports suggest possible association between the long-term use (3+ years) of estrogens and the development of cancer of the lining of the uterus. Further studies are needed to establish a definite cause-and-effect relationship (see Glossary). Prudence dictates that women with uterus intact should use estrogens only when symptoms justify it and with proper supervision.

Suggested Periodic Examinations While Taking This Drug (at physician's discretion)

Regular (every 6 months) evaluation of the breasts and pelvic organs, including Pap smears. Liver function tests as indicated.

▷ **While Taking This Drug, Observe the Following**

Foods: Avoid excessive use of salt if fluid retention occurs. Combined use of calcium can be a further step to help avoid osteoporosis.

Beverages: No restrictions. May be taken with milk.

▷ *Alcohol:* No interactions expected.

Tobacco Smoking: Recent studies indicate that heavy smoking (15 or more cigarettes daily) in association with the use of estrogen-containing oral contraceptives significantly increases the risk of heart attack (coronary thrombosis). Avoid heavy smoking during long-term estrogen therapy.

▷ *Other Drugs*

Estrogens *taken concurrently* with

- antidiabetic drugs may cause unpredictable fluctuations of blood sugar.
- oral hypoglycemic agents (see Drug Classes) or oral blood sugar lowering medicines may cause loss of glucose control and high blood sugars.
- thyroid hormones may increase the bound (inactive) drug and require an increase in thyroid dose.
- tricyclic antidepressants (Elavil, Sinequan, etc.) may enhance their adverse effects and reduce their antidepressant effectiveness.
- vitamin C (ascorbic acid, various brands) in higher doses may result in in-

creased estrogen effects. A lower dose of estrogens may be indicated if ongoing higher dose vitamin C will be taken.
- warfarin (Coumadin) may cause alterations of prothrombin activity. Increased doses may be needed.

The following drugs may **decrease** the effects of estrogens
- carbamazepine (Tegretol).
- phenobarbital.
- phenytoin (Dilantin).
- primidone (Mysoline).
- rifampin (Rifadin, Rimactane).

▷ *Driving, Hazardous Activities:* Usually no restrictions. Consult your physician
for assessment of individual risk and for guidance regarding specific restrictions.

Aviation Note: Usually no restrictions. However, watch for the rare occurrence
of disturbed vision and restrict activities accordingly. Consult a designated
Aviation Medical Examiner.

Exposure to Sun: Use caution—these drugs can cause photosensitivity (see Glossary).

Discontinuation: Best to stop estrogens periodically to see if they are still
needed. The dose is reduced gradually to prevent acute withdrawal hot
flushes. Avoid continual, uninterrupted use of large doses. Stop altogether
when a definite need for replacement therapy has ended. Ask your doctor
for help.

ETHAMBUTOL (eth AM byu tohl)

Introduced: 1971   **Prescription:** USA: Yes; Canada: Yes   **Available as
Generic:** USA: No; Canada: No   **Class:** Anti-infective, antituberculosis drug
Controlled Drug: USA: No; Canada: No
Brand Names: ♣Etibi, Myambutol

BENEFITS versus RISKS	
Possible Benefits	*Possible Risks*
EFFECTIVE ADJUNCTIVE TREATMENT OF PULMONARY TUBERCULOSIS	RARE OPTIC NEURITIS WITH IMPAIRMENT OR LOSS OF VISION
EFFECTIVE ADJUNCTIVE TREATMENT OF AIDS-RELATED M. AVIUM-INTRACELLULARE INFECTIONS	Rare peripheral neuritis (see Glossary) Activation of gout
Possibly effective treatment of tuberculous meningitis	

▷ **Principal Uses**
As a Single Drug Product: Uses currently included in FDA approved labeling:
Treatment of pulmonary tuberculosis, in combination with other an-
titubercular drugs (currently three other medicines are added to etham-
butol).
Other (unlabeled) generally accepted uses: (1) Treatment of tuberculous men-

ingitis; (2) treatment of AIDS-related Mycobacterium avium-intracellulare (MAI) infections, in combination with other antimycobacterial drugs.

How This Drug Works: It enters mycobacterial cells that are actively dividing, and keeps them from reproducing by interfering with nuclear material (RNA).

Available Dosage Forms and Strengths

Tablets — 100 mg, 400 mg

▷ **Recommended Dosage Ranges** (Actual dosage and administration schedule must be determined by the physician for each patient individually.)

Infants and Children: Dosage not established. Some authorities recommend that children under 6 years of age not be given this drug.

13 to 60 Years of Age: For initial treatment of tuberculosis—15 mg/kg of body weight, once daily. The total daily dose should not exceed 500–1500 mg.

For retreatment of tuberculosis—25 mg/kg of body weight, once daily for 60 days; then 15 mg/kg of body weight. The total daily dose should not exceed 900–2500 mg.

For tuberculous meningitis or AIDS-related MAI infections—15 to 25 mg/kg of body weight, once daily.

Over 60 Years of Age: Same as 13 to 60 years of age.

Conditions Requiring Dosing Adjustments

Liver function: No dose decreases are anticipated in mild to moderate liver compromise.

Kidney function: For mild to moderate kidney failure, the usual dose can be given every 24–36 hours. Severe kidney failure only requires a dose every 48 hours.

▷ **Dosing Instructions:**   The tablet may be crushed and taken with food to reduce stomach irritation. Take full course prescribed.

Usual Duration of Use: Use on a regular schedule for 4 to 6 weeks is necessary to determine this drug's effectiveness in controlling infections. Long-term use (6 months to 2 or more years) requires periodic physician evaluation.

▷ **This Drug Should Not Be Taken If**
- you have had an allergic reaction to it previously.
- you currently have optic neuritis or peripheral neuritis.
- you currently have active gout.

▷ **Inform Your Physician Before Taking This Drug If**
- you have a history of gout.
- you have a history of optic neuritis or peripheral neuritis.
- you have diabetes or a history of alcoholism; these conditions predispose to eye problems (optic neuritis).
- you have impaired kidney function.
- you have a history of low blood platelets.

Possible Side Effects (natural, expected, and unavoidable drug actions)
Increased blood level of uric acid (50–66% of users).

▷ **Possible Adverse Effects** (unusual, unexpected, and infrequent reactions)
If any of the following develop, consult your physician promptly for guidance.

Mild Adverse Effects
    Allergic Reactions: Skin rash, itching, fever.
    Headache, confusion, disorientation.
    Loss of appetite, nausea, vomiting, stomach pain.
Serious Adverse Effects
    Allergic Reactions: Severe skin reactions, painful joints.
    Optic neuritis (one or both eyes): Eye pain, blurred vision, red–green color blindness.
    Peripheral neuritis (see Glossary): Numbness, tingling, burning, pain, and/or weakness in hands or feet.
    Low blood platelets or white blood cells (rare).
    Hallucinations.
    Porphyria (rare). Rare kidney problems (interstitial nephritis).
    Gouty arthritis.

▷ **Possible Effects on Sexual Function:** None reported.

Possible Delayed Adverse Effects: Optic neuritis may not happen until many months of therapy. Visual loss may continue for up to a year after stopping this drug, and may be permanent.

Natural Diseases or Disorders That May Be Activated by This Drug
    Latent gout.

Possible Effects on Laboratory Tests
    Complete blood cell counts: decreased white cells and platelets.
    Blood uric acid levels: increased.
    Liver function tests: increased liver enzymes (ALT/GPT, AST/GOT).
    Kidney function tests: increased blood urea nitrogen (BUN) and creatinine (rare kidney damage).

CAUTION
    1. Promptly report any vision changes; this could be the start of optic neuritis. Immediate evaluation is mandatory.
    2. Report promptly any unusual sensations in the hands or feet; these could indicate the onset of peripheral neuritis.

Precautions for Use
    By Infants and Children: Safety and effectiveness for those under 13 years of age not established.
    By Those over 60 Years of Age: Confusion or disorientation more likely. Age-related decrease in kidney function may require decreased doses.

▷ **Advisability of Use During Pregnancy**
    Pregnancy Category: B. See Pregnancy Code at the back of this book.
    Animal studies: Mouse and rabbit studies confirm multiple drug-induced birth defects.
    Human studies: Adequate studies of pregnant women are not available.
    Use this drug only if clearly needed. Ask your physician for guidance.

Advisability of Use if Breast-Feeding
    Presence of this drug in breast milk: Yes.
    Avoid drug or refrain from nursing.

Habit-Forming Potential: None.

Effects of Overdosage: Nausea, vomiting, stomach discomfort, confusion, possible blurred vision.

Possible Effects of Long-Term Use: Optic neuritis with significant visual impairment.

Suggested Periodic Examinations While Taking This Drug (at physician's discretion)
Complete eye examinations (including visual fields and color vision) should be performed before treatment is started and monthly during therapy.
Blood uric acid levels.
Liver and kidney function tests.

▷ **While Taking This Drug, Observe the Following**
Foods: Follow physician's advice regarding high-purine foods.
Beverages: Avoid excessive caffeine containing beverages such as coffee or some sodas.
▷ *Alcohol:* No interactions expected.
Tobacco Smoking: No interactions expected.
▷ *Other Drugs*
The following drugs may ***decrease*** the effects of ethambutol
• antacids containing aluminum salts can slow and reduce absorption.
Ethambutol ***taken concurrently*** with
• BCG vaccine may blunt the immune response which could have been given by the vaccine.
▷ *Driving, Hazardous Activities:* This drug may cause confusion, disorientation and impaired vision. Restrict activities as necessary.
Aviation Note: The use of this drug ***is a disqualification*** for piloting. Consult a designated Aviation Medical Examiner.
Exposure to Sun: No restrictions.
Discontinuation: This drug is generally used for long-term treatment—months to years. Ask your doctor about the appropriate time to stop this medicine.

ETHANOL (ETH an all)

Other Names: Prescription: None
nonprescription: Moonshine, alcohol, jack, white lightning, wine, beer, whiskey, vodka, others.

Introduced: 1980 (Prescription), 10 BC (nonprescription—perhaps earlier)
Prescription: USA: Yes (IV); Canada: Yes (IV) Canada: No   **Available as Generic:** USA: Yes; Canada: Yes   **Class:** Antianxiety drug (nonprescription form)   **Controlled Drug:** USA:No

Brand Names: Prescription: Tuss-Ornade (5%), Vicks Formula 44D, Temaril (5.7%), Nyquil Nightime Cold Medicine, Novahistine DMX Liquid, Eskaphen B, ✦Dilusol (38.7%), nonprescription: Robert Alison Chardonnay (12% by volume), Bud Dry, Glenlivet, Smirnoff (40% by volume), others,

Warning: The clinical use of this medication is limited to intravenous treatment of methanol and antifreeze (ethylene glycol) poisoning, and as a preservative. There are a huge number of products containing alcohol. Ask your pharmacist for help with ingredients if alcohol is forbidden for you. Past use has included treatment of premature labor (tocolytic).

This drug is widely used in its nonprescription form as an anti-anxiety agent. Recent data appear to show this as a benefit of moderate use. Some people may not experience any mental or physical changes even though a breath or blood alcohol says they are "legally drunk."

BENEFITS versus RISKS	
Possible Benefits	*Possible Risks*
EFFECTIVE TREATMENT OF POISONING	WITHDRAWAL SYMPTOMS SEIZURES
MODERATE use may decrease heart disease/heart attack risk	LIVER DAMAGE (with prolonged use)
	Pancreatitis
	Encephalopathy
	Low white blood cell counts and anemia
	Myopathy

▷ **Principal Uses**

As a Single Drug Product: Uses currently included in FDA approved labeling: (1) Supplementation of caloric intake intravenously in very specific cases.

Other (unlabeled) generally accepted uses: (1) Treatment of methanol or anti-freeze (ethylene glycol) poisoning; (2) adjunctive treatment of cancer pain; (3) intravenous treatment of DTs (delirium tremens); (4) used to sclerose esophageal varicies and stop bleeding; (5) treatment of hepatocellular cancer where severe liver problems preclude surgery; (6) used to sclerose thyroid cysts; (7) used to destroy nerve tissue (neurolytic block) in chronic pain therapy; (8) widely used in nonprescription form as an antianxiety agent; (9) recent data appears to show that use ranging up to moderate (and NO GREATER than 0.7 mg per kg for three days in a row) may actually help prevent coronary heart disease and heart attacks.

As a Combination Drug Product [CD]: Uses currently included in FDA approved labeling: (1) Widely present in elixirs and other liquid vehicles for drugs as a preservative, and partial drug action enhancer.

How This Drug Works: In overdose situations, this drug provides a less toxic alternative, and lets the body remove the antifreeze or methanol. When used in its nonprescription form in excess, it depresses nerve function and leads to emotional changes and disturbances of perception, coordination and intoxication.

Nonprescription use of up to moderate amounts appears to decrease risk of heart and blood vessel disease, but the way in which it does this is not known.

Available Dosage Forms and Strengths

Intravenous — 5%, 10% and 95%

nonprescription — Each ounce of 100 proof whiskey has 15 ml of ethanol
— 6 ounces (12%) wine has 22 ml of ethanol
— 12 ounces of beer (4.9%) has 18 ml of ethanol

▷ **Recommended Dosage Ranges (Actual dosage and administration schedule must be determined by the physician for each patient individually.)**

Infants and Children: Methanol or ethylene glycol poisoning: 40 ml per kg per day.

18 to 60 Years of Age: Methanol or ethylene glycol poisoning: A loading dose of 0.6 mg per kg is given, and followed by 109 to 125 mg per kg per hour to maintain a blood level of 100 mg/dl.

Coronary heart disease or heart attack prevention: It APPEARS THAT: use of moderate amounts (up to 0.8 g/kg per day or no more than 0.7 mg per kg per day for three days in a row) of alcohol may help in preventing risk of this kind of blood vessel disease and myocardial infarctions.

Over 60 Years of Age: Same as 12 to 60 years of age for poisonings. The amount consumed versus the collective mental and physical effects may decrease in older people for the nonprescription products. It will generally take less of a dose to cause an equal or greater change in coordination or mental ability. There is also an increased risk of hypothermia.

Conditions Requiring Dosing Adjustments

Liver function: Ethanol is extensively metabolized in the liver to acetaldehyde and acetyl co-A. The drug is also a clear cause of liver toxicity. The dose must be decreased in liver compromise.

Kidney function: Minimal involvement of the kidney in the elimination of this drug.

▷ **Dosing Instructions:**   If methanol or ethylene glycol poisoning is suspected— the nearest poison control center should be contacted, and oral dosing (use of a strong vodka mixed in orange juice) may be of benefit depending on your distance from a hospital or freestanding emergency center.

For nonprescription antianxiety use, the specific dose of this drug and the resulting blood level of alcohol depends on many factors, however, the more important ones are: the weight of the person, the metabolic activity of the liver, food content in the stomach, the strength of the alcohol in the consumed beverage, the number of "drinks" consumed over a given period of time, and how well hydrated (has there been extreme exercise and fluid loss) you are. Again, although a blood or breath alcohol may be a marker for mental or physical changes, some people may not have physical or mental changes and have a blood or breath alcohol which is in the state-defined range that constitutes being "legally drunk." Specific levels of blood or breath alcohol do not absolutely predict impairment.

Each 10 ml of ethanol increases the blood ethanol level of an average 150 lb (70 kg) man by 16.6 mg percent (3.6 mm/liter). The legal definition of intoxication is a blood alcohol level of 0.10 or 100 mg/dl. "Under the influence" in Maryland is .07 or 70 mg/dl. Driving impairment **may** occur at blood levels of 0.05% (50 mg/dl) or lower.

Usual Duration of Use: Use on a regular schedule for 48 hours determines effectiveness in methanol overdose. Long-term excessive use as an antianxiety agent is NOT recommended.

▷ **This Drug Should Not Be Taken If**
- you have had an allergic reaction to any dosage form of it previously.
- you have epilepsy.
- you have a history of alcohol addiction.

- you have a urinary tract infection.
- you are pregnant.
- you are in diabetic coma.

▷ **Inform Your Physician Before Taking This Drug If**
- you have liver or kidney compromise.
- you have gout.
- you are prone to low blood sugars.
- you are a diabetic.
- you have congestive heart failure.

Possible Side Effects (natural, expected, and unavoidable drug actions)
Intoxication, perception, coordination, and mood changes.

▷ **Possible Adverse Effects** (unusual, unexpected, and infrequent reactions)
If any of the following develop, consult your physician promptly for guidance.

Mild Adverse Effects
Allergic Reactions: Itching, rash, hives, and flushing.
Headache.
"Hangover": Nausea, headache, malaise.
Sedation (dose-dependent).
Disorientation.
Color blindness (with chronic use).
Neuropathy (tingling, burning, or numbness).
Memory loss.
Vitamin deficiency.
Stomach irritation.
Myopathy (with chronic use).

Serious Adverse Effects
Allergic Reactions: Anaphylaxis: rash, swelling of tongue, breathing problems, flushing.
Bronchospasm (asthmatics at increased risk).
Respiratory depression.
Elevated or decreased white blood cell count.
Increased or decreased platelets.
Anemia (megaloblastic with chronic use).
Heart dysfunction (myopathy with chronic use).
High blood pressure.
Abnormal heart rhythms (atrial and ventricular).
Chest pain (angina).
Liver toxicity (cirrhosis with chronic use).
Osteoporosis (with chronic use).
Pancreatitis.
Encephalopathy (with chronic use).
Cerebrovascular bleeding (dose-dependent).
Low blood sugar (especially if meals are missed).
Ketoacidosis (with chronic use).
Vitamin deficiency with chronic use (folic acid, vitamins B1 and B6).
Low magnesium (with chronic use).
Low potassium (especially with acute intoxication in children).
Gout (precipitated by alcohol use in those with gout).

Tolerance (with chronic use).

Withdrawal: Nausea, fever, rapid heart rate, hallucinations.

May progress to DTs (5%): profound confusion, hallucinations, etc.

▷ **Possible Effects on Sexual Function:**   Decreased libido, impotence (with excessive chronic use). Difficulty achieving an erection in males and decreased vaginal dilation in females. Chronic alcohol use may lead to tenderness and swelling of male and female breast tissue, testicular atrophy, low sperm counts, decreased menstrual blood flow and diminished capability for orgasm in females.

Possible Delayed Adverse Effects: Liver toxicity, anemia, low or high platelets, vitamin deficiency.

▷ **Adverse Effects That May Mimic Natural Diseases or Disorders**

Alcoholic cirrhosis may mimic hepatitis.

Natural Diseases or Disorders That May Be Activated by This Drug

Peptic ulcer disease.

Possible Effects on Laboratory Tests

Liver function tests: elevated ALT.

Complete blood count: decreased white blood cells, decreased hemoglobin, increased or decreased platelets.

Amylase: elevated.

Sperm count: decreased with chronic use.

Magnesium: decreased with chronic use.

CAUTION

1. This drug in its nonprescription form may cause fatal increases in blood pressure if combined with cocaine.
2. With high doses (nearly pure "grain" alcohol) or many drinks (frequent dosing) over a short period of time, fatal blood alcohol levels may be reached with the nonprescription form.

Precautions for Use

By Infants and Children: Safety and effectiveness for those under 12 years of age not established. Accidental and unsupervised drinking of the nonprescription form may result in severe consequences in children. Seriously low blood sugar may happen and be delayed up to 6 hours after drinking. Low potassium may also occur with high ethanol levels. Therapy is guided by blood sugar, potassium and blood alcohol (ethanol) levels. Fatality caused by low blood sugar was reported in a 4 year old child who drank 12 ounces of a mouthwash which contained 10% ethanol.

By Those over 60 Years of Age: Poisoning with methanol or ethylene glycol is an emergency situation, and while there may be an increased sensitivity to effects, dosing is adjusted to blood levels. The nonprescription form dosing (number of drinks) tolerated would be expected to decrease with increasing age.

▷ **Advisability of Use During Pregnancy**

Pregnancy Category: D, X if used for long periods. See Pregnancy Code at the back of this book.

Human studies: Fetal alcohol syndrome, a collection of limb, neurological and behavioral defects occur with excessive alcohol use.

Avoid use of this drug during your **entire** pregnancy.

Advisability of Use if Breast-Feeding
Presence of this drug in breast milk: Yes.
Avoid drug or refrain from nursing.

Habit-Forming Potential: Clearly defined alcoholism exists and occurs.

Effects of Overdosage: Toxic levels result in ataxia, loss of consciousness progressing to coma, anesthesia, respiratory failure and death. Levels of 150 to 300 mg/dl may result in exaggerated emotional states, confusion and incoordination. Fatalities most often result with blood concentrations greater than 400 mg/dl. Fatal blood levels vary greatly, however, and death has been reported following levels as low as 260 mg/dl. Once again, some people will not have any mental or physical changes with an alcohol level that is in the "legally drunk" range and even with higher levels.

Possible Effects of Long-Term Use: Liver toxicity, anemia, esophageal varicies, low white blood cell counts, compromised heart function, high blood pressure, arrhythmias, depression, peripheral neuropathy, seizures, cerebrovascular accident (with acute high levels), water intoxication, vitamin deficiency, electrolyte disturbances, gastritis or ulcers, pancreatitis, muscle pain, osteoporosis, tolerance and withdrawal on discontinuation.

Suggested Periodic Examinations While Taking This Drug (at physician's discretion)
Blood alcohol levels and methanol or ethylene glycol levels guide therapy in poisonings.
Chronic alcohol abuse: Complete blood counts, liver function tests, amylase and lipase, electrocardiograms.

▷ **While Taking This Drug, Observe the Following**
Foods: Food may decrease the absorption of ethanol from the stomach.
Nutritional Support: Vitamin support, particularly thiamin (B1), folic acid and B6 are needed with chronic use. Magnesium replacement is also needed. Vitamin C may help eliminate ethanol.
Tobacco Smoking: No interactions expected.
Marijuana Smoking: Additive central nervous system depression.
▷ *Other Drugs*
Ethanol may ***increase*** the effects of
- Central nervous system depressants such as benzodiazepines, barbiturates, opioids and anesthetic agents.
- chlorpromazine (Thorazine) will result in increased sedation.
- cocaine and result in dangerous increases in blood pressure.
- cyclosporine (Sandimune) if the ethanol is taken in large doses.
- diphenhydramine (Benadryl, others) will increase sedation.
- warfarin (Coumadin) and require more frequent INR testing and possible dose changes.
Ethanol may ***decrease*** the effects of
- phenytoin (Dilantin) by reducing blood phenytoin levels.
- propranolol (Inderal) by increasing propranolol elimination.
Ethanol ***taken concurrently*** with
- acetaminophen (Tylenol) poses an increased risk of liver damage.
- some antihistamines may increase sedation.
- aspirin may result in increased blood loss from the stomach.
- cefamandole (Mandol), cefotetan (Cefotan), metronidazole (Flagyl) and

cefoperazone (Cefobid) may result in disulfiramlike reaction (see Glossary).

- cimetidine may decrease the amount of alcohol that it takes to make you drunk (intoxicated).
- disulfiram (Antabuse) will result in severe vomiting and intolerance.
- griseofulvin can increase the effects of alcohol.
- insulin may result in potential severe hypoglycemia.
- isoniazid may result in elevated isoniazid levels.
- ketoconazole may result in disulfiramlike reactions.
- lithium (Lithobid) may result in worsened impairment of coordination and intoxication.
- methotrexate (especially with long term ethanol use) may increase risk of liver damage.
- metronidazole (Flagyl) may result in a disulfiramlike reaction.
- nitroglycerin (Nitrostat, others) may result in excessive decreases in blood pressure.
- oral hypoglycemic agents pose an increased risk of seriously low glucose levels.
- tricyclic antidepressants may result in increased antidepressant levels and toxicity.
- verapamil may increase the amount of time ethanol stays in the body and may pose an increased risk of intoxication.

▷ *Driving, Hazardous Activities:* This drug may cause drowsiness, mental impairment and coordination problems.

Driving skill may be impaired at very low blood levels with the perception that capabilities are **not** reduced. Drinking and driving is **not** recommended. Restrict activities as necessary.

Aviation Note: The use of this drug *is a disqualification* for piloting. Consult a designated Aviation Medical Examiner.

Exposure to Sun: May result in additive dehydration.

Heavy Exercise or Exertion: May worsen the adverse effects of this drug.

Discontinuation: Abrupt discontinuation after chronic use may result in a serious withdrawal syndrome known as DTs or delirium tremens.

ETHOSUXIMIDE (eth oh SUX i mide)

Introduced: 1960   **Prescription:** USA: Yes; Canada: Yes   **Available as Generic:** Yes   **Class:** Anticonvulsant   **Controlled Drug:** USA: No; Canada: No

Brand Name: Zarontin

BENEFITS versus RISKS	
Possible Benefits	*Possible Risks*
EFFECTIVE CONTROL OF ABSENCE SEIZURES (PETIT MAL EPILEPSY) in 70% of cases	RARE APLASTIC ANEMIA (see Aplastic Anemia and Bone Marrow Depression in Glossary)
EFFECTIVE CONTROL OF MYOCLONIC AND AKINETIC EPILEPSY in some individuals	Rare decrease in white blood cells and blood platelets

▷ **Principal Uses**

As a Single Drug Product: Uses currently included in FDA improved labeling: (1) Used to treat petit mal epilepsy and is a drug of choice in absence seizures Other (unlabeled) generally accepted uses: None at present.

How This Drug Works: By altering certain nerve impulses, this drug suppresses abnormal electrical activity that causes absence seizures of petit mal epilepsy.

Available Dosage Forms and Strengths

Capsules — 250 mg
Syrup — 250 mg per 5-ml

▷ **Usual Adult Dosage Range:** 20 to 30 mg per kilogram of body weight/24 hours. Initially 500 mg/24 hours.

Dosage may be increased cautiously by 250 mg every 4 to 7 days until satisfactory control is achieved. The total daily dosage should not exceed 1500 mg. IMPORTANT: Blood levels increase more quickly dose to dose in females than males.

For children 3 to 6 years old: Usual starting dose is 250 mg per day. The dose is then increased by 250 doses every 4 to 7 days as needed. Usually 20–30 mg per kg per 24 hours is used as a once daily dose.

Those more than 6 years old with absence seizures: same as adult dose.

Note: Actual dosage and administration schedule must be determined by the physician for each patient individually.

Conditions Requiring Dosing Adjustments

Liver function: Blood levels are recommended if this medication is used in liver compromise.

Kidney function: In severe kidney failure, 75% of the usual dose should be given at the usual interval.

▷ **Dosing Instructions:** Capsule may be opened and taken with food to reduce stomach irritation.

Usual Duration of Use: Use on a regular schedule for 1 to 2 weeks is usually needed to see this drug's effectiveness in reducing the frequency of absence seizures. Long-term use requires physician supervision.

▷ **This Drug Should Not Be Taken If**

• you are allergic to this or any succinimide (see Drug Classes).
• you have active liver disease.
• you currently have a blood cell or bone marrow disorder.

▷ **Inform Your Physician Before Taking This Drug If**

• you have a history of liver or kidney disease.
• you have any type of blood disorder, especially one caused by drugs.
• you have a history of serious depression or other mental illness.

Possible Side Effects (natural, expected, and unavoidable drug actions)

Drowsiness, lethargy, fatigue.

▷ **Possible Adverse Effects** (unusual, unexpected, and infrequent reactions)

If any of the following develop, consult your physician promptly for guidance.

Mild Adverse Effects

Allergic Reactions: Skin rash, hives.

Headache, dizziness, unsteadiness, euphoria, impaired vision, numbness and tingling in extremities.

Loss of appetite, nausea, vomiting, hiccups, stomach pain, diarrhea.
Excessive growth of hair.
Serious Adverse Effects
Allergic Reaction: Swelling of tongue.
Thickening and overgrowth of gums.
Nervousness, hyperactivity, disturbed sleep, night terrors.
Aggravation of emotional depression and paranoid mental disorders.
Severe bone marrow depression—fatigue, weakness, fever, sore throat, abnormal bleeding or bruising.
Porphyria (rare).
Myasthenia gravis (rare).
Systemic lupus erythematosus (rare).

▷ **Possible Effects on Sexual Function:**   Increased libido (questionable); nonmenstrual vaginal bleeding.

Natural Diseases or Disorders That May Be Activated by This Drug
Latent psychosis, systemic lupus erythematosus.

Possible Effects on Laboratory Tests
Complete blood cell counts: decreased red cells, hemoglobin, white cells and platelets; increased eosinophils.
Blood aspartate aminotransferase (AST) level: increased in 33% of users.
Blood bilirubin level: increased (rare liver damage).
Blood lupus erythematosus (LE) cells: positive (rare).
Kidney function tests: increased blood urea nitrogen (BUN) level, increased urine protein content.

CAUTION
1. May increase the frequency of grand mal seizures in people with mixed seizure disorders.
2. Periodic blood counts and other tests are mandatory.

Precautions for Use
By Infants and Children: If a single daily dose causes nausea or vomiting, give in 2 or 3 divided doses 8 to 12 hours apart. Large differences in response occur, and require blood levels. Watch for a lupuslike reaction: Fever, rash, arthritis.
By Those over 60 Years of Age: Rarely used in this age group.

▷ **Advisability of Use During Pregnancy**
Pregnancy Category: C. See Pregnancy Code at the back of this book.
Animal studies: Bone defects reported in rodents.
Human studies: Three instances of birth defects have been reported. Adequate studies of pregnant women are not available.
Avoid during first 3 months. Use only if clearly needed during the last 6 months.

Advisability of Use if Breast-Feeding
Presence of this drug in breast milk: Yes.
Watch nursing infant closely and discontinue drug or nursing if adverse effects develop. If mother requires high doses, refrain from nursing. Ask doctor for help.

Habit-Forming Potential: None.

Effects of Overdosage: Increased drowsiness, lethargy, weakness, dizziness, unsteadiness, nausea, vomiting, stupor progressing to coma.

Possible Effects of Long-Term Use: Systemic lupus erythematosus.

Suggested Periodic Examinations While Taking This Drug (at physician's discretion)

Complete blood counts every 2 weeks during the first months of use, then monthly thereafter; liver and kidney function tests.

▷ **While Taking This Drug, Observe the Following**

Foods: No restrictions.

Beverages: No restrictions. May be taken with milk.

▷ *Alcohol:* Use caution—this drug may increase the sedative effects of alcohol. Excessive alcohol may precipitate seizures.

Tobacco Smoking: No interactions expected.

▷ *Other Drugs*

Ethosuximide may *increase* the effects of

• phenytoin (Dilantin), by slowing its elimination.

Ethosuximide *taken concurrently* with

• carbamazepine (Tegretol) may change ethosuximide blood levels.
• phenobarbital may decrease seizure control success.
• valproic acid (Depakene) may unpredictably alter ethosuximide effects.

The following drugs may *increase* the effects of ethosuximide

• isoniazid (INH, Niconyl, etc.).

▷ *Driving, Hazardous Activities:* This drug may cause drowsiness, dizziness, unsteadiness and impaired vision. Restrict activities as necessary.

Aviation Note: Seizure disorders and the use of this drug *are disqualifications* for piloting. Consult a designated Aviation Medical Examiner.

Exposure to Sun: No restrictions.

Discontinuation: Do not stop taking this drug abruptly. Ask your physician for help with gradual dose reduction.

ETIDRONATE (e ti DROH nate)

Introduced: 1976   **Prescription:** USA: Yes; Canada: Yes   **Available as**
Generic: USA: No; Canada: No   **Class:** Antiosteoporotic   **Controlled**
Drug: USA: No; Canada: No

Brand Name: Didronel

BENEFITS versus RISKS	
Possible Benefits	*Possible Risks*
PARTIAL RELIEF OF SYMPTOMS OF PAGET'S DISEASE OF BONE	Increased bone pain
	Bone fractures
EFFECTIVE PREVENTION AND TREATMENT OF ABNORMAL CALCIFICATION	Kidney failure
	Focal osteomalacia
Effective adjunctive treatment of abnormally high blood calcium levels (associated with malignant disease)	
Treatment of postmenopausal osteoporosis	

▷ **Principal Uses**

As a Single Drug Product: Uses currently included in FDA approved labeling: (1) treatment of symptomatic Paget's disease of bone (excessive bone growth of skull, spine and long bones); (2) prevention and treatment of abnormal bone formation (ossification) following total hip replacement or spinal cord injury; (3) adjunctive treatment of excessively high blood calcium levels due to malignant bone disease.

Other (unlabeled) generally accepted uses: (1) treatment of Paget's disease of bone that is not yet causing symptoms; (2) treatment of postmenopausal osteoporosis; (3) treatment of abnormal calcium levels which may result from prolonged immobilization; (4) helps hyperparathyroidism; (5) helps pulmonary alveolar microlithiasis (PAM).

How This Drug Works: This drug attaches to the surface of bone and slows the abnormally accelerated processes of "bone turnover" that occur in Paget's disease. In malignant bone disease, this drug slows bone destruction and reduces excessive transfer of calcium from bone to blood.

Available Dosage Forms and Strengths

Injection — 50 mg per ml

Tablets — 200 mg, 400 mg

▷ **Recommended Dosage Ranges** (Actual dosage and administration schedule must be determined by the physician for each patient individually.)

Infants and Children: Dosage not established.

12 to 60 Years of Age: For Paget's disease—Initially 5 mg/kg of body weight daily, as a single dose, for up to 6 months. Discontinue for a drug-free period of 6 months. As needed, repeat alternating 6 month courses of drug treatment and abstention. Doses above 10 mg per kg per day are only used if there is a critical need to decrease increased work output of the heart or to quickly slow down increased bone turnover. For ossification associated with hip replacement—20 mg/kg of body weight daily for 1 month before and 3 months after surgery.

For ossification associated with spinal cord injury—Initially 20 mg/kg of body weight daily for 2 weeks after injury; then decrease dose to 10 mg/kg of body weight daily for an additional 10 weeks.

For high blood calcium associated with malignant bone disease—20 mg/kg of body weight daily for 30 days; if needed and tolerated, continue for a maximum of 90 days.

The total daily dose should not exceed 20 mg/kg of body weight.

Over 60 Years of Age: Same as 12 to 60 years of age.

Conditions Requiring Dosing Adjustments

Liver function:

This drug is not known to be metabolized in the liver.

Kidney function: The drug should be used with caution if at all in patients with steady state creatinines (a measure of kidney function) greater than 2.5. Etidronate should never be used in patients with steady state creatinines greater than 5.0.

▷ **Dosing Instructions:**   The tablet may be crushed and taken with water on an empty stomach, 2 hours before or after food; suggested times—

on arising, midmorning, or at bedtime. Do not take with milk. If nausea or diarrhea occurs, the daily dose may be divided into 2 or 3 portions.

Usual Duration of Use: Use on a regular schedule for 1 to 3 months will determine this drug's effectiveness in relieving the symptoms of Paget's disease. If effective, the standard course of treatment is 6 months. Long-term use (months to years) requires periodic physician evaluation.

Possible Advantages of This Drug
Effective orally, with once-a-day dosage.
Less expensive than calcitonin.

Currently a "Drug of Choice"
for managing Paget's disease of bone.

▷ **This Drug Should Not Be Taken If**
- you have had an allergic reaction to it previously.
- you recently fractured a bone that has not healed completely.

▷ **Inform Your Physician Before Taking This Drug If**
- you have a history of heart disease, especially congestive heart failure.
- you have impaired kidney function.
- you are subject to enterocolitis, or recurrent diarrhea.

Possible Side Effects (natural, expected, and unavoidable drug actions)
Increased bone pain or tenderness (usually starts 4 to 6 weeks after beginning treatment).

▷ **Possible Adverse Effects** (unusual, unexpected, and infrequent reactions)
If any of the following develop, consult your physician promptly for guidance.
Mild Adverse Effects
Allergic Reactions: Skin rash, hives, itching.
Nausea, diarrhea.
Taste disorders.
Serious Adverse Effects
Allergic Reactions: Angioedema (swelling of face, lips, tongue, throat, and/or vocal cords); may be life-threatening.
Osteomalacia (thinning and weakening of bone) with fractures.
Pseudomembranous colitis.
Ulcers (rare).
Kidney failure.

▷ **Possible Effects on Sexual Function:** None reported.

Natural Diseases or Disorders That May Be Activated by This Drug
Senile osteomalacia.

Possible Effects on Laboratory Tests
Blood alkaline phosphatase levels: decreased.
Blood calcium levels: decreased.
Blood phosphate levels: increased.
Urine hydroxyproline values: decreased.

CAUTION
1. Maintain a well-balanced diet with adequate calcium and vitamin D.
2. Mineral supplements and drugs containing aluminum, calcium, iron, or magnesium can prevent etidronate absorption; separate doses by at least 2 hours.

3. Tell your doctor if nausea or diarrhea persists; dosage adjustment (multiple small doses) can help.
4. Call your physician if bone pain persists or increases.

Precautions for Use

By Infants and Children: Avoid large doses or prolonged use to reduce the risk of inducing rickets.

By Those over 60 Years of Age: Watch fluid balance carefully if this drug is given intravenously to lower blood calcium levels.

▷ **Advisability of Use During Pregnancy**

Pregnancy Category: C. See Pregnancy Code at the back of this book.
Animal studies: Rat and rabbit studies reveal no drug-induced birth defects.
Human studies: Adequate studies of pregnant women are not available.
Use this drug only if clearly needed. Ask your doctor for help.

Advisability of Use if Breast-Feeding

Presence of this drug in breast milk: Unknown.
Avoid drug or refrain from nursing.

Habit-Forming Potential: None.

Effects of Overdosage: Nausea, vomiting, diarrhea.

Possible Effects of Long-Term Use: Development of osteomalacia (softening and weakening of bone structure).

Suggested Periodic Examinations While Taking This Drug (at physician's discretion)

Measurements of blood calcium, phosphate, and alkaline phosphatase levels.
Measurement of urine hydroxyproline content.
Kidney function tests.

▷ **While Taking This Drug, Observe the Following**

Foods: Avoid all foods, especially dairy products, for 2 hours before and after taking this drug.
Nutritional Support: Ensure adequate intake of calcium and vitamin D.
Beverages: Take this drug with water. Avoid all forms of milk for 2 hours before and after taking this drug.
▷ *Alcohol:* No interactions expected.
Tobacco Smoking: No interactions expected.
▷ *Other Drugs*
The following drugs may *decrease* the effects of etidronate
- all antacids containing aluminum, calcium, or magnesium.
- all iron preparations.
Etidronate *taken concurrently* with
- foscarnet (Foscavir) may lead to additive decreases in calcium.
- plicamycin can lead to additive calcium decreases.
▷ *Driving, Hazardous Activities:* No restrictions.
Aviation Note: The use of this drug *may be a disqualification* for piloting. Consult a designated Aviation Medical Examiner.
Exposure to Sun: No restrictions.
Discontinuation: Take this medicine exactly as prescribed. Your doctor should decide when to stop this drug.

ETODOLAC (E TOE do lak)

Introduced: 1986   **Prescription:** USA: Yes   **Available as Generic:** USA: No   **Class:** NSAID, mild analgesic   **Controlled Drug:** USA: No
Brand Names: Lodine

BENEFITS versus RISKS	
Possible Benefits	*Possible Risks*
EFFECTIVE TREATMENT OF MILD TO MODERATE INFLAMMATION AND PAIN DECREASED GASTROINTESTINAL BLEEDING RISK	Gastrointestinal pain, ulceration or bleeding (rare) Rare blood cell disorders: Low platelet counts, anemia Fluid retention Rare kidney damage Rare liver damage Hearing toxicity (ototoxicity) (rare)

Please see the acetic acid nonsteroidal anti-inflammatory drug profile for further information.

ETRETINATE (e TRET i nayt)

Introduced: 1976   **Prescription:** USA: Yes; Canada: Yes   **Available as Generic:** USA: No; Canada: No   **Class:** Antipsoriasis   **Controlled Drug:** USA: No; Canada: No
Brand Name: Tegison

BENEFITS versus RISKS	
Possible Benefits	*Possible Risks*
EFFECTIVE TREATMENT FOR SEVERE, RESISTANT PSORIASIS	MAJOR DRUG-INDUCED BIRTH DEFECTS RARE DRUG-INDUCED HEPATITIS Adverse effects on eyes and vision Adverse effects on musculoskeletal structures Adverse effects on blood cholesterol and triglycerides Increased intracranial pressure (very rare) Extended PTT Increased triglycerides

▷ **Principal Uses**

As a Single Drug Product: Uses currently included in FDA approved labeling: (1) Treatment of severe, generalized forms of psoriasis (and related skin disorders) that have failed to respond to conventional, less hazardous treatments.

Other (unlabeled) generally accepted uses: (1) Treatment of acne; (2) local treatment of warts; (3) treatment of cutaneous neoplasia in kidney transplant patients; (4) eases symptoms of Darier's disease; (5) can help symptoms in a variety of abnormal keratin conditions; (6) eases cutaneous systemic lupus erythematosus; (7) helps Reiter's syndrome in AIDS patients.

How This Drug Works: Regulates cell differentiation in the skin; this results in a more normal pattern of cell growth, with reduction of inflammation and scale formation.

Available Dosage Forms and Strengths
Capsules — 10 mg, 25 mg

▷ **Usual Adult Dosage Range:**   Initially 1 mg/kg/day, in divided doses, until satisfactory response is obtained (usually 8 to 16 weeks). Maintenance: 0.5 to 0.75 mg/kg/day, beginning after initial response. Total daily dosage should not exceed 1.5 mg per kg per day. **Note: Actual dosage and administration schedule must be determined by the physician for each patient individually.**

Conditions Requiring Dosing Adjustments
Liver function: This drug is a rare cause of hepatitis. It should be used with caution in liver compromise, and the dose should be decreased.
Kidney function: The kidneys are not a significant factor in the elimination of this drug. Etretinate is a rare cause of kidney toxicity, and it should be used with caution in patients with compromised kidneys.

▷ **Dosing Instructions:**   Take with or immediately following meals, preferably with whole milk. Do not suck or chew the capsule; swallow it whole.

Usual Duration of Use: Use on a regular schedule for 2 to 4 weeks is usually necessary to see this drug's benefit in reversing the skin changes of psoriasis. The full effect of treatment may not be apparent for 2 to 3 months of continual use. Long-term use (months to years) requires periodic physician evaluation. Due to the potential for accumulation and toxicity with long-term use, this drug should be temporarily discontinued after 18 months of treatment; it may be resumed as needed. Consult your physician on a regular basis.

Possible Advantages of This Drug: When used in conjunction with other antipsoriasis drugs and procedures, this drug can enhance the therapeutic response and reduce the total dosage and length of treatment required for satisfactory management.

▷ **This Drug Should Not Be Taken If**
• you have had an allergic reaction to any dosage form of it previously.
• you are pregnant or breast-feeding.
• you currently take vitamin A therapy.
• you plan to donate blood in the near future.

▷ **Inform Your Physician Before Taking This Drug If**
• you are allergic to vitamin A or other vitamin A derivatives: isotretinoin (Accutane), tretinoin (Retin-A).
• you are allergic to parabens (preservatives).
• you have cerebral or coronary artery disease.
• you have high blood cholesterol or triglyceride levels.
• you have diabetes.
• your night vision is of critical use to you.

- you have impaired liver or kidney function.
- you have alcoholism.
- you have a history of Crohn's disease or ulcerative colitis.

Possible Side Effects (natural, expected, and unavoidable drug actions)

Dry nose, nosebleed, dry lips, sore mouth and tongue, bleeding gums.

Loss of hair, skin peeling of hands and feet, dry skin, itching, bruising, nail deformities.

Thickening of bone (hyperostosis), calcification of tendons and ligaments, bone and joint pain.

▷ **Possible Adverse Effects** (unusual, unexpected, and infrequent reactions)

If any of the following develop, consult your physician promptly for guidance.

Mild Adverse Effects

Allergic Reactions: Skin rash, hives, itching.

Headache, dizziness, fatigue, fever, emotional irritability.

Eye irritation, blurred or double vision, sensitivity to bright light, decreased night vision, decreased tolerance for contact lenses, earache, impaired hearing.

Altered taste, loss of appetite, nausea, stomach pain, constipation, diarrhea.

Muscle cramps.

Painful urination.

Serious Adverse Effects

Increased intracranial pressure (rare): Headache, nausea, vomiting, visual disturbances.

Hepatitis (rare); 4 reported deaths worldwide.

Kidney damage (nephrotoxicity) (very rare).

Eye reactions: corneal erosion, abrasion, staining; cataract; retinal hemorrhage; visual field defects; reduced night vision.

Inflammatory bowel disease (Crohn's disease) (rare).

Altered blood fat levels: increased triglycerides (45%), increased total cholesterol (16%), decreased HDL cholesterol (37%); any of these changes may increase the risk for the development of atherosclerotic heart disease.

Muscle damage (rare).

Abnormal bone changes: premature epiphyseal closure, periosteal thickening.

Ototoxicity.

Extended PTT (a measure of blood clotting).

Low blood platelets (rare).

▷ **Possible Effects on Sexual Function:**   Altered timing and pattern of menstruation. Loss of libido. Erectile dysfunctions.

Possible Delayed Adverse Effects: This drug has been found in the blood 2.9 years following termination of its use and has the potential for inducing birth defects during this time. It has not been determined how long pregnancy should be avoided after therapy has been stopped.

▷ **Adverse Effects That May Mimic Natural Diseases or Disorders**

Increased intracranial pressure may suggest brain tumor.

Liver reactions may suggest viral hepatitis.

Joint pains due to calcification of ligaments and tendons may suggest the onset of arthritis.

Natural Diseases or Disorders That May Be Activated by This Drug
Angina may start in the people with coronary artery heart disease. Heart attack (myocardial infarction) has been associated with this drug.

Possible Effects on Laboratory Tests
Red blood cell counts: decreased.

Blood eosinophil counts: increased.

Blood total cholesterol, LDL cholesterol and triglyceride levels: increased.

Liver function tests: increased liver enzymes (ALT/GPT, AST/GOT and alkaline phosphatase.

PTT: increased.

CAUTION
1. ***This drug should not be taken during pregnancy.*** A pregnancy test should be performed within 2 weeks prior to taking this drug. In the absence of pregnancy, the drug should be started on the second or third day of the next normal menstrual period. An effective form of contraception should be used for 1 month before the drug is started, during the entire period of treatment, and for an indefinite period (minimum of 3 years) after the drug is discontinued. If pregnancy does occur, stop this drug immediately and consult your physician.

2. ***Do not donate blood to a blood bank if you are taking this drug.*** Blood containing this drug could pose a serious risk to the developing fetus of a pregnant patient who received it. Avoid blood donation for a minimum of 3 years if use of the blood is beyond your control.

3. ***Comply fully with your physician's recommendations for periodic examinations before, during and following treatment with this drug.*** These are mandatory for safe and effective use.

4. Avoid concurrent use of vitamin A supplements.

5. Call your doctor promptly if you have significant eye reactions or altered vision.

6. Your psoriasis may appear to worsen during the early period of treatment with this drug. Call your doctor if symptoms become severe or prolonged.

7. If dry mouth or sore and bleeding gums persist, consult your dentist.

Precautions for Use
By Infants and Children: This drug should be used only after all less hazardous treatments have failed. Best to obtain pretreatment X-rays to determine bone age and to monitor bone growth and development by yearly X-ray studies. This drug can impair normal bone maturation.

By Those over 60 Years of Age: Watch for development of anemia, impaired kidney function and fluctuation of blood potassium levels.

▷ **Advisability of Use During Pregnancy**
Pregnancy Category: X. See Pregnancy Code at the back of this book.

Animal studies: No information available.

Human studies: Major birth defects occur in association with the use of this drug: Malformations of the skull, vertebrae, face, extremities, brain and spinal cord.

Avoid this drug completely during entire pregnancy. See *CAUTION.*

Advisability of Use if Breast-Feeding
Presence of this drug in breast milk: Unknown.

Avoid drug or refrain from nursing.

Habit-Forming Potential: None.

Effects of Overdosage: Severe headache, irritability, drowsiness, itching, nausea, vomiting.

Possible Effects of Long-Term Use: Hyperostosis (84%): abnormal thickening of bone (pelvis), calcification of ligaments and tendons (knees and ankles).

Suggested Periodic Examinations While Taking This Drug (at physician's discretion)
Complete blood counts; tests of blood sugar, potassium, sodium and chloride. Blood cholesterol profiles, before and during treatment.
Liver and kidney function tests.
Complete eye examinations.
Bone X-rays, especially for children.

▷ **While Taking This Drug, Observe the Following**
Foods: No restrictions. High-fat foods increase absorption of this drug.
Beverages: No restrictions. Whole milk increases absorption of this drug.
▷   *Alcohol:* No interactions expected. Use moderately; excessive intake can increase blood triglyceride levels.
Tobacco Smoking: No interactions expected.
▷   *Other Drugs*
Etretinate may ***increase*** the effects of
• vitamin A and its derivatives (isotretinoin and tretinoin) and increase the risk of vitamin A toxicity.
Etretinate ***taken concurrently*** with
• carbamazepine (Tegretol) may result in decreased etretinate effectiveness.
• methotrexate may increase the risk of liver toxicity.
• tetracyclines may increase the risk of elevated intracranial pressure.
• warfarin (Coumadin) may cause a decreased effectiveness of warfarin.
▷   *Driving, Hazardous Activities:* This drug may cause dizziness and blurred vision. Limit activities as necessary.
Aviation Note: The use of this drug ***may be a disqualification*** for piloting. Consult a designated Aviation Medical Examiner.
Exposure to Sun: Use caution. This drug can cause photosensitivity (see Glossary).
Discontinuation: If this drug is not significantly beneficial after 4 months of continual use, it should be stopped. If response is adequate to justify its long-term use, it should be discontinued temporarily ("drug holiday") after 18 months of continual treatment. Once the skin has cleared satisfactorily, this drug should be stopped. Most people have some degree of recurrence by the end of 2 months. Subsequent treatment courses of 4 to 9 months can be started as required.

FAMCICLOVIR (fam SEYE klo veer)

Introduced: 1994   **Prescription:** USA: Yes   **Available as Generic:** USA: No   **Class:** Antiviral   **Controlled Drug:** USA: No
Brand Names: Famvir

> **BENEFITS versus RISKS**
>
> | *Possible Benefits* | *Possible Risks* |
> |---|---|
> | EFFECTIVE TREATMENT OF HERPES ZOSTER (SHINGLES) | Diarrhea |
> | TREATS AN INFECTION WHICH MAY BE LIFE-THREATENING IN AIDS AND MARROW TRANSPLANT PATIENTS | Purpura |
> | TREATS RECURRENT GENITAL HERPES | Paresthesias |

▷ **Principal Uses**

As a Single Drug Product: Uses currently included in FDA approved labeling: (1) Treatment of acute herpes zoster (shingles); (2) recently approved for treatment of recurrent genital herpes.

Other (unlabeled) generally accepted uses: May have a role in treating hepatitis B.

How This Drug Works: This drug is changed in the body to the active penciclovir. Penciclovir inhibits the virus by blocking DNA synthesis and viral reproduction (replication).

Available Dosage Forms and Strengths

Tablets — 250 mg (Germany) and 500 mg

▷ **Recommended Dosage Ranges (Actual dosage and administration schedule must be determined by the physician for each patient individually.)**

Infants and Children: Safety and efficacy for those under 18 not established.

18 to 60 Years of Age: Shingles (herpes zoster): 500 mg is given every 8 hours for seven days. It is important to start this medicine promptly after the diagnosis is made.

Recurrent genital herpes: 125 mg twice a day for 5 days.

Over 60 Years of Age: Same as 12 to 60 years of age, except for those with compromised livers or kidneys.

Conditions Requiring Dosing Adjustments

Liver function: No dose changes are needed in well-compensated liver impairment.

Kidney function: In people with mild kidney compromise (creatinine clearance greater than 60), 500 mg is given every 8 hours. People with mild to moderate compromise (creatinine clearance 40 to 59) receive 500 mg every 12 hours. Patients with moderate to severe kidney compromise (creatinine clearance 20 to 39) receive 500 mg every 24 hours.

Usual Duration of Use: Use on a regular schedule for two days usually determines effectiveness in treating Herpes zoster, and the medicine is typically continued for seven days. Physician evaluation is needed to determine when this medicine should be stopped. For recurrent genital herpes: Dosing is started at the first sign of recurrence and dosing is continued for 5 days.

▷ **This Drug Should Not Be Taken If**

• you have had an allergic reaction to any dosage form of it previously.

▷ **Inform Your Physician Before Taking This Drug If**
  - you are uncertain how much famciclovir to take or how often to take it.
  - you have a history of kidney or liver problems.
  - your immune system is compromised.

▷ **Possible Adverse Effects** (unusual, unexpected, and infrequent reactions)
  If any of the following develop, consult your physician promptly for guidance.
  Mild Adverse Effects
  Allergic Reactions: Itching.
  Diarrhea.
  Fever.
  Headache.
  Nausea.
  Fatigue.
  Serious Adverse Effects
  Allergic Reactions: Unknown.
  Not defined at present.
  Purpura.
  Paresthesias.
  Rigors (rare).

▷ **Possible Effects on Sexual Function:**   None reported.

Possible Delayed Adverse Effects: Unknown.

Possible Effects on Laboratory Tests
  Unknown.

CAUTION
  1. The best effect is achieved with this medicine if it is started very soon after the condition is diagnosed. If used for recurrent genital herpes, it is best started as soon as signs of recurrence occur.

Precautions for Use
  By Infants and Children: Safety and effectiveness for those under 18 years of age are not established.
  By Those over 60 Years of Age: Specific adjustments or precautions are not defined except for those with compromised livers or kidneys.

▷ **Advisability of Use During Pregnancy**
  Pregnancy Category: B. See Pregnancy Code at the back of this book.
  Human studies: Adequate studies of pregnant women are not available.
  Ask your doctor for guidance.

Advisability of Use if Breast-Feeding
  Presence of this drug in breast milk: Unknown.
  Stop nursing or discontinue the drug.

Effects of Overdosage: Unknown.

▷ **While Taking This Drug, Observe the Following**
  Foods: No restrictions.
  Tobacco Smoking: No interactions expected to date.

▷ *Other Drugs*
  No interactions reported.

▷ *Driving, Hazardous Activities:* This drug may cause dizziness or fatigue. Restrict activities as necessary.

Aviation Note: The use of this drug *may be a disqualification* for piloting. Consult a designated Aviation Medical Examiner.

Exposure to Sun: No restrictions.

FAMOTIDINE (fa MOH te deen)

Introduced: 1986   **Prescription:** USA: Yes   **Available as Generic:** USA: No   **Class:** H-2 receptor blocker   **Controlled Drug:** USA: No
Author's note: This drug was approved in 1995 as Pepcid AC. This is a nonprescription form of famotidine used to treat heartburn.

Brand Name: Pepcid, Pepcid AC (nonprescription)

BENEFITS versus RISKS	
Possible Benefits	*Possible Risks*
EFFECTIVE TREATMENT OF PEPTIC ULCER DISEASE: relief of symptoms, acceleration of healing, prevention of recurrence	Headache, dizziness
CONTROL OF HYPERSECRETORY STOMACH DISORDERS	
Beneficial in treatment of reflux esophagitis	

Please see the new histamine (H2) blocking drug profile for further information.

FELODIPINE (fe LOH di peen)

Introduced: 1986   **Prescription:** USA: Yes   **Available as Generic:** No   **Class:** Antihypertensive, calcium channel blocker   **Controlled Drug:** USA: No

Brand Name: Plendil

Controversies In Medicine: Study data indicates that medicines in this class should NOT be used in some patients with extremely compromised hearts. There have also been several FDA hearings held on the calcium channel blocker class. Be certain to ask your doctor about your cardiac output and if the benefits of this medicine outweigh the risks of its use. A recent FDA panel found medicines in this class to be safe and effective. A retrospective chart review yielded data that showed increased risks for nifedipine immediate release forms in those over 71, and cautioned physicians against using the immediate release form for indications other than angina. The immediate release form in question had never been approved for other uses. Most recently, a study of nearly 6,000 patients at Tel Aviv Medical Center found that there was no statistically significant increased risk of death in the patients who took calcium channel blockers versus those who did not.

```
┌────────────────────────────────────────────────────────────┐
│                    BENEFITS versus RISKS                     │
│    Possible Benefits              Possible Risks             │
│ EFFECTIVE TREATMENT OF MILD   Peripheral edema (fluid retention in │
│   TO MODERATE HYPERTENSION      feet and ankles)             │
└────────────────────────────────────────────────────────────┘
```

▷ **Principal Uses**
  As a Single Drug Product: Uses currently included in FDA approved labeling:
  Treatment of mild to moderate hypertension.
  Other (unlabeled) generally accepted uses: (1) Treatment of angina; (2) treatment of arrhythmias; (3) adjunctive treatment of congestive heart failure; (4) useful in inhibiting the progression of atherosclerosis.

How This Drug Works: Controversial, however, by blocking the normal passage of calcium through certain cell walls (which is necessary for the function of nerve and muscle tissue), this drug slows the spread of electrical activity and reduces contraction of peripheral arterial walls, lowering the blood pressure.

Available Dosage Forms and Strengths
  Tablets (sustained release) — 5 mg, 10 mg

▷ **Recommended Dosage Ranges** (Actual dosage and administration schedule must be determined by the physician for each patient individually.)
  Infants and Children: Dosage not established.
  12 to 60 Years of Age: High blood pressure: Initially 5 mg, once daily. Increase dose as needed and tolerated at intervals of 2 weeks. The usual dosage range is 5 to 10 mg, once daily. The total daily dose should not exceed 10 mg, once daily.
  Over 65 Years of Age: Starting dose is 2.5 mg per day. The total daily dose should not exceed 10 mg, once daily.

Conditions Requiring Dosing Adjustments
  Liver function: When felodipine is used in patients with liver compromise, the starting dose should be 2.5 mg per day with a maximum of 10 mg per day.
  Kidney function: The kidneys are not significantly involved in elimination of felodipine.

▷ **Dosing Instructions:** May be taken with or following food to reduce stomach irritation. The tablet should be swallowed whole; do not crush or chew.

Usual Duration of Use: Use on a regular schedule for 2 to 4 weeks is needed to determine this drug's effectiveness in controlling hypertension. The smallest effective dose should be used in long-term (months to years) therapy. Supervision and periodic physician visits are essential.

Possible Advantages of This Drug
  Gradual onset and prolonged duration of action, permitting effective once-a-day treatment.

▷ **This Drug Should Not Be Taken If**
  • you have had an allergic reaction to it or similar medicines previously.
  • you have active liver disease.
  • you have severe lowering of the blood pressure.
  • you have severe problems (dysfunction) in the left side of your heart.

- you have atrioventricular blockade or sick sinus syndrome (talk with your doctor).
- you have uncorrected congestive heart failure.

▷ **Inform Your Physician Before Taking This Drug If**
- you have had an unfavorable response to any calcium blocker drug.
- you currently take any form of digitalis or a beta blocker drug (see Drug Classes).
- you are taking any other drugs that lower blood pressure.
- you have a history of congestive heart failure, heart attack or stroke.
- you are subject to disturbances of heart rhythm.
- you have Duschenne muscular dystrophy.
- you have developed a skin reaction while taking this medicine.
- you have circulatory impairment to the fingers.
- you have muscular dystrophy.
- you have a history of atrial fibrillation.
- you have myasthenia gravis.
- you have a history of impaired liver or kidney function.

Possible Side Effects (natural, expected, and unavoidable drug actions)
Swelling of feet and ankles, flushing and sensation of warmth.

▷ **Possible Adverse Effects** (unusual, unexpected, and infrequent reactions)
If any of the following develop, consult your physician promptly for guidance.
Mild Adverse Effects
Allergic Reactions: Skin rash (rare).
Headache, dizziness, fatigue.
Indigestion, nausea, stomach pain, constipation, or diarrhea (all rare).
Palpitations.
Dose-related flushing.
Cough.
Increased urination (rare).
Peripheral edema.
Sleep disorders (rare).
Pharyngitis (rare).
Abnormal growth of the gums (gingival hyperplasia) (rare).
Serious Adverse Effects
Allergic Reactions: None reported.
Idiosyncratic Reactions: None reported.
Tachycardia.
Aggravation of angina.
Decreased hemoglobin, hematocrit, and red blood cell count (extremely rare).

▷ **Possible Effects on Sexual Function:**   Impotence (0.5–1.5%).

▷ **Adverse Effects That May Mimic Natural Diseases or Disorders**
An allergic rash and swelling of the legs may resemble erysipelas.

Possible Effects on Laboratory Tests
Liver function tests: minor and short term increases.

CAUTION
1. Tell all of your health care providers that you are taking this drug. Carry a note that says you take felodipine.

2. You may use nitroglycerin and other nitrate drugs as needed to relieve acute episodes of angina pain. However, if your angina attacks are becoming more frequent or intense, call your doctor promptly.

Precautions for Use

By Infants and Children: Safety and effectiveness for those under 12 years of age not established.

By Those over 60 Years of Age: You may be more susceptible to the development of weakness, dizziness, fainting and falling. Take necessary precautions to prevent injury.

▷ **Advisability of Use During Pregnancy**

Pregnancy Category: C. See Pregnancy Code at the back of this book.

Animal studies: No information available.

Human studies: Adequate studies of pregnant women are not available.

Avoid this drug during the first 3 months. Use during the last 6 months only if clearly needed. Ask physician for guidance.

Advisability of Use if Breast-Feeding

Presence of this drug in breast milk: Unknown.

Avoid drug or refrain from nursing.

Habit-Forming Potential: None.

Effects of Overdosage: Weakness, light-headedness, fainting, fast pulse, low blood pressure, shortness of breath, flushed and warm skin, tremors.

Possible Effects of Long-Term Use: None reported.

Suggested Periodic Examinations While Taking This Drug (at physician's discretion)

Evaluations of heart function, including electrocardiograms; measurements of blood pressure in supine, sitting and standing positions.

▷ **While Taking This Drug, Observe the Following**

Foods: No restrictions. Avoid excessive salt intake.

Beverages: Grapefruit juice can cause **a serious increase** in the absorption of this drug. Levels may be increased by over 400%. Do **not** take this drug with grapefruit juice. May be taken with milk or water.

▷ *Alcohol:* Use with caution—alcohol may exaggerate the drop in blood pressure experienced by some individuals.

Tobacco Smoking: Nicotine may reduce the effectiveness of this drug. Follow your physician's advice regarding smoking.

▷ *Other Drugs*

Felodipine *taken concurrently* with

- adenosine may result in an extended slowing of the heart.
- beta blocker drugs or digitalis preparations (see Drug Classes) may affect heart rate and rhythm adversely. Careful monitoring by your physician is necessary if these drugs are taken concurrently.
- carbamazepine (Tegretol) may result in decreased felodipine effectiveness.
- digoxin may increase digoxin levels and result in toxicity.
- magnesium (particularly in high doses) may cause low blood pressure (not specifically reported for felodipine, but another drug in the calcium blocker class does this).
- phenobarbital can cause decreased felodipine benefits.
- phenytoin (Dilantin) may cause decreased phenytoin levels.

- rifampin may cause decreased felodipine benefits. (not specifically reported for felodipine, but has been reported with other calcium blockers).

The following drug may *increase* the effects of felodipine
- cimetidine (Tagamet).
- erythromycin—may also occur with clarithromycin since it is structurally similar.

▷ *Driving, Hazardous Activities:* Usually no restrictions. This drug may cause dizziness. Restrict activities as necessary.

Aviation Note: Hypertension *is a disqualification* for piloting. Consult a designated Aviation Medical Examiner.

Exposure to Sun: No restrictions.

Exposure to Heat: Caution advised. Hot environments can exaggerate the blood-pressure-lowering effects of this drug. Observe for light-headedness or weakness.

Discontinuation: Do not stop this drug abruptly. Ask your physician about gradual withdrawal. Watch for development of rebound hypertension.

FENAMATES
(Nonsteroidal Antiinflammatory Drugs)

Meclofenamate (MEK low fen a mate)   **Mefenamic acid** (MEF en amik a sid)

Introduced: 1977, 1966   **Prescription:** USA: Yes; Canada: Yes   **Available as Generic:** Yes   **Class:** Analgesic, mild; NSAID   **Controlled Drug:** USA: NO; Canada: No

Brand Names: Meclodium, Meclomen, MeclodiumPonstel, ✦Ponstan

BENEFITS versus RISKS	
Possible Benefits	*Possible Risks*
EFFECTIVE RELIEF OF MILD TO MODERATE PAIN AND INFLAMMATION	Gastrointestinal pain, ulceration, bleeding (rare)
	Rare kidney damage
	Rare fluid retention
	Rare bone marrow depression (mefenamic acid)
	Rare hemolytic anemia (mefenamic acid)
	Rare systemic lupus erythematosus (mefenamic acid)
	Rare pancreatitis (mefenamic acid)

▷ **Principal Uses**

As a Single Drug Product: Uses currently included in FDA approved labeling: (1) Meclofenamate is used to relieve pain of osteoarthritis and rheumatoid arthritis; (2) Mefenamic acid is used to relieve chronic pain; painful menstruation (dysmenorrhea) and postoperative pain.

Other (unlabeled) generally accepted uses: (1) Meclofenamate is used to treat temporal arteritis and the nephrotic syndrome; (2) Mefenamic acid is used to treat PMS, osteoarthritis (maximum one week) and temporal arteritis.

How These Drugs Work: These drugs reduce tissue levels of prostaglandins (and related substances), chemicals involved in the production of inflammation and pain.

Available Dosage Forms and Strengths
Meclofenamate (Meclomen):
Capsules — 50 mg, 100 mg
Mefenamic acid (Ponstel)
Capsule — 250 mg

▷ **Usual Adult Dosage Range:**   Meclofenamate: (osteoarthritis or rheumatoid arthritis)
200 to 400 mg daily, in 3 or 4 divided doses. Total daily dosage should not be more than 400 mg.
Mefenamic acid:
500 mg initially, then 250 mg every 6 hours taken with food.
Note: Actual dosage and administration schedule must be determined by the physician for each patient individually.

Conditions Requiring Dosing Adjustments
Liver function: Changes in dosing are not presently recommended in liver compromise.
Kidney function: Meclofenamate is kidney eliminated, however specific dosing guidelines have not been elaborated. Mefenamic acid should **not** be used in patients with compromised kidneys.

▷ **Dosing Instructions:**   Take with food or milk to prevent stomach irritation. Take with a full glass of water and remain upright (do not lie down) for 30 minutes. The capsule may be opened for administration.

Usual Duration of Use: Meclofenamate: Use on a regular schedule for 2 to 3 weeks usually determines effectiveness in arthritis therapy. Long-term use (months to years) requires physician supervision and periodic evaluation.
Mefenamic acid: Peak levels occur in up to 4 hours. Use beyond seven days is **not recommended**.

▷ **These Drugs Should Not Be Taken If**
• you have had an allergic reaction to them previously.
• you are subject to asthma or nasal polyps caused by aspirin.
• you have active peptic ulcer disease, regional enteritis, ulcerative colitis or any form of gastrointestinal bleeding.
• you have a bleeding disorder or a blood cell disorder.
• you have severe impairment of kidney function (mefanamic acid).
• you have systemic lupus erythematosus (mefenamic acid)
• you have recently had pancreatitis (mefenamic acid).

▷ **Inform Your Physician Before Taking These Drugs If**
• you are allergic to aspirin or to other aspirin substitutes.
• you have a history of peptic ulcer disease, regional enteritis or ulcerative colitis.
• you have a history of any type of bleeding disorder.
• you have impaired liver or kidney function.
• you have high blood pressure or a history of heart failure.
• you take: acetaminophen, aspirin or other aspirin substitutes, anticoagulants, oral antidiabetic drugs or cortisonelike drugs.

Possible Side Effects (natural, expected, and unavoidable drug actions)
Ringing in ears, fluid retention.

▷ **Possible Adverse Effects** (unusual, unexpected, and infrequent reactions)
If any of the following develop, consult your physician promptly for guidance.

Mild Adverse Effects
Allergic Reactions: Skin rash, hives, itching.
Headache, dizziness, altered or blurred vision, depression.
Mouth sores, indigestion, nausea, vomiting, diarrhea (10% to 33%, sometimes severe).

Serious Adverse Effects
Allergic Reactions: Severe skin reactions, drug fever (see Glossary).
Active peptic ulcer, with or without bleeding.
Kidney damage with painful urination, bloody urine, reduced urine formation.
Rare bone marrow depression (see Glossary) (mefenamic acid)—fatigue, weakness, fever, sore throat, abnormal bleeding or bruising.
Mefenamic acid: Also causes rare hemolytic anemia, seizures, porphyria, liver damage, pancreatitis, and systemic lupus erythematosus.

▷ **Possible Effects on Sexual Function**
None reported.

Possible Delayed Adverse Effects: Mild anemia due to "silent" blood loss from the stomach (less than that caused by aspirin).

Natural Diseases or Disorders That May Be Activated by These Drugs
Peptic ulcer disease, ulcerative colitis.

Possible Effects on Laboratory Tests
Complete blood cell counts: decreased red cells, hemoglobin, white cells and platelets (all rare). For mefenamic acid also add SLE test.

CAUTION
1. Dosage should always be limited to the smallest amount that produces reasonable improvement.
2. This drug may mask early indications of infection. Inform your physician if you think you are developing an infection of any kind.
3. Mefenamic acid should be used for a maximum of seven days.

Precautions for Use
By Infants and Children: Safety and effectiveness for those under 14 years of age have not been established for meclofenamate and 18 years of age for mefenamic acid.
By Those over 60 Years of Age: Small doses are advisable until tolerance is determined. Observe for any indications of liver or kidney toxicity, fluid retention, dizziness, confusion, impaired memory, stomach bleeding or diarrhea.

▷ **Advisability of Use During Pregnancy**
Pregnancy Category: Meclofenamate: B normally and D in the last three months of pregnancy. Mefenamic acid: C. See Pregnancy Code at the back of this book.
Animal studies: Some minor birth defects reported in rodents for meclofenamate. Increased fetal resorption in rabbits with 2.5 times the human mefenamic acid dose.

Human studies: Adequate studies of pregnant women are not available.

Avoid meclofenamate during the first and last 3 months. Ask physician for guidance regarding use during the second 3 months.

The manufacturer does not recommend the use of meclofenamate during pregnancy.

Use of mefenamic acid in late pregnancy should be avoided. Ask your doctor for help regarding mefenamic acid use in pregnancy.

Advisability of Use if Breast-Feeding

Presence of these drugs in breast milk: Yes.

Avoid drug or refrain from nursing.

Habit-Forming Potential: None.

Effects of Overdosage: Drowsiness, nausea, vomiting, diarrhea, marked agitation, irrational behavior, metabolic acidosis and seizures.

Possible Effects of Long-Term Use: None identified.

Suggested Periodic Examinations While Taking These Drugs (at physician's discretion)

Complete blood cell counts, kidney function tests, complete eye examinations if vision is altered in any way.

▷ **While Taking These Drugs, Observe the Following**

Foods: No restrictions.

Beverages: No restrictions. May be taken with milk.

▷ *Alcohol:* Use with caution. The irritant action of alcohol on the stomach lining, added to the irritant action of this drug in sensitive individuals, can increase the risk of stomach ulceration and/or bleeding.

Tobacco Smoking: No interactions expected.

▷ *Other Drugs*

Meclofenamate may *increase* the effects of

• acetaminophen (Tylenol, etc.), and increase the risk of kidney damage; avoid prolonged use of this combination.

• anticoagulants (Coumadin, etc.), and increase the risk of bleeding; monitor prothrombin time, adjust dose accordingly.

Meclofenamate *taken concurrently* with the following drugs may increase the risk of bleeding; avoid these combinations:

• aspirin.

• dipyridamole (Persantine).

• sulfinpyrazone (Anturane).

• valproic acid (Depakene).

Mefenamic acid *taken concurrently with*

• cyclosporine (Sandimmune) may result in increased cyclosporine levels and toxicity.

• magnesium containing antacids may result in rapid mefenamic acid toxicity.

• anticoagulants (Coumadin, etc.) will displace the drugs from binding sites and increase bleeding risk.

• aspirin, dipyridamole or sulfinpyrazone may result in increased bleeding risk.

Meclofenamate or mefenamic acid *taken concurrently with*

• diuretics (see Drug Classes) may result in decreased effectiveness of the diuretic in controlling blood pressure.

- enoxaparin may result in increased surgical blood loss if patients receiving this combination undergo surgery.
- lithium will increase blood lithium levels over time and may result in toxicity.
- methotrexate can result in serious methotrexate toxicity.

▷ *Driving, Hazardous Activities:* This drug may cause dizziness or altered vision. Restrict activities as necessary.

Aviation Note: The use of these drugs **may be a disqualification** for piloting. Consult a designated Aviation Medical Examiner.

Exposure to Sun: No restrictions.

FENOPROFEN (fen oh PROH fen)

Introduced: 1976   **Prescription:** USA: Yes; Canada: Yes   **Available as Generic:** Yes   **Class:** Analgesic, mild, NSAID   **Controlled Drug:** USA: No; Canada: No
Brand Name: Nalfon

BENEFITS versus RISKS	
Possible Benefits	*Possible Risks*
EFFECTIVE RELIEF OF MILD TO MODERATE PAIN AND INFLAMMATION	Gastrointestinal pain, ulceration, bleeding (rare)
	Rare liver or kidney damage
	Rare fluid retention
	Rare bone marrow depression

Please see the propionic-acid, nonsteroidal anti-inflammatory drug profile for further information.

FENTANYL (FEN ta nil)

Introduced: 1991   **Prescription:** USA: Yes; Canada: Yes   **Available as Generic:** USA: No; Canada: No   **Class:** Analgesic, strong   **Controlled Drug:** USA:C-ll*
Brand Names: Duragesic, Oralet

BENEFITS versus RISKS	
Possible Benefits	*Possible Risks*
EFFECTIVE PAIN RELIEF	Habit-forming potential with prolonged use
SKIN PATCH APPLICATION NEEDED ONLY ONCE EVERY THREE DAYS	Impairment of mental function
	Methemoglobinemia (rare)
	Respiratory depression

▷ **Principal Uses**

As a Single Drug Product: Uses currently included in FDA approved labeling: (1) Treatment of chronic pain.

Other (unlabeled) generally accepted uses: None.

*See schedules of Controlled Drugs at the back of this book.

How This Drug Works: This drug acts at specific pain receptors (Mu agonist) to block pain.

Available Dosage Forms and Strengths

Transdermal patch — 2.5 mg, 5 mg, 7.5 mg, 10 mg
Lozenge on a handle (has been likened to a lollipop) — 200 mcg, 300 mcg and 400 mcg

▷ **Recommended Dosage Ranges (Actual dosage and administration schedule must be determined by the physician for each patient individually.)**

Infants and Children: Safety and efficacy for those under 12 years of age are not established.

18 to 60 Years of Age: Patch: Not indicated for patients 18 years old who weigh less than 50 kg (110 lbs).

In patients who have not been using opioids such as morphine, the 25 mcg/hr (2.5 mg) patch should be used.

In people who have been given opioids previously, the amount needed to control pain on a 24 hour basis is calculated, converted to an equal amount of morphine (morphine equianalgesic dose), and then converted to fentanyl.

Lozenge (sucker): Used to treat pain and control anxiety prior to surgery 400 micrograms is suggested for those 50 kgs or more.

Over 60 Years of Age: These people should receive the 25 mcg/hr (2.5 mg) patch, unless they were already receiving the equivalent of 135 mg of oral morphine daily. Intravenous fentanyl has been cleared more slowly in this population than in younger patients, and careful observation for overdose should be made.

Conditions Requiring Dosing Adjustments

Liver function: The dose **must be decreased** in liver compromise.

Kidney function: In moderate to severe kidney failure, 75% of the usual dose should be given.

In severe kidney failure, the dose should be reduced by 50%. Patients in end-stage kidney disease may be more sensitive to this medicine.

▷ **Dosing Instructions:** Take the patch from its protective pouch, and remove the stiff protective liner from the sticky side of the patch. Do not cut or damage the system. Put the stick side of the patch on a nonhairy, dry area such as the back, chest, flank or upper arm. Avoid any skin which is burned, irritated or excessively oily. Wash your hands once you have successfully applied the patch. Once the patch has been worn for three days, a new patch should be applied to a different area. The exhausted patch should be folded onto itself and flushed down the toilet. Avoid exposing the patch to external heat sources such as electric blankets or heating pads.

The lozenge or sucker should be allowed to slowly dissolve in the mouth. It should not be bitten or chewed.

Usual Duration of Use: Use on a regular schedule for one to three days usually determines effectiveness in controlling pain. An immediate release form of morphine or similar opioid should be available for pain control while this drug reaches its peak effect. Long-term use (months) requires periodic physician evaluation of response and dosage adjustment of both the patch and an immediate release form of morphine or similar drug.

Possible Advantages of This Drug

Effective pain relief with patch placement once every three days and no injections.

▷ **This Drug Should Not Be Taken If**
- you have had an allergic reaction to any dosage form of it previously.
- you have had an allergic reaction to the adhesive in the patch before.
- you are less than 12 years old.
- you weigh less than 50 kg and are less than 18 years old.
- you have mild or intermittent pain.
- you have acute or postoperative pain without opportunity for proper dose adjustment.

▷ **Inform Your Physician Before Taking This Drug If**
- you have liver or kidney compromise.
- you have chronic lung disease (such as COPD).
- you have an abnormally slow heart beat or other heart disease.
- you develop a high fever.
- you have not taken narcotic pain medicines before and you are given a dose more than 25 mcg per hour.
- you take an MAO inhibitor (see Drug Classes).
- you have a brain tumor.
- you are anemic.
- you have a history of alcoholism or drug abuse.
- you take other prescription or nonprescription medicines which were not discussed with your doctor when transdermal fentanyl was prescribed.

Possible Side Effects (natural, expected, and unavoidable drug actions)

Constipation, dry mouth, and sleepiness.

▷ **Possible Adverse Effects** (unusual, unexpected, and infrequent reactions)

If any of the following develop, consult your physician promptly for guidance.

Mild Adverse Effects

Allergic Reactions: Skin rash and itching.
Nausea and vomiting.
Sleepiness and confusion.
Sweatiness and constipation.
Blurred vision.
Tremor or muscular rigidity.
Amblyopia (rare).

Serious Adverse Effects

Allergic Reactions: Exfoliative dermatitis and/or anaphylactoid reactions.
Arrhythmias (rare).
Paranoid reaction (rare).
Depersonalization and stupor (dose-related or rare).
Seizures (rare).
Hallucinations.
Methemoglobinemia.
Paresthesias (rare).
Urinary retention.
Porphyrias (rare).
Respiratory depression. This effect may last longer than the pain-relieving effect.

▷ **Possible Effects on Sexual Function:**   Impotence and blunted orgasm sensation in men. Irregular menstrual periods and blunted orgasm sensation in women.

Possible Delayed Adverse Effects: Dependence and tolerance.

Possible Effects on Laboratory Tests
   Methemoglobinemia.

CAUTION
   1. Extreme caution should be used if this drug is combined with other opioids, narcotic drugs, benzodiazepines or alcohol.
   2. May cause serious constipation in older patients.
   3. Do not expose the patch site to external sources of heat such as heating pads or electric blankets as an increased rate of drug release may occur.

Precautions for Use
   By Infants and Children: Safety and effectiveness for those under 12 years of age are not established.
   By Those over 60 Years of Age: The 25 mcg patch should **NOT** be used as a starting dose unless you are already taking more than 135 mg of morphine daily. Those with cardiac, respiratory, kidney or liver compromise should be given low doses and be carefully monitored.

▷ **Advisability of Use During Pregnancy**
   Pregnancy Category: C, D if used in high doses when the baby is born or for prolonged periods. See Pregnancy Code at the back of this book.
   Animal studies: Some fetal death data with intravenous use in rats.
   Human studies: Adequate studies of pregnant women are not available.
   Ask your doctor for guidance.

Advisability of Use if Breast-Feeding
   Presence of this drug in breast milk: Yes.
   Avoid drug or refrain from nursing.

Habit-Forming Potential: Fentanyl is a schedule two narcotic and can cause dependence resembling morphine dependence. Physical and psychological dependence and tolerance can occur with repeated use.

Effects of Overdosage: Dizziness, amnesia and stupor. Respiratory depression and apnea may occur.

Possible Effects of Long-Term Use: Tolerance and physical or psychological dependence.

Suggested Periodic Examinations While Taking This Drug   (at physician's discretion)
   Liver function tests.

▷ **While Taking This Drug, Observe the Following**
   Foods: No restrictions.
   Beverages: No restrictions.
▷   *Alcohol:* **DO NOT DRINK ALCOHOL** while you are taking this drug. Leads to additive loss of mental status, respiratory depression and confusion.
   Tobacco Smoking: No interactions expected.
   Marijuana Smoking: Additive adverse effects, however, marijuana may block the vomiting effect of fentanyl.
▷   *Other Drugs*
      Fentanyl may *increase* the effects of
      • benzodiazepines such as diazepam (Valium) and alprazolam (Xanax).

- central nervous system depressants such as opiates, barbiturates, tranquilizers, and tricyclic antidepressants.

Fentanyl *taken concurrently* with

- amiodarone (Codarone) may result in heart (cardiac) toxicity.
- clonidine (Catapres, others) may result in greater than expected fentanyl effects. The fentanyl dose may need to be decreased if these medicines are to be combined.
- MAO inhibitors (see Drug Classes) may worsen the lowering of blood pressure and depression of breathing seen with fentanyl.

▷ *Driving, Hazardous Activities:* This drug may cause drowsiness, sedation and respiratory depression. Restrict activities as necessary.

Aviation Note: The use of this drug *is a disqualification* for piloting. Consult a designated Aviation Medical Examiner.

Exposure to Sun: No restrictions.

Discontinuation: The patch may be removed if the drug is not tolerated or is to be stopped. Once the patch is removed, fentanyl will still continue to be released from the patch site for 17 hours or more. Ideally, if pain medicine is still needed, the chosen alternative should be substituted, and fentanyl transdermal slowly tapered.

FILGRASTIM (fil GRA stem)

Other Names: Recombinant G-CSF

Introduced: 1991   **Prescription:** USA: Yes; Canada: Yes   **Available as Generic:** USA: No; Canada: No   **Class:** Hematopoietic agent   **Controlled Drug:** USA: No; Canada: No

Brand Names: Neupogen

BENEFITS versus RISKS	
Possible Benefits	*Possible Risks*
PREVENTION OF INFECTIONS DUE TO LOWERED WHITE BLOOD CELL COUNTS: FOLLOWING CHEMOTHERAPY FOLLOWING BONE MARROW TRANSPLANT IN PATIENTS WITH CHRONIC OR CYCLIC NEUTROPENIA INCREASED BLOOD CELLS IN AIDS PATIENTS CORRECTION OF DRUG-INDUCED LOWERING OF WHITE BLOOD CELLS	Bone pain Changes in heart waves (rare)

▷ **Principal Uses**

As a Single Drug Product: Uses currently included in FDA approved labeling: (1) Used to help white blood cell counts recover after chemotherapy and bone marrow transplants; (2) used subcutaneously or intravenously to reduce or prevent low white blood cell counts which occur after cancer chemotherapy; (3) treats patients who have an absence of white blood cells at birth; (4) used to help patients with Kostman's syndrome have improved white blood cell counts; (5) used to help patients who have low white blood cell counts (neutropenia) of unknown cause (idiopathic).

Other (unlabeled) generally accepted uses: (1) Helps patients recover from a particular kind of lack of white blood cells (agranulocytosis) which has been caused by medications (drug-induced); (2) used in AIDS patients to help restore white blood cell counts; (3) used to treat patients with severe long-term (chronic) low white blood cell counts; (4) used to treat patients with abnormally low white blood cell and neutrophil counts (myelodysplastic syndrome).

How This Drug Works: This drug is made by recombinant technology and is one of the many acknowledged hematopoietic growth factors. Filgrastin regulates the proliferation and release of early (progenitor) forms of white blood cells. This medicine also can tell the bone marrow to increase the rate at which it makes white blood cells. Filgrastim may also work with other factors to increase the production of blood platelets.

Available Dosage Forms and Strengths

Solution for injection — 300 mcg per ml (supplied as a 300 or 480 mcg vial)

How To Store

The prepared solution should be stored at 36 to 46 degrees Fahrenheit (2 to 8 degrees Centigrade). This medicine **should not** be frozen. Some centers draw up a seven-day supply of syringes which are then stored in a refrigerator.

▷ **Recommended Dosage Ranges (Actual dosage and administration schedule must be determined by the physician for each patient individually.)**

Infants and Children: The medicine has been studied in this population and doses of 0.6 to 120 mcgs per kilogram per day for up to three years have been well tolerated. These doses have been used in children 3 months to 18 years of age. In chronic low white blood cell counts (chronic neutropenia), doses of 5 to 10 mcg per kilogram per day have been used.

18 to 60 Years of Age: Patients receiving therapy which destroys the bone marrow (myeloablative treatment) and then receive a bone marrow transplant: Should wait 24 hours after the chemotherapy was given and 24 hours after bone marrow transplant, then are given 10 mcg per kg per day as a starting dose. This dose is adjusted depending on the degree of increase of white blood cells (absolute neutrophil count).

Patients receiving medicine which suppresses the bone marrow should wait until 24 hours after or 24 hours before the chemotherapy is given. In this population, filgrastim therapy is started with 5 mcg per kilogram per day. Doses may be increased by 5 mcg per kg per day for each cycle of chemotherapy based on the severity of the lowering of white blood cell count (nadir) and how long the lowered white cell (absolute neutrophil) count lasts. This drug can be given daily for up to 14 days.

Over 60 Years of Age: Same as 12 to 60 years of age.

Conditions Requiring Dosing Adjustments

Liver function: Not significantly involved in the elimination of this drug.

Kidney function: Roughly 90% of a given filgrastim dose is eliminated by the kidneys. Changes in dosing are not defined.

▷ **Dosing Instructions:**   The solution in the reconstituted vial should be colorless and clear. Once your doctor or nurse has taught you how to inject the medicine:
1. Make certain the solution has not expired (check the expiration date).
2. Make certain you have the correct kind of syringe (insulin syringes are commonly used).
3. Follow the provided patient instructions carefully.
4. If you are using a syringe, make certain you inject the medicine under the skin, not into a vein.
5. This medicine can also be given intravenously over a period of 15 to 30 minutes.

Usual Duration of Use: Continual use on a regular schedule for up to two weeks (10 to 14 days) may be needed to determine this drug's effectiveness in correcting low white blood (absolute neutrophil) count after chemotherapy. Bone marrow transplant patients may take still longer to respond. Long-term problems with white blood cells (such as chronic neutropenia) may require years of therapy. Long-term use requires periodic evaluation of response and dosage adjustment. Consult your physician on a regular basis.

Possible Advantages of This Drug
Effective recombinant product with few side effects.

▷ **This Drug Should Not Be Taken If**
• you have had an allergic reaction to any dosage form of it previously.
• known allergy to E. coli (a bacteria) derived products.

▷ **Inform Your Physician Before Taking This Drug If**
• you have a history of gout.
• you have a history of psoriasis.
• you have received chemotherapy within the last 24 hours.
• you have a history of heart problems (heart rhythm should be closely monitored).
• you have a history of leukemia (myeloid type). The safety and efficacy of this medicine is not established in that condition.
• you have a history of cancer (with myeloid characteristics). There is a possibility that this drug may act as a growth factor for these tumors. Use, however, in a small number of leukemia patients has not resulted in worsening of their leukemia.
• you are uncertain of how much filgrastim to take or how often to take it.

Possible Side Effects (natural, expected, and unavoidable drug actions)
Pain on injection.
Bone pain (up to 22% in Phase Three studies).

▷ **Possible Adverse Effects** (unusual, unexpected, and infrequent reactions)
If any of the following develop, consult your physician promptly for guidance.
Mild Adverse Effects
Allergic Reactions: Skin rash or itching.
Mild decreases in blood pressure.
Mild increases in uric acid.
Drug-induced fever.

Nausea and anorexias (rare).
Irritation of the eye (iridocyclitis, conjunctival erythema).
Bone pain (mild to moderate).
Enlargement of the spleen—reported in patients with chronic lowering of the white blood cells (chronic neutropenia).
Serious Adverse Effects
Allergic Reactions: Anaphylaxis (rare).
Depression of part of the heart action (ST depression) (rare).
Sweet syndrome (acute neutrophilic dermatosis).
Worsening of psoriasis.
Low oxygen in the blood (hypoxemia) (very rare).
Potential (though not yet reported) for this medicine to act as a growth factor for certain cancers (malignancies of the myeloid type).
Potential (though not yet reported) breathing problems (respiratory distress syndrome) in patients with serious (septic) infections because white blood cells may travel to the infected area.

▷ **Possible Effects on Sexual Function:**   None reported.

Possible Delayed Adverse Effects: Increased uric acid.

▷ **Adverse Effects That May Mimic Natural Diseases or Disorders**
None reported.

Natural Diseases or Disorders That May Be Activated by This Drug
Gout.

Possible Effects on Laboratory Tests
Absolute neutrophil count: increased.
Alkaline phosphatase: increased markedly.
Uric acid: increased mildly.
Lactate dehydrogenase (LDH): increased.

CAUTION
1. Bone pain may be prevented by taking acetaminophen (Tylenol, others) before this medicine is injected.
2. Call your doctor if you have chills, fever or any other sign of infection.
3. Be certain to follow up with your laboratory testing as scheduled.
4. The solution in the vial should be clear. Do **not** inject any discolored or cloudy solution.
5. Make sure you have the correct kind of syringe before you inject this medicine.
6. This medicine can be given intravenously when it is appropriately prepared. If your doctor has instructed you on how to give yourself an injection using a syringe, the medicine should be given under the skin. Be certain you understand the technique.
7. Always change the site in which you inject this medicine as your doctor instructed.

Precautions for Use
By Infants and Children: This medicine has been used in children with long-term lowering of white blood cell counts (chronic neutropenia) in doses of 5 to 10 mcg per kg per day.
By Those over 60 Years of Age: No specific precautions.

▷ **Advisability of Use During Pregnancy**
   Pregnancy Category: C. See Pregnancy Code at the back of this book.
   Animal studies: In rabbits given 80 mcg per kg per day (very high doses), increased abortion and death of embryos were observed.
   Human studies: Information from adequate studies of pregnant women is not available. Ask your doctor for help with this benefit to risk decision.

Advisability of Use if Breast-Feeding
   Presence of this drug in breast milk: Unknown.
   Ask your doctor for guidance.

Habit-Forming Potential: None.

Effects of Overdosage: No maximum tolerated dose has been identified.

Possible Effects of Long-Term Use: Enlarged spleens may occur in up to 25% of patients (splenomegaly) with severe chronic neutropenia. Skin rashes may occur in up to 6% of patients.

Suggested Periodic Examinations While Taking This Drug (at physician's discretion)
   Complete blood cell counts and platelet counts should be obtained prior to chemotherapy and twice weekly during filgrastim therapy.

▷ **While Taking This Drug, Observe the Following**
   Foods: No restrictions.
   Beverages: No restrictions.
▷ *Alcohol:* No restrictions.
   Tobacco Smoking: No interactions expected.
▷ *Other Drugs*
      Filgrastim *taken concurrently* with
      • lithium (Lithobid, others) may (in theory) result in additive release of white blood cells.
▷ *Driving, Hazardous Activities:* No restrictions presently attributed to this medicine.
   Aviation Note: The use of this drug *is probably not a disqualification* for piloting. Consult a designated Aviation Medical Examiner.
   Exposure to Sun: SEVERE intolerance of sunlight (photophobia) has been a treatment limiting factor.
   Occurrence of Unrelated Illness: Report development of chills, fever or other signs or symptoms of infection immediately to your doctor.
   Discontinuation: In patients receiving medicine which suppresses the bone marrow: the drug is usually stopped if a white count (absolute neutrophil count) reaches 10,000 per cubic millimeter after the expected lowest white blood cell count is reached specific to the chemotherapy which was given.
   In people receiving medicine which destroys the bone marrow and subsequently have a bone marrow transplant: The drug is started as described earlier. If the white blood cell count reaches 1,000 per cubic millimeter, the dose is decreased to 5 mcg per kilogram per day. Once the white blood cell count reaches 1,000 per cubic millimeter for six consecutive days, filgrastim can be stopped.
   Special Storage Instructions: This drug should be stored at 36 to 46 degrees Fahrenheit once it has been reconstituted. Care should be taken **not to shake** the prepared drug as it may lose activity. Care should also be taken

not to freeze the prepared medicine as it will clump and lose therapeutic activity.

Observe the Following Expiration Times: Once the medicine is prepared, it is stable for one day (24 hours) if it is refrigerated. If the drug is stored at room temperature, it is stable for 24 hours. Medicine left at room temperature for more than 24 hours should be returned.

FINASTERIDE (fin ES tur ide)

Introduced: 1992   **Prescription:** USA: Yes; Canada: Yes   **Available as Generic:** USA: No; Canada: No   **Class:** 5-alpha reductase inhibitor   **Controlled Drug:** USA: No; Canada: No

Brand Name: Proscar

BENEFITS versus RISKS	
Possible Benefits	*Possible Risks*
NON-SURGICAL TREATMENT OF SYMPTOMATIC BENIGN PROSTATIC HYPERPLASIA. Shrinkage of prostatic tissue and increase in urine flow.	Impotence (small percentage) Decreased libido (small percentage)

▷ **Principal Uses**

As a Single Drug Product: Uses currently included in FDA approved labeling: Treatment of symptomatic benign prostatic hyperplasia (BPH). Maximum shrinkage of the prostate has occurred after six months of therapy.

Other (unlabeled) generally accepted uses: A study of 200 men showed 58% had clinically significant hair growth after one year of use.

How This Drug Works: Finasteride blocks an enzyme (chemical responsible for helping a chemical reaction take place) called 5-alpha reductase. This effect blocks the conversion of testosterone to dihydrotestosterone in the liver and tissues; when the dihydrotestosterone hormone is not available, the prostate shrinks. When the prostate shrinks, symptoms such as urgency and difficulty in urination improve.

Available Dosage Forms and Strengths

Finasteride (Proscar) tablets — 5 mg

How To Store

Keep at room temperature. Avoid exposure to extreme humidity.

▷ **Recommended Dosage Ranges (Actual dosage and administration schedule must be determined by the physician for each patient individually.)**

Infants and Children: **not indicated**.

12 to 60 Years of Age: Symptomatic benign prostatic hyperplasia often does not occur in the younger end of this adult dosing range; however, the dose for this age range is—5 (five) mg each day taken by mouth.

Over 60 Years of Age: Same as 12 to 60 years of age, unless liver function has decreased.

Conditions Requiring Dosing Adjustments

Liver function: Extensive metabolism occurs in the liver, however, specific guidelines for decreases in doses are not available. People with abnormal liver function tests should be followed more closely by their physicians.

Kidney function: No dose decreases needed for mild to moderate kidney failure.

▷ **Dosing Instructions:**   This medicine is best taken on an empty stomach. Food changes the peak blood concentration that is reached, and may decrease the total amount absorbed.

Usual Duration of Use: Use on a regular schedule for at least 6 (six) months is needed to see this drug's peak benefit in shrinking the prostate and decreasing symptoms.

Possible Advantages of This Drug

May give you symptomatic relief of benign prostatic hyperplasia (BPH) without surgery.

▷ **This Drug Should Not Be Taken If**

• you have had an allergic reaction to any dosage form of it previously.
• you are a woman or a child.

▷ **Inform Your Physician Before Taking This Drug If**

• have a history of impaired liver function or liver disease.
• you have kidney problems of any nature.
• your sexual partner is pregnant.

Possible Side Effects (natural, expected, and unavoidable drug actions)

Usually increases testosterone levels; however, the significance of this effect is not known.

▷ **Possible Adverse Effects** (unusual, unexpected, and infrequent reactions)

If any of the following develop, consult your physician promptly for guidance.

Mild Adverse Effects

Allergic Reactions: Rare skin rash, hives.

Increased plasma testosterone.

Serious Adverse Effects

Allergic Reactions: Rare hypersensitivity reactions.

▷ **Possible Effects on Sexual Function:**   Impotence (3.7%).

Decreased libido (3.3%). Gynecomastia.

Decreased volume of ejaculate (2.8%).

Adverse sexual effects may resolve in more than 60% of patients who continue this medication.

Possible Delayed Adverse Effects: Not defined at present.

Possible Effects on Laboratory Tests

Decreased PSA (prostate specific antigen).

CAUTION

1. You should have a digital rectal examination and other examinations for prostate cancer before this medicine is started.
2. If you have a change in liver function, inform your doctor.
3. If your sexual partner is pregnant, avoid exposing your partner to your semen. Exposure to finasteride containing semen may cause genital abnormalities in male offspring.

Precautions for Use

> *By Infants and Children:* Safety and effectiveness for infants and children not established.

> *By Those over 60 Years of Age:* No specific precautions other than changes related to decreased liver function.

▷ **Advisability of Use During Pregnancy**

> *Pregnancy Category:* X. See Pregnancy Code at the back of this book.

> Animal studies: When administered to pregnant rats, the male offspring developed hypospadias. The offspring experienced decreased prostatic and seminal vesicular weight, slow preputial separation and transient nipple problems.

> Human studies: Contraindicated in women who are pregnant or who plan to become pregnant. Women who are pregnant must avoid exposure to crushed tablets, and exposure to semen of a sexual partner who is on finasteride.

> Ask your physician for guidance.

Advisability of Use if Breast-Feeding

> Refrain from nursing if you have been exposed to finasteride or finasteride containing semen.

Habit-Forming Potential: None.

Effects of Overdosage: Multiple doses of up to 80 mg per day have been taken without adverse effect.

Possible Effects of Long-Term Use: Adverse effects of long term use are similar to short-term use effects.

Suggested Periodic Examinations While Taking This Drug (at physician's discretion)

> Patients should be monitored for signs and symptoms of hypersensitivity.

> Patients should be monitored for improvement in symptoms of BPH.

▷ **While Taking This Drug, Observe the Following**

> *Foods:* This medicine is best taken on an empty stomach.

> *Beverages:* No restrictions.

▷ *Alcohol:* No restrictions.

> *Tobacco Smoking:* No interactions expected.

> *Marijuana Smoking:* No interactions expected.

▷ *Other Drugs*

> Finasteride may ***decrease*** the effects of

> • theophylline.

> *Driving, Hazardous Activities:* No restrictions.

> *Aviation Note:* No restrictions.

> *Exposure to Sun:* No restrictions.

FLUCONAZOLE (flu KOHN a zohl)

Introduced: 1985   **Prescription:** USA: Yes; Canada: Yes   **Available as**
Generic: USA: No; Canada: No   **Class:** Antifungal (triazole)   **Controlled**
Drug: USA: No; Canada: No
Brand Name: Diflucan

BENEFITS versus RISKS

Possible Benefits	*Possible Risks*
EFFECTIVE TREATMENT AND SUPPRESSION OF CRYPTOCOCCAL MENINGITIS	Severe skin reactions (rare)
	Possible liver damage (rare)
EFFECTIVE TREATMENT OF CANDIDA INFECTIONS OF THE MOUTH, THROAT, AND ESOPHAGUS	
EFFECTIVE TREATMENT OF SYSTEMIC CANDIDA INFECTIONS	
Effective one-dose treatment of vaginal yeast infections	

▷ **Principal Uses**

As a Single Drug Product: Uses currently included in FDA approved labeling: (1) Treatment of Candida (yeast) infections of the mouth, throat and esophagus (may be AIDS-related); (2) therapy of systemic Candida infections—pneumonia, peritonitis, urinary tract infections (may be AIDS-related).

Other (unlabeled) generally accepted uses: (1) Prevention of yeast infections in patients with low white blood cell counts, cancer or those taking steroids; (2) treatment and suppression of Cryptococcal meningitis; (3) treatment of some fungal eye infections (endophthalmitis); (4) one dose treatment of vaginal yeast infections; (5) treatment of Aspergillus pneumonia; (6) treatment of candidal urinary tract infections; (7) used to treat some fungal infections which may occur in people who have received transplanted organs.

How This Drug Works: By damaging cell walls and blocking essential cell enzymes, this drug inhibits cell growth and reproduction (with low drug concentrations) and destroys fungal cells (with high drug concentrations).

Available Dosage Forms and Strengths

Injection — 200 mg in 100 ml and 400 mg in 200 ml

Tablets — 50 mg, 100 mg, 200 mg

Oral suspension — 50 mg per 5 ml

— 200 mg per 5 ml

▷ **Recommended Dosage Ranges** (Actual dosage and administration schedule must be determined by the physician for each patient individually.)

Infants and Children: From 3 to 13 years of age—3–6 mg per kg of body weight daily, depending on the kind and site of infection.

Cryptococcal meningitis has a recommendation for 12 mg per kg on the first day followed by 6 mg per kg once daily for 10 to 12 weeks after the CSF culture becomes negative.

13 to 60 Years of Age: For treatment of Cryptococcal meningitis—400 mg once daily until significant improvement occurs; then 200 to 400 mg once daily for 10 to 12 weeks after the cerebrospinal fluid (CSF) culture becomes negative.

For suppression of Cryptococcal meningitis—200 mg once daily.

For treatment of Candida infections of mouth and throat—200 mg on the first day; then 100 mg once daily for 2 weeks.

For treatment of Candida infection of the esophagus—200 mg on the first day; then 100 mg once daily for at least 3 weeks; continue treatment for 2 weeks after all signs of infection are gone. If needed, doses up to 400 mg once daily may be used.

Some AIDS patients with chronic mucocutaneous Candida infections have benefited from 50 mg per day of this medicine. For treatment of systemic Candida infections—400 mg once daily for at least 4 weeks; continue treatment for 2 weeks after clearance of all symptoms of infection.

Over 60 Years of Age: Same as 13 to 60 years of age. Dose must be adjusted for impaired kidneys.

Conditions Requiring Dosing Adjustments

Liver function: This drug is a rare cause of hepatitis and should be used with caution in patients with liver compromise.

Kidney function: In mild to moderate kidney failure, the usual dose should be given every 48 hours. In severe kidney failure, half (50%) of the usual dose should be given every 48 hours.

▷ **Dosing Instructions:** The tablet may be crushed, may be taken with or after food to reduce stomach upset.

Usual Duration of Use: Use on a regular schedule for 2 to 4 weeks is usually needed to see this drug's benefit in controlling Candidal or Cryptococcal infections. Actual cures or long-term suppression often require continual treatment for many months. May be continuous therapy in AIDS patients.

Currently a "Drug of Choice"

for maintenance therapy to prevent relapse following control of AIDS-related Candidal esophagitis.

▷ **This Drug Should Not Be Taken If**
- you have had an allergic reaction to it previously.
- you have active liver disease.

▷ **Inform Your Physician Before Taking This Drug If**
- you are allergic to: clotrimazole, itraconazole, ketoconazole or miconazole.
- you have impaired liver or kidney function.
- you are taking any other drugs currently.
- you tend to have low blood potassium.

▷ **Possible Adverse Effects** (unusual, unexpected, and infrequent reactions)
If any of the following develop, consult your physician promptly for guidance.

Mild Adverse Effects

Allergic Reactions: Skin rash (rare).

Hair loss (very rare with usual doses). Reversible hair loss (alopecia) may be more common with high doses of fluconazole given for two months or longer.

Headache (rare).

Nausea, vomiting , stomach pain, diarrhea, or loss of appetite.

Serious Adverse Effects

Allergic Reactions: Severe dermatitis (Stevens-Johnson syndrome) (very rare). Anaphylactoid reactions.

Liver toxicity (rare).

Abnormally low blood platelet counts: Abnormal bruising or bleeding (rare).

Low white blood cell counts (rare).
Seizures (rare).
Adrenal suppression (rare).
Low blood potassium.

▷ **Possible Effects on Sexual Function:**   Amenorrhea (very rare and of questionable cause).

Possible Delayed Adverse Effects: Liver toxicity.

▷ **Adverse Effects That May Mimic Natural Diseases or Disorders**
Possible liver reaction may suggest viral hepatitis.

Possible Effects on Laboratory Tests
Blood platelet counts: decreased.
Liver function tests: increased liver enzymes (ALT/GPT, AST/GOT and alkaline phosphatase), increased bilirubin.

Precautions for Use
By Infants and Children: Safety and effectiveness for those under 13 years of age not established.
By Those over 60 Years of Age: Age-related decrease in kidney function may require adjustment of dosage.

▷ **Advisability of Use During Pregnancy**
Pregnancy Category: C. See Pregnancy Code at the back of this book.
Animal studies: Rat studies revealed significant abnormalities in bone growth and development.
Human studies: Adequate studies of pregnant women not available.
Use this drug only if clearly needed. Ask your doctor for help.

Advisability of Use if Breast-Feeding
Presence of this drug in breast milk: Unknown.
Avoid drug or refrain from nursing.

Habit-Forming Potential: None.

Effects of Overdosage: Possible nausea, vomiting, diarrhea.

Possible Effects of Long-Term Use: None reported.

Suggested Periodic Examinations While Taking This Drug (at physician's discretion)
Liver and kidney function tests.

▷ **While Taking This Drug, Observe the Following**
Foods: No restrictions.
Beverages: No restrictions. May be taken with milk.
▷ *Alcohol:* No interactions expected.
Tobacco Smoking: No interactions expected.
▷ *Other Drugs*
Fluconazole may *increase* the effects of
• oral antidiabetic drugs (chlorpropamide, glipizide, glyburide, tolbutamide), and cause hypoglycemia; check glucose levels carefully.
• cyclosporine (Sandimmune).
• phenytoin (Dilantin, etc.), and cause phenytoin toxicity; monitor phenytoin blood levels.
• trimetrexate (Neutrexin).
• warfarin (Coumadin), and cause unwanted bleeding; monitor prothrombin times as necessary.

- zidovudine (AZT) and result in toxicity. The zidovudine dose may need to be decreased if this combination is to be continued.

The following drug may *decrease* the effects of fluconazole
- cimetidine (Tagamet).
- rifampin (Rifadin, Rimactane, etc.).

Fluconazole *taken concurrently* with
- astemizole (Hismanal) may result in fatal toxicity to the heart.
- hydrochlorothiazide (Esidrex, others) may increase potassium loss.
- loratadine (Claritin) may result in increased blood levels of loratadine, but to date, toxicity to the heart has not been reported. Since blood levels may be increased if combined use is undertaken, it is prudent to decrease the dose of loratadine.
- oral hypoglycemic agents (see Drug Classes) may result in increased lowering of blood sugar.
- terfenadine (Seldane) may result in toxicity to the heart.
- trimexate may increase trimexate toxicity.

▷ *Driving, Hazardous Activities:* No restrictions.

Aviation Note: The use of this drug *is probably not a disqualification* for piloting. Consult a designated Aviation Medical Examiner.

Exposure to Sun: No restrictions.

Discontinuation: Take the full course prescribed. Continual treatment for several months may be necessary. Consult your physician regarding the appropriate time to consider discontinuation.

FLUCYTOSINE (flu SI toh seen)

Other Names: 5-fluorocytosine, 5-FC

Introduced: 1977   **Prescription:** USA: Yes; Canada: Yes   **Available as Generic:** USA: No; Canada: No   **Class:** Antifungal   **Controlled Drug:** USA: No; Canada: No

Brand Names: Ancobon, ✛Ancotil

BENEFITS versus RISKS	
Possible Benefits	*Possible Risks*
EFFECTIVE ADJUNCTIVE TREATMENT OF CERTAIN INFECTIONS CAUSED BY CANDIDA, CRYPTOCOCCUS FUNGI and Aspergillus	BONE MARROW DEPRESSION DRUG-INDUCED LIVER DAMAGE Peripheral neuritis
Effective adjunctive treatment of chromomycosis infection	

▷ **Principal Uses**

As a Single Drug Product: Uses currently included in FDA approved labeling: (1) Treatment of endocarditis, osteomyelitis, arthritis, meningitis, pneumonia, septicemia and urinary tract infections caused by Candida; (2) treatment of meningitis, pneumonia, septicemia, endocarditis and urinary tract infections caused by Cryptococcus. These infections are often AIDS-related.

Other (unlabeled) generally accepted uses: (1) Treatment of disseminated Candidiasis, Chromomycosis and Cryptococcosis. These infections may be AIDS-related; (2) treatment of general fungal infections.

Note: Flucytosine is usually used together with amphotericin B to treat disseminated fungal infections.

How This Drug Works: This drug goes into fungal cells and blocks production of RNA and DNA, thus inhibiting fungal development and reproduction.

Available Dosage Forms and Strengths
Capsules — 250 mg, 500 mg

▷ **Recommended Dosage Ranges** (Actual dosage and administration schedule must be determined by the physician for each patient individually.)

Infants and Children: 50 to 150 mg/kg of body weight, divided into 4 equal doses and given every 6 hours.

12 to 60 Years of Age: 50 to 150 mg per kg of body weight, divided into equal doses and given every 6 hours. In some severe infections, 250 mg per kg per day have been given.

Over 60 Years of Age: Same as 12 to 60 years of age. If kidney function is impaired, dosage reduction is mandatory.

Conditions Requiring Dosing Adjustments
Liver function: In mild to moderate liver compromise, changes in dosage do not presently appear to be needed. Flucytosine has been associated with liver toxicity (especially with blood levels greater than 100 mcg/ml), and should be used with caution in patients with liver compromise.

Kidney function: In mild to moderate kidney failure, the usual dose can be given every 12–24 hours. In severe kidney failure, the usual dose can be given every 24–48 hours.

▷ **Dosing Instructions:**   If a single dose requires more than one capsule, space administration over a period of 15 minutes to reduce stomach irritation and nausea. The capsule may be opened and taken with or after food.

Usual Duration of Use: Use on a regular schedule for 4 to 6 weeks is needed to see effectiveness in controlling Candida or Cryptococcal infection. Long-term use (months to years) requires periodic physician evaluation.

▷ **This Drug Should Not Be Taken If**
• you have had an allergic reaction to it previously.
• you have an active blood cell or bone marrow disorder.
• you have active liver disease.

▷ **Inform Your Physician Before Taking This Drug If**
• you have a history of drug-induced bone marrow depression.
• you have a history of peripheral neuritis.
• you have impaired liver or kidney function.

Possible Side Effects (natural, expected, and unavoidable drug actions)
None.

▷ **Possible Adverse Effects** (unusual, unexpected, and infrequent reactions)
If any of the following develop, consult your physician promptly for guidance.

Mild Adverse Effects
Allergic Reactions: Skin rash, itching.
Headache, dizziness, drowsiness, confusion, hallucinations (infrequent).
Loss of appetite, nausea, vomiting, stomach pain, diarrhea.

Serious Adverse Effects
   Allergic Reactions: Anaphylactoid reactions.
   Bone marrow depression (see Glossary): fatigue, weakness, fever, sore throat,
      abnormal bleeding or bruising.
   Liver damage, with or without jaundice (see Glossary).
   Peripheral neuritis (see Glossary).
   Bowel perforation (rare).
   Kidney damage (rare).

▷ **Possible Effects on Sexual Function:**   None reported.

▷ **Adverse Effects That May Mimic Natural Diseases or Disorders**
   Drug-induced hepatitis may suggest viral hepatitis.

Natural Diseases or Disorders That May Be Activated by This Drug
   Crohn's disease, ulcerative colitis.

Possible Effects on Laboratory Tests
   Complete blood counts: decreased red cells, hemoglobin, white cells and
      platelets.
   Liver function tests: increased liver enzymes (ALT/GPT, AST/GOT and alka-
      line phosphatase), increased bilirubin.
   Kidney function tests: increased blood urea nitrogen (BUN) and creatinine.
   Serum creatinine: may be falsely increased if tested by some methods.

CAUTION
   1. When this drug is used alone, resistance can occur rapidly; it is usually
      used concurrently with amphotericin B (given intravenously).

Precautions for Use
   By Infants and Children: No information available.
   By Those over 60 Years of Age: If necessary, adjust dosage for age-related de-
      crease in kidney function.

▷ **Advisability of Use During Pregnancy**
   Pregnancy Category: C. See Pregnancy Code at the back of this book.
   Animal studies: Rat studies reveal drug-induced birth defects.
   Human studies: Adequate studies of pregnant women not available.
   Use this drug only if clearly needed. Ask your physician for guidance.

Advisability of Use if Breast-Feeding
   Presence of this drug in breast milk: Yes.
   Avoid drug or refrain from nursing.

Habit-Forming Potential: None.

Effects of Overdosage: Nausea, vomiting, stomach pain, diarrhea, confusion.

Possible Effects of Long-Term Use: Bone marrow depression, liver or kidney
   damage.

Suggested Periodic Examinations While Taking This Drug (at physician's dis-
   cretion)
   Measurement of blood levels of flucytosine.
   Complete blood cell counts.
   Liver and kidney function tests.

▷ **While Taking This Drug, Observe the Following**
   Foods: No restrictions.
   Beverages: No restrictions. May be taken with milk.
▷ *Alcohol:* No interactions expected.

Tobacco Smoking: No interactions expected.

▷ *Other Drugs*

The following drug may ***decrease*** the effects of flucytosine
- cytarabine (Cytosar).
- antacids.

Flucytosine ***taken concurrently*** with
- amphotericin B may result in increased risk of kidney toxicity.
- zidovudine (AZT) may result in additive and serious blood (hematological) toxicity.

▷ *Driving, Hazardous Activities:* This drug may cause dizziness, drowsiness or confusion. Limit activities as necessary.

Aviation Note: The use of this drug ***may be a disqualification*** for piloting. Consult a designated Aviation Medical Examiner.

Exposure to Sun: Use caution—this drug may cause photosensitivity (see Glossary).

Discontinuation: This drug may be needed for an extended period of time. Your physician should decide the appropriate time to stop it.

FLUNISOLIDE (flu NIS oh lide)

Introduced: 1980   **Prescription:** USA: Yes; Canada: Yes   **Available as Generic:** No   **Class:** Antiasthmatic, cortisonelike drugs   **Controlled Drug:** USA: No; Canada: No

Brand Names: Aerobid, Aerobid-M, ✦Bronalide, Nasalide, Nasarel, ✦Rhinalar

BENEFITS versus RISKS	
Possible Benefits	*Possible Risks*
EFFECTIVE CONTROL OF SEVERE, CHRONIC BRONCHIAL ASTHMA	Yeast infections of mouth and throat (inhaler form)
	Increased susceptibility to respiratory tract infections (inhaler form)
	Localized areas of "allergic" pneumonia (inhaler form)

▷ **Principal Uses**

As a Single Drug Product: Uses currently included in FDA approved labeling: (1) Treats chronic bronchial asthma in people who require cortisonelike drugs for asthma control. This inhalation form is better than cortisone taken by mouth (swallowed) or by injection as it works locally on the respiratory tract; (2) treatment of various kinds of hay fever (seasonal or perennial allergic rhinitis).

Other (unlabeled) generally accepted uses: (1) Treatment of nasal polyps; (2) treatment of bronchopulmonary dysplasia; (3) may have a role in acute or chronic sinusitis in combination with an antibiotic (amoxicillin/clavulanate in one study).

How This Drug Works: By increasing cyclic AMP, this drug may increase epinephrine, which is an effective bronchodilator and antiasthmatic. An additional benefit is reduction of local allergic reaction and inflammation.

Available Dosage Forms and Strengths
> Inhalation aerosol — 0.25 mg (250 mcg) per metered spray
> Nasal solution — 25 mcg per actuation

▷ **Recommended Dosage Ranges** (Actual dosage and administration schedule must be determined by the physician for each patient individually.)

Infants and Children: Oral inhalation:

Up to 6 years of age—not recommended.

6–15 years old—2 inhalations or 500 micrograms twice a day. Maximum daily dose is 1 mg.

Nasal inhalation:

Up to 6 years of age—not recommended.

6 to 15 years of age—0.25 mcg (1 spray in each nostril) 3 times a day. Once the peak effect is seen, the dose should be reduced to the smallest dose and frequency that works. Maximum is 4 sprays in each nostril (200 mcg per day).

Aqueous nasal form: Up to 6 years of age—not recommended.

6 to 14 years of age: 2 sprays in each nostril twice daily or one spray in each nostril three times a day. Once the peak effect is seen, the dose should be reduced to the smallest dose and frequency that works.

15 to 60 Years of Age: Oral inhalation: 0.5 to 1 mg (2 to 4 metered sprays) 2 times a day, morning and evening. Limit total daily dose to 2 mg. Once the peak effect is seen, the dose should be reduced to the smallest dose and frequency that works.

Nasal inhalation: 2 sprays per nostril twice daily. The dose may be increased to 2 sprays in each nostril 3 times a day (300 mcg per day). Maximum dose with this route is 8 sprays in each nostril (400 mcgs) per day.

Once the peak effect is seen, the dose should be reduced to the smallest dose and frequency that works.

Aqueous nasal form: Two sprays in each nostril twice daily to start. Maintenance dosing is continued with the lowest dose that is effective. This may be as low as one spray in each nostril daily.

Over 60 Years of Age: Same as 15 to 60 years of age.

Conditions Requiring Dosing Adjustments

Liver function: Specific guidelines not available for dosage adjustment in liver compromise.

Kidney function: No specific changes are recommended in patients with compromised kidneys.

▷ **Dosing Instructions:** May be used as needed without regard to eating. Shake the container well before using. Carefully follow the printed patient instructions provided with the inhaler; rinse the mouth and throat (gargle) with water thoroughly after each inhalation.

Usual Duration of Use: Use on a regular schedule for 1 to 4 weeks is necessary to see effectiveness in controlling severe, chronic asthma. Long-term use requires physician supervision and guidance.

▷ **This Drug Should Not Be Taken If**
- you have had an allergic reaction to it previously.
- you are experiencing severe acute asthma or status asthmaticus that requires more intense treatment for prompt relief.
- you have a form of nonallergic bronchitis with asthmatic features.

▷ **Inform Your Physician Before Taking This Drug If**
  • you are now taking or have recently taken any cortisone-related drug (including ACTH by injection) for any reason (see Drug Classes).
  • you have a history of tuberculosis (inhalation form).
  • you have herpes simplex infection of the eye.
  • you have chicken pox.
  • if you have had recent surgery of the nose, have ulcers of the nose or nose bleeds, this medicine should be used cautiously until the site has healed.
  • you have chronic bronchitis or bronchiectasis.
  • you think you may have an active infection of any kind, especially a respiratory infection.

Possible Side Effects (natural, expected, and unavoidable drug actions)
  Yeast infections (thrush) of the mouth and throat.
  Unpleasant taste. Orally inhaled flunisolide can cause flu-like symptoms occasionally in people taking the drug by oral inhalation.

▷ **Possible Adverse Effects** (unusual, unexpected, and infrequent reactions)
  If any of the following develop, consult your physician promptly for guidance.

  Mild Adverse Effects
  Allergic Reactions: Skin rash, hives, itching.
  Headache, dizziness, nervousness, loss of smell or taste.
  Aftertaste (nasal form).
  Moodiness.
  Upper respiratory infections, cough.
  Heart palpitation, increased blood pressure, swelling of feet and ankles (inhalation form).
  Loss of appetite, indigestion, nausea, vomiting, stomach pain, diarrhea.
  Sore throat (20%; 3–9% with aqueous form), stinging of the nose (up to 44%).
  Nasal irritation (33%; 13% with the aqueous form).
  Insomnia.

  Serious Adverse Effects
  Allergic Reaction: Localized areas of "allergic" pneumonitis (lung inflammation).
  Bronchospasm, asthmatic wheezing (rare with the inhalation form).
  Tachycardia (rare with the inhalation form).
  Hypertension (rare with the inhalation form).

▷ **Possible Effects on Sexual Function:**   None reported.

Natural Diseases or Disorders That May Be Activated by This Drug
  Cortisone-related drugs (used by inhalation) that produce systemic effects can impair immunity and lead to reactivation of "healed" or quiescent tuberculosis. People with a history of tuberculosis should be watched closely during use of cortisonelike drugs by inhalation.

Possible Effects on Laboratory Tests
  None reported.

CAUTION
  1. This drug does not act primarily as a brochodilator and **should not be used** for immediate relief of acute asthma.
  2. If you were using any cortisone-related drugs for treatment of your

asthma *before* changing to this inhaler, you may need to restart the cortisone-related drug if you are injured, have an infection or if you require surgery. Be sure to tell your doctor about prior use of cortisone-related drugs taken either by mouth or by injection.

3. If severe asthma returns while using this drug, call your physician immediately so that supportive treatment can be provided as needed.

4. If you have used cortisone-related drugs in the past year, carry a card that says this has happened. During periods of stress it may be necessary to resume cortisone treatment in adequate dosage.

5. Five to 10 minutes should separate the inhalation of bronchodilators such as albuterol, epinephrine, pirbuterol, etc., (which should be used first) and the inhalation of this drug. This lets more flunisolide reach the bronchial tubes, and reduces risk of adverse effects from the propellants used in the two inhalers.

6. A decongestant may be a good idea in people with blocked nasal passages. Talk with your doctor or pharmacist.

Precautions for Use
By Infants and Children: Safety and effectiveness for those under 4 years of age not established. To obtain maximal benefit, the use of a spacer device is recommended for inhalation therapy in children.

By Those over 60 Years of Age: People with chronic bronchitis or bronchiectasis should be watched closely for the development of lung infections.

▷ **Advisability of Use During Pregnancy**
Pregnancy Category: C. See Pregnancy Code at the back of this book.
Animal studies: Rat and rabbit studies reveal significant birth defects due to this drug.
Human studies: Adequate studies of pregnant women not available.
Avoid drug during the first 3 months. Use infrequently and only as clearly needed during the last 6 months.

Advisability of Use if Breast-Feeding
Presence of this drug in breast milk: Unknown.
Avoid drug or refrain from nursing.

Habit-Forming Potential: With recommended dosage, a state of functional dependence (see Glossary) is not likely to develop.

Effects of Overdosage: Indications of cortisone excess (due to systemic absorption)—fluid retention, flushing of the face, stomach irritation, nervousness.

Possible Effects of Long-Term Use: Development of acne, cataracts, altered menstrual pattern.

Suggested Periodic Examinations While Taking This Drug (at physician's discretion)
Inspection of mouth and throat for evidence of yeast infection.
Check of adrenal function in people who have used cortisone-related drugs for an extended period of time before using this drug.
X-ray of the lungs of people with a prior history of tuberculosis.

▷ **While Taking This Drug, Observe the Following**
Foods: No specific restrictions beyond those advised by your physician.
Beverages: No specific restrictions.

▷ *Alcohol:* No interactions expected.

Tobacco Smoking: No interactions expected. However, smoking can worsen asthma and reduce the effectiveness of this drug. Follow your physician's advice.

▷ *Other Drugs*

The following drugs may ***increase*** the effects of flunisolide
- inhalant bronchodilators—albuterol, bitolterol, epinephrine, etc.
- oral bronchodilators—aminophylline, ephedrine, terbutaline, theophylline, etc.

Flunisolide ***taken concurrently*** with
- Stanazolol may result in increased risk of acne or edema.

▷ *Driving, Hazardous Activities:* No restrictions.

Aviation Note: The use of this drug and the disorder for which this drug is prescribed ***may be disqualifications*** for piloting. Consult a designated Aviation Medical Examiner.

Exposure to Sun: No restrictions.

Occurrence of Unrelated Illness: Acute infections, serious injuries or surgical procedures can create an urgent need for cortisone-related drugs given by mouth and/or injection. Call your doctor immediately in the event of new illness or injury.

Discontinuation: If this drug has made it possible to reduce or discontinue cortisonelike drugs by mouth, ***do not*** stop this drug abruptly. If you must stop this drug, call your doctor promptly. Cortisone preparations and other measures may be necessary.

Special Storage Instructions: Store at room temperature. Avoid exposure to temperatures above 120 degrees F (49 degrees C). Do not store or use this inhaler near heat or open flame.

FLUOXETINE (flu OX e teen)

Introduced: 1978   **Prescription:** USA: Yes   **Available as Generic:** USA: No   **Class:** Antidepressant   **Controlled Drug:** USA: No
Brand Name: Prozac

BENEFITS versus RISKS	
Possible Benefits	*Possible Risks*
EFFECTIVE TREATMENT OF MAJOR DEPRESSIVE DISORDERS	Serious allergic reactions
Possibly effective in relieving the symptoms of obsessive-compulsive disorder	Conversion of depression to mania in manic-depressive (bipolar) disorders (rare)

▷ **Principal Uses**

As a Single Drug Product: Uses currently included in FDA approved labeling: (1) Treatment of major forms of depression. This drug should not be used to treat the symptoms of mild and transient (reactive) depression; (2) obsessive-compulsive disorder.

Author's note: The FDA granted approvable status for use of fluoxetine in the treatment of bulimia in 1994. Final approval is still pending.

Other (unlabeled) generally accepted uses: (1) Refractory bulimia; (2) refractory diabetic neuropathy; (3) may help control kleptomania; (4) can be of help in treating obesity, especially when obesity is accompanied by depression; (5) eases symptoms of panic attacks, (6) may be given only during the premenstrual period to treat premenstrual syndrome (PMS); (7) used to treat seasonal affective disorder (such as depression limited to winter months).

How This Drug Works: It slowly restores normal levels of a nerve transmitter (serotonin).

Available Dosage Forms and Strengths
Capsules — 10 mg, 20 mg
Syrup — 20 mg per 5 ml

▷ **Usual Adult Dosage Range:**   Started at 20 mg as a single morning dose; if no improvement occurs after several weeks of treatment, the dose may be increased by 20 mg/day as needed and tolerated. Doses over 20 mg/day should be divided into two equal doses and taken twice daily. Maximum daily dosage is 80 mg. **Note: Actual dosage and administration schedule must be determined by the physician for each patient individually.**

Conditions Requiring Dosing Adjustments
Liver function: The dose should be decreased or the dosing interval lengthened in patients with liver compromise. Some clinicians decrease the dose by 50% in compensated cirrhosis. This drug is also a rare cause of hepatotoxicity, and should be used with caution in this patient population.
Kidney function: The dose should be decreased or the time between doses increased in severe kidney (renal) compromise.

▷ **Dosing Instructions:**   The capsule may be opened and the contents mixed with any convenient food. To make smaller doses, the contents may be mixed with orange juice or apple juice and refrigerated; doses of 5 mg to 10 mg may prove effective and better tolerated.

Usual Duration of Use: Use on a regular schedule for as little as 1 to 2 weeks may reveal the beginning of improvement in depression. Up to 4 to 8 weeks may be needed to determine (1) this drug's effectiveness in relieving depression; (2) the pattern of both favorable and unfavorable effects. Since there is an active metabolite and a long half life, it may take several weeks before the benefits of a change in dose is seen. Long-term use (months to years) requires periodic physician evaluation.

Possible Advantages of This Drug
Does not cause weight gain, a common side effect of tricyclic antidepressants. May actually cause weight loss.
Less likely to cause dry mouth, constipation, urinary retention, orthostatic hypotension (see Glossary) and heart rhythm disturbances than tricyclic antidepressants.
Does not cause Parkinson-like reactions.

▷ **This Drug Should Not Be Taken If**
- you have had an allergic reaction to any dosage form of it previously.
- you currently take or have taken within the past 14 days any monoamine oxidase (MAO) type A inhibitor (see Drug Classes).

▷ **Inform Your Physician Before Taking This Drug If**
- you have had any adverse effects from antidepressant drugs.
- you have impaired liver or kidney function.
- you have Parkinson's disease.
- you have a seizure disorder.
- you have a history of psychosis.
- you have a history of SIADH (talk with your doctor).
- you are pregnant or plan pregnancy while taking this drug.

Possible Side Effects (natural, expected, and unavoidable drug actions)
Decreased appetite, weight loss.

▷ **Possible Adverse Effects** (unusual, unexpected, and infrequent reactions)
If any of the following develop, consult your physician promptly for guidance.

Mild Adverse Effects
Allergic Reactions: Skin rash, hives (rare), itching.
Headache, nervousness, insomnia, drowsiness, tremor, dizziness, fatigue, impaired concentration (rare).
Excessive lowering of blood pressure upon standing (orthostatic hypotension) (rare).
Altered taste (rare), nausea, vomiting, diarrhea.
Hair loss (rare).
Fast heart rate (tachycardia) or palpitations (rare).
Blurred vision.
Excessive sweating.

Serious Adverse Effects
Allergic Reactions: Serum-sickness-like syndrome: fever, weakness, joint pain and swelling, swollen lymph glands, fluid retention, skin rash and/or hives.
Drug-induced seizures (rare).
Worsening of Parkinson's disease.
Intense suicidal preoccupation in severe depression that does not respond to this drug (see Current Controversies at the end of this Profile).
Mania or hypomania (rare).
Psychosis or hallucinations (rare).
Abnormal and excessive urination (SIADH).
Liver toxicity (rare).

▷ **Possible Effects on Sexual Function:** Impaired erection (1.9%), inhibition of ejaculation, and inhibited orgasm in men and women.

Natural Diseases or Disorders That May Be Activated by This Drug
Latent epilepsy.

Possible Effects on Laboratory Tests
Blood glucose level: decreased.
Blood sodium level: decreased.

CAUTION
1. If any skin reaction develops (rash, hives, etc.), stop this drug and inform your physician promptly.
2. If dry mouth develops and persists for more than 2 weeks, consult your dentist for help.

3. Ask your doctor or pharmacist before taking any other prescription or over-the-counter drug while taking fluoxetine.
4. If you must start any monoamine oxidase (MAO) type A inhibitor (see Drug Classes), allow an interval of 5 weeks after stopping this drug before starting the MAO inhibitor.
5. This drug should be withheld if electroconvulsive therapy (ECT, "shock" treatment) is to be used.

Precautions for Use

By Infants and Children: Safety and effectiveness for those under 12 years of age not established.

By Those over 60 Years of Age: Total daily dosage should not exceed 60 mg.

▷ **Advisability of Use During Pregnancy**

Pregnancy Category: B. See Pregnancy Code at the back of this book.

Animal studies: No birth defects due to this drug found in rat or rabbit studies.

Human studies: Adequate studies of pregnant women are not available.

Use this drug only if clearly needed.

Advisability of Use if Breast-Feeding

Presence of this drug in breast milk: Yes.

Avoid drug or refrain from nursing.

Habit-Forming Potential: Reports of patients using excess doses of fluoxetine or combining the drug with alcohol have surfaced. It appears possible that a euphoric effect and abuse potential exists.

Effects of Overdosage: Agitation, restlessness, excitement, nausea, vomiting, seizures.

Possible Effects of Long-Term Use: None reported.

Suggested Periodic Examinations While Taking This Drug (at physician's discretion)

None.

▷ **While Taking This Drug, Observe the Following**

Foods: No restrictions.

Beverages: No restrictions. May be taken with milk.

▷ *Alcohol:* Does not appear to increase the central nervous system effects of fluoxetine or change the metabolism of alcohol.

Tobacco Smoking: No interactions expected.

▷ *Other Drugs*

Fluoxetine may *increase* the effects of

- diazepam (Valium).
- digitalis preparations (digitoxin, digoxin).
- phenytoin (Dilantin) by increasing the drug level.
- warfarin (Coumadin) and related oral anticoagulants.

Fluoxetine *taken concurrently* with

- antidiabetic drugs (insulin, oral hypoglycemics) may increase the risk of hypoglycemic reactions; monitor blood sugar levels carefully.
- astemizole (Hismanal), or terfenadine (Seldane), or similar drugs may result in increased terfenadine levels and risk of heart arrhythmias. **Avoid** combining.

- buspirone (Buspar) may increase underlying anxiety. **Avoid** the combination.
- carbamazepine (Tegretol) will increase the carbamazepine level. Drug levels are critical if the drugs are combined.
- clozapine (Clozaril) may result in increased levels of clozapine. The clozapine dose may need to be decreased if both medicines are to be used at the same time.
- dextromethorphan (a cough suppressant in many "DM" labeled nonprescription cough medicines) may result in visual hallucinations if these drugs are combined. **DO NOT** combine these medicines.
- haloperidol (Haldol) will increase haloperidol levels. Dosage decrease and blood levels are needed.
- ketorolac (Toradol) may result in hallucinations. **DO NOT** take these medicines at the same time.
- lithium (Lithobid, etc.) will result in increased lithium levels and increased risk of neurotoxicity. **Avoid** the combination.
- loratidine (Claritin) may result in increased loratadine levels. It may be prudent to decrease the dose if these medicines are to be combined. Unlike some of the other nonsedating antihistamines (see Drug Classes), loratadine has not (to date) resulted in abnormal heart rhythms.
- monoamine oxidase (MAO) type A inhibitor drugs may cause confusion, agitation, high fever, seizures and dangerous elevations of blood pressure. Avoid combining these drugs.
- tryptophan will result in central nervous system toxicity. **Avoid** the combination.
- any tricyclic antidepressant (amitriptyline, nortriptyline, etc.) will result in increased antidepressant drug levels that will persist for weeks. **Avoid** the combination.
- selegiline (Eldepryl) can result in serotonin toxicity syndrome. **Avoid** this Combination.

▷ *Driving, Hazardous Activities:* This drug may cause drowsiness, dizziness, impaired judgment and delayed reaction time. Restrict activities as necessary.

Aviation Note: The use of this drug *is a disqualification* for piloting. Consult a designated Aviation Medical Examiner.

Exposure to Sun: No restrictions.

Discontinuation: Slow drug elimination makes withdrawal effects unlikely. However, call your doctor if you plan to stop this drug for any reason.

Current Controversies in Drug Management

In 1990 it was reported that six patients being treated with fluoxetine experienced the onset of intense and violent suicidal preoccupation. All six had severe depression that had not responded to the use of fluoxetine for 2 to 7 weeks. For most of them, suicidal mentality persisted for 2 to 3 months after discontinuation of the drug.

The resultant adverse publicity suggested that this experience may be somewhat characteristic of fluoxetine in contrast to other antidepressant drugs. A review of relevant literature on this subject reveals that the development or intensification of suicidal thoughts during treatment (regardless of the severity of depression) has been documented repeatedly for many antidepressant drugs in wide use. Suicidal thinking may emerge during treatment with any antidepressant. Recent reports establish that some patients who become suicidal while taking one antidepressant can be switched to fluoxetine and experience cessation of suicidal thinking and satisfactory relief of depression.

This is another example of the marked variability of individual response to drug therapy. The choice of a drug to treat many serious disorders remains an experiment of trial and error. Successful management requires clinical judgment (based on experience), close monitoring and appropriate doses.

FLUPHENAZINE (flu FEN a zeen)

Introduced: 1959   **Prescription:** USA: Yes; Canada: Yes   **Available as Generic:** USA: No; Canada: Yes   **Class:** Strong tranquilizer, phenothiazines
Controlled Drug: USA: No; Canada: No
Brand Names: ✦Apo-Fluphenazine, ✦Modecate, ✦Moditen, Permitil, PMS-Fluphenazine, Prolixin

---

BENEFITS versus RISKS

Possible Benefits	*Possible Risks*
EFFECTIVE CONTROL OF ACUTE MENTAL DISORDERS	SERIOUS TOXIC EFFECTS ON BRAIN with long-term use
Beneficial effects on thinking, mood, and behavior	Liver damage with jaundice (very rare)
	Rare blood cell disorders: abnormally low white blood cell counts

---

▷ **Principal Uses**

As a Single Drug Product: Uses currently included in FDA approved labeling: (1) Treatment of schizophrenia.

Other (unlabeled) currently accepted uses: (1) Combination treatment of refractory neuropathy; (2) an alternative neuroleptic drug in treating Tourette's syndrome in combination with clonidine; (3) therapy of Alzheimer's disease symptoms; (4) may help control sexual aggressiveness.

How This Drug Works: By inhibiting the action of dopamine, this drug acts to correct an imbalance of nerve impulse transmissions.

Available Dosage Forms and Strengths

Concentrate — 5 mg per ml (1% alcohol)
     Elixir — 2.5 mg per 5-ml (14% alcohol)
     Injection — 2.5 mg per ml
     Tablets — 1 mg, 2.5 mg, 5 mg 10 mg

▷ **Usual Adult Dosage Range:** 2.5 to 10 mg given 3 to 4 times daily. The dose is adjusted as needed and tolerated. Total daily dosage should not exceed 40 mg. **Note: Actual dosage and administration schedule must be determined by the physician for each patient individually.**

Conditions Requiring Dosing Adjustments

Liver function: Used with caution in patients with both liver and kidney compromise.

Kidney function: Used with caution in patients with compromised kidneys and livers.

▷ **Dosing Instructions:**   Regular tablets can be crushed and taken with or following meals to reduce stomach irritation. Prolonged-action tablets should be swallowed whole (not crushed). The concentrate must be diluted in 4 to 6 ounces of water, milk, fruit juice or carbonated beverage.

Usual Duration of Use: Use on a regular schedule for several weeks is needed to determine effectiveness in controlling psychotic disorders. If not of benefit in 6 weeks, it should be stopped. Long-term use (months to years) requires periodic physician evaluation.

▷ **This Drug Should Not Be Taken If**
  • you are allergic to any of the drugs bearing the brand names listed.
  • you have a history of brain damage.
  • you have active liver disease.
  • you have cancer of the breast.
  • you have an active blood dyscrasia.
  • you are taking large doses of other medicines which can depress the central nervous system.
  • you have a current blood cell or bone marrow disorder.

▷ **Inform Your Physician Before Taking This Drug If**
  • you are allergic or sensitive to any phenothiazine (see Drug Classes).
  • you have impaired liver or kidney function.
  • you have any type of seizure disorder.
  • you have diabetes, glaucoma, heart disease or chronic lung disease.
  • you have a history of lupus erythematosus.
  • you have a history of depressed white blood cell counts of the granulocytic series (agranulocytosis).
  • you have a history of neuroleptic malignant syndrome.
  • you are taking any drug with sedative effects.
  • you will have surgery under general or spinal anesthesia soon.

Possible Side Effects (natural, expected, and unavoidable drug actions)
  Drowsiness (usually during the first 2 weeks), orthostatic hypotension (see Glossary), blurred vision, dry mouth, nasal congestion, constipation, impaired urination (all mild).

▷ **Possible Adverse Effects** (unusual, unexpected, and infrequent reactions)
  If any of the following develop, consult your physician promptly for guidance.
  Mild Adverse Effects
  Allergic Reactions: Skin rash, hives, itching.
  Lowering of body temperature, especially in the elderly.
  Headache, dizziness, weakness, excitement, restlessness, unusual dreaming.
  Increased appetite and weight gain.
  Serious Adverse Effects
  Allergic Reactions: Hepatitis with jaundice (see Glossary), usually between second and fourth week; anaphylactic reaction (see Glossary).
  Idiosyncratic Reaction: Neuroleptic malignant syndrome (see Glossary).
  Impaired production of white blood cells—fever, sore throat, infections.
  Parkinson-like disorders (see Glossary); muscle spasms of face, jaw, neck, back, extremities.
  Liver toxicity.
  Depression.

Porphyria.
Pituitary tumors (extremely rare).
Abnormal heart beats (rare).
Seizures (rare).
Prolonged drop in blood pressure with weakness, perspiration, and fainting.

▷ **Possible Effects on Sexual Function**
Decreased male libido; increased female libido.
Impaired erection (38% to 42%); complete impotence.
Inhibited male orgasm (58%); inhibited female orgasm (22% to 33%).
Inhibited ejaculation (46%).
Altered timing and pattern of menstruation (frequent).
Female breast enlargement and milk production (galactorrhea).
Prolonged and painful erection.
Male breast enlargement and tenderness (gynecomastia).
May help treat sexual hyperactivity.

▷ **Adverse Effects That May Mimic Natural Diseases or Disorders**
Nervous system reactions may suggest Parkinson's disease.
Liver reactions may suggest viral hepatitis.
Reactions resembling systemic lupus erythematosus may occur.

Natural Diseases or Disorders That May Be Activated by This Drug
Latent epilepsy, glaucoma, prostatism (see Glossary).

Possible Effects on Laboratory Tests
Complete blood counts: decreased red cells, hemoglobin, white cells and platelets; increased eosinophils (allergic reaction).
Blood sugar (glucose): decreased.
Liver function tests: increased liver enzymes (ALT/GPT, AST/GOT and alkaline phosphatase), increased bilirubin.
Urine pregnancy tests: false positive results.
Urine screening test for drug abuse: initial test may be falsely *positive* for barbiturates; the confirmatory test will be *negative*.

CAUTION
1. Many over-the-counter medications (see OTC Drugs in Glossary) for allergies, colds and coughs can interact unfavorably with this drug. Ask your physician or pharmacist for help before using any such medications.
2. Antacids containing aluminum and/or magnesium can prevent absorption.
3. Obtain prompt evaluation of any change or disturbance of vision.

Precautions for Use
By Infants and Children: Do not use this drug in infants under 6 months of age, or in children of any age with symptoms suggestive of Reye syndrome (see Glossary). Monitor carefully for blood cell changes.
Children with psychosis have been given 0.25 to 0.75 mg from one to four times daily.
By Those over 60 Years of Age: Small starting doses are advisable. Increased risk of drowsiness, lethargy, constipation, lowering of body temperature (hypothermia) and orthostatic hypotension (see Glossary). This drug can enhance existing prostatism (see Glossary). You may also be more susceptible

to the development of Parkinson-like reactions and/or tardive dyskinesia (see discussion of these terms in Glossary).

▷ **Advisability of Use During Pregnancy**
Pregnancy Category: C. See Pregnancy Code at the back of this book.
Animal studies: Significant birth defects reported in mice.
Human studies: Adequate studies of pregnant women are not available.
Avoid drug during the first 3 months and during the last month because of possible effects on the newborn infant.

Advisability of Use if Breast-Feeding
Presence of this drug in breast milk: Yes.
They do not usually accumulate in high enough concentrations to effect the infant. Watch the infant closely and discuss the situation with your doctor.

Habit-Forming Potential: None.

Effects of Overdosage: Marked drowsiness, weakness, tremor, agitation, unsteadiness, deep sleep, coma, convulsions.

Possible Effects of Long-Term Use: Tardive dyskinesia (see Glossary); eye changes—cataracts and pigmentation of retina; gray to violet pigmentation of skin in exposed areas, more common in women.

Suggested Periodic Examinations While Taking This Drug (at physician's discretion)
Complete blood counts.
Liver function tests, electrocardiograms.
Complete eye examinations—eye structures and vision.
Careful tongue exam for evidence of fine, involuntary, wavelike movements that could be the beginning of tardive dyskinesia.

▷ **While Taking This Drug, Observe the Following**
Foods: No restrictions.
Beverages: No restrictions. May be taken with milk.
▷   *Alcohol:* Avoid completely. Alcohol can increase phenothiazine sedation and accentuate depressant effects on brain function and blood pressure. Phenothiazines can increase the intoxicating effects of alcohol.
Tobacco Smoking: Possible increased removal of fluphenazine and need for dose increase.
Marijuana Smoking: Moderate increase in drowsiness; accentuation of orthostatic hypotension; increased risk of precipitating latent psychoses, confusing the interpretation of mental status and drug responses.
▷   *Other Drugs*
Fluphenazine may *increase* the effects of
• all sedative drugs, and cause excessive sedation.
• all atropinelike drugs, and cause nervous system toxicity.
Fluphenazine may *decrease* the effects of
• guanethidine (Ismelin, Esimil), and reduce its effectiveness in lowering blood pressure.
Fluphenazine *taken concurrently* with
• beta blocker drugs (see Drug Classes) may cause increased effects of both drugs; watch drug effects—may need smaller doses.
• clonidine (Catapress, others) may result in an acute organic brain syndrome (disorientation, agitation, delirium). These medicines should not be combined.

- lithium can cause increase toxicity to the nerves.
- MAO inhibitors (see Drug Classes) can cause very low blood pressure and worsening of the central nervous system and respiratory depression effects.
- oral hypoglycemic agents (see Drug Classes) may result in lower blood sugar levels than expected. Doses of the oral hypoglycemic agents may need to be decreased.
- vitamin C (ascorbic acid) may decrease the therapeutic benefits of fluphenazine.

The following drugs may *decrease* the effects of fluphenazine

- antacids containing aluminum and/or magnesium.
- benztropine (Cogentin).
- trihexyphenidyl (Artane).

▷ *Driving, Hazardous Activities:* This drug can impair mental alertness, judgment and physical coordination. Avoid hazardous activities.

Aviation Note: The use of this drug *is a disqualification* for piloting. Consult a designated Aviation Medical Examiner.

Exposure to Sun: Use caution—some phenothiazines can cause photosensitivity (see Glossary).

Exposure to Heat: Use caution and avoid excessive heat. This drug may impair the regulation of body temperature and increase heat stroke risk.

Exposure to Cold: Use caution and dress warmly. Increased risk of hypothermia in the elderly.

Discontinuation: After long-term use, do not stop this drug suddenly. Gradual withdrawal over 2 to 3 weeks under physician supervision is needed. Do not stop this drug without your doctor's knowledge and approval. The relapse rate of schizophrenia after discontinuation is 50–60%.

FLURAZEPAM (flur AZ e pam)

Introduced: 1970   **Prescription:** USA: Yes; Canada: Yes   **Available as Generic:** USA: Yes; Canada: Yes   **Class:** Hypnotic, benzodiazepines
Controlled Drug: USA: C-IV*; Canada: No

Brand Names: ✦Apo-Flurazepam, Dalmane, Durapam, ✦Novo-flupam, ✦Somnol

BENEFITS versus RISKS	
Possible Benefits	*Possible Risks*
EFFECTIVE HYPNOTIC	Habit-forming potential with
NO SUPPRESSION OF REM (RAPID EYE MOVEMENT) SLEEP	long-term use
NO REM SLEEP REBOUND after discontinuation	Minor impairment of mental functions ("hangover" effect)
Wide margin of safety with therapeutic doses	Very rare jaundice
	Very rare blood cell disorder
	Suppression of stage-4 sleep with reduced "quality" of sleep

*See Schedules of Controlled Drugs at the back of this book.

▷ **Principal Uses**

As a Single Drug Product: Uses currently included in FDA approved labeling: Short-term treatment of insomnia consisting of difficulty in falling asleep, frequent nighttime awakenings, and/or early morning awakenings.

Other (unlabeled) generally accepted uses: May be of benefit in patients who have undergone herniorrhaphy in helping them sleep.

How This Drug Works: By enhancing the action of the nerve transmitter gamma-aminobutyric acid (GABA), arousal of higher brain centers is blocked and helps sleep occur.

Available Dosage Forms and Strengths

Capsules — 15 mg, 30 mg (US, Canada)
Tablets — 15 mg, 30 mg (Canada)

▷ **Recommended Dosage Ranges** (Actual dosage and administration schedule must be determined by the physician for each patient individually.)

Infants and Children: Up to 15 years of age—use not recommended.

15 to 60 Years of Age: Initially 15 mg at bedtime; increase to 30 mg only if needed and tolerated.

Over 60 Years of Age: Same as 15 to 60 years of age. Usually 15 mg is adequate; use higher doses with caution.

Conditions Requiring Dosing Adjustments

Liver function: The dose **must** be decreased in patients with liver compromise. Flurazepam is also a rare cause of hepatocellular and cholestatic jaundice, and must be used as a benefit to risk decision in patients with compromised livers.

Kidney function: Changes in dosage are not usually needed.

▷ **Dosing Instructions:**   The capsule may be opened and taken on an empty stomach or with food or milk. Do not stop this drug abruptly if taken for more than 4 weeks.

Usual Duration of Use: Use for 3 nights is usually needed to see this drug's benefit in relieving insomnia. If possible, this drug should be used for periods of 3 to 5 nights intermittently, repeated as needed with appropriate dosage adjustment. Avoid uninterrupted and prolonged use. Duration of use should not exceed 2 weeks without reappraisal of continued need.

▷ **This Drug Should Not Be Taken If**
- you have had an allergic reaction to it previously.
- you are pregnant.
- you have sleep apnea.
- you have acute narrow-angle glaucoma.

▷ **Inform Your Physician Before Taking This Drug If**
- you are allergic to any benzodiazepine (see Drug Classes).
- you have a history of alcoholism or drug abuse.
- you are planning pregnancy.
- you have impaired liver or kidney function.
- you are an alcoholic.
- you have a history of serious depression or mental disorder.
- you are taking other drugs with sedative effects.
- you have: asthma, emphysema, epilepsy, or myasthenia gravis.

Possible Side Effects (natural, expected, and unavoidable drug actions)
"Hangover" effects on arising: drowsiness, lethargy, and unsteadiness.

▷ **Possible Adverse Effects** (unusual, unexpected, and infrequent reactions)
If any of the following develop, consult your physician promptly for guidance.

Mild Adverse Effects
Allergic Reactions: Skin rash, hives, burning eyes, swelling of tongue.
Dizziness, fainting, blurred vision, double vision, slurred speech, nausea, indigestion.
Taste disorders.
Ringing in the ears.
Increased heart rate.

Serious Adverse Effects
Allergic Reactions: Rare liver damage with jaundice (see Glossary).
Idiosyncratic Reactions: Nervousness, talkativeness, irritability, apprehension, euphoria, excitement, hallucinations.
Rare bone marrow depression—impaired production of white blood cells, fever, sore throat.
Liver toxicity (rare).
Intraocular pressure increase.
Sleep apnea.
Increased risk of hip fracture (from falls) if used in those over 60.

▷ **Possible Effects on Sexual Function:**   None reported.

▷ **Adverse Effects That May Mimic Natural Diseases or Disorders**
Liver reaction with jaundice may suggest viral hepatitis.

Possible Effects on Laboratory Tests
Liver function tests: increased liver enzymes (ALT/GPT, AST/GOT and alkaline phosphatase, increased bilirubin.
Urine sugar tests: no drug effect with TesTape; false low results with Clinistix and Diastix; false positive result with Benedict's solution.
Urine screening tests for drug abuse: may be *positive*. (Test results depend upon amount of drug taken and testing method used.)

CAUTION
1. This drug should not be stopped abruptly if it has been taken continually for more than 4 weeks.
2. Some over-the-counter drug products that contain antihistamines (allergy and cold preparations, sleep aids) can cause excessive sedation.
3. Regular nightly use of any hypnotic drug should be avoided.
4. This drug is transformed by the liver into long-acting forms that can persist in the body for 24 hours or more. With continual use of this drug daily, these active drug forms accumulate and produce increasing sedation. If you experience a "hangover" effect, avoid hazardous activities (driving, etc.) and the use of alcohol.

Precautions for Use
By Infants and Children: Safety and effectiveness for those under 15 years of age not established.
By Those over 60 Years of Age: Starting doses are reduced and given less often. Watch for lethargy, indifference, fatigue, weakness, unsteadiness, disturb-

ing dreams, nightmares and paradoxical reactions (excitement, agitation, anger and rage.)

Because this is a long-acting benzodiazepine, it may cause residual sluggishness and unsteadiness with increased risk of falls. This drug may also increase the number of periods of sleep apnea in this age group.

▷ **Advisability of Use During Pregnancy**

Pregnancy Category: X. See Pregnancy Code at the back of this book.

Animal studies: No birth defects reported in rat and rabbit studies.

Human studies: Adequate studies of pregnant women are not available.

Several studies indicate an increased risk of birth defects if drugs of this class (benzodiazepines) are used during the first 3 months.

Frequent use in late pregnancy can cause the "floppy infant" syndrome in the newborn: weakness, lethargy, unresponsiveness, depressed breathing, low body temperature.

Avoid use during entire pregnancy.

Advisability of Use if Breast-Feeding

Presence of this drug in breast milk: Probably yes.

Avoid drug or refrain from nursing.

Habit-Forming Potential: This drug can produce psychological and/or physical dependence (see Glossary) if used in large doses for an extended period of time. Avoid continual use.

Effects of Overdosage: Marked drowsiness, weakness, feeling of drunkenness, staggering gait, tremor, stupor progressing to deep sleep or coma.

Possible Effects of Long-Term Use: Psychological and/or physical dependence, impaired liver function.

Suggested Periodic Examinations While Taking This Drug (at physician's discretion)

Complete blood cell counts and liver function tests during long-term use.

▷ **While Taking This Drug, Observe the Following**

Foods: No restrictions.

Beverages: Avoid excessive intake of caffeine-containing beverages (coffee, tea, cola) within 4 hours of taking this drug. May be taken with milk.

▷ *Alcohol:* Use with extreme caution—alcohol may increase the absorption of this drug and add to its depressant effects on the brain. It is advisable to avoid alcohol completely—throughout the day and night—if it is necessary to drive or to engage in any hazardous activity.

Tobacco Smoking: Heavy smoking may reduce the hypnotic action of this drug.

Marijuana Smoking: Increased sedation and significant impairment of intellectual and physical performance.

▷ *Other Drugs*

Flurazepam may *increase* the effects of

• digoxin (Lanoxin), and cause digoxin toxicity.

• lithium and cause additive drowsiness.

• phenytoin (Dilantin), and cause phenytoin toxicity.

Flurazepam may *decrease* the effects of

• levodopa (Sinemet, etc.), and reduce its effectiveness in treating Parkinson's disease.

Fluphenazine *taken concurrently* with

- narcotics, other benzodiazepines, phenothiazines or antihistamines (see Drug Classes section) or other medicines with sedating properties may result in additive sedation.

The following drugs may *increase* the effects of flurazepam

- cimetidine (Tagamet).
- disulfiram (Antabuse).
- isoniazid (INH, Rifamate, etc.).
- omeprazole (Prilosec).
- oral contraceptives.
- valproic acid (Depakene).

The following drugs may *decrease* the effects of flurazepam

- rifampin (Rimactane, etc.).
- theophylline (aminophylline, Theo-Dur, etc.).

▷ *Driving, Hazardous Activities:* This drug can impair mental alertness, judgment, physical coordination and reaction time. Avoid hazardous activities accordingly.

Aviation Note: The use of this drug *is a disqualification* for piloting. Consult a designated Aviation Medical Examiner.

Exposure to Sun: No restrictions.

Exposure to Heat: Use caution until the effect of excessive perspiration is determined. Because of reduced urine volume, this drug may accumulate in the body and produce effects of overdosage.

Discontinuation: Avoid sudden discontinuation if this drug has been taken for over 4 weeks without interruption. Dosage should be tapered gradually to prevent a withdrawal syndrome that could include depression, confusion, hallucinations, tremor, seizures, muscle cramping, sweating and vomiting.

FLURBIPROFEN (flur BI proh fen)

Introduced: 1977 **Prescription:** USA: Yes; Canada: Yes **Available as Generic:** USA: No; Canada: No **Class:** Analgesic, mild; NSAID **Controlled Drug:** USA: No; Canada: No

Brand Names: Ansaid, ♣Apo-flurbiprofen, ♣Froben, ♣Froben-SR, Ocufen

BENEFITS versus RISKS	
Possible Benefits	*Possible Risks*
EFFECTIVE RELIEF OF SYMPTOMS ASSOCIATED WITH MAJOR TYPES OF ARTHRITIS	PEPTIC ULCER DISEASE, with associated bleeding and perforation
Effective relief of symptoms associated with bursitis, tendonitis, and related conditions	Liver toxicity with jaundice (rare)
Effective relief of menstrual cramps	Water retention
	Rare kidney toxicity
	Rare aplastic anemia (see Glossary)

Please see the propionic acid nonsteroidal antiinflammatory drug profile for further information.

FLUTAMIDE (FLU ta mide)

Introduced: 1983   **Prescription:** USA: Yes; Canada: Yes   **Available as Generic:** USA: No; Canada: No   **Class:** Anticancer (antineoplastic)   **Controlled Drug:** USA: No; Canada: No

Brand Names: ✦Euflex, Eulexin, Flutamex (Germany)

BENEFITS versus RISKS	
Possible Benefits	*Possible Risks*
EFFECTIVE ADJUNCTIVE	Rare drug-induced hepatitis
TREATMENT OF PROSTATE	Breast enlargement and tenderness
CANCER	Hot flashes

▷ **Principal Uses**

As a Single Drug Product: Uses currently included in FDA approved labeling: Treatment of metastatic prostate cancer, used concurrently with leuprolide (given by injection).

Other (unlabeled) generally accepted uses: There has been some isolated use as a 2% alcoholic gel in treating acne.

How This Drug Works: Flutamide is an antiandrogenic drug; it suppresses the biological effects of the male sex hormone (testosterone, an androgen) by blocking its uptake and binding in target tissues (such as the prostate gland). It is used in conjunction with leuprolide, a hormonelike drug that suppresses the production of testosterone by the testicles (by damping the pituitary gland's stimulation of the testicles). The combination of these two drug actions—chemical castration by leuprolide and testosterone blockage by flutamide)—significantly reduces hormonal stimulation of cancerous prostate tissue.

Available Dosage Forms and Strengths

Capsules — 125 mg (US)
Tablets — 250 mg (Canada, Germany)

▷ **Recommended Dosage Ranges** (Actual dosage and administration schedule must be determined by the physician for each patient individually.)

Infants and Children: Not used in this age group.

12 to 60 Years of Age: 250 mg every 8 hours. Flutamide is to be taken concurrently with leuprolide; the usual dose of leuprolide is 7.5 mg given by injection once a month.

Over 60 Years of Age: Same as 12 to 60 years of age.

Conditions Requiring Dosing Adjustments

Liver function: It should be used with caution in patients with liver compromise. It is also a rare cause of cholestatic jaundice.

Kidney function: Primarily eliminated by the kidneys. Used with caution in kidney compromise.

▷ **Dosing Instructions:** May be taken without regard to food. The capsule may be opened and the tablet may be crushed for administration.

Warning: Since this medicine is an antineoplastic agent, proper disposal (ask your doctor) of urine or vomit MUST be undertaken.

Usual Duration of Use: Use on a regular schedule for 2 to 3 months is usually needed to see this drug's effectiveness in controlling prostate cancer. Long-term use (months to years) requires periodic physician evaluation.

Possible Advantages of This Drug
Ease of use.
Significantly less toxicity than chemotherapeutic drugs.

Currently a "Drug of Choice"
for the management of prostate cancer (in combination with leuprolide).

▷ **This Drug Should Not Be Taken If**
• you have had an allergic reaction to it previously.

▷ **Inform Your Physician Before Taking This Drug If**
• you have a history of liver disease or impaired liver function.
• you have high blood pressure (hypertension).
• you have a history of anemia, low white blood cells or low blood platelets.
• you have a history of lupus erythematosus.

Possible Side Effects (natural, expected, and unavoidable drug actions)
Hot flashes (61%), loss of libido (with combination LHRH therapy), impotence, breast enlargement and tenderness.

▷ **Possible Adverse Effects** (unusual, unexpected, and infrequent reactions)
If any of the following develop, consult your physician promptly for guidance.
Mild Adverse Effects
Allergic Reactions: Skin rash.
Drowsiness, confusion, nervousness (rare).
Indigestion, nausea/vomiting, diarrhea.
Blurred vision (rare).
Fluid retention (edema) of legs.
Serious Adverse Effects
Drug-induced hepatitis with jaundice (see Glossary) (rare).
Low blood platelets (rare).
Low white blood cells.
Anemia.
Lupus-erythematosus-like skin rash (rare).
Rare heart attack.

▷ **Possible Effects on Sexual Function**
See Possible Side Effects above. Flutamide itself does not presently appear to change libido, sexual performance or the ability to have an erection. Combination therapy does appear to carry the risks of these adverse effects.

▷ **Adverse Effects That May Mimic Natural Diseases or Disorders**
Drug-induced hepatitis may suggest viral hepatitis.

Possible Effects on Laboratory Tests
Complete blood counts: decreased red and white cells, hemoglobin and platelets.
Liver function tests: increased liver enzymes (ALT/GPT, AST/GOT and alkaline phosphatase), increased bilirubin.
Sperm counts: decreased.
Testosterone levels: decreased.

CAUTION
1. For best results, flutamide and leuprolide should be started together and continued for the duration of therapy.
2. During combination therapy with flutamide and leuprolide, symptoms of prostate cancer (difficult urination, bone pain, etc.) may worsen temporarily; these are transient and not significant.

Precautions for Use
By Those over 60 Years of Age: This drug is more slowly excreted. If digestive symptoms or edema are troublesome, ask your doctor about adjusting your dose.

▷ **Advisability of Use During Pregnancy**
Pregnancy Category: D. See Pregnancy Code at the back of this book.
Animal studies: Rat studies reveal malformation of bone structures and feminization of male fetuses.
Human studies: Adequate studies of pregnant women are not available.

Habit-Forming Potential: None.

Effects of Overdosage: Possible drowsiness, unsteadiness, nausea, vomiting.

Possible Effects of Long-Term Use: None reported.

Suggested Periodic Examinations While Taking This Drug (at physician's discretion)
Prostatic specific antigen (PSA) assays.
Complete blood cell counts.
Liver function tests.

▷ **While Taking This Drug, Observe the Following**
Foods: No restrictions.
Beverages: No restrictions. May be taken with milk.
▷ *Alcohol:* No interactions expected.
Tobacco Smoking: No interactions expected.
Marijuana Smoking: Animal studies have shown this combination to result in additive suppression of the immune system. The combination therefore is not advisable.
▷ *Other Drugs:* Flutamide *taken concurrently* with
  • influenza, pneumococcal or yellow fever vaccine may result in blunting of immune response to the vaccine.
▷ *Driving, Hazardous Activities:* This drug may cause drowsiness. Restrict activities as necessary.
Aviation Note: The use of this drug *may be a disqualification* for piloting. Consult a designated Aviation Medical Examiner.
Exposure to Sun: This drug may cause photosensitivity (see Glossary).
Discontinuation: To be determined by your physician.

FLUTICASONE (flu TIC a zone)

Introduced: 1994   **Prescription:** USA: Yes; Canada: Yes   **Available as Generic:** USA: No; Canada: No   **Class:** adrenocorticosteroid   **Controlled Drug:** USA: No; Canada: No

Brand Names: Flonase, Flovent, Cutivate
   Author's note: This profile will focus on the aqueous nasal form of this medicine.

Warning: Even though this medicine is a nasal spray, there is still a remote risk of suppression of the hypothalamic pituitary adrenal (HPA) axis.

BENEFITS versus RISKS	
Possible Benefits	*Possible Risks*
EFFECTIVE, ONCE-A-DAY RELIEF OF SEASONAL ALLERGIC RHINITIS	Reversible adrenal gland suppression Irritation of the nose

▷ **Principal Uses**
   As a Single Drug Product: Uses currently included in FDA approved labeling: (1) Management of perennial and seasonal (hay fever) allergic or nonallergic rhinitis in adults or children who are 12 years of age or older; (2) the topical form is used for a variety of skin conditions from sunburn to lupus erythematosus; (3) the inhaler form was approved in 1996 for treatment of asthma. Other (unlabeled) generally accepted uses: None at present.

How This Drug Works: This medicine belongs to a new class of corticosteroids. The exact mechanism of action of this medicine is not known, however, halomethyl carbothionates have very potent antiinflammatory and blood vessel contracting (vasoconstrictive) activity.

Available Dosage Forms and Strengths
                Amber Glass Bottle — 16 gram (120 actuations) and 9 gram (60 actuations)
                Cream (Germany) — 0.05 mg per gram
         Inhalation powder (Germany) — 50, 100 and 250 mcg per actuation

▷ **Recommended Dosage Ranges (Actual dosage and administration schedule must be determined by the physician for each patient individually.)**
   Infants and Children: Safety and efficacy for those less than 12 years of age have not yet been defined.
   12 to 60 Years of Age: Dosing is started with two sprays (50 mcg in each spray) in each nostril once daily. The same dose can also be given as 100 mcg twice daily (8 AM and 8 PM). After a few days, the dose can often be decreased to 100 mcg (one spray in each nostril) daily.
   Over 60 Years of Age: Same as 12 to 60 years of age.

Conditions Requiring Dosing Adjustments
   Liver function: This drug is extensively changed in the liver, however, no specific dosing changes are defined in patients with compromised livers.
   Kidney function: No changes in dosing needed.

▷ **Dosing Instructions:**   A patient instruction sheet will always accompany this medicine. The instructions should be followed closely. Your doctor should be called if the condition worsens or does not improve.

Usual Duration of Use: Continual use on a regular schedule for several days is usually necessary to determine this drug's effectiveness in treating seasonal and perennial allergic rhinitis. Long-term use (months to years) requires periodic evaluation of response and dosage adjustment. Consult your physician on a regular basis.

Possible Advantages of This Drug
Once a day dosing.

▷ **This Drug Should Not Be Taken If**
• you have had an allergic reaction to any dosage form of it previously.

▷ **Inform Your Physician Before Taking This Drug If**
• you are already taking systemic prednisone.
• you are exposed to measles or chicken pox.
• you are uncertain of how much fluticasone to take or how often to take it.
• you take other prescription or nonprescription medicines which were not discussed with your doctor when fluticasone was prescribed.
• you have signs or symptoms of an infection in your nose.
• you have damage from an accident or surgery to your nose while you are taking this medicine.
• your allergic rhinitis does not improve or worsens.

Possible Side Effects (natural, expected, and unavoidable drug actions)
Irritation of the nose. Systemic steroid effects (possible).

▷ **Possible Adverse Effects** (unusual, unexpected, and infrequent reactions)
If any of the following develop, consult your physician promptly for guidance.
Mild Adverse Effects
Allergic Reactions: Contact dermatitis.
Nosebleeds.
Nasal burning.
Dizziness.
Unpleasant taste, nausea, or vomiting (rare).
Serious Adverse Effects
Allergic Reactions: Anaphylaxis.
Suppression of the HPA axis (rare).
Increased risk from viral infections.
Yeast infections of the nose (rare).
Cushing's syndrome (with excessive doses or very sensitive patients).

▷ **Possible Effects on Sexual Function:**   None defined.

Possible Delayed Adverse Effects: Yeast infections of the nose (rare).

▷ **Adverse Effects That May Mimic Natural Diseases or Disorders**
None defined.

Natural Diseases or Disorders That May Be Activated by This Drug
If systemic effects occur, the patient may be more susceptible to infections, or dormant infections may become active.

Possible Effects on Laboratory Tests
Cortisol levels: decreased.

CAUTION
1. Call your doctor if you are exposed to measles or chicken pox.
2. Long-term use requires periodic evaluation for yeast infection of the nose.
3. Call your doctor if your condition does not improve or worsens.

Precautions for Use

By Infants and Children: Safety and effectiveness for use by those under 12 years of age have not been established for the intranasal form. Many adolescents can be started successfully with one spray in each nostril per day (100 mcgs). Maximum total daily dosage should not exceed 200 mcgs.

By Those over 60 Years of Age: No specific precautions.

▷ **Advisability of Use During Pregnancy**

Pregnancy Category: C. See Pregnancy Code at the back of this book.

Animal studies: High dose studies in rats revealed fetal toxicity consistent with changes caused by other steroids.

Human studies: Information from adequate studies of pregnant women is not available. Ask your doctor for guidance.

Advisability of Use if Breast-Feeding

Presence of this drug in breast milk: Unknown.

Monitor nursing infant closely and discontinue drug or nursing if adverse effects develop.

Habit-Forming Potential: Not defined.

Effects of Overdosage: Not defined.

Possible Effects of Long-Term Use: Rare nasal yeast infections.

Suggested Periodic Examinations While Taking This Drug (at physician's discretion)

Nasal exams.

▷ **While Taking This Drug, Observe the Following**

Foods: No restrictions.

Beverages: No restrictions.

▷ *Alcohol:* No interactions expected.

Tobacco Smoking: No interactions expected.

▷ *Other Drugs*

Fluticasone *taken concurrently* with

• Systemic steroids (such as prednisone) may increase the likelihood of suppression of the HPA axis.

▷ *Driving, Hazardous Activities:* This drug may cause dizziness. Restrict activities as necessary.

Aviation Note: The use of this drug *may be a disqualification* for piloting. Consult a designated Aviation Medical Examiner.

Exposure to Sun: No restrictions.

Discontinuation: This medicine should not be stopped abruptly. Talk with your doctor before stopping this drug.

FLUVASTATIN (flu va STAT in)

Introduced: 1994   **Prescription:** USA: Yes; Canada: Yes   **Available as Generic:**   USA: No; Canada: No   **Class:** Cholesterol reducing drug, HMG-CoA reductase inhibitor.   **Controlled Drug:** USA: No; Canada: No

Brand Names: Lescol

```
┌──────────────────────────────────────────────────────────────┐
│                    BENEFITS versus RISKS                       │
│        Possible Benefits              Possible Risks           │
│  EFFECTIVE REDUCTION OF TOTAL    Increased liver enzymes (rare)│
│     BLOOD CHOLESTEROL           Muscle pain or weakness (rare) │
│  SLOWS PROGRESSION OF                                          │
│     CORONARY ATHEROSCLEROSIS                                   │
└──────────────────────────────────────────────────────────────┘
```

▷ **Principal Uses**

As a Single Drug Product: Uses currently included in FDA approved labeling: (1) Management of abnormally high cholesterol in people with II hypercholesterolemia; (2) slows the progression of atherosclerosis in patients with coronary heart disease.

Other (unlabeled) generally accepted uses: Not fully defined at present.

How This Drug Works: This medicine is changed (hydrolyzed) in the body to the beta-hydroxy acid form. The beta-hydroxy acid form inhibits an enzyme (HMG-CoA reductase) which is the (rate controlling) enzyme in the process the body uses to make cholesterol.

Available Dosage Forms and Strengths

Tablets — 10 mg, 20 mg and 40 mg

▷ **Recommended Dosage Ranges (Actual dosage and administration schedule must be determined by the physician for each patient individually.)**

Infants and Children: Safety and efficacy for those less than 12 years of age have not yet been defined.

18 to 60 Years of Age: Dosing is started with 20 mg a day, taken with the evening meal. This dose is increased as needed and tolerated to 80 mg with each evening (24 hours apart) meal. Any needed increases are made at intervals of 4 weeks.

Patients who take immunosuppressant medicines are started on 10 mg of lovastatin daily and should not receive more than 20 mg daily with the evening meal.

Over 60 Years of Age: Same as 12 to 60 years of age.

Conditions Requiring Dosing Adjustments

Liver function: This drug is extensively changed in the liver, however, no specific dosing changes are defined in patients with compromised livers.

Kidney function: Patients with severe kidney failure (creatinine clearance less then 30 ml/ min.) should be given more than 20 milligrams a day only with great caution.

▷ **Dosing Instructions:**   This medicine is best taken with the evening meal as it produces the best cholesterol lowering results or outcomes. **Author's note: This profile will be further developed in subsequent editions of this book.**

FLUVOXAMINE (FLU vox a meen)

Introduced: 1995   **Prescription:** USA: Yes; Canada: Yes   **Available as Generic:** USA: No; Canada: No   **Class:** Antidepressant, selective serotonin reuptake inhibitor   **Controlled Drug:** USA: No; Canada: No
Brand Names: Luvox

Warning: Do not combine this medicine with terfenadine (Seldane) or astemizole (Hismanal).

BENEFITS versus RISKS	
Possible Benefits	*Possible Risks*
TREATMENT OF OBSESSIVE-COMPULSIVE DISORDER	Nausea and vomiting (often resolves with time)

▷ **Principal Uses**

As a Single Drug Product: Uses currently included in FDA approved labeling: (1) Treatment of obsessive compulsive disorder.

Other (unlabeled) generally accepted uses: (1) May have a role in helping compulsive exhibitionism; (2) can have a role in treating depression; (3) may be useful in eating problems where bingeing is a key difficulty; (4) can help panic attacks; (5) could have a role in long standing (chronic) tension headaches.

How This Drug Works: This medicine inhibits the reuptake of the neurotransmitter 5-HT effecting a beneficial change in the treated behaviors or conditions.

Available Dosage Forms and Strengths

Tablets — 50 mg 100 mg

▷ **Recommended Dosage Ranges (Actual dosage and administration schedule must be determined by the physician for each patient individually.)**

Infants and Children: Safety and efficacy have not been established in those under 18 years old.

18 to 60 Years of Age: Therapy is started with 50 mg taken at bedtime. The dose may then be increased as needed and tolerated by 50 mg intervals every 4 to 7 days to a maximum dose of 300 mg daily. The prescriber should remember that the drug may take from 4 to 14 days to begin to work. If a patient does need a daily dose greater than 100 mg, the dose should be divided in half and taken twice daily.

Over 60 Years of Age: This medicine is removed half as slowly as in younger patients. Plasma concentrations are also roughly 40% higher than in younger patients. Slower time frames for any increases beyond the starting dose and lower maintenance doses are indicated.

Conditions Requiring Dosing Adjustments

Liver function: This drug is extensively changed by the liver. If it is used in patients with liver disease, lower starting doses, slow dose increases and careful patient monitoring is indicated.

Kidney function: A lower starting dose and careful patient monitoring is needed.

▷ **Dosing Instructions:**   Take this medicine exactly as prescribed and at the same time. This medicine may be taken with or without food. Call your doctor if vomiting (a possible side effect) continues for more than two days after you start treatment.

Usual Duration of Use: Continual use on a regular schedule for 4 to 14 days is usually necessary to determine this drug's effectiveness in helping obsessive-compulsive disorder. Long-term use (months to years) requires periodic evaluation of response and dosage adjustment. Consult your physician on a regular basis.

Possible Advantages of This Drug
Requires one daily dosing and has a good side effect profile.

▷ **This Drug Should Not Be Taken If**
- you have had an allergic reaction to any dosage form of it previously.
- you have taken or are taking terfenadine or astemizole.

▷ **Inform Your Physician Before Taking This Drug If**
- you have continued to have a problem with vomiting two days after starting this medicine.
- you feel light headed when you get up from a sitting position.
- you have a history of seizures.
- you are uncertain of how much fluvoxamine to take or how often to take it.
- you have taken a MAO inhibitor (see Drug Classes) within the last 14 days.
- you have a history of heart problems.
- you take other prescription or nonprescription medicines which were not discussed with your doctor when fluvoxamine was prescribed.

Possible Side Effects (natural, expected, and unavoidable drug actions)
Nausea and vomiting (usually stops after a few days of treatment).

▷ **Possible Adverse Effects** (unusual, unexpected, and infrequent reactions)
If any of the following develop, consult your physician promptly for guidance.
Mild Adverse Effects
Allergic Reactions: Skin rash.
Somnolence and dry mouth.
Headache or agitation.
Sleep disorders.
Liver toxicity (rare).
Constipation.
Anorexia.
Serious Adverse Effects
Allergic Reactions: Anaphylactoid reaction.
Liver toxicity (rare).
Seizures (rare).
Mania (rare).
Tourette's syndrome (very rare).
Excessive urination (rare).
Serious skin rash (rare).

▷ **Possible Effects on Sexual Function:**   Delayed or absent orgasm, failure to ejaculate.

Possible Delayed Adverse Effects: Not reported.

▷ **Adverse Effects That May Mimic Natural Diseases or Disorders**
Not reported.

Natural Diseases or Disorders That May Be Activated by This Drug
None defined.

Possible Effects on Laboratory Tests
Liver function tests: increased.
Melatonin level: increased.

CAUTION

1. This medicine has several important drug-drug interactions. Be certain to tell any health care professionals who provide care for you that you take this medicine.
2. If nausea and vomiting continue for more than two days after you start this medicine, call your doctor.

Precautions for Use

By Infants and Children: Safety and effectiveness for use by those under 18 years of age have not been established.

By Those over 60 Years of Age: Lowering starting and maintenance doses are indicated.

▷ **Advisability of Use During Pregnancy**

Pregnancy Category: C. See Pregnancy Code at the back of this book.

Animal studies: Consistent with category C.

Human studies: Information from adequate studies of pregnant women is not available. Ask your doctor for help.

Advisability of Use if Breast-Feeding

Presence of this drug in breast milk: Yes, in small amounts.

Monitor nursing infant closely and discontinue drug or nursing if adverse effects develop.

Habit-Forming Potential: None, but a withdrawal syndrome has been reported if the medicine is stopped abruptly.

Effects of Overdosage: Nausea, vomiting, seizures.

Possible Effects of Long-Term Use: Not defined.

Suggested Periodic Examinations While Taking This Drug (at physician's discretion)

Liver function tests.

▷ **While Taking This Drug, Observe the Following**

Foods: No restrictions.

Beverages: No restrictions.

▷ *Alcohol:* No significant interaction. Ask your doctor for guidance.

Tobacco Smoking: Fluvoxamine stays in the body of smokers up to one-quarter less time than in nonsmokers. Smokers may need higher than typical doses to get the same benefit as nonsmokers.

Marijuana Smoking: Additive somnolence.

▷ *Other Drugs*

Fluvoxamine *taken concurrently* with

- amitriptyline (Elavil others) can result in amitriptyline toxicity.
- astemizole (Hismanal) may cause **serious heart arrhythmias**. Do not combine.
- benzodiazepines (see Drug Classes) may result in benzodiazepine toxicity.
- beta blockers (see Drug Classes) may result in decreased drug clearance and toxicity.
- carbamazepine (Tegretol) may cause toxicity.
- clomipramine (Anafranil) may cause toxicity.
- clozapine (Clozaril) can result in higher clozapine levels and toxicity.
- imipramine (Tofranil, others) may result in imipramine toxicity.
- lithium (Lithobid) can cause serotonin syndrome.

- MAO inhibitors (see Drug Classes) can cause toxicity. Do **not** combine.
- maprotiline can cause maprotiline toxicity.
- methadone may result in increased opioid effects.
- oral hypoglycemic agents (see Drug Classes) may remain in the body longer than expected, requiring a dosage decrease. This has not been reported with fluvoxamine, but has been reported with sertraline, a medicine in the same pharmacologic family.
- phenytoin (Dilantin) may lead to phenytoin toxicity. Patients should be watched closely for problems walking (ataxia) or drowsiness (early toxicity signs) and their doctor notified at once if these occur.
- terfenadine (Seldane) may cause **serious heart arrhythmias**. Do not combine.
- theophylline may result in theophylline toxicity.
- warfarin (Coumadin) can result in increased warfarin concentrations and may lead to bleeding. More frequent INR testing is needed.

▷ *Driving, Hazardous Activities:* This drug may cause drowsiness. Restrict activities as necessary.

 Aviation Note: The use of this drug *is probably a disqualification* for piloting. Consult a designated Aviation Medical Examiner.

Exposure to Sun: No restrictions.

Discontinuation: A withdrawal syndrome has been reported if this medicine is abruptly stopped. The doses should be slowly tapered.

FOSINOPRIL (FOH sin oh pril)

Introduced: 1986   **Prescription:** USA: Yes   **Available as Generic:** No   **Class:** Antihypertensive, ACE inhibitor   **Controlled Drug:** USA: No
Brand Name: Monopril

BENEFITS versus RISKS	
Possible Benefits	*Possible Risks*
EFFECTIVE CONTROL OF MILD TO MODERATE HIGH BLOOD PRESSURE	Low blood pressure (rare) Allergic swelling of face, tongue, throat, vocal cords (rare)

▷ **Principal Uses**

  As a Single Drug Product: Uses currently included in FDA approved labeling: Treats mild to moderate high blood pressure, alone or in combination with other medicines.

  Other (unlabeled) generally accepted uses: (1) Combination with other drugs (digoxin and diuretics) to treat congestive heart failure; (2) may help decrease enlargement of the left side of the heart; (3) reduces abnormal elimination of protein by the kidneys; (4) helps survival after a heart attack.

How This Drug Works: By blocking an enzyme system (angiotensin-converting enzyme, ACE), this drug relaxes arterial walls and lowers blood pressure. This, in turn, reduces the workload of the heart and improves its performance.

Available Dosage Forms and Strengths

  Tablets — 10 mg, 20 mg

▷ **Recommended Dosage Ranges** (Actual dosage and administration schedule must be determined by the physician for each patient individually.)

Infants and Children: Dosage not established.

18 to 60 Years of Age: Initially 10 mg once daily. Usual maintenance dose is 20 to 40 mg/day taken in a single dose. Total daily dosage should not exceed 80 mg.

Over 60 Years of Age: Same as 18 to 60 years of age.

Conditions Requiring Dosing Adjustments

Liver function: Fosinopril is a prodrug, and is changed into fosinoprilat (the active form) by the liver. It should be used with caution and in lower doses in patients with liver compromise. Fosinopril can also be a rare cause of hepatitis.

Kidney function: This drug undergoes liver and bile (dual hepatobiliary) and kidney (renal) elimination. Patients with renal compromise (especially those with renal artery stenosis) should be started on a decreased dose, and the dose should be increased slowly and only if needed.

▷ **Dosing Instructions:**   The tablet may be crushed, and taken on an empty stomach or with food, at the same time each day.

Usual Duration of Use: Use on a regular schedule for 2 to 3 weeks determines effectiveness in controlling high blood pressure. Long-term use of effective medicines and periodic physician evaluation is needed in high blood pressure.

Possible Advantages of This Drug

Usually controls blood pressure effectively with one daily dose.

Relatively low incidence of adverse effects.

No adverse influence on asthma, cholesterol blood levels or diabetes.

Sudden withdrawal does not result in a rapid increase in blood pressure.

▷ **This Drug Should Not Be Taken If**
- you have had an allergic reaction to it previously.
- you are pregnant (last 6 months).
- you have an abnormally high level of blood potassium.

▷ **Inform Your Physician Before Taking This Drug If**
- you have had an allergic reaction (or other adverse effect) to any ACE inhibitor (see Drug Classes).
- you are planning pregnancy.
- you plan to breast feed your baby.
- you have a history of kidney disease or impaired kidney function.
- you have scleroderma or systemic lupus erythematosus.
- you currently have a blood cell or bone marrow disorder.
- you have cerebral artery disease.
- you have any form of heart disease.
- you are taking: other antihypertensives, diuretics, nitrates or potassium supplements.
- you plan to have surgery under general anesthesia in the near future.

Possible Side Effects (natural, expected, and unavoidable drug actions)

Dizziness (rare), orthostatic hypotension (rare) (see Glossary), increased blood potassium level.

▷ **Possible Adverse Effects** (unusual, unexpected, and infrequent reactions)
If any of the following develop, consult your physician promptly for guidance.
Mild Adverse Effects
Allergic Reactions: Skin rash, hives, itching (rare).
Headache, fatigue (rare), drowsiness, numbness and tingling, weakness (rare).
Chest pain, palpitation (rare), cough.
Indigestion, nausea and vomiting (rare), diarrhea (rare).
Serious Adverse Effects
Allergic Reactions: Swelling (angioedema) of face, tongue, and/or vocal cords (rare); can be life-threatening.
Impairment of kidney function (rare).
Decreased white blood cells (uncommon).
Pancreatitis (not reported for this drug—only with members of the same pharmacological family) (rare).
Symptomatic lowering of the blood pressure (hypotension) (rare).
Compromise of kidney function, especially in those with severe congestive heart failure.

▷ **Possible Effects on Sexual Function:**   Decreased libido (less than 1%). Abnormal swelling of male breast tissue (rare). Impotence has been reported with other members of the same pharmacologic family.

Possible Effects on Laboratory Tests
Blood potassium level: increased.
Liver function tests: increased liver enzymes (ALT/GPT, AST/GOT and alkaline phosphatase), increased bilirubin.
Kidney function tests: increased blood urea nitrogen (BUN) and creatinine.
May give a falsely low test for digoxin levels.

CAUTION
1. Ask your doctor if you should stop other antihypertensive drugs (especially diuretics) for 1 week before starting this drug.
2. **Inform your physician immediately if you become pregnant.** This drug should not be taken beyond the first 3 months of pregnancy.
3. *Report promptly* any indications of infection (fever, sore throat), or water retention (weight gain, puffiness, swollen feet or ankles).
4. Do not use a salt substitute without your physician's knowledge and approval. (Many salt substitutes contain potassium.)
5. It is advisable to obtain blood cell counts and urine analyses *before* starting this drug.

Precautions for Use
By Infants and Children: Safety and effectiveness for those under 18 years of age not established.
By Those over 60 Years of Age: Small starting doses are advisable. Sudden and excessive lowering of blood pressure can predispose to stroke or heart attack in impaired brain circulation or coronary artery heart disease.

▷ **Advisability of Use During Pregnancy**
Pregnancy Category: C during the first three months (trimester). D during the second and third trimesters (4–9th month). See Pregnancy Code at the back of this book.

Animal studies: Significant birth defects associated with this drug.

Human studies: The use of ACE inhibitor drugs during the last 6 months of pregnancy is known to possibly cause very serious injury and possible death to the fetus; skull and limb malformations, lung defects, and kidney failure have been reported in over 50 cases worldwide.

Avoid this drug completely during the last 6 months. During the first 3 months of pregnancy, use this drug only if clearly needed. Ask your physician for guidance.

Advisability of Use if Breast-Feeding

Presence of this drug in breast milk: Yes.

Avoid drug or refrain from nursing.

Habit-Forming Potential: None.

Effects of Overdosage: Excessive drop in blood pressure, light-headedness, dizziness, fainting.

Possible Effects of Long-Term Use: Gradual increase in blood potassium level.

Suggested Periodic Examinations While Taking This Drug (at physician's discretion)

Before starting drug: Complete blood counts; urine analysis with measurement of protein content; blood potassium level. During use of drug: Blood cell counts; measurements of blood potassium.

▷ **While Taking This Drug, Observe the Following**

Foods: Consult physician regarding salt intake.

*Nutritional Support: **Do not take*** potassium supplements unless directed by your physician.

Beverages: No restrictions. May be taken with milk.

▷ *Alcohol:* Use caution—alcohol may enhance the blood-pressure-lowering effect.

Tobacco Smoking: No interactions expected.

▷ *Other Drugs*

Fosinopril ***taken concurrently*** with

- chlorpromazine (thorazine) can cause large and undesirable decreases in blood pressure. Avoid this combination.
- cyclosporine (Sandimmune) can cause a large decrease in kidney function.
- lithium causes increased lithium blood levels and toxicity; blood levels and dosage decreases are critical.
- loop diuretics—furosemide or bumetanide (Lasix, Bumex) can cause marked lowering of blood pressure on standing (postural hypotension).
- nonsteroidal antiinflammatory drugs (NSAIDS) such as aspirin or ketorolac (Toradol).
- potassium preparations (K-Lyte, Slow-K, etc.) may cause increased blood levels of potassium with risk of serious heart rhythm disturbances.
- potassium-sparing diuretics: amiloride (Moduretic), spironolactone (Aldactazide), triamterene (Dyazide) may cause increased blood levels of potassium with risk of serious heart rhythm disturbances.

▷ *Driving, Hazardous Activities:* Usually no restrictions. Be aware of possible drops in blood pressure with resultant dizziness or faintness.

Aviation Note: The use of this drug ***may be a disqualification*** for piloting. Consult a designated Aviation Medical Examiner.

Exposure to Sun: Caution advised. A similar drug of this class can cause photosensitivity.

Exposure to Heat: Caution advised. Avoid excessive perspiring with resultant loss of body water and drop in blood pressure.

Occurrence of Unrelated Illness: Promptly report any nausea, vomiting or diarrhea. Fluid and chemical imbalances must be corrected as soon as possible.

Discontinuation: This drug may be stopped abruptly without causing a sudden increase in blood pressure. However, you should ask your physician before stopping this drug for any reason.

FUROSEMIDE (fur OH se mide)

Introduced: 1964   **Prescription:** USA: Yes; Canada: Yes   **Available as Generic:** USA: Yes; Canada: Yes   **Class:** Antihypertensive, diuretic   **Controlled Drug:** USA: No; Canada: No

Brand Names: ✦Albert Furosemide, ✦Apo-Furosemide, Fumide MD, Furomide MD, Furocot, Furosemide-10, ✦Furoside, Lasaject, Lasimide, Lasix, ✦Lasix special, Lo-Aqua, Luramide, Myrosemide, Ro-Semide, SK-Furosemide, ✦Uritol

BENEFITS versus RISKS	
Possible Benefits	*Possible Risks*
PROMPT, EFFECTIVE, RELIABLE DIURETIC	WATER AND ELECTROLYTE DEPLETION with excessive use
MODEST ANTIHYPERTENSIVE IN MILD TO MODERATE HYPERTENSION	Excessive potassium and magnesium loss
ENHANCES EFFECTIVENESS OF OTHER ANTIHYPERTENSIVES	Increased blood sugar level
	Increased blood uric acid level
	Decreased blood calcium level
	Rare liver damage
	Rare blood cell disorder

▷ **Principal Uses**

As a Single Drug Product: Uses currently included in FDA approved labeling: (1) Used to increase urine and remove excessive water (edema) that is seen in: (a) congestive heart failure (b) some forms of liver, lung and kidney disease; (2) it is used in the treatment of high blood pressure, but usually is combined with other drugs.

Other (unlabeled) generally accepted uses: (1) Inhaled furosemide may help protect the lungs in people with asthma; (2) can have a role in helping infants with lung problems (chronic bronchopulmonary dysplasia).

How This Drug Works: By increasing the elimination of salt and water through increased urine production, this drug reduces fluid in the blood and body tissues. These changes also contribute to lowering blood pressure.

Available Dosage Forms and Strengths

Injection — 10 mg per ml
Solution — 10 mg per ml
Tablets — 20 mg, 40 mg, 80 mg

▷ **Usual Adult Dosage Range:**   As antihypertensive: 40 mg/12 hours initially; increase dose as needed and tolerated. As diuretic: 20 to 80 mg in a single dose initially; if necessary, increase the dose by 20 to 40 mg/6 to 8 hours. The smallest effective dose should be used, and total daily dose should not exceed 640 mg. In general, other medicines effective in treating high blood pressure should be added on before the daily oral dose is increased beyond 80 mg per day. **Note: Actual dosage and administration schedule must be determined by the physician for each patient individually.**

Conditions Requiring Dosing Adjustments
Liver function: Larger doses may be needed in patients with liver compromise, and extreme care must be used to maintain critical electrolytes.
Kidney function: Larger initial doses may be needed before any benefit is seen. Furosemide is also capable of causing kidney stones and protein in urine.
Cystic fibrosis: Patients with this disease may be more sensitive to the drug, and smaller starting doses are indicated.

▷ **Dosing Instructions:**   The tablet may be crushed and taken with or following meals to reduce stomach irritation. Best taken in the morning to avoid nighttime urination.

Usual Duration of Use: Use on a regular schedule for 2 to 3 weeks is best to see effectiveness in lowering high blood pressure. Long-term use (months to years) requires periodic physician evaluation of response.

▷ **This Drug Should Not Be Taken If**
- you have had an allergic reaction to any dosage form of it previously.
- your kidneys are not making urine.

▷ **Inform Your Physician Before Taking This Drug If**
- you are allergic to any form of "sulfa" drug.
- you are pregnant or planning pregnancy.
- you have a history of kidney or liver disease.
- you have diabetes, gout or lupus erythematosus.
- you have impaired hearing.
- you have low blood potassium or other electrolytes (talk with your doctor).
- you take any form of cortisone, digitalis, oral antidiabetic drug or insulin.
- you plan to have surgery under general anesthesia in the near future.

Possible Side Effects (natural, expected, and unavoidable drug actions)
Light-headedness on arising from sitting or lying position (see Orthostatic Hypotension in Glossary).
Increase in blood sugar level, affecting control of diabetes.
Increase in blood uric acid level, affecting control of gout.
Decrease in blood potassium level, causing muscle weakness and cramping.

▷ **Possible Adverse Effects** (unusual, unexpected, and infrequent reactions)
If any of the following develop, consult your physician promptly for guidance.
Mild Adverse Effects
Allergic Reactions: Skin rashes, hives, drug fever.
Headache, dizziness, blurred or yellow vision, ringing in ears, numbness and tingling.
Reduced appetite, indigestion, nausea, vomiting, diarrhea.
Metabolic alkalosis.

Serious Adverse Effects

Allergic Reactions: Hepatitis with jaundice (see Glossary), anaphylactic reaction (see Glossary), severe skin reactions.

Idiosyncratic Reaction: Fluid accumulation in lungs.

Temporary hearing loss.

Inflammation of the pancreas—severe abdominal pain.

Bone marrow depression (see Glossary)—fatigue, weakness, fever, sore throat, abnormal bleeding or bruising.

Low blood pressure on standing.

Abnormal heartbeat (arrhythmias).

Drug-induced porphyria (rare).

Excessive activity of the parathyroid gland (hyperparathyroidism).

Low blood potassium or magnesium.

Vitamin deficiency (thiamine).

Pancreatitis (rare).

Kidney stones (calcium-containing) (rare).

Liver toxicity (cholestatic jaundice).

Skin lesions (erythema multiforme).

Skin syndromes (Stevens-Johnson syndrome).

Hip fractures (may increase risk).

▷ **Possible Effects on Sexual Function:** Impotence (5%) using recommended dosage of 20 to 80 mg/day.

▷ **Adverse Effects That May Mimic Natural Diseases or Disorders**

Liver reaction may suggest viral hepatitis.

Natural Diseases or Disorders That May Be Activated by This Drug

Diabetes, gout, systemic lupus erythematosus.

Possible Effects on Laboratory Tests

Complete blood counts: reduced red cells, hemoglobin, white cells and platelets.

Blood amylase and lipase levels: increased (possible pancreatitis).

Blood sodium and chloride levels: decreased.

Blood levels of total cholesterol, LDL and VLDL cholesterol, and triglycerides: increased.

Blood glucose level: increased.

Glucose tolerance test (GTT): decreased.

Blood potassium level: decreased.

Blood thyroid hormone (T_3 and T_4) levels: decreased.

Blood uric acid level: increased.

Blood urea nitrogen (BUN): increased.

Urine sugar tests: no drug effect with TesTape; false low results with Clinistix and Diastix.

CAUTION

1. Take exactly the dose which was prescribed. Increased doses can cause serious loss of sodium and potassium, with resultant loss of appetite, nausea, fatigue, weakness, confusion and tingling in the extremities.
2. If you take a digitalis preparation (digitoxin, digoxin), ensure an ade-

quate intake of high-potassium foods to prevent potassium deficiency. (See Table of High Potassium Foods)

Precautions for Use

By Infants and Children: Avoid overdosage that could cause serious dehydration. Significant potassium loss can occur within the first 2 weeks of drug use.

By Those over 60 Years of Age: Small starting doses are critical. Increased risk of impaired thinking, orthostatic hypotension, potassium loss and blood sugar increase. Overdosage and extended use of this drug can cause excessive loss of body water, thickening (increased viscosity) of the blood and an increased tendency for the blood to clot—predisposing to stroke, heart attack or thrombophlebitis (vein inflammation with blood clot).

▷ **Advisability of Use During Pregnancy**

Pregnancy Category: C. See Pregnancy Code at the back of this book.

Animal studies: Significant birth defects have been reported.

Human studies: Adequate studies of pregnant women are not available.

It should not be used during pregnancy unless a very serious complication occurs for which this drug is significantly beneficial. Avoid completely during the first 3 months. Ask physician for guidance.

Advisability of Use if Breast-Feeding

Presence of this drug in breast milk: Yes.

Avoid drug or refrain from nursing.

Habit-Forming Potential: None.

Effects of Overdosage: Dry mouth, thirst, lethargy, weakness, muscle cramping, nausea, vomiting, drowsiness progressing to stupor or coma.

Possible Effects of Long-Term Use: Impaired water, salt and potassium balance; dehydration and increased blood coagulability, with risk of blood clots. Development of diabetes in predisposed individuals.

Suggested Periodic Examinations While Taking This Drug (at physician's discretion)

Complete blood counts, measurements of blood levels of sodium, potassium, chloride, sugar and uric acid.

Kidney and liver function tests.

▷ **While Taking This Drug, Observe the Following**

Foods: Ask your doctor about eating foods rich in potassium. If so advised, see the Table of High Potassium Foods. Follow physician's advice regarding the use of salt. Food decreases absorption of furosemide by up to 30%. Take this medicine 1 hour before or 2 hours after a meal.

Beverages: No restrictions. This drug may be taken with milk.

▷ *Alcohol:* Use with caution—alcohol may exaggerate the blood-pressure-lowering effects of this drug and cause orthostatic hypotension.

Tobacco Smoking: No interactions expected. Follow physician's advice.

▷ *Other Drugs*

Furosemide may ***increase*** the effects of

- other antihypertensive drugs; dosage adjustments may be necessary to prevent excessive lowering of blood pressure.
- digoxin and result in digoxin toxicity.
- lithium, and cause lithium toxicity.

Furosemide may *decrease* the effects of
- oral antidiabetic drugs (sulfonylureas); dosage adjustments may be necessary for proper control of blood sugar.

Furosemide *taken concurrently* with
- amikacin, gentamicin, tobramycin or other aminoglycosides may cause hearing toxicity (ototoxicity).
- cephalosporin antibiotics may increase the risk of kidney problems (nephrotoxicity).
- cholestyramine (Questran) may cause loss of furosemide effectiveness.
- colestipol (Colestid) may cause loss of furosemide effectiveness.
- corticosteroids (see Drug Classes) may cause additive loss of potassium.
- cyclosporine (Sandimmune) may cause elevated uric acid levels (hyperuricemia) and gout.
- digitalis preparations (digitoxin, digoxin) require blood tests or dose changes to maintain potassium levels and avoid heart rhythm problems.
- NSAIDs (see Drug Classes) may cause loss of diuretic effectiveness.

The following drug may *decrease* the effects of furosemide
- indomethacin (Indocin).

▷ *Driving, Hazardous Activities:* Use caution until the possible occurrence of orthostatic hypotension, dizziness or impaired vision has been determined.

Aviation Note: The use of this drug *may be a disqualification* for piloting. Consult a designated Aviation Medical Examiner.

Exposure to Sun: Use caution—this drug may cause photosensitivity (see Glossary).

Exposure to Heat: Avoid excessive perspiring, which could cause additional loss of salt and water from the body.

Heavy Exercise or Exertion: Avoid exertion that produces light-headedness, excessive fatigue or muscle cramping. Isometric exercises—the "overload" technique for strengthening individual muscles—can raise blood pressure significantly. Ask physician for guidance regarding participation in this form of exercise.

Occurrence of Unrelated Illness: Vomiting or diarrhea can produce a serious imbalance of important body chemistry. Ask your doctor for guidance.

Discontinuation: It may be advisable to discontinue this drug 5 to 7 days before major surgery. Ask your physician, surgeon and/or anesthesiologist for guidance regarding dosage adjustment or drug withdrawal.

GANCICLOVIR (ganz EYE klo veer)

Introduced: 1995 (tablet)   **Prescription:** USA: Yes; Canada: Yes   **Available as Generic:** USA: No; Canada: No   **Class:** Antiviral   **Controlled Drug:** USA: No; Canada: No

Brand Names: Cytovene, Vitrasert

Warning: The oral form of this medicine should only be used in patients who are not candidates for intravenous administration and in whom the risk of more rapid disease progression of CMV retinitis is outweighed by the benefit of avoiding the intravenous route.

BENEFITS versus RISKS	
Possible Benefits	*Possible Risks*
Oral, intravenous, or implanted treatment of CMV retinitis	More rapid progression of CMV disease (capsules)
Decreased side effects with the oral form	Bone marrow suppression
Transition to an oral form following intravenous induction	

▷ **Principal Uses**

As a Single Drug Product: Uses currently included in FDA approved labeling: (1) Treatment of Cytomegalovirus retinitis; (2) prevention of CMV retinitis in a variety of patients such as: Liver, kidney, lung, bone marrow and heart transplant patients; (3) implantation of the ocular implant into the diseased area. This form may work for 6 months or more; (4) prevention of CMV disease in patients with advanced HIV infection.

Other (unlabeled) generally accepted uses: (1) Treatment of pediatric CMV; (2) may have a role in treating Epstein Barr virus infection; (3) can have a role in leukoplakia.

How This Drug Works: This medicine is changed into an active triphosphate form by cells infected with cytomegalovirus. This active form interferes with synthesis of DNA and the ability of the virus to survive.

Available Dosage Forms and Strengths

Capsules — 250 mg
Intravenous — 500 mg per 10 ml

How To Store

The intravenous solution should be stored at 4 degrees centigrade and used within 12 hours after it has been reconstituted.

▷ **Recommended Dosage Ranges (Actual dosage and administration schedule must be determined by the physician for each patient individually.)**

Infants and Children: **Author's note—this drug has potential for reproductive toxicity and the risk of causing cancer. It is used in children only after careful evaluation and with extreme caution.**

Induction: 2.5 mg per kg given intravenously three times daily.

Maintenance: 6.5 mg per kg given intravenously once daily 5 to 7 times a week.

12 to 60 Years of Age: Induction: 5 mg per kg intravenously (infused over one hour) every 12 hours for 14 to 21 days.

Maintenance dose: 5 mg per kg infused into a vein over 1 hour each day. Some centers have used 6 mg per kg given once daily 5 days weekly. If retinitis progresses, the patient can be restarted on the twice daily dosing approach. Maximum dose is 6 milligrams per kilogram infused over one hour.

Oral: Once the intravenous induction dosing has been accomplished, oral ganciclovir is given 1000 mg 3 times daily. Some centers have opted for 500 mg 6 times per day, given every 3 hours while the patient is awake. If retinitis progresses, intravenous induction therapy should be given. Intravitreous: An experimental slow release device was used in a small number of patients with good results. This used a 6 mg pellet which lasted 4 months.

Over 60 Years of Age: Kidney function must be assessed and the dose appropriately adjusted.

Conditions Requiring Dosing Adjustments

Liver function: The liver is only minimally involved in the elimination of this drug, and dosing changes in liver compromise are not needed.

Kidney function: The dose **must** be decreased in kidney compromise. This adjustment is accomplished based on creatinine clearance (see Glossary):

Induction—70 or higher: 5 mg per kg every 12 hours; 50–69: 2.5 mg per kg every 12 hours; 25–49: 2.5 mg per kg every 24 hours; 10–24: 1.25 mg per kg every 24 hours; less than 10: 1.25 mg per kg 3 times weekly.

Maintenance:—70 or higher: 5 mg per kg every 24 hours; 50–69: 2.5 mg per kg every 24 hours; 25–49: 1.25 mg per kg every 24 hours; 10–24: 0.625 mg per kg every 24 hours; less than 10: 0.625 mg per kg 3 times weekly.

▷ **Dosing Instructions:** This medicine should be taken with food if taken by mouth (orally). It is best to take the medicine at the same time each day. If you are taking the capsule form and your vision declines, call your doctor immediately.

Usual Duration of Use: Continual use on a regular schedule for up to 16 days is usually needed to determine this drug's effectiveness in treating retinitis. Because of a very high frequency of relapse, most centers recommend ongoing maintenance therapy. Long-term use (months to years) requires periodic evaluation of response and dosage adjustment. The new ocular implant form may work for 6 months or more. Consult your physician on a regular basis.

Possible Advantages of This Drug

Transition from the intravenous form to the oral form (if successful in treatment) offers a clear quality of life advantage.

Currently a "Drug of Choice"

for patients with kidney failure.

▷ **This Drug Should Not Be Taken If**

- you have had an allergic reaction to any dosage form of it previously.
- your absolute neutrophil count (a specific kind of white blood cell) is less than 500 per cubic millimeter.
- your platelet count is less than 25,000 per cubic millimeter.

▷ **Inform Your Physician Before Taking This Drug If**

- you think you are dehydrated (this drug is primarily removed by the kidneys).
- you have a sore throat or fever.
- you have a history of blood cell disorders.
- you are planning pregnancy.
- you are male and are planning pregnancy (attempted conception should be avoided for at least 3 months after ganciclovir therapy).
- you are uncertain of how much ganciclovir to take, how often to take it or how to handle the intravenous solution.
- you take other prescription or nonprescription medicines which were not discussed with your doctor when ganciclovir was prescribed. This includes natural extracts or herbal remedies and underground therapies for AIDS.

Possible Side Effects (natural, expected, and unavoidable drug actions)

Pain at the injection site with the IV form.

▷ **Possible Adverse Effects** (unusual, unexpected, and infrequent reactions)
If any of the following develop, consult your physician promptly for guidance.

Mild Adverse Effects
Allergic Reactions: Skin rash and itching.
Confusion, headache, and nervousness.
Tremor, somnolence, abnormal dreams, and ataxia.
Rapid heart rate (tachycardia) (rare)."Pins-and-needles" sensations of the hands (paresthesias).
Fever (up to 38% with oral therapy).
Decreased blood glucose (rare).
Nausea, vomiting, or diarrhea.
Phlebitis.

Serious Adverse Effects
Allergic Reactions: Anaphylactoid reaction.
Bone marrow suppression.
Arrhythmias (rare).
Coma or psychosis.
Phlebitis.
Neuropathy.
Lowered white blood cell (neutropenia) counts (up to 54% with oral and 65% with intravenous therapy).
Seizures (rare).
Liver toxicity (rare).
Retinal detachment (occasional with oral therapy).
This drug is a potential cancer-causing (carcinogenic) agent (no percentage defined).

▷ **Possible Effects on Sexual Function:** Reversible infertility in men.

Possible Delayed Adverse Effects: Lowered white blood cell counts.

▷ **Adverse Effects That May Mimic Natural Diseases or Disorders**
Increased liver enzymes may mimic hepatitis.

Natural Diseases or Disorders That May Be Activated by This Drug
None defined.

Possible Effects on Laboratory Tests
Liver enzymes: increased.
Serum bilirubin: increased.
Serum creatinine: increased.
Blood glucose: decreased.

CAUTION
1. The oral form may be less effective than the intravenous form. Call your doctor immediately if your vision declines.
2. This drug can cause bone marrow suppression. Call your doctor if you develop a sore throat, start to bruise easily or develop a fever.

Precautions for Use
By Infants and Children: Safety and effectiveness for use by those under 18 years of age have not been established. The drug has been used selectively in patients as young as 36 weeks.
By Those over 60 Years of Age: Because of the age-related decline in kidney function, a creatinine clearance should be obtained and dosing adjusted appropriately.

▷ **Advisability of Use During Pregnancy**
  Pregnancy Category: C. See Pregnancy Code at the back of this book.
    Animal studies: Rabbits have developed cleft palate, exhibited poorly developed organs and have experienced fetal death.
    Human studies: Information from adequate studies of pregnant women is not available. Use of this drug during pregnancy is not recommended.

Advisability of Use if Breast-Feeding
  Presence of this drug in breast milk: Unknown.
  Avoid drug or refrain from nursing.

Habit-Forming Potential: None.

Effects of Overdosage: Nausea and vomiting, excessive salivation, increased liver function tests, bone marrow suppression and kidney failure.

Possible Effects of Long-Term Use: Not defined.

Suggested Periodic Examinations While Taking This Drug   (at physician's discretion)
  Platelet counts and complete blood counts: every 2 days during induction and weekly thereafter.
  Liver function tests: monthly.
  Kidney function tests: every two weeks.
  Eye (ophthalmologic) exams: weekly during induction and every two weeks thereafter. These exams may be needed more frequently if the optic nerve or macula of the eye is involved.

▷ **While Taking This Drug, Observe the Following**
  Foods: No restrictions—the oral form should be taken with food.
  Beverages: No restrictions.
▷ *Alcohol:* No restrictions, however, alcohol may blunt the immune system.
  Tobacco Smoking: No interactions expected.
  Marijuana Smoking: May increase somnolence.
▷ *Other Drugs*
  Ganciclovir *taken concurrently* with
  • amphotericin B (Fungizone) may result in increased bone marrow suppression.
  • cancer chemotherapy may result in additive bone marrow suppression.
  • cotrimoxazole may result in added bone marrow suppression problems.
  • cyclosporine (Sandimmune) can result in increased kidney toxicity.
  • dapsone is a benefit to risk decision as additive bone marrow suppression may occur.
  • flucytosine (Ancobon) can cause additive bone marrow toxicity.
  • imipenem/cilastatin (Primaxin) can cause seizures.
  • pentamidine may result in additive bone marrow suppression.
  • zidovudine (AZT) will cause a serious increase in bone marrow suppression.
  The following drugs may *increase* the effects of ganciclovir
  • probenecid (Benemid), by interfering with elimination by the kidney.
▷ *Driving, Hazardous Activities:* This drug may cause somnolence. Restrict activities as necessary.
  Aviation Note: The use of this drug *may be a disqualification* for piloting. Consult a designated Aviation Medical Examiner.

Exposure to Sun: Caution is advised. Photosensitivity has been reported.

Discontinuation: Talk with your doctor before stopping this medicine.

Special Storage Instructions: The intravenous form should be stored at 4 degrees centigrade.

Observe the Following Expiration Times: The intravenous form will be stamped or labeled with a specific expiration time if this has been provided by a home infusion company.

GEMFIBROZIL (jem FI broh zil)

Introduced: 1976 **Prescription:** USA: Yes; Canada: Yes **Available as Generic:** USA: Yes; Canada: No **Class:** Anticholesterol **Controlled Drug:** USA: No; Canada: No

Brand Name: Lopid, Gemcor

BENEFITS versus RISKS	
Possible Benefits	*Possible Risks*
EFFECTIVE REDUCTION OF TRIGLYCERIDE BLOOD LEVELS	Gallstone formation with long-term use
INCREASE IN HIGH-DENSITY LIPOPROTEIN (HDL) BLOOD LEVELS	Decreased white blood cell counts

▷ **Principal Uses**

As a Single Drug Product: Uses currently included in FDA approved labeling: (1) Reduces abnormally high blood levels of triglycerides in Types II and IV blood lipid (fat) disorders; (2) decreases risk for developing coronary artery heart disease.

Other (unlabeled) generally accepted uses: (1) Used in diabetics as combination therapy with oral hypoglycemic agents to further increase desirable HDLs.

How This Drug Works: Reduces blood levels of triglycerides by inhibiting their production in the liver. Decreases VLDL and LDL. Causes a larger increase in desirable HDL than clofibrate.

Available Dosage Forms and Strengths

Capsules — 300 mg

Tablets — 600 mg

▷ **Usual Adult Dosage Range:** 1200 to 1600 daily in 2 divided doses. The average dose is 1200 mg/24 hours. Dose increases should be made gradually over a period of 2 to 3 months. **Note: Actual dosage and administration schedule must be determined by the physician for each patient individually.**

Conditions Requiring Dosing Adjustments

Liver function: This drug is contraindicated in primary biliary cirrhosis and severe liver failure.

Kidney function: In patients with moderate kidney failure, 50% of the usual dose should be given at the usual interval. Patients with severe kidney failure should be given 25% of the usual dose at the usual dosing interval.

▷ **Dosing Instructions:**   The capsule may be opened and taken 30 minutes before the morning and evening meals.

Usual Duration of Use: Use on a regular schedule for 4 to 8 weeks determines effectiveness in reducing blood levels of triglycerides. Long-term use (months to years) requires periodic physician evaluation.

▷ **This Drug Should Not Be Taken If**
  • you have had an allergic reaction to it previously.
  • you have biliary cirrhosis of the liver.
  • you have severe kidney compromise.

▷ **Inform Your Physician Before Taking This Drug If**
  • you have impaired liver or kidney function.
  • you have gallbladder disease or gallstones.
  • you are a diabetic.
  • you have an underactive thyroid (hypothyroidism).

Possible Side Effects (natural, expected, and unavoidable drug actions)
Moderate increase in blood sugar levels.

▷ **Possible Adverse Effects** (unusual, unexpected, and infrequent reactions)
If any of the following develop, consult your physician promptly for guidance.
Mild Adverse Effects
Allergic Reactions: Skin rash, hives, itching.
Headache, dizziness, blurred vision, fatigue, muscle aches, and cramps.
Indigestion, excessive gas, stomach discomfort, nausea, vomiting (rare), diarrhea.
Paresthesias (very rare).
Serious Adverse Effects
Abnormally low white blood cell count: Fever, chills, sore throat (rare).
Formation of gallstones with long-term use.
Raynaud's phenomenon (rare).
Low blood potassium.
Liver toxicity.
Myopathy (muscle weakness and tenderness).
Rhabdomyolysis (inability to walk, muscle weakness).

▷ **Possible Effects on Sexual Function:**   Decreased libido (rare). Impotence (rare).

Natural Diseases or Disorders That May Be Activated by This Drug
Latent diabetes, latent urinary tract infections.

Possible Effects on Laboratory Tests
Complete blood counts: decreased red cells, hemoglobin, white cells and platelets.
Blood HDL cholesterol levels: increased.
Blood triglyceride levels: decreased.
Liver function tests: increased liver enzymes (ALT/GPT, AST/GOT and alkaline phosphatase), increased bilirubin.

CAUTION
  1. Gemfibrozil is used only after diet has NOT worked to lower triglyceride levels.

2. If you used the drug clofibrate (Atromid-S) in the past, inform your physician fully regarding your experience.
3. Periodic triglyceride and cholesterol levels are critical.

Precautions for Use

By Infants and Children: Safety and effectiveness for those under 12 years of age not established.

By Those over 60 Years of Age: Watch for increased tendency to infection; treat all infections promptly.

▷ **Advisability of Use During Pregnancy**

Pregnancy Category: C. See Pregnancy Code at the back of this book.

Animal studies: Produces adverse effects in rabbits and rats.

Human studies: Adequate studies of pregnant women are not available.

Ask your physician for guidance.

Advisability of Use if Breast-Feeding

Presence of this drug in breast milk: Yes.

Avoid drug or refrain from nursing.

Habit-Forming Potential: None.

Effects of Overdosage: Abdominal pain, nausea, vomiting, diarrhea.

Possible Effects of Long-Term Use: Formation of gallstones.

Suggested Periodic Examinations While Taking This Drug (at physician's discretion)

Complete blood cell counts.

Measurements of blood levels of total cholesterol, HDL and LDL cholesterol fractions, triglycerides and sugar.

Liver function tests.

▷ **While Taking This Drug, Observe the Following**

Foods: Follow the diet prescribed by your physician.

Beverages: No restrictions. May be taken with milk.

▷ *Alcohol:* No interactions expected.

Tobacco Smoking: No interactions expected.

▷ *Other Drugs*

Gemfibrozil may *increase* the effects of
• glyburide and other oral hypoglycemic agents (see Drug Classes).
• lovastatin if taken at the same time and results in myopathy.
• warfarin (Coumadin), and increase the risk of bleeding. Increased frequency of INR (prothrombin time or 'protime') measurements and dose changes based on results are critical.

Gemfibrozil may *decrease* the effects of
• chenodiol (Chenix), reducing its benefit in gallstone therapy.

▷ *Driving, Hazardous Activities:* This drug may cause dizziness and blurred vision. Restrict activities as necessary.

Aviation Note: The use of this drug *is usually not a disqualification* for piloting. Consult a designated Aviation Medical Examiner.

Exposure to Sun: No restrictions.

Discontinuation: If triglyceride lowering does not occur after 3 months, this drug should be stopped.

GLIMEPIRIDE (glim EP er ide)

Introduced: 1996   **Prescription:** USA: Yes   **Available as Generic:** No   **Class:** Antidiabetic, sulfonylureas   **Controlled Drug:** USA: No
Brand Name: Amaryl

BENEFITS versus RISKS	
Possible Benefits	*Possible Risks*
TIGHTER CONTROL OF BLOOD SUGAR (adjunctive to appropriate diet and weight control)	Allergic skin reactions
DECREASED RISK OF HEART DISEASE, KIDNEY DISEASE, ETC., BY ATTAINING TIGHTER CONTROL OF BLOOD SUGAR	
ONCE-A-DAY DOSING	
DECREASED RISK OF INCREASED INSULIN LEVELS	
DECREASED RISK OF HYPOGLYCEMIA	

▷ **Principal Uses**

As a Single Drug Product: Uses currently included in FDA approved labeling: (1) Better control of mild to moderate type II diabetes mellitus (adult, maturity-onset) that does not require insulin, but is not adequately controlled by diet alone; (2) approved for combination use with insulin if diet and exercise and glimepiride are not adequate and in secondary failures.

Other (unlabeled) generally accepted uses: None at present.

How This Drug Works: This drug (1) stimulates the secretion of insulin; and (2) enhances the utilization of insulin by appropriate tissues (increased sensitivity); and (3) may bind to a different receptor site than other sulfonylureas.

Available Dosage Forms and Strengths

Tablets — 1 mg, 2 mg and 4 mg

▷ **Usual Adult Dosage Range (Actual dosage and administration schedule must be determined by the physician for each patient individually):** Treatment is started with 1 or 2 mg once daily, given with breakfast or the first meal. Once a dose of 2 mg is reached, any further dose increases should be made as needed and tolerated at one to two week intervals in increments of no more than 2 mg; the maximum daily dose is 8 mg. Typical ongoing doses have ranged from 1 to 4 mg a day. Some clinicians advocate the Type II patients with secondary failure may be considered for combined glimepiride and insulin therapy. If the fasting blood sugar (glucose) is greater than 150 mg/dl, and this is undertaken, 8 mg administered with the first main meal is recommended. Low dose insulin is started, and increased as needed and tolerated on a weekly basis consistent with blood glucose measurements.

Conditions Requiring Dosing Adjustments
Liver function: Since glimepiride is removed by the liver, it appears prudent that patients with mild liver failure should be given small starting doses. Data regarding use in patients with moderate to severe compromised livers is not available, and use should probably be avoided.
Kidney function: Patients with kidney compromise may be given 1 mg of glimepiride a day. Any further dose changes should be based on results of blood sugar testing.

▷ **Dosing Instructions:** The tablet may be crushed for administration. Follow your doctor's instructions regarding dosing and diet closely. If meals are skipped after this medicine is taken, hypoglycemia may result. Be certain you know the signs and symptoms of hypoglycemia.

Usual Duration of Use: Use on a regular schedule for 1 to 2 weeks determines effectiveness in controlling diabetes. Failure to respond to maximal doses within 1 month constitutes a primary failure. Blood sugars must be measured, and your doctor will decide if the drug should be continued.

Possible Advantages of This Drug
Effective with once-daily dosing.
May be less likely to cause excessive lowering of the blood sugar (hypoglycemia).
May cause less excessive insulin in the blood stream (hyperinsulinemia).

▷ **This Drug Should Not Be Taken If**
• you have had an allergic reaction to it previously.
• you have severe impairment of liver or kidney function.
• you have diabetic ketoacidosis for which insulin is the drug of choice.

▷ **Inform Your Physician Before Taking This Drug If**
• you are allergic to other sulfonylurea drugs or to "sulfa" drugs.
• you have been experiencing prolonged vomiting.
• you do not know how to recognize or treat hypoglycemia (see Glossary).
• you are pregnant.
• you have a history of congestive heart failure, peptic ulcer disease, cirrhosis of the liver or hypothyroidism.
• you are malnourished, have a high fever or pituitary or adrenal insufficiency.

Possible Side Effects (natural, expected, and unavoidable drug actions)
Hypoglycemia will occur if drug dosage is excessive or if meals are missed or inadequate. The risk of hypoglycemia may be increased if this medicine is combined with insulin.

▷ **Possible Adverse Effects** (unusual, unexpected, and infrequent reactions)
If any of the following develop, consult your physician promptly for guidance.
Mild Adverse Effects
Allergic Reactions: Skin rash, hives, itching (may subside over time).
Headache or dizziness (rare).
Nausea (rare).
Blurred vision (rare).

Serious Adverse Effects
    Allergic Reactions: None reported.
    Rare lowering of blood sodium reported with other medicines in this drug class.
    Rare porphyria reported with other medicines in this drug class.

▷ **Possible Effects on Sexual Function:** None reported.

▷ **Adverse Effects That May Mimic Natural Diseases or Disorders**
    Increased liver enzymes may suggest viral hepatitis.

Possible Effects on Laboratory Tests
    Hemoglobin A1C (glycosylated hemoglobin): trending toward normal if tight control of blood sugar has been achieved.
    Blood glucose levels: decreased.
    Liver function tests: increased liver enzymes (ALT/GPT, AST/GOT and alkaline phosphatase), increased bilirubin.

CAUTION
    1. This drug is only one part of a total diabetes program. It is not a substitute for a proper diet and regular exercise.
    2. Over time (usually several months), this drug may not work. Periodic follow-up examinations are necessary.

Precautions for Use
    By Infants and Children: Safety and effectiveness in pediatrics have not been established.
    By Those over 60 Years of Age: Used with caution, and started with 1 mg/day. Dose is increased slowly as needed and tolerated and glucose checked often. Repeated hypoglycemia in the elderly can cause brain damage.

▷ **Advisability of Use During Pregnancy**
    Pregnancy Category: C. See Pregnancy Code at the back of this book.
    Human studies: Adequate studies of pregnant women are not available.
    Because uncontrolled blood sugar levels during pregnancy are associated with a higher incidence of birth defects, many experts recommend that insulin instead of an oral agent be used as necessary to control diabetes during pregnancy.

Advisability of Use if Breast-Feeding
    Presence of this drug in breast milk: Yes in animal data, unknown in humans.
    Avoid drug or refrain from nursing.

Habit-Forming Potential: None.

Effects of Overdosage: Symptoms of mild to severe hypoglycemia: Headache, light-headedness, faintness, nervousness, confusion, tremor, sweating, heart palpitation, weakness, hunger, nausea, vomiting, stupor progressing to coma.

Possible Effects of Long-Term Use: Increased frequency and severity of heart and blood vessel diseases with long-term use of this class of drugs are highly controversial and inconclusive. A direct cause-and-effect relationship (see Glossary) is tenuous. Ask your physician for help.

Suggested Periodic Examinations While Taking This Drug (at physician's discretion)
    Hemoglobin A1C, liver function tests, evaluation of heart and circulatory system, blood sugar levels.

▷ **While Taking This Drug, Observe the Following**

Foods: Follow the diabetic diet prescribed by your physician.

Beverages: As directed in the diabetic diet. May be taken with milk.

▷ *Alcohol:* Use with extreme caution—alcohol can prolong this drug's hypoglycemic effect. Other drugs in this class can also cause a disulfiramlike reaction
(see Glossary).

Tobacco Smoking: No interactions expected.

▷ *Other Drugs*

The following drugs may ***increase*** the effects of glimepiride
- aspirin, and other salicylates.
- cimetidine (Tagamet).
- clofibrate (Atromid S).
- fenfluramine (Pondimin).
- monoamine oxidase (MAO) type A inhibitors (see Drug Classes).
- NSAIDs (see Drug Classes).
- ranitidine (Zantac).
- sulfa drugs such as Septra.

The following drugs may ***decrease*** the effects of glimepiride
- beta blocker drugs (see Drug Classes).
- bumetanide (Bumex).
- conjugated estrogens (Premarin).
- diazoxide (Proglycem).
- ethacrynic acid (Edecrin).
- furosemide (Lasix).
- phenytoin (Dilantin).
- rifampin (Rifadin, others).
- steroids (betamethasone, prednisone, others).
- thiazide diuretics (see Drug Classes).

Glimepiride ***taken concurrently*** with
- antacids (magnesium hydroxide containing) may result in increased risk of
excessively lowered blood sugar.
- antifungal agents (such as itraconazole or other azoles) may result in severe
lowering of blood sugar.
- calcium channel blockers (see Drug Classes) may cause excessive lowering
of blood glucose.
- cyclosporine (Sandimmune) may result in cyclosporine toxicity.
- warfarin (Coumadin) can cause an increased hypoglycemic effect.

▷ *Driving, Hazardous Activities:* Dosing schedule, eating schedule and physical
activities must be coordinated to prevent hypoglycemia. Know the early
symptoms of hypoglycemia so you can avoid hazardous activities and take
corrective measures.

Aviation Note: Diabetes ***is a disqualification*** for piloting. Consult a designated
Aviation Medical Examiner.

Exposure to Sun: Some drugs of this class can cause photosensitivity (see Glossary).

Occurrence of Unrelated Illness: Acute infections, vomiting or diarrhea, serious
injuries and surgical procedures can worsen diabetic control and may require insulin. If any of these conditions occur, call your doctor.

Discontinuation: Because of secondary failures, the continued benefit of this
drug should be evaluated every 6 months.

GLIPIZIDE (GLIP i zide)

Introduced: 1972   **Prescription:** USA: Yes   **Available as Generic:**
No   **Class:** Antidiabetic, sulfonylureas   **Controlled Drug:** USA: No
Brand Name: Glucotrol, Glucotrol XL

BENEFITS versus RISKS	
Possible Benefits	*Possible Risks*
Help in regulating blood sugar in noninsulin-dependent diabetes (adjunctive to appropriate diet and weight control)	HYPOGLYCEMIA, severe and prolonged INCREASED CARDIOVASCULAR MORTALITY Allergic skin reactions (some severe) Rare blood cell and bone marrow disorders

▷ **Principal Uses**
   As a Single Drug Product: Uses currently included in FDA approved labeling: (1) Better control of mild to moderate type II diabetes mellitus (adult, maturity-onset) that does not require insulin, but is not adequately controlled by diet alone.
   Other (unlabeled) generally accepted uses: (1) Delay of abnormal metabolism and blood vessel disease if given early in diabetes.

How This Drug Works: This drug (1) stimulates the secretion of insulin; and (2) enhances the utilization of insulin by appropriate tissues.

Available Dosage Forms and Strengths
                    Tablets — 5 mg, 10 mg
         Extended Release tablets — 5 mg, 10 mg

▷ **Usual Adult Dosage Range:** Initially 5 mg daily before a meal. At 3 to 7-day intervals the dose may be increased by increments of 2.5 to 5 mg daily as needed and tolerated. Total daily dosage should not exceed 40 mg. The extended release form is started at 5 mg given with breakfast. If the dose needs to be increased, it is done so at 7 day intervals. Most patients have a favorable response to 10 mg daily. The maximum daily extended release form dose is 20 mg. **Note: Actual dosage and administration schedule must be determined by the physician for each patient individually.**

Conditions Requiring Dosing Adjustments
   Liver function: Patients with liver failure should be given a starting dose of 2.5 mg, and closely followed.
   Kidney function: Some clinicians DO NOT recommend use of glipizide in severe renal compromise. Patients should be monitored closely if the drug is used in mild to moderate renal (kidney) compromise. It is a rare cause of kidney stones.

▷ **Dosing Instructions:** If the daily maintenance dose is found to be 15 mg or more, the total dose should be divided into 2 equal doses—the first taken with the morning meal, the second with the evening meal. The tablet may be crushed for administration.

Usual Duration of Use: Use on a regular schedule for 1 to 2 weeks determines effectiveness in controlling diabetes. Failure to respond to maximal doses within 1 month constitutes a primary failure. Up to 10% of those who respond initially may develop secondary failure. Blood sugars must be measured, and your doctor will decide if the drug should be continued.

Possible Advantages of This Drug
Effective with once-daily dosing.
Onset of action within 30 minutes.
Near-normal insulin response to eating.
Well tolerated by the elderly diabetic.

Currently a "Drug of Choice"
for starting therapy in noninsulin-dependent diabetes when diet and weight control fail.

▷ **This Drug Should Not Be Taken If**
- you have had an allergic reaction to it previously.
- you have severe impairment of liver or kidney function.
- you have diabetic ketoacidosis.
- you are pregnant.

▷ **Inform Your Physician Before Taking This Drug If**
- you are allergic to other sulfonylurea drugs or to "sulfa" drugs.
- your diabetes has been unstable or "brittle" in the past.
- you do not know how to recognize or treat hypoglycemia (see Glossary).
- you are pregnant.
- you have a history of congestive heart failure, peptic ulcer disease, cirrhosis of the liver, bone marrow depression, hypothyroidism or porphyria.

Possible Side Effects (natural, expected, and unavoidable drug actions)
If drug dosage is excessive or if meals are missed or inadequate, abnormally low blood sugar (hypoglycemia) will occur as a drug effect.

▷ **Possible Adverse Effects** (unusual, unexpected, and infrequent reactions)
If any of the following develop, consult your physician promptly for guidance.
Mild Adverse Effects
Allergic Reactions: Skin rash, hives, itching.
Headache (rare), drowsiness (rare), dizziness, fatigue, sweating (rare).
Indigestion, nausea (rare), vomiting, diarrhea (rare).
Serious Adverse Effects
Allergic Reactions: Hepatitis with jaundice (see Glossary), severe skin reactions.
Idiosyncratic Reaction: Hemolytic anemia (see Glossary).
Disulfiramlike reaction with concurrent use of alcohol (see Glossary) (infrequent with this drug).
Low blood sodium.
Drug-induced urinary stones.
Bone marrow depression (see Glossary)—fatigue, weakness, fever, sore throat, abnormal bleeding or bruising (rare).
Potential increased risk of cardiovascular mortality (based on the University Group Diabetes Program [UGDP]).

▷ **Possible Effects on Sexual Function:** None reported.

▷ **Adverse Effects That May Mimic Natural Diseases or Disorders**
Liver reactions may suggest viral hepatitis.

Possible Effects on Laboratory Tests

Complete blood counts: decreased red cells, hemoglobin, white cells and platelets.

Blood glucose levels: decreased.

Liver function tests: increased liver enzymes (ALT/GPT, AST/GOT and alkaline phosphatase), increased bilirubin.

CAUTION

1. This drug is only one part of a total diabetes program. It is not a substitute for a proper diet and regular exercise.
2. Over time (usually several months), this drug may not work. Periodic follow-up examinations are necessary.

Precautions for Use

By Infants and Children: This drug does not work in type (juvenile, growth-onset) insulin-dependent diabetes.

By Those over 60 Years of Age: Used with caution, and started with 2.5 mg/day. Dose is increased slowly and glucose checked often. Repeated hypoglycemia in the elderly can cause brain damage.

▷ **Advisability of Use During Pregnancy**

Pregnancy Category: C. See Pregnancy Code at the back of this book.

Animal studies: No birth defects reported in rats and rabbits.

Human studies: Adequate studies of pregnant women are not available.

Because uncontrolled blood sugar levels during pregnancy are associated with a higher incidence of birth defects, many experts recommend that insulin (instead of an oral agent) be used as necessary to control diabetes during the entire pregnancy.

Advisability of Use if Breast-Feeding

Presence of this drug in breast milk: Unknown.

Avoid drug or refrain from nursing.

Habit-Forming Potential: None.

Effects of Overdosage: Symptoms of mild to severe hypoglycemia: Headache, light-headedness, faintness, nervousness, confusion, tremor, sweating, heart palpitation, weakness, hunger, nausea, vomiting, stupor progressing to coma.

Possible Effects of Long-Term Use: Reduced thyroid function (hypothyroidism). Increased frequency and severity of heart and blood vessel diseases with long-term use of this class of drugs are highly controversial and inconclusive. A direct cause-and-effect relationship (see Glossary) is tenuous. Ask your physician for help.

Suggested Periodic Examinations While Taking This Drug (at physician's discretion)

Complete blood cell counts, liver function tests, thyroid function tests, periodic evaluation of heart and circulatory system.

▷ **While Taking This Drug, Observe the Following**

Foods: Follow the diabetic diet prescribed by your physician.

Beverages: As directed in the diabetic diet. May be taken with milk.

▷   *Alcohol:* Use with extreme caution—alcohol can prolong this drug's hypoglycemic effect. This drug can also cause a disulfiramlike reaction (see Glossary): Facial flushing, sweating, palpitation.

Tobacco Smoking: No interactions expected.

▷ *Other Drugs*

The following drugs may ***increase*** the effects of glipizide

- aspirin, and other salicylates.
- cimetidine (Tagamet).
- clofibrate (Atromid S).
- fenfluramine (Pondimin).
- monoamine oxidase (MAO) type A inhibitors (see Drug Classes).
- NSAIDs (see Drug Classes).
- ranitidine (Zantac).
- sulfa drugs such as Septra.

The following drugs may ***decrease*** the effects of glipizide

- beta blocker drugs (see Drug Classes).
- bumetanide (Bumex).
- conjugated estrogens (Premarin).
- diazoxide (Proglycem).
- ethacrynic acid (Edecrin).
- furosemide (Lasix).
- phenytoin (Dilantin).
- rifampin (Rifadin, others).
- steroids (betamethasone, prednisone, others).
- thiazide diuretics (see Drug Classes).

Glipizide ***taken concurrently*** with

- antacids (magnesium hydroxide containing) may result in increased risk of excessively lowered blood sugar.
- antifungal agents (such as itraconazole or other azoles) may result in severe lowering of blood sugar.
- calcium channel blockers (see Drug Classes) may cause excessive lowering of blood glucose.
- cyclosporine (Sandimmune) may result in cyclosporine toxicity.
- warfarin (Coumadin) can cause an increased hypoglycemic effect.

▷ *Driving, Hazardous Activities:* Dosing schedule, eating schedule and physical activities must be coordinated to prevent hypoglycemia. Know the early symptoms of hypoglycemia so you can avoid hazardous activities and take corrective measures.

Aviation Note: Diabetes ***is a disqualification*** for piloting. Consult a designated Aviation Medical Examiner.

Exposure to Sun: Some drugs of this class can cause photosensitivity (see Glossary).

Occurrence of Unrelated Illness: Acute infections, vomiting or diarrhea, serious injuries and surgical procedures can worsen diabetic control and may require insulin. If any of these conditions occur, call your doctor.

Discontinuation: Because of secondary failures, the continued benefit of this drug should be evaluated every 6 months.

GLYBURIDE (GLI byoor ide)

Other Name: Glibenclamide

Introduced: 1970   **Prescription:** USA: Yes; Canada: Yes   **Available as Generic:** Yes   **Class:** Antidiabetic, sulfonylureas   **Controlled Drug:** USA: No; Canada: No

Brand Names: ✦Albert-Glyburide, ✦Apo-Glyburide, DiaBeta, ✦Euglucon, ✦Gen-Glybe, Glubate, Glynase Prestab, Micronase, ✦Novo-Glyburide

BENEFITS versus RISKS	
Possible Benefits	*Possible Risks*
Help in regulating blood sugar in noninsulin-dependent diabetes (adjunctive to appropriate diet and weight control)	HYPOGLYCEMIA, severe and prolonged INCREASED RISK OF CARDIOVASCULAR MORTALITY Allergic skin reactions (some severe) Rare liver damage Rare blood cell and bone marrow disorders

▷ **Principal Uses**

As a Single Drug Product: Uses currently included in FDA approved labeling: (1) Helps control mild to moderate type II diabetes mellitus (adult, maturity-onset) that does not require insulin, but can't be adequately controlled by diet alone.

Other (unlabeled) generally accepted uses: None.

How This Drug Works: This drug (1) stimulates the secretion of insulin, (2) decreases glucose production in the liver, and (3) enhances insulin use.

Available Dosage Forms and Strengths

Tablets — 1.25 mg, 1.5 mg, 2.5 mg, 3 mg, 5 mg, 6 mg

▷ **Usual Adult Dosage Range:** Initially 2.5 to 5 mg daily with breakfast. At 7-day intervals the dose may be increased by increments of 2.5 mg daily as needed and tolerated. Total daily dosage should not exceed 20 mg. Some patients respond to 1.25 mg daily. **Note: Actual dosage and administration schedule must be determined by the physician for each patient individually.**

Conditions Requiring Dosing Adjustments

Liver function: Glyburide may cause catastrophic hypoglycemia (low blood sugar) if it is used in patients with liver disease. Very low starting doses should be given and the patient closely followed. It is also a rare cause of hepatitis and cholestatic jaundice.

Kidney function: Glyburide should be used with caution in mild renal compromise, with low initial doses and careful patient monitoring. The drug SHOULD NOT be used in patients with moderate kidney failure (creatinine clearances less than 50 ml per minute) or in severe kidney failure.

▷ **Dosing Instructions:** If the daily maintenance dose is found to be 10 mg or more, the total dose should be divided into 2 equal doses: the first taken with the morning meal, the second with the evening meal. The tablet may be crushed for administration.

Usual Duration of Use: Use on a regular schedule for 1 to 2 weeks determines effectiveness in controlling diabetes. No response to peak doses in 1 month constitutes a primary failure. Up to 10% of those who respond initially may develop secondary failure. The duration of effective use can only be determined by periodic measurement of the blood sugar.

▷ **This Drug Should Not Be Taken If**
  - you have had an allergic reaction to it previously.
  - you have severe impairment of liver and kidney function.
  - you have diabetic ketoacidosis.
  - you are pregnant.

▷ **Inform Your Physician Before Taking This Drug If**
  - you are allergic to other sulfonylurea drugs or to "sulfa" drugs.
  - your diabetes has been unstable or "brittle" in the past.
  - you do not know how to recognize or treat hypoglycemia (see Glossary).
  - you have a history of problems with blood clotting.
  - you have G6PD deficiency.
  - you have a history of congestive heart failure, peptic ulcer disease, cirrhosis of the liver, hypothyroidism or porphyria.

Possible Side Effects (natural, expected, and unavoidable drug actions)
  If drug dosage is excessive or food intake is delayed or inadequate, abnormally low blood sugar (hypoglycemia) will occur as a predictable drug effect.

▷ **Possible Adverse Effects** (unusual, unexpected, and infrequent reactions)
  If any of the following develop, consult your physician promptly for guidance.
  Mild Adverse Effects
  Allergic Reactions: Skin rash, hives, itching.
  Headache, drowsiness, dizziness, fatigue.
  Indigestion, heartburn, nausea.
  Bed-wetting at night (nocturnal enuresis) (especially in young adults).
  Abnormally frequent urination.
  Serious Adverse Effects
  Allergic Reactions: Hepatitis with jaundice (see Glossary), severe skin reactions (exfoliative dermatitis).
  Idiosyncratic Reaction: Hemolytic anemia (see Glossary).
  Disulfiramlike reaction with concurrent use of alcohol (see Glossary) (infrequent with this drug).
  Bone marrow depression (see Glossary)—fatigue, weakness, fever, sore throat, abnormal bleeding or bruising.
  Liver toxicity (cholestatic jaundice).
  Blood clotting defects (coagulation).
  Cardiovascular mortality (increased) (based on the University Group Diabetes Program [UGDP]).
  Drug-induced urinary tract stones.

▷ **Possible Effects on Sexual Function:**   None reported.

▷ **Adverse Effects That May Mimic Natural Diseases or Disorders**
  Liver reactions may suggest viral hepatitis.

Possible Effects on Laboratory Tests

Blood platelet counts: decreased.

Blood cholesterol and triglyceride levels: decreased.

Blood glucose levels: decreased.

Liver function tests: increased liver enzymes (ALT/GPT, AST/GOT and alkaline phosphatase), rare and transient.

CAUTION

1. This drug is only part of the program for management of your diabetes. It is not a substitute for a proper diet and regular exercise.
2. Over time (usually several months), this drug may not work. Periodic follow-up examinations are necessary.

Precautions for Use

By Infants and Children: This drug does not work in type (juvenile, growth-onset) insulin-dependent diabetes.

By Those over 60 Years of Age: Used with caution and started with 1.25 mg/day. Dose is slowly increased and glucose closely followed. Repeated hypoglycemia in the elderly can cause brain damage.

▷ **Advisability of Use During Pregnancy**

Pregnancy Category: C. See Pregnancy Code at the back of this book.

Animal studies: No birth defects reported in rats and rabbits.

Human studies: Adequate studies of pregnant women are not available.

Uncontrolled blood sugar levels during pregnancy are associated with a higher incidence of birth defects, so many experts recommend insulin (instead of an oral agent) to control diabetes during the entire pregnancy.

Advisability of Use if Breast-Feeding

Presence of this drug in breast milk: Unknown.

Avoid drug or refrain from nursing.

Habit-Forming Potential: None.

Effects of Overdosage: Symptoms of mild to severe hypoglycemia: headache, light-headedness, faintness, nervousness, confusion, tremor, sweating, heart palpitation, weakness, hunger, nausea, vomiting, stupor progressing to coma.

Possible Effects of Long-Term Use: Reduced thyroid gland function (hypothyroidism). Reports of increased frequency and severity of heart and blood vessel diseases associated with long-term use of this class of drugs are highly controversial and inconclusive. A direct cause-and-effect relationship (see Glossary) is tenuous. Ask your physician for guidance.

Suggested Periodic Examinations While Taking This Drug (at physician's discretion)

Complete blood cell counts, liver function tests, thyroid function tests, periodic evaluation of heart and circulatory system.

▷ **While Taking This Drug, Observe the Following**

Foods: Follow the diabetic diet prescribed by your physician.

Beverages: As directed in the diabetic diet. May be taken with milk.

▷ *Alcohol:* Use with extreme caution—alcohol can exaggerate this drug's hypoglycemic effect. This drug can cause a disulfiramlike reaction (see Glossary): facial flushing, sweating, palpitation.

Tobacco Smoking: No interactions expected.

▷   *Other Drugs*
  The following drugs may *increase* the effects of glyburide
  • aspirin, and other salicylates.
  • cimetidine (Tagamet).
  • clofibrate (Atromid S).
  • fenfluramine (Pondimin).
  • gemfibrozil (Lopid)
  • monoamine oxidase (MAO) type A inhibitors (see Drug Classes).
  • phenylbutazone (Butazolidin).
  • ranitidine (Zantac).
  • sulfa drugs such as Septra.
  The following drugs may *decrease* the effects of glyburide
  • beta blocker drugs (see Drug Classes).
  • bumetanide (Bumex).
  • diazoxide (Proglycem).
  • ethacrynic acid (Edecrin).
  • furosemide (Lasix).
  • phenytoin (Dilantin).
  • rifampin (Rifadin, others).
  • thiazide diuretics (see Drug Classes).
  • thyroid hormones.
  Glyburide *taken concurrently* with
  • antacids (magnesium hydroxide containing) may result in increased risk of excessively lowered blood sugar.
  • antifungal agents (such as itraconazole or other azoles) may result in severe lowering of blood sugar.
  • enalapril (Vasotec) changes effects.
  • steroids (betamethasone, prednisone, others) blunts benefits.
  • Warfarin (Coumadin) may result in bleeding. Checking INR (prothrombin time or protime) more often is prudent.

▷   *Driving, Hazardous Activities:* Regulate dosing, eating and physical activities carefully to prevent hypoglycemia. Know the early symptoms of hypoglycemia so you can avoid hazardous activities and take corrective measures.

Aviation Note: Diabetes *is a disqualification* for piloting. Consult a designated Aviation Medical Examiner.

Exposure to Sun: Use caution until sensitivity has been determined. Some drugs of this class can cause photosensitivity (see Glossary).

Occurrence of Unrelated Illness: Acute infections, vomiting or diarrhea, serious injuries and surgical procedures can worsen diabetic control and may require insulin. If any of these conditions occur, consult your physician promptly.

Discontinuation: Because of the possibility of secondary failure, it is advisable to evaluate the continued benefit of this drug every 6 months.

GUANFACINE (GWAHN fa seen)

Introduced: 1980   **Prescription:** USA: Yes   **Available as Generic:**
USA: No   **Class:** Antihypertensive   **Controlled Drug:** USA: No
Brand Name: Tenex

BENEFITS versus RISKS	
Possible Benefits	*Possible Risks*
EFFECTIVE ANTIHYPERTENSIVE in mild to moderate high blood pressure	Amnesia (uncommon)
EFFECTIVE in high blood pressure of pregnancy	

▷ **Principal Uses**

   As a Single Drug Product: Uses currently included in FDA approved labeling: (1) Used to treat mild to moderate high blood pressure; (2) used alone or in combination to treat high blood pressure caused by kidney problems. Other (unlabeled) generally accepted uses: (1) Heroin withdrawal; (2) may be useful in problem pregnancies.

How This Drug Works: By reducing sympathetic nervous system output (by affecting brain alpha two receptors), this drug causes relaxation of blood vessel walls and lowering of blood pressure.

Available Dosage Forms and Strengths

   Tablets — 1 mg and 2 mg

▷ **Usual Adult Dosage Range:** Initially 1 mg once daily taken at bedtime. The dose may be increased after 3 to 4 weeks to 2 mg daily, as needed and tolerated. If needed, the dose may be increased again after 3 to 4 weeks to 3 mg daily. The total daily requirement may be taken in 2 divided doses if necessary for stable blood pressure control. Use of up to 40 mg daily has been reported, but in general, combination therapy is used before such doses are reached. **Note: Actual dosage and administration schedule must be determined by the physician for each patient individually.**

Conditions Requiring Dosing Adjustments

   Liver function: It should be used with caution in patients with liver compromise.
   Kidney function: Used with caution, but can be removed by non-kidney mechanisms.

▷ **Dosing Instructions:** Tablets may be crushed and taken without regard to eating. It is recommended that the daily dose be taken at bedtime to reduce the side effect of daytime drowsiness.

Usual Duration of Use: Continual use on a regular schedule for 4 to 6 weeks is usually necessary to determine this drug's effectiveness in controlling high blood pressure. Peak benefit may not be seen for 12 weeks. Long-term use (months to years) requires supervision and guidance by the physician. Consult your physician on a regular basis.

▷ **This Drug Should Not Be Taken If**

   • you have had an allergic reaction to it previously.

▷ **Inform Your Physician Before Taking This Drug If**
- you have a circulatory disorder of the brain.
- you have angina or coronary artery disease.
- you have or have had serious emotional depression.
- you have impaired liver or kidney function.
- you are a diabetic.
- you have a history of orthostatic hypotension.
- you are taking any sedative or hypnotic drugs or an antidepressant.
- you plan to have surgery under general anesthesia in the near future.

Possible Side Effects (natural, expected, and unavoidable drug actions)
Drowsiness, dry nose and mouth, constipation, decreased heart rate, mild orthostatic hypotension (see Glossary).

▷ **Possible Adverse Effects** (unusual, unexpected, and infrequent reactions)
If any of the following develop, consult your physician promptly for guidance.
Mild Adverse Effects
Allergic Reactions: Skin rash, itching.
Headache, dizziness, fatigue, insomnia.
Sedation.
Indigestion, nausea, diarrhea.
Edema (rare).
Leg cramps.
Serious Adverse Effects
Abnormally low blood pressure on standing (orthostatic hypotension).
Slow heartbeat (bradycardia).
Liver toxicity (rare).
Amnesia.
Rebound hypertension (if abruptly stopped).

▷ **Possible Effects on Sexual Function:** Dose-related decreased libido, impotence.

Possible Effects on Laboratory Tests
Liver function tests: increased.

CAUTION
1. ***Do not stop this drug suddenly.*** Sudden withdrawal can produce anxiety, nervousness, tremors, fast or irregular heart action, nausea, stomach cramps, vomiting and rebound hypertension.
2. Hot weather and fever can reduce blood pressure significantly. Dosage adjustments may be necessary.
3. Report the development of any tendency to emotional depression.

Precautions for Use
By Infants and Children: Safety and effectiveness for use by those under 12 years of age have not been established.
*By Those over 60 Years of Age: **Proceed cautiously**.* Pressure should be reduced without creating the risks associated with excessively low blood pressure. Watch for light-headedness, dizziness, unsteadiness, fainting and falling. Sedation and dry mouth occur commonly in elderly users. Report promptly any changes in mood or behavior: depression, delusions, hallucinations.

▷ **Advisability of Use During Pregnancy**
 Pregnancy Category: B. See Pregnancy Code at the back of this book.
  Animal studies: No birth defects due to this drug reported in rat and rabbit studies.
  Human studies: Adequate studies of pregnant women are not available.
  Use this drug only if clearly needed. Ask your physician for guidance.

Advisability of Use if Breast-Feeding
 Presence of this drug in breast milk: Probably yes.
 Avoid drug or refrain from nursing.

Habit-Forming Potential: None.

Effects of Overdosage: Marked drowsiness, weakness, dry mouth, slow pulse, low blood pressure, vomiting, stupor progressing to coma.

Possible Effects of Long-Term Use: Development of tolerance (see Glossary) with loss of drug effectiveness.

Suggested Periodic Examinations While Taking This Drug (at physician's discretion)
 Blood pressure measurements.

▷ **While Taking This Drug, Observe the Following**
 Foods: Avoid excessive salt, and ask your doctor about degree of salt restriction.
 Beverages: No restrictions. May be taken with milk.
▷ *Alcohol:* Use with extreme caution—combined effects can cause marked drowsiness and exaggerated reduction of blood pressure.
 Tobacco Smoking: No interactions expected. Follow your physician's advice about tobacco.
▷ *Other Drugs:* Guanfacine **taken concurrently** with
  • amitriptyline (Elavil) can cause decreased effectiveness as an antihypertensive.
  • desipramine and other tricyclic antidepressants can cause loss of therapeutic benefits of guanfacine.
  • phenobarbital can lead to loss of therapeutic effect of guanfacine.
▷ *Driving, Hazardous Activities:* Use caution. This drug can cause drowsiness and can impair mental alertness, judgment and coordination.
 Aviation Note: Hypertension (high blood pressure) *is a disqualification* for piloting. Consult a designated Aviation Medical Examiner.
 Exposure to Sun: No restrictions.
 Exposure to Heat: Use caution. Hot environments may reduce the blood pressure significantly; be alert to the possibility of orthostatic hypotension (see Glossary).
 Heavy Exercise or Exertion: Use caution. Isometric exercises can raise blood pressure significantly. This drug may intensify the hypertensive response to isometric exercise. Ask physician for guidance.
 Occurrence of Unrelated Illness: Fever may lower blood pressure significantly. Vomiting may prevent regular use of this drug and result in acute withdrawal reactions. Call your doctor.
 Discontinuation: **Do not stop this drug suddenly.** Withdrawal reactions occur within 2 to 7 days after the last dose. Best to reduce dose gradually (over 3 to 4 days), with periodic monitoring of the blood pressure.

HALOPERIDOL (hal oh PER i dohl)

Introduced: 1958   **Prescription:** USA: Yes; Canada: Yes   **Available as**
Generic: USA: Yes; Canada: Yes   **Class:** Antipsychotic; tranquilizer, strong
Controlled Drug: USA: No; Canada: No

Brand Names: ✦Apo-Haloperidol, Haldol, ✦Haldol LA, Halperon, ✦Novo-Peri-
dol, ✦Peridol, ✦PMS-haloperidol

BENEFITS versus RISKS

Possible Benefits	*Possible Risks*
EFFECTIVE CONTROL OF PSYCHOSES	FREQUENT PARKINSON-LIKE side effects
BENEFICIAL EFFECTS ON THINKING, MOOD, AND BEHAVIOR	SERIOUS TOXIC EFFECTS ON BRAIN with long-term use
EFFECTIVE CONTROL OF SOME CASES OF TOURETTE'S DISORDER	Rare blood cell disorders
Beneficial in management of some hyperactive children	Abnormally low white blood cell count

---

▷ **Principal Uses**

As a Single Drug Product: Uses currently included in FDA approved labeling: (1)
Helps control psychotic thinking and abnormal behavior associated with
acute psychosis of unknown nature, acute schizophrenia, paranoid states
and the manic phase of manic-depressive disorders; (2) helps control out-
bursts of aggression and agitation; (3) used to treat Gilles de la Tourette's
syndrome.

Other (unlabeled) generally accepted uses: (1) Helps control refractory hiccups; (2) used to lessen delirium in LSD flashbacks and phencyclidine intoxication; (3) used as combination (adjuvant) therapy in chronic pain syndromes; (4) may be helpful in autistic patients; (5) may have a role in
refractory vomiting caused by cancer chemotherapy; (6) can ease symptoms in refractory sneezing; (5) may be helpful as adjunctive therapy in
stuttering.

How This Drug Works: By interfering with a nerve impulse transmitter (dopamine) in the brain, this drug reduces anxiety and agitation, improves coher-
ence and organization of thinking and abolishes delusions and hallucinations.

Available Dosage Forms and Strengths

Concentrate — 2 mg per ml
Injection — 5 mg, 50 mg and 100 mg per ml
Tablets — 0.5 mg, 1 mg, 2 mg, 5 mg, 10 mg, 20 mg

▷ **Usual Adult Dosage Range:** Initially 0.5 to 2 mg 2 or 3 times daily. Dose may be
increased by 0.5 mg/day at 3- to 4-day intervals as needed and tolerated. The
usual dosage range is 0.5 to 30 mg/24 hours. The total daily dosage should
not exceed 100 mg. **Note: Actual dosage and administration schedule**
must be determined by the physician for each patient individually.

Conditions Requiring Dosing Adjustments

Liver function: The dose, dosing interval and titration interval (time taken to adjust the medication to the desired effect) should be adjusted with liver compromise.

Kidney function: High doses of haloperidol should be used with caution in kidney compromise.

▷ **Dosing Instructions:**   The tablet may be crushed and taken with or following food to reduce stomach irritation. The concentrate may be diluted in 2 ounces of water or fruit juice; do not add it to coffee or tea.

Usual Duration of Use: Use on a regular schedule for several weeks determines this drug's effectiveness in controlling psychotic behavior. If it doesn't provide significant benefit in 6 weeks, it should be stopped. Long-term use requires supervision and periodic physician evaluation.

▷ **This Drug Should Not Be Taken If**
- you have had an allergic reaction to any dosage form of it previously.
- you are experiencing severe mental depression.
- you have any form of Parkinson's disease.
- you have cancer of the breast.
- you have severe active liver disease.
- you are presently experiencing central nervous system (CNS) depression due to alcohol or narcotics.
- you currently have a bone marrow or blood cell disorder.

▷ **Inform Your Physician Before Taking This Drug If**
- you are allergic or abnormally sensitive to phenothiazine drugs.
- you have a history of mental depression.
- you have any type of heart disease.
- you have impaired liver or kidney function.
- you have thyroid disease.
- you are allergic to the dye tartrazine.
- you are pregnant or are planning pregnancy.
- you have a history of neuroleptic malignant syndrome.
- you have low blood pressure, epilepsy or glaucoma.
- you are taking any drugs with a sedative effect.
- you plan to have surgery and general or spinal anesthesia soon.

Possible Side Effects (natural, expected, and unavoidable drug actions)
Mild drowsiness, low blood pressure, blurred vision, dry mouth, constipation, marked and frequent Parkinson-like reactions (see Glossary).

▷ **Possible Adverse Effects** (unusual, unexpected, and infrequent reactions)
If any of the following develop, consult your physician promptly for guidance.

Mild Adverse Effects
Allergic Reactions: Skin rash, hives.
Dizziness, weakness, agitation, insomnia.
Loss of appetite, indigestion, nausea, vomiting, diarrhea.
Urinary retention.

Serious Adverse Effects
Allergic Reactions: Rare liver reaction with jaundice, asthma, spasm of vocal cords.

Idiosyncratic Reactions: Neuroleptic malignant syndrome (see Glossary).
Depression, disorientation, eye damage (deposits in cornea, lens, and retina).
Blood cell disorders: anemia, fluctuation in number of white blood cells.
Nervous system reactions: rigidity of extremities, tremors, restlessness, constant movement, facial grimacing, eye-rolling, spasm of neck muscles, tardive dyskinesia (see Glossary).
Abnormal heartbeat (premature ventricular contractions).
Seizures.
Worsening of psychosis.
Low blood sugar.
Abnormal and frequent urination (SIADH).
Liver toxicity.
Abnormal eye orientations (oculogyric crisis).
Bronchospasm (rare).
Myasthenia gravis (rare).

▷ **Possible Effects on Sexual Function**
Decreased libido; impotence (10–20%); painful ejaculation; priapism (see Glossary).
Tender and enlarged breast tissue in men; breast enlargement with milk production in women.
Altered timing and pattern of menstruation.

▷ **Adverse Effects That May Mimic Natural Diseases or Disorders**
Liver reaction may suggest viral hepatitis.
Nervous system reactions may suggest Parkinson's disease or Reye syndrome.

Natural Diseases or Disorders That May Be Activated by This Drug
Latent epilepsy, glaucoma, diabetes.

Possible Effects on Laboratory Tests
Complete blood counts: decreased red cells, hemoglobin and white cells; increased eosinophils.
INR (prothrombin time): decreased.
Blood cholesterol level: decreased.
Blood glucose level: increased.
Liver function tests: increased liver enzymes (ALT/GPT, AST/GOT and alkaline phosphatase), increased bilirubin.

CAUTION
1. The smallest effective dose should be used for long-term therapy.
2. Used with extreme caution in epilepsy; can alter seizure patterns.
3. People with lupus erythematosus and those taking prednisone are more susceptible to nervous system reactions.
4. Levodopa should **not** be used to treat Parkinson-like reactions; it can cause agitation and worsening of the psychotic disorder.
5. Obtain prompt evaluation of any change or disturbance in vision.

Precautions for Use
By Infants and Children: This drug should not be used in children under 3 years of age or 15 kg in weight. Avoid this drug in the presence of symptoms suggestive of Reye syndrome. Children are quite susceptible to nervous system reactions induced by this drug.

By Those over 60 Years of Age: Small doses are indicated when therapy is started. This drug can cause significant changes in mood and behavior; watch for confusion, disorientation, agitation, restlessness, aggression and paranoia. You may be more susceptible to the development of drowsiness, lethargy, orthostatic hypotension (see Glossary), hypothermia (see Glossary), Parkinson-like reactions and prostatism (see Glossary).

▷ **Advisability of Use During Pregnancy**
   Pregnancy Category: C. See Pregnancy Code at the back of this book.
    Animal studies: Cleft palate reported in mouse studies.
    Human studies: No increase in birth defects reported in 100 exposures. Adequate studies of pregnant women are not available.
    Avoid during the first three months (trimester). Use only if clearly needed. Ask physician for guidance.

Advisability of Use if Breast-Feeding
   Presence of this drug in breast milk: Yes.
   Monitor nursing infant closely and discontinue drug or nursing if adverse effects develop.

Habit-Forming Potential: Reports of recreational use have been filed. If the drug is stopped suddenly, patient may experience a withdrawal syndrome.

Effects of Overdosage: Marked drowsiness, weakness, tremor, unsteadiness, agitation, stupor, coma, convulsions.

Possible Effects of Long-Term Use: Eye damage—deposits in cornea, lens or retina; tardive dyskinesia (see Glossary).

Suggested Periodic Examinations While Taking This Drug (at physician's discretion)
   Complete blood counts, liver function tests, eye examinations, electrocardiograms.
   The tongue should be watched for fine, involuntary, wavelike movements that could be the beginning of tardive dyskinesia.

▷ **While Taking This Drug, Observe the Following**
   Foods: No restrictions.
   Beverages: No restrictions. May be taken with milk.
▷   *Alcohol:* Avoid completely. Alcohol can increase the sedative action of haloperidol and accentuate its depressant effects on brain function. Haloperidol can increase the intoxicating effects of alcohol.
   Tobacco Smoking: Combination with nicotine actually increased suppression of tics in Tourette's disorder in one study.
   Marijuana Smoking: Moderate increase in drowsiness; accentuation of orthostatic hypotension; increased risk of precipitating latent psychosis, confusing interpretation of mental status and of drug response.
▷   *Other Drugs*
   Haloperidol may *increase* the effects of
    • all drugs with sedative actions, and cause excessive sedation.
    • fluvoxamine (Luvox) and result in toxicity (altered mental status, GI side effects).
    • some antihypertensive drugs and cause excessive lowering of blood pressure; monitor the combined effects carefully.

Haloperidol may *decrease* the effects of
- guanethidine (Esimil, Ismelin), and reduce its antihypertensive effect.

Haloperidol *taken concurrently* with
- anticholinergic drugs (see Drug Classes) can cause additive anticholinergic effects (dry mouth, constipation or sedation.)
- beta blocker drugs may cause excessive lowering of blood pressure.
- fluoxetine (Prozac) can result in an increased risk of haloperidol toxicity.
- lithium may cause toxic effects on the brain and nervous system.
- methyldopa (Aldomet) may cause serious dementia.

The following drugs may *decrease* the effects of haloperidol
- antacids containing aluminum and/or magnesium may reduce its absorption.
- barbiturates.
- benztropine (Cogentin).
- carbamazepine (Tegretol).
- phenytoin (Dilantin).
- rifampin (Rifater, others).
- trihexyphenidyl (Artane).

▷ *Driving, Hazardous Activities:* This drug may impair mental alertness, judgment and physical coordination. Restrict activities as necessary.

Aviation Note: The use of this drug *is a disqualification* for piloting. Consult a designated Aviation Medical Examiner.

Exposure to Sun: Use caution—this drug can cause photosensitivity.

Exposure to Heat: Use caution in hot environments. This drug may impair the regulation of body temperature and increase the risk of heat stroke.

Exposure to Cold: This drug can increase the risk of hypothermia (see Glossary) in the elderly.

Discontinuation: This drug should not be stopped abruptly following long-term use. Gradual withdrawal over a period of 2 to 3 weeks is advised. Ask doctor for help.

HISTAMINE (H-2) BLOCKING DRUGS

Cimetidine (si MET i deen)   **Ranitidine** (ra NI te deen)   **Famotidine** (fa MOH te deen)   **Nizatidine** (ni ZA te deen)

Introduced: 1977, 1983, 1986, 1988   **Prescription:**   USA: Yes; Canada: Yes
Available as Generic: USA: No; Canada: Yes   **Class:**   Histamine (H-2) Blocking Drugs   **Controlled Drug:**   USA: No; Canada: No

Brand Names: ✦Apo-Cimetidine, ✦Enlon, ✦Novo-Cimetine, ✦Nu-Cimet ✦Peptol, Tagamet, Tagamet HB (nonprescription form), Zantac, ✦Zantac-C, ✦Apo-Ranitidine, Novo-Ranidine, Nu-Ranit and Xantac 75 (nonprescription form), Pepcid, Pepcid AC (nonprescription form), Axid, Axid AR (nonprescription form)

Warning: The brand names Zantac and Xanax are similar and can be mistaken. These are very different drugs, and can lead to serious problems. Check the color chart and verify that you are taking the correct drug.

BENEFITS versus RISKS

Possible Benefits	*Possible Risks*
EFFECTIVE TREATMENT OF PEPTIC ULCER DISEASE: relief of symptoms, acceleration of healing, prevention of recurrence	Drug-induced hepatitis (rare)
	Bone marrow depression (lowered white blood cells or hemoglobin) (rare)
CONTROL OF HYPERSECRETORY STOMACH DISORDERS	Confusion (particularly in compromised elderly with some of these drugs) (rare)
TREATMENT OF REFLUX ESOPHAGITIS	Low blood platelet counts (rare)
TREATMENT OF HEARTBURN	
Pepcid AC nonprescription form is approved for prevention of heartburn	

Author's note: The nonprescription heartburn preventing or treating forms of these medicines have, in general because of episodic use and lower doses, side effects or adverse effects that occur even less frequently than the already well tolerated prescription forms.

▷ **Principal Uses**

As a Single Drug Product: Uses currently included in FDA approved labeling: (1) Treatment and prevention of recurrence of peptic ulcer; (2) all are used for both duodenal and gastric ulcers; (3) cimetidine, ranitidine, and famotidine are used in conditions where extreme production (Zollinger-Ellison syndrome) of stomach acid occurs; (4) all four medications are used to control excess acid moving from the stomach into the lower throat (gastroesophageal reflux disease—GERD); (5) Cimetidine is approved for use in preventing upper stomach/intestinal bleeding; (6) cimetidine, ranitidine, famotidine and nizatidine have been used as combination treatment with antibiotics and bismuth compounds (Pepto Bismol and others) in refractory ulcers where the organism Helicobacter pylori has been found; (7) cimetidine is approved to prevent ulcers caused by stress (stress ulcer prophylaxis); (8) all of these medicines are approved in nonprescription forms for treatment of heartburn. Famotidine (Pepcid AC) and Nizatidine (Axid AR) are also approved for *prevention* of heartburn.

Other (unlabeled) generally accepted uses: (1) Ranitidine, famotidine and nizatidine have been used in the prevention of upper stomach/intestinal bleeding; (2) cimetidine has been used prior to surgery to prevent aspiration pneumonitis caused by anesthesia, and ranitidine has shown some benefit here as well; (3) ranitidine and famotidine have been used to help prevent ulcers which may occur in acutely and seriously ill patients; (4) cimetidine appears to have a role in helping patients with colorectal cancer live longer, but further research is needed; (5) cimetidine also may have a role in helping recurrent and resistant warts in some children.

How These Drugs Work: These drugs block the action of histamine, and by doing this, inhibit the ability of the stomach to make acid. Once the acid production is decreased, the body is able to heal itself. Ulcers which are resistant to healing have now been shown to have an infectious component

(Helicobacter pylori), and antibiotics combined with a histamine (H-2) blocking drug can work.

Available Dosage Forms and Strengths

Cimetidine (Tagamet):

Injection — 300 mg per 2 ml
— 300 mg per 50 ml (single dose in 0.9% sodium chloride)
Liquid — 300 mg per 5 ml (2.8% alcohol)
Oral solution — 300 mg per 5 ml
Tablets — 200 mg, 300 mg, 400 mg, 600 mg, 800 mg
Tablets (nonprescription) — 100 mg

Ranitidine (Zantac):

GELdose Capsules — 150 mg, 300 mg
Injection — 0.5 mg per ml (single dose in 100 ml)
— 25 mg per ml (in 2, 10 and 40 ml vials and 2 ml syringes)
Oral solution (Canada) — 84 mg per 5 ml
Syrup — 15 mg per ml (7.5% alcohol)
Tablets — 150 mg, 300 mg
Tablets (effervescent) — 150 mg
Tablets (nonprescription) — 75 mg

Famotidine (Pepcid):

Injection — 10 mg per ml (in 2 ml and 4 ml vials)
Oral Suspension — 40 mg per 5 ml
Tablets — 20 mg, 40 mg
Tablets (nonprescription) — 10 mg

Nizatidine (Axid):

Pulvules (capsules) — 150 and 300 mg
Tablets (nonprescription) — 75 mg

▷ **Recommended Dosage Ranges (Actual dosage and administration schedule must be determined by the physician for each patient individually.)**

Infants and Children: Cimetidine: routine use not recommended in those less than 16 years old. Doses of 20 to 40 mg per kilogram per day have been used. Ranitidine: for those 2 to 18 years old: 1.25 to 2 milligrams per kilogram per dose, given every 12 hours or 37.5 milligrams per dose.

Famotidine: 0.5 mg per kilogram twice a day for 8 weeks in those 6–15 years old. Nizatidine: No data.

16 to 60 Years of Age: Peptic ulcer and hypersecretory states:

cimetidine: 300 mg by mouth four times daily—taken with meals and at bedtime. A maintenance dose of 400 mg at bedtime is useful in some patients.

ranitidine: 150 mg by mouth twice daily, or 300 mg at bedtime. Maintenance doses of 150 g at bedtime may be of benefit in some patients. Up to 6 grams in hypersecretory states.

famotidine: 40 mg by mouth at bedtime for 4 or up to 8 weeks. Maintenance doses of 20 mg at bedtime have been used. Up to 640 mg daily for hypersecretory states.

nizatidine: 300 mg by mouth at bedtime, or 150 mg twice a day for up to 8 weeks. A maintenance dose of 150 mg at bedtime is useful for some patients. Not used for hypersecretory states.

Heartburn (nonprescription forms):
cimetidine: 100 mg by mouth. ranitidine: 75 mg by mouth.
famotidine: 10 mg by mouth before eating foods or drinking liquids that cause you problems.
nizatidine: 75 mg up to twice daily.

Over 60 Years of Age: Cimetidine: Half the usual adult dose to start. Ranitidine, famotidine and nizatidine: Same dose as 16 to 60 years of age. All pose a risk for formation of masses (phytobezoars) of undigested vegetable fibers. Watch for nervousness, confusion, loss of appetite, stomach fullness, nausea and vomiting.

Conditions Requiring Dosing Adjustments:
Liver function: Cimetidine and famotidine are most dependent on the liver for elimination. Dose must be decreased in liver failure.
Kidney function: All of these H2 blockers are primarily eliminated by the kidneys. Doses **must** be decreased in moderate kidney failure.

▷ **Dosing Instructions:** Cimetidine and ranitidine should be taken immediately after meals to obtain the longest decrease in stomach acid when treating peptic ulcers. Cimetidine, ranitidine and famotidine should be taken after meals when used in hypersecretory states.

Usual Duration of Use: Use on a regular schedule for 4 to 6 weeks usually determines effectiveness in healing active peptic ulcer disease. Long-term use (months to years) for prevention requires periodic individualized consideration by your physician. Continual use for 6 to 12 weeks is needed to heal the esophagus when cimetidine, ranitidine, famotidine or nizatidine is used in GERD. Since nonprescription forms are available for heartburn, if heartburn relief has not occurred in two hours, call your doctor as there may be another reason for your symptoms.

Possible Advantages of These Drugs
Famotidine, ranitidine and nizatidine offer effective treatment of peptic ulcer disease with once a day dosing. Nonprescription forms offer relief of heartburn discomfort. Famotidine is approved for nonprescription *prevention* of heartburn.

▷ **These Drugs Should Not Be Taken If**
• you have had an allergic reaction to any dosage form of it previously.

▷ **Inform Your Physician Before Taking This Drug If**
• you have impaired liver or kidney function.
• you have a low sperm count (cimetidine).
• you are taking any anticoagulant drug.
• you do not tolerate or should not take phenylalanine (ranitidine efferdose tablets or granules).
• you have had low white blood cell counts.
• you have a history of acute porphyria (ranitidine).
• you are taking medicines listed in the drug interactions section.

Possible Side Effects (natural, expected, and unavoidable drug actions)
None reported.

▷ **Possible Adverse Effects** (unusual, unexpected, and infrequent reactions)
If any of the following develop, consult your physician promptly for guidance.

Mild Adverse Effects

Allergic Reactions: Skin rash and hives.

Headache: ranitidine (rare), cimetidine (rare), famotidine (4.7 %), and nizatidine (up to 20%).

Diarrhea: ranitidine, nizatidine, cimetidine, and famotidine (all rare).

Joint pain (arthralgia): cimetidine, ranitidine, and famotidine (all rare).

Depression: cimetidine (very rare).

Muscle pain: cimetidine, nizatidine, and famotidine (rare). Abnormal dreams: nizatidine (rare).

Serious Adverse Effects

Allergic Reactions: Cimetidine and ranitidine can be rare causes of pancreatitis and anemia. Cimetidine and nizatidine can cause exfoliative dermatitis. There have been some reports of serious skin rashes with cimetidine, nizatidine, and famotidine.

Anaphylactoid reactions: cimetidine, nizatidine (rare). Idiosyncratic Reactions: Nervousness, confusion, hallucinations.

Liver damage: cimetidine, ranitidine, and nizatidine (rare).

Abnormal heart rhythm changes (slow heartbeat or atrioventricular block): cimetidine, ranitidine, famotidine, and nizatidine (rare).

Bone marrow depression: cimetidine, ranitidine, and famotidine (all rare).

Decreased platelets: cimetidine, ranitidine, and nizatidine (rare). Famotidine may be a very rare and questionable cause.

Bronchospasm: cimetidine and ranitidine (rare) and famotidine (rare and questionable).

▷ **Possible Effects on Sexual Function:** Impotence: ranitidine, famotidine, cimetidine and nizatidine (rare).

Decreased libido: cimetidine, ranitidine, famotidine and nizatidine (rare).

Male breast enlargement (gynecomastia): nizatidine and cimetidine (rare).

Possible Delayed Adverse Effects: Male breast enlargement (ranitidine, nizatidine and cimetidine).

Famotidine may impair vitamin B-12 absorption and lead to deficiency.

▷ **Adverse Effects That May Mimic Natural Diseases or Disorders**

Liver changes may mimic viral hepatitis.

Possible Effects on Laboratory Tests

Blood platelet counts: may be decreased by all histamine (H-2) blockers.

Complete blood counts: rare white blood cell (granulocytes) decrease by cimetidine, ranitidine and famotidine.

Urine protein tests (Multistix): False-positive with ranitidine use.

Urine urobilinogen: False-positive with nizatidine.

Thyroid hormones: T4 and free T4 are decreased with ranitidine use.

Liver enzymes (SGPT, OT etc.): Can be increased with liver damage.

Sperm count: Decreased with cimetidine.

CAUTION

1. Ulcer rebound/perforation may occur if you stop these drugs abruptly when they are being used to treat ulcers.

2. Once medicines are stopped, call your doctor promptly if symptoms recur.

3. Use of these medicines and symptom relief does not absolutely remove possibility of cancer of the stomach (gastric malignancy).

4. The nonprescription forms of these medicines should NOT be used to treat ulcers.

5. Some of cimetidine is removed by hemodialysis. Redose is needed.

Precautions for Use

By Infants and Children: Cimetidine: Routine use not recommended in those less than 16 years old. Doses of 20 to 40 mg per kilogram per day have been used. Ranitidine: for those 2 to 18 years old: 1.25 to 2 milligrams per kilogram per dose, given every 12 hours or 37.5 milligrams per dose.

Famotidine: 0.5 mg per kilogram twice a day for 8 weeks in those 6–15 years old. Nizatidine : No data.

By Those over 60 Years of Age: Increased risk of masses of partially digested vegetable fibers (phytobezoars), especially in people who can't chew well. Watch closely for decreased appetite, stomach fullness, nausea and vomiting.

▷ **Advisability of Use During Pregnancy**

Pregnancy Category: B for cimetidine, ranitidine and famotidine. C for nizatidine. See Pregnancy Code at the back of this book.

Animal studies: No birth defects for cimetidine, ranitidine and famotidine. Rabbit studies of nizatidine showed heart, brain/spinal cord defects.

Human studies: Adequate studies of pregnant women are not available.

Use cimetidine, ranitidine or famotidine only if clearly needed. Ask your doctor for advice.

Nizatidine should be avoided during the first 3 months of pregnancy. Ask your doctor for guidance.

Advisability of Use if Breast-Feeding

Presence of this drug in breast milk: Yes.

Avoid drugs or refrain from nursing.

Habit-Forming Potential: None.

Effects of Overdosage: Cimetidine (rarely documented): Confusion, tachycardia, sweating, drowsiness, muscle twitching, seizures, respiratory failure, severe CNS symptoms such as coma (after 20–40 grams). Nizatidine (rarely documented): Increased tearing of the eyes, salivation, vomiting and diarrhea.

Ranitidine and famotidine: No documentation of overdose changes. Transient changes would be expected that are consistent with adverse effects of the usual dose. Symptomatic and supportive care would be indicated.

(nonprescription forms do not have documentation of overdoses).

Possible Effects of Long-Term Use: Rare liver damage with cimetidine, ranitidine and nizatidine. Swelling and tenderness of breast tissue with cimetidine, ranitidine and nizatidine.

Suggested Periodic Examinations While Taking This Drug (at physician's discretion)

Complete blood counts, liver and kidney function tests, more frequent tests of INR (prothrombin times) if an anticoagulant is also taken, and sperm counts (cimetidine).

▷ **While Taking This Drug, Observe the Following**

Foods: Protein-rich foods increase stomach acid secretion. Garlic, onions, citrus fruits and tomatoes may also increase acid secretion. Many people know the kinds of foods that are likely to result in significant heartburn.

Ask your doctor or pharmacist for help in timing the dose of a nonprescription agent for heartburn. Only one of the nonprescription agents is FDA approved for prevention of heartburn.

Nutritional Support: Cimetidine may decrease vitamin B-12 over time and require supplements.

Beverages: The caffeine in caffeine containing beverages such as coffee, tea and some sodas may stay in the body up to 50% longer usual with cimetidine (Tagamet) use. Milk may increase acid secretion.

▷ *Alcohol:* Stomach acidity is increased by alcohol—avoid use. Cimetidine may produce a drug interaction with higher than expected levels.

Tobacco Smoking: Smoking is a clear risk factor for peptic ulcer disease. Stop if possible.

Marijuana Smoking: Possible additive reduction in sperm counts with cimetidine use.

▷ *Other Drugs*

Cimetidine may ***increase*** the effects of
- amiodarone (Codarone).
- amitriptyline (Elavil) and perhaps other tricyclic antidepressants (see Drug Classes). Decreased doses may be needed if the medicines are to be combined.
- oral anticoagulants—with increased risk of bleeding. Increased frequency of INR testing recommended.
- benzodiazepines (Librium, etc.)—see Drug Class Section.
- carbamazepine (Tegretol) with increased toxicity risk. Blood levels are recommended and ongoing carbamazepine doses adjusted to blood levels.
- flecainide (Tambocor) and require dosing changes and more frequent blood level checks.
- loratadine (Claritin) by causing a large increase in blood levels. A study did NOT report any adverse effects on the heart from these levels, but since excessive blood levels of any medicine may be more likely to cause undesirable effects, it appears prudent to lower loratadine doses if these medicines are to be combined.
- meperidine (Demerol, others) and result in toxicity with potential respiratory depression and low blood pressure.
- metoprolol (Lopressor, others) (and perhaps other beta blockers—see Drug Classes) and result in very slow heartbeat and excessively low blood pressure.
- morphine (MS Contin, MSIR others) and result in central nervous system depression and respiratory depression.
- phenytoin (Dilantin).
- procainamide (Procan, Pronestyl).
- propranolol (Inderal).
- quinidine (Quiniglute).
- theophylline (Theo-Dur, etc.).
- venlafaxine (Effexor).
- warfarin (Coumadin).

Ranitidine may ***increase*** the effects of
- diazepam (Valium).
- glipizide (Glucotrol) and perhaps other oral hypoglycemic agents (see drug classes).

- midazolam (Versed).
- procainamide (Procan, Pronestyl).
- theophylline (Theo-Dur, etc.).
- warfarin (Coumadin) rarely. Increased INR testing is recommended.

Nizatidine, ranitidine and famotidine (prescription forms) may *increase* the effects of

- amoxicillin.
- high dose aspirin (may increase level and toxicity risk).
- pentoxiphylline (Trental); however this interaction has only been documented with cimetidine.

Nizatidine, ranitidine and famotidine (prescription forms) may *increase* the effects of

- theophylline (Theodur, others). Ongoing theophylline dosing should be based on more frequent blood levels if these medicines are to be taken together.

Cimetidine *taken concurrently* with

- most calcium channel blockers (see Drug Classes) may result in increased blood levels of the calcium channel blockers and potential toxicity. Decreased calcium channel blocker doses may be needed. This may also occur with other H2 blockers and caution is advised.
- carmustine (BCNU) may cause severe bone marrow depression.
- chloroquine may result in toxicity and may cause cardiac arrest.
- cisapride (Propulcid) may result in increased cisapride levels and a potential serious increase in heart rate.
- clozapine (Clozaril) may result in increased blood levels and clozapine toxicity.
- digoxin (Lanoxin) may result in changes in digoxin levels.
- oral hypoglycemic agents such as glipizide (Glucotrol), glyburide (DiaBeta, Micronase), and tolbutamide (Tolinase, others) may result in severe low blood sugars and seizures.
- paroxetine (Paxil) and perhaps other SSRIs (see Drug Classes) may result in increased blood levels of the SSRI and require dosing changes.
- pentoxifylline (Trental) may result in increases in blood levels of pentoxifylline. Pentoxifylline dose changes may be needed.
- zalcitabine (Hivid) may result in increased blood levels of zalcitabine and result in toxicity. Decreased doses of zalcitabine may be needed.

Cimetidine, ranitidine, famotidine and nizatidine *taken concurrently* with

- antacids will result in a decreased histamine blocker level. May be prudent to separate the dosing of these medicines (prescription forms).

Cimetidine *may decrease the effects of*

- iron salts, by decreasing absorption.
- indomethacin, by decreasing absorption.
- ketoconazole, itraconazole and fluconazole.
- tetracyclines, by decreasing absorption.

Ranitidine, nizatidine and famotidine may *decrease* the effects of

- indomethacin, by decreasing absorption.
- ketoconazole, itraconazole and fluconazole.
- sucralfate (Carafate).

▷ *Driving, Hazardous Activities:* Use caution until the degree of confusion, dizziness or other effect is seen.

Aviation Note: The use of these drugs (prescription forms) *may be a disqualification* for piloting. Consult a designated Aviation Medical Examiner.

Exposure to Sun: Rare and questionable association with ranitidine, use caution
with sun exposure when first starting this medicine.

Occurrence of Unrelated Illness: Idiopathic thrombocytopenic purpura (ITP), a
rare lowering of blood platelets is a contraindication for use of any of these
medications. Aplastic anemia, whatever the cause, may be worsened by
cimetidine. If symptoms of heartburn get worse, and you are experiencing
unexplained weight loss, and are over 45 years old, talk with your doctor
. . . this may be an indication of stomach cancer.

Discontinuation: **Do not** stop these medicines suddenly if they are being taken
for peptic ulcer disease. Ask your doctor for withdrawal instructions. Be
alert to the recurrence of ulcers any time after these drugs are stopped.
Recurrent or refractory ulcers may also represent an infectious disease
caused by Helicobacter pylori. If this is the case, combination therapy with
an antibiotic may be indicated.

HYDRALAZINE (hi DRAL a zeen)

Introduced: 1950   **Prescription:** USA: Yes; Canada: Yes   **Available as
Generic:** USA: Yes; Canada: No   **Class:** Antihypertensive   **Controlled
Drug:** USA: No; Canada: No

Brand Names: Alazine, Apo-Hydralazine, Apresazide [CD], Apresoline, Apresoline-Esidrix [CD], Cam-Ap-Es, Dralserp, Dralzine, H-H-R, H.H.R., Hydroserpine [CD], Lo-Ten, Novo-Hylazin, Nu-Hydral, Ser-Ap-Es [CD], Serpasil-
Apresoline [CD], Tri-Hydroserpine, Unipres [CD]

BENEFITS versus RISKS	
Possible Benefits	*Possible Risks*
EFFECTIVE ADJUNCT IN MODERATE TO SEVERE HYPERTENSION	DRUG-INDUCED LUPUS-ERYTHEMATOSUS-LIKE SYNDROME
Possibly beneficial in the management of severe congestive heart failure	Intensification of angina pectoris Rare blood cell disorders Rare liver damage

▷ **Principal Uses**

As a Single Drug Product: Uses currently included in FDA approved labeling: (1)
Treats (in combination with other drugs) moderate to severe high blood
pressure or hypertensive crisis; (2) therapy of hypertension caused by abnormal changes in kidney blood vessels.

Other (unlabeled) generally accepted uses: (1) Therapy for aortic or mitral
heart valve insufficiency—providing support until surgery can be performed; (2) treatment of acute congestive heart failure in combination with
dobutamine; (3) help in anorexia or cachexia; (4) therapy of high blood
pressure in pregnancy; (5) painful erections which may occur in sickle disease (sickle cell priapism).

As a Combination Drug Product [CD]: Available combined with hydrochlorothiazide (a diuretic) and with reserpine (another type of antihypertensive).

When used in combination, several different types of drug action occur at the same time and result in a more beneficial decrease in blood pressure.

How This Drug Works: By causing direct relaxation of arterial walls (mechanism unknown), this drug lowers blood pressure. The dilation of blood vessels can also help in some cases of heart failure by reducing the workload and increasing the output of the heart. Combination therapy with a diuretic reduces the amount of sodium and water in the body, and combination with reserpine reduces the rate and force of contraction of the heart and increases blood vessel expansion.

Available Dosage Forms and Strengths

Tablets — 10 mg, 25 mg, 50 mg, 100 mg

▷ **Usual Adult Dosage Range:**   Initially 10 mg 4 times daily for 2 to 4 days; then increase to 25 mg 4 times daily for the balance of the first week. During the second week the dose may be increased to 50 mg 4 times daily if needed and tolerated. The total daily dosage should not exceed 300 mg for fast acetylators or 200 mg for slow acetylators. Ask your physician for guidance. **Note: Actual dosage and administration schedule must be determined by the physician for each patient individually.**

Conditions Requiring Dosing Adjustments

Liver function: Hydralazine can cause hepatitis, hepatic necrosis and non-cancerous growths. It should be used with caution in patients with liver compromise.

Kidney function: In mild to moderate kidney failure the usual dose can be given every eight hours. In severe kidney failure and people with slow hydralazine metabolism, the usual dose is given every 12 to 24 hours and 200 mg per day is a maximum. This medication should be used with caution.

▷ **Dosing Instructions:**   The tablet may be crushed and the capsule [CD] may be opened and best taken with or following meals to help absorption and reduce stomach upset.

Usual Duration of Use: Use on a regular schedule for several weeks determines effectiveness in lowering blood pressure. Long-term use requires physician supervision.

▷ **This Drug Should Not Be Taken If**

- you have had an allergic reaction to it previously.
- you have rheumatic heart disease.
- you have coronary artery disease.
- you have a dissecting aneurysm of the aorta.
- you have mitral valvular heart disease.

▷ **Inform Your Physician Before Taking This Drug If**

- you have a history of any type of heart disease.
- you have lupus erythematosus.
- you have active angina pectoris.
- you have impaired brain circulation, or have had a stroke.
- you are subject to migraine headaches.
- you have impaired kidney function.
- you have systemic lupus erythematosus.

- you have a history of liver sensitivity to other drugs.
- you plan to have surgery under general anesthesia in the near future.

Possible Side Effects (natural, expected, and unavoidable drug actions)
Orthostatic hypotension (see Glossary), nasal congestion, constipation, delayed or impaired urination, increased heartrate of 10 to 25 beats/minute.

▷ **Possible Adverse Effects** (unusual, unexpected, and infrequent reactions)
If any of the following develop, consult your physician promptly for guidance.

Mild Adverse Effects
Allergic Reactions: Skin rash, hives, itching, drug fever.
Headache, dizziness, flushing of face, palpitation.
Loss of appetite, nausea, vomiting, diarrhea.
Taste or smell disorders.
Arthritis.
Tremors, muscle cramps.
Reflex tachycardia.

Serious Adverse Effects
Allergic Reactions: Liver reaction, with or without jaundice.
Idiosyncratic Reactions: Behavioral changes: nervousness, confusion, emotional depression. Asthma, bleeding into lung tissue: densities found on X ray. A syndrome resembling rheumatoid arthritis or lupus erythematosus (see Glossary).
Intensification of coronary artery disease.
Peripheral neuropathy (see Glossary): weakness, numbness, and/or pain in extremities (may be corrected by pyridoxine [vitamin B6] replacement).
Serious skin rashes (Stevens-Johnson syndrome).
Drug-induced periarteritis nodosa.
Drug-induced porphyria.
Drug-induced gastrointestinal bleeding.
Kidney problems (glomerulonephritis).
Drug-induced gallstones.
Congestive heart failure (rare).
ST segment depression on ECG.
Excessive lowering of the blood pressure.
Rare bone marrow depression (see Glossary): fatigue, weakness, fever, sore throat, abnormal bleeding or bruising.

▷ **Possible Effects on Sexual Function:** Rare reports of impotence and priapism (see Glossary).

▷ **Adverse Effects That May Mimic Natural Diseases or Disorders**
Drug fever may suggest systemic infection. Liver reaction may suggest viral hepatitis. Skin and joint symptoms may suggest lupus erythematosus.

Natural Diseases or Disorders That May Be Activated by This Drug
Latent coronary artery disease.

Possible Effects on Laboratory Tests
Complete blood cell counts: decreased red cells, hemoglobin, white cells and platelets.

Blood antinuclear antibodies (ANA): positive.

Blood cholesterol level: decreased.

Blood lupus erythematosus (LE) cells: positive.

Blood urea nitrogen (BUN) level: increased (kidney damage).

Liver function tests: increased liver enzymes (ALT/GPT, AST/GOT and alkaline phosphatase), increased bilirubin.

CAUTION

1. Increased risk of toxicity with large doses. Follow prescribed doses exactly and keep appointments for follow-up examinations.
2. Report the development of any tendency to emotional depression.
3. May cause salt and water retention if not taken with a diuretic.
4. This drug can provoke migraine headache.

Precautions for Use

By Infants and Children: Dosage is based upon age, weight and kidney function status. For high blood pressure: 0.75 to 1 mg per kilogram daily. This dose is divided into 2 to 4 equal doses and given every 6 to 12 hours. This is gradually increased as needed and tolerated to a maximum of 200 mg per day. Watch for development of a lupus erythematosuslike reaction.

By Those over 60 Years of Age: Low doses are indicated. Unacceptably high blood pressure should be slowly reduced, avoiding the risks associated with excessively low blood pressure. Sudden, rapid and excessive reduction of blood pressure can predispose to stroke or heart attack. Watch for dizziness, unsteadiness, fainting or falling. Headache, palpitation and rapid heart rates are more common in the elderly and can mimic acute anxiety states.

▷ Advisability of Use During Pregnancy

Pregnancy Category: C. See Pregnancy Code at the back of this book.

Animal studies: Birth defects of head and facial bones reported in mice.

Human studies: Adequate studies of pregnant women are not available.

Avoid use during the first and last 3 months; if taken late in pregnancy, this drug can cause low blood platelets (see Glossary) in the newborn.

Advisability of Use if Breast-Feeding

Presence of this drug in breast milk: Yes.

Avoid drug or refrain from nursing.

Habit-Forming Potential: None, but sudden stopping of this medicine may result in congestive heart failure.

Effects of Overdosage: Marked light-headedness, dizziness, headache, flushing of skin, nausea, vomiting, collapse of circulation; loss of consciousness, cold and sweaty skin, weak and rapid pulse, irregular heart rhythm.

Possible Effects of Long-Term Use: An acute or subacute syndrome resembling rheumatoid arthritis or lupus erythematosus, usually seen in slow acetylators taking daily doses of over 200 mg. Tolerance to the therapeutic benefits may develop.

Suggested Periodic Examinations While Taking This Drug (at physician's discretion)

Complete blood counts, liver function tests, blood tests for evidence of lupus erythematosus.

▷ **While Taking This Drug, Observe the Following**

Foods: May decrease hydralazine absorption and lessen its therapeutic effect.

Nutritional Support: Watch for peripheral neuropathy and take pyridoxine (vitamin B-6) as needed. Ask physician for guidance.

Beverages: No restrictions. May be taken with milk.

▷ *Alcohol:* Use with extreme caution—alcohol can exaggerate the blood-pressure-lowering effect of this drug and cause excessive reduction.

Tobacco Smoking: Avoid completely. Nicotine can contribute significantly to this drug's ability to intensify angina in susceptible individuals.

▷ *Other Drugs*

Hydralazine may *increase* the effects of
- metoprolol (Lopressor) and other beta blocking medicines.
- oxprenolol (Trasicor).
- propranolol (Inderal).

Hydralazine *taken concurrently* with
- clonidine (Catapress) may result in additive lowering of blood pressure. This may be used to therapeutic benefit.
- furosemide (Lasix) can result in decreased furosemide levels and a need to increase the dose in order to get the same therapeutic benefit if these two drugs are combined.
- nitrates (isosorbide dinitrate, others) may result in increased benefits in patients with heart failure.
- NSAIDs (see Drug Classes) may blunt hydralazine's benefit in lowering blood pressure.

▷ *Driving, Hazardous Activities:* May cause light-headedness or dizziness. Limit activities as necessary.

Aviation Note: Hypertension and the use of this drug *are disqualifications* for piloting. Consult a designated Aviation Medical Examiner.

Exposure to Sun: No restrictions.

Exposure to Heat: Caution advised. Hot environments may reduce blood pressure significantly.

Exposure to Cold: Caution advised. Cold environments may increase this drug's ability to cause angina in susceptible individuals.

Heavy Exercise or Exertion: Caution advised. Exertion can increase this drug's ability to cause angina. Also, isometric exercises can raise blood pressure significantly.

HYDROCHLOROTHIAZIDE (hi droh klor oh THI a zide)

Introduced: 1959   **Prescription:** USA: Yes; Canada: Yes   **Available as Generic:** USA: Yes; Canada: Yes   **Class:** Antihypertensive, diuretic, thiazides   **Controlled Drug:** USA: No; Canada: No

Brand Names: Aldactazide [CD], Aldoril-15/25 [CD], Aldoril D30/D50 [CD], Amiloride, ✦Apo-Hydro, ✦Apo-Methazide [CD], ✦Apo-Spirozide, ✦Apo-Triazide [CD], Apresazide [CD], Apresoline-Esidrix [CD], Cam-AP-Es, Capozide [CD], ✦Co-Betaloc [CD], Diaqua, Dyazide [CD], Esidrix, Esimil, H-H-R, H.H.R., Hydrodiuril, Hydro-Chlor, Hydromal, Hydropres [CD],

Hydro-T, Hydro-Z-50, Inderide [CD], Inderide LA [CD], ✦Ismelin-Esidrix [CD], Lopressor HCT [CD], Lo-Ten, Lotensin-HCT, Maxzide [CD], Maxzide-25 [CD], M Dopazide, Mictrin, ✦Moduret [CD], Moduretic [CD], ✦Natrimax, ✦Neo-Codema, Normozide [CD], ✦Novo-Noparil [CD], ✦Novohydrazide, ✦Novospirozine [CD], ✦Novotriamzide [CD], ✦Nu-Amilzide, ✦Nu-Triazide, Oretic, Oreticyl [CD], ✦PMS Dopazide [CD], Prinzide [CD], Ser-Ap-Es [CD], Serpasil-Esidrix [CD], SK-Hydrochlorothiazide, Thiuretic, Timolide [CD], Trandate HCT [CD], Unipres [CD], ✦Urozide, Vaseretic [CD], ✦Viskazide [CD], Zestoretic [CD], Zide, Ziac

Warning: Studies have shown that doses of 50 mg may increase risk of sudden heart (cardiac) death by 70%. Doses greater than 100 mg may increase risk of sudden cardiac death by 400%. This effect is thought to be due to loss of magnesium and potassium from the body. Ask your doctor for guidance.

BENEFITS versus RISKS	
Possible Benefits	*Possible Risks*
EFFECTIVE, WELL-TOLERATED DIURETIC	LOSS OF BODY POTASSIUM AND MAGNESIUM, especially with
POSSIBLY EFFECTIVE IN MILD HYPERTENSION	doses over 25 mg
ENHANCES EFFECTIVENESS OF OTHER ANTIHYPERTENSIVES	SUDDEN CARDIAC DEATH FROM ELECTROLYTE LOSS
Beneficial in treatment of diabetes insipidus	Increased blood sugar, uric acid, and calcium
	Rare blood cell disorders

Please see the thiazide diuretic profile for further information.

HYDROCODONE (hi droh KOH dohn)

Other Name: Dihydrocodeinone

Introduced: 1951   **Prescription:** USA: Yes; Canada: Yes   **Available as Generic:** USA: Yes; Canada: No   **Class:** Analgesic, strong; cough suppressant, opioid drug   **Controlled Drug:** USA:C-III*

Brand Names: Allay [CD], Anaplex, Anexsia [CD], Anexsia 7.5 [CD], Anolor DH5, Azdone [CD], Ban-Tuss-HC [CD], ✦Biohisdex DHC [CD], ✦Biohisdine DHC [CD], Chemdal-HD [CD], Codone, Detussin [CD], DHC Plus, Dicoril, Dimetane Expectorant-DC [CD], Duocet [CD], Duratuss HD [CD], Endagen HD [CD], Endal-HD, Entuss-D, Histinex-HC [CD], Histussin HC [CD], ✦Hycodan, Hycodan [CD], ✦Hycomine [CD], Hycomine Compound [CD], Hycomine Pediatric Syrup [CD], ✦Hycomine-S [CD], Hycomine Syrup [CD], Hycotuss Expectorant [CD], Lorcet-HD [CD], Lorcet Plus [CD], Lortab [CD], Lortab ASA [CD], Medipain 5, Norcet 7 [CD], ✦Novahistex DH [CD], ✦Novahistine DH [CD], Polygesic, Protuss, ✦Robidone, T-Gesic [CD], Triaminic Expectorant DH [CD], ✦Tussaminic Expectorant DH [CD], Tussend [CD], Tussend Expectorant [CD], Tussionex [CD], Tycolet [CD], Vanex [CD], Vicodin [CD], Vicodin ES [CD], Zydone [CD]

*See Schedules of Controlled Drugs at the back of this book.

BENEFITS versus RISKS	
Possible Benefits	*Possible Risks*
EFFECTIVE RELIEF OF MILD TO MODERATE PAIN	Mild allergic reactions (infrequent)
	Nausea, constipation
EFFECTIVE CONTROL OF COUGH	Potential for addiction

▷ **Principal Uses**

As a Single Drug Product: Uses currently included in FDA approved labeling: (1) Controls cough; (2) relieves mild to moderate pain.

Other (unlabeled) generally accepted uses: May be a benefit in some patients with chronic obstructive lung disease.

As a Combination Drug Product [CD]: Hydrocodone is often added to cough mixtures containing antihistamines, decongestants and expectorants to make these "shotgun" preparations more effective in reducing cough. It is also combined with milder analgesics, such as acetaminophen and aspirin, to enhance pain relief.

How This Drug Works: Depresses some brain functions, decreasing pain perception, calming emotional responses to pain and reducing cough reflex sensitivity.

Available Dosage Forms and Strengths

Syrup — 5 mg per 5-ml

Tablets — 5 mg

▷ **Usual Adult Dosage Range:** As analgesic—5 to 10 mg every 6 hours—scheduled to start and may later be reduced as needed. Maximum for pain is 40 mg. For cough—5 mg per 6 to 8 hours as needed. Total daily dosage should not exceed 20 mg. **Note: Actual dosage and administration schedule must be determined by the physician for each patient individually.**

Conditions Requiring Dosing Adjustments

Liver function: Used with caution in patients with severe liver compromise with decreases in dose or longer time between doses.

Kidney function: This drug may cause urinary retention, and a benefit to risk decision should be made in patients with renal (kidney) outflow problems. Up to 20% of this drug is eliminated by the kidneys. Consideration for reduced doses should be given, especially for longer term therapy.

▷ **Dosing Instructions:** Tablet may be crushed and taken with or following food to reduce stomach irritation or nausea.

Usual Duration of Use: As required, to control pain or cough. Continual use should not exceed 5 to 7 days without interruption and reassessment of need.

▷ **This Drug Should Not Be Taken If**
- you have had an allergic reaction to any dosage form of it previously.
- you have a lesion in your head (intracranial) which causes increased pressure.
- you are having an acute attack of asthma.

▷ **Inform Your Physician Before Taking This Drug If**
- you have had an unfavorable reaction to any narcotic drug in the past.
- you have a history of drug abuse or alcoholism.
- you have chronic lung disease with impaired breathing.

- you have impaired liver or kidney function.
- you have gallbladder disease, a seizure disorder or an underactive thyroid gland.
- you have difficulty emptying the urinary bladder.
- you are allergic to sulfites (some preparations contain sulfites).
- you are taking any other drugs that have a sedative effect.
- you plan to have surgery under general anesthesia in the near future.

Possible Side Effects (natural, expected, and unavoidable drug actions)
Drowsiness, light-headedness, dry mouth, urinary retention, constipation.

▷ **Possible Adverse Effects** (unusual, unexpected, and infrequent reactions)
If any of the following develop, consult your physician promptly for guidance.
Mild Adverse Effects
Allergic Reactions: Skin rash, hives, itching.
Dizziness, impaired concentration, sensation of drunkenness, confusion, depression, blurred or double vision, facial flushing, sweating.
Nausea, vomiting.
Abnormal constriction of the pupils of the eye (miosis).
Serious Adverse Effects
Allergic Reactions: Anaphylaxis (rare), severe skin reactions.
Idiosyncratic Reactions: Delirium, hallucinations, excitement, increased sensitivity to pain after the analgesic effect has worn off.
Seizures (rare).
Impaired breathing (respiratory depression).
Refractory constipation.
Liver toxicity.
Kidney toxicity.
Psychological and physical dependence.

▷ **Possible Effects on Sexual Function:**   Blunting of sexual response or drive.

▷ **Adverse Effects That May Mimic Natural Diseases or Disorders**
Paradoxical behavioral disturbances may suggest psychotic disorder.

Possible Effects on Laboratory Tests
Blood amylase and lipase levels: increased (natural side effect).
Urine screening tests for drug abuse: *initial* test result may be falsely *positive*; *confirmatory* test result will be *negative*. (Test results depend upon amount of drug taken and testing method used.)

CAUTION
1. Patients with asthma, chronic bronchitis or emphysema may have significant respiratory problems with excessive use of this drug because of thickening of bronchial secretions and suppression of coughing.
2. Combination of this drug with atropinelike drugs can increase the risk of urinary retention and reduced intestinal function.
3. Do not take this drug following acute head injury.

Precautions for Use
By Infants and Children: Do not use this drug in children under 2 years of age because of their vulnerability to life-threatening respiratory depression.
By Those over 60 Years of Age: Small doses and short-term treatment are indicated. May be increased susceptibility to drowsiness, dizziness, unsteadi-

ness, falling, urinary retention and constipation (often leading to fecal impaction).

▷ **Advisability of Use During Pregnancy**
Pregnancy Category: C. See Pregnancy Code at the back of this book.
Animal studies: Birth defects reported in hamster studies.
Human studies: Adequate studies of pregnant women are not available. Hydrocodone taken repeatedly during the last few weeks before delivery may cause withdrawal symptoms in the newborn infant.
Use this drug only if clearly needed and in small, infrequent doses.

Advisability of Use if Breast-Feeding
Presence of this drug in breast milk: Unknown.
Monitor nursing infant closely and discontinue drug or nursing if adverse effects develop. Ask physician for guidance.

Habit-Forming Potential: Psychological and/or physical dependence can develop with use of large doses for an extended period of time. True dependence is infrequent and unlikely with prudent use.

Effects of Overdosage: Drowsiness, restlessness, agitation, nausea, vomiting, dry mouth, vertigo, weakness, lethargy, stupor, coma, seizures.

Possible Effects of Long-Term Use: Psychological and physical dependence, chronic constipation.

Suggested Periodic Examinations While Taking This Drug (at physician's discretion)
Liver function tests.

▷ **While Taking This Drug, Observe the Following**
Foods: No restrictions.
Beverages: No restrictions. May be taken with milk.
▷ *Alcohol:* Use extreme caution. Hydrocodone can intensify the intoxicating effects of alcohol, and alcohol can intensify the depressant effects of hydrocodone on brain function, breathing and circulation.
Tobacco Smoking: No interactions expected.
Marijuana Smoking: Increased drowsiness and pain relief; impaired mental and physical status.
▷ *Other Drugs*
Hydrocodone may *increase* the effects of
• other drugs with sedative effects.
• atropinelike drugs, and increase the risk of constipation and urinary retention.
Hydrocodone *taken concurrently* with
• cimetidine (Tagamet) may result in increased risk of breathing problems and central nervous system suppression.
• MAO inhibitors (see Drug Classes) may result in an increased effect and the need to decrease the dose of hydrocodone.
▷ *Driving, Hazardous Activities:* This drug can impair mental alertness, judgment, reaction time and physical coordination. Avoid hazardous activities accordingly.
Aviation Note: The use of this drug *is a disqualification* for piloting. Consult a designated Aviation Medical Examiner.
Exposure to Sun: No restrictions.

Discontinuation: Best limited to short-term use. If used for extended periods, discontinuation should be gradual to minimize withdrawal (usually mild with this drug).

HYDROXYCHLOROQUINE (hi drox ee KLOR oh kwin)

Introduced: 1967   **Prescription:** USA: Yes; Canada: Yes   **Available as Generic:** USA: Yes; Canada: No   **Class:** Antimalarial, immunosuppressant **Controlled Drug:** USA: No; Canada: No
Brand Name: ✦Dermoplast, Plaquenil

BENEFITS versus RISKS	
Possible Benefits	*Possible Risks*
EFFECTIVE PREVENTION AND TREATMENT OF CERTAIN FORMS OF MALARIA	INFREQUENT BUT SERIOUS DAMAGE OF CORNEAL AND RETINAL EYE TISSUES
Possibly effective in the management of acute and chronic rheumatoid arthritis and juvenile arthritis	RARE BUT SERIOUS BONE MARROW DEPRESSION
Possibly effective in the management of chronic discoid and systemic lupus erythematosus	Rare heart muscle damage
Rare ear damage: hearing loss, ringing in ears

▷ **Principal Uses**

As a Single Drug Product: Uses currently included in FDA approved labeling: (1) Prevention and therapy of acute attacks of certain types of malaria; (2) reduces disease activity in rheumatoid arthritis; (3) suppresses disease activity in chronic discoid and systemic lupus erythematosus.

Other (unlabeled) generally accepted uses: (1) Treatment of Sjogren's syndrome which is characterized by marked immune problems; (2) treatment of refractory Lyme arthritis; (3) therapy of sarcoidosis, polymorphous light eruption, porphyria, solar urticaria and chronic vasculitis; (4) may have a role in helping decrease steroid requirements in patients with asthma; (5) can help decrease insulin needs in patients who take an oral hypoglycemic agent with insulin; (6) part of a combination regimen in treating Weber-Christian Syndrome.

How This Drug Works: As an anti-infective in treating malaria, it is thought that this drug impairs the function of DNA in the organisms.

As an antiarthritic and antilupus drug, it is thought to act as a mild immunosuppressant. It accumulates in white blood cells and inhibits many enzymes involved in tissue destruction.

Available Dosage Forms and Strengths

Tablets — 200 mg

▷ **Usual Adult Dosage Range:**   For malaria suppression: 400 mg once every 7 days.

For malaria treatment: (1) 800 mg as a single dose; or (2) initially 800 mg, followed by 400 mg in 6 to 8 hours; then 400 mg once a day on the second and third days.

For pediatric malaria treatment: 10 mg per kg followed in 6 hours by 5 mg per kg with 5 mg per kg given 18 hours after the second dose and then 5 mg per kg taken 24 hours after the first dose was given.

For rheumatoid arthritis: Up to 6.5 mg per kilogram of lean body weight daily.

For lupus erythematosus: Up to 6.5 mg per kilogram of lean body weight daily.

Note: Actual dosage and administration schedule must be determined by the physician for each patient individually.

Conditions Requiring Dosing Adjustments

Liver function: It should be used with caution and as a benefit to risk decision in patients with liver compromise or who are already taking liver toxic drugs.

Kidney function: Used with caution in kidney compromise.

▷ **Dosing Instructions:**   Take with food or milk to reduce stomach irritation. The tablet may be crushed and mixed with jam, jelly or jello for administration. Take full course of treatment as prescribed.

Note: For malaria prevention, begin medication 2 weeks before entering malarious area; continue medication while in the area and for 4 weeks after leaving the area.

For treating arthritis and lupus, take medication on a regular schedule daily; continual use for 6 months may be necessary to determine maximal benefit.

Usual Duration of Use: Use on a regular schedule for 2 weeks before exposure, during period of exposure, and 4 weeks after exposure determines this drug's effectiveness in preventing attacks of malaria. Use on a regular schedule for up to 6 months may be required to evaluate benefits in reducing rheumatoid arthritis and lupus erythematosus. If significant improvement is not achieved, this drug should be stopped. Long-term use (months to years) requires periodic physician evaluation of response and dosage adjustment.

Possible Advantages of This Drug

Considered to have less potential for retinal toxicity than chloroquine.

Currently a "Drug of Choice"

for the treatment of chronic discoid and systemic lupus erythematosus.

▷ **This Drug Should Not Be Taken If**

- you have had an allergic reaction to chloroquine or hydroxychloroquine.
- you have an active bone marrow or blood cell disorder.
- should not be used for long-term treatment in children.

▷ **Inform Your Physician Before Taking This Drug If**

- you are pregnant or planning pregnancy.
- you have had bone marrow depression or a blood cell disorder.
- you have a deficiency of glucose-6-phosphate dehydrogenase (talk with your doctor).
- you have any disorder of the eyes, especially disease of the cornea or retina, or visual field changes.
- you have impaired hearing or ringing in the ears.
- you have a seizure disorder of any kind.
- you have a history of peripheral neuritis.

- you have low blood pressure or a heart rhythm disorder.
- you have peptic ulcer disease, Crohn's disease or ulcerative colitis.
- you have impaired liver or kidney function.
- you have a history of porphyria.
- you have any form of psoriasis.
- you are taking antacids, cimetidine, digoxin or penicillamine.

Possible Side Effects (natural, expected, and unavoidable drug actions)
Light-headedness (low blood pressure); blue-black discoloration of skin, fingernails, or mouth lining with long-term use.

▷ **Possible Adverse Effects** (unusual, unexpected, and infrequent reactions)
If any of the following develop, consult your physician promptly for guidance.

Mild Adverse Effects
Allergic Reactions: Skin rash, itching (more common in African-Americans).
Loss of hair color, loss of hair.
Headache, blurring of near vision (reading), ringing in ears.
Loss of appetite, nausea, vomiting, stomach cramps, diarrhea.
Dizziness.

Serious Adverse Effects
Allergic Reactions: Severe skin rash, exfoliative dermatitis.
Idiosyncratic Reactions: Hemolytic anemia in those with glucose-6-phosphate dehydrogenase deficiency in red blood cells.
Emotional or psychotic mental changes; seizures.
Loss of hearing.
Porphyria.
Excessive muscle weakness.
Eye tissue damage, specifically cornea and retina, with significant impairment of vision.
Heart rhythm abnormalities.
Aplastic anemia (see Glossary): abnormally low red blood cell counts (fatigue and weakness); abnormally low white blood cell counts (fever, sore throat, infections); abnormally low platelet counts (abnormal bruising or bleeding).

▷ **Possible Effects on Sexual Function:**   None reported.

Possible Delayed Adverse Effects: Irreversible retinal damage has developed 7 years after discontinuation of chloroquine, a closely related drug. Retinal damage is more likely to occur following high-dose and/or long-term use.

▷ **Adverse Effects That May Mimic Natural Diseases or Disorders**
Central nervous system toxicity may suggest unrelated neuropsychiatric disorder. Seizures may suggest the onset of epilepsy.

Natural Diseases or Disorders That May Be Activated by This Drug
Porphyria, psoriasis.

Possible Effects on Laboratory Tests
Complete blood cell counts: decreased red cells, hemoglobin, white cells and platelets.
Liver function tests: increased liver enzymes (ALT/GPT, AST/GOT and alkaline phosphatase), increased bilirubin.
Electrocardiogram: conduction abnormalities, prolonged QRS interval,

T-wave changes, and heart block have all been reported for chloroquine, a closely related drug.

CAUTION
1. This drug does not prevent relapses in certain types of malaria.
2. High-dose and/or long-term use of this drug may cause irreversible retinal damage, significant visual impairment or hearing loss due to nerve damage. Report promptly any changes in vision or hearing so appropriate evaluation can be made.

Precautions for Use

By Infants and Children: This age group is very sensitive to the effects of this drug. Dosages should be determined and therapy should be monitored by a qualified pediatrician.

By Those over 60 Years of Age: Tolerance for this drug may be reduced. Watch for behavioral changes, low blood pressure, heart rhythm disturbances, muscle weakness and changes in vision or hearing.

▷ **Advisability of Use During Pregnancy**

Pregnancy Category: D. See Pregnancy Code at the back of this book.

Animal studies: No information available.

Human studies: Adequate studies of pregnant women are not available. However, closely related drugs of this class are known to cause abnormal retinal pigmentation and hemorrhage and congenital deafness in the fetus.

Avoid use during pregnancy except for the suppression or treatment of malaria.

Advisability of Use if Breast-Feeding

Presence of this drug in breast milk: Yes.

Avoid drug or refrain from nursing.

Habit-Forming Potential: None.

Effects of Overdosage: Drowsiness, headache, blurred vision, excitability, low blood pressure, seizures, coma.

Possible Effects of Long-Term Use: Irreversible eye damage (cornea and retina), hearing loss, muscle weakness, aplastic anemia.

Suggested Periodic Examinations While Taking This Drug (at physician's discretion)

Complete blood cell counts; liver and kidney function tests.

Serial blood pressure readings and electrocardiograms.

Neurological examinations for significant muscle weakness.

Complete eye examinations before starting high-dose and/or long-term treatment and every 3 to 6 months during drug use.

Hearing tests as indicated.

▷ **While Taking This Drug, Observe the Following**

Foods: No restrictions.

Beverages: No restrictions. May be taken with milk.

▷ *Alcohol:* Use sparingly to minimize stomach irritation.

Tobacco Smoking: No interactions expected.

▷ *Other Drugs*

Hydroxychloroquine may ***increase*** the effects of
• digoxin (Lanoxin), and increase its toxic potential.
• penicillamine (Cuprimine, Depen), and increase its toxic potential.

The following drug may *increase* the effects of hydroxychloroquine
- cimetidine (Tagamet).

The following drugs may *decrease* the effects of hydroxychloroquine
- magnesium salts and antacids.

▷ *Driving, Hazardous Activities:* This drug may cause light-headedness, blurred vision or impaired hearing. Restrict activities as necessary.

Aviation Note: The use of this drug *may be a disqualification* for piloting. Consult a designated Aviation Medical Examiner.

Exposure to Sun: Use caution until sensitivity has been determined. Closely related drugs of this class may cause photosensitivity (see Glossary).

Discontinuation: This drug should be stopped and prompt evaluation should be made if any of the following develop—any changes in vision or hearing, seizures, unusual muscle weakness, indications of infection (fever, sore throat, etc.), abnormal bruising or bleeding.

HYDROXYUREA (hi DROXEE yur ia)

Introduced: 1995 (AIDS or Sickle Cell)   **Prescription:** USA: Yes; Canada: No   **Available as Generic:** USA: No; Canada: No   **Class:** Anti-AIDS, anticancer, antisickle-cell   **Controlled Drug:** USA:No

Brand Names: Hydrea

Warning: This drug is a cytotoxic agent. Appropriate precautions must be taken as with other chemotherapy.

BENEFITS versus RISKS	
Possible Benefits	*Possible Risks*
COMBINATION TREATMENT OF AIDS	BONE MARROW SUPPRESSION
DECREASED SEVERITY AND FREQUENCY OF SICKLE CELL CRISES	Hepatitis
Treatment of chronic myelocytic leukemia, melanoma, and other cancers	

▷ **Principal Uses**

As a Single Drug Product: Uses currently included in FDA approved labeling: (1) Blast crisis; (2) chronic myelogenous leukemia; (3) head and neck cancers; (4) chronic leukemias; (5) cancers of certain cell types (squamous cell).

Other (unlabeled) generally accepted uses: (1) Used to decrease the frequency and severity of sickle cell crises; (2) used to treat certain diseases of the red blood cells (Polycythemia vera); (3) used in combination with didanosine to treat AIDS patients.

How This Drug Works: When used in cancer, this medicine is a cell cycle-specific drug. It works in the S phase of mitosis.

When used in AIDS patients, the exact mechanism of action is not fully understood.

When used in sickle cell patients, the specific mechanism has not been identified.

Available Dosage Forms and Strengths

Capsule — 500 mg

▷ **Recommended Dosage Ranges (Actual dosage and administration schedule must be determined by the physician for each patient individually.)**

Infants and Children: Safety and effectiveness have not been defined in this age group.

18 to 60 Years of Age: All doses are decided based on ideal or actual weight, whichever is less.

Oral dosing: Usual oral doses range from 20 to 30 mg per kg per day which is given as a single daily dose. Some centers give 80 mg per kg every third day. If a patient is in blast crisis, up to 12 grams per day has been given to rapidly decrease white blood cell counts.

In the sickle cell studies: Patients were started on 15 mg per kg and had their dose increased by 5 mg per kg every 12 weeks unless toxicity occurred or the maximum dose of 35 mg per kg per day was reached.

In AIDS: the protocols are still changing.

Over 60 Years of Age: Same as 18 to 60 years of age.

Conditions Requiring Dosing Adjustments

Liver function: No changes in dosing are anticipated.

Kidney function: The dose must be decreased in patients with kidney compromise. Decreases of up to 80% are needed in severe compromise.

▷ **Dosing Instructions:** This medicine is best taken on an empty stomach. Call your doctor if you vomit after taking this medicine.

Usual Duration of Use: Continual use on a regular schedule for up to 16 weeks may be needed to treat cancers of the head and neck. Treatment in sickle cell disease is ongoing, using the lowest effective dose. Treatment in AIDS is yet to be defined.

Long-term use (months to years) requires periodic evaluation of response and dosage adjustment. Consult your physician on a regular basis.

Currently a "Drug of Choice"

for reducing the frequency and severity of sickle cell crises in patients with sickle cell disease.

▷ **This Drug Should Not Be Taken If**

- you have had an allergic reaction to any dosage form of it previously.
- you have severely depressed bone marrow. This is seen in very low white blood cell, platelet or hemoglobins.

▷ **Inform Your Physician Before Taking This Drug If**

- you have signs or symptoms of cancer.
- you are considering pregnancy (males or females).
- you have had chemotherapy or radiation therapy previously.
- you have compromised kidneys.
- you have Herpes zoster (shingles).
- you have recently been exposed to chicken pox.
- you are having unusual bruising or bleeding.
- you are unsure of how to appropriately dispose of urine or vomit.
- you are uncertain of how much hydroxyurea to take or how often to take it.
- you take other prescription or nonprescription medicines which were not discussed with your doctor when hydroxyurea was prescribed.

Possible Side Effects (natural, expected, and unavoidable drug actions)
Hair loss, painful mouth sores, sensitivity to the sun.

▷ **Possible Adverse Effects** (unusual, unexpected, and infrequent reactions)
If any of the following develop, consult your physician promptly for guidance.
Mild Adverse Effects
Allergic Reactions: Skin rash and itching.
Headaches (rare).
Fever (rare).
Nausea, vomiting, or diarrhea.
Dizziness or disorientation (rare).
Loss of appetite.
Difficulty urinating (rare).
Ulceration of the skin (rare).
Serious Adverse Effects
Allergic Reactions: Skin ulceration.
Idiosyncratic Reactions: Not reported.
Bone marrow depression.
Convulsions (rare).
Kidney problems (rare).
Hepatitis (rare).
Drug-induced lupus erythematosus (rare).
Lung problems (acute interstitial lung disease) (rare).
Hallucinations (rare).

▷ **Possible Effects on Sexual Function:**   None reported.

Possible Delayed Adverse Effects: Bone marrow suppression.

▷ **Adverse Effects That May Mimic Natural Diseases or Disorders**
Liver toxicity may be similar to acute hepatitis.

Natural Diseases or Disorders That May Be Activated by This Drug
Not defined.

Possible Effects on Laboratory Tests
Liver function tests: increased.
Complete blood counts: decreases in several components.

CAUTION
1. This medicine is toxic to cells. Be certain your doctor has carefully explained how to dispose of urine or vomit.
2. Call your doctor at once if you have a seizure.
3. Both women and men should avoid conception for several months after taking this medicine.
4. Wash your hands after taking this medicine **before** you touch your eyes or your nose.

Precautions for Use
By Infants and Children: Safety and effectiveness for use by those under 18 years of age have not been established.
By Those over 60 Years of Age: Natural declines in kidney function may require decreases in doses.

▷ **Advisability of Use During Pregnancy**
  Pregnancy Category: D. See Pregnancy Code at the back of this book.
    Animal studies: This drug is known to cause birth defects in animals.
    Human studies: Information from adequate studies of pregnant women is not
      available. Ask your doctor for help in making this benefit to risk decision.

Advisability of Use if Breast-Feeding
  Presence of this drug in breast milk: Yes.
  Avoid drug or refrain from nursing.

Habit-Forming Potential: None.

Effects of Overdosage: Bone marrow depression, increased heart rate, liver cell
    damage, testicular damage.

Possible Effects of Long-Term Use: Bone marrow depression.

Suggested Periodic Examinations While Taking This Drug (at physician's
    discretion)
  Dental exams, complete blood counts.

▷ **While Taking This Drug, Observe the Following**
  Foods: No restrictions.
  Beverages: No restrictions.
▷ *Alcohol:* Do not drink alcohol.
  Tobacco Smoking: No interactions expected.
▷ *Other Drugs*
    Hydroxyurea *taken concurrently* with
    • fluorouracil may increase toxicity to nerves.
    • other medicines which cause bone marrow suppression (see Drug Tables)
      may result in additive bone marrow suppression.
▷ *Driving, Hazardous Activities:* This drug may cause dizziness or hallucinations.
    Restrict activities as necessary.
  Aviation Note: The use of this drug *is probably a disqualification* for piloting.
    Consult a designated Aviation Medical Examiner.
  Exposure to Sun: Use extreme caution. Extreme reactions to the sun have been
    reported.
  Occurrence of Unrelated Illness: Call your doctor at once if you develop fever or
    chills.
  Discontinuation: Do not stop this medicine without first discussing this with
    your doctor.

IBUPROFEN (i byu PROH fen)

Introduced: 1969   **Prescription:** USA: Varies; Canada: Yes   **Available as
Generic:** Yes   **Class:** analgesic, mild; NSAID   **Controlled Drug:** USA:
No; Canada: No

Brand Names: Aches-N-Pain, ✦Actiprofen, Advil, ✦Amersol, ✦Apo-Ibuprofen,
  Bayer Select, Children's Advil, Children's Motrin Suspension (nonprescrip-
  tion form), Children's Motrin Drops (nonprescription form), CoAdvil [CD],
  Dimetapp Sinus [CD], Direct formulary ibuprofen, Dologesic, Dristan
  Sinus, Excedrin IB, Genpril, Guildprofen, Haltran, Ibuprin, Ibuprohm,
  Ibutab, Junior Strength Motrin Caplets (nonprescription), Medipren,

Medi-Profen, Midol-IB, Motrin, Motrin IB, ♣Novoprofen, Nuprin, Pedia-Profen, Profen-IB, Rufen, Superior Pain Medicine, Supreme Pain Medicine, Tab-Profen

BENEFITS versus RISKS	
Possible Benefits	*Possible Risks*
EFFECTIVE RELIEF OF MILD TO MODERATE PAIN AND INFLAMMATION	Gastrointestinal pain, ulceration, bleeding (rare) Rare kidney damage Rare fluid retention Rare bone marrow depression

Please see the propionic acid nonsteroidal anti-inflammatory drug profile for further information.

IMIPRAMINE (im IP ra meen)

Introduced: 1955   **Prescription:** USA: Yes; Canada: Yes   **Available as Generic:** USA: Yes; Canada: Yes   **Class:** Antidepressant   **Controlled Drug:** USA: No; Canada: No

Brand Names: Antipress, ♣Apo-Imipramine, ♣Impril, Janimine, ♣Novopramine, ♣PMS Imipramine, Sk-pramine, Tipramine, Tofranil, Tofranil-PM

BENEFITS versus RISKS	
Possible Benefits	*Possible Risks*
EFFECTIVE RELIEF OF VARIOUS NEUROTIC AND PSYCHOTIC DEPRESSIVE STATES EFFECTIVE TREATMENT FOR CHILDHOOD BED-WETTING (enuresis) Helps manage chronic, severe pain Aids cocaine withdrawal Relieves symptoms of attention deficit disorder Helps prevent panic attacks Helps control binge eating and purging in bulimia	ADVERSE BEHAVIORAL EFFECTS CONVERSION OF DEPRESSION TO MANIA in manic-depressive (bipolar) disorders Aggravation of schizophrenia and paranoia Induction of serious heart rhythm abnormalities Abnormally low white blood cell and platelet counts (rare)

▷ **Principal Uses**

As a Single Drug Product: Uses currently included in FDA approved labeling: (1) Relieves severe emotional depression and to initiate gradual restoration of normal mood; (2) aids in the prevention of childhood bed-wetting in children over 6 years of age; (3) used to treat delusions.

Other (unlabeled) generally accepted uses: (1) Helps treat agoraphobia; (2) some case evidence of help in treating aspermia; (3) can be of help in chronic pain syndromes; (4) eases diabetic neuropathy; (5) inappropriate emotionalism (such as pathological crying) can be controlled by this drug; (6) of use in globus hystericus syndrome; (7) may have a role in treating panic disorder; (8) can help post traumatic stress disorder; (9) may help control retrograde ejaculation; (10) can be of adjunctive benefit in helping control schizophrenia; (11) shows some benefit in patients who fail ENT surgery or weight reduction as treatment of sleep apnea; (12) may be of help as a second line agent in attention deficit hyperactivity disorder.

How This Drug Works: Not completely established. It is thought that by increasing brain tissue concentrations of certain nerve impulse transmitters (norepinephrine and seratonin), this drug relieves the symptoms associated with depression. Beneficial effects in treating bedwetting are thought to be due partially to this drug's atropinelike action.

Available Dosage Forms and Strengths

Capsules — 75 mg, 100 mg, 125 mg, 150 mg
Injection — 25 mg per 2 ml
Tablets — 10 mg, 25 mg, 50 mg, 75 mg

▷ **Usual Adult Dosage Range:** Initially 75 mg daily, divided into 3 doses. Dose may be increased cautiously as needed and tolerated by 10 mg to 25 mg daily at intervals of 1 week. The usual maintenance dose is 50 mg to 150 mg/24 hours. The total daily dosage should not exceed 200 mg for outpatient therapy. (When determined, the optimal daily requirement may be given at bedtime as a single dose.) **Note: Actual dosage and administration schedule must be determined by the physician for each patient individually.**

Conditions Requiring Dosing Adjustments

Liver function: This drug is significantly metabolized in the liver to active and inactive metabolites. It should be used with caution and in decreased dose in patients with liver compromise. It is also a rare cause of hepatic necrosis.
Kidney function: No changes in dosing are anticipated in kidney compromise.

▷ **Dosing Instructions:** May be taken without regard to meals. If necessary, may be taken with food to reduce stomach irritation. The capsule may be opened and the tablet may be crushed for administration. Note: Tofranil-PM capsules should not be used to treat childhood bedwetting.

Usual Duration of Use: Continual use on a regular schedule for 3 to 4 weeks is usually necessary to determine this drug's effectiveness in relieving depression; optimal response may require 3 or more months of use. Long-term use (months to years) requires periodic evaluation of response and dosage adjustment. Consult your physician on a regular basis.

Possible Advantages of This Drug

Less likely to increase the heart rate than other tricyclic antidepressants.
Less hazardous and more easily managed than monoamine oxidase (MAO) inhibitor antidepressants.

Currently a "Drug of Choice"

for adjunctive use in treating childhood bedwetting when organic causes for this disorder have been eliminated.

▷ **This Drug Should Not Be Taken If**
  • you have had an allergic reaction to it previously.
  • you are taking, or have taken within the past 14 days, any monoamine oxidase (MAO) type A inhibitor drug (see Drug Classes).
  • you have had a recent heart attack (myocardial infarction).

- you have angina, abnormal heart beats or congestive heart failure.
- you are pregnant.

▷ **Inform Your Physician Before Taking This Drug If**
- you have had an adverse reaction to any other antidepressant drug.
- you have any type of seizure disorder.
- you have increased internal eye pressure.
- you have narrow-angle glaucoma.
- you have any type of heart disease, especially coronary artery disease or a heart rhythm disorder.
- you are subject to bronchial asthma.
- you have impaired liver or kidney function.
- you have any type of thyroid disorder or are taking thyroid medication.
- you have diabetes or sugar intolerance.
- you have prostatism (see Glossary).
- you have a history of alcoholism.
- you plan to have surgery under general anesthesia in the near future.

Possible Side Effects (natural, expected, and unavoidable drug actions)
Moderate drowsiness, light-headedness (low blood pressure), blurred vision, dry mouth, constipation, impaired urination.

▷ **Possible Adverse Effects** (unusual, unexpected, and infrequent reactions)
If any of the following develop, consult your physician promptly for guidance.
Mild Adverse Effects
Allergic Reactions: Skin rash, hives, swelling of face or tongue, drug fever (see Glossary).
Headache, dizziness, nervousness, weakness, unsteadiness, tremors, fainting.
Increased appetite, weight gain.
Sleep disturbances, ringing in the ears.
Irritation of tongue or mouth, dry mouth (xerostomia), dental cavities, altered taste, indigestion, nausea.
Fluctuations of blood sugar.

Serious Adverse Effects
Allergic Reactions: Drug-induced hepatitis, with or without jaundice; anaphylactoid reaction (see terms in Glossary).
Idiosyncratic Reactions: Neuroleptic malignant syndrome (see Glossary).
Adverse behavioral effects: confusion, delirium, disorientation, delusions, hallucinations.
Abnormally low blood pressure on standing (orthostatic hypotension).
Tourette's syndrome (rare).
Porphyria (rare).
Liver or kidney toxicity (rare).
Drug-induced myasthenia gravis (rare).
Abnormal urine excretion (SIADH).
Spasm of blood vessels.
Seizures; reduced control of epilepsy.
Eye changes (glaucoma, ophthalmoplegia).
Aggravation of paranoid psychoses and schizophrenia.
Heart rhythm disturbances.

Abnormally low white blood cell and platelet counts: Fever, sore throat, infections, abnormal bleeding or bruising.

▷ **Possible Effects on Sexual Function**

Decreased libido, increased libido (antidepressant effect), impaired erection (43%), impaired ejaculation (28%), impotence, inhibited male orgasm (20%), inhibited female orgasm (27%), male breast enlargement and tenderness, female breast enlargement with milk production, swelling of testicles.

▷ **Adverse Effects That May Mimic Natural Diseases or Disorders**

Liver toxicity may suggest viral hepatitis.

Natural Diseases or Disorders That May Be Activated by This Drug

Latent diabetes, epilepsy, glaucoma, prostatism.

Possible Effects on Laboratory Tests

Complete blood cell counts: decreased white cells and platelets; increased eosinophils (allergic reaction).

Blood glucose levels: increased and decreased (fluctuations).

Liver function tests: increased liver enzymes (ALT/GPT, AST/GOT and alkaline phosphatase), increased bilirubin.

CAUTION

1. Look for early signs of toxicity or overdosage: confusion, agitation, rapid heart rate, heart irregularity. Measurement of the drug blood level will clarify the situation.
2. Use with caution in treating depression associated with schizophrenia. Observe closely for any deterioration of thinking or behavior.
3. It is advisable to withhold this drug if electroconvulsive therapy is to be used to treat the depression in the near future.

Precautions for Use

By Infants and Children: Safety and effectiveness for use by those under 6 years of age have not been established. Recent experience indicates that children (6 to 12 years of age) may be more susceptible than adults to heart toxicity from this and related drugs. Dosage and management should be supervised by a properly trained pediatrician.

By Those over 60 Years of Age: Treatment is started with 25 mg at bedtime. Dosage may be increased gradually as needed and tolerated to 100 mg daily in divided doses. During the first 2 weeks of treatment, observe for behavioral reactions: Restlessness, agitation, forgetfulness, disorientation, delusions or hallucinations. Also observe for unsteadiness and instability that may predispose to falling. This drug may aggravate prostatism.

▷ **Advisability of Use During Pregnancy**

Pregnancy Category: D. See Pregnancy Code at the back of this book.

Animal studies: Skeletal defects reported in rabbit studies. No defects reported in mouse, rat and monkey studies.

Human studies: Information from adequate studies of pregnant women is not available. Case reports of fetal respiratory distress, convulsions.

Ask your doctor for guidance.

Advisability of Use if Breast-Feeding

Presence of this drug in breast milk: Yes, in small amounts.

Monitor nursing infant closely and discontinue drug or nursing if adverse effects develop.

Habit-Forming Potential: Psychological or physical dependence is possible. A withdrawal syndrome has been described.

Effects of Overdosage: Confusion, hallucinations, drowsiness, tremors, heart irregularity, seizures, stupor, hypothermia (see Glossary) early, fever later.

Possible Effects of Long-Term Use: Neuroleptic malignant syndrome (see Glossary): Fever, fast or irregular heartbeat, fast breathing, sweating, weakness, muscle stiffness, seizures, loss of bladder control.

Suggested Periodic Examinations While Taking This Drug (at physician's discretion)

Monitoring of blood drug levels as appropriate.

Complete blood cell counts; liver and kidney function tests.

Serial blood pressure readings and electrocardiograms.

Measurement of internal eye pressure.

▷ **While Taking This Drug, Observe the Following**

Foods: No specific restrictions. May need to limit food intake to avoid excessive weight gain.

Beverages: No restrictions. May be taken with milk.

▷ *Alcohol:* Avoid completely. This drug can markedly increase the intoxicating effects of alcohol; the combination can depress brain function significantly.

Tobacco Smoking: May accelerate the elimination of this drug and require increased dosage.

Marijuana Smoking: Increased drowsiness and mouth dryness; possible reduced effectiveness of this drug. Excessive increases in heart rate.

▷ *Other Drugs*

Imipramine may ***increase*** the effects of

• all drugs with sedative effects; observe for excessive sedation.
• all drugs with atropinelike effects (see Drug Classes).
• norepinephrine.
• phenytoin (Dilantin).
• warfarin (Coumadin) and require more frequent INR testing.

Imipramine may ***decrease*** the effects of

• clonidine (Catapres).
• guanadrel (Hylorel).
• guanethidine (Ismelin, Esimil).
• guanfacine (Tenex).

Imipramine ***taken concurrently*** with

• anticonvulsants requires careful monitoring for changes in seizure patterns and need to adjust anticonvulsant dosage.
• antihistamines (see Drug Classes) may result in urinary retention, acute glaucoma or excessive anticholinergic actions.
• ethchlorvynol (Placidyl) may cause delirium; avoid concurrent use.
• meperidine (Demerol) may result in increased meperidine caused depression of breathing.
• monoamine oxidase (MAO) type A inhibitor drugs (see Drug Classes) may cause high fever, seizures and excessive rise in blood pressure; avoid concurrent use of these drugs and provide periods of 14 days between administration of either.

- stimulant drugs (amphetamine, cocaine, epinephrine, phenylpropanola-mine, etc.) may cause severe high blood pressure and/or high fever.
- thyroid preparations may increase the risk of heart rhythm disorders.

The following drugs may *increase* the effects of imipramine

- cimetidine (Tagamet).
- estrogens.
- fluoxetine (Prozac)
- fluvoxamine (Luvox)
- labetalol.
- methylphenidate (Ritalin).
- oral contraceptives.
- phenothiazines (see Drug Classes).
- quinidine.
- ranitidine (Zantac).

The following drugs may *decrease* the effects of imipramine

- barbiturates (see Drug Class, Section Four).
- carbamazepine (Tegretol).
- chloral hydrate (Noctec, Somnos, etc.).
- lithium (Lithobid, Lithotab, etc.).
- reserpine (Serpasil, Ser-Ap-Es, etc.).
- vitamin C (if more than 2 grams per day are taken).

▷ *Driving, Hazardous Activities:*
This drug may impair mental alertness, judgment, physical coordination and reaction time. Restrict activities as necessary.

Aviation Note: The use of this drug *is a disqualification* for piloting. Consult a designated Aviation Medical Examiner.

Exposure to Sun: Use caution until sensitivity has been determined. This drug may cause photosensitivity (see Glossary).

Exposure to Heat: Use caution. This drug can inhibit sweating and impair the body's adaptation to hot environments, increasing the risk of heat stroke. Avoid saunas.

Exposure to Cold: The elderly should use caution and avoid conditions condu-cive to hypothermia (see Glossary).

Exposure to Environmental Chemicals: This drug may mask the symptoms of poisoning due to handling certain insecticides (organophosphorus types). Read their labels carefully.

Discontinuation: It is advisable to discontinue this drug gradually over a period of 3 to 4 weeks. Abrupt withdrawal after prolonged use may cause nausea, vomiting, diarrhea, headache, malaise, disturbed sleep and vivid dreaming. When this drug is stopped, it may be necessary to adjust the dosages of other drugs taken concurrently.

INDAPAMIDE (in DAP a mide)

Introduced: 1974   **Prescription:** USA: Yes; Canada: Yes   **Available as Generic:** Yes   **Class:** Antihypertensive, diuretic   **Controlled Drug:** USA: No; Canada: No

Brand Names: ✦Lozide, Lozol

BENEFITS versus RISKS

Possible Benefits	*Possible Risks*
EFFECTIVE ONCE-A-DAY TREATMENT OF MILD TO MODERATE HYPERTENSION EFFECTIVE, MILD DIURETIC	Excessive loss of blood potassium Increased blood sugar level Increased blood uric acid level

---

▷ **Principal Uses**

As a Single Drug Product: Uses currently included in FDA approved labeling: (1) Increases urine output (diuresis) to correct fluid retention seen in congestive heart failure (edema); (2) used as starting therapy in high blood pressure (hypertension).

Other (unlabeled) generally accepted uses: (1) Helps ease the excessive elimination of calcium in the urine (hypercalciuria); (2) may help protect the heart after blood-flow problems (preserves ischemic heart from reperfusion injury).

How This Drug Works: Increases elimination of salt and water (through increased urine production). Relaxes the walls of smaller arteries and decreases pressure reactions (angiotensin two). The combined effects lower blood pressure.

Available Dosage Forms and Strengths

Tablets — 1.25 mg and 2.5 mg

▷ **Usual Adult Dosage Range:**   Started with 2.5 mg/day, as a single dose in the morning. If needed, the dose may be increased to 5 mg/day after 1 week (for diuresis) or after 4 weeks (for hypertension). Maximum total daily dose is 5 mg. (In Canada, the total daily dosage limit is given as 2.5 mg.) **Note: Actual dose and dosing schedule must be individually determined by your doctor.**

Conditions Requiring Dosing Adjustments

Liver function: Used with caution and in decrease dose in patients with liver problems. Blood chemistry (electrolytes) should be closely followed.

Kidney function: Must be stopped if kidney failure progresses after indapamide is started.

▷ **Dosing Instructions:**   The tablet may be crushed and taken with or following food to reduce stomach upset. Take in the morning to avoid nighttime urination.

Usual Duration of Use: Use on a regular schedule for 2 to 4 weeks determines peak effect in lowering blood pressure. Long-term use (months to years) requires periodic physician evaluation.

Possible Advantages of This Drug

Causes no significant increase in blood cholesterol levels.

Less likely to cause significant loss of potassium.

▷ **This Drug Should Not Be Taken If**

- you have had an allergic reaction to it previously.
- your kidneys are not making any urine.

▷ **Inform Your Physician Before Taking This Drug If**

- you are allergic to any form of "sulfa" drug.
- you are pregnant or planning pregnancy.

- you presently have an excessively low blood potassium.
- you have a history of kidney or liver disease.
- you have diabetes, gout or lupus erythematosus.
- you take any form of cortisone, digoxin, oral antidiabetic drug or insulin.
- you have had a sympathectomy.
- you plan to have surgery under general anesthesia in the near future.

Possible Side Effects (natural, expected, and unavoidable drug actions)
Light-headedness on arising from sitting or lying position (see Orthostatic Hypotension in Glossary).
Increase in blood sugar level, affecting control of diabetes.
Increase in blood uric acid level, affecting control of gout.
Decrease in blood potassium level, causing muscle weakness and cramping.
Low blood sodium and magnesium.

▷ **Possible Adverse Effects** (unusual, unexpected, and infrequent reactions)
If any of the following develop, consult your physician promptly for guidance.
Mild Adverse Effects
Allergic Reactions: Skin rashes, hives, itching.
Headache, dizziness, drowsiness, weakness, lethargy, visual disturbance.
Reduced appetite, indigestion, nausea, vomiting, diarrhea.
Paresthesias.
Increased uric acid may blunt gout control.
Urination at night.
Serious Adverse Effects
Abnormally low blood pressure on standing (orthostatic hypotension).
Abnormal heartbeat (premature ventricular contractions) (rare).
Worsening of glucose intolerance.
Low blood potassium or chloride.
Low blood sodium.
Liver or kidney toxicity (rare).
Serious skin rashes (Stevens-Johnson syndrome, toxic epidermal necrolysis).

▷ **Possible Effects on Sexual Function:** Decreased libido (4%); impotence (less than 1%).

Natural Diseases or Disorders That May Be Activated by This Drug
Diabetes, gout, systemic lupus erythematosus.

Possible Effects on Laboratory Tests
Total cholesterol and LDL cholesterol levels: no effect or slightly increased.
Blood HDL cholesterol level: no effect or slightly decreased.
Blood potassium level: slightly decreased.
Blood uric acid level: increased.

CAUTION
1. Take exactly as prescribed—excessive doses can cause excessive sodium and potassium loss, with decrease in appetite, nausea, fatigue, weakness, confusion and tingling in the extremities.
2. If you take a digitalis preparation (digitoxin, digoxin), ensure intake of high-potassium foods to help avoid digitalis toxicity. (See Table of High Potassium Foods.)

Precautions for Use

By Infants and Children: Safety and effectiveness for those under 12 years of age not established.

By Those over 60 Years of Age: Best to start with small doses. You may be more susceptible to impaired thinking, orthostatic hypotension, potassium loss and blood sugar increase. Overdosage or extended use causes excessive loss of body water, thickening (increased viscosity) of blood and an increased tendency for the blood to clot—predisposing to stroke, heart attack or thrombophlebitis (vein inflammation with blood clot).

▷ **Advisability of Use During Pregnancy**

Pregnancy Category: B. See Pregnancy Code at the back of this book.

Animal studies: No birth defects reported.

Human studies: Data from studies of pregnant women is not available.

This drug should not be used during pregnancy unless a very serious complication occurs for which this drug is significantly beneficial. Ask physician for guidance.

Advisability of Use if Breast-Feeding

Presence of this drug in breast milk: Unknown.

Avoid drug or refrain from nursing.

Habit-Forming Potential: None.

Effects of Overdosage: Dry mouth, thirst, lethargy, weakness, muscle cramping, nausea, vomiting, drowsiness progressing to stupor or coma.

Possible Effects of Long-Term Use: Impaired balance of water, salt and potassium in blood and body tissues. Development of diabetes in predisposed individuals.

Suggested Periodic Examinations While Taking This Drug (at physician's discretion)

Measurements of blood levels of sodium, potassium, chloride, sugar and uric acid.

▷ **While Taking This Drug, Observe the Following**

Foods: Ask about a high potassium diet. If so advised, see the Table of High Potassium Foods in Section Six. Follow doctor's advice about salt use.

Beverages: No restrictions. This drug may be taken with milk.

▷ *Alcohol:* Alcohol may exaggerate the blood-pressure-lowering effects of this drug and cause orthostatic hypotension.

Tobacco Smoking: No interactions expected. Follow physician's advice.

▷ *Other Drugs*

Indapamide may *increase* the effects of

• other antihypertensive drugs; dosage adjustments may be necessary to prevent excessive lowering of blood pressure.

• lithium (Lithobid, others), and cause lithium toxicity.

Indapamide may *decrease* the effects of

• oral antidiabetic drugs (sulfonylureas); dose adjustments may be needed for proper control of blood sugar.

Indapamide *taken concurrently* with

• digitalis preparations (digitoxin, digoxin) must be followed closely and adjustments made to prevent fluctuations of blood potassium levels and serious disturbances of heart rhythm.

- NSAIDs (see Drug Classes) may blunt the therapeutic benefit of indapamide.

The following drugs may **decrease** the effects of indapamide

- cholestyramine (Cuemid, Questran) may interfere with its absorption.
- colestipol (Colestid) may interfere with its absorption.

Take cholestyramine and colestipol 1 hour before any oral diuretic.

▷   *Driving, Hazardous Activities:* Use caution until the possible occurrence of orthostatic hypotension, drowsiness, dizziness or impaired vision has been determined.

Aviation Note: The use of this drug **may be a disqualification** for piloting. Consult a designated Aviation Medical Examiner.

Exposure to Sun: No restrictions.

Exposure to Heat: Excessive perspiring could cause additional loss of salt and water.

Heavy Exercise or Exertion: Isometric exercises can raise blood pressure significantly. Ask physician for help.

Occurrence of Unrelated Illness: Vomiting or diarrhea can produce a serious imbalance of important body chemistry. Consult your physician for guidance.

Discontinuation: It may be advisable to discontinue this drug 5 to 7 days before major surgery. Ask your physician, surgeon and/or anesthesiologist for guidance.

INDOMETHACIN (in doh METH a sin)

Introduced: 1963   **Prescription:** USA: Yes; Canada: Yes   **Available as Generic:** USA: Yes; Canada: No   **Class:** analgesic, mild; NSAID   **Controlled Drug:** USA: No; Canada: No

Brand Names: ✦Apo-Indomethacin, Indameth, ✦Indocid, ✦Indocid PDA, Indocin, Indocin-SR, Indo-Lemmon, ✦Novomethacin, ✦Nu-Indo, Zendole

BENEFITS versus RISKS	
Possible Benefits	*Possible Risks*
EFFECTIVE RELIEF OF MILD TO MODERATE PAIN AND INFLAMMATION	Gastrointestinal pain, ulceration, bleeding (rare)
	Rare liver or kidney damage
	Rare fluid retention
	Rare bone marrow depression
	Mental depression, confusion

Please see acetic acid nonsteroidal anti-inflammatory drug profile for further information.

INFLUENZA VACCINE (IN flu en za vax ceen)

Other Names: Flu vaccine

Introduced: Specific formulation for each year   **Prescription:** USA: Yes; Canada: Yes   **Available as Generic:** USA: No; Canada: No   **Class:** Antiviral   **Controlled Drug:** USA: No; Canada: No

Brand Names: Fluogen, Flu-immune, Flu-Shield, Fluzone
Author's note: The three virus strains for the 1996/1997 flu season vaccines are: A/Texas, A/Wuhan and B/Beijing.

Warning: Since the vaccine is formulated to contain the viral strains expected to cause the most serious problems in a given year, the side effects or adverse effects may differ annually.

BENEFITS versus RISKS

Possible Benefits	*Possible Risks*
PREVENTION OF INFLUENZA CAUSED BY THE MOST SERIOUS OR PREVALENT VIRAL STRAINS IDENTIFIED FOR A GIVEN YEAR	GUILLAIN-BARRE SYNDROME (questionable causation) Hypersensitivity (rare)

▷ **Principal Uses**

As a Single Drug Product: Uses currently included in FDA approved labeling: (1) Prevention of influenza.

Other (unlabeled) generally accepted uses: (1) Used in patients with compromised immune systems (such as HIV positive, cancer patients and bone marrow transplant patients); (2) can be of use in isolated outbreaks such as in nursing homes or military camps; (3) may decrease the number of middle ear infections in children who attend day-care centers.

How This Drug Works: This vaccine is made of purified parts of the surface of the virus, split virus or whole virus which has been inactivated. When it is injected, it stimulates the immune system to make antibodies. These antibodies (which are created and the production knowledge stored in immune cells roughly two weeks after vaccination) act to reduce disease severity or decrease the probability of infection by the expected flu viruses.

Available Dosage Forms and Strengths

Typical split virus: 15 mcg per 0.5 ml of each of the three selected strains

How To Store

This vaccine is ideally stored in the refrigerator. If this is how storage is accomplished, the outdate specified by the manufacturer is valid. If the vaccine is stored at room temperature, it is stable for up to seven days.

▷ **Recommended Dosage Ranges (Actual dosage and administration schedule must be determined by the physician for each patient and each flu season individually.)**

Infants and Children: Those 6 to 35 months old should be given 0.25 ml of a split dose vaccine. If this is the first vaccination, two doses should be given one month apart. Split dose is suggested for children because it tends to cause fewer undesirable effects. For infants and young children, the vaccine is usually given in the thigh muscle.

Children 3 to 8 years old should be given 0.5 ml of the selected split virus vaccine. Children in this age range who have not been previously vaccinated should be given two vaccinations, one month apart.

Children 9 years old or older should be given a single vaccination of 0.5 ml of split virus vaccine in the deltoid muscle.

13 to 60 Years of Age: Should be given 0.5 ml of whole or split virus vaccine in the deltoid muscle.

Over 60 Years of Age: Same as 13 to 60 years of age.

Conditions Requiring Dosing Adjustments

Liver function: Not involved.

Kidney function: Not involved.

▷ **Dosing Instructions:** Prior vaccination **does not** mean you are immune to the current year virus strains. Some tenderness at the injection site is possible. Fever and muscular aches or pains are also possible and may be treated with acetaminophen (Tylenol, others).

Usual Duration of Use: Single vaccination confers relative immunity to the expected viral strains in two weeks. This does **not** confer immunity to all strains of virus capable of causing an influenza-like (flu-like) syndrome. Annual vaccination is strongly suggested.

Possible Advantages of This Drug

Allows the prevention of a viral syndrome which can cause loss of several weeks of work in younger otherwise healthy patients or serious illness in older or compromised patients.

Currently a "Drug of Choice"

for prevention of type A influenza due to the viral strains which are of the greatest concern in the current flu season.

▷ **This Drug Should Not Be Taken If**
- you have had an allergic reaction to any dosage form of it previously.
- you are allergic to eggs (the virus is grown on eggs).
- you have an acute illness and a fever.

▷ **Inform Your Physician Before Taking This Drug If**
- you are HIV positive.
- you have a history of blood disorders.
- you have had Guillain-Barre syndrome.
- you have a history of seizures.
- you have been receiving cancer therapy (chemotherapy).

Possible Side Effects (natural, expected, and unavoidable drug actions)

Pain at the vaccination site. Muscle aches, fever, or bothersome tiredness (malaise). This is **not** the flu. The vaccine contains viral fragments or non-infectious virus. These symptoms are a reaction to the components of the vaccine.

▷ **Possible Adverse Effects** (unusual, unexpected, and infrequent reactions)

If any of the following develop, consult your physician promptly for guidance.

Mild Adverse Effects

Allergic Reactions: Swelling and redness.

Muscle aches or fever.

Fatigue, nausea, and headache.

Vasculitis (joint pain, weakness, fever, and rash) (rare).

Serious Adverse Effects

Allergic Reactions: Anaphylactoid reactions.

Low blood platelets (extremely rare).

Pericarditis (very rare).
Guillain-Barre syndrome (only reported during the 1976–1977 flu season and of questionable causation).
Kidney toxicity (very rare).
Vision changes (very rare).

▷ **Possible Effects on Sexual Function:**   None reported.

Possible Delayed Adverse Effects: None reported.

▷ **Adverse Effects That May Mimic Natural Diseases or Disorders**
Reaction to vaccine contents may mimic the flu.

Natural Diseases or Disorders That May Be Activated by This Drug
None reported.

Possible Effects on Laboratory Tests
Hepatitis B test: false positive.
Hepatitis C test: false positive.
HTLV-1 test: false positive.

CAUTION
1. The fact that a patient has had the vaccine in the previous year does **not** confer immunity to the flu in following years.
2. The flu vaccine typically confers immunity to the virus types that are predicted to cause the most problems in a particular flu season. The vaccine does not confer immunity to all strains of virus which are capable of causing a flu-like syndrome.
3. If muscle aches or fever occur after vaccination, acetaminophen (Tylenol, others) is recommended. **Do not** take aspirin to address these symptoms if they occur after vaccination.
4. Call your doctor immediately if you develop hives, facial swelling or difficulty breathing after the vaccination.

Precautions for Use
By Infants and Children: Safety and effectiveness for use by those under 6 months of age have not been established.
By Those over 60 Years of Age: The vaccine may be especially valuable in this age group as the effects of the flu may be very challenging.

▷ **Advisability of Use During Pregnancy**
Pregnancy Category: C. See Pregnancy Code at the back of this book.
Animal studies: Animal studies have not been conducted.
Human studies: Information from adequate studies of pregnant women is not available. Ask your doctor for guidance.

Advisability of Use if Breast-Feeding
Presence of this drug in breast milk: Not defined.
Monitor nursing infant closely and contact your doctor if adverse effects develop. The CDC has **not** listed breast-feeding as a precaution against receiving this vaccine.

Habit-Forming Potential: None.

Effects of Overdosage: No specific cases reported. Treatment would be consistent with any symptoms which the patient presents with.

Possible Effects of Long-Term Use: Not indicated for long-term use.

Suggested Periodic Examinations While Taking This Drug (at physician's discretion)

None indicated.

▷ **While Taking This Drug, Observe the Following**

Foods: No restrictions.

Beverages: No restrictions.

▷ *Alcohol:* No restrictions.

Tobacco Smoking: No interactions expected.

▷ *Other Drugs*

Influenza vaccine may *increase* the effects of
- carbamazepine (Tegretol) by decreasing the elimination of the drug.
- phenobarbital by increasing the half life of the drug.
- theophylline (Theo-Dur, others) by increasing the blood level of the drug.
- warfarin (Coumadin) and pose an increased risk of bleeding. More frequent INR (protime or prothrombin time) testing is suggested.

Influenza vaccine *taken concurrently* with
- cyclosporine (Sandimmune) can cause blunting of the immune response to the vaccine.
- immunosuppressive agents (chemotherapy, corticosteroids) may be associated with an impaired or blunted immune response to the vaccine.
- methotrexate can result in blunting of the immune response to this vaccine
- phenytoin (Dilantin) has had variable effects on the blood levels of this drug.

▷ *Driving, Hazardous Activities:* This drug may cause excessive tiredness and muscle aches. Restrict activities as necessary.

Aviation Note: The use of this drug *may be a short-term disqualification* for piloting. Consult a designated Aviation Medical Examiner.

Exposure to Sun: No restrictions.

Exposure to Heat: Since this vaccine may cause short duration fevers, it is wise to avoid hot environments for a day after vaccination.

Heavy Exercise or Exertion: A fever may result from this vaccination and it is wise to avoid strenuous exercise for a day after vaccination.

Author's note: There is now a Vaccine Adverse Event Reporting System (VAERS). The toll free number is 1-800-822-7967.

INSULIN (IN suh lin)

Introduced: 1922   **Prescription:** USA: No; Canada: No   **Available as Generic:** Yes   **Class:** Antidiabetic   **Controlled Drug:** USA: No; Canada: No

Brand Names: Humulin BR, Humulin L, Humulin N, Humulin R, Humulin U, Humulin U Ultralente, Humulin 70/30, Humulin 30/70, Iletin I NPH, Iletin II Pork, ✦Initard, Insulatard NPH, ✦Insulin Human, ✦Insulin-Toronto, Lente Iletin I, Lente Iletin II Beef, Lente Iletin II Pork, Lente Insulin, Lente Purified Pork, Mixtard, Mixtard Human 70/30, Novolin L, Novolin N, NovolinPen, Novolin R, Novolin 30/70, Novolin 70/30, ✦Novolin-Lente, ✦Novolin-NPH, Novolin-70/30, ✦Novolin-Toronto, ✦Novolin-Ultralente, ✦Novolinset, ✦Novolinset 30/70, ✦Novolinset NPH, ✦Novolinset Toronto, NPH Iletin I, NPH Iletin II Beef, NPH Iletin II Pork, NPH Insulin, NPH Purified Pork, Protamine, Zinc & Iletin I, Protamine, Zinc & Iletin II Beef, Protamine, Zinc & Iletin II Pork, Regular Concentrated Iletin II, Regular Iletin I, Regular Iletin II Beef, Regular Iletin II Pork, Regular Iletin II U-500, Regular Insulin, Regular Purified Pork Insulin, Semilente Iletin I, Semilente Insulin, Semilente Purified Pork, Ultralente Iletin I, Ultralente Insulin, Ultralente Purified Beef, Velosulin, ✦Velosulin Cartridge, Velosulin Human

BENEFITS versus RISKS	
Possible Benefits	*Possible Risks*
EFFECTIVE CONTROL OF TYPE I (INSULIN-DEPENDENT) DIABETES MELLITUS	HYPOGLYCEMIA WITH EXCESSIVE DOSAGE Infrequent allergic reactions

▷ **Principal Uses**

As a Single Drug Product: Uses currently included in FDA approved labeling: (1) Used in diabetes mellitus which is insulin-dependent, and in people who have noninsulin-dependent diabetes who are experiencing stress such as illness; (2) used to control blood sugar in critically ill patients who are being fed by intravenous nutrient mixtures.

Other (unlabeled) generally accepted uses: (1) Controls blood sugar in pregnancy (gestational diabetes); (2) insulin in combination with glucagon has been used in alcoholic hepatitis; (3) may have a role in combination therapy with an oral hypoglycemic agent in some diabetics; (4) helps diabetic ketoacidosis; (5) can help diabetic neuropathy and retinopathy; (6) can be of help in critically ill patients with maple syrup urine disease.

How This Drug Works: Insulin helps sugar through the cell wall to the inside of the cell (by direct action on cell membranes) where it is used for energy.

Available Dosage Forms and Strengths

Injections — 40 units, 100 units and 500 units per ml
PenFil cartridges — 150 units

▷ **Usual Adult Dosage Range:**   According to individual requirements for the best regulation of blood sugar on a 24-hour basis. **Note: Actual dosage and administration schedule must be determined by the physician for each patient individually.**

Conditions Requiring Dosing Adjustments

Liver function: Specific adjustment guidelines are not available.
Kidney function: Caution should be used in patients with compromised kidneys. Requirements become extremely variable.
Thyrotoxicosis: Glucose utilization is typically increased and insulin requirements may actually decrease.

▷ **Dosing Instructions:**   Inject insulin subcutaneously according to the schedule prescribed by your physician. The timing and frequency of injections will vary with the type of insulin prescribed. The following table of insulin actions (according to type) will help you understand the treatment schedule prescribed for you.

Insulin Type	Action Onset	Peak	Duration
Regular	0.5–1 hr	2–4 hrs	5–7 hrs
Isophane (NPH)	3–4 hrs	6–12 hrs	18–28 hrs
Regular 30%/NPH 70%	0.5 hr	4–8 hrs	24 hrs
Semilente	1–3 hrs	2–8 hrs	12–16 hrs
Lente	1–3 hrs	8–12 hrs	18–28 hrs
Ultralente	4–6 hrs	18–24 hrs	36 hrs
Protamine Zinc	4–6 hrs	14–24 hrs	36 hrs

Usual Duration of Use: In Type I insulin-dependent (juvenile-onset) diabetes mellitus, insulin therapy is usually required for life. Type II noninsulin-dependent (maturity-onset) diabetes may be controlled by oral antidiabetic drugs and/or diet but can require insulin for adequate control. Such occasions include serious infections, injuries, burns, surgical procedures and other physical stress. Insulin is used as needed on a temporary basis to regulate the body's use of sugar until recovery is complete. Consult your physician on a regular basis.

▷ **This Drug Should Not Be Taken If**
  • the need for insulin and its correct dosage schedule has not been established by a properly qualified physician.

▷ **Inform Your Physician Before Taking This Drug If**
  • you have an insulin allergy.
  • you do not know how to recognize and treat abnormally low blood sugar (see Hypoglycemia in Glossary).
  • you are pregnant.
  • you take: aspirin, beta blockers, fenfluramine (Pondimin), monoamine oxidase (MAO) type A inhibitors (see Drug Classes Section).

Possible Side Effects (natural, expected, and unavoidable drug actions)
  In stable diabetes, no side effects occur when insulin dose, diet, and physical activity are correctly balanced and maintained. In unstable ("brittle") diabetes, unexpected drops in blood sugar levels can occur, resulting in hypoglycemia (see Glossary).

▷ **Possible Adverse Effects** (unusual, unexpected, and infrequent reactions)
  If any of the following develop, consult your physician promptly for guidance.
  Mild Adverse Effects
  Allergic Reactions: Local redness, swelling, and itching at site of injection.
  Occasional hives.
  Taste disorders.
  Thinning of subcutaneous tissue at sites of injection.
  Serious Adverse Effects
  Allergic Reaction: Anaphylactic reactions (see Glossary).
  Severe, prolonged hypoglycemia.
  Inflammation of the parotid (parotitis).
  Hemolytic anemia (rare).
  Arrhythmias (associated with hypoglycemia).
  Very fast heart rate (with intravenous use).
  Porphyria (rare).

▷ **Possible Effects on Sexual Function:**   May resolve sexual dysfunction in patients who have this prior to starting insulin therapy. May also cause decrease in libido and erective dysfunction.

▷ **Adverse Effects That May Mimic Natural Diseases or Disorders**
The early signs of hypoglycemia may be mistaken for alcoholic intoxication.

Possible Effects on Laboratory Tests
Blood cholesterol level: decreased.
Blood glucose level: decreased.
Blood potassium level: decreased.

CAUTION
1. Carry with you a card of personal identification with a notation that you have diabetes and are taking insulin.
2. Know how to recognize hypoglycemia and how to treat it. Always carry a readily available form of sugar, such as hard candy or sugar cubes. Report all episodes of hypoglycemia to your doctor.
3. Your vision may improve during the first few weeks of insulin therapy. Postpone eye exams for glasses for 6 weeks after starting insulin.
4. Insulin is absorbed more quickly or slowly depending on where it is injected. Absorption is 80% greater from the abdominal wall than from the leg, and 30% greater than from the arm. It is advisable to rotate the injection site within the same body region than from one site to another.

Precautions for Use
By Infants and Children: Insulin dosages and schedules are modified according to patient size. Adhere strictly to the physician's prescribed routine.
By Those over 60 Years of Age: Insulin needs may change with age. Periodic individual evaluation is needed to identify the best dose and schedule. The aging brain adapts well to higher blood sugar levels. Rigid attempts at "tight" sugar control may result in hypoglycemia that shows as confusion and abnormal behavior. Repeated hypoglycemia (especially if severe) may cause brain damage.

▷ **Advisability of Use During Pregnancy**
Pregnancy Category: B. See Pregnancy Code at the back of this book.
Animal studies: Inconclusive.
Human studies: Adequate studies of pregnant women are not available. Birth defects occur 2 to 4 times more frequently in infants of diabetic mothers than in infants of mothers who do not have diabetes. The exact causes of this are not known. Insulin is the drug of choice for managing diabetes during pregnancy. To preserve the health of the mother and fetus, every effort must be made to establish the best dose of insulin necessary for "good control" and to prevent episodes of hypoglycemia.

Advisability of Use if Breast-Feeding
Presence of this drug in breast milk: No.
Insulin treatment of the mother has no adverse effect on the nursing infant.
Breast-feeding may decrease insulin requirements; dosage adjustment may be necessary.

Habit-Forming Potential: None; however cases of surreptitious insulin injection have been reported.

Effects of Overdosage: Hypoglycemia: fatigue, weakness, headache, nervousness, irritability, sweating, tremors, hunger, confusion, delirium, abnormal behavior (resembling alcoholic intoxication), loss of consciousness, seizures.

Possible Effects of Long-Term Use: Thinning of subcutaneous fat tissue at sites of insulin injection. Insulin resistance.

Suggested Periodic Examinations While Taking This Drug (at physician's discretion)

Historically, estimates of blood sugar were obtained by checking urine sugar. This method has been replaced by fingerstick testing of blood glucose. Fingerstick testing accurately reflects the blood sugar and helps ensure better control (tighter control) of blood glucose. If you are ill, increased frequency of fingerstick blood glucose testing may be indicated. Routine testing of blood sugar levels at intervals recommended by physician is prudent.

▷ **While Taking This Drug, Observe the Following**

Foods: Follow your diabetic diet conscientiously. Do not omit snack foods in mid-afternoon or at bedtime if they help prevent hypoglycemia.

Beverages: According to prescribed diabetic diet.

▷ *Alcohol:* Used excessively, alcohol can cause severe hypoglycemia, resulting in brain damage.

Tobacco Smoking: Regular smoking can decrease insulin absorption and increase insulin requirements by 30%. It is advisable to stop smoking altogether.

Marijuana Smoking: Possible increase in blood sugar levels.

▷ *Other Drugs*

The following drugs may ***increase*** the effects of insulin

- aspirin, and other salicylates.
- some beta blocker drugs (especially the nonselective ones) may prolong insulin-induced hypoglycemia (see Drug Classes).
- clofibrate (Atromid-S).
- fenfluramine (Pondimin).
- monoamine oxidase (MAO) type A inhibitors (see Drug Classes).
- oral hypoglycemic agents (see Drug Classes) result in additive hypoglycemia.

The following drugs may ***decrease*** the effects of insulin (by raising blood sugar levels)

- chlorthalidone (Hygroton).
- cortisonelike drugs (see Drug Classes).
- furosemide (Lasix).
- oral contraceptives.
- phenytoin (Dilantin, etc.).
- thiazide diuretics (see Drug Classes).
- thyroid preparations.

▷ *Driving, Hazardous Activities:* Be prepared to stop and take corrective action if hypoglycemia develops.

Aviation Note: Diabetes and the use of this drug ***are disqualifications*** for piloting. Consult a designated Aviation Medical Examiner.

Exposure to Sun: No restrictions.

Exposure to Heat: Use caution. Sauna baths can significantly increase the rate of insulin absorption and cause hypoglycemia.

Heavy Exercise or Exertion: Use caution. Periods of unusual or unplanned heavy physical activity will use up sugar more quickly and predispose to hypoglycemia.

Occurrence of Unrelated Illness: Omission of meals as a result of nausea, vomiting or injury may lead to hypoglycemia. Infections can increase insulin needs. Ask doctor for help.

Discontinuation: Do not stop this drug without asking your doctor. Omission of insulin may result in life-threatening coma.

Special Storage Instructions: Keep in a cool place, preferably in the refrigerator. Protect from freezing. Protect from strong light and high temperatures when not refrigerated.

Observe the Following Expiration Times: Do not use this drug if it is older than the expiration date on the vial. Always use fresh, "within date" insulin.

IPRATROPIUM (i pra TROH pee um)

Introduced: 1975   **Prescription:** USA: Yes; Canada: Yes   **Available as Generic:** USA: No; Canada: No   **Class:** Bronchodilator   **Controlled Drug:** USA: No; Canada: No

Brand Name: Atrovent, Atrovent nasal spray, Combivent

BENEFITS versus RISKS	
Possible Benefits	*Possible Risks*
EFFECTIVE BRONCHODILATOR FOR TREATMENT OF CHRONIC BRONCHITIS AND EMPHYSEMA	Mild and infrequent adverse effects (see below)
EFFECTIVE TREATMENT OF RUNNY NOSE (RHINORRHEA)	
Possibly effective as adjunctive treatment in some cases of bronchial asthma	

▷ **Principal Uses**

As a Single Drug Product: Uses currently included in FDA approved labeling: (1) Helps prevent or relieve episodes of difficult breathing in chronic bronchitis and emphysema. Should not be used to treat acute attacks of asthma because it takes a while to work; (2) used in nasal spray form to relieve symptoms of runny nose (rhinorrhea) that comes from allergic or nonallergic perennial rhinitis (this includes runny nose from the common cold) in adults and children more than 12 years old. Other (unlabeled) generally accepted uses: None.

How This Drug Works: This drug is a derivative of atropine. Through its atropinelike (anticholinergic) action, it blocks bronchial constriction and opens up the bronchi. In the nasal form, it keeps acetylcholine from working (antagonizes it) and decreases production and secretion of mucous.

Available Dosage Forms and Strengths
Inhalation aerosol — 14 gram metered dose inhaler; 18 mcg per inhalation
Nebulizer — 250 mcg/ml solution
Nasal inhaler — 20 mcg per actuation
Nasal spray — 0.03 and 0.06%

▷ **Usual Adult Dosage Range:** Initially 2 inhalations (36 mcg) 4 times a day, 4 hours apart. If needed, the dose may be increased to 4 inhalations (80 mcg) at one time to get optimal relief. Maintain 4 hour intervals between doses. Maximum daily dose is 12 inhalations (216 mcg). The nasal spray is used as: 0.03% two sprays (21 micrograms each) in each nostril two to three times a day for up to four days. 0.06% two sprays (42 micrograms each) in each nostril three to four times a day for up to four days. **Note: Actual dose and dosing schedule must be determined by the physician for each patient individually.**

Conditions Requiring Dosing Adjustments
Liver function: Specific guidelines for dosage decreases have not been elaborated.
Kidney function: Used with caution in patients with bladder neck obstructions.

▷ **Dosing Instructions:** Carefully follow the patient instructions provided with the inhaler. Shake well before using. Many people do NOT take the time to learn the best inhaler technique for them. Make the time to do this. The pump of the nasal form must be primed before the unit is used. Read the package insert carefully, and ask your pharmacist for help if you don't understand the directions that come with this medicine.

Usual Duration of Use:
Inhalation form: Continual use on a regular schedule for 48 to 72 hours is usually necessary to determine this drug's effectiveness. Long-term use (months to years) requires check of response and dosage adjustment. See your doctor.
Nasal Spray: The nasal form does NOT relieve sneezing or nasal congestion that may happen with a cold. The nasal spray may only be used for up to four (4) days.

Possible Advantages of This Drug
Inhalation form: Produces a greater degree of bronchodilation than theophylline in patients with chronic bronchitis and emphysema. Causes minimal adverse effects. Repeated use does not lead to tolerance and loss of effectiveness.
Suitable for long-term maintenance therapy.
Nasal spray: Eases a very annoying symptom of the common cold.

Currently a "Drug of Choice"
for difficult breathing associated with chronic bronchitis and emphysema.

▷ **This Drug Should Not Be Taken If**
- you have had an allergic reaction to it previously.
- you are allergic to soybeans or peanuts (inhalation form).
- you are allergic to atropine or to aerosol propellants (fluorocarbons) (inhalation form).
- you are allergic to benzalkonium chloride or edetate disodium (nasal spray).

▷ **Inform Your Physician Before Taking This Drug If**
- you have had an adverse effect from any belladonna derivative previously.
- you have a history of glaucoma.
- you have any form of urinary retention or prostatism (see Glossary).

Possible Side Effects (natural, expected, and unavoidable drug actions)
Throat dryness, cough, irritation from aerosol (rare), blurred vision (rare), dry mouth.

▷ **Possible Adverse Effects** (unusual, unexpected, and infrequent reactions)
If any of the following develop, consult your physician promptly for guidance.

Mild Adverse Effects
Allergic Reactions: Skin rash (rare), hives (rare).
Headache (rare), dizziness (rare), nervousness.
Lip and mouth ulcers, unpleasant taste, indigestion, nausea.
Palpitations (rare).
Nosebleeds (with nasal spray, occasional).

Serious Adverse Effects
Allergic reactions: Rare first-dose angioedema or bronchospasm.
Author's note: Other than the rare allergic reactions, the nasal spray does not have any serious adverse effects.
Abnormal heartbeat (supraventricular tachycardia) (rare).
Intraocular pressure changes (rare).
Bronchospasm or difficulty breathing (dyspnea) (nebulized form).

Possible Effects on Sexual Function
None reported.

Natural Diseases or Disorders That May Be Activated by This Drug
Angle-closure glaucoma, prostatism (see Glossary).

Possible Effects on Laboratory Tests
None reported.

CAUTION
1. Won't start to work for 5 to 15 minutes. It should **not** be used alone to treat acute attacks of asthma needing a fast result.
2. When used as combination therapy with beta-adrenergic antiasthmatic drugs (albuterol, terbutaline, metaproterenol, etc.), the beta-adrenergic aerosol should be used about 5 minutes before using ipratropium to prevent fluorocarbon toxicity.
3. When used as an adjunct to steroid or cromolyn aerosols (beclomethasone, Intal), ipratropium should be used about 5 minutes before using the steroid or cromolyn aerosol to prevent fluorocarbon toxicity.
4. Contact with the eyes can cause temporary blurring of vision.
5. Call your doctor if you are using the nasal spray and your runny nose (rhinorrhea) continues or gets worse and you develop a fever.

Precautions for Use
By Infants and Children: Safety and effectiveness for those under 12 years of age not established.
By Those over 60 Years of Age: Watch for possible development of prostatism and adjust dosage as necessary.

▷ **Advisability of Use During Pregnancy**
Pregnancy Category: B. See Pregnancy Code at the back of this book.
Animal studies: No drug-induced birth defects in mice, rat or rabbit studies.
Human studies: Adequate studies of pregnant women are not available.
Use this drug during pregnancy only if clearly needed.

Advisability of Use if Breast-Feeding
Presence of this drug in breast milk: Possibly yes, but in very small amounts.
Watch nursing infant closely and stop drug or nursing if adverse effects start.

Habit-Forming Potential: None.

Effects of Overdosage: This drug is not well absorbed into the circulation when it is taken by aerosol inhalation. No systemic effects of overdose are expected.

Possible Effects of Long-Term Use: Drying of the nose.

Suggested Periodic Examinations While Taking This Drug (at physician's discretion)
Internal eye pressure measurements if appropriate.

▷ **While Taking This Drug, Observe the Following**
Foods: No restrictions.
Beverages: No restrictions.
▷ *Alcohol:* No interactions expected.
Tobacco Smoking: No interactions expected. However, smoking should be avoided completely if you have chronic bronchitis or emphysema.
Marijuana Smoking: Possible excessive increase in heart rate (tachycardia).
▷ *Other Drugs*
Ipratropium may *increase* the effects of
• albuterol (Proventil, others).
• other atropinelike drugs (see Drug Classes).
Ipratropium *taken concurrently* with
• tricyclic antidepressants (see Drug Classes) may result in additive anticholinergic effects.
▷ *Driving, Hazardous Activities:*
May cause dizziness or blurred vision. Restrict activities as necessary.
Aviation Note: The use of this drug *may be a disqualification* for piloting. Consult a designated Aviation Medical Examiner.
Exposure to Sun: No restrictions.
Exposure to Cold: Inhaling cold air may cause bronchospasm and induce asthmatic breathing and cough; dosage adjustment of this drug may be necessary.
Heavy Exercise or Exertion: This drug is not considered to be consistently effective in preventing or treating exercise-induced asthma.
Discontinuation: Ask your doctor for help. Substitute medication may be advisable.

ISONIAZID (i soh NI a zid)

Other Names: Isonicotinic acid hydrazide, INH
Introduced: 1956   **Prescription:** USA: Yes; Canada: Yes   **Available as Generic:** USA: Yes; Canada: Yes   **Class:** Antituberculosis   **Controlled Drug:** USA: No; Canada: No
Brand Names: INH, ✦Isotamine, Laniazid, Nydrazid, P-I-N Forte [CD], ✦PMS Isoniazid, Rifamate [CD], Rifater [CD], Rimactane/INH Dual Pack [CD], Teebaconin, Teebaconin and Vitamin B-6 [CD]

BENEFITS versus RISKS	
Possible Benefits	*Possible Risks*
EFFECTIVE PREVENTION AND TREATMENT OF ACTIVE TUBERCULOSIS	ALLERGIC LIVER REACTION (RARE) Peripheral neuropathy (see Glossary) Bone marrow depression (see Glossary) Mental and behavioral disturbances

▷ **Principal Uses**
  As a Single Drug Product: Uses currently included in FDA approved labeling: (1) Used alone to prevent the development of tuberculous infection in people who are at high risk because of exposure to infection or recent conversion of a negative tuberculin skin test to positive; (2) used **in combination** with other drugs to treat tuberculosis in a variety of body sites.
    Other (unlabeled) generally accepted uses: (1) May have a role in treating atypical mycobacteria which can be associated with Crohn's disease.
  As a Combination Drug Product [CD]: Available in combination with rifampin, another antitubercular drug that works in a different way. This combination is more effective than either drug used alone. Isoniazid can cause low pyridoxine (vitamin B-6); for this reason, a combination of the two drugs is available in tablet form.
  How This Drug Works: By interfering with metabolism or cell walls, this drug kills (bactericidal) or inhibits (bacteristatic) susceptible tuberculosis organisms.

Available Dosage Forms and Strengths
  Injection — 100 mg per ml
    Syrup — 50 mg per 5 ml
  Tablets — 50 mg, 100 mg, 300 mg
▷ **Usual Adult Dosage Range:**   For prevention: 300 mg once daily (usually for 6 to 12 months). For treatment: 5 mg per kilogram of body weight daily. The total daily dosage should not exceed 300 mg. **Note: Actual dose and dosing schedule must be determined on an individual basis by the physician.**

Conditions Requiring Dosing Adjustments
  Liver function: Should **not** be used in acute liver disease. It should be discontinued if the liver function tests become increased to three times the normal value.
  Kidney function: Should be used with caution in kidney compromise—a rare

cause of nephrosis. In severe kidney failure (CCl <10 ml per minute), the daily dose should be decreased by 50%.

▷ **Dosing Instructions:**   The tablet may be crushed and taken with food to prevent stomach irritation.

Usual Duration of Use: Use on a regular schedule for 1 or more years is often necessary, depending upon the nature of the infection. Shorter courses of intermittent high doses may work. See your doctor on a regular basis.

▷ **This Drug Should Not Be Taken If**
- you have had an allergic reaction (especially a liver reaction) to any dosage form of it previously.
- you have active liver disease.

▷ **Inform Your Physician Before Taking This Drug If**
- you have serious impairment of liver or kidney function.
- you drink an alcoholic beverage daily.
- you are an alcoholic.
- your are pregnant or are nursing your baby.
- you have a seizure disorder.
- you take other drugs on a long-term basis, especially phenytoin (Dilantin).
- you plan to have surgery under general anesthesia in the near future.

Possible Side Effects (natural, expected, and unavoidable drug actions)
Toxic fever (rare).

▷ **Possible Adverse Effects** (unusual, unexpected, and infrequent reactions)
If any of the following develop, consult your physician promptly for guidance.
Mild Adverse Effects
Allergic Reactions: Skin rash, fever, swollen glands, painful muscles and joints.
Dizziness, indigestion, nausea, vomiting.
Serious Adverse Effects
Allergic Reactions: Drug-induced hepatitis (see Glossary): loss of appetite, nausea, fatigue, fever, itching, dark-colored urine, yellow discoloration of eyes and skin, hypersensitivity, meningitis.
Severe skin reactions (Stevens-Johnson syndrome, pellagra).
Peripheral neuritis (see Glossary): numbness, tingling, pain, weakness in hands and/or feet.
Acute mental and behavioral disturbances, psychosis, impaired vision, increase in epileptic seizures.
High or low blood sugars (hyperglycemia or hypoglycemia).
Porphyria (rare).
Lupus-erythematosus-like syndrome.
Pellagra (rare).
Kidney toxicity (nephrotoxicity) (very, very rare).
Bone marrow depression (see Glossary): fatigue, weakness, fever, sore throat, abnormal bleeding or bruising.
Abnormal muscle changes (rhabdomyolysis) (very, very rare).

▷ **Possible Effects on Sexual Function:**   Male breast enlargement and tenderness in men (gynecomastia).

Possible Delayed Adverse Effects: An increase in the frequency of cirrhosis of the liver has been reported.

▷ **Adverse Effects That May Mimic Natural Diseases or Disorders**
Drug-induced hepatitis may suggest viral hepatitis. Collagen vascular changes may mimic rheumatoid arthritis or systemic lupus erythematosus. Pseudolymphoma may occur.

Natural Diseases or Disorders That May Be Activated by This Drug
Latent epilepsy, systemic lupus erythematosus (questionable).

Possible Effects on Laboratory Tests
Complete blood cell counts: decreased red cells, hemoglobin, white cells and platelets; increased eosinophils (allergic reaction).
Blood amylase level: increased (possible pancreatitis).
Blood antinuclear antibodies (ANA): positive.
Blood lupus erythematosus (LE) cells: positive.
Blood glucose level: increased (with large doses).
Liver function tests: increased liver enzymes (ALT/GPT, AST/GOT and alkaline phosphatase), increased bilirubin.
Urine sugar tests: increased; false positive results with Benedict's solution and Clinitest.

CAUTION
1. Ask your doctor about determining if you are a "slow" or "rapid" inactivator (acetylator) of isoniazid. This has a bearing on your predisposition to developing adverse effects.
2. Copper sulfate tests for urine sugar may give a false positive test result. (Diabetics please note.)

Precautions for Use
By Infants and Children: Use with caution in children with seizure disorders. "Slow acetylators" are more prone to adverse drug effects. It is advisable to give supplemental pyridoxine (vitamin B-6).
By Those over 60 Years of Age: There is a greater incidence of liver damage in this age group; and liver status should be closely watched. Observe for any indications of an "acute brain syndrome" consisting of confusion, delirium and seizures.

▷ **Advisability of Use During Pregnancy**
Pregnancy Category: C. See Pregnancy Code at the back of this book.
Animal studies: No birth defects reported in mice, rats or rabbits.
Human studies: Data from adequate studies of pregnant women is not available.
If clearly needed, this drug is now used at any time during pregnancy. Ask your physician for guidance.

Advisability of Use if Breast-Feeding
Presence of this drug in breast milk: Yes.
Avoid drug or refrain from nursing.

Habit-Forming Potential: None.

Effects of Overdosage: Nausea, vomiting, dizziness, blurred vision, hallucinations, slurred speech, stupor, coma, seizures.

Possible Effects of Long-Term Use: Peripheral neuritis due to a deficiency of pyridoxine (vitamin B-6).

Suggested Periodic Examinations While Taking This Drug (at physician's discretion)

Complete blood cell counts, liver function tests, complete eye examinations.

▷ **While Taking This Drug, Observe the Following**

Foods: Eat the following foods cautiously until your tolerance is determined: Swiss and Cheshire cheeses, tuna fish, skipjack fish and Sardinella species. These may interact with the drug to produce skin rash, itching, sweating, chills, headache, light-headedness or rapid heart rate. Taking this drug with food also acts to decrease absorption and lessen therapeutic benefits. Some red wines and aged cheeses also contain high levels of tyramine. This may result in an undesirable increase in blood pressure if consumed. Avoid this combination.

Nutritional Support: It is advisable to take a supplement of pyridoxine (vitamin B-6) to prevent peripheral neuritis. Ask your physician for dosage.

Beverages: No restrictions. May be taken with milk.

▷ *Alcohol:* Alcohol may reduce the effectiveness of this drug and increase the risk of liver toxicity.

Tobacco Smoking: No interactions expected.

▷ *Other Drugs*

Isoniazid may *increase* the effects of
- carbamazepine (Tegretol), and cause toxicity.
- phenytoin (Dilantin), and cause toxicity.

The following drugs may *decrease* the effects of isoniazid
- cortisonelike drugs (see Drug Classes).

Isoniazid *taken concurrently* with
- acetaminophen (Tylenol) may increase the risk of hepatoxicity.
- antacids may decrease the absorption of this medicine. Separate antacid dosing by two hours from dosing of this medicine.
- BCG vaccine will result in decreased vaccine effectiveness.
- diazepam and perhaps other benzodiazepines (see Drug Classes) may result in increased blood levels and toxicity.
- ketoconazole, itraconazole or related compounds may result in decreased therapeutic benefit of the antifungal.
- meperidine (Demerol) may result in excessive lowering of blood pressure.
- oral hypoglycemic agents (see Drug Classes) may result in loss of control of blood glucose.
- rifampin (Rifadin, others) can result in a serious increased risk of liver toxicity.
- theophylline may result in theophylline toxicity.
- valproic acid (Depakene) can result in isoniazid or valproic acid toxicity.
- warfarin (Coumadin) may result in increased bleeding risk. More frequent INR (protime) testing is needed.

▷ *Driving, Hazardous Activities:* This drug may cause dizziness. Restrict activities as necessary.

Aviation Note: The use of this drug *may be a disqualification* for piloting. Consult a designated Aviation Medical Examiner.

Exposure to Sun: No restrictions.

Discontinuation: Long-term treatment is required. Do not stop this drug without asking your physician.

ISOSORBIDE DINITRATE (i soh SOHR bide di NI trayt)

Other Name: Sorbide nitrate

Introduced: 1959   **Prescription:** USA: Yes; Canada: No   **Available as**
Generic: USA: Yes; Canada: No   **Class:** Antianginal, nitrates   **Controlled**
Drug: USA: No; Canada: No

Brand Names: ✤Apo-ISDN, ✤Cedocard-SR, ✤Coradur, ✤Coronex, Dilatrate-SR, Iso-BID, Isonate, Isordil, Isordil Tembids, Isordil Titradose, Isotrate Timecelles, ✤Novosorbide, Sorbitrate-SA, Sorbitrate

Warning: The brand names Isordil and Isuprel are similar and can be mistaken for each other; this can lead to serious medication errors. These names represent very different drugs. Isordil is the generic drug isosorbide dinitrate; used to treat angina. Isuprel is the generic drug isoproterenol; used for asthma. Verify that you are taking the correct drug.

BENEFITS versus RISKS	
Possible Benefits	*Possible Risks*
EFFECTIVE RELIEF AND PREVENTION OF ANGINA	Orthostatic hypotension (see Glossary)
EFFECTIVE ADJUNCTIVE TREATMENT IN SELECTED CASES OF CONGESTIVE HEART FAILURE	Rare skin reactions (severe peeling)

▷ **Principal Uses**

As a Single Drug Product: Uses currently included in FDA approved labeling: (1) The sublingual (under-the-tongue) tablets and the chewable tablets are used to prevent and to relieve acute attacks of anginal pain; (2) the longer-acting tablets and capsules are used to prevent the development of angina, but are not effective in relieving acute episodes of anginal pain.

Other (unlabeled) generally accepted uses: (1) This drug is also used to improve heart function in selected cases of congestive heart failure; (2) can help ease the pressure in esophageal varices in alcoholics; (3) can help painful leg cramping (intermittent claudication); used after a heart attack intravenously to help address congestive heart failure.

How This Drug Works: By direct action on the muscle in blood vessel walls, this drug relaxes and dilates both arteries and veins. Its beneficial effects in treating angina and heart failure are due to (1) dilation of coronary arteries, and (2) dilation of systemic veins. The net effects are improved blood flow to the heart muscle and reduced work load of the heart.

Available Dosage Forms and Strengths

Capsules — 40 mg
Capsules, prolonged-action — 40 mg
Tablets — 5 mg, 10 mg, 20 mg, 30 mg, 40 mg
Tablets, chewable — 5 mg, 10 mg
Tablets, prolonged-action — 20 mg, 40 mg
Tablets, sublingual — 2.5 mg, 5 mg, 10 mg

▷ **Recommended Dosage Ranges** (Actual dosage and administration schedule must be determined by the physician for each patient individually.)

Infants and Children: Dosage not established.

12 to 60 Years of Age: Sublingual tablets: 5 to 10 mg dissolved under tongue every 2 to 3 hours; use for relief of acute attack and for prevention of anticipated attack.

Chewable tablets: Initially, 5 mg chewed to evaluate tolerance; increase dose to 5 or 10 mg every 2 to 3 hours as needed and tolerated; use for relief of acute attack and for prevention of anticipated attack.

Tablets: 5 to 20 mg 4 times daily to prevent acute attack; usual dose is 10 to 40 mg 4 times/day.

Prolonged-action capsules and tablets: 40 mg to start, then 40–80 mg every 8 to 12 hours as needed to prevent acute attacks.

The total daily dosage should not exceed 120 mg.

Over 60 Years of Age: Same as 12 to 60 years of age, however excessive lowering of the blood pressure on standing (postural hypotension) may be more likely in this population.

Conditions Requiring Dosing Adjustments

Liver function: It should be used with caution and in decreased dose in patients with liver compromise, as increased blood levels will occur.

Kidney function: No specific dosing changes are needed in compromised kidneys. This drug can discolor (brown to black) urine.

▷ **Dosing Instructions:**   Capsules and tablets to be swallowed are best taken on an empty stomach to achieve maximal blood levels. Regular tablets may be crushed for administration; prolonged-action capsules and tablets should be taken whole, NOT chewed.

Usual Duration of Use: Use on a regular schedule for 3 to 7 days is needed to (1) identify this drug's peak effect in preventing or relieving acute anginal pain, and (2) to find the optimal dosage schedule. Long-term use (months to years) requires physician supervision.

▷ **This Drug Should Not Be Taken If**
- you have had an allergic reaction to any dosage form of it previously.
- you have severe anemia.
- you have increased intraocular pressure.
- you have suffered trauma to the head.
- you have an overactive thyroid gland.
- you have abnormal growth of the heart muscle (hypertrophic cardiomyopathy).
- you have had a very recent heart attack (myocardial infarction) and have elevated blood pressure or very rapid heart rate (tachycardia).

▷ **Inform Your Physician Before Taking This Drug If**
- you have had an unfavorable response to other nitrate drugs or vasodilators in the past.
- you have a history of low blood pressure.
- you have any form of glaucoma.
- you have had a cerebral hemorrhage recently.
- you are pregnant or are planning pregnancy.
- you are allergic to the dye tartrazine.
- you have a G6PD deficiency (talk with your doctor).

Possible Side Effects (natural, expected, and unavoidable drug actions)
Flushing of face, throbbing in head, palpitation, rapid heart rate, orthostatic hypotension (see Glossary).

▷ **Possible Adverse Effects** (unusual, unexpected, and infrequent reactions)
If any of the following develop, consult your physician promptly for guidance.
Mild Adverse Effects
Allergic Reaction: Skin rash.
Headache (may be severe and persistent), dizziness, fainting.
Nausea, vomiting.
Urine discoloration.
Serious Adverse Effects
Allergic Reaction: Severe dermatitis with peeling of skin.
Transient ischemic attacks (TIAs) in presence of impaired circulation within the brain: dizziness, fainting, impaired vision or speech, localized numbness or weakness.
Anemia (in those with G6PD deficiency).
Abnormal heart rates or conduction.
Abnormally low blood pressure on standing (postural hypotension).

▷ **Possible Effects on Sexual Function:**   None reported.

▷ **Adverse Effects That May Mimic Natural Diseases or Disorders**
Spells of low blood pressure (due to this drug) may mimic late-onset epilepsy.

Possible Effects on Laboratory Tests
None reported.

CAUTION
1. Tolerance (see Glossary) to long-acting forms of nitrates may cause sublingual tablets of nitroglycerin to be less effective in relieving acute anginal attacks. Antianginal effectiveness is restored after 1 week of abstinence from long-acting nitrates.
2. Many over-the-counter (OTC) medications for allergies, colds and coughs contain drugs that may counteract the desired drug effects. Ask your physician or pharmacist for help before using such medications.

Precautions for Use
By Those over 60 Years of Age: Small starting doses are advisable. You may be more susceptible to the development of low blood pressure and associated "blackout" spells, fainting and falling. Throbbing headaches and flushing may be more apparent.

▷ **Advisability of Use During Pregnancy**
Pregnancy Category: C. See Pregnancy Code at the back of this book.
Animal studies: No information available.
Human studies: Adequate studies of pregnant women are not available.
Use this drug only if clearly needed.

Advisability of Use if Breast-Feeding
Presence of this drug in breast milk: Unknown.
If drug is thought to be necessary, monitor the nursing infant for low blood pressure and poor feeding.

Habit-Forming Potential: None.

Effects of Overdosage: Headache, dizziness, marked flushing of face and skin, vomiting, weakness, fainting, difficult breathing, coma.

Possible Effects of Long-Term Use: Development of tolerance with temporary loss of effectiveness at recommended doses. Development of abnormal hemoglobin (red blood cell pigment).

Suggested Periodic Examinations While Taking This Drug (at physician's discretion)
Measurement of internal eye pressure. Red cell counts and hemoglobin tests.

▷ **While Taking This Drug, Observe the Following**
Foods: Oral doses are best taken on an empty stomach to insure quick absorption.
Beverages: No restrictions. May be taken with milk.
▷ *Alcohol:* Use extreme caution and avoid alcohol completely in the presence of any side effects or adverse effects of this drug. Alcohol may exaggerate the blood-pressure-lowering effect of this drug.
Tobacco Smoking: Nicotine can reduce the benefits of this drug. Avoid all forms of tobacco.
Marijuana Smoking: Possible reduced effectiveness of this drug; mild to moderate increase in angina; possible changes in electrocardiogram, confusing interpretation.
▷ *Other Drugs*
Isosorbide dinitrate *taken concurrently* with
• antihypertensive drugs may cause excessive lowering of blood pressure; dosage adjustments may be necessary.
• hydralazine (Apresoline) may work well to help control angina.
• propranolol (Inderal) can help improve exercise time without angina.
▷ *Driving, Hazardous Activities:* Usually no restrictions. This drug may cause dizziness or spells of low blood pressure. Restrict activities as necessary.
Aviation Note: Coronary artery disease *is a disqualification* for piloting. Consult a designated Aviation Medical Examiner.
Exposure to Sun: No restrictions.
Exposure to Heat: Use caution. Hot environments can cause significant drop in blood pressure.
Exposure to Cold: Cold environments can increase the need for this drug and limit its benefits.
Heavy Exercise or Exertion: This drug may improve your ability to be more active without anginal pain. Use caution and avoid excessive exertion.
Discontinuation: It is advisable to gradually withdraw this drug after long-term use. Dose and frequency of prolonged-action dosage forms should be reduced gradually over a period of 4 to 6 weeks.

ISOSORBIDE MONONITRATE (i soh SOHR bide mon oh NI trayt)

Introduced: 1983 **Prescription:** USA: Yes **Available as Generic:** USA: No **Class:** Antianginal, nitrates **Controlled Drug:** USA: No
Brand Name: Elan (Italy), Elantan, Imdur, Ismo, Monoket

BENEFITS versus RISKS

Possible Benefits	*Possible Risks*
EFFECTIVE PREVENTION OF ANGINA	Orthostatic hypotension (see Glossary)
	Headache

▷ **Principal Uses**

As a Single Drug Product: Uses currently included in FDA approved labeling: To reduce the frequency and severity of recurrent angina; not effective in acute anginal pain.

Other (unlabeled) generally accepted uses: (1) May have a role in treating congestive heart failure; (2) can help in decreasing the number and time spent in silent myocardial ischemia; (3) may be of help in heart attacks (myocardial infarction).

How This Drug Works: By direct action on the muscle in blood vessel walls, this drug relaxes and dilates both arteries and veins. Beneficial effects in treating angina are due to (1) dilation of coronary arteries, and (2) dilation of systemic veins. The net effects are improved blood flow to the heart muscle and reduced work load of the heart.

Available Dosage Forms and Strengths

Tablets — 10 mg and 20 mg
Tablets sustained release — 60 mg
Capsules sustained release — 50 mg (Italy)

▷ **Recommended Dosage Ranges** (Actual dosage and administration schedule must be determined by the physician for each patient individually.)

Infants and Children: Dosage not established.

12 to 60 Years of Age: Regular release: 20 mg (1 tablet), taken twice daily: take the first tablet on arising; take the second tablet 7 hours later. Do not take additional doses during the balance of the day.

The total daily dosage should not exceed 40 mg.

Sustained release: 30 mg (one half tablet) or 60 mg (a whole tablet) once daily, taken in the morning when you get up.

The total daily dose should not exceed 240 mg.

Over 60 Years of Age: Same as 12 to 60 years of age.

Conditions Requiring Dosing Adjustments

Liver function: This drug should be used with caution in patients with liver compromise, however, no specific guidelines for dosage reduction are available.

Kidney function: No dosing changes are recommended in renal compromise. Isosorbide mononitrate may turn the urine brown to black in color.

▷ **Dosing Instructions:** The tablet may be crushed and is preferably taken on an empty stomach to achieve the best blood levels. Sustained release forms should not be chewed or crushed.

Usual Duration of Use: Use on a regular schedule for 3 to 7 days determines this drug's effectiveness in preventing episodes of acute anginal pain. Long-term use (months to years) requires physician supervision.

Possible Advantages of This Drug

Designed to provide the best possible prevention of acute angina with minimal development of tolerance (loss of effectiveness). See Tolerance in the

Glossary. The nitrate-free interval during the evening and night prevents the development of tolerance.

▷ **This Drug Should Not Be Taken If**
- you have had an allergic reaction to it previously.
- you have had a very recent heart attack (myocardial infarction) and your heart is beating quickly (tachycardia) or your blood pressure is excessively high.
- you currently have congestive heart failure.
- you have a severe anemia.
- your thyroid is overactive.
- you have a hypertrophic cardiomyopathy.

▷ **Inform Your Physician Before Taking This Drug If**
- you have had an unfavorable response to other nitrate drugs or vasodilators in the past.
- you have a history of low blood pressure.
- you have had a cerebral hemorrhage recently.
- you are pregnant or are planning pregnancy or you are nursing your baby.
- you have any form of glaucoma.

Possible Side Effects (natural, expected, and unavoidable drug actions)
Flushing of face, throbbing in head, palpitation, rapid heart rate, orthostatic hypotension (see Glossary).

▷ **Possible Adverse Effects** (unusual, unexpected, and infrequent reactions)
If any of the following develop, consult your physician promptly for guidance.
Mild Adverse Effects
Allergic Reactions: Skin rash, itching (rare).
Headache, dizziness (rare), fainting (rare).
Blurred vision.
Nausea, vomiting.
Bad breath (halitosis).
Serious Adverse Effects
Transient ischemic attacks (TIAs) in presence of impaired circulation within the brain: dizziness, fainting, impaired vision or speech, localized numbness or weakness.
Bone marrow depression (less than 5% and of uncertain relationship).
Anemia (in patients with G6PD deficiency).
Abnormally low blood pressure.
Abnormal heartbeat (rare).

▷ **Possible Effects on Sexual Function:** Decreased libido and impotence (less than 5%).

▷ **Adverse Effects That May Mimic Natural Diseases or Disorders**
Spells of low blood pressure with fainting (due to this drug) may be mistaken for late-onset epilepsy.

Possible Effects on Laboratory Tests
Liver function tests: increased.

CAUTION
1. Take this drug exactly as prescribed. If headaches are frequent or troublesome, call your doctor. Aspirin or acetaminophen may be taken to relieve headaches.

2. Many over-the-counter (OTC) medications for allergies, colds and coughs contain drugs that may counteract the desired effects of this drug. Ask your doctor or pharmacist for help before using such medications.

Precautions for Use

By Those over 60 Years of Age: Small starting doses are advisable. Increased risk of low blood pressure and associated "blackout" spells, fainting and falling. Throbbing headaches and flushing may be more apparent.

▷ **Advisability of Use During Pregnancy**

Pregnancy Category: C—Ismo. See Pregnancy Code at the back of this book. B—Imdur.

Animal Studies: Rat and rabbit studies reveal embryo deaths due to large doses of Ismo. Rat and rabbit studies did not reveal embryo deaths from Imdur.

Human studies: Adequate studies of pregnant women are not available.

Use this drug only if clearly needed. Ask your physician for guidance.

Advisability of Use if Breast-Feeding

Presence of this drug in breast milk: Unknown.

If drug is thought to be necessary, watch the nursing infant for low blood pressure and poor feeding.

Habit-Forming Potential: None.

Effects of Overdosage: Headache, dizziness, marked flushing of face and skin, vomiting, weakness, fainting, difficult breathing, coma.

Possible Effects of Long-Term Use: Development of abnormal hemoglobin (red blood cell pigment).

Suggested Periodic Examinations While Taking This Drug (at physician's discretion)

Measurement of internal eye pressure.

▷ **While Taking This Drug, Observe the Following**

Foods: No restrictions.

Beverages: No restrictions. May be taken with milk.

▷ *Alcohol:* Use extreme caution. Avoid alcohol completely in the presence of any side effects or adverse effects of this drug. Alcohol may exaggerate the blood-pressure-lowering effect of this drug.

Tobacco Smoking: Nicotine can reduce the effectiveness of this drug. Avoid all forms of tobacco.

Marijuana Smoking: Possible reduced effectiveness of this drug; mild to moderate increase in angina; possible changes in electrocardiogram, confusing interpretation.

▷ *Other Drugs*

Isosorbide mononitrate *taken concurrently* with

• antihypertensive drugs may cause excessive lowering of blood pressure; dosage adjustments may be necessary.

• calcium channel-blocking drugs (see Drug Classes) may cause marked orthostatic hypotension (see Glossary).

• hydralazine (Apresoline) may work well to help control angina.

• propranolol (Inderal) can help improve exercise time without angina.

▷ *Driving, Hazardous Activities:* Usually no restrictions. This drug may cause dizziness or spells of low blood pressure. Restrict activities as necessary.

Aviation Note: Coronary artery disease *is a disqualification* for piloting. Consult a designated Aviation Medical Examiner.

Exposure to Sun: No restrictions.

Exposure to Heat: Use caution. Hot environments can cause significant drop in blood pressure.

Exposure to Cold: Cold environments can increase the need for this drug and limit effectiveness.

Heavy Exercise or Exertion: This drug may improve your ability to be more active without anginal pain. Use caution and avoid excessive exertion.

Discontinuation: It is best to withdraw this drug gradually (over a period of 2 to 4 weeks) after long-term use.

ISOTRETINOIN (i soh TRET i noin)

Introduced: 1979   **Prescription:** USA: Yes; Canada: Yes   **Available as Generic:** No   **Class:** Antiacne   **Controlled Drug:** USA: No; Canada: No

Brand Name: Accutane

BENEFITS versus RISKS	
Possible Benefits	*Possible Risks*
EFFECTIVE TREATMENT OF SEVERE CYSTIC ACNE	MAJOR BIRTH DEFECTS
	Initial worsening of acne (transient)
	Inflammation of lips
	Dry skin, nose, and mouth
	Musculoskeletal discomfort
	Corneal opacities (rare)

▷ **Principal Uses**

As a Single Drug Product: Uses currently included in FDA approved labeling: (1) Reserved to treat severe, disfiguring nodular and cystic acne that has failed to respond to all other forms of therapy. *It should not be used to treat mild forms of acne;* (2) It is also used to treat some less common conditions of the skin that are due to disorders of keratin production.

Other (unlabeled) generally accepted uses: (1) May be helpful in refractory hypertrophic lupus erythematosus; (2) can help control resistant oral leukoplakia; (3) Apert syndrome facial treatment; (4) used adjunctively to surgery in some cervical cancers; (5) treats mycosis fungoides; (6) eases symptoms in Darier's disease; (7) may have a role in treating dysplastic nevi; (8) eases symptoms of Grover's disease; (9) can help treat the abnormal gum growth (gingival hyperplasia) which can occur with Phenytoin therapy; (10) treats severe and refractory rosacea; (11) has been combined with interferon alpha treatment in squamous cell skin cancer.

How This Drug Works: By an unknown action, this drug reduces the size of sebaceous glands and inhibits sebum (skin oil) production. This helps to correct the major feature of acne and its complications.

Available Dosage Forms and Strengths

Capsules — 10 mg, 20 mg, 40 mg

▷ **Usual Adult Dosage Range:**   Starting dose is based on the patient's weight and severity of acne; the usual dose is 0.5 to 2 mg per kilogram of body weight daily, taken in 2 divided doses for 15 to 20 weeks. After weeks of treatment, the dose should be adjusted according to response of the acne and the development of adverse effects. **Note: Actual dosage and administration schedule must be determined by the physician for each patient individually.**

Conditions Requiring Dosing Adjustments
Liver function: The dose should be decreased when isotretinoin is used in patients with compromised livers.
Kidney function: Isotretinoin is used with caution in kidney compromise.

▷ **Dosing Instructions:**   Begin treatment only on the second or third day of your next normal menstrual period. Take with meals (morning and evening) to achieve optimal blood levels. The capsule should not be opened for administration.

Usual Duration of Use: Use on a regular schedule for 15 to 20 weeks best determines effectiveness in clearing or improving severe cystic acne. The drug may be stopped earlier if the total cyst count is reduced by more than 70%. If a repeat course of treatment is necessary, it should not be started for 2 months. Long-term use (months to years) requires physician supervision.

▷ **This Drug Should Not Be Taken If**
• you have had an allergic reaction to it previously.
• you are allergic to parabens, preservatives used in this drug product.
• you are pregnant, or planning pregnancy.

▷ **Inform Your Physician Before Taking This Drug If**
• you have had an allergic reaction to any form of vitamin A in the past.
• you routinely take a nonprescription form of vitamin A.
• you have diabetes mellitus.
• you are considering giving blood (you will NOT be eligible for one month after the last isotretinoin dose).
• you have a cholesterol or triglyceride disorder.
• you are considering having a child.
• you wear contact lenses (your tolerance for these may decrease while you take this medicine).
• you have a history of liver or kidney disease.

Possible Side Effects (natural, expected, and unavoidable drug actions)
Frequent dryness of the nose and mouth, inflammation of the lips, dryness of the skin with itching, peeling of the palms and soles. Dose-related increase in triglycerides.

▷ **Possible Adverse Effects** (unusual, unexpected, and infrequent reactions)
If any of the following develop, consult your physician promptly for guidance.
Mild Adverse Effects
Allergic Reaction: Skin rash—may resemble pityriasis rosea.
Thinning of hair, conjunctivitis, intolerance of contact lenses, decreased night vision, muscular and joint aches, headache, fatigue, indigestion.
Serious Adverse Effects
Skin infections, worsening of arthritis, inflammatory bowel disorders.
Abnormal acceleration of bone development in children.

Development of opacities in the cornea of the eye.

Reduced red blood cell and white blood cell counts; increased blood platelet count.

Seizures.

Kidney toxicity (rare).

Pancreatitis (rare).

Abnormal blood glucose control.

Increased pressure within the head, with associated headache, visual disturbances, nausea, and vomiting.

Drug-induced hepatitis.

▷ **Possible Effects on Sexual Function**

Decreased male libido (7%), decreased female libido (13%) beginning after 1 month of drug use.

Impotence (3%) beginning after 3 months of drug use.

Decreased vaginal secretions (43%).

Altered timing and pattern of menstruation (22%).

Female breast discharge (rare).

Possible Effects on Laboratory Tests

Complete blood cell counts: infrequently decreased red cells and white cells.

Blood total cholesterol, LDL cholesterol, VLDL cholesterol and triglyceride levels: increased.

Blood HDL cholesterol levels: decreased.

Blood thyroid hormones (T_3, T_4 and free T_4 index): decreased.

Liver function tests: infrequently increased liver enzymes (ALT/GPT, AST/GOT and alkaline phosphatase), increased bilirubin.

Blood calcium level: increased.

CAUTION

1. This drug should not be used to treat mild forms of acne.
2. Worsening of your acne may occur during the first few weeks of treatment; this will subside with continued use of the drug.
3. Do not take any other form of vitamin A while taking this drug. (Observe contents of multiple vitamin preparations.)
4. Women with potential for pregnancy should have a ***blood*** pregnancy test within 2 weeks before taking this drug and should use 2 effective forms of contraception simultaneously during its use. Contraception should be continued until normal menstruation resumes after discontinuing this drug.
5. This drug may cause increased blood levels of cholesterol and triglycerides.
6. If repeated courses of this drug are prescribed, wait a minimum of 2 months between courses before resuming medication.

Precautions for Use

By Infants and Children: Long-term use (6 to 12 months) may cause abnormal acceleration of bone growth and development. Your physician can monitor this possibility by periodic X-ray examination of long bones.

▷ **Advisability of Use During Pregnancy**

Pregnancy Category: X. See Pregnancy Code at the back of this book.

Animal studies: Birth defects of skull, brain and vertebral column found in rats; skeletal birth defects found in rabbits.

Human studies: Adequate studies of pregnant women are not available. How-

ever, many serious birth defects (thought to be due to this drug) have been reported. These include major abnormalities of the head, brain, heart, blood vessels and hormone-producing glands.
Avoid this drug completely during entire pregnancy.

Advisability of Use if Breast-Feeding
Presence of this drug in breast milk: Unknown.
Avoid drug or refrain from nursing.

Habit-Forming Potential: None.

Effects of Overdosage: Increased blood pressure, lethargy, nausea, vomiting, mild gastrointestinal bleeding, elevated blood calcium, hallucinations and psychosis.

Suggested Periodic Examinations While Taking This Drug (at physician's discretion)
Complete blood cell counts, including platelet counts.
Measurements of blood cholesterol and triglyceride levels.
Complete eye examinations.
Liver and kidney function tests.

▷ **While Taking This Drug, Observe the Following**
Foods: Increases absorption and may be a good mechanism to maintain blood levels.
Beverages: No restrictions.
▷ *Alcohol:* No interactions expected.
Tobacco Smoking: No interactions expected.
▷ *Other Drugs:* Isotretinoin **taken concurrently** with
   • carbamazepine (Tegretol) may cause subtherapeutic carbamazepine levels.
   • minocycline may increase risk of severe headache, papilledema and visual changes.
   • tetracyclines may cause increased risk of pseudotumor cerebri.
▷ *Driving, Hazardous Activities:* No restrictions.
Exposure to Sun: Caution, this drug can cause photosensitivity (see Glossary).

ISRADIPINE (is RA di peen)

Introduced: 1984   **Prescription:**   USA: Yes   **Available as Generic:** USA: No   **Class:**   Antihypertensive, calcium channel blocker   **Controlled Drug:**   USA: No

Brand Name: DynaCirc

Controversies In Medicine: Study data indicates that medicines in this class should NOT be used in some patients with extremely compromised hearts. There have also been several FDA hearings held on the calcium channel blocker class. Be certain to ask your doctor about your cardiac output and if the benefits of this medicine outweigh the risks of its use. A recent FDA panel found medicines in this class to be safe and effective. A retrospective chart review yielded data that showed increased risks for nifedipine immediate release forms in those over 71, and cautioned physicians against using the immediate release form for indications other than angina. The immediate release form in question had never been approved for other uses. Most recently, a study of nearly 6,000 patients at Tel Aviv Medical Center found that there was no statistically significant increased risk of death in the patients who took calcium channel blockers versus those who did not.

BENEFITS versus RISKS	
Possible Benefits	*Possible Risks*
EFFECTIVE TREATMENT OF MILD TO MODERATE HYPERTENSION	Headache Dizziness Fluid retention Palpitations

▷ **Principal Uses**

As a Single Drug Product: Uses currently included in FDA approved labeling: (1) Treats mild to moderate hypertension, alone or in combination with thiazide-type diuretics.

Other (unlabeled) generally accepted uses: (1) Treatment of chronic, stable angina; (2) combination therapy of congestive heart failure; (3) may help resolve atherosclerosis; (4) could have a role in premature labor.

How This Drug Works: By blocking passage of calcium through cell walls (which is necessary for the function of nerve and muscle tissue), this drug inhibits the contraction of coronary arteries and peripheral arterioles. As a result of these effects, this drug

- promotes dilation of the coronary arteries (antianginal effect).
- reduces the degree of contraction of peripheral arterial walls, resulting in relaxation and consequent lowering of blood pressure. This further reduces the work load of the heart and helps prevent angina.

Available Dosage Forms and Strengths

Capsules — 2.5 mg, 5 mg

▷ **Usual Adult Dosage Range:** Initially 2.5 mg 2 times daily, 12 hours apart, for a trial period of 2 to 4 weeks. If needed, the dose may be increased by 5 mg per day at intervals of 2 to 4 weeks. The usual maintenance dose is 5 to 10 mg daily. The total daily dosage should not exceed 20 mg. **Note: Actual dose and dosing schedule must be determined by the physician for each patient individually.**

Conditions Requiring Dosing Adjustments

Liver function: Specific guidelines for dosage reduction are not available, yet empiric decreases in dosing are prudent in patients with compromised livers.

Kidney function: Used with caution in kidney compromise. Initial dose should be 2.5 mg twice a day.

▷ **Dosing Instructions:** May be taken with or following food to reduce stomach irritation. The capsule may be opened; mixed with food and swallowed promptly.

Usual Duration of Use: Use on a regular schedule for 2 to 4 weeks determines this drug's effectiveness in controlling hypertension or in reducing the frequency and severity of angina. The smallest effective dose should be used for long-term (months to years) therapy. Periodic physician evaluation is essential.

Possible Advantages of This Drug
Does not cause orthostatic hypotension (see Glossary).
No adverse effects on heart or kidney function.
No adverse effects on blood cholesterol levels.

▷ **This Drug Should Not Be Taken If**
- you have had an allergic reaction to it previously.
- you have symptomatic low blood pressure (hypotension).
- you have advanced narrowing of the aorta.

▷ **Inform Your Physician Before Taking This Drug If**
- you have had an unfavorable response to any calcium blocker drug in the past (see Drug Classes).
- you are currently taking any beta blocker drug (see Drug Classes).
- you are taking any drugs that lower blood pressure.
- you have a history of congestive heart failure, heart attack or stroke.
- you are subject to disturbances of heart rhythm.
- you have muscular dystrophy.
- you have myasthenia gravis.
- you develop a skin reaction while taking this drug.
- you have impaired liver or kidney function.
- you plan to have surgery under general anesthesia in the near future.

Possible Side Effects (natural, expected, and unavoidable drug actions)
Rapid heart rate (rare), swelling of the feet and ankles, cough, flushing and sensation of warmth.

▷ **Possible Adverse Effects** (unusual, unexpected, and infrequent reactions)
If any of the following develop, consult your physician promptly for guidance.
Mild Adverse Effects
Allergic Reactions: Skin rash (rare), hives, itching.
Headache, dizziness, weakness (rare), nervousness (rare), blurred vision (rare).
Decreased skin sensation (rare).
Palpitation, shortness of breath (rare).
Indigestion, nausea, vomiting, constipation (all rare).
Cramps in legs and feet (rare).
Increased urination (rare).
Abnormal growth of the gums (gingival hyperplasia).
Serious Adverse Effects
Allergic Reactions: Erythema multiforme, exfoliative dermatitis.
Rare heart rhythm disturbances.
Increased frequency or severity of angina (when therapy is started or following an increase in dose).
Marked drop in blood pressure with fainting (rare).
Low white blood cell counts (very rare).

▷ **Possible Effects on Sexual Function:** Decreased libido, impotence (less than 1%).

▷ **Adverse Effects That May Mimic Natural Diseases or Disorders**
Flushing and warmth may resemble menopausal "hot flushes."

Possible Effects on Laboratory Tests
White blood cell counts: decreased (less than 1% of users).

Liver function tests: increased enzyme levels (infrequent).

Electrocardiogram: slight increase in QT interval

CAUTION

1. If you are monitoring your own blood pressure, check it just before each dose and 2 to 3 hours after each dose. This will detect excessive fluctuations between high and low readings.
2. Tell all physicians and dentists who care for you that you take this drug. Note the use of this drug on your personal identification card.
3. Nitroglycerin and other nitrate drugs may be used as needed to relieve acute episodes of angina pain. However, if your angina attacks are becoming more frequent or intense, notify your physician promptly.

Precautions for Use

By Infants and Children: Safety and effectiveness for those under 18 years of age not established.

By Those over 60 Years of Age: Usually well tolerated by this age group. However, watch for weakness, dizziness, fainting and falling. Take necessary precautions to prevent injury.

▷ **Advisability of Use During Pregnancy**

Pregnancy Category: C. See Pregnancy Code at the back of this book.

Animal studies: Embryo and fetal toxicity reported in small animals, but no birth defects due to this drug.

Human studies: Adequate studies of pregnant women are not available.

Avoid this drug during the first 3 months. Use during the last 6 months only if clearly needed. Ask physician for guidance.

Advisability of Use if Breast-Feeding

Presence of this drug in breast milk: Unknown.

Avoid drug or refrain from nursing.

Habit-Forming Potential: None.

Effects of Overdosage: Weakness, light-headedness, fainting, fast pulse, low blood pressure, shortness of breath, flushed and warm skin, tremors and abnormal heart beats.

Possible Effects of Long-Term Use: None reported.

Suggested Periodic Examinations While Taking This Drug (at physician's discretion)

Evaluations of heart function, including electrocardiograms; measurements of blood pressure in supine, sitting and standing positions.

▷ **While Taking This Drug, Observe the Following**

Foods: No restrictions. Avoid excessive salt intake.

Beverages: No restrictions. May be taken with milk.

▷ *Alcohol:* Use caution. Alcohol may exaggerate the drop in blood pressure in some people.

Tobacco Smoking: Nicotine may reduce the effectiveness of this drug. Follow your physician's advice regarding smoking.

Marijuana Smoking: Possible reduced effectiveness; mild to moderate increase in angina; possible changes in electrocardiogram, confusing interpretation.

▷ *Other Drugs*

Isradipine *taken concurrently* with

• beta blocker drugs or digitalis preparations (see Drug Classes) may affect heart rate and rhythm adversely. Careful monitoring by your physician is needed if these drugs are taken concurrently.

- carbamazepine (Tegretol) has resulted in decreased blood levels of carbamazepine with calcium channel blockers from the same pharmacologic family. Caution is advised.
- digoxin may cause an increased blood level. Laboratory testing of blood levels should be performed more often if these drugs are combined.
- magnesium, especially in doses used in premature labor can cause very low and abnormal blood pressure.
- phenytoin (Dilantin) may result in loss of isradipine effectiveness. Caution is advised.
- propranolol (Inderal, others) can result in increased blood levels of isradipine and excessive lowering of blood pressure and slowing of the heart.
- rifampin (Rifadin, others) may result in a decreased therapeutic benefit from isradipine.

▷ ⱶ *Driving, Hazardous Activities:* Usually no restrictions. This drug may cause drowsiness or dizziness. Restrict activities as necessary.

Aviation Note: Coronary artery disease and hypertension *are disqualifications* for piloting. Consult a designated Aviation Medical Examiner.

Exposure to Sun: No restrictions.

Exposure to Heat: Caution advised. Hot environments can exaggerate the blood-pressure-lowering effects of this drug. Observe for light-headedness or weakness.

Heavy Exercise or Exertion: This drug may improve your ability to be more active without resulting angina pain. Use caution and avoid excessive exercise that could impair heart function in the absence of warning pain.

Discontinuation: Do not stop this drug abruptly. Ask your doctor about gradual withdrawal. Watch for the development of rebound angina.

KETOCONAZOLE (kee toh KOHN a zohl)

Introduced: 1981   **Prescription:** USA: Yes; Canada: Yes   **Available as Generic:** USA: No; Canada: No   **Class:** Antifungal   **Controlled Drug:** USA: No; Canada: No

Brand Name: Nizoral

BENEFITS versus RISKS	
Possible Benefits	*Possible Risks*
EFFECTIVE TREATMENT OF THE FOLLOWING FUNGUS INFECTIONS: Blastomycosis, candidiasis, chromomycosis, coccidioidomycosis, histoplasmosis, paracoccidioidomycosis, tinea (ringworm)	SERIOUS DRUG-INDUCED LIVER DAMAGE (1 in 10,000) Rare but serious allergic reactions Low blood platelets and anemia (rare)
Beneficial short-term treatment of advanced prostate cancer	
Beneficial auxiliary treatment of Cushing's syndrome	

▷ **Principal Uses**

As a Single Drug Product: Uses currently included in FDA approved labeling: (1) Treatment of lung and systemic blastomycosis; (2) treatment of Candida (yeast) infections of the skin, mouth, throat and esophagus (may be AIDS-related); (3) treatment of systemic Candida infections—pneumonia, peritonitis, urinary tract infections (may be AIDS-related); (4) auxiliary treatment of chromomycosis; (5) treatment of lung and systemic coccidioidomycosis; (6) treatment of lung and systemic histoplasmosis; (7) treatment of para-coccidioidomycosis; (8) treatment of Tinea infections of the body, groin (jock itch), and feet (athlete's foot).

Other (unlabeled) generally accepted uses: (1) Treatment of Candida infections of the vulva and vagina; (2) short-term treatment of prostate cancer; (3) treatment of Cushing's syndrome (excessive adrenal hormones); (4) treatment of systemic sporotrichosis; (5) topical treatment of fungal dandruff; (6) therapy of fungal infections of the toe nails; (7) designated as an orphan drug in therapy kidney toxicity caused by cyclosporine; (8) treats visceral leishmaniasis.

How This Drug Works: As an antifungal: By damaging cell walls and impairing critical cell enzymes, this drug inhibits cell growth and reproduction (with low drug levels) and destroys fungal cells (with high drug concentrations).

In treating prostate cancer: This drug decreases testosterone (male hormone) levels; and prostate cancer cells need testosterone to grow.

In treating Cushing's syndrome: This drug suppresses the excessive production of adrenal corticosteroid hormones.

Available Dosage Forms and Strengths

Cream — 2% (For local application to Candida or Tinea skin infections)

Shampoo — 2% (For topical therapy of fungal dandruff)

Oral suspension — 100 mg per 5-ml (Canada)

Tablets — 200 mg (US and Canada)

▷ **Recommended Dosage Ranges** (Actual dosage and administration schedule must be determined by the physician for each patient individually.)

Infants and Children: Up to 2 years of age: Dosage not established.

Over 2 years of age: 3.3 to 6.6 mg/kg of body weight, once daily; the dosage depends upon the nature of the infection.

12 to 60 Years of Age: For fungus infections—200 to 400 mg once daily; 800 mg maximum daily dose.

For prostate cancer—400 mg 3 times a day; 1,200 mg maximum daily dose.

For Cushing's syndrome—600 to 1200 mg once daily; total daily dosage should not exceed 1200 mg.

Over 60 Years of Age: Same as 12 to 60 years of age.

Conditions Requiring Dosing Adjustments

Liver function: The dose should be empirically decreased in patients with liver compromise.

Kidney function: Decreased doses are not needed in kidney compromise.

Achlorhydria (lack of acid in the stomach):   This medicine requires an acid environment in the stomach to be absorbed. Talk with your doctor about making a dilute acid solution to drink prior to taking the tablet form.

▷ **Dosing Instructions:**   The tablet may be crushed and is best taken with or after food to enhance absorption and reduce stomach irritation. Do not take with antacids. Take the full course prescribed.

Usual Duration of Use: Use on a regular schedule for 2 to 4 weeks determines effectiveness in controlling fungal infections. Actual cures or long-term suppression often require continual treatment for many months. Periodic physician evaluation of response and dosage adjustment are essential.

▷ **This Drug Should Not Be Taken If**
  • you have had an allergic reaction to it previously.
  • you have active liver disease.
  • you take astemizole or terfenadine.

▷ **Inform Your Physician Before Taking This Drug If**
  • you are allergic to related antifungal drugs: clotrimazole, fluconazole, itraconazole or miconazole.
  • you have a history of liver disease or impaired liver function.
  • you take loratadine (heart problems have not been reported as with other nonsedating antihistamines, but the blood level does increase if the drugs are combined and the dose of loratadine may need to be decreased.
  • you have a history of adrenal gland problems (adrenal insufficiency).
  • you have a history of low blood platelets or anemia.
  • you have a history of alcoholism.
  • you have a deficiency of stomach hydrochloric acid.
  • you are taking any other drugs currently.

Possible Side Effects (natural, expected, and unavoidable drug actions)
  Suppression of testosterone and adrenal corticosteroid hormone production (more pronounced with high drug doses).

▷ **Possible Adverse Effects** (unusual, unexpected, and infrequent reactions)
  If any of the following develop, consult your physician promptly for guidance.
  Mild Adverse Effects
  Allergic Reactions: Skin rash, hives, itching (rare).
  Headache, dizziness, drowsiness, photophobia (all rare).
  Nausea and vomiting, stomach pain (rare), diarrhea (rare).
  Increased blood pressure.
  Hair loss.
  Tinnitus.
  Muscle and joint aches.
  Serious Adverse Effects
  Allergic Reactions: Anaphylactic reaction (see Glossary).
  Severe liver toxicity (very rare): loss of appetite, nausea, fatigue, yellow skin and eyes, dark urine, light-colored stools (see jaundice in Glossary).
  Suppression of the adrenal gland.
  Low thyroid activity.
  Rare mental depression.
  Hemolytic anemia (rare).
  Abnormally low blood platelet counts: abnormal bruising or bleeding (rare).

▷ **Possible Effects on Sexual Function:**   Decreased testosterone blood levels: Reduced sperm counts, decreased libido, impotence, male breast enlargement and tenderness (gynecomastia). Altered menstrual patterns.

Possible Delayed Adverse Effects: Deficiency of adrenal corticosteroid hormones (cortisone-related); this could be serious during stress resulting from illness or injury.

▷ **Adverse Effects That May Mimic Natural Diseases or Disorders**
Drug-induced liver reaction may suggest viral hepatitis.

Possible Effects on Laboratory Tests
Complete blood cell counts: decreased red cells, white cells and platelets.
Liver function tests: increased liver enzymes (ALT/GPT, AST/GOT and alkaline phosphatase), increased bilirubin.
Adrenal corticosteroid blood levels: decreased.
Testosterone blood levels: decreased.

Precautions for Use
By Infants and Children: Safety and effectiveness for those under 2 years of age not established.
By Those over 60 Years of Age: No information available. It is advisable to avoid high doses.

▷ **Advisability of Use During Pregnancy**
Pregnancy Category: C. See Pregnancy Code at the back of this book.
Animal studies: Rat studies revealed significant embryo toxicity and birth defects due to this drug.
Human studies: Adequate studies of pregnant women are not available.
Use this drug only if clearly needed. Ask your physician for guidance.

Advisability of Use if Breast-Feeding
Presence of this drug in breast milk: Yes.
Avoid drug or refrain from nursing.

Habit-Forming Potential: None.

Effects of Overdosage: Possible nausea, vomiting, diarrhea.

Possible Effects of Long-Term Use: Suppression of adrenal corticosteroid hormone production, requiring replacement therapy during periods of stress.

Suggested Periodic Examinations While Taking This Drug (at physician's discretion)
Liver function tests should be obtained BEFORE long-term therapy is started and checked monthly during treatment.
Sperm counts.

▷ **While Taking This Drug, Observe the Following**
Foods: No restrictions.
Beverages: No restrictions. May be taken with milk.
▷ *Alcohol:* Avoid completely. Alcohol can cause a disulfiramlike reaction (see Glossary). In addition, alcohol may cause liver toxicity.
Tobacco Smoking: No interactions expected.
▷ *Other Drugs*
Ketoconazole may *increase* the effects of
- cortisonelike drugs (prednisone, etc.).
- cyclosporine (Sandimmune).
- oral hypoglycemic agents (see Drug Classes) and result in very low blood sugars.
- nonsedating antihistamines such as astemizole (Hismanal) and terfenadine (Seldane) and may cause large increases in blood levels and result in serious heart rhythm problems. Do not combine these medicines.
- loratadine (Claritin) is also a nonsedating antihistamine, but **HAS NOT**

been associated with heart rhythm problems when combined. The blood level does appear to increase, and lower doses of loratadine are prudent if these medicines are to be combined.

- quinidine (Quinaglute) and cause toxicity. Blood levels are needed.
- sucralfate (Carafate) may decrease the blood levels of ketoconazole.
- warfarin (Coumadin), and cause bleeding. Increased testing of INR (protimes) are needed.

Ketoconazole may *decrease* the effects of

- didanosine (Videx).
- theophyllines (Aminophyllin, Theo-Dur, etc.).

The following drugs may *decrease* the effects of ketoconazole

- antacids; if needed, take antacids 2 hours after ketoconazole.
- histamine H-2 blocking drugs: cimetidine, famotidine, nizatidine, ranitidine; if needed, take 2 hours after ketoconazole.
- isoniazid (Laniazid, Nydrazid, etc.).
- rifampin (Rifadin, Rifater, Rimactane, etc.).

Ketoconazole *taken concurrently* with

- cisapride (Propulcid).
- miconazole (Monistat) may increase the blood levels of ketoconazole or miconazole.
- phenytoin (Dilantin) may change the levels of both drugs.

▷ *Driving, Hazardous Activities:* This drug may cause dizziness or drowsiness. Restrict activities as necessary.

Aviation Note: The use of this drug *may be a disqualification* for piloting. Consult a designated Aviation Medical Examiner.

Exposure to Sun: This drug may cause photophobia; wear sun glasses if appropriate.

Discontinuation: Take the full course prescribed. Continual treatment for several months may be needed. Ask your doctor when the drug should be stopped.

KETOPROFEN (kee toh PROH fen)

Introduced: 1973   **Prescription:** USA: Yes; Canada: Yes   **Available as Generic:** Yes   **Class:** analgesic, mild; NSAID   **Controlled Drug:** USA: No; Canada: No

Brand Names: Actron (Nonprescription form), ✦Apo-Keto, ✦Apo-keto-E, Orudis, Orudis KT (nonprescription), Orudis SR, ✦Orudis E-50, ✦Orudis E-100, Oruvail ER, ✦Oruvail SR, ✦Rhodis, ✦Rhodis EC

BENEFITS versus RISKS	
Possible Benefits	*Possible Risks*
EFFECTIVE RELIEF OF MILD TO MODERATE PAIN AND INFLAMMATION	Gastrointestinal pain, ulceration, bleeding (rare)
	Rare congestive heart failure
	Rare liver or kidney damage
	Rare fluid retention
	Rare bone marrow depression

Please see the propionic acid nonsteroidal anti-inflammatory drug profile for further information.

LABETALOL (la BET a lohl)

Introduced: 1978 **Prescription:** USA: Yes; Canada: Yes **Available as Generic:** No **Class:** Antihypertensive, alpha- and beta-adrenergic blocker **Controlled Drug:** USA: No; Canada: No

Brand Names: Normodyne, Normozide [CD], Trandate, Trandate HCT [CD]

BENEFITS versus RISKS	
Possible Benefits	*Possible Risks*
EFFECTIVE, WELL-TOLERATED ANTIHYPERTENSIVE in mild to moderate high blood pressure PROLONGS LIFE AFTER A HEART ATTACK	CONGESTIVE HEART FAILURE in advanced heart disease Worsening of angina in coronary heart disease (if drug is abruptly withdrawn) Masking of low blood sugar (hypoglycemia) in drug-treated diabetes Liver toxicity

▷ **Principal Uses**

As a Single Drug Product: Uses currently included in FDA approved labeling: (1) Therapy of mild to moderate high blood pressure. May be used alone or in combination.

Other (unlabeled) generally accepted uses: (1) Combination therapy of hypertension in heart attacks (acute MI), beta blockers have also been shown to decrease the risk of repeat heart attacks, limit the size of the original heart attack damage and help control arrhythmias; (2) treatment of cocaine overdose; (3) therapy of phobic anxiety reactions; (4) treatment of angina; (5) therapy of pheochromocytoma, a tumor that releases compounds which increase blood pressure.

As a Combination Drug Product [CD]: This drug has been combined with hydrochlorothiazide (a thiazide diuretic) to attack high blood pressure through the combination benefit of two different medicines.

How This Drug Works: By blocking part of the sympathetic nervous system, this drug
- reduces the rate and contraction force of the heart, thus lowering the ejection pressure of blood leaving the heart.
- reduces the degree of contraction of blood vessel walls, resulting in their expansion and lowering of blood pressure.

Available Dosage Forms and Strengths

Injection — 5 mg per ml
Tablets — 100 mg, 200 mg, 300 mg

▷ **Usual Adult Dosage Range:** Initially, 100 mg twice daily, 12 hours apart; the dose may be increased by 100 mg twice daily every 2 to 3 days as needed to reduce blood pressure. The usual maintenance dose is 200 to 400 mg twice daily. Maximum daily dose is 2400 mg/24 hours, given as 800 mg 3 times daily. **Note: Actual dose and dosing schedule must be determined individually by your doctor.**

Conditions Requiring Dosing Adjustments

Liver function: The dose **must** be decreased in patients with compromised livers. The average dose in patients with long standing liver disease is about half that of patients with healthy livers. It is also a rare cause of severe liver (hepatocellular) injury.

Kidney function: Decreased doses are not thought to be needed in kidney compromise.

▷ **Dosing Instructions:**   The tablet may be crushed and is best taken at the same times daily, ideally following morning and evening meals. Do not abruptly stop this drug.

Usual Duration of Use: Use on a regular schedule for 10 to 14 days determines effectiveness in lowering blood pressure. Long-term use (months to years) of this drug will be determined by your individual response to an overall treatment program (weight reduction, salt restriction, smoking cessation, etc.).

Possible Advantages of This Drug

Decreases blood pressure more promptly than other beta blocker drugs.
Can be used to treat hypertensive emergencies.

▷ **This Drug Should Not Be Taken If**

- you have had an allergic reaction to it previously.
- you have active bronchial asthma.
- you have congestive heart failure.
- you are in cardiogenic shock.
- you have an abnormally slow heart rate or a serious form of heart block.

▷ **Inform Your Physician Before Taking This Drug If**

- you have had an adverse reaction to any beta blocker drug (see Drug Classes).
- you have a history of serious heart disease.
- you have a history of hay fever (allergic rhinitis), asthma, chronic bronchitis or emphysema.
- you have a history of overactive thyroid function (hyperthyroidism).
- you have a history of low blood sugar (hypoglycemia).
- you are a diabetic.
- you have sporadic cramping of the leg muscles (intermittent claudication).
- you have a history of spasms of the bronchi of the lungs.
- you have impaired liver or kidney function.
- you have intermittent claudication.
- you have diabetes or myasthenia gravis.
- you take any form of digitalis, quinidine or reserpine, or any calcium blocker drug (see Drug Classes).
- you plan to have surgery under general anesthesia in the near future.

Possible Side Effects (natural, expected, and unavoidable drug actions)
Lethargy and fatigability, light-headedness in upright position (see Orthostatic Hypotension in Glossary).

▷ **Possible Adverse Effects** (unusual, unexpected, and infrequent reactions)
If any of the following develop, consult your physician promptly for guidance.

Mild Adverse Effects
　Allergic Reactions: Skin rash, itching.
　Headache, drowsiness, dizziness, scalp tingling (during early treatment).
　Urine retention, difficulty urinating.
　Vivid dreams, nightmares, depression.
　Indigestion, nausea, diarrhea.
　Joint and muscle discomfort, fluid retention (edema).

Serious Adverse Effects
　Allergic Reactions: Anaphylaxis.
　Chest pain, shortness of breath, precipitation of congestive heart failure.
　Induction of bronchial asthma (in asthmatic individuals).
　Elevated blood glucose.
　Lichen planus.
　Abnormally low blood pressure on standing (postural hypotension).
　Muscle toxicity (toxic myopathy, worsening of intermittent claudication).
　Drug-induced systemic lupus erythematosus.
　Aggravation of myasthenia gravis.
　Liver damage with jaundice (rare).
　Difficult urination (urinary bladder retention).

▷ **Possible Effects on Sexual Function**
　Impotence (10%), inhibited ejaculation (10%), prolonged erection following orgasm (related to higher doses), Peyronie's disease (see Glossary).
　Decreased vaginal secretions (with low doses), inhibited female orgasm (related to higher doses).

Possible Effects on Laboratory Tests
　Blood potassium: slight increase.

CAUTION
　1. ***Do not stop this drug suddenly*** without the knowledge and help of your doctor. Carry a note or wear a labetalol drug identification bracelet.
　2. Ask your physician or pharmacist before using nasal decongestants usually present in over-the-counter cold preparations and nose drops. These can cause sudden increases in blood pressure if combined with labetalol.
　3. Report the development of any tendency to emotional depression.

Precautions for Use
　By Infants and Children: Safety and effectiveness for those under 12 years of age not established. However, if this drug is used, watch for low blood sugar (hypoglycemia) during periods of reduced food intake.
　By Those over 60 Years of Age: Proceed ***cautiously*** with all antihypertensive drugs. Therapy should be started with small doses, with frequent checks of blood pressure. Sudden, rapid or excessive lowering of blood pressure can increase stroke or heart attack risk. Watch for dizziness, unsteadiness, tendency to fall, confusion, hallucinations, depression or urinary frequency.

▷ **Advisability of Use During Pregnancy**
　Pregnancy Category: C. See Pregnancy Code at the back of this book.
　Animal studies: No significant increase in birth defects found in rats or rabbits; some increase in fetal deaths reported.
　Human studies: Adequate studies of pregnant women are not available.
　Use this drug only if clearly needed. Ask physician for guidance.

Advisability of Use if Breast-Feeding
>Presence of this drug in breast milk: Yes, in very small amounts.
>Avoid drug or refrain from nursing.

Habit-Forming Potential: None.

Effects of Overdosage: Weakness, slow pulse, low blood pressure, fainting, cold and sweaty skin, congestive heart failure, possible coma and convulsions.

Possible Effects of Long-Term Use: Reduced heart reserve and eventual heart failure in susceptible individuals with advanced heart disease.

Suggested Periodic Examinations While Taking This Drug (at physician's discretion)
>Measurements of blood pressure, evaluation of heart function.

▷ **While Taking This Drug, Observe the Following**

Foods: May increase the absorption of labetalol and result in a larger than expected blood level. Patients taking this medicine should also avoid excessive salt intake.

Beverages: No restrictions. May be taken with milk.

▷   *Alcohol:* Use with caution. Alcohol may exaggerate this drug's ability to lower blood pressure and may increase its mild sedative effect.

Tobacco Smoking: Nicotine may reduce this drug's effectiveness in treating high blood pressure, and increase bronchial constriction seen in regular smokers.

▷   *Other Drugs*

Labetalol may *increase* the effects of
- oral hypoglycemic agents (see Drug Classes) and prolong recovery from any hypoglycemia (low blood sugar) which may occur.
- other antihypertensive drugs and cause excessive lowering of blood pressure. Dosage adjustments may be necessary.

Labetalol *taken concurrently* with
- amiodarone (Codarone) may result in extremely slow heart rates and cardiac arrest.
- cimetidine (Tagamet) can cause elevated labetalol levels and low blood pressure or heart rate.
- clonidine (Catapres) must be closely watched for rebound high blood pressure if clonidine is withdrawn while labetalol is still being taken.
- epinephrine may result in severe increases in blood pressure.
- fluvoxamine (Luvox) may result in excessive lowering of the blood pressure or excessive slowing of the heart.
- imipramine and other tricyclic antidepressants (TCAs) may result in increases in antidepressant blood levels and toxicity.
- insulin must be watched for development of hypoglycemia (see Glossary).
- NSAIDs may result in blunting of the therapeutic effect of labetalol.
- phenothiazines (see Drug Classes) may cause additive lowering of the blood pressure.
- ritodrine (Yutopar) may blunt the beneficial effects of ritodrine.

▷   *Driving, Hazardous Activities:* Use caution until the full extent of fatigue, dizziness and blood pressure change has been determined.

Aviation Note: The use of this drug *is a disqualification* for piloting. Consult a designated Aviation Medical Examiner.

Exposure to Sun: No restrictions.

Exposure to Heat: Caution advised. Hot environments can lower the blood pressure and exaggerate the effects of this drug.

Exposure to Cold: Caution advised. Cold environments can increase blood flow problems in the extremities that may occur with beta blocker drugs. The elderly should take precautions to prevent hypothermia (see Glossary).

Heavy Exercise or Exertion: It is advisable to avoid exertion that produces light-headedness, excessive fatigue or muscle cramping. The use of this drug may intensify the hypertensive response to isometric exercise.

Occurrence of Unrelated Illness: Fever can lower the blood pressure and require decreased doses. Nausea or vomiting may interrupt scheduled doses. Ask your doctor for help.

Discontinuation: If possible, gradual reduction of dose over a period of 2 to 3 weeks is recommended—otherwise, rebound increases in blood pressure may occur. Ask your physician for specific guidance.

LAMIVUDINE (LAMB iv u deen)

Introduced: 1995   **Prescription:** USA: Yes   **Available as Generic:** No   **Class:** Antiviral, antiretroviral, reverse transcriptase inhibitor, nucleoside analog   **Controlled Drug:** USA: No
Brand Name: Epivir

BENEFITS versus RISKS	
Possible Benefits	*Possible Risks*
IMPRESSIVE SUPPRESSION OF VIRAL LOAD WHEN USED IN COMBINATION THERAPY TREATING AIDS DOES NOT LEAD TO SUPPRESSION OF THE BONE MARROW EFFECTIVE EARLY DATA IN TREATING HEPATITIS B	DECREASED WHITE BLOOD CELL COUNTS Peripheral neuropathy Pancreatitis

▷ **Principal Uses**

As a Single Drug Product: Uses currently included in FDA approved labeling: Used in combination with zidovudine (Retrovir) to treat HIV infection. Other (unlabeled) generally accepted uses: One significant study found that single agent therapy with lamivudine cleared hepatitis B virus from the blood of some of the test patients.

How This Drug Works: This medicine is a potent reverse transcriptase inhibitor, and as such, interferes with the ability of the HIV virus to create genetic material. The exact mechanism of action in treating hepatitis B is not clear.

Available Dosage Forms and Strengths
Solution — 10 mg per milliliter
Tablets — 150 mg

▷ **Recommended Dosage Ranges: (Actual dosage and administration schedule must be determined by the physician or clinical pharmacist for each patient individually.)**

Infants and Children: 3 months to 12 years old: 4 mg per kg twice daily (300 mg maximum a day). Used in combination with zidovudine (Retrovir).

18 to 65 Years of Age: Usual dose is 150 mg twice daily in combination with zidovudine (Retrovir).

Adults weighing less than 110 lb. or 50 kg: 2 mg per kilogram twice daily in combination with zidovudine (Retrovir).

Over 65 Years of Age: Not studied in those over 65.

Conditions Requiring Dosing Adjustments

Liver function: Metabolism is a minor (less than 5% of a given dose) route of elimination.

Kidney function: Up to 70% of a given dose is removed by the kidneys. Dosing must be adjusted in kidney compromise. For example, those with creatinine clearances (see Glossary) of 5 to 14 ml per minute should be given a first dose of 150 mg and then 50 mg once daily.

▷ **Dosing Instructions:**   Lamivudine tablets and solution can be given without regard to meals. Studies have NOT been conducted to test the effects of crushing the tablets and mixing them with food. A solution is available for patients who can't swallow the tablets.

Usual Duration of Use: The present indication is based on surrogate endpoints; no data is available on clinical HIV progression. Measurement of viral load (burden) and/or CD4 counts are now used by many clinicians to decide the effectiveness of treatment and help in the decision to continue or change medications.

Possible Side Effects (natural, expected, and unavoidable drug actions)
Not defined.

▷ **Possible Adverse Effects** (unusual, unexpected, and infrequent reactions)
If any of the following develop, consult your physician promptly for guidance.

Mild Adverse Effects
Dizziness.
Nausea.
Sleep disorders.
Paresthesias and/or peripheral neuropathy (13% in a study in children taking lamivudine monotherapy).

Serious Adverse Effects
Lowered white blood cell counts (7.2% used in combination with zidovudine).
Increased amylase (4.2% in combination with zidovudine).
Pancreatitis (up to 14% in a study of children receiving lamivudine monotherapy).

▷ **Possible Effects on Sexual Function:**   None reported
Author's note: This profile will be further developed in the next edition of this book once more information is available.

LAMOTRIGINE (la MOH tri jean)

Introduced: 1995   **Prescription:** USA: Yes; Canada: Yes   **Available as**
Generic: USA: No   **Class:** Anticonvulsant, phenyltriazine   **Controlled**
Drug: USA: No; Canada: No
Brand Names: Lamictal

BENEFITS versus RISKS	
Possible Benefits	*Possible Risks*
EFFECTIVE MANAGEMENT OF SEIZURES THAT RESIST THERAPY INCREASE IN SEIZURE-FREE DAYS	Rashes Visual changes Dizziness

▷ **Principal Uses**

As a Single Drug Product: Uses currently included in FDA approved labeling: (1) Adjunctive combination therapy of partial seizures in adults which have not responded to treatment with other medicines.

Other (unlabeled) generally accepted uses: (1) May have a role in epilepsy in children that has not responded to more established treatment; (2) could have a role in status epilepticus; (3) of use in Lennox-Gastaut syndrome.

How This Drug Works: The exact mechanism of action is not known, but animal models appear to show that this medicine blocks voltage-dependent sodium channels. This causes a decreased amount of glutamate and aspartate transmitters, and a decreased likelihood of seizures.

Available Dosage Forms and Strengths

Tablets — 25 mg, 100 mg, 150 mg, 200 mg

▷ **Recommended Dosage Ranges: (Actual dosage and administration schedule must be determined by the physician or clinical pharmacist for each patient individually.)**

Infants and Children: Safety and efficacy in those less than 16 years old have not been established. Some researcher use in intractable epilepsy: 2–15 mg per kg divided into two equal doses and given every 12 hours.

16 to 65 Years of Age: In patients receiving medicines known to interact (phenytoin, primidone, cabamazepine or phenobarbital)—but not valproic acid: the starting dose is 50 mg a day for two weeks, and then 50 mg twice a day as needed or tolerated, and then the dose can be increased as needed and tolerated by 100 mg a day every week. Most patients end up taking 300–500 mg a day divided into two equal doses. Some centers have used doses as high as 700 mg a day. Patients only taking valproic acid are expected to need still lower doses, but studies have not been done.

Over 65 Years of Age: Same dosing as 18 to 65 (single dose pharmacokinetics were similar to younger adults). Few patients over 65 were included during premarket studies, so specific statements can't presently be made.

Conditions Requiring Dosing Adjustments

Liver function: This drug is primarily glucuronidated in the liver, but guidelines are not available for adjusting the dose in liver failure. Specific studies in this population have not been made.

Kidney function: Most of this medicine is removed by the kidneys, but guidelines for decreases the dose or interval are not available. Used with caution and decreased doses are suggested.

▷ **Dosing Instructions:**   Take this medicine exactly as prescribed. Food does not effect how much medicine gets into your body. Talk with your doctor immediately if you develop a rash with swollen lymph glands and fever.

Usual Duration of Use: Use on a regular schedule for three months in children with resistant seizures may be needed to see the peak benefits. Long-term use (months to years) of this drug will be determined by your individual response to therapy. Long-term use requires periodic physician follow up. Be sure to keep appointments with your doctor.

Possible Advantages of This Drug
Generally well tolerated medicine effective where single medicines have failed.

▷ **This Drug Should Not Be Taken If**
- you have developed a rash with swollen lymph glands while taking this medicine.
- you are allergic to this medicine or to ones similar to it.

▷ **Inform Your Physician Before Taking This Drug If**
- you develop a rash.
- you do not understand how much or how often to take this medicine.

Possible Side Effects (natural, expected, and unavoidable drug actions)
Somnolence.

▷ **Possible Adverse Effects** (unusual, unexpected, and infrequent reactions)
If any of the following develop, consult your physician promptly for guidance.
Mild Adverse Effects
Allergic Reactions: Skin rash (should be reported to your doctor), itching.
Dizziness and headache (most common adverse effects).
Problems coordinating moving (ataxia).
Nausea and vomiting.
Blurred vision (dose-related).
Weight gain.
Serious Adverse Effects
Allergic Reactions: Anaphylaxis.
Serious rashes (Stevens-Johnson syndrome; toxic epidermal necrolysis [TEN]).
Hostility (rare).
One case report of lowered blood platelets (thrombocytopenia) in a 15-year-old.
One case report of sudden (acute) liver (hepatic) failure.
Rare disseminated intravascular coagulation.
Blood in the urine (infrequent).
Peripheral neuropathy (rare and of questionable cause).
Rare sudden unexplained death (SUDEP). The rate of SUDEP was similar to that of another agent also tested, and appears to be a population effect.

▷ **Possible Effects on Sexual Function:**   None reported.

Possible Effects on Laboratory Tests
  Blood levels of interacting medicines may be changed.

CAUTION
  1. **DO NOT** stop this medicine suddenly as seizures may occur.

Precautions for Use
  By Infants and Children: This medicine is approved for add-on therapy in children over 16 years of age.
  By Those over 60 Years of Age: No specific changes.

▷ **Advisability of Use During Pregnancy**
  Pregnancy Category: C. See pregnancy code at the back of this book.
    Animal studies: No evidence of drug related changes were found in mice or rabbits who were given up to 1.2 times the human dose.
    Human studies: This medicine has been shown to cause toxicity to the mother and because of this, toxicity to the fetus. Adequate studies of pregnant women are not available.
    Discuss the benefits to risk balance with your doctor.

Advisability of Use if Breast-Feeding
  Presence of this drug in breast milk: Probably yes.
  Avoid drug or refrain from nursing.

Habit-Forming Potential: None.

Effects of Overdosage: Sleepiness, changes in muscular reflexes, coma. Seizure diary to check for decrease in seizure frequency.

Possible Effects of Long-Term Use: Weight gain.

Suggested Periodic Examinations While Taking This Drug (at physician's discretion)
    Examinations for nystagmus, muscular coordination.

▷ **While Taking This Drug, Observe the Following**
  Foods: No restrictions.
  Beverages: No restrictions. May be taken with milk.
▷   *Alcohol:* Avoid alcohol use, unless you discuss this with your doctor.
  Tobacco Smoking: No interactions expected, but smoking does not enhance your health.
▷   *Other Drugs*
    Lamotrigine *taken concurrently* with: Long-standing use of acetaminophen (Tylenol, others) may result in decreases in blood levels of this medicine and a potential decrease in seizure control. Periodic use should not cause problems. Carbamazepine (Tegretol) may increase the removal of lamotrigine from the body and require dosing adjustments. Phenobarbital may result in a faster removal of lamotrigine from the body and require dosing changes. Phenytoin (Dilantin) may result in a faster removal of lamotrigine from the body and require dosing changes. Primidone (Mysoline) may result in a faster removal of lamotrigine from the body and require dosing changes. Valproic acid (Depakene) may result in slower removal of lamotrigine from the body and require decreases in lamotrigine doses in order to avoid toxicity.
▷   *Driving, Hazardous Activities:* Use caution until the full extent of fatigue, dizziness, coordination or vision changes have been determined.

Aviation Note: The use of this drug *is a disqualification* for piloting. Consult a designated Aviation Medical Examiner.

Exposure to Sun: No restrictions.

Exposure to Heat: Use caution, muscular coordination problems may be worsened by excessive heat.

Discontinuation: DO NOT stop this medicine abruptly without talking with your doctor first. Abrupt discontinuation of lamotrigine without first starting another antiseizure medicine may result in seizures.

LANSOPRAZOLE (lan SO pra sole)

Introduced: 1995   **Prescription:** USA: Yes; Canada: Yes   **Available as**
Generic: USA: No; Canada: No   **Class:** Antiulcer, proton pump inhibitor
Controlled Drug: USA: No; Canada: No
Brand Names: Prevacid

BENEFITS versus RISKS	
Possible Benefits	*Possible Risks*
VERY EFFECTIVE TREATMENT OF CONDITIONS ASSOCIATED WITH EXCESSIVE PRODUCTION OF STOMACH (GASTRIC) ACID: ZOLLINGER-ELLISON SYNDROME, MASTOCYTOSIS ENDOCRINE ADENOMA	Rare liver enzyme increases Rare protein in the urine
VERY EFFECTIVE TREATMENT OF REFLUX ESOPHAGITIS	
VERY EFFECTIVE TREATMENT OF DUODENAL ULCER	

▷ **Principal Uses**

As a Single Drug Product: Uses currently included in FDA approved labeling: (1) Used to treat duodenal ulcers; (2) treats erosive esophagitis; (3) used in syndromes (such as Zollinger-Ellison) where excessive amounts of stomach acid are produced.

Other (unlabeled) generally accepted uses: (1) Treatment of stomach (gastric) ulcers; (2) helps refractory reflux esophagitis.

How This Drug Works: This drug inhibits a specific enzyme system (the H/K adenosine triphosphate) in the stomach (parietal cells) lining and stops the production of stomach acid. By doing this it eliminates the principal cause of ulcers or esophagitis and also creates an environment conducive to healing.

Available Dosage Forms and Strengths

Capsules — 15 mg 30 mg

▷ **Recommended Dosage Ranges (Actual dosage and administration schedule must be determined by the physician for each patient individually.)**

Infants and Children: Not studied in this age group.

18 to 60 Years of Age: For duodenal ulcer: 15 mg daily, taken before a meal. Four weeks of therapy are indicated.

For erosive esophagitis: 30 mg daily, taken before a meal. Up to eight weeks of treatment can be given. If healing does not occur, an additional 8 weeks may be considered.

For excessive acid production syndromes: Dosing is started at 60 mg daily. The dose is increased as needed and tolerated. Doses up to 90 mg twice daily have been used. Once the condition is under control, the dose is usually reduced in stepwise fashion to 30 mg a day.

Over 60 Years of Age: Same as 18 to 60 years of age.

Conditions Requiring Dosing Adjustments

Liver function: Decreases in doses should be considered. The manufacturer strongly suggests a dose of 15 mg daily in people with significant liver problems.

Kidney function: No dosing changes needed.

▷ **Dosing Instructions:**   The capsules contain enteric coated granules which protect the medicine in the stomach's acid. Take the capsules whole. Some studies have found that taking lansoprazole in the morning worked the best in controlling stomach acid. Take this medicine exactly as prescribed.

Usual Duration of Use: Use on a regular schedule for seven days resulted in a 90–94% decrease in stimulated acid release. Patients with stomach (gastric) or duodenal ulcers had a decrease in symptoms in about one week. People with reflux esophagitis had significant decreases in heartburn after 7 to 28 days. Some esophagitis patients needed a second 8 week course to bring symptoms under control. Long-term use requires periodic physician follow up.

▷ **This Drug Should Not Be Taken If**
- you are allergic to the medicine or any of its components.

▷ **Inform Your Physician Before Taking This Drug If**
- you have a history of liver disease.
- you smoke and expect to continue smoking (worsens acid secretion).

Possible Side Effects (natural, expected, and unavoidable drug actions)
Increased serum gastrin levels (clinical significance is unknown).

▷ **Possible Adverse Effects** (unusual, unexpected, and infrequent reactions)
If any of the following develop, consult your physician promptly for guidance.

Mild Adverse Effects
Allergic reactions: Skin rash.
Headache, dizziness, or tiredness.
Diarrhea.
Ringing in the ears (rare).

Serious Adverse Effects
Allergic reaction:
Protein in the urine (rare).
Liver toxicity (rare and of uncertain cause).
Low blood platelets (rare and of questionable cause).

▷ **Possible Effects on Sexual Function:**   None reported.

▷ **Adverse Effects That May Mimic Natural Diseases or Disorders**
Drug-induced liver reaction may suggest viral hepatitis.

Possible Effects on Laboratory Tests
  Liver function tests: increased.

CAUTION
  1. Follow your doctor's advice as to how long to take this medicine.
  2. This drug effectively treats ulcers, but does not preclude the chance of cancer of the stomach.

Precautions for Use
  By Infants and Children: Not indicated in this age group.
  By Those over 60 Years of Age: This medicine may cause dizziness. Use caution until you've seen the effects it has on you.

▷ **Advisability of Use During Pregnancy**
  Pregnancy Category: B. See Pregnancy Code at the back of this book.

Advisability of Use if Breast-Feeding
  Presence of this drug in breast milk: Unknown.
  Avoid drug or refrain from nursing.

Habit-Forming Potential: None.

Effects of Overdosage: Possible nausea, vomiting, dizziness, lethargy, and abdominal pain.

Possible Effects of Long-Term Use: Serum gastrin levels are increased by this medicine, but the clinical significance is not known. Presently, it is indicated for a maximum of two 8 week courses in erosive esophagitis.

Suggested Periodic Examinations While Taking This Drug (at physician's discretion)
  Complete blood counts, liver function tests.

▷ **While Taking This Drug, Observe the Following**
  Foods: Lansoprazole is best taken on an empty stomach. Please follow your doctor's instructions regarding the types of foods you eat.
  Beverages: No restrictions.
▷ *Alcohol:* No specific interactions, however; alcohol stimulates the secretion of stomach acid and may lessen the therapeutic benefits of this medicine.
  Tobacco Smoking: Smoking does not enhance your health and is not advisable. Smoking can also stimulate the production of stomach acid and may lessen the benefits of this medicine.
▷ *Other Drugs*
  Lansoprazole *taken concurrently* with
  • sucralfate (Carafate) may decrease the absorption of lansoprazole. Separate doses of the two medicines by two hours.
  • theophylline (Theodur, others) may decrease the blood theophylline level and require dosing adjustments.
▷ *Driving, Hazardous Activities:* Caution. This medicine may cause drowsiness. Limit activities as necessary.
  Aviation Note: The use of this drug **may be a disqualification** for piloting. Consult a designated Aviation Medical Examiner.
  Exposure to Sun: No restrictions.
  Discontinuation: Talk with your doctor before stopping this medicine for any reason. Taking the medicine for a shorter time than needed may result in incomplete ulcer healing and continuation of the original problem.

LEVODOPA (lee voh DOH pa)

Introduced: 1967   **Prescription:** USA: Yes; Canada: Yes   **Available as
Generic:** USA: Yes; Canada: No   **Class:** Antiparkinsonism   **Controlled
Drug:** USA: No; Canada: No

Brand Names: Bendopa, Dopar, Larodopa, ✦Prolopa [CD], Sinemet [CD], Sinemet CR [CD]

BENEFITS versus RISKS

Possible Benefits	*Possible Risks*
EFFECTIVE SYMPTOM RELIEF IN IDIOPATHIC PARKINSON'S DISEASE	Emotional depression, confusion, abnormal thinking and behavior Abnormal involuntary movements Heart rhythm disturbance Urinary bladder retention Induction of peptic ulcer (rare) Blood abnormalities: hemolytic anemia, reduced white blood cell count (both rare)

▷ **Principal Uses**

As a Single Drug Product: Uses currently included in FDA approved labeling: (1) Treats the major types of Parkinson's disease: paralysis agitans ("shaking palsy" of unknown cause), the type that follows encephalitis, the parkinsonism that develops with aging (associated with hardening of the brain arteries), and the forms of parkinsonism that follow poisoning by carbon monoxide or manganese.

Other (unlabeled) generally accepted uses: (1) May have a limited role in treating catatonic stupor; (2) can improve conscious level in coma caused by liver failure; (2) can help restless leg or periodic limb movements in sleep.

As a Combination Drug Product [CD]: This drug is available in combination with carbidopa, a chemical that prevents the breakdown of levodopa before it reaches its site of action. The addition of carbidopa reduces levodopa requirements by 75%, and also decreases the frequency and severity of adverse effects.

How This Drug Works: Levodopa enters the brain tissue and is converted to dopamine. After sufficient dosage, this corrects the dopamine deficiency (thought to be the cause of parkinsonism) and restores a more normal brain chemistry.

Carbidopa blocks an enzyme (decarboxylase) that degrades levodopa before it reaches the brain. This allows a lower dose to have a greater benefit. Products containing carbidopa also have fewer adverse effects.

Available Dosage Forms and Strengths

Capsules — 100 mg, 250 mg, 500 mg
Tablets — 100 mg, 250 mg, 500 mg
Tablets, Sinemet — 10–100 mg, 25–100 mg, 25–250 mg
Tablets, Sinemet CR, sustained-release — 25–100 mg, 50–200 mg

▷ **Usual Adult Dosage Range:**   Initially, 250 mg 2 to 4 times/day. The dose may be increased cautiously by increments of 100 to 750 mg at 3- to 7-day intervals as needed and tolerated. The total dosage should not exceed 8000 mg/24 hours. If the combination drug Sinemet is used, the total levodopa requirement will be considerably less: Someone who has not taken levodopa before (levodopa naive): One 25/100 tablet three times daily. The dose is then increased as needed and tolerated by either daily or every other day dosing of one tablet to a maximum of eight tablets daily. **Note: Actual dosage and administration schedule must be determined by the physician for each patient individually.**

Conditions Requiring Dosing Adjustments
Liver function: Dosing changes are not indicated in liver compromise. This medicine is degraded (decarboxylated) in the stomach, kidney and liver.
Kidney function: Possible urine retention requires that patients with urine outflow problems should be closely watched. No dose decreases needed in kidney failure.

Intestinal parasites: A recent report of large increases in doses needed in patients with Strongyloides stercoralis has been filed. Cure of this intestinal parasite allowed the levodopa dose to be decreased by 33%.

▷ **Dosing Instructions:**   The tablet may be crushed and is best taken with or following carbohydrate foods to reduce stomach upset; when possible, do not take this drug with high-protein foods. Sustained-release tablet (Sinemet CR) may be cut in half, but it should not be crushed or chewed. The last daily dose should be taken before 7 PM in order to avoid problems with normal sleeping patterns. Drug holidays or periods where no medicine is taken are controversial, and not all patients benefit from this approach to therapy.

Usual Duration of Use: Use on a regular schedule for 3 to 6 weeks determines effectiveness in relieving the major symptoms of parkinsonism. Maximal effectiveness may require continual use for 6 months. Long-term use (months to years) requires physician supervision and periodic evaluation.

Possible Advantages of This Drug
The slow-release formulation of Sinemet CR allows a 25% to 50% reduction in dosing frequency. The wearing-off phenomenon and end-of-dose failure seen with standard Sinemet may be reduced or eliminated.

▷ **This Drug Should Not Be Taken If**
 • you are allergic to any of the drugs bearing the brand names listed.
 • you have narrow-angle glaucoma (inadequately controlled).
 • you have a history of melanoma.
 • you are taking, or have taken within the past 14 days, any monoamine oxidase (MAO) type A inhibitor drug (see Drug Classes).

▷ **Inform Your Physician Before Taking This Drug If**
 • you have diabetes, epilepsy, heart disease, high blood pressure or chronic lung disease.
 • you have impaired liver or kidney function.
 • you have problems making blood (hematopoiesis).
 • you are taking medicines for blood pressure.
 • you have had a heart attack and have some abnormal heart rhythms.

- you have a history of depression or other mental illness.
- you have a history of peptic ulcer disease or malignant melanoma.
- you plan to have surgery under general anesthesia in the near future.

Possible Side Effects (natural, expected, and unavoidable drug actions)

Fatigue, lethargy, altered taste, offensive body odor, orthostatic hypotension (see Glossary).

Pink- to red-colored urine, which turns black on exposure to air (of no significance). Gout.

▷ **Possible Adverse Effects** (unusual, unexpected, and infrequent reactions)

If any of the following develop, consult your physician promptly for guidance.

Mild Adverse Effects

Allergic Reactions: Skin rash, itching.

Headache, dizziness, numbness, unsteadiness, insomnia, nightmares, blurred vision, double vision.

Loss of appetite, nausea, vomiting, dry mouth, difficult swallowing, excessive gas, diarrhea, constipation.

Loss of hair (rare).

Serious Adverse Effects

Idiosyncratic Reactions: Hemolytic anemia (see Glossary). Neuroleptic malignant syndrome (see Glossary).

Confusion, delusions, hallucinations, agitation, paranoia, depression, psychotic episodes, seizures.

Low blood pressure on standing (orthostatic hypotension).

Increased blood pressure.

Congestive heart failure (rare).

Mania (rare).

Seizures (rare).

Abnormal involuntary movements of the head, face, and extremities.

Disturbances of heart rhythm, high blood pressure (rare).

Development of peptic ulcer, gastrointestinal bleeding.

Urinary bladder retention.

Low blood platelets (rare).

Low white blood cell count—increased infection risk, fever, sore throat (transient, but may require you to stop taking this medicine until the condition clears).

▷ **Possible Effects on Sexual Function:**   Increased libido reported by both males and females (24% to 36%); inhibited ejaculation (rare); priapism (see Glossary), postmenopausal bleeding (rare).

▷ **Adverse Effects That May Mimic Natural Diseases or Disorders**

Mental reactions may resemble idiopathic psychosis.

Natural Diseases or Disorders That May Be Activated by This Drug

Latent peptic ulcer, gout.

Possible Effects on Laboratory Tests

Complete blood cell counts: occasionally decreased white cells; occasionally increased eosinophils (without symptoms).

Blood thyroxine (T_4) level: increased.

Urine sugar tests: no effect with TesTape; false negative with Clinistix; false positive with Clinitest.

Urine ketone tests: false positive with Ketostix and Phenistix.
Blood uric acid: increased.
Blood potassium: may be decreased.
Blood sodium: may be decreased.

CAUTION

1. Advisable to begin treatment with small doses, and to increase dosage gradually until the desired response is achieved.
2. As improvement occurs, avoid excessive and hurried activity (which often causes falls and injury).

Precautions for Use

By Infants and Children: This drug can cause precocious puberty in prepubertal boys. Watch for hypersexual behavior and for premature growth of genital organs.

By Those over 60 Years of Age: Therapy should start with half the usual adult dose; and dose increases should be made in small increments as needed and tolerated. Watch for significant behavioral changes: Depression or inappropriate elation, acute confusion, agitation, paranoia, dementia, nightmares and hallucinations. Abnormal involuntary movements may also occur.

▷ Advisability of Use During Pregnancy

Pregnancy Category: C. See Pregnancy Code at the back of this book.
Animal studies: Significant birth defects reported in rodent studies.
Human studies: Adequate studies of pregnant women are not available.
Avoid use of drug during the first 3 months. Use only if clearly needed during the last 6 months.

Advisability of Use if Breast-Feeding

Presence of this drug in breast milk: Yes.
Avoid drug or refrain from nursing.

Habit-Forming Potential: None.

Effects of Overdosage: Muscle twitching, spastic closure of eyelids, nausea, vomiting, diarrhea, weakness, fainting, confusion, agitation, hallucinations.

Possible Effects of Long-Term Use: Development of abnormal involuntary movements involving the head, face, mouth and extremities. May be reversible and gradually subside as the drug is withdrawn.

Suggested Periodic Examinations While Taking This Drug (at physician's discretion)

Complete blood cell counts; measurements of internal eye pressure; blood pressure measurements in lying, sitting and standing positions.

▷ While Taking This Drug, Observe the Following

Foods: Insofar as possible, do not take concurrently with protein foods; proteins compete for absorption.

Nutritional Support: If taken alone (without carbidopa), watch for tingling of the extremities (peripheral neuritis). Small (10 mg or less) doses of pyridoxine (vitamin B-6) may help. Larger doses can decrease the effectiveness of levodopa. If taking Sinemet, supplemental pyridoxine is not required. Rare reports of vitamin C (ascorbic acid) decreasing nausea and other side effects have been made.

Beverages: No restrictions. May be taken with milk.

▷ *Alcohol:* No interactions expected.

Tobacco Smoking: No interactions expected.

Marijuana Smoking: Increased fatigue and lethargy; possible accentuation of orthostatic hypotension (see Glossary).

▷ *Other Drugs*

Levodopa *taken concurrently* with

- benzodiazepines (see Drug Classes) may blunt the therapeutic benefit of levodopa.
- bromocriptine (Parlodel) may result in decreased blood levels of bromocriptine.
- clonidine (Catapres) can result in decreased therapeutic benefit of levodopa. Avoid this combination.
- fentanyl/droperidol (Innovar) can cause muscular rigidity.
- isoniazid (INH) may cause flushing, worsening of Parkinson's symptoms and increased blood pressure. Do not combine.
- monoamine oxidase (MAO) type A inhibitor drugs (see Drug Classes) can cause a dangerous rise in blood pressure and body temperature. Do not combine these drugs.
- phenothiazines (see Drug Classes) may result in loss of therapeutic benefits of levodopa. Avoid this combination.
- reserpine (Naquival, others) may blunt the therapeutic benefits of levodopa. Avoid this combination.
- risperidone (Risperdal) can blunt the therapeutic benefits of levodopa. Avoid this combination.
- tricyclic antidepressants (see Drug Classes) may decrease the therapeutic effect of levodopa by interfering with the absorption of levodopa.

The following drugs may *decrease* the effects of levodopa

- chlordiazepoxide (Librium) or other benzodiazepines (see Drug Classes).
- iron salts.
- papaverine (Cerespan, Pavabid, Vasospan, etc.).
- phenytoin (Dilantin, etc.).
- pyridoxine (vitamin B-6).

▷ *Driving, Hazardous Activities:* This drug may cause dizziness, impaired vision and orthostatic hypotension. Restrict activities as necessary.

Aviation Note: Parkinson's disease *is a disqualification* for piloting. Consult a designated Aviation Medical Examiner.

Exposure to Sun: No restrictions.

Exposure to Heat: Use caution. This drug can cause flushing and excessive sweating and predispose to heat exhaustion.

Occurrence of Unrelated Illness: Dark-colored skin lesions should be evaluated carefully by your doctor as they may be malignant melanoma. White blood cell counts should be closely followed if you develop an infection.

LEVOTHYROXINE (lee voh thi ROX een)

Other Names: L-thyroxine, thyroxine, T-4

Introduced: 1953   **Prescription:** USA: Yes; Canada: Yes   **Available as**
Generic: USA: Yes; Canada: No   **Class:** Thyroid hormones   **Controlled**
Drug: USA: No; Canada: No

Brand Names: Armour Thyroid, ✦Eltroxin, Euthroid [CD], L-Thyroxine, Levothroid, Levoxine, Synthroid, Synthrox, Syroxine, Thyroid USP, Thyrolar [CD]

BENEFITS versus RISKS

Possible Benefits	*Possible Risks*
EFFECTIVE REPLACEMENT THERAPY IN STATES OF THYROID HORMONE DEFICIENCY (HYPOTHYROIDISM) EFFECTIVE TREATMENT OF SIMPLE GOITER, CHRONIC THYROIDITIS, AND THYROID GLAND CANCER	Intensification of angina in presence of coronary artery disease Drug-induced hyperthyroidism (with excessive dosage) Spasm of the coronary vessels (rare)

▷ **Principal Uses**

As a Single Drug Product: Uses currently included in FDA approved labeling: (1) Replacement therapy to correct thyroid deficiency (hypothyroidism); (2) treatment of simple (nonendemic) goiter and benign thyroid nodules; (3) treatment of Hashimoto's thyroiditis; (4) adjunctive prevention and treatment of thyroid cancer.

Other (unlabeled) generally accepted uses: (1) Helps amenorrhea caused by (secondary to) low thyroid function; (2) may be helpful in helping fetal lung tissue mature in babies expected to be premature; (3) treatment of Grave's disease.

As a Combination Drug Product [CD]: This thyroid hormone is available in combination with the other principal thyroid hormone, liothyronine, in a preparation (generic name: liotrix) that resembles the natural hormone material produced by the thyroid gland.

How This Drug Works: By altering cellular chemistry that stores energy in an inactive (reserve) form, this drug makes more energy available and increases the rate of cellular metabolism of all tissues throughout the body. Thyroid hormones are essential to normal growth and development, especially the development of the infant's brain and nervous system.

Available Dosage Forms and Strengths

Injections — 100 mcg per ml, 200 mcg per ml and 500 mcg per ml

Tablets — 0.0125 mg, 0.025 mg, 0.05 mg, 0.075 mg, 0.088 mg, 0.1 mg, 0.112 mg, 0.125 mg, 0.037 mg, 0.15 mg, 0.175 mg, 0.2 mg, 0.3 mg

▷ **Recommended Dosage Ranges** (Actual dosage and administration schedule must be determined by the physician for each patient individually.)

Infants and Children: Up to 6 months of age—8 to 10 mcg/kg of body weight, in a single daily dose.

6 to 12 months of age—6 to 8 mcg/kg of body weight, in a single daily dose.

1 to 5 years of age—5 to 6 mcg/kg of body weight, in a single daily dose.

6 to 12 years of age—4 to 5 mcg/kg of body weight, in a single daily dose.

Over 12 years of age—2 to 3 mcg/kg of body weight, in a single daily dose, until the usual adult daily dose is reached: 150 to 200 mcg.

12 to 60 Years of Age: Starts at 0.05 mg as a single daily dose; increased by 0.025 to 0.05 mg at intervals of 2 to 3 weeks as needed and tolerated. Usual maintenance dose is 0.17 mg/day. Total daily dosage should not exceed 0.3 mg. If response is not seen at this level, absorption problems or misunderstanding in taking the medicine should be evaluated.

Over 60 Years of Age: Initially 0.0125 to 0.025 mg as a single daily dose; increase gradually at intervals of 3 to 4 weeks, as needed and tolerated. The usual maintenance dose is approximately 0.075 mg daily.

Conditions Requiring Dosing Adjustments

Liver function: Dosing changes are not indicated in patients with liver compromise.

Kidney function: Dosing changes are not indicated in kidney compromise.

▷ **Dosing Instructions:** The tablets may be crushed and are best taken in the morning on an empty stomach to ensure maximal absorption and uniform results.

Usual Duration of Use: Use on a regular schedule for 4 to 6 weeks determines effectiveness in correcting the symptoms of thyroid deficiency. Long-term use (months to years, possibly for life) requires physician supervision.

Currently a "Drug of Choice"

for the treatment of hypothyroidism.

▷ **This Drug Should Not Be Taken If**

- you have had an allergic reaction to it previously.
- you are recovering from a heart attack; ask your doctor for help.
- you have an adrenal insufficiency which has not been corrected.
- you are using it to lose weight and your thyroid function is normal (no deficiency).

▷ **Inform Your Physician Before Taking This Drug If**

- you have high blood pressure, any form of heart disease or diabetes.
- you have a history of Addison's disease or adrenal gland deficiency.
- you are taking any antiasthmatic medications.
- you are taking an anticoagulant.

Possible Side Effects (natural, expected, and unavoidable drug actions)

None if dosage is adjusted correctly.

▷ **Possible Adverse Effects** (unusual, unexpected, and infrequent reactions)

If any of the following develop, consult your physician promptly for guidance.

Mild Adverse Effects

Allergic Reactions: Skin rash, hives.

Headache in sensitive individuals, even with proper dosage adjustment.

Serious Adverse Effects
> Increased frequency or intensity of angina in people with coronary artery disease.
> Spasm of the arteries which supply blood to the heart (rare).
> Seizures.
> Pseudotumor cerebri (rare).
> Drug-induced porphyria (rare).
> Decrease in IgA immune concentration (rare).
> May be a part of the development of osteoporosis. Bone mineral density testing is recommended.
> Drug-induced myasthenia gravis (rare).
> Note: Other adverse effects are manifestations of excessive dosage. See Effects of Overdosage category.

▷ **Possible Effects on Sexual Function**
> Altered menstrual pattern during dosage adjustments.
> Possibly beneficial in treating impaired sexual function that is associated with true hypothyroidism.

Natural Diseases or Disorders That May Be Activated by This Drug
> Latent coronary artery insufficiency (angina), diabetes.

Possible Effects on Laboratory Tests
> Prothrombin time: increased (when taken concurrently with warfarin).
> Blood total cholesterol, HDL and LDL cholesterol levels: decreased.
> Blood triglyceride levels: no effect.
> Blood glucose level: increased.
> Blood thyroid hormone levels: increased T_3, T_4 and free T_4.
> Blood thyroid stimulating hormone (TSH) level: decreased.

CAUTION
> 1. Careful supervision of individual response is needed to identify correct dosage. Do not change dosing without asking your physician.
> 2. This drug should not be used to treat nonspecific fatigue, obesity, infertility or slow growth. Such use is inappropriate and could be harmful.

Precautions for Use
> *By Infants and Children:* Thyroid-deficient children often require higher doses than adults. Transient hair loss may occur during the early months of treatment. Follow the child's response to thyroid therapy by periodic measurements of bone age, growth, mental and physical development.
> *By Those over 60 Years of Age:* Usually, requirements for thyroid hormone replacement are about 25% lower than in younger adults. Watch closely for any indications of toxicity.

▷ **Advisability of Use During Pregnancy**
> *Pregnancy Category:* A. See Pregnancy Code at the back of this book.
> Animal studies: Cataract formation reported in rat studies. Other defects reported in rabbit and guinea pig studies.
> Human studies: Thyroid hormones do not reach the fetus (cross the placenta) in significant amounts. Clinical experience has shown that appropriate use of thyroid hormones causes no adverse effects on the fetus.
> Use this drug only if clearly needed and with carefully adjusted dosage.

Advisability of Use if Breast-Feeding
Presence of this drug in breast milk: Yes, in minimal amounts.
Breast-feeding is considered safe with correctly adjusted dosage.

Habit-Forming Potential: None.

Effects of Overdosage: Headache, sense of increased body heat, nervousness, increased sweating, hand tremors, insomnia, rapid and irregular heart action, diarrhea, muscle cramping, weight loss, heart attack.

Possible Effects of Long-Term Use: Bone loss (osteoporosis) in the lumbar vertebrae (spine).

Suggested Periodic Examinations While Taking This Drug (at physician's discretion)
Measurement of thyroid hormone levels in blood. Bone mineral density testing

▷ **While Taking This Drug, Observe the Following**
Foods: Enteral formulas for nutrition support which contain soybeans may increase the fecal elimination of thyroxine.
Beverages: No restrictions.
▷ *Alcohol:* No interactions expected.
Tobacco Smoking: No interactions expected.
▷ *Other Drugs*
Levothyroxine may ***increase*** the effects of
• warfarin (Coumadin), and increase the risk of bleeding; decreased anticoagulant dosage is usually needed. More frequent INR testing ("protimes" or prothrombin times) are needed.
Levothyroxine may ***decrease*** the effects of
• digoxin (Lanoxin), when correcting hypothyroidism; a larger dose of digoxin may be needed.
Levothyroxine ***taken concurrently*** with
• antacids may cause decreased levothyroxine absorption and a decreased therapeutic effect.
• all antidiabetic drugs (insulin and oral hypoglycemic agents) may require an increased dose to obtain proper control of blood sugar levels. Once correct doses of both drugs have been identified, a reduction in the dose of thyroid may require a simultaneous reduction in the antidiabetic drug.
• benzodiazepines (Librium and others) can enhance the toxic or therapeutic effects of both drugs.
• conjugated estrogens (Premarin) may require an increased levothyroxine dose.
• tricyclic antidepressants (see Drug Classes) may cause an increase in the activity of both drugs; watch for signs of overdosage.
The following drug may ***decrease*** the effects of levothyroxine
• cholestyramine (Cuemid, Questran) may reduce its absorption; intake of the two drugs should be separated by 5 hours.
• colestipol (Colestid).
• iron salts by decreasing absorption.
• lovastatin (Mevacor).
• phenytoin (Dilantin) can increase levothyroxine clearance.
• sodium polystyrene sulfonate (Kayexalate).
• sucralfate (Carafate).

▷ *Driving, Hazardous Activities:* No restrictions.

   Aviation Note: The use of this drug *is probably not a disqualification* for piloting. Consult a designated Aviation Medical Examiner.

   Exposure to Sun: No restrictions.

   Exposure to Heat: This drug may decrease individual tolerance to warm environments, increasing discomfort due to heat. Consult your physician if you
   develop symptoms of overdosage during the warm months of the year.

   Heavy Exercise or Exertion: Use caution if you have angina (coronary artery
   disease). This drug may increase the frequency or severity of angina during
   physical activity.

   Discontinuation: This drug must be taken continually on a regular schedule to
   correct thyroid deficiency. Do not stop it without consulting your physician.

LIOTHYRONINE (li oh THI roh neen)

Other Names: triiodothyronine, T-3

Introduced: 1956   **Prescription:** USA: Yes; Canada: Yes   **Available as
Generic:** USA: Yes; Canada: No   **Class:** Thyroid hormones   **Controlled
Drug:** USA: No; Canada: No

Brand Names: Armour thyroid, Cyronine, Cytomel, Euthroid [CD], Thyroid
USP, Thyrolar [CD], Triostat

BENEFITS versus RISKS	
Possible Benefits	*Possible Risks*
EFFECTIVE REPLACEMENT THERAPY IN STATES OF THYROID HORMONE DEFICIENCY (HYPOTHYROIDISM) EFFECTIVE TREATMENT OF SIMPLE GOITER, CHRONIC THYROIDITIS, AND THYROID GLAND CANCER	Intensification of angina in presence of coronary artery disease Drug-induced hyperthyroidism (with excessive dosing) Rapid heartbeat Heart attack (rare)

▷ **Principal Uses**

   As a Single Drug Product: Uses currently included in FDA approved labeling: (1)
   Replacement therapy to correct thyroid deficiency (hypothyroidism); (2)
   treatment of simple (nonendemic) goiter and benign thyroid nodules; (3)
   treatment of Hashimoto's thyroiditis; (4) adjunctive prevention and treatment of thyroid cancer; (5) therapy of cretinism; (6) used to help diagnose
   different kinds of thyroid problems.

   Other (unlabeled) generally accepted uses: (1) Can help infertility caused by
   low thyroid function; (2) thyroid replacement of choice in thyroid cancer.

   As a Combination Drug Product [CD]: This thyroid hormone is available in combination with the other principal thyroid hormone, levothyroxine, in a
   preparation (generic name: liotrix) that resembles the natural hormone
   material produced by the thyroid gland.

How This Drug Works: By altering cellular chemistry that stores energy reserves, this drug makes more energy available and increases cellular metabolism in all tissues of the body. Thyroid hormones are essential to normal growth and development, especially the development of the infant's brain and nervous system.

Available Dosage Forms and Strengths
> Injection — 10 mcg per ml
> Tablets — 5 mcg, 25 mcg and 50 mcg

▷ **Recommended Dosage Ranges** (Actual dosage and administration schedule must be determined by the physician for each patient individually.)

Infants and Children: Infants several months old may need 20 micrograms a day. When they reach one year, 50 micrograms a day may be needed. Children more than 3 years old may need the full adult dose.

12 to 60 Years of Age: For mild hypothyroidism—Initially 25 mcg daily; increased by 12.5 to 25 mcg every 1 to 2 weeks as needed and tolerated. The usual maintenance dose is 20 to 50 mcg daily.

For severe hypothyroidism—Initially 2.5 to 5 mcg daily; increased by 5 to 10 mcg at intervals of 1 to 2 weeks. When a dose of 25 mcg is reached, increase by 12.5 to 25 mcg at intervals of 1 to 2 weeks, as needed and tolerated. The usual maintenance dose is 25 to 50 mcg daily.

For simple goiter—Initially 5 mcg daily; increase by 5 to 10 mcg at intervals of 1 to 2 weeks. When a dose of 25 mcg is reached, increase by 12.5 to 25 mcg at intervals of 1 week, as needed and tolerated. The usual maintenance dose is 50 to 100 mcg daily.

Over 60 Years of Age: Initially 5 mcg as a single daily dose; increase by 5 mcg at intervals of 1 to 2 weeks, as needed and tolerated. The usual maintenance dose is 12.5 to 37.5 mcg daily.

Conditions Requiring Dosing Adjustments

Liver function: Dosing changes are not indicated in patients with liver compromise.

Kidney function: Dosing changes are not indicated in renal compromise. Caution is used when increasing the dose of this medicine in those with kidney problems.

▷ **Dosing Instructions:** The tablets may be crushed and are preferably taken in the morning on an empty stomach to ensure maximal absorption and uniform results.

Usual Duration of Use: Use on a regular schedule for 2 to 4 days determines effectiveness in correcting the symptoms of thyroid deficiency. Long-term use (months to years, possibly for life) requires physician supervision.

▷ **This Drug Should Not Be Taken If**
- you have had an allergic reaction to it previously.
- you are recovering from a heart attack; ask your doctor for guidance.
- you have an uncorrected adrenal cortical deficiency.
- you are using it to lose weight and your thyroid function is normal (no deficiency).

▷ **Inform Your Physician Before Taking This Drug If**
- you have high blood pressure, any form of heart disease or diabetes.
- you have a history of Addison's disease or adrenal gland deficiency.

- you are taking any antiasthmatic medications.
- you take digoxin.
- you are taking an anticoagulant.

Possible Side Effects (natural, expected, and unavoidable drug actions)
None if dosage is adjusted correctly.

▷ **Possible Adverse Effects** (unusual, unexpected, and infrequent reactions)
If any of the following develop, consult your physician promptly for guidance.

Mild Adverse Effects
Allergic Reactions: Skin rash, hives.
Headache in sensitive individuals, even with proper dosage adjustment.
Rapid heart rate (tachycardia).
Hair loss.

Serious Adverse Effects
Allergic Reactions: Erythema, bullae, and papules.
Increased frequency or intensity of angina in the presence of coronary artery disease.
Abnormal heartbeat.
Lowering of blood pressure (rare).
Heart attack (rare).
Osteoporosis. Bone mineral density testing is recommended.
Hyperthyroidism.
Drug fever (rare).
Drug-induced myasthenia gravis (rare).
Note: Other adverse effects are manifestations of excessive dosage. See Effects of Overdosage category.

▷ **Possible Effects on Sexual Function**
Altered menstrual pattern during dosage adjustments.
Possibly beneficial in treating impaired sexual function that is associated with true hypothyroidism.

Natural Diseases or Disorders That May Be Activated by This Drug
Latent coronary artery insufficiency (angina), diabetes.

Possible Effects on Laboratory Tests
Prothrombin time: increased (when taken concurrently with warfarin).
Blood total cholesterol, HDL and LDL cholesterol levels: decreased.
Blood triglyceride levels: no effect.
Blood glucose level: increased.
Blood thyroid hormone levels: increased T_3.
Blood thyroid stimulating hormone (TSH) level: decreased.

CAUTION
1. Careful supervision of individual response is needed to identify correct dose. Do not change dosing schedule without asking your doctor.
2. This drug should not be used to treat nonspecific fatigue, obesity, infertility or slow growth. Such use is inappropriate and could be harmful.

Precautions for Use
By Infants and Children: **Not** recommended for treatment of this age group. It must reach the brain and nervous system, and this drug may not do that.

Levothyroxine is the drug of choice to treat thyroid deficiency in infants and children.

By Those over 60 Years of Age: Requirements for thyroid hormone replacement are usually about 25% lower than in younger adults. Watch closely for any toxicity.

▷ **Advisability of Use During Pregnancy**

Pregnancy Category: A. See Pregnancy Code at the back of this book.

Animal studies: No information available.

Human studies: Thyroid hormones do not reach the fetus (cross the placenta) in significant amounts. Clinical experience has shown that appropriate use of thyroid hormones causes no adverse effects on the fetus.

Use this drug only if clearly needed and with carefully adjusted dosage.

Advisability of Use if Breast-Feeding

Presence of this drug in breast milk: Yes, in minimal amounts.

Breast-feeding is considered safe with correctly adjusted dosage.

Habit-Forming Potential: None.

Effects of Overdosage: Headache, sense of increased body heat, nervousness, increased sweating, hand tremors, insomnia, rapid and irregular heart action, diarrhea, muscle cramping, weight loss, heart attack.

Possible Effects of Long-Term Use: Bone loss (osteoporosis) in the lumbar vertebrae (spine). Bone mineral density testing is recommended.

Suggested Periodic Examinations While Taking This Drug (at physician's discretion)

Measurement of thyroid hormone levels in blood.

▷ **While Taking This Drug, Observe the Following**

Foods: No restrictions.

Beverages: No restrictions.

▷ *Alcohol:* No interactions expected.

Tobacco Smoking: No interactions expected.

▷ *Other Drugs*

Liothyronine may *increase* the effects of
- warfarin (Coumadin), and increase the risk of bleeding; decreased anticoagulant doses and more frequent INR (prothrombin times or protime) tests are needed.

Liothyronine may *decrease* the effects of
- digoxin (Lanoxin), when correcting hypothyroidism; a larger dose of digoxin may be needed.

Liothyronine *taken concurrently* with
- all antidiabetic drugs (insulin and oral hypoglycemic agents) may require an increased dose to obtain proper control of blood sugar. Once correct doses of both drugs have been determined, if thyroid dose is decreased, a simultaneous reduction in the antidiabetic drug may be needed.
- estrogens (including birth control pills and Premarin) may result in the need for increased doses of liothyronine.
- monoamine oxidase inhibitors (MAO inhibitors—see Drug Classes) may increase the therapeutic benefits of the antidepressant
- tricyclic antidepressants (see Drug Classes) may cause an increase in the activity of both drugs; watch for signs of toxicity.

The following drug may *decrease* the effects of liothyronine
- cholestyramine (Cuemid, Questran) and perhaps other cholesterol lowering resins may reduce its absorption; intake of the two drugs should be separated by 5 hours.

▷ *Driving, Hazardous Activities:* No restrictions.

Aviation Note: The use of this drug *is probably not a disqualification* for piloting. Consult a designated Aviation Medical Examiner.

Exposure to Sun: No restrictions.

Exposure to Heat: This drug may decrease individual tolerance to warm environments, increasing discomfort due to heat. Consult your physician if you develop symptoms of overdosage during the warm months of the year.

Heavy Exercise or Exertion: Use caution if you have angina (coronary artery disease). This drug may increase the frequency or severity of angina during physical activity.

Discontinuation: This drug must be taken continually on a regular schedule to correct thyroid deficiency. Do not stop it without consulting your physician.

LISINOPRIL (li SIN oh pril)

Introduced: 1988   **Prescription:** USA: Yes   **Available as Generic:** No   **Class:** Antihypertensive, ACE inhibitor   **Controlled Drug:** USA: No
Brand Names: Prinivil, Prinzide [CD], Zestoretic [CD], Zestril

BENEFITS versus RISKS	
Possible Benefits	*Possible Risks*
EFFECTIVE CONTROL OF MILD TO SEVERE HIGH BLOOD PRESSURE	Headache, dizziness, fatigue
	Low blood pressure
IMPROVES PATIENT SURVIVAL AFTER A HEART ATTACK	Allergic swelling of face, tongue, throat, vocal cords (rare)
	Kidney compromise
	Possible lowering of white blood cell counts

▷ **Principal Uses**

As a Single Drug Product: Uses currently included in FDA approved labeling: (1) Treats all degrees of high blood pressure. Mild to moderate high blood pressure usually responds to low doses; severe high blood pressure may require higher doses and the concurrent use of a thiazide or other class of antihypertensive drug; (2) helps improve survival in congestive heart failure; (3) the first drug in this class approved by the FDA to help improve survival and symptoms after a heart attack in hemodynamically stable patients.

Other (unlabeled) generally accepted uses: (1) May be of benefit in slowing or reducing atherosclerosis; (2) helps patients with some kidney problems (nephrotic syndrome); (3) can be of marked help in preventing migraines in some patients.

As a Combination Drug Product [CD]: Combined with the diuretic hydrochlorothiazide to enhance antihypertensive action.

How This Drug Works: By blocking certain enzyme systems, this drug helps relax arterial walls throughout the body and lowers the resistance to blood flow that causes high blood pressure. This, in turn, reduces the work load of the heart and improves its performance.

Available Dosage Forms and Strengths
Tablets — 5 mg, 10 mg, 20 mg, 40 mg
Prinzide Zestoretic — 20 mg lisinopril with 12.5 or 25 mg of hydrochlorothiazide

▷ **Recommended Dosage Ranges** (Actual dosage and administration schedule must be determined by the physician for each patient individually.)

Infants and Children: Dosage not established.

12 to 60 Years of Age: Initially 10 mg once daily for those not taking a diuretic; 5 mg once daily for those taking a diuretic. Usual maintenance dose is 20 to 40 mg/day taken in a single dose. Maximum total daily dosage is 80 mg. After a heart attack in patients who are hemodynamically stable: 5 milligrams may be given within 24 hours after symptoms started. If this dose is tolerated, a repeat dose is given 24 hours later and then increased to 10 mg a day. Therapy continues for at least 6 weeks.

Over 60 Years of Age: Exercise tolerance was improved by 2.5 to 20 mg daily. Any needed dose increases should be made at longer intervals between adjustments.

Conditions Requiring Dosing Adjustments

Liver function: The liver is minimally involved in the elimination of this drug.

Kidney function: Patients with moderate kidney failure should be started on 5 mg daily. In severe kidney failure, the patient can be given 2.5 mg of lisinopril daily. Contraindicated in kidney blood flow problems (renal artery stenosis).

▷ **Dosing Instructions:** The tablet may be crushed and taken on an empty stomach or with food, at same time each day.

Usual Duration of Use: Use on a regular schedule for several weeks determines effectiveness in controlling high blood pressure. The proper treatment of high blood pressure usually requires the long-term use of effective medications.

Possible Advantages of This Drug
Controls blood pressure effectively with one daily dose.
Relatively low incidence of adverse effects.
No adverse influence on asthma, cholesterol blood levels or diabetes.
Sudden withdrawal does not result in a rapid increase in blood pressure.

▷ **This Drug Should Not Be Taken If**
• you have had an allergic reaction to it previously.
• you currently have a blood cell or bone marrow disorder.
• you are pregnant.
• you have an abnormally high level of blood potassium.

▷ **Inform Your Physician Before Taking This Drug If**
• you have a history of kidney disease or impaired kidney function.
• you have Myasthenia Gravis or a specific autoimmune disease.
• you have scleroderma or systemic lupus erythematosus.
• you have cerebral artery disease.

- you are taking another drug which can suppress the immune system.
- you have any form of heart disease.
- you are breast-feeding your infant.
- you have swelling of the face, glottis or tongue. Call your doctor immediately if this occurs after starting this medicine.
- you have a history of elevated potassium.
- you are taking any of the following drugs: other antihypertensives, diuretics, nitrates or potassium supplements.
- you plan to have surgery under general anesthesia in the near future.

Possible Side Effects (natural, expected, and unavoidable drug actions)

Dizziness, orthostatic hypotension (rare) (see Glossary), increased blood potassium level. Feeling of a scalded mouth has been reported with other medicines in this class.

▷ **Possible Adverse Effects** (unusual, unexpected, and infrequent reactions)

If any of the following develop, consult your physician promptly for guidance.

Mild Adverse Effects

Allergic Reactions: Skin rash (rare), itching (rare).
Headache, fatigue, numbness and tingling (rare), weakness (rare), insomnia.
Blurred vision (rare).
Psoriasis (rare).
Ringing in the ears (rare).
Joint pain with positive ANA titer (rare).
Chest pain (rare), palpitation (rare), cough.
Indigestion (rare), nausea, vomiting (rare), diarrhea.

Serious Adverse Effects

Allergic Reactions: Swelling (angioedema) of face, tongue, and/or vocal cords (rare); can be life-threatening.
Purpura (rare).
Heart attack (myocardial infarction) (rare).
Impairment of kidney function (rare).
Orthostatic hypotension (rare).
Hepatitis (rare).
Bone marrow depression (rare).
Neutropenia (uncommon except in vascular collagen disease or kidney failure).
Abnormal heartbeat (rare).
Hyperkalemia.
Hyperuricemia and gout (rare).
Hyperthermia, arthralgia, and positive ANA titer (rare).
Pancreatitis (rare).

▷ **Possible Effects on Sexual Function:** Decreased libido (0.2%), impotence (0.7%), swelling and tenderness of male breast tissue (rare).

Possible Effects on Laboratory Tests

Blood potassium: increased.
Blood uric acid: increased.
ANA titer: positive.

CAUTION

1. Ask your doctor about the advisability of stopping other antihypertensive drugs (especially diuretics) for 1 week before starting this drug.

2. **Report promptly** any signs of infection (fever, sore throat), or water retention (weight gain, puffiness, swollen feet or ankles).
3. Do not use a salt substitute without your physician's knowledge and approval. (Many salt substitutes contain potassium.)
4. It is advisable to obtain blood cell counts and urine analyses **before** starting this drug.

Precautions for Use

By Infants and Children: Safety and effectiveness for use by those in this age group have not been established.

By Those over 60 Years of Age: Small starting doses indicated. Sudden and excessive lowering of blood pressure can predispose to stroke or heart attack in those with impaired brain circulation or coronary artery heart disease.

▷ **Advisability of Use During Pregnancy**

Pregnancy Category: D during the first three months of pregnancy. D during the second and third trimester. See Pregnancy Code at the back of this book.

Animal studies: No birth defects found in mouse or rat studies. Impaired bone formation found in rabbit studies.

Human studies: May cause fetal or neonatal injury or death. May cause fetal death or injury if used during the last six months of pregnancy.

Advisability of Use if Breast-Feeding

Presence of this drug in breast milk: Unknown.

Avoid drug or refrain from nursing.

Habit-Forming Potential: None.

Effects of Overdosage: Excessive drop in blood pressure, light-headedness, dizziness, fainting.

Possible Effects of Long-Term Use: Gradual increase in blood potassium level.

Suggested Periodic Examinations While Taking This Drug (at physician's discretion)

Before starting drug: Complete blood cell counts; urine analysis with measurement of protein content; blood potassium level.

During use of drug: Blood cell counts; measurements of blood potassium. ANA titer.

▷ **While Taking This Drug, Observe the Following**

Foods: Consult physician regarding salt intake.

Nutritional Support: **Do not take** potassium supplements unless directed by your physician.

Beverages: No restrictions. May be taken with milk.

▷ *Alcohol:* Use caution until combined effect has been determined. Alcohol may enhance the blood-pressure-lowering effect of this drug.

Tobacco Smoking: No interactions expected.

▷ *Other Drugs*

Lisinopril *taken concurrently* with

- acetaminophen may cause increased blood pressure.
- allopurinol (Zyloprim) can result increased risk of hypersensitivity reactions.
- chlorpromazine (Thorazine) may cause low blood pressure.
- cyclosporine (Sandimmune) can cause acute kidney (renal) failure.
- lithium (Lithobid, others) may cause lithium toxicity.
- loop diuretics (bumetanide-Bumex) increases effect.

- NSAIDs (see drug Classes) can cause blunting of the therapeutic effect of lisinopril.
- potassium preparations (K-Lyte, Slow-K, etc.) may cause increased blood levels of potassium with risk of serious heart rhythm disturbances.
- potassium-sparing diuretics: amiloride (Moduretic), spironolactone (Aldactazide), triamterene (Dyazide) may cause increased blood levels of potassium with risk of serious heart rhythm disturbances.

▷ *Driving, Hazardous Activities:* Usually no restrictions. Be aware of possible drops in blood pressure with resultant dizziness or faintness.

Aviation Note: The use of this drug *may be a disqualification* for piloting. Consult a designated Aviation Medical Examiner.

Exposure to Sun: Caution advised. A similar drug of this class can cause photosensitivity.

Exposure to Heat: Caution advised. Avoid excessive perspiring with resultant loss of body water and drop in blood pressure.

Occurrence of Unrelated Illness: Report promptly any disorder that causes nausea, vomiting or diarrhea. Fluid and chemical imbalances must be corrected as soon as possible.

Discontinuation: This drug may be stopped abruptly without causing a sudden increase in blood pressure. However, ask your doctor before stopping this drug for any reason.

LITHIUM (LITH i um)

Introduced: 1949   **Prescription:** USA: Yes; Canada: Yes   **Available as Generic:** USA: Yes; Canada: No   **Class:** Antidepressant   **Controlled Drug:** USA: No; Canada: No

Brand Names: ✦Carbolith, Cibalith-S, ✦Duralith, Eskalith, Eskalith CR, Lithane, ✦Lithizine, Lithobid, Lithonate, Lithotabs

BENEFITS versus RISKS	
Possible Benefits	*Possible Risks*
RAPID REVERSAL OF ACUTE MANIA	VERY NARROW MARGIN OF TREATMENT
STABILIZATION OF MOOD	POTENTIALLY FATAL TOXICITY with inadequate monitoring
Prevention of recurrent depression in "responders"	Infrequent induction of diabetes mellitus, hypothyroidism
	Diabetes-insipidus-like syndrome (excessive dilute urine without sugar)

▷ **Principal Uses**

As a Single Drug Product: Uses currently included in FDA approved labeling: (1) Management of bipolar disorder. Promptly corrects acute mania, and also stabilizes these disorders by reducing the frequency and severity of recurrent manic-depressive mood swings; (2) used to treat mania; (3) helps control mania.

Other (unlabeled) generally accepted uses: (1) May be helpful in chronic hair pulling (trichotillomania); (2) can help prevent cluster headaches; (3) may help control aggressive behavior; (4) can have a role in Fanconi aplastic anemia; (5) could have an adjunctive role in AIDS patients who have low platelet and white blood cells; (6) may help patients who have mood problems which also affects their sex drive.

How This Drug Works: It is thought that lithium changes the way nerve signals are transmitted and interpreted, influencing emotional status and behavior.

Available Dosage Forms and Strengths

> Capsules — 150 mg, 300 mg, 600 mg
> Syrup — 8 mEq per 5-ml
> Tablets — 300 mg
> Tablets, prolonged-action — 300 mg, 450 mg

▷ **Usual Adult Dosage Range:**   First day: 900 to 1200 milligrams per day. This is divided into three equal doses. This dose is then increased as needed and tolerated by 300 mg increments to attain a blood level of 1–1.5 millimole/liter. The usual maintenance dose is 1200 to 1800 mg/24 hours taken in 3 divided doses. The total daily dosage should not exceed 3600 mg. **Note: Actual dose and dosing schedule must be determined by the physician for each patient individually.**

Conditions Requiring Dosing Adjustments

Liver function: The liver is minimally involved in the elimination of lithium.

Kidney function: If the decision is made to use lithium in this patient population, frequent and careful monitoring and decreased dosing must be provided. Doses are usually decreased and blood levels obtained more often. In moderate to severe kidney failure (CCl 10–50 ml/min.), 50–75 % of the usual dose is given. In severe kidney failure, 25–50% of the usual dose is given.

▷ **Dosing Instructions:**   The capsules may be opened and the regular tablets crushed and taken with or after meals to reduce stomach upset. The prolonged-action tablets should be swallowed whole and not altered.

Usual Duration of Use: Use on a regular schedule for 1 to 3 weeks determines effectiveness in correcting acute mania; several months of continual treatment may be required to correct depression. Long-term use (months to years) requires physician supervision and periodic evaluation.

Currently a "Drug of Choice"

for the treatment of acute mania in bipolar manic-depressive disorders.

▷ **This Drug Should Not Be Taken If**
- you have had an allergic reaction to any dosage form of it previously.
- you have uncontrolled diabetes or uncorrected hypothyroidism.
- you are breast-feeding your infant.
- you will be unable to comply with the need for regular monitoring of lithium blood levels.
- you have severe kidney failure.

▷ **Inform Your Physician Before Taking This Drug If**
- you have a history of a schizophreniclike thought disorder.
- you have any type of organic brain disease, or a history of grand mal epilepsy.

- you have diabetes, heart disease, hypothyroidism or impaired kidney function.
- you are on a salt-restricted diet.
- you are pregnant or planning pregnancy.
- you are taking any diuretic drug or a cortisonelike steroid preparation.
- you plan to have surgery under general anesthesia in the near future.

Possible Side Effects (natural, expected, and unavoidable drug actions)

Increased thirst and urine volume may occur in 60% of initial users and in 20% of long-term maintenance users. Weight gain may occur in first few months of use. Drowsiness and lethargy may occur in sensitive individuals.

▷ **Possible Adverse Effects** (unusual, unexpected, and infrequent reactions)

If any of the following develop, consult your physician promptly for guidance.

Mild Adverse Effects

Allergic Reactions: Skin rashes, generalized itching.

Skin dryness, loss of hair.

Headache, dullness, joint pain, dizziness, weakness, blurred vision, ringing in ears, fine hand tremor, unsteadiness.

Metallic taste, loss of appetite, stomach irritation, nausea, vomiting, diarrhea.

Edema.

Incontinence.

Increased white blood cells—**not** a sign of infection, but an effect of lithium.

Serious Adverse Effects

"Blackout" spells, confusion, stupor, slurred speech, spasmodic movements of extremities, epilepticlike seizures.

Abnormal fixed eye position (oculogyric crisis).

Abnormal changes in heart rate, rhythm, and wave forms.

Loss of bladder or rectal control.

Diabetes-insipidus-like syndrome: loss of kidney concentrating power, excessive dilute urine.

Abnormal movements (may be a sign of toxicity).

Cerebellar atrophy (rare).

Increased blood platelets.

Inflammation of the heart muscle (myocarditis) (rare).

Abnormal heart rhythms.

Pseudotumor cerebri.

Drug-induced myasthenia gravis or systemic lupus erythematosus.

Low thyroid function.

Abnormally high thyroid function.

Elevated blood calcium (rare).

Elevated blood sugar.

Hyperparathyroidism.

Porphyria (rare).

Seizures.

Inflammation of the parotid gland.

Drug-induced low potassium.

Neuroleptic malignant syndrome (rare).

▷ **Possible Effects on Sexual Function:** Decreased libido (blood level of 0.7 to 0.9 mEq/L); inhibited erection: 30% of users (0.6 to 0.8 mEq/L); male infertility; female breast swelling with milk production.

▷ **Adverse Effects That May Mimic Natural Diseases or Disorders**
> Painful discoloration and coldness of the hands and feet may resemble Raynaud's syndrome.

Natural Diseases or Disorders That May Be Activated by This Drug
> Diabetes mellitus may be worsened. Psoriasis may be intensified. Myasthenia gravis may be induced (1 case).

Possible Effects on Laboratory Tests
> White blood cell and platelet counts: increased.
> Blood alkaline phosphatase (bone isoenzyme): markedly increased in 66% of users.
> Blood cholesterol level: increased.
> Blood parathyroid hormone level: increased.
> Blood thyroid stimulating hormone (TSH) level: increased.
> Blood thyroid hormone (T_3 and T_4) levels: decreased.
> Blood uric acid level: decreased.
> Blood bromide levels: increased.
> Blood calcium: increased.
> Blood glucose: increased.
> Blood potassium level: increased or decreased.

CAUTION
> 1. The blood level of drug required to be effective is quite close to the level that can cause toxic effects. Periodic measurements of blood lithium levels are mandatory for appropriate adjustments of dosage. Follow instructions exactly regarding drug dosage and periodic blood tests.
> 2. Lithium should be stopped at the first signs of toxicity: drowsiness, sluggishness, unsteadiness, tremor, muscle twitching, vomiting or diarrhea.
> 3. The major causes of lithium toxicity are
>   • accidental overdose (may be due to inadequate blood level checks).
>   • impaired kidney function.
>   • salt restriction.
>   • inadequate fluid intake, dehydration.
>   • concurrent use of diuretics.
>   • intercurrent illness.
>   • childbirth (rapid decrease in kidney clearance of lithium).
>   • initiation of treatment with a new drug.
> 4. Over-the-counter preparations that contain iodides (some cough products and vitamin-mineral supplements) should be avoided because of the added antithyroid effect when taken with lithium.

Precautions for Use
> *By Infants and Children:* Safety and effectiveness for those under 12 years of age not established. Follow physician's instructions exactly.
> *By Those over 60 Years of Age:* Treatment should start with a "test" dose of 75 to 150 mg daily. Observe closely for early indications of toxic effects, especially if on a low-salt diet and using diuretics. Increased risk of Parkinsonian reactions (abnormal gait and movements); coma can develop without warning symptoms.

▷ **Advisability of Use During Pregnancy**
> *Pregnancy Category:* D. See Pregnancy Code at the back of this book.
> Animal studies: Cleft palate reported in mice; eye, ear and palate defects reported in rats.

Human studies: Adequate studies of pregnant women are not available. However, cardiovascular defects and goiter in newborn infants (of mothers using lithium) have been reported. If the infant's blood level of lithium approaches the toxic range before delivery, the newborn may suffer the "floppy infant" syndrome: weakness, lethargy, unresponsiveness, low body temperature, weak cry and poor feeding ability.

Avoid use of drug during the first 3 months. Use only if clearly necessary during the last 6 months. Monitor mother's blood lithium levels carefully to avoid possible toxicity.

Advisability of Use if Breast-Feeding
Presence of this drug in breast milk: Yes, in significant amounts.
Avoid drug or refrain from nursing.

Habit-Forming Potential: None.

Effects of Overdosage: Drowsiness, weakness, lack of coordination, nausea, vomiting, diarrhea, muscle spasms, blurred vision, dizziness, staggering gait, slurred speech, confusion, stupor, coma, seizures.

Possible Effects of Long-Term Use: Hypothyroidism (5%), goiter, reduced sugar tolerance, diabetes insipiduslike syndrome, serious kidney damage.

Suggested Periodic Examinations While Taking This Drug (at physician's discretion)
Regular determinations of blood lithium levels are absolutely essential.
Time to sample blood for lithium level: 12 hours after evening dose, or in the morning, just before next dose.
Recommended therapeutic range: 0.8 to 1.5 mEq/L acute and 0.6 to 1.2 maintenance.
Periodic evaluation of thyroid gland size and function.
Complete blood cell counts; kidney function tests.

▷ **While Taking This Drug, Observe the Following**
Foods: Maintain a normal diet; **do not** restrict your use of salt.
Beverages: No restrictions. Drink at least 8 to 12 glasses of liquids/24 hours. This drug may be taken with milk.
▷ *Alcohol:* Used with caution. May have an increased intoxicating effect. Avoid alcohol completely if any symptoms of lithium toxicity develop.
Tobacco Smoking: When taking lithium may increase sensitivity to nicotine.
Marijuana Smoking: Possible increase in apathy, lethargy, drowsiness or sluggishness; accentuation of lithium-induced tremor; possible increased risk of precipitating psychotic behavior.
▷ *Other Drugs*
Lithium may *increase* the effects of
• tricyclic antidepressants (see Drug Classes).
Lithium *taken concurrently* with
• ACE inhibitors such as captopril (Capoten) may increase lithium levels by as much as three times the level prior to combination therapy.
• calcium channel blockers such as Diltiazem (see Drug Classes) may cause neurotoxicity or psychosis.
• carbamazepine (Tegretol) may result in neurotoxicity.
• chlorpromazine (Thorazine, etc.), and other phenothiazines (see Drug Classes) may result in decreased lithium or phenothiazine therapeutic effects.

- clozapine (Clozaril) may result in serious agranulocytosis, delirium, and neuroloeptic malignant syndrome. Do not combine these medicines.
- diazepam (Valium) may cause hypothermia.
- fludrocortisone (Florinef) may result in loss of the mineralocorticoid benefits of fludrocortisone.
- fluoxetine (Prozac) may result in neurotoxicity.
- fluvoxamine (Luvox) may result in increased lithium levels and toxicity.
- haloperidol (Haldol) or with other neuroleptics may result in decreased beneficial effects from both medicines.
- methyldopa (Aldomet, etc.) is usually well tolerated; however, it may cause a severe neurotoxic reaction in susceptible individuals. These combinations should be used very cautiously.
- metronidazole (Flagyl) may lead to lithium toxicity.
- monoamine oxidase inhibitors (MAO inhibitors-see Drug Classes) may result in the serotonin syndrome and potential fatality.
- nicotine (Nicorette gum or nicotine patches) may cause supersensitivity to nicotine.
- verapamil (Calan, Isoptin) may cause unpredictable effects; both lithium toxicity and decreased lithium blood levels have been reported.

The following drugs may *increase* the effects of lithium
- bumetanide (Bumex).
- ethacrynic acid (Edecrin).
- fluoxetine (Prozac).
- furosemide (Lasix, etc.).
- indomethacin (Indocin).
- piroxicam (Feldene) or any nonsteroidal anti-inflammatory drug (NSAID-see Drug Classes).
- thiazide diuretics (see Drug Classes).

The following drugs may *decrease* the effects of lithium
- acetazolamide (Diamox, etc.).
- sodium bicarbonate.
- theophylline (Theo-Dur, etc.) and related drugs.

▷ Driving, Hazardous Activities: This drug may impair mental alertness, judgment, physical coordination and reaction time. Restrict activities as necessary.

Aviation Note: The use of this drug *is a disqualification* for piloting. Consult a designated Aviation Medical Examiner.

Exposure to Sun: No restrictions.

Exposure to Heat: Excessive sweating can cause significant depletion of salt and water and resultant lithium toxicity. Avoid sauna baths.

Occurrence of Unrelated Illness: Fever, sweating, vomiting or diarrhea can result in significant alterations of blood and tissue lithium concentrations. Close monitoring of your physical condition and blood lithium levels is needed to prevent serious toxicity.

Discontinuation: Sudden discontinuation does not cause withdrawal symptoms. Avoid premature discontinuation; some individuals may require continual treatment for up to a year to achieve maximal response. Discontinuation by "responders" may result in recurrence of either mania or depression. Lithium should be discontinued if symptoms of brain toxicity appear or if an uncorrectable diabetes insipiduslike syndrome develops.

LOMEFLOXACIN (loh me FLOX a sin)

Introduced: 1992   **Prescription:** USA: Yes   **Available as Generic:**
USA: No   **Class:** Anti-infective, fluoroquinolone   **Controlled Drug:** USA:
No

Brand Name: Maxaquin

Warning: Reports are being made for some drugs in this class which find tendon rupture as a rare adverse effect. Ask your doctor about limits on strenuous exercise while you are taking this medicine. A rare idiosyncratic reaction has also been reported which presents as mental confusion and disorientation. Use of this medicine after head trauma may be a risk factor. If you have suffered a fall, ask your doctor if a medicine in a different antibiotic class should be substituted. If you are taking this drug and notice a change in your thinking, call your doctor.

BENEFITS versus RISKS

Possible Benefits	*Possible Risks*
HIGHLY EFFECTIVE TREATMENT FOR SOME INFECTIONS OF THE LOWER RESPIRATORY AND URINARY TRACTS	Rare but serious allergic reactions
	Rare seizures
	Neurological reactions (rare)
	Tendon rupture (rare)
Effective prevention of postoperative infection of the lower urinary tract	Headache, dizziness, nausea, diarrhea

---

▷ **Principal Uses**

As a Single Drug Product: Uses currently included in FDA approved labeling: Used primarily to treat responsive infections (in adults) of: (1) the lower respiratory tract (lungs and bronchial tubes); (2) the urinary tract (kidneys, bladder, urethra). Also used to prevent post-operative infection following transurethral surgical procedures.

Other (unlabeled) generally accepted uses: (1) Limited use in dermatologic infections.

How This Drug Works: By blocking the bacterial enzyme DNA gyrase (which is required for DNA synthesis and cell reproduction), this drug arrests bacterial growth (in low concentrations) and destroys bacteria (in high concentrations).

Available Dosage Forms and Strengths

Tablets — 400 mg

▷ **Recommended Dosage Ranges** (Actual dosage and administration schedule must be determined by the physician for each patient individually.)

Infants and Children: Use not recommended.

18 to 60 Years of Age: For bronchitis—400 mg daily for 10 days.

For bladder infections (cystitis)—400 mg daily for 10 days.

For complicated urinary tract infections—400 mg daily for 14 days.

For preoperative prevention of urinary tract infection—400 mg (single dose) taken 2 to 6 hours before surgery.

Over 60 Years of Age: Same as 18 to 60 years of age.

Conditions Requiring Dosing Adjustments

Liver function: No changes in dosing are indicated in patients with compromised livers.

Kidney function: Patients with mild to moderate kidney failure can be given a 400 mg loading dose to be followed by 200 mg daily. The same doses and less frequent dosing should be used in severe kidney failure.

▷ **Dosing Instructions:** The tablet may be crushed and taken without regard to food. Drink fluids liberally during the entire course of treatment. Avoid antacids containing aluminum or magnesium and supplements containing iron or zinc for 2 hours before and after dosing.

Usual Duration of Use: Use on a regular schedule for up to 10 days determines effectiveness in eradicating infection. The drug should be continued for at least 2 days after all indications of infection have disappeared.

Possible Advantages of This Drug

Broad spectrum of antibacterial activity.

No significant effect on kidney function.

▷ **This Drug Should Not Be Taken If**

- you have had an allergic reaction to it previously.
- you are pregnant or breast-feeding.
- you have a seizure disorder that is not adequately controlled.
- it is prescribed for a person under 18 years of age.

▷ **Inform Your Physician Before Taking This Drug If**

- you are allergic to cinoxacin (Cinobac), nalidixic acid (NegGram), ciprofloxacin (Cipro), norfloxacin (Noroxin), ofloxacin (Floxin), or other related quinolone drugs.
- you have a seizure disorder or a circulatory disorder of the brain.
- you have a history of psychosis.
- you have a history of tendon disease.
- you develop inflammation or pain in a tendon (it is best to stop the drug in these cases). Call your doctor immediately.
- you have impaired kidney function.
- you are taking any form of probenecid, sucralfate, antacids or warfarin.

Possible Side Effects (natural, expected, and unavoidable drug actions)

Superinfections (see Glossary): yeast vaginitis (rare).

▷ **Possible Adverse Effects** (unusual, unexpected, and infrequent reactions)

If any of the following develop, consult your physician promptly for guidance.

Mild Adverse Effects

Allergic Reactions: Rash, hives, itching (rare).

Headache, dizziness, weakness, drowsiness, anxiety, nervousness, insomnia, visual disturbances (rare).

Nausea, vomiting, indigestion, diarrhea (rare).

Serious Adverse Effects

Allergic Reactions: Anaphylactoid reactions (see Glossary).

Idiosyncratic Reactions: Rare and unpredictable central nervous system problems ranging from sleep disorders to extreme confusion to seizures have been reported.

Central nervous system stimulation: restlessness, tremor, hallucinations, aphasia, and seizures (all very rare).
Tendon rupture (rare).

▷ **Possible Effects on Sexual Function:**   Intermenstrual bleeding.

▷ **Natural Diseases or Disorders That May Be Activated by This Drug**
Latent epilepsy.

Possible Effects on Laboratory Tests
Liver function tests: rarely increased liver enzymes (ALT/GPT, AST/GOT).
Blood urea nitrogen (BUN): rarely increased.

CAUTION
1. With high doses or prolonged use of other drugs of this class, crystal formation in the kidney may occur. This can be prevented by drinking large amounts of water, up to 2 quarts/24 hours.
2. May decrease the formation of saliva and predispose to dental cavities or gum disease. Consult your dentist if dry mouth persists.
3. If a skin rash, hives or other indications of allergy develop, stop this drug and inform your physician promptly.
4. Avoid the use of iron and mineral supplements while taking this drug.
5. Experience with a drug in the same class says that it should be stopped immediately at the first sign of lightheadedness, restlessness or confusion. Call your doctor immediately if these problems develop.

Precautions for Use
By Infants and Children: Avoid the use of this drug completely. It can impair normal bone growth and development in immature animals.
By Those over 60 Years of Age: Impaired kidney function may require dosage reduction.

▷ **Advisability of Use During Pregnancy**
Pregnancy Category: C. See Pregnancy Code at the back of this book.
Animal studies: Mild skeletal defects due to this drug were found in rabbit studies; toxic effects on the fetus were shown in monkey studies. This drug can impair normal bone development in immature dogs.
Human studies: adequate studies of pregnant women are not available. However, the potential for adverse effects on fetal bone development contraindicates the use of this drug during entire pregnancy.

Advisability of Use if Breast-Feeding
Presence of this drug in breast milk: Unknown.
Avoid drug or refrain from nursing.

Habit-Forming Potential: None.

Effects of Overdosage: Hallucinations, nausea, vomiting, interstitial nephritis, seizures, precipitation of drug crystals in the kidney, joint and tendon toxicity, cerebellar dysfunction.

Possible Effects of Long-Term Use: Superinfections (see Glossary).

Suggested Periodic Examinations While Taking This Drug (at physician's discretion)
None.

▷ **While Taking This Drug, Observe the Following**
Foods: Food prolongs the time it takes to reach the peak blood level, but the same amount of medicine goes into your body. No restrictions.

Beverages: No restrictions. May be taken with milk.
▷ *Alcohol:* No interactions expected.
Tobacco Smoking: No interactions expected.
▷ *Other Drugs*

Lomefloxacin may ***increase*** the effects of
- warfarin (Coumadin), and increase the risk of bleeding. More frequent INR testing (prothrombin times or protimes) should be carefully followed and warfarin doses adjusted appropriately.

The following drug may ***increase*** the effects of lomefloxacin
- furosemide (lasix).
- probenecid (Benemid).

The following drugs may ***decrease*** the effects of lomefloxacin
- antacids containing aluminum or magnesium can reduce the absorption of lomefloxacin and lessen its effectiveness.
- iron salts.
- sucralfate (Carafate) can impair absorption of lomefloxacin. Take antacids and sucralfate 4 hours before or 2 hours after taking lomefloxacin.

▷ *Driving, Hazardous Activities:* This drug may cause drowsiness, dizziness and impaired vision. Restrict activities as necessary.
Aviation Note: The use of this drug ***may be a disqualification*** for piloting. Consult a designated Aviation Medical Examiner.
Exposure to Sun: This drug may cause moderate to severe skin photosensitivity (see Glossary). Sunglasses are advised if eyes are overly sensitive to bright light.
Discontinuation: If you experience no adverse effects from this drug, take the full course prescribed for best results. Ask your doctor when to stop the drug.

LOPERAMIDE (loh PER a mide)

Introduced: 1977   **Prescription:** USA: Yes; Canada: No   **Available as Generic:** Yes   **Class:** Antidiarrheal   **Controlled Drug:** USA: No; Canada: No

Brand Names: Anti-Diarrheal, Imodium, Imodium AD, Kaopectate 1-D, Maalox A/D, Pepto Diarrhea Control

BENEFITS versus RISKS	
Possible Benefits	*Possible Risks*
EFFECTIVE RELIEF OF INTESTINAL CRAMPING AND DIARRHEA	Drowsiness Constipation Induction of toxic megacolon

▷ **Principal Uses**

As a Single Drug Product: Uses currently included in FDA approved labeling: (1) Control of cramping and diarrhea associated with acute gastroenteritis and chronic enteritis and colitis; (2) used to reduce the volume of discharge from ileostomies.

Other (unlabeled) generally accepted uses: (1) Used in irritable bowel syndrome which has failed to respond to dietary supplements; (2) combination therapy of travelers diarrhea; (3) decreases unformed stools in Shigella diarrhea.

How This Drug Works: This drug acts directly on the nerve supply of the gastrointestinal tract, decreases secretions and helps relieve cramping and diarrhea.

Available Dosage Forms and Strengths

Capsules — 2 mg

Liquid — 1 mg per 5-ml (alcohol 5.25%)

— 0.2 mg per 5 ml (alcohol 4.07 %)

Tablets — 2 mg

▷ **Usual Adult Dosage Range:**   For acute diarrhea: 4 mg initially, then 2 mg after each unformed stool until diarrhea is controlled. For chronic diarrhea: 4 to 8 mg/day in divided doses, taken 8 to 12 hours apart. Maximum daily dosage is 16 mg. Pediatric dosing: NOT recommended for children under two years old. 2 to 5 year olds can be given 1 mg three times a day on the first day (13–20 kg); 6 to 8 year olds can have 2 mg twice daily on the first day (20–30 kg); those 8–12 years old can have 2 mg three times daily (greater than 30 kg). Follow up doses on the next day are 1 mg per each 10 kilograms up the maximum daily doses on day one. If diarrhea persists, call your doctor. **Note: Actual dosage and administration schedule must be determined by the physician for each patient individually.**

Conditions Requiring Dosing Adjustments

Liver function: Dosing adjustments in patients with liver compromise are not needed as half of a given dose is removed unchanged in the feces.

Kidney function: Changes in dosing are not indicated in kidney compromise.

▷ **Dosing Instructions:**   The capsule may be opened and taken on an empty stomach or with food if stomach upset occurs.

Usual Duration of Use: Use on a regular schedule for 48 hours determines effectiveness in controlling acute diarrhea; continual use for 10 days may be needed to evaluate its effectiveness in controlling chronic diarrhea. If diarrhea persists, consult your physician.

▷ **This Drug Should Not Be Taken If**

• you have had an allergic reaction to it previously.

• it is prescribed for a child under 2 years of age.

▷ **Inform Your Physician Before Taking This Drug If**

• you have a history of liver disease or impaired liver function.

• you have regional enteritis or ulcerative colitis.

• you develop swelling (distension) of the abdomen while taking this medicine.

• you have acute dysentery.

Possible Side Effects (natural, expected, and unavoidable drug actions)

Drowsiness, constipation.

▷ **Possible Adverse Effects** (unusual, unexpected, and infrequent reactions)

If any of the following develop, consult your physician promptly for guidance.

Mild Adverse Effects

Allergic Reaction: Skin rash.

Fatigue, dizziness (rare).

Reduced appetite, cramps, dry mouth, nausea, vomiting, stomach pain, bloating.

Serious Adverse Effects
"Toxic megacolon" (distended, immobile colon with fluid retention) may develop while treating acute ulcerative colitis.
Necrotizing enterocolitis (rare).
Paralytic ileus (rare).

▷ **Possible Effects on Sexual Function:** None reported.

Possible Effects on Laboratory Tests
None reported.

CAUTION
1. Do not exceed recommended doses.
2. If treating chronic diarrhea, promptly report development of bloating, abdominal distension, nausea, vomiting, constipation or abdominal pain.

Precautions for Use
By Infants and Children: Do not use in those under 2 years of age. Follow physician's instructions exactly regarding dosage. Watch for drowsiness, irritability, personality changes and altered behavior.
By Those over 60 Years of Age: Small starting doses are needed as you may be more sensitive to the sedative and constipating effects of this drug.

▷ **Advisability of Use During Pregnancy**
Pregnancy Category: B. See Pregnancy Code at the back of this book.
Animal studies: No birth defects found in rat and rabbit studies.
Human studies: Adequate studies of pregnant women are not available.
Use sparingly and only if clearly needed. Ask physician for guidance.

Advisability of Use if Breast-Feeding
Presence of this drug in breast milk: Small, clinically insignificant amounts. Talk with your doctor about the benefits versus risks of using this medicine and nursing.

Habit-Forming Potential: Physical dependence has occurred in monkeys, but there have been no reports in humans.

Effects of Overdosage: Drowsiness, lethargy, depression, dry mouth.

Possible Effects of Long-Term Use: None identified.

Suggested Periodic Examinations While Taking This Drug (at physician's discretion)
Decreased frequency of stools within 48 hours.

▷ **While Taking This Drug, Observe the Following**
Foods: No restrictions. Follow prescribed diet.
Beverages: No restrictions, other than your doctor's recommendations regarding diet.
▷ *Alcohol:* Use with caution. This drug may increase the depressant action of alcohol on the brain.
Tobacco Smoking: No interactions expected.
▷ *Other Drugs:* No significant drug interactions reported.
▷ *Driving, Hazardous Activities:* This drug may cause drowsiness or dizziness. Restrict activities as necessary.
Aviation Note: The use of this drug *is a disqualification* for piloting. Consult a designated Aviation Medical Examiner.
Exposure to Sun: No restrictions.

LORATADINE (lor AT a deen)

Introduced: 1992   **Prescription:** USA: Yes; Canada: Yes   **Available as Generic:** USA: No; Canada: No   **Class:** antihistamines, nonsedating
Controlled Drug: USA: No; Canada: No

Brand Names: ✤Chlor-Tripolon ND [CD], Claritin, Claritin D [CD], ✤Claritin Extra [CD]

Author's note: Some other drugs in this class have some life-threatening drug interactions with some antibiotics and some antifungal drugs. This medicine **HAS NOT** shown the same effect on the heart (in some studies of otherwise healthy young and subsequently older subjects), but does undergo an increased blood level if combined with these medicines. It would appear prudent to decrease the dose of loratadine if it is to be combined with these medicines. Current FDA labeling **DOES NOT** require a warning found in package inserts for some other nonsedating antihistamines.

BENEFITS versus RISKS

Possible Benefits	*Possible Risks*
EFFECTIVE AND LONG-LASTING RELIEF OF ALLERGIC RHINITIS	Headache Mild sedation
EFFECTIVE RELIEF OF SOME ALLERGIC SKIN DISORDERS	

▷ **Principal Uses**

As a Single Drug Product: Uses currently included in FDA approved labeling: (1) Used to treat non-nasal and nasal symptoms of seasonal rhinitis (hay fever); (2) helps ease symptoms of rhinitis; used to treat swellings of unknown origin (chronic idiopathic urticaria).

Other (unlabeled) generally accepted uses: (1) None at present.

How This Drug Works: Medications in this class block the action of histamine, thereby stopping the development of symptoms (which are caused by histamine) such as swelling and itching of the eyes.

Available Dosage Forms and Strengths

Tablet — 10 mg
Repeat action tablet — 5 mg loratadine, 120 mg pseudoephedrine

▷ **Recommended Dosage Ranges (Actual dosage and administration schedule must be determined by the physician for each patient individually.)**

Infants and Children: Safety and efficacy in those less than 12 years old have not been established. Two earlier studies of children 3–12 years old found loratadine to be well tolerated. Children who weighed less than 30 kg were given 5 mg once a day (of the nonrepeat action noncombination product). Those weighing more than 30 kilograms (kg) were given 10 mg (of the nonrepeat action noncombination product) once daily.

12 to 60 Years of Age: A single 10 mg (of the nonrepeat action noncombination product) tablet is taken once daily on an empty stomach.

Over 60 Years of Age: This medicine may be more slowly removed by patients in this age range. Consideration should be given to a lower dose or less frequent dosing if symptoms of accumulation of this drug occur.

Conditions Requiring Dosing Adjustments

Liver function: Patients with liver compromise are given a dose of 10 mg (of the nonrepeat action noncombination product) every other day. This medicine is best taken on an empty stomach.

Kidney function: Patients with moderate kidney failure (CrCl of less than 30 ml per min.) should be given a starting dose of 10 mg (of the nonrepeat action noncombination product) every other day.

▷ **Dosing Instructions:**   This medicine is best taken on an empty stomach.

Usual Duration of Use:

Continual use on a regular schedule for 3 days is usually necessary to see substantial improvement in allergic symptoms. Long-term use (months to years) requires periodic evaluation of response and dosage adjustment. See your doctor on a regular basis.

Possible Advantages of This Drug

Less sedating than previously available antihistamines.

Once a day dosing.

Interaction with certain antifungals and macrolide antibiotics (see Drug Classes) does not appear to cause side effects on the heart or to change the safety profile of this medicine.

Tachyphylaxis or tolerance to the beneficial effects of this medicine has NOT been shown to date.

Currently a "Drug of Choice"

In those patients who must take chronic doses of certain antifungal medicines or macrolide antibiotics. Since there is still a drug interaction which increases the blood level, the dose of loratadine should be reduced if these medicines are to be combined and the patient develops undesirable effects.

▷ **This Drug Should Not Be Taken If**

- you have had an allergic reaction to any dosage form of or any of the ingredients in it previously.
- you are presently being tested (using skin tests) for allergies.

▷ **Inform Your Physician Before Taking This Drug If**

- you have asthma.
- you are at risk for drowsiness or fainting.
- you have a history of a heart rhythm disorder.
- you are taking ketoconazole, itraconazole, fluconazole or macrolide (see Drug Classes) antibiotics. The blood level of loratadine may be increased by these medicines, and decreases in loratadine doses may be prudent if the medicines are to be combined.
- you have a history of liver or kidney compromise.
- you are uncertain of how much loratadine to take or how often to take it.

Possible Side Effects (natural, expected, and unavoidable drug actions)

Dry nose, mouth, or throat.

▷ **Possible Adverse Effects** (unusual, unexpected, and infrequent reactions)

If any of the following develop, consult your physician promptly for guidance.

Mild Adverse Effects

Allergic Reactions: Skin rash, itching.

Headache, drowsiness, or dizziness.

Dry mouth.
Leg cramps (rare).
Tachycardia (rare).
Lowering of the blood pressure (rare).
Serious Adverse Effects
Allergic Reactions: Anaphylaxis (rare).
Idiosyncratic Reactions: Not reported.
Tachycardia (rare).
Abnormal liver function (rare).
Depression, confusion, paresthesias (rare).
Passing out (syncope) (rare).

▷ **Possible Effects on Sexual Function:**   Rare reports of vaginitis, painful menses (dysmenorrhea), breast enlargement, menorrhagia or breast pain have been made. Rare impotence has been reported.

Possible Delayed Adverse Effects: None reported.

▷ **Adverse Effects That May Mimic Natural Diseases or Disorders**
Increased liver enzymes may mimic hepatitis of infectious origin.

Natural Diseases or Disorders That May Be Activated by This Drug
None reported.

Possible Effects on Laboratory Tests
Skin tests for allergies will be blunted and less diagnostic.
Liver function tests: may be increased.

CAUTION
1. This medicine does interact with some antifungals and some macrolide antibiotics—but appears to be free of the heart (cardiac) effects, even though blood levels of loratadine may increase if it is given with these interacting medicines. Talk to your doctor or pharmacist before taking any medicines which were not discussed when loratadine was prescribed.
2. Report dizziness, heart palpitation or chest pain promptly.

Precautions for Use
By Infants and Children: Safety and effectiveness for use by those under 12 years of age have not been established.
By Those over 60 Years of Age: Smaller starting and maintenance doses are needed. Longer dosing intervals may be needed as well.

▷ **Advisability of Use During Pregnancy**
Pregnancy Category: B. See Pregnancy Code at the back of this book.
Animal studies: No birth defects reported.
Human studies: Information from adequate studies of pregnant women is not available.
This medicine should be used during pregnancy only if clearly needed. Discuss the benefits versus risks with your doctor.

Advisability of Use if Breast-Feeding
Presence of this drug in breast milk: Yes.
Ask your doctor for guidance regarding stopping the drug or stopping nursing.

Habit-Forming Potential: None.

Effects of Overdosage: With overdoses greater than 10 mg (40–80 mg): Tachycardia, somnolence and headache.

Possible Effects of Long-Term Use: None defined.

Suggested Periodic Examinations While Taking This Drug (at physician's discretion)
Examination for relief of rhinitis or idiopathic urticaria. Electrocardiogram (ECG), especially for those with heart conditions.

▷ **While Taking This Drug, Observe the Following**
Foods: No restrictions, but food may delay the time it takes to achieve the peak blood level. In a single dose study, food actually increased the amount of this medicine that was absorbed into the body.
Beverages: No restrictions.
▷ *Alcohol:* May cause excessive drowsiness (central nervous system depression).
Tobacco Smoking: No interactions expected.
Marijuana Smoking: Additive drowsiness or lethargy.
▷ *Other Drugs*
Loratadine *taken concurrently* with
- cimetidine (Tagamet) may produce a significant increase in loratadine blood levels. No serious drug effects have been reported, but since in general, the frequency of adverse effects increases with increasing blood levels, it appears prudent to decrease the dose of loratadine if these medicines are to be taken at the same time because of possible loratadine toxicity. The loratadine dose should certainly be decreased if increased frequency of adverse effects occur if these medicines are combined in usual doses.
- ketoconazole (and perhaps other similar structure antifungals) may cause increased blood levels of this medicine. While no serious heart rhythm toxicity has been reported to date with this medicine, caution is advised as other nonsedating antihistamines have been associated with heart problems with this interaction. It appears prudent to lower the dose of loratadine if these medicines are to be combined.
- macrolide antibiotics such as azithromycin, clarithromycin or erythromycin. Other nonsedating antihistamines have been reported to have toxic interactions with these medicines. While no serious heart rhythm toxicity has been reported to date with this loratadine, caution is advised as excessive blood levels of any medicine may increase the risk of adverse effects. It appears prudent to lower the dose of loratadine if these medicines are to be combined.
- quinidine (Quinaglute, others) may result in a change in the effect of quinidine and result in undesirable effects on the heart. There is only one case report of this, but caution is advised.
▷ *Driving, Hazardous Activities:* While it is much less likely than earlier antihistamines to cause drowsiness, caution should be used until your individual reaction to this medicine is determined. Restrict activities as necessary.
Aviation Note: The use of this drug *is probably not a disqualification* for piloting. Consult a designated Aviation Medical Examiner.
Exposure to Sun: Rare cases of photosensitivity have been reported with other medicines in this class. Use Caution.

LORAZEPAM (lor A za pam)

Introduced: 1977   **Prescription:** USA: Yes; Canada: Yes   **Available as Generic:** USA: Yes; Canada: Yes   **Class:** Mild tranquilizer, benzodiazepines
Controlled Drug: USA: C-IV*; Canada: No

Brand Names: ✦Apo-Lorazepam, Ativan, Lorazepam Intensol, ✦Novo-Loraze-pam, ✦Nu-Loraz

---

BENEFITS versus RISKS

Possible Benefits	*Possible Risks*
RELIEF OF ANXIETY AND NERVOUS TENSION	Habit-forming potential with prolonged use
NOT CHANGED SIGNIFICANTLY INTO ACTIVE DRUG FORMS IN THE LIVER	Minor impairment of mental functions
Wide margin of safety with therapeutic doses	Very rare blood cell disorders
	Very rare movement disorders
	Very rare liver disorders
	Dose-related respiratory depression
	Withdrawal symptoms if abruptly stopped

▷ **Principal Uses**

As a Single Drug Product: Uses currently included in FDA approved labeling: (1) Helps treat anxiety; (2) used to relieve insomnia; (3) used in surgical cases to help in delivering effective anesthesia; (4) used intravenously as a sedative.

Other (unlabeled) generally accepted uses: (1) Used to help prevent the severe symptoms of alcohol detoxification (Delirium tremens or DTs); (2) used under the tongue to treat serial seizures in children; (3) can be used to promote amnesia in patients who must take chemotherapy and have suffered vomiting.

How This Drug Works: This drug attaches to a specific site (GABA-A receptor) in the brain and enables gamma-aminobutyric acid to inhibit activity of nervous tissue. Drugs in this class also reduce the time it takes to fall asleep and the number of times people awaken during the night.

Available Dosage Forms and Strengths

Tablet — 0.5 mg, 1 mg, 2 mg
Sublingual tablet — 0.5 mg, 1 mg, 2 mg
Oral Solution — 2 mg per ml
Injection — 2 mg, 4 mg per ml

▷ **Recommended Dosage Ranges (Actual dose and dosing schedule must be determined by the physician for each patient individually.)**

Infants and Children: Safety and effectiveness in those under 18 years of age not established. Has been used in 1 to 4 mg doses under the tongue for treatment of serial seizures in children.

18 to 60 Years of Age: Sedation and anxiety: Therapy is started with 1 to 2 mg per day in 2 to 3 divided doses. Doses may be increased as needed and tolerated

---

*See schedules of Controlled Drugs at the back of this book.

to the usual maintenance dose of 2 to 6 mg daily in divided doses. The maximum dose is 10 mg daily in two to three divided doses.

Insomnia: 2 to 4 mg at bedtime.

Over 60 Years of Age: Sedation and anxiety: therapy is started with 0.5 to 1 mg in divided doses. The initial dose should **not** exceed two mg daily.

Insomnia: 0.5 to 1 mg at bedtime.

Conditions Requiring Dosing Adjustments

Liver function: The dose **must** be decreased in liver compromise, and the drug should **not** be used in liver failure. Use of the lowest effective dose is recommended in those with mild to moderate liver failure.

Kidney function: The drug should **not** be used in kidney failure. In mild to moderate kidney compromise, the dose **must** be decreased, and the lowest effective dose is recommended.

▷ **Dosing Instructions:** The tablet may be crushed and taken on an empty stomach or with milk or food. Do **not** stop this drug abruptly if it has been taken for more than 4 weeks.

Usual Duration of Use:

Use on a regular schedule for 3 to 5 days usually determines effectiveness in relieving moderate anxiety or insomnia. Continual use should be limited to 1 to 3 weeks. Consult your physician on a regular basis.

Possible Advantages of This Drug

More direct elimination and lack of active forms may be of benefit in the elderly. Increased lipid solubility is of benefit when the drug is used to treat acute alcohol withdrawal.

▷ **This Drug Should Not Be Taken If**
- you have had an allergic reaction to any dosage form of it or any component of the dosage form previously.
- you have a primary depression or psychosis.
- you have excessively low blood pressure.
- you have narrow-angle glaucoma.

▷ **Inform Your Physician Before Taking This Drug If**
- you are allergic to any benzodiazepine (see Drug Classes).
- you have a history of alcoholism or drug abuse.
- you are prone to respiratory depression.
- you are pregnant or planning pregnancy.
- you have impaired liver or kidney function.
- you have a history of low white blood cell counts.
- you have: asthma, emphysema, epilepsy or myasthenia gravis.
- you take other prescription or nonprescription medicines which were not discussed with your doctor when lorazepam was prescribed.

Possible Side Effects (natural, expected, and unavoidable drug actions)

Sedation, dizziness, unsteadiness, "hangover" effects on the day following bedtime use.

▷ **Possible Adverse Effects** (unusual, unexpected, and infrequent reactions)
If any of the following develop, consult your physician promptly for guidance.

Mild Adverse Effects

Allergic Reactions: Rashes (rare), hives.

Dizziness, insomnia, fainting, confusion, blurred vision, slurred speech, constipation, and sweating.

Amnesia.

Sedation.

Ringing in the ears (associated with withdrawal), decreased hearing ability (infrequent).

Serious Adverse Effects

Allergic Reactions: Liver damage with jaundice (see Glossary) (rare).

Low white blood cell counts (leukopenia—rare).

Paradoxical excitement and rage (rare).

Low blood pressure (rare).

Hallucinations (1% and transient).

Porphyria (rare).

Respiratory depression (dose-related).

Abnormal body movements (rare).

Seizures (rare).

▷ **Possible Effects on Sexual Function:**   Extremely rare decreased male libido or impotence.

Possible Effects on Laboratory Tests

White blood cell counts: decreased.

Liver function tests: increased SGPT, SGOT and LDH.

CAUTION

1. This drug should **not** be stopped abruptly if it has been taken continually for more than 4 weeks.
2. Some over-the-counter medications containing antihistamines can cause excessive sedation if taken with lorazepam.
3. Lorazepam should **not** be combined with alcohol. This combination will worsen adverse mental and coordination decreases, and increase lorazepam levels.

Precautions for Use

By Infants and Children: Safety and effectiveness for those under 18 years of age not established. Lorazepam has been used under the tongue in children with serial seizures.

By Those over 60 Years of Age: Small doses are indicated. Watch for lethargy, fatigue, weakness and paradoxical agitation, anger, hostility and rage.

▷ **Advisability of Use During Pregnancy**

Pregnancy Category: D. See Pregnancy Code at the back of this book.

Animal studies: Cleft palate has been reported in mice; skeletal defects in rats with similar drugs in this class.

Human studies: Adequate studies of pregnant women are not available.

Frequent use in late pregnancy can result in "floppy infant" syndrome in the newborn: Weakness, lethargy, depressed breathing and low body temperature.

Avoid use during the entire pregnancy

Advisability of Use if Breast-Feeding

Presence of this drug in breast milk: Yes.

Avoid drug or refrain from nursing.

Habit-Forming Potential: This drug can cause psychological and/or physical dependence (see Glossary).

Effects of Overdosage: Marked drowsiness, weakness, feeling of drunkenness, staggering gait, depression of breathing, stupor progressing to coma.

Possible Effects of Long-Term Use: Psychological or physical dependence, rare liver toxicity.

Suggested Periodic Examinations While Taking This Drug (at physician's discretion)
Liver function tests and complete blood cell counts.

▷ **While Taking This Drug, Observe the Following**
Foods: No restrictions.
Beverages: Avoid excessive caffeine-containing beverages: coffee, tea and cola.
▷   *Alcohol:* Avoid this combination. Alcohol increases depression of mental function, further worsens coordination and causes increased lorazepam levels.
Tobacco Smoking: Heavy smoking may reduce the calming action of this drug.
Marijuana Smoking: Additive drowsiness, and impaired physical performance.
▷   *Other Drugs*
Lorazepam **taken concurrently** with
- clozapine (Clozaril) may result in marked sedation and muscular incoordination.
- heparin may result in increased effects of lorazepam (increased free fraction).
- lithium (Lithobid, others) may result in a lowering of body temperature (hypothermic reaction).
- oxycodone (Percocet, others) and other central nervous system depressants may result in additive CNS or respiratory depression.
- phenytoin (Dilantin) may result in altered phenytoin or lorazepam levels.
The following drugs may **increase** the effects of lorazepam
- probenecid (Benemid)—and result in a 50% increased lorazepam level. Decreased lorazepam doses or an increased time between doses is indicated.
- valproic acid (Depakene). Decreased doses or an increased time between doses may be needed.
The following drugs may **decrease** the effects of lorazepam
- birth control pills (oral contraceptives).
- caffeine, amphetamines or other stimulants.
- theophylline (Theodur, others).
▷   *Driving, Hazardous Activities:* This drug can impair alertness and coordination. Restrict activities as necessary.
Aviation Note: The use of this drug **is a disqualification** for piloting. Consult a designated Aviation Medical Examiner.
Exposure to Sun: No restrictions.
Discontinuation: Do **not** stop this drug suddenly if it has been taken for over 4 weeks. Consult your doctor about a gradual tapering of dosage.

LOSARTAN (loh SAR tan)

Other Names: None.

Introduced: 1995   **Prescription:**   USA: Yes; Canada: Yes   **Available as Generic:**   USA: No; Canada: No   **Class:**   Angiotensin II antagonist   **Controlled Drug:**   USA: No; Canada: No

Brand Names: Cozaar, Hyzaar

BENEFITS versus RISKS	
Possible Benefits	*Possible Risks*
EFFECTIVE CONTROL OF HIGH BLOOD PRESSURE	Generally well tolerated
Decreased cough versus ACE inhibitors	

▷ **Principal Uses**

As a Single Drug Product: Uses currently included in FDA approved labeling: (1) Treatment of high blood pressure.

Other (unlabeled) generally accepted uses: May have a role in treating congestive heart failure.

As a Combination Drug Product [CD]: This drug has been combined with hydrochlorothiazide in a new fixed dosage form. The drug is called Hyzaar, and it contains 12.5 mg of hydrochlorothiazide and 50 mg of losartan. The different ways in which these drugs work complement each other, making the combination a more effective antihypertensive.

How This Drug Works: This drug and its active metabolite block the effects of angiotensin II by binding to a specific site (the AT1) receptor. This helps the blood vessels stay more open and thereby controls blood pressure. This drug and its metabolite also block the secretion of aldosterone.

Available Dosage Forms and Strengths

Tablet — 25 mg, 50 mg

▷ **Recommended Dosage Ranges (Actual dosage and administration schedule must be determined by the physician for each patient individually.)**

Infants and Children: Not recommended for use in this age group.

18 to 60 Years of Age: A starting dose of 50 mg daily is used. If the blood pressure response is not sufficient, the same dose may be divided into two equal doses and given twice daily. The dose may also be increased as needed and tolerated and is then given in two divided doses daily. Consideration should be given to the fact that peak effects may not be seen for 3 to 6 weeks before dosing changes are made. The maximum daily dose is 100 mg.

Over 60 Years of Age: Patients who are dehydrated or who have a decreased intravascular volume should be given 25 mg once daily as a starting dose.

Conditions Requiring Dosing Adjustments

Liver function: This drug is extensively changed (metabolized) in the liver to an active metabolite. The drug is given here as a starting dose of 25 mg. Dosing is then increased as needed and tolerated at weekly intervals. The fixed dose Hyzaar should not be used in patients with liver failure.

Kidney function: No dosing changes appear to be needed. The fixed dose combination Hyzaar should not be used in patients with creatinine clearances (see Glossary) less than 30 ml per minute.

▷ **Dosing Instructions:** Food slows the absorption of losartan, but does not decrease the total absorption of this medicine.

Usual Duration of Use: Continual use on a regular schedule for three to six weeks is usually necessary to determine this drug's effectiveness in controlling high blood pressure. Long-term use (months to years) requires periodic evaluation of response and dosage adjustment. Consult your physician on a regular basis.

Possible Advantages of This Drug
A completely new mechanism of action.
Appears to avoid the cough effect typical of ACE inhibitors.

▷ **This Drug Should Not Be Taken If**
- you have had an allergic reaction to any dosage form of it previously.
- you are pregnant.

▷ **Inform Your Physician Before Taking This Drug If**
- you have a history of liver or kidney disease.
- you have a history of circulation problems in the brain.
- you are breast feeding your infant.
- you have a history of aspirin or penicillin allergy. (Some cases of reactions to losartan have been reported in this population.)
- you have a history of disease in the blood vessels which supply the heart (coronary artery disease).
- you are uncertain of how much losartan to take or how often to take it.

Possible Side Effects (natural, expected, and unavoidable drug actions)
Taste disorders.

▷ **Possible Adverse Effects** (unusual, unexpected, and infrequent reactions)
If any of the following develop, consult your physician promptly for guidance.
Mild Adverse Effects
Allergic Reactions: Skin rash.
Dizziness or insomnia (infrequent).
Fatigue or muscle cramps.
Sleep disturbances.
Nausea and headache.
Serious Adverse Effects
Allergic Reactions: Not defined.
Swelling of the face and lips (angioedema) (rare).
Migraine headaches (rare).
Gout (rare and of questionable cause).
Liver toxicity (rare).
Dose-related increase in blood potassium (hyperkalemia).
Anemia (rare and of minimal clinical significance).

▷ **Possible Effects on Sexual Function:** Decreased libido, impotence (both rare and of questionable causation).

Possible Delayed Adverse Effects: None reported.

▷ **Adverse Effects That May Mimic Natural Diseases or Disorders**
Increases in liver function tests may mimic infectious hepatitis.

Natural Diseases or Disorders That May Be Activated by This Drug
None reported.

Possible Effects on Laboratory Tests
Liver function tests: increased.

CAUTION
1. This drug should **not** be taken in pregnancy.

Precautions for Use
By Infants and Children: Safety and effectiveness for use by those under 18 years of age have not been established.

By Those over 60 Years of Age: People in this age group may be more sensitive to the effects of medicines which lower blood pressure. Lower starting doses are indicated in patients who are dehydrated.

▷ **Advisability of Use During Pregnancy**
Pregnancy Category: C in the first three months, D in the fourth month through birth. See Pregnancy Code at the back of this book.

Animal studies: Rat studies have produced kidney toxicity and death in fetuses.

Human studies: Information from adequate studies of pregnant women is not available. If pregnancy is detected, this medicine should be stopped as soon as possible.

Advisability of Use if Breast-Feeding
Presence of this drug in breast milk: Unknown, but expected.
Avoid drug or refrain from nursing.

Habit-Forming Potential: None.

Effects of Overdosage: Severe decreases in blood pressure. Increased heart rate.

Possible Effects of Long-Term Use: Not defined.

Suggested Periodic Examinations While Taking This Drug   (at physician's discretion)
Periodic checks of blood pressure and liver function tests.

▷ **While Taking This Drug, Observe the Following**
Foods: Follow the diet that your doctor has prescribed.
Nutritional Support: Specific measures not indicated.
Beverages: Avoid excessive caffeine intake.
▷ *Alcohol:* Alcohol may intensify the blood pressure lowering effects of this medicine. Ask your doctor for guidance.
Tobacco Smoking: No interactions expected, however, tobacco smoke lessens the oxygen available to your body.
Marijuana Smoking: May increase the blood pressure lowering effects of this drug.
▷ *Other Drugs*
Losartan **taken concurrently** with
• moxonidine (Cynt available in Germany) may result in additive lowering of blood pressure.
▷ *Driving, Hazardous Activities:* This drug may cause confusion. Restrict activities as necessary.
Aviation Note: The use of this drug **may be a disqualification** for piloting. Consult a designated Aviation Medical Examiner.

Exposure to Sun: Caution is advised. Isolated cases of photosensitivity have been reported.

Exposure to Heat: Caution. Excessive sweating (perspiration) may lead to dehydration and to an excessive blood pressure lowering effect of this drug.

Discontinuation: Talk with your doctor before stopping this medicine for any reason.

LOVASTATIN (loh vah STA tin)

Introduced: 1987   **Prescription:** USA: Yes   **Available as Generic:** USA: No   **Class:** Anticholesterol   **Controlled Drug:** USA: No
Brand Name: Mevacor

BENEFITS versus RISKS	
Possible Benefits	*Possible Risks*
EFFECTIVE REDUCTION OF TOTAL BLOOD CHOLESTEROL	Drug-induced hepatitis (without jaundice)
SLOWS PROGRESSION OF CORONARY ATHEROSCLEROSIS	Drug-induced myositis (muscle inflammation)
	Drug-induced stomach ulceration (rare)

▷ **Principal Uses**

As a Single Drug Product: Uses currently included in FDA approved labeling: (1) Reduces abnormally high total blood cholesterol levels in people with Type II hypercholesterolemia. It should not be used until a trial of nondrug methods for lowering cholesterol has proved to be inadequate; (2) recently approved for use in *slowing the progression* of coronary (heart) atherosclerosis in patients with coronary heart disease. It also showed a reduction in the number of heart attacks. Other (unlabeled) generally accepted uses: (1) May help decrease hypercholesterolemia in cholesterol ester storage disease prior to liver transplant; (2) could have a role in helping blue toe syndrome (peripheral atheroembolism); (3) could help lower cholesterol in secondary hyperlipidemia; (4) may help (low dose) in the nephrotic syndrome; (5) could help hyperlipidemia in transplant recipients.

How This Drug Works: This drug is converted in the body to mevolinic acid, which inhibits the liver enzyme that starts to make cholesterol. It decreases low-density lipoproteins (LDL), the fraction of total blood cholesterol that increases the risk of coronary heart disease. This drug also increases high-density lipoproteins (HDL), the cholesterol fraction that is thought to reduce the risk of heart disease.

Available Dosage Forms and Strengths

Tablets — 10 mg, 20 mg, 40 mg

▷ **Usual Adult Dosage Range:** Initially 20 mg once a day with the evening meal. Dose may be increased up to 40 mg twice a day as needed and tolerated. Dosage adjustments should be made at 4-week intervals. Limited data supports low dose therapy where some patients responded to 20 mg as a single evening dose. Maximum daily dosage should not exceed 80 mg. **Note: Ac-**

tual dose and dosing schedule must be determined by the physician for each patient individually.

Conditions Requiring Dosing Adjustments

Liver function: It should be used with caution in patients with liver compromise. 83% of a dose is removed in the feces.

Kidney function: Great caution should be used in considering doses above 20 mg per day in patients with severe kidney problems (creatinine clearance less than 30 ml per minute).

▷ **Dosing Instructions:** Take with food, preferably with the evening meal for maximal effectiveness. (The highest rates of cholesterol production occur between midnight and 5 a.m.). The tablet may be crushed for administration.

Usual Duration of Use: Use on a regular schedule for 4 to 6 weeks determines effectiveness in reducing blood levels of total and LDL cholesterol. Long-term use (months to years) requires periodic physician evaluation of response.

Possible Advantages of This Drug: Recent studies indicate that this drug is more effective and better tolerated than other drugs currently available for reducing total and LDL cholesterol. Its long-term effects are yet to be determined.

▷ **This Drug Should Not Be Taken If**
  • you have had an allergic reaction to it previously.
  • you have active liver disease.
  • you are pregnant or breast-feeding.

▷ **Inform Your Physician Before Taking This Drug If**
  • you have a history of liver disease or impaired liver function.
  • you have had peptic ulcer disease or upper gastrointestinal bleeding.
  • you are not using any method of birth control, or you are planning pregnancy.
  • you have a history of kidney compromise.
  • you regularly consume substantial amounts of alcohol.
  • you have cataracts or impaired vision.
  • you have any type of chronic muscular disorder.

Possible Side Effects (natural, expected, and unavoidable drug actions)

Development of abnormal liver function tests without associated symptoms.

▷ **Possible Adverse Effects** (unusual, unexpected, and infrequent reactions)

If any of the following develop, consult your physician promptly for guidance.

Mild Adverse Effects

Allergic Reactions: Skin rash, itching.

Headache, dizziness (rare), blurred vision (rare), altered taste (rare).

Indigestion, stomach pain, nausea, excessive gas, constipation, diarrhea.

Insomnia.

Muscle cramps or pain.

Serious Adverse Effects

Marked and persistent abnormal liver function tests with focal hepatitis (without jaundice) occurred in 1.9% after 1 year of use.

Acute myopathy (muscle pain and tenderness) occurred in 0.1% during long-term use.

Rhabdomyolysis (rare).

Cataracts were a concern based on some early data; however, long-term information fails to demonstrate any adverse effect on the lens of the eye.

Neuropathy (rare).

Systemic lupus-erythematosus-like syndrome (rare).

▷ **Possible Effects on Sexual Function:** None reported.

Possible Delayed Adverse Effects: Myopathy.

Natural Diseases or Disorders That May Be Activated by This Drug

Latent liver disease.

Possible Effects on Laboratory Tests

Blood alanine aminotransferase (ALT) enzyme level: increased (with higher doses of drug).

Blood total cholesterol, LDL cholesterol and triglyceride levels: decreased.

Blood HDL cholesterol level: increased.

CAUTION

1. Stop the drug immediately and call your doctor if you become pregnant.
2. Promptly report development of muscle pain or tenderness, especially if accompanied by fever or malaise.
3. Report promptly the development of altered or impaired vision so that appropriate evaluation can be made.

Precautions for Use

By Infants and Children: Safety and effectiveness for those under 20 years of age not established.

By Those over 60 Years of Age: Tell your doctor about any personal or family history of cataracts. Comply with periodic eye examinations. Promptly report any alterations in vision.

▷ **Advisability of Use During Pregnancy**

Pregnancy Category: X. See Pregnancy Code at the back of this book.

Animal studies: Mouse and rat studies reveal skeletal birth defects due to this drug.

Human studies: Adequate studies of pregnant women are not available.

This drug should be avoided during entire pregnancy.

Advisability of Use if Breast-Feeding

Presence of this drug in breast milk: Probably yes.

Avoid drug or refrain from nursing.

Habit-Forming Potential: None.

Effects of Overdosage: Increased indigestion, stomach distress, nausea, diarrhea.

Possible Effects of Long-Term Use: Abnormal liver function with focal hepatitis. Studies in rats with 3 to 4 times the human dose has resulted in increases in hepatocellular carcinoma (cancer). The clinical significance in humans is not known.

Suggested Periodic Examinations While Taking This Drug (at physician's discretion)

Blood cholesterol studies: total cholesterol, HDL and LDL fractions.

Liver function tests every 4 to 6 weeks during the first 15 months of use and periodically thereafter.

Complete eye examination at beginning of treatment and periodically thereafter. Ask your physician for guidance.

▷ **While Taking This Drug, Observe the Following**

Foods: Follow a standard low-cholesterol diet.

Beverages: No restrictions. May be taken with milk.

▷ *Alcohol:* No interactions expected. Use sparingly.

Tobacco Smoking: No interactions expected.

Other Drugs

Lovastatin *taken concurrently* with

- clofibrate (Atromid-S, others) may result in a severe rhabdomyolosis.
- cyclosporine (Sandimmune) can cause a severe myopathy.
- erythromycin (EES) and perhaps other macrolide antibiotics (azithromycin and clarithromycin) may result in severe rhabdomyolysis.
- gemfibrozil (Lopid) may cause myopathy.
- niacin can cause myopathy.
- warfarin may result in bleeding. Increased frequency of INR (prothrombin
time or protime) testing is suggested.

▷ *Driving, Hazardous Activities:* This drug may cause dizziness or impaired vision.
Restrict activities as necessary.

Aviation Note: The use of this drug *may be a disqualification* for piloting. Consult a designated Aviation Medical Examiner.

Exposure to Sun: No restrictions.

Discontinuation: Do not stop this drug without your physician's knowledge and
guidance.

MAPROTILINE (ma PROH ti leen)

Introduced: 1974   **Prescription:** USA: Yes; Canada: Yes   **Available as**
Generic: Yes   **Class:** Antidepressant   **Controlled Drug:** USA: No; Canada: No

Brand Name: Ludiomil

BENEFITS versus RISKS	
Possible Benefits	*Possible Risks*
EFFECTIVE RELIEF OF ALL TYPES OF DEPRESSION	ADVERSE BEHAVIORAL EFFECTS CONVERSION OF DEPRESSION TO MANIA in manic-depressive (bipolar) disorders
	Irregular heart rhythms
	Rare liver toxicity with jaundice
	Rare seizures with therapeutic doses
	Low white blood cells (rare)

▷ **Principal Uses**

As a Single Drug Product: Uses currently included in FDA approved labeling: (1)
Relieves spontaneous (endogenous) depression and reactive depressions,
and helps restore normal mood. This drug should be used only when a diagnosis of true depression of significant degree has been established. It
should not be used to treat mild and transient despondency.

Other (unlabeled) generally accepted uses: (1) Adjunctive use in chronic pain;

(2) helps decrease and control bed wetting; (3) may have a role in the combination therapy of bulimia and other eating disorders; (4) can help cocaine craving.

How This Drug Works: It is thought that this drug relieves depression by slowly restoring the nerve impulse transmitter norepinephrine to normal levels within brain tissue.

Available Dosage Forms and Strengths

Tablets — 10 mg (in Canada), 25 mg, 50 mg, 75 mg

▷ **Usual Adult Dosage Range:** Initially 25 mg 3 times daily. Dose may be increased cautiously as needed and tolerated (after the starting dose has been maintained for two weeks) by 25 mg daily at intervals of 1 week. Usual maintenance dose is 50 to 100 mg/24 hours. The total daily dose should not exceed 150 mg. When the optimal requirement is determined, it may be taken at bedtime as one dose. Bedwetting (children 6–14): therapy is started at 10 mg a day and gradually increased as needed and tolerated to 75 mg daily. **Note: Actual dosage and administration schedule must be determined by the physician for each patient individually.**

Conditions Requiring Dosing Adjustments

Liver function: It should be used with caution, and the dose empirically decreased in patients with liver compromise.

Kidney function: Dosage adjustments not indicated in kidney failure. The drug should be used with caution in patients with urine outflow problems as maprotiline may worsen the problem.

▷ **Dosing Instructions:** The tablet may be crushed and taken without regard to meals.

Usual Duration of Use: Some benefit may be apparent within 1 to 2 weeks, but adequate response may require continual use for 4 to 6 weeks or longer. Long-term use should not exceed 6 months without reevaluation for continued use.

▷ **This Drug Should Not Be Taken If**
- you have had an allergic reaction to it previously.
- you are taking or have taken within the past 14 days any monoamine oxidase (MAO) type A inhibitor drug (see Drug Classes).
- you are recovering from a recent heart attack.

▷ **Inform Your Physician Before Taking This Drug If**
- you are allergic or overly sensitive to any tricyclic antidepressant (see Drug Classes).
- you have a history of any of the following: Alcoholism, asthma, epilepsy, glaucoma, heart disease, paranoia, prostate gland enlargement, schizophrenia or overactive thyroid function.
- you have impaired liver or kidney function.
- you are taking an adrenergic blocking agent (talk with your doctor).
- you plan to have surgery under general anesthesia in the near future.
- you have had a heart attack.
- you are nursing your infant.

Possible Side Effects (natural, expected, and unavoidable drug actions)
Drowsiness, blurred vision, dry mouth, constipation, impaired urination. Weight gain and craving for sugar.

▷ **Possible Adverse Effects** (unusual, unexpected, and infrequent reactions)
   If any of the following develop, consult your physician promptly for guidance.
   Mild Adverse Effects
   Allergic Reactions: Skin rash, itching.
   Insomnia, nervousness, palpitations, dizziness, unsteadiness, tremors, fainting, weakness.
   Blurred vision.
   Rapid heart rate (tachycardia).
   Cavities.
   Delayed urination.
   Nausea, vomiting, acid indigestion, diarrhea.
   Increased sweating.
   Serious Adverse Effects
   Behavioral effects: Anxiety, confusion, hallucinations.
   Aggravation of paranoid psychosis and schizophrenia.
   Aggravation of seizure disorders (epilepsy).
   Abnormally low blood pressure.
   Vasculitis.
   Myoclonus (rare).
   Liver toxicity with jaundice (see Glossary).
   Decreased white blood cells (rare).

▷ **Possible Effects on Sexual Function:**   Decreased libido, increased libido (antidepressant effect), impotence, male breast enlargement and tenderness, female breast enlargement with milk production, swelling of testicles.

▷ **Adverse Effects That May Mimic Natural Diseases or Disorders**
   The development of jaundice may suggest viral hepatitis.

Natural Diseases or Disorders That May Be Activated by This Drug
   Latent epilepsy, glaucoma, prostatism (see Glossary).

Possible Effects on Laboratory Tests
   Liver function tests: Rarely increased liver enzymes (ALT/GPT and AST/GOT).

CAUTION
   1. Dose must be individualized. Report for follow-up evaluation and laboratory tests as directed by your physician.
   2. Observe for early indications of toxicity: confusion, agitation, rapid heartbeat.
   3. It is advisable to withhold this drug if electroconvulsive therapy (ECT, "shock" treatment) is to be used to treat your depression.

Precautions for Use
   By Infants and Children: Safety and effectiveness for use as an antidepressant by those under 18 years of age have not been established.
   By Those over 60 Years of Age: Lower starting doses are indicated. During the first 2 weeks of treatment, watch for confusion, agitation, forgetfulness, disorientation, delusions and hallucinations. Reduction of dosage or discontinuation may be necessary. Unsteadiness may predispose to falling and injury. This drug can increase the degree of impaired urination associated with prostate gland enlargement (prostatism).

▷ **Advisability of Use During Pregnancy**

Pregnancy Category: B. See Pregnancy Code at the back of this book.

Animal studies: No birth defects found in mouse, rat or rabbit studies.

Human studies: Adequate studies of pregnant women are not available.

Avoid use of drug during first 3 months. Use during the last 6 months only if clearly needed.

Advisability of Use if Breast-Feeding

Presence of this drug in breast milk: Yes.

Watch nursing infant closely for drowsiness or failure to feed properly; discontinue drug or nursing if adverse effects develop.

Habit-Forming Potential: None.

Effects of Overdosage: Confusion, hallucinations, marked drowsiness, heart palpitations, dilated pupils, tremors, stupor, respiratory depression, deep sleep, coma, convulsions.

Suggested Periodic Examinations While Taking This Drug (at physician's discretion)

Complete blood cell counts, liver function tests, serial blood pressure readings and electrocardiograms.

▷ **While Taking This Drug, Observe the Following**

Foods: No restrictions.

Beverages: No restrictions. May be taken with milk.

▷ *Alcohol:* Avoid completely. This drug can markedly increase the intoxicating effects of alcohol and accentuate its depressant action on brain function.

Tobacco Smoking: No interactions expected.

Marijuana Smoking: Increased drowsiness and dryness of mouth; possible reduced effectiveness.

▷ *Other Drugs*

Maprotiline may ***increase*** the effects of

• atropinelike drugs (see Drug Classes).

• all drugs with sedative effects, and cause excessive sedation.

Maprotiline may ***decrease*** the effects of

• clonidine (Catapres).

• guanethidine (Ismelin).

• methyldopa (Aldomet).

• reserpine (Serpasil, Ser-Ap-Es, etc.).

Maprotiline ***taken concurrently*** with

• amphetaminelike drugs may cause severe high blood pressure and/or high fever (see Drug Classes).

• antiseizure drugs requires careful monitoring for change in seizure patterns; dosage adjustments may be necessary.

• carbamazepine (Tegretol) may increase the level of the carbamazepine (potential toxicity) and decrease the level of the maprotiline (blunting of therapeutic benefit).

• ethchlorvynol (Placidyl) may cause delirium; avoid concurrent use.

• monoamine oxidase (MAO) type A inhibitor drugs may cause high fever, delirium and convulsions (see Drug Classes).

• quinidine (Quinaglute, others) may result in maprotiline toxicity (dry mouth, blurred vision, lowered blood pressure). Maprotiline doses may need to be decreased.

- thyroid preparations may impair heart rhythm and function.
- tricyclic antidepressants (TCAs) may result in increased antidepressant levels and maprotiline toxicity.

Ask physician for guidance regarding adjustment of thyroid dose.

The following drugs may *decrease* the effects of maprotiline

- estrogens.
- oral contraceptives.

▷ *Driving, Hazardous Activities:* This drug may impair mental alertness, judgment, physical coordination and reaction time. Avoid hazardous activities.

Aviation Note: The use of this drug *is a disqualification* for piloting. Consult a designated Aviation Medical Examiner.

Exposure to Sun: Use caution. This drug may cause photosensitivity (see Glossary).

Exposure to Heat: This drug can inhibit sweating and impair the body's adaptation to hot environments, increasing the risk of heat stroke. Avoid saunas.

Exposure to Cold: The elderly should use caution and avoid conditions conducive to hypothermia (see Glossary).

Discontinuation: It is advisable to discontinue this drug gradually. Abrupt withdrawal after long-term use may cause headache, malaise and nausea.

MECLOFENAMATE (me kloh fen AM ayt)

Introduced: 1977   **Prescription:** USA: Yes   **Available as Generic:** Yes   **Class:** analgesic, mild; NSAID   **Controlled Drug:** USA: No

Brand Names: Meclodium, Meclomen

BENEFITS versus RISKS	
Possible Benefits	*Possible Risks*
EFFECTIVE RELIEF OF MILD TO MODERATE PAIN AND INFLAMMATION	Gastrointestinal pain, ulceration, bleeding (rare)
	Rare kidney damage
	Rare fluid retention
	Rare bone marrow depression

Please see the fenamate nonsteroidal anti-inflammatory drug profile for further information.

MEDROXYPROGESTERONE (me DROX e proh jess te rohn)

Introduced: 1959   **Prescription:** USA: Yes; Canada: Yes   **Available as Generic:** Yes   **Class:** Female sex hormones, progestins   **Controlled Drug:** USA: No; Canada: No

Brand Names: Amen, Cycrin, Curretab, Depo-Provera, Premphase, Prempro, Provera

---

BENEFITS versus RISKS

Possible Benefits	*Possible Risks*
EFFECTIVE TREATMENT OF ABSENT OR ABNORMAL MENSTRUATION due to hormone imbalance	Thrombophlebitis (rare)
	Pulmonary embolism (rare)
	Liver reaction with jaundice (rare)
	Drug-induced birth defects
EFFECTIVE CONTRACEPTION when given by injection	
Useful adjunctive therapy in selected cases of uterine and kidney cancer	

▷ **Principal Uses**

As a Single Drug Product: Uses currently included in FDA approved labeling: (1) Used to initiate and regulate menstruation and to correct abnormal patterns of menstrual bleeding caused by hormonal imbalance (and not by organic disease); (2) used in combination to treat metastatic, inoperable or recurrent endometrial carcinoma; (3) treatment of renal cell carcinoma; (4) used as a contraceptive injected into the muscle once every three months; (5) helps dysfunctional uterine bleeding.

Other (unlabeled) generally accepted uses: (1) Used as a part of combination therapy in breast, refractory prostate, lung and ovarian cancer; (2) therapy of endometriosis; (3) used in osteoporosis to help increase bone mineral density; (4) helps abnormal hair growth in women (hirsutism); (5) can help breast pain (mastalgia); (6) used in combination with estrogen to help symptoms of menopause; (7) can be of use in pelvic congestion and Pickwickian syndrome; (8) may help severe PMS; (9) can be of use in male hypersexuality.

How This Drug Works: By inducing and maintaining a lining in the uterus that resembles pregnancy, this drug can prevent uterine bleeding until it is withdrawn. By suppressing the release of the pituitary gland hormone that induces ovulation, and by stimulating the secretion of mucus by the uterine cervix (to resist the passage of sperm), this drug can prevent pregnancy.

Available Dosage Forms and Strengths

Injection — 150 mg (single dose vials)
— 100 mg, 150 mg and 400 mg per ml
Tablets — 2.5 mg, 5 mg, 10 mg

▷ **Usual Adult Dosage Range:**   To initiate menstruation: 5 to 10 mg/day for 5 to 10 days, started at any time; to correct abnormal bleeding: 5 to 10 mg/day for 5 to 10 days, started on the sixteenth or twenty-first day of the menstrual cycle. Withdrawal bleeding usually begins within 3 to 7 days after stopping the drug.

As a contraceptive: Intramuscular injections of 150 mg every 3 months are needed. **Note: Actual dosage and administration schedule must be determined by the physician for each patient individually.**

Conditions Requiring Dosing Adjustments

Liver function: It should be used with caution, and the dose empirically decreased in patients with liver compromise.

Kidney function: The kidneys are not involved in the elimination of this medication.

▷ **Dosing Instructions:**   The tablet may be crushed and taken on an empty stomach or with food to prevent nausea.

Usual Duration of Use: Use on a regular schedule for 2 or 3 menstrual cycles determines effectiveness in correcting abnormal patterns of menstrual bleeding. Consult your physician on a regular basis.

▷ **This Drug Should Not Be Taken If**
- you have had an allergic reaction to it previously.
- you are pregnant.
- you have experienced a missed abortion.
- you have seriously impaired liver function.
- you have a history of cancer of the breast or reproductive organs.
- you have a history of thrombophlebitis, embolism or stroke.
- you have abnormal and unexplained vaginal bleeding.

▷ **Inform Your Physician Before Taking This Drug If**
- you have impaired kidney function.
- you have any of the following disorders: asthma, diabetes, emotional depression, epilepsy, heart disease, migraine headaches.

Possible Side Effects (natural, expected, and unavoidable drug actions)
Fluid retention, weight gain, changes in menstrual timing and flow, spotting between periods.

▷ **Possible Adverse Effects** (unusual, unexpected, and infrequent reactions)
If any of the following develop, consult your physician promptly for guidance.
Mild Adverse Effects
Allergic Reactions: Skin rash, hives, itching.
Fatigue, weakness, nausea.
Acne, excessive hair growth.
Serious Adverse Effects
Liver toxicity with jaundice (see Glossary): yellow eyes and skin, dark-colored urine, light-colored stools.
Thrombophlebitis (inflammation of a vein with blood clot formation): pain or tenderness in thigh or leg, with or without swelling of the foot, ankle, or leg.
Pulmonary embolism (movement of blood clot to lung): sudden shortness of breath, chest pain, cough, bloody sputum.
Stroke (blood clot in the brain): sudden headache, blackouts, sudden weakness or paralysis of any part of the body, severe dizziness, double vision, slurred speech, inability to speak.
Retinal thrombosis (blood clot in principal blood vessel to the eye): sudden impairment or loss of vision.
Drug-induced pseudotumor cerebri.
Pneumonitis, especially in patients who have received radiation therapy.

▷ **Possible Effects on Sexual Function**
Altered timing and pattern of menstruation. Female breast tenderness and secretion.
Decreased vaginal secretions. Infertility.

▷ **Adverse Effects That May Mimic Natural Diseases or Disorders**
Liver toxicity may suggest viral hepatitis.

Possible Effects on Laboratory Tests

Blood total cholesterol, HDL cholesterol, LDL cholesterol and triglyceride levels: decreased.

Glucose tolerance test (GTT): decreased.

CAUTION

1. There is an increased risk of birth defects in children whose mothers take this drug during the first 4 months of pregnancy.
2. Inform your physician promptly if you think you may be pregnant.
3. This drug should not be used as a test for pregnancy.

Precautions for Use

By Infants and Children: Not used in this age group.

By Those over 60 Years of Age: Used selectively as adjunctive therapy in treating cancer of the breast, uterus, prostate and kidney. Observe for excessive fluid retention.

▷ **Advisability of Use During Pregnancy**

Pregnancy Category: D. See Pregnancy Code at the back of this book.

Animal studies: Genital defects reported in rat and rabbit studies; masculinization of the female rodent fetus; various defects in chick embryo and rabbit.

Human studies: In a study of 1016 pregnancies, oral doses of 80–120 mg daily used from the 5th to 7th week of pregnancy to the 18th week was not associated with teratogenic effects. Other data show masculinization of the female genitals: enlargement of the clitoris, fusion of the labia. Increased risk of heart, nervous system and limb defects when used in the second and third trimesters of pregnancy.

The drug is used as a benefit to risk decision in the first three months of pregnancy. Avoid this drug completely during the last six months of pregnancy.

Advisability of Use if Breast-Feeding

Presence of this drug in breast milk: Yes.

Avoid drug or refrain from nursing.

Habit-Forming Potential: None.

Effects of Overdosage: Nausea, vomiting, fluid retention, breast enlargement and discomfort, abnormal vaginal bleeding.

Possible Effects of Long-Term Use: There has been considerable controversy regarding use of this drug and cancer. The most recent large patient studies do not show an increased relative risk that is statistically significant.

Suggested Periodic Examinations While Taking This Drug (at physician's discretion)

Regular examinations (every 6 to 12 months) of the breasts and reproductive organs (pelvic examination of the uterus and ovaries, including Pap smear).

▷ **While Taking This Drug, Observe the Following**

Foods: No restrictions.

Beverages: No restrictions.

▷ *Alcohol:* No interactions expected.

Tobacco Smoking: It is advisable to smoke lightly or not at all.

▷ *Other Drugs*

The following drugs may **decrease** the effects of medroxyprogesterone
- rifampin (Rifadin, Rimactane, etc.) may hasten its elimination.

Medroxyprogesterone **taken concurrently** with
- digitoxin may result in slightly higher than expected digoxin levels.
- tamoxifen (Nolvadex) may result in blunting of the therapeutic benefits of tamoxifen.
- warfarin (Coumadin) may increase the length of time needed to remove the warfarin by up to 71%. Increased lab INR (protime) testing is needed.

▷ *Driving, Hazardous Activities:* Usually no restrictions. Ask your doctor about your individual risk and for guidance regarding specific restrictions.

Aviation Note: The use of this drug **may be a disqualification** for piloting. Consult a designated Aviation Medical Examiner.

Exposure to Sun: No restrictions.

MEFENAMIC ACID (me FEN am ik a sid)

Introduced: 1966   **Prescription:** USA: Yes; Canada: Yes   **Available as Generic:** USA: Yes; Canada: Yes   **Class:** NSAID, mild analgesic   **Controlled Drug:** USA: No; Canada: No

Brand Names: ✤Ponstan, Ponstel

Warning: The use of mefenamic acid beyond one week is **not** recommended.

BENEFITS versus RISKS	
Possible Benefits	*Possible Risks*
Effective relief of mild to moderate pain and inflammation	Hemolytic anemia
	Low white blood cell counts (rare)
	Gastrointestinal pain, ulceration, and bleeding (rare)
	Rare kidney damage
	Rare systemic lupus erythematosus
	Rare pancreatitis

Please see the fenamate nonsteroidal anti-inflammatory drug profile for further information.

MEPERIDENE (me PER i deen)

Other Name: Pethidine

Introduced: 1939   **Prescription:** USA: Yes; Canada: Yes   **Available as Generic:** Yes   **Class:** Strong analgesic, opioids   **Controlled Drug:** USA: C-II*; Canada: No

Brand Names: Demerol, Demerol APAP [CD], Mepergan, Pethadol

*See Schedules of Controlled Drugs at the back of this book.

```
┌─────────────────────────────────────────────────────────────────┐
│                    BENEFITS versus RISKS                          │
│      Possible Benefits                    Possible Risks          │
│   EFFECTIVE RELIEF OF              POTENTIAL FOR HABIT             │
│     MODERATE TO SEVERE PAIN         FORMATION (DEPENDENCE)         │
│                                    Weakness, fainting             │
│                                    Disorientation, hallucinations │
│                                    Interference with urination    │
└─────────────────────────────────────────────────────────────────┘
```

▷ **Principal Uses**

As a *Single Drug Product:* Uses currently included in FDA approved labeling: (1) This potent analgesic is used by mouth or injection to relieve moderate to severe pain of any cause.

Other (unlabeled) generally accepted uses: (1) Used to treat fevers caused by amphotericin-B; (2) can help porphyrias; (3) eases postanesthesia chills; (4) used in sickle cell disease pain.

As a *Combination Drug Product* [CD]: This drug is available in combination with acetaminophen (APAP) to create a dosage form that utilizes two pain relievers, and also reduces fever.

How This Drug Works: Acting primarily as a depressant of certain brain functions, this drug suppresses the perception of pain and calms the emotional response to pain.

Available Dosage Forms and Strengths

Injection — 10 mg per ml, 25 mg per ml, 50 mg per ml, 75 mg per ml and 100 mg per ml

Syrup — 50 mg per 5-ml teaspoonful

Tablets — 50 mg, 100 mg

▷ **Usual Adult Dosage Range:**   Taken by mouth: 50 to 150 mg every 3 to 4 hours as needed to relieve pain. The usual dose is 100 mg. The total daily dosage should not exceed 900 mg. **Note: Actual dosage and dosing schedule must be determined by the physician for each patient individually.**

Conditions Requiring Dosing Adjustments

Liver function: The initial dose should be the same in liver compromise, however, subsequent doses should be decreased by 50% or the dosing interval doubled. Some clinicians report that doses of 25 to 50 mg have produced acceptable effects in some patients with severe liver disease.

Kidney function: Patients with mild to moderate kidney failure should be given 75% of the usual dose at the usual interval. Patients with severe kidney failure should be given 50% of the usual dose at the usual time. **Multiple doses should be avoided** as a toxic (normeperidine) metabolite may accumulate and can cause severe central nervous system reactions.

▷ **Dosing Instructions:**   The tablet may be crushed and taken with or following food to reduce stomach irritation or nausea. The syrup may be diluted in 4 ounces of water to reduce the numbing effect on the tongue and mouth tissues.

Usual Duration of Use: As required to control pain. Current pain therapy often uses timed or scheduled doses to prevent pain rather than treat it. Continual use should not exceed 5 to 7 days without interruption and reassessment of need.

▷ **This Drug Should Not Be Taken If**
- you have had an allergic reaction to any dosage form of it previously.
- you are having an acute attack of asthma.
- you have increased intracranial pressure (talk with your doctor).
- you have an abnormal heart rhythm (atrioventricular flutter).
- you have a history of convulsions or seizures.
- you have a history of kidney failure and multiple doses are scheduled.
- you have significant respiratory depression.
- you are taking, or have taken within the past 14 days, any monoamine oxidase (MAO) type A inhibitor drug (see Drug Classes).

▷ **Inform Your Physician Before Taking This Drug If**
- you have a history of drug abuse or alcoholism.
- you have impaired liver or kidney function.
- you have a history of asthma, epilepsy or glaucoma.
- you are taking any other drugs that have a sedative effect.
- you plan to have surgery under general anesthesia in the near future.

Possible Side Effects (natural, expected, and unavoidable drug actions)
Drowsiness, light-headedness, weakness, euphoria, dry mouth, urinary retention, constipation.

▷ **Possible Adverse Effects** (unusual, unexpected, and infrequent reactions)
If any of the following develop, consult your physician promptly for guidance.
Mild Adverse Effects
Allergic Reactions: Skin rash, hives, itching.
Headache, dizziness, impaired concentration, sensation of drunkenness, confusion, depression, blurred or double vision.
Facial flushing, sweating, heart palpitation.
Nausea, vomiting, taste disorders.
Constipation.
Serious Adverse Effects
Allergic Reactions: Anaphylactic reactions.
Drop in blood pressure, causing severe weakness and fainting.
Disorientation, hallucinations, unstable gait, tremor, muscle twitching.
Slow heartbeat.
Drug-induced myasthenia gravis.
Respiratory depression.
Urinary retention.
Kidney failure (rare).
Seizures, especially in patients with kidney failure who are given multiple doses (normeperidine accumulates).

▷ **Possible Effects on Sexual Function:**   Blunting of sexual response. Retrograde ejaculation.

▷ **Adverse Effects That May Mimic Natural Diseases or Disorders**
Paradoxical behavioral disturbances may suggest psychotic disorder.

Possible Effects on Laboratory Tests
Blood alanine aminotransferase (ALT) and aspartate aminotransferase (AST) levels: increased (natural side effects).
Blood amylase and lipase levels: increased (natural Side Effects).

CAUTION

1. If you have asthma, chronic bronchitis or emphysema, excessive use of this drug may cause significant respiratory difficulty, thickening of bronchial secretions and suppression of coughing.
2. The concurrent use of this drug with atropinelike drugs can increase the risk of urinary retention and reduced intestinal function.
3. Do not take this drug following acute head injury.

Precautions for Use

By Infants and Children: Do not use this drug in infants under 1 year of age because of their vulnerability to life-threatening respiratory depression.

By Those over 60 Years of Age: Small doses initially and slow increases as needed and tolerated. Limit use to short-term treatment only if possible. There may be increased risk of drowsiness, dizziness, unsteadiness, falling, urinary retention and constipation (often leading to fecal impaction).

▷ **Advisability of Use During Pregnancy**

Pregnancy Category: B, D if used in higher doses or for a longer period of time, especially when the baby is due to be born. See Pregnancy Code at the back of this book.

Animal studies: Significant birth defects reported in hamster studies.

Human studies: Adequate studies of pregnant women are not available. However, no significant increase in birth defects was found in 1100 drug exposures.

Avoid during the first 3 months. Use sparingly and in small doses during the last 6 months only if clearly needed as it has clear effects on the breathing capabilities of the infant.

Advisability of Use if Breast-Feeding

Presence of this drug in breast milk: Yes.

Avoid drug or refrain from nursing.

Habit-Forming Potential: This drug can cause psychological and physical dependence (see Glossary).

Effects of Overdosage: Marked drowsiness, confusion, tremors, convulsions, stupor leading to coma.

Possible Effects of Long-Term Use: Psychological and physical dependence, chronic constipation.

Suggested Periodic Examinations While Taking This Drug (at physician's discretion)

Should assess bowel status if prone to constipation.

▷ **While Taking This Drug, Observe the Following**

Foods: No restrictions.

Beverages: No restrictions. May be taken with milk.

▷ *Alcohol:* Opioid analgesics can intensify the intoxicating effects of alcohol, and alcohol can intensify the depressant effects of opioids on brain function, breathing and circulation. Alcohol is best avoided.

Tobacco Smoking: No interactions expected.

Marijuana Smoking: Increase in drowsiness and pain relief; impairment of mental and physical performance.

▷ *Other Drugs*

Meperidine may ***increase*** the effects of

- other drugs with sedative effects.
- atropinelike drugs, and increase the risk of constipation and urinary retention.

Meperidine ***taken concurrently*** with

- cimetidine (Tagamet), famotidine (Pepcid), nizatidine (Axid), ranitidine (Zantac) and omeprazole (Prilosec) act to increase alkalinity of the stomach and may result in increased meperidine levels and toxicity.
- intravenous acyclovir (Zovirax) can result in kidney and nerve problems.
- monoamine oxidase (MAO) type A inhibitor drugs (see Drug Classes) can cause the equivalent of an acute narcotic overdose: unconsciousness; severe breathing depression; slowed heart action and circulation. Can also cause excitability, convulsions, high fever and rapid heart action.
- phenothiazines (see Drug Classes) can cause excessive and prolonged depression of brain functions, breathing and circulation.
- phenytoin (Dilantin) can result in decreased therapeutic effect of meperidine.
- tricyclic antidepressants (amitriptyline, others) may result in worsening of meperidine's respiratory depression side effect.

▷ *Driving, Hazardous Activities:* This drug can impair mental alertness, judgment, reaction time and physical coordination. Avoid hazardous activities.

Aviation Note: The use of this drug ***is a disqualification*** for piloting. Consult a designated Aviation Medical Examiner.

Exposure to Sun: No restrictions.

Discontinuation: Best limited to short-term use. If used for extended periods of time, discontinuation should be gradual to minimize withdrawal effects.

MERCAPTOPURINE (mer kap toh PYUR een)

Other Names: 6-mercaptopurine, 6-MP

Introduced: 1960   **Prescription:**   USA: Yes; Canada: Yes   **Available as Generic:**   USA: No; Canada: No   **Class:**   Anticancer (antineoplastic), immunosuppressant   **Controlled Drug:**   USA: No; Canada: No

Brand Name: Purinethol

BENEFITS versus RISKS	
Possible Benefits	*Possible Risks*
EFFECTIVE TREATMENT OF CERTAIN ACUTE AND CHRONIC LEUKEMIAS AND LYMPHOMAS	BONE MARROW DEPRESSION (see Glossary)
Effective treatment of polycythemia vera	DRUG-INDUCED LIVER DAMAGE
Possibly effective treatment of Crohn's disease and ulcerative colitis	Rare gastrointestinal ulceration
Possibly effective treatment of severe psoriatic arthritis	

▷ **Principal Uses**

> *As a Single Drug Product:* Uses currently included in FDA approved labeling: Combination treatment of (1) acute lymphocytic leukemia; (2) acute non-lymphocytic leukemia.
>
> Other (unlabeled) generally accepted uses: Treatment of (1) inflammatory bowel diseases (Crohn's disease and ulcerative colitis); (2) certain cases of severe psoriatic arthritis; (3) may help in cases of autoimmune hepatitis.

How This Drug Works: This drug interferes with specific stages of cell reproduction (tissue growth) by inhibiting the formation of DNA and RNA.

Available Dosage Forms and Strengths

> Tablets — 50 mg

▷ **Recommended Dosage Ranges** (Actual dosage and administration schedule must be determined by the physician for each patient individually.)

> *Infants and Children:* For leukemia—2.5 mg/kg of body weight (to the nearest 25 mg) daily (roughly 50 mgs for the average five year old), in single or divided doses. If the platelets and white blood cells do not fall, and clinical improvement is not acceptable after four weeks of the induction dosing, the dose may be increased to 5 milligrams per kilogram per day. If there is still not response, some centers give mercaptopurine as 75 mg per square meter on days 29 to 42. This is combined with vincristine, prednisone and methotrexate. Maintenance therapy then occurs as in adult dosing.
>
> *12 to 60 Years of Age:* For leukemia—Induction: initially 2.5 mg/kg of body weight (to the nearest 25 mg) daily, in single or divided doses, for 4 weeks. If the white blood cells or platelet counts do not fall and there is no clinical improvement, the dose may be increased as needed and tolerated to 5 mg/kg of body weight daily. For maintenance, 1.5 to 2.5 mg/kg of body weight daily.
>
> For inflammatory bowel disease—1.5 mg/kg of body weight daily. The dose is subsequently adjusted to keep the platelet count above 100,000 and the white blood cell count above 4500.
>
> *Over 60 Years of Age:* Same as 12 to 60 years of age.

Conditions Requiring Dosing Adjustments

> *Liver function:* Used with caution and in decreased doses in patients with liver compromise. It is also a rare cause of liver hepatoxicity.
>
> *Kidney function:* The dose should be decreased in patients with renal (kidney) compromise to avoid accumulation of drug. It is a rare cause of drug crystals in urine.
>
> *TPMT negatives:* Some patients do not have an enzyme called thiopurine methyltransferase (TPMT). The mercaptopurine dose is decreased by 10% in these patients.

▷ **Dosing Instructions:** The tablet may be crushed and taken with or following food to reduce stomach upset.

Usual Duration of Use:

> Use on a regular schedule for 4 to 6 weeks determines effectiveness in inducing remission in leukemia; continual use for 2 to 3 months to determine benefit in treating inflammatory bowel disease. Long-term use (months to years) requires periodic physician evaluation.

▷ **This Drug Should Not Be Taken If**
- you have had an allergic reaction to it previously.
- you have a solid tumor or lymphoma (this drug is **not** indicated).
- have leukemia that has spread to the central nervous system.
- you are pregnant. (Ask your physician for guidance.)

▷ **Inform Your Physician Before Taking This Drug If**
- you have a history of drug-induced bone marrow depression.
- you have impaired liver or kidney function.
- you are not using any contraception.
- you have gout.
- you are taking allopurinol. (the mercaptopurine dose must be reduced).
- you have inflammatory bowel disease.
- you do not understand the steps needed to dispose of any vomit or urine.
- you have been exposed recently to chicken pox or herpes zoster (shingles).
- you are taking any of the following drugs: allopurinol, probenecid, sulfinpyrazone, anticoagulants, immunosuppressants.

Possible Side Effects (natural, expected, and unavoidable drug actions)
Bone marrow depression (see Glossary).
Abnormally increased blood uric acid levels; possible urate kidney stones, hyperpigmentation of the skin.

▷ **Possible Adverse Effects** (unusual, unexpected, and infrequent reactions)
If any of the following develop, consult your physician promptly for guidance.
Mild Adverse Effects
Allergic Reactions: Skin rash, itching.
Headache, weakness.
Joint pain.
Loss of appetite, mouth and lip sores, nausea, vomiting, diarrhea.
Serious Adverse Effects
Liver damage with jaundice (see Glossary).
Kidney damage: fever, cloudy or bloody urine.
Drug fever.
Pancreatitis (especially in those patients taking this medicine for inflammatory bowel disease).
Gastrointestinal ulceration: stomach pain, bloody or black stools.

▷ **Possible Effects on Sexual Function:** Suppression of sperm production; cessation of menstruation.

Possible Delayed Adverse Effects: Bone marrow depression may not be apparent during early treatment.

▷ **Adverse Effects That May Mimic Natural Diseases or Disorders**
Drug-induced liver damage may suggest viral hepatitis.

Natural Diseases or Disorders That May Be Activated by This Drug
Latent gout, peptic ulcer disease, inflammatory bowel disease.

Possible Effects on Laboratory Tests
Complete blood cell counts: decreased red cells, hemoglobin, white cells and platelets.
Blood glucose levels: falsely increased with SMA testing.
Blood uric acid levels: increased.

Liver function tests: increased liver enzymes (ALT/GPT, AST/GOT and alkaline phosphatase), increased bilirubin.

Kidney function tests: increased blood urea nitrogen (BUN) and creatinine.

Sperm counts: decreased.

CAUTION
1. Comply fully with all requests for periodic laboratory tests.
2. Call your doctor at the first sign of infection or abnormal bleeding or bruising.
3. Inform your physician promptly if you become pregnant.
4. It is best to avoid immunizations while taking this drug, and to avoid contact with people who have recently taken oral poliovirus vaccine.

Precautions for Use
By Infants and Children: No specific problems anticipated.

By Those over 60 Years of Age: Increased risk of bone marrow depression. Periodic blood counts are mandatory.

▷ **Advisability of Use During Pregnancy**

Pregnancy Category: D. See Pregnancy Code at the back of this book.

Animal studies: Rat studies reveal toxic effects on the embryo.

Human studies: Adequate studies of pregnant women are not available. This drug is known to cause abortions and premature births.

Avoid drug during entire pregnancy if possible. Use a nonhormonal method of contraception.

Advisability of Use if Breast-Feeding
Presence of this drug in breast milk: Unknown.

Avoid drug or refrain from nursing.

Habit-Forming Potential: None.

Effects of Overdosage: Headache, dizziness, abdominal pain, nausea.

Possible Effects of Long-Term Use: Development of new malignant diseases.

Suggested Periodic Examinations While Taking This Drug (at physician's discretion)

Complete blood cell counts.

Blood uric acid levels.

Liver and kidney function tests.

▷ **While Taking This Drug, Observe the Following**

Foods: No restrictions.

Beverages: No restrictions. Drink liquids liberally, up to 2 quarts daily.

▷ *Alcohol:* Avoid completely.

Tobacco Smoking: No interactions expected.

▷ *Other Drugs*

Mercaptopurine may *decrease* the effects of
- warfarin (Coumadin); the INR (protime or prothrombin time) should be checked more frequently.

The following drug may *increase* the effects of mercaptopurine
- allopurinol (Zyloprim). Doses must be reduced to 33% or even as low as 25% of the usual dose if these two medicines are to be combined.

Mercaptopurine *taken concurrently* with
- methotrexate (Mexate) can result in mercaptopurine toxicity.

▷ *Driving, Hazardous Activities:* No restrictions.

Aviation Note: The use of this drug *may be a disqualification* for piloting. Consult a designated Aviation Medical Examiner.

Exposure to Sun: No restrictions.

Discontinuation: To be determined by your physician.

MESALAMINE (me SAL a meen)

Other Names:
Mesalazine
5-aminosalicylic acid
5-ASA

Introduced: 1982   **Prescription:** USA: Yes; Canada: Yes   **Available as Generic:** USA: No; Canada: No   **Class:** Bowel anti-inflammatory   **Controlled Drug:** USA: No; Canada: No

Brand Names: Asacol, Pentasa, Rowasa, ✦Salofalk

BENEFITS versus RISKS	
Possible Benefits	*Possible Risks*
EFFECTIVE SUPPRESSION OF INFLAMMATORY BOWEL DISEASE	Allergic reactions: acute intolerance syndrome, drug-induced kidney damage (very rare)

▷ **Principal Uses**

As a Single Drug Product: Uses currently included in FDA approved labeling: (1) Treatment of active mild to moderate ulcerative colitis, proctosigmoiditis, and proctitis.

Other (unlabeled) generally accepted uses: (1) May help improve semen quality which had been damaged by prior sulfasalazine treatment; (2) can ease canker sores (aphthous ulcers); (3) has a steroid sparing effect in Crohn's disease; (4) used to maintain remission in ulcerative colitis.

How This Drug Works: This drug suppresses the formation of prostaglandins (and related compounds), tissue substances that induce inflammation, tissue destruction and diarrhea—the main problems in ulcerative colitis and proctitis.

Available Dosage Forms and Strengths

Rectal suspension — 4 grams per 60-ml unit

Suppositories — 250 mg (Canada) and 500 mg (US and Canada)

Tablets, delayed release — 250 mg, 400 mg and 500 mg

Capsules, controlled release — 250 mg

▷ **Recommended Dosage Ranges** (Actual dosage and administration schedule must be determined by the physician for each patient individually.)

Infants and Children: Dosage not established.

12 to 60 Years of Age: Rectal suspension—4 grams (as a retention enema) every night for 3 to 6 weeks.

Suppositories—500 mg (inserted into rectum) 2 or 3 times daily.

Tablets—400 to 800 mg (1 or 2 tablets by mouth) 3 times daily for 6 weeks. The total daily dose should not exceed 2400 mg.

Over 60 Years of Age: Same as 12 to 60 years of age.

Conditions Requiring Dosing Adjustments
Liver function: Specific guidelines for dosage adjustment in liver compromise not available. The drug is changed by the liver and colon wall to Ac-5-ASA.
Kidney function: This drug should be used with caution in kidney compromise.

▷ **Dosing Instructions:**   Rectal suspension—Use as a retention enema at bedtime; if possible, empty the rectum before inserting suspension; try to retain the suspension all night.

Tablets—Best taken with 8 ounces of water on an empty stomach, 1 hour before or 2 hours after eating. However, it may be taken with or following food to reduce stomach upset. The sustained-release tablet should be swallowed whole without alteration.

Usual Duration of Use: Use on a regular schedule for 1 to 3 weeks determines effectiveness in controlling ulcerative colitis. Long-term use (months to years) requires supervision and periodic physician evaluation.

Possible Advantages of This Drug
Does not cause bone marrow or blood cell disorders.
Does not inhibit sperm production or function.

▷ **This Drug Should Not Be Taken If**
- you have had an allergic reaction to it previously.
- you have severely impaired kidney function.
- you have a known sulfite allergy. (Rectal suspension should NOT be used.)
- you have active ulcer disease.

▷ **Inform Your Physician Before Taking This Drug If**
- you are allergic to aspirin (or other salicylates), olsalazine or sulfasalazine.
- you are allergic by nature: History of hay fever, asthma, hives, eczema.
- you have impaired liver or kidney function.
- you have a history of a blood clotting (coagulation) disorder.
- you have a history of low white blood cell counts.
- you are taking other medicines that effect the bone marrow. Discuss this with your doctor.
- you are currently taking sulfasalazine (Azulfidine).

Possible Side Effects (natural, expected, and unavoidable drug actions)
Anal irritation (with use of rectal suspension or suppositories). Flu-like syndrome with oral mesalamine use.

▷ **Possible Adverse Effects** (unusual, unexpected, and infrequent reactions)
If any of the following develop, consult your physician promptly for guidance.
Mild Adverse Effects
Allergic Reactions: Skin rash.
Headache, hair loss (rare).
Blurred vision, ringing in the ears.
Paresthesias, neck and joint pain, dizziness, cough.
Nausea, stomach pain, excessive gas.
Serious Adverse Effects
Allergic Reactions: Acute intolerance syndrome: fever, skin rash, severe headache, severe stomach pain, bloody diarrhea.
Kidney damage (nephrosis, interstitial nephritis) (rare).
Peripheral neuropathy (rare).
Pancreatitis (rare).

Peptic ulcers (rare).

Low white blood cell, anemia and platelet counts (rare).

Myocarditis, pericarditis, or pericardial effusions (rare).

Hepatitis (rare).

▷ **Possible Effects on Sexual Function:**   Oligospermia and infertility has been reported with other forms of mesalamine, but NOT with the oral form.

Possible Effects on Laboratory Tests

Increased liver function tests.

CAUTION

1. Report promptly any signs of acute intolerance syndrome. Stop drug.
2. Shake the rectal suspension thoroughly before administering.
3. This medicine is a salicylate and as such is a cousin of aspirin. Avoid taking this medicine in combination with other medicines or during other conditions in which aspirin is contraindicated.

Precautions for Use

By Infants and Children: Safety and effectiveness by those under 12 years of age not established.

By Those over 60 Years of Age: None.

▷ **Advisability of Use During Pregnancy**

Pregnancy Category: B. See Pregnancy Code at the back of this book.

Animal studies: No drug-induced birth defects found in rat or rabbit studies.

Human studies: Adequate studies of pregnant women are not available.

Use this drug only if clearly needed. Ask your physician for guidance.

Advisability of Use if Breast-Feeding

Presence of this drug in breast milk: Yes.

Avoid drug or refrain from nursing.

Habit-Forming Potential: None.

Effects of Overdosage: Headache, dizziness, nausea, vomiting, abdominal cramping.

Possible Effects of Long-Term Use: None reported.

Suggested Periodic Examinations While Taking This Drug (at physician's discretion)

Kidney function tests, urinalysis.

▷ **While Taking This Drug, Observe the Following**

Foods: Decreased mesalamine levels. Follow prescribed diet.

Beverages: No restrictions. May be taken with milk.

▷   *Alcohol:* No interactions expected.

Tobacco Smoking: No interactions expected.

▷   *Other Drugs:* Mercaptopurine *taken concurrently* with

Varicella vaccine (Varivax) may result in Reye's syndrome. Avoid taking this medicine for 6 weeks following varicella vaccine.

No interactions expected.

▷   *Driving, Hazardous Activities:* No restrictions.

Aviation Note: The use of this drug *is probably not a disqualification* for piloting. Consult a designated Aviation Medical Examiner.

Exposure to Sun: No restrictions.

METAPROTERENOL (met a proh TER e nohl)

Other Name: Orciprenaline

Introduced: 1964   **Prescription:** USA: Yes; Canada: Yes   **Available as Generic:** Yes   **Class:** Antiasthmatic, bronchodilator   **Controlled Drug:** USA: No; Canada: No

Brand Names: Alupent, Arm-a-Med, Dey-Dose, Dey-Lute, Metaprel, Prometa

BENEFITS versus RISKS	
Possible Benefits	*Possible Risks*
VERY EFFECTIVE RELIEF OF BRONCHOSPASM	Increased blood pressure
	Fine hand tremor
	Fast heart rate
	Irregular heart rhythm (with excessive use)

▷ **Principal Uses**

As a Single Drug Product: Uses currently included in FDA approved labeling: (1) Relieves acute bronchial asthma and reduces the frequency and severity of chronic, recurrent asthmatic attacks; (2) used to relieve reversible bronchospasm associated with chronic bronchitis and emphysema; (3) eases symptoms in obstructive bronchial disease.

Other (unlabeled) generally accepted uses: (1) Has been used in threatened abortion.

How This Drug Works: This drug acts to dilate those bronchial tubes that are in sustained constriction, thereby increasing the size of the airway and improving the ability to breathe.

Available Dosage Forms and Strengths

Oral suspension — 10 mg per 5 ml
Powder for inhalation — 0.65 mg/inhalation
Solution for nebulizer — 0.4%, 0.6% and 5%
Syrup — 10 mg per 5-ml
Tablets — 10 mg, 20 mg

▷ **Usual Adult Dosage Range:** Inhaler: 2 or 3 inhalations as often as every 3 to 4 hours; do not exceed 12 inhalations/day. Hand nebulizer: 5 to 15 inhalations every 4 hours; do not exceed 40 inhalations per day. Syrup and tablets: 20 mg up to every 6 to 8 hours. **Note: Actual dosage and administration schedule must be determined by the physician for each patient individually.**

Conditions Requiring Dosing Adjustments

Liver function: Specific guidelines for dosing adjustment in patients with liver compromise are not usually indicated.

Kidney function: Dosing changes are not indicated in kidney compromise.

▷ **Dosing Instructions:** May be taken on empty stomach or with food or milk. Tablets should not be crushed for administration. For aerosol and nebulizer, follow the written instructions carefully. Do not overuse. If symptoms are not controlled with the most frequent dosing allowed, call your doctor immediately.

Usual Duration of Use: According to individual requirements. Do not use beyond the time necessary to terminate episodes of asthma.

▷ **This Drug Should Not Be Taken If**
- you have had an allergic reaction to any dosage form of it previously.
- you currently have an irregular heart rhythm.
- you are taking, or have taken within the past 2 weeks, any monoamine oxidase (MAO) type A inhibitor drug (see Drug Classes).

▷ **Inform Your Physician Before Taking This Drug If**
- you are overly sensitive to other sympathetic stimulant drugs.
- you currently use epinephrine (Adrenalin, Primatene Mist, etc.) to relieve asthmatic breathing.
- you have any type of heart or circulatory disorder, especially high blood pressure or coronary heart disease.
- you have diabetes or an overactive thyroid gland (hyperthyroidism).
- you are taking any form of digitalis or any stimulant drug.

Possible Side Effects (natural, expected, and unavoidable drug actions)
Aerosol—dryness or irritation of mouth or throat, altered taste.
Tablet—nervousness, palpitation.

▷ **Possible Adverse Effects** (unusual, unexpected, and infrequent reactions)
If any of the following develop, consult your physician promptly for guidance.
Mild Adverse Effects
Headache, dizziness, restlessness, insomnia, fine tremor of hands.
Rapid, pounding heartbeat; increased sweating; muscle cramps in arms and legs.
Nausea, heartburn, vomiting.
Serious Adverse Effects
Rapid or irregular heart rhythm, intensification of angina, increased blood pressure.
Hallucinations and psychosis (rare).
Paradoxical spasm of the bronchi (bronchospasm) (rare).

▷ **Possible Effects on Sexual Function:** None reported.

Natural Diseases or Disorders That May Be Activated By This Drug
Latent coronary artery disease, diabetes or high blood pressure.

Possible Effects on Laboratory Tests
Urine sugar tests: positive (unreliable results with Benedict's solution).

CAUTION
1. Combined use of this drug by aerosol inhalation with beclomethasone aerosol (Beclovent, Vanceril) may increase the risk of toxicity due to fluorocarbon propellants. Use this aerosol 20 to 30 minutes *before* beclomethasone aerosol as this will reduce the risk of toxicity and will enhance the penetration of beclomethasone.
2. *Avoid excessive use of aerosol inhalation.* Excessive or prolonged use of this drug by inhalation can reduce its effectiveness and cause serious heart rhythm disturbances, including cardiac arrest.
3. Do not combine this drug with epinephrine. These two drugs may be used alternately if an interval of 4 hours is allowed between doses.
4. If you do not respond to your usually effective dose, ask your doctor for

help. Do not increase the size or frequency of the dose without your physician's approval.

Precautions for Use

By Infants and Children: Safety and effectiveness of the aerosol and nebulized solution not established for children under 12 years of age. Oral dosing in children less than 6 years old: 1.3 to 2.6 milligrams per kilogram per day divided into equal doses and given three to four times a day. In children 6 to 9 years old or less than 60 pounds: 10 mgs per dose 3 to 4 times a day. For children more than 9 years old or over 60 pounds are given 20 mgs three or four times a day.

Safety and effectiveness of the syrup and tablet not established for children under 6 years of age.

By Those over 60 Years of Age: Avoid excessive and continual use. If acute asthma is not relieved promptly, other drugs will have to be tried. Watch for nervousness, palpitations, irregular heart rhythm and muscle tremors. Use with extreme caution if you have hardening of the arteries, heart disease or high blood pressure.

▷ **Advisability of Use During Pregnancy**

Pregnancy Category: C. See Pregnancy Code at the back of this book.
Animal studies: Significant birth defects reported in rabbit studies.
Human studies: Adequate studies of pregnant women are not available.
Avoid use during first 3 months. Use during the last 6 months only if clearly needed.

Advisability of Use if Breast-Feeding

Presence of this drug in breast milk: Unknown.
Avoid drug or refrain from nursing.

Habit-Forming Potential: None.

Effects of Overdosage: Nervousness, palpitation, rapid heart rate, sweating, headache, tremor, vomiting, chest pain.

Possible Effects of Long-Term Use: Loss of effectiveness. See *CAUTION* category.

Suggested Periodic Examinations While Taking This Drug (at physician's discretion)

Blood pressure measurements, evaluation of heart status.

▷ **While Taking This Drug, Observe the Following**

Foods: No restrictions.
Beverages: Avoid excessive use of caffeine-containing beverages: coffee, tea, cola, chocolate.

▷ *Alcohol:* No interactions expected.
Tobacco Smoking: No interactions expected.

▷ *Other Drugs*

Metaproterenol *taken concurrently* with

- albuterol (Proventil, others) may result in increased heart (cardiovascular side effects).
- monoamine oxidase (MAO) type A inhibitor drugs may cause excessive increase in blood pressure and undesirable heart stimulation.
- phenothiazines (see Drug Classes) may blunt the central effects of this medicine.

▷ *Driving, Hazardous Activities:* Usually no restrictions. Use caution if excessive nervousness or dizziness occurs.

Aviation Note: The use of this drug *is a disqualification* for piloting. Consult a designated Aviation Medical Examiner.

Exposure to Sun: No restrictions.

Heavy Exercise or Exertion: Use caution. Excessive exercise can induce asthma in sensitive individuals.

METFORMIN (met FOR min)

Other Names: None

Introduced: 1995   **Prescription:** USA: Yes; Canada: Yes   **Available as Generic:** USA: No; Canada: No   **Class:** Antidiabetes drug, oral; biguanide **Controlled Drug:** USA: No; Canada: No

Brand Names: Glucophage

Warning: Avoid excessive alcohol intake with this drug. Alcohol can cause lactic acidosis, a condition which metformin can also rarely cause. All oral hypoglycemic agents may carry the risk of increased cardiovascular death based on a 1975 study of tolbutamide and phenformin.

BENEFITS versus RISKS

Possible Benefits	*Possible Risks*
EFFECTIVE GLUCOSE CONTROL WITHOUT INSULIN INJECTIONS MAY BE USED CONCURRENTLY WITH A SULFONYLUREA DOES NOT LEAD TO WEIGHT GAIN TAKEN BY MOUTH VERSUS INJECTION OF INSULIN Usually avoids excessive lowering of blood sugar Favorable effects on lipids	LACTIC ACIDOSIS (RARE) Possible anemia with long-term use

---

▷ **Principal Uses**

As a Single Drug Product: Uses currently included in FDA approved labeling: (1) Used in combination with diet restrictions to treat noninsulin-dependent diabetes; (2) can be combined with a sulfonylurea (see Drug Classes) in those patients who do not have an adequate response to diet restrictions plus a sulfonylurea.

Other (unlabeled) generally accepted uses: (1) May be used as single agent therapy to overcome insulin resistance; (2) could have a use in nondiabetic, obese women with high blood pressure in helping improve blood pressure and lipid profile; (3) may have a role in insulin-dependent diabetics in helping decrease their insulin requirements.

How This Drug Works: This biguanide decreases sugar (glucose) production in the liver. It also increases sensitivity of the body to insulin.

Available Dosage Forms and Strengths

Tablets — 500 mg, 850 mg

▷ **Recommended Dosage Ranges (Actual dosage and administration schedule must be determined by the physician for each patient individually.)**

Infants and Children: Not approved for use in this population.

12 to 60 Years of Age: Dosing is started at 500 mg twice daily. It is best to take this medicine with the morning and evening meal. Typical effective dosages are 850 mg twice daily. Maximum dose is 850 mg three times daily.

Over 60 Years of Age: Lower doses are used. Some patients may have acceptable blood sugar control with as little as 500 mg daily. If this dose is used, it should be taken with the morning meal. The dose may be slowly increased as needed and tolerated.

Conditions Requiring Dosing Adjustments

Liver function: This drug should **not** be used in patients with liver compromise. This is a risk factor for lactic acidosis.

Kidney function: This drug should **not** be used in patients who have kidney problems (renal dysfunction) which is defined as females with steady state creatinine levels greater than 1.4 or in males with steady state creatinine levels greater than 1.5.

▷ **Dosing Instructions:**   This drug should be taken with the morning and evening meal if it has been prescribed on a twice daily basis.

Usual Duration of Use:

Continual use on a regular schedule for a week is usually necessary to determine this drug's effectiveness in establishing tight glucose control. A month of continuous use will be needed before an effect on glycosylated hemoglobin (a measure of past success of glucose control) is seen. Long-term use (months to years) requires periodic evaluation of response and dosage adjustment. Consult your physician on a regular basis.

Possible Advantages of This Drug

Does not lead to weight gain.

Can be used (because of its mechanism of action) in combination with a sulfonylurea.

Can be used to overcome insulin resistance.

Does not cause excessive lowering of blood sugar (hypoglycemia) when used as monotherapy.

Currently a "Drug of Choice"

for treatment of hyperglycemia in the elderly.

▷ **This Drug Should Not Be Taken If**

- you have had an allergic reaction to any dosage form of it or related medicines previously.
- you have impaired kidneys (serum creatinine greater than 1.4 for females or 1.5 for males).
- you have liver disease.
- you have a serious infection (increases risk of lactic acidosis).
- you are an alcoholic.
- you have a heart or lung insufficiency (increased lactic acidosis risk).
- you are going to have a radiology test that uses iodinated contrast media (ask your doctor).
- you have chronic metabolic acidosis or ketoacidosis.
- you are breast-feeding your infant.

▷ **Inform Your Physician Before Taking This Drug If**
- you are planning to have surgery soon.
- you have a history of megaloblastic anemia.
- you have seen another physician and a diagnosis of ketoacidosis has been made.
- you are uncertain of how much metformin to take or how often to take it.

Possible Side Effects (natural, expected, and unavoidable drug actions)
Lactic acidosis (rare).

▷ **Possible Adverse Effects** (unusual, unexpected, and infrequent reactions)
If any of the following develop, consult your physician promptly for guidance.
Mild Adverse Effects
Allergic Reactions: Rash.
Metallic taste.
Anorexia, nausea, vomiting, or diarrhea (up to 30% when the drug is started, then these effects subside).
Headache, nervousness, dizziness, or tiredness (occasional).
Serious Adverse Effects
Allergic Reactions: Not reported.
Idiosyncratic Reactions: None reported.
Lactic acidosis (rare).
Lowered vitamin B12 levels and resultant anemia (megaloblastic) (rare).
Drug-induced porphyria.
All oral hypoglycemic agents carry a label indicating that they may increase risk of cardiovascular death (based on a 1975 study of tolbutamide and phenformin).

▷ **Possible Effects on Sexual Function:**   None reported.

Possible Delayed Adverse Effects: Low vitamin B12 levels and anemia (megaloblastic).

▷ **Adverse Effects That May Mimic Natural Diseases or Disorders**
Acidosis may mimic (ketoacidosis), which is seen in diabetics.

Natural Diseases or Disorders That May Be Activated by This Drug
None reported.

Possible Effects on Laboratory Tests
Blood glucose: decreased.

CAUTION
1. This drug may cause lactic acidosis. Ask your doctor for signs or symptoms which may occur.
2. Drugs in this class (phenformin) or tolbutamide were reported to increase risk of cardiovascular death. While there is no data to support that effect for this medicine, patients should be closely followed.

Precautions for Use
By Infants and Children: Safety and effectiveness for use by those under 18 years of age have not been established.
By Those over 60 Years of Age: Smaller starting doses (500 mg daily) are indicated. People in this age group tend to have an age-related decline in kidney function as well as a more compromised ability to tolerate lower blood sugar levels.

▷ **Advisability of Use During Pregnancy**
Pregnancy Category: B. See Pregnancy Code at the back of this book.
Animal studies: No birth defects in rats at two times the typical human dose.
Human studies: Information from adequate studies of pregnant women is not available. The manufacturer does not recommend the use of this drug in pregnancy. Insulin is still considered the drug of choice to control blood sugar in pregnancy.

Advisability of Use if Breast-Feeding
Presence of this drug in breast milk: Yes.
Avoid drug or refrain from nursing.

Habit-Forming Potential: None.

Effects of Overdosage: Nausea and vomiting, pulmonary edema, hemorrhage from the stomach, lactic acidosis, seizures, intractable lowering of the blood pressure, coma.

Possible Effects of Long-Term Use: Lowering of vitamin B12 and resultant anemia (megaloblastic). Possible malabsorption of folic acid and amino acids.

Suggested Periodic Examinations While Taking This Drug (at physician's discretion)
Vitamin B12 levels, tests of kidney and liver function.

▷ **While Taking This Drug, Observe the Following**
Foods: No restrictions.
Nutritional Support: Diet as prescribed by your doctor.
Beverages: No restrictions.
▷ *Alcohol:* Use with extreme caution. Alcohol worsens the effect of metformin on lactate. Avoid alcohol in excessive amounts.
Tobacco Smoking: No interactions expected.
Marijuana Smoking: May worsen dizziness.
▷ *Other Drugs*
Metformin may *increase* the effects of
  • insulin in the sense that the lowering of blood sugar will be increased. This may be used to therapeutic advantage in some insulin dependent diabetics.
Metformin *taken concurrently* with
  • ACE inhibitors (see Drug Classes) may increase lowering of blood sugar to an undesirable extent.
  • beta blockers (see Drug Classes) may slow recovery from any hypoglycemia which occurs and can also block symptoms of low blood sugar.
  • itraconazole or other azole antifungal agents can result in severe lowering of the blood sugar.
  • thyroid hormones (see Drug Classes) can result in blunting of metformin's therapeutic effect.
The following drugs may *increase* the effects of metformin
  • cimetidine (Tagamet) and result in toxicity.
  • oral hypoglycemic agents (see Drug Classes). This effect may be used to therapeutic advantage.
▷ *Driving, Hazardous Activities:* This drug may cause drowsiness or dizziness. Restrict activities as necessary.

Aviation Note: Diabetes *is a disqualification* for piloting. Consult a designated Aviation Medical Examiner.

Exposure to Sun: Use caution. Some medicines which are similar in chemical structure can cause increased sensitivity to the sun.

Heavy Exercise or Exertion: Heavy exercise will tend to use up sugar faster than usual. This drug will have an effect on lowering the blood sugar. Be alert to the symptoms of low blood sugar.

Occurrence of Unrelated Illness: Infections or other illness may still require use of insulin to achieve acceptable blood sugar control.

Discontinuation: Periodic physician evaluations of the continued benefit of this medicine are needed.

METHOTREXATE (meth oh TREX ayt)

Other Names: Amethopterin, MTX

Introduced: 1948   **Prescription:** USA: Yes; Canada: Yes   **Available as Generic:** Yes   **Class:** Anticancer drugs, antipsoriasis   **Controlled Drug:** USA: No; Canada: No

Brand Names: Abitrexate, Folex, Folex PFS, Mexate, Mexate AQ, Rheumatrex Dose Pack

BENEFITS versus RISKS	
Possible Benefits	*Possible Risks*
EFFECTIVE TREATMENT OF SOME CASES OF SEVERE DISABLING PSORIASIS	GASTROINTESTINAL ULCERATION AND BLEEDING
EFFECTIVE TREATMENT OF CERTAIN ADULT AND CHILDHOOD CANCERS	MOUTH AND THROAT ULCERATION
PREVENTION OF REJECTION OF BONE MARROW TRANSPLANTS	SEVERE BONE MARROW DEPRESSION
Helpful adjunctive therapy in severe, refractory rheumatoid arthritis and related disorders	DAMAGE TO LUNGS, LIVER, OR KIDNEYS
	Loss of hair

▷ **Principal Uses**

As a Single Drug Product: Uses currently included in FDA approved labeling: (1) Combination therapy of acute lymphocytic leukemia; (2) combination therapy of various types of adult and childhood cancer; (3) severe and widespread forms of disabling psoriasis that have failed to respond to all standard treatment procedures; (4) various types of both adult and childhood cancer; (5) used to prevent rejection of transplanted bone marrow; (6) used in the treatment of connective tissue disorders such as rheumatoid arthritis and related conditions. Its use in rheumatoid arthritis is restricted to the treatment of selected adults with severe active disease that has failed to respond to conventional therapy.

Other (unlabeled) generally accepted uses: (1) Used in a variety of neoplastic syndromes in combination therapy; (2) may have a role in helping decrease steroid use in steroid-dependent asthma; (3) helps lessen neutropenia in

Felty's syndrome; (4) used in combination with misoprostol to cause abortion; (5) can be of help in chronic granulomatous hepatitis of unknown cause (idiopathic).

How This Drug Works: By interfering with the normal utilization of folic acid in tissue cell reproduction, this drug retards abnormally rapid tissue growth (as in psoriasis and cancer).

Available Dosage Forms and Strengths

Injections — 2.5 mg per ml, 10 mg per ml and 25 mg per ml

Intrathecal cryodessicated powder — 20 mg, 50 mg, 100 mg

Injections (preservative-free) — 25 mg, 50 mg, 100 mg, 250 per ml

Tablets — 2.5 mg

▷ **Usual Adult Dosage Range**

For psoriasis (alternate schedules): (1) 10 to 50 mg once/week; (2) 2.5 to 5 mg/12 hours for 3 doses, or every 8 hours for 4 doses, once a week up to a maximum of 30 mg/week; (3) 2.5 mg/day for 5 days, followed by 2 days without drug, with gradual increase in dosage to a maximum of 6.25 mg/day.

For rheumatoid arthritis (alternate schedules): (1) single oral dose of 7.5 mg once weekly; (2) divided doses of 2.5 mg every 12 hours for 3 doses per week. Dosage may be increased gradually as needed and tolerated. Do not exceed a weekly dose of 20 mg.

For acute lymphocytic leukemia (ALL): induction: 3.3 milligrams per square meter in combination with corticosteroid treatment is usually given daily for 4 to 6 weeks. Maintenance: a total weekly dose of 30 milligrams per square meter is given as two divided oral or intramuscular injections. Some centers also use 2.5 milligrams per kilogram intravenously every 14 days.

Note: Actual dosage and administration schedule must be determined by the physician for each patient individually.

Conditions Requiring Dosing Adjustments

Liver function: It should be used with caution and in decreased dose in patients with liver compromise. One researcher used some laboratory tests as a guide: When the dose is due, if the bilirubin is less than 3 mg % and the AST (SGOT) is less than 180 IU, 100% of the scheduled dose can be given. If the bilirubin is 3.1 to 5.0 mg % or AST is greater then 180 IU—

75% of the scheduled dose should be given. If the bilirubin is greater than 5.0 mg %, the dose SHOULD NOT be given.

Kidney function: Methotrexate should be used as a result of a benefit to risk decision. Increased systemic adverse effects may occur if this medication is used in patients with compromised kidneys. This drug should **not** be given to patients with severe kidney failure (creatinine clearances less than 10 ml/min). In patients with moderate kidney failure, 50% of the usual dose should be given in the usual dosing interval.

▷ **Dosing Instructions:** The tablet may be crushed and taken with food to reduce stomach irritation. Drink at least 2 to 3 quarts of liquids daily. Many clinicians who give methotrexate to their patients to treat rheumatoid arthritis also give folic acid in order to minimize methotrexate toxicity.

Usual Duration of Use: Use on a regular schedule for several weeks determines benefit in reducing the severity and extent of psoriasis. Response in rheumatoid arthritis usually begins after 3 to 6 weeks of treatment. When a favorable response has been achieved, the dosage should be reduced to the smallest amount that will maintain acceptable improvement. Long-term use (months to years) requires physician supervision.

▷ **This Drug Should Not Be Taken If**
- you have had an allergic reaction to it previously.
- you currently have, or have had a recent exposure to, either chicken pox or shingles (herpes zoster).
- you are pregnant or planning pregnancy in the near future, and you are taking this drug to treat psoriasis or rheumatoid arthritis.
- you are nursing your infant.
- you have alcoholic liver disease.
- you have an immune deficiency.
- you have fluid in the pleura of the lung (pleural effusions).
- you have active liver disease, peptic ulcer, regional enteritis or ulcerative colitis.
- your white blood cell count is less than 3,000 or your platelet count is less than 100,000.
- you are making very small amounts of urine or your creatinine clearance (see Glossary) is less than 40 ml/minute.
- you currently have a blood cell or bone marrow disorder.

▷ **Inform Your Physician Before Taking This Drug If**
- you have a chronic infection of any kind.
- you do not understand how to handle vomit or urine while taking chemotherapy.
- you have impaired liver or kidney function.
- you have a history of bone marrow impairment of any kind, especially drug-induced bone marrow depression.
- you are dehydrated.
- you have a history of gout, peptic ulcer disease, regional enteritis or ulcerative colitis.

Possible Side Effects (natural, expected, and unavoidable drug actions)
The following are due to the pharmacological actions of this drug. **Report such developments to your physician promptly.**
Sores on the lips, in the mouth or throat; vomiting; intestinal cramping; diarrhea (may be bloody); painful urination; bloody urine.
Reduced resistance to infection, fatigue, weakness, fever, abnormal bleeding or bruising (bone marrow depression).

▷ **Possible Adverse Effects** (unusual, unexpected, and infrequent reactions)
If any of the following develop, consult your physician promptly for guidance.
Mild Adverse Effects
Allergic Reactions: Skin rash, hives, itching.
Headache, drowsiness, blurred vision, conjunctivitis.
Loss of appetite, nausea, vomiting.
Muscle pain.
Loss of hair, loss of skin pigmentation, acne.

Serious Adverse Effects

Allergic Reactions: Drug-induced pneumonia: cough, chest pain, shortness of breath. Anaphylaxis.

Nervous system toxicity: speech disturbances, paralysis, seizures.

Liver toxicity with jaundice (see Glossary).

Kidney toxicity: reduced urine volume, kidney failure.

Colitis or toxic megacolon.

Tumor lysis syndrome: uric acid nephropathy; excessively low potassium, magnesium, and calcium.

Bone marrow depression.

Fluid buildup in the lung pleura (pleural effusion).

Immune suppression and subsequent infection with Pneumocystis carinii pneumonia.

Severe skin reactions (toxic epidermal necrolysis).

Chromosomal damage (from occupational exposure).

▷ **Possible Effects on Sexual Function:** Altered timing and pattern of menstruation. Swelling and tenderness of the male breast tissue (gynecomastia).

Possible Delayed Adverse Effects: Some reports suggest that methotrexate therapy may contribute to the later development of secondary cancers. Other studies have not confirmed this.

Possible Effects on Laboratory Tests

Complete blood cell counts: decreased red cells, hemoglobin, white cells and platelets.

Blood uric acid level: increased.

Liver function tests: increased liver enzymes (ALT/GPT, AST/GOT and alkaline phosphatase), increased bilirubin.

Kidney function tests: increased blood urea nitrogen (BUN) level; increased urine creatinine content (kidney damage).

Fecal occult blood test: positive.

Sperm count: decreased.

CAUTION

1. This drug must be monitored carefully by a physician who is skilled in its proper administration. Request the Patient Package Insert that is available with this drug (Rheumatrex Dose Pack) and read it thoroughly.
2. Many clinicians who use methotrexate to treat rheumatoid arthritis also use folic acid to help minimize methotrexate toxicity.
3. Appropriate laboratory examinations, performed before and during the use of this drug, are mandatory.
4. Women with potential for pregnancy should have a pregnancy test before taking this drug and should use an effective form of contraception during its use and for 8 weeks following its discontinuation.
5. Live virus vaccines should be avoided during use of this drug. Live virus vaccines could actually produce infection rather than stimulate an immune response.

Precautions for Use

By Those over 60 Years of Age: Careful evaluation of kidney function should be made before starting treatment and during the entire course of therapy.

▷ **Advisability of Use During Pregnancy**

Pregnancy Category: X. See Pregnancy Code at the back of this book.

Animal studies: Skull and facial defects reported in mice.

Human studies: This drug is known to cause fetal deaths and birth defects.

Its use during pregnancy to treat psoriasis or rheumatoid arthritis cannot be justified.

Advisability of Use if Breast-Feeding

Presence of this drug in breast milk: Yes.

Avoid drug or refrain from nursing.

Habit-Forming Potential: None.

Effects of Overdosage: The Side Effects and Adverse Effects listed previously develop earlier and with greater severity.

Possible Effects of Long-Term Use: Liver compromise (fibrosis and cirrhosis) occurs in 3–5% of long-term users (35 to 49 months).

Suggested Periodic Examinations While Taking This Drug (at physician's discretion)

Complete blood cell counts, liver and kidney function tests, blood uric acid levels, chest X-ray examinations.

▷ **While Taking This Drug, Observe the Following**

Foods: Avoid highly seasoned foods that could be irritating. Between courses of treatment, eat liberally of the following foods: beef, chicken, lamb and pork liver, asparagus, navy beans, kale and spinach. Any food will reduce the peak methotrexate level obtained.

Beverages: No restrictions. This drug may be taken with milk.

▷ *Alcohol:* Avoid completely.

Tobacco Smoking: No interactions expected.

Marijuana Smoking: May cause additional impairment of immunity.

▷ *Other Drugs*

Methotrexate may *decrease* the effects of

• digoxin (Lanoxin).

• phenytoin (Dilantin).

The following drugs may *increase* the effects of methotrexate and enhance its toxicity

• aspirin and other salicylates.

• NSAIDs (see Drug Classes).

• probenecid (Benemid).

Methotrexate *taken concurrently* with

• bismuth subsalicylate (Pepto Bismol, others) may result in methotrexate toxicity.

• carbenicillin (Geocillin, others) may lead to methotrexate toxicity.

• cholestyramine (Questran, others) and other cholesterol lowering resins may result in decreased methotrexate effectiveness.

• cotrimoxazole (Bactrim) may result in lowering of all blood cells (pancytopenia).

• cyclosporine (Sandimune) can result in increased toxicity from both drugs. The combination should be avoided.

• etretinate (Tegison) results in increased liver toxicity.

- pneumococcal or smallpox vaccine may result in decreased immune response to the vaccine.
- sulfa drugs such as sulfamethoxazole can result in increased hematologic toxicity.
- thiazide diuretics (see Drug Classes) may increase risk of myelosuppression.
- theophylline (Theodur, others) may result in theophylline toxicity. Decreased theophylline doses may be needed.
- yellow fever vaccine can result in blunted response and benefit from the vaccine.

▷ *Driving, Hazardous Activities:* This drug may cause drowsiness, dizziness or blurred vision. Restrict activities as necessary.

Aviation Note: The use of this drug *is a disqualification* for piloting. Consult a designated Aviation Medical Examiner.

Exposure to Sun: Use caution. This drug can cause photosensitivity. Avoid ultraviolet lamps.

METHYCLOTHIAZIDE (METH i kloh thi a zide)

Introduced: **Prescription:** USA: Yes; Canada: No   **Available as Generic:** USA: Yes; Canada: Yes   **Class:** Thiazide Diuretic   **Controlled Drug:** USA: No; Canada: No

Brand Names: Aquatensen, ✦Duretic, ✦Dureticyl, Enduron

BENEFITS versus RISKS	
Possible Benefits	*Possible Risks*
Effective, well-tolerated diuretic Enhances the effectiveness of other antihypertensives	Loss of blood potassium and magnesium Abnormal heartbeat caused by loss of electrolytes Increased blood sugar, uric acid, and calcium Rare blood cell disorders

Please see the combined thiazide diuretic profile for further information.

METHYLPHENIDATE (meth il FEN i dayt)

Introduced: 1956   **Prescription:** USA: Yes; Canada: Yes   **Available as Generic:** USA: Yes; Canada: Yes   **Class:** amphetaminelike drug, anti-attention deficit disorder drug   **Controlled Drug:** USA:C-II*

Brand Names: ✦PMS-Methylphenidate, Ritalin, Ritalin-SR

*See Schedules of Controlled Drugs at the back of this book.

BENEFITS versus RISKS

Possible Benefits	*Possible Risks*
EFFECTIVE CONTROL OF NARCOLEPSY	POTENTIAL FOR SERIOUS PSYCHOLOGICAL DEPENDENCE
USEFUL AS ADJUNCTIVE TREATMENT IN THE ATTENTION-DEFICIT DISORDERS OF CHILDHOOD	SUPPRESSION OF GROWTH IN CHILDHOOD
Useful in treatment of mild to moderate depression	Abnormal behavior
Useful in some cases of emotional withdrawal in the elderly	Rare blood cell disorders

---

▷ **Principal Uses**

As a Single Drug Product: Uses currently included in FDA approved labeling: (1) Treats narcolepsy, recurrent spells of uncontrollable drowsiness and sleep; and (2) attention-deficit disorders of childhood, formerly known as the hyperactive child syndrome, minimal brain damage and minimal brain dysfunction.

Other (unlabeled) generally accepted uses: (1) Treatment of mild to moderate depression; (2) management of apathetic and withdrawal states in the elderly; (3) combination therapy of chronic pain, particularly cancer pain; (4) could have a role in helping autism.

How This Drug Works: This activates the brain stem, improves alertness and concentration, and increases learning ability and attention span.

Available Dosage Forms and Strengths

Tablets — 5 mg, 10 mg, 20 mg

Tablets, prolonged-action — 20 mg

▷ **Usual Adult Dosage Range:**   Narcolepsy: 10 to 60 mg daily. This is divided into equal doses and given two to three times daily. Ideally, this is given 30 minutes before meals.

Pediatric dosing: In children over six years old: Regular release form: Five milligrams before breakfast and lunch (twice daily). This dose is increased as needed and tolerated at weekly intervals to a maximum recommended dose of 60 mgs. **Note: Actual dosage and administration schedule must be determined by the physician for each patient individually.**

Conditions Requiring Dosing Adjustments

Liver function: Used with caution and in decreased dose in patients with liver compromise.

Kidney function: The kidney does not appear to be involved in the elimination of this drug.

▷ **Dosing Instructions:**   The regular tablet may be crushed and taken 30 to 45 minutes before meals. The prolonged-action tablet should be taken whole, not crushed.

Usual Duration of Use: Use on a regular schedule for 3 to 4 weeks determines effectiveness in controlling the symptoms of narcolepsy or improving the behavior of attention-deficit children. If there is no improvement after this time, the drug should be stopped. Long-term use (months to years) requires physician supervision and periodic evaluation.

▷ **This Drug Should Not Be Taken If**
- you have had an allergic reaction to it previously.
- you have glaucoma (inadequately treated).
- you have Tourette's Syndrome.
- you are experiencing a period of severe anxiety, nervous tension or emotional depression.

▷ **Inform Your Physician Before Taking This Drug If**
- you have high blood pressure, angina or epilepsy.
- you are taking, or have taken within the past 14 days, any monoamine oxidase (MAO) type A inhibitor drug (see Drug Class Section).

Possible Side Effects (natural, expected, and unavoidable drug actions)
Nervousness, insomnia.

▷ **Possible Adverse Effects** (unusual, unexpected, and infrequent reactions)
If any of the following develop, consult your physician promptly for guidance.
Mild Adverse Effects
Allergic Reactions: Skin rash, hives, drug fever, joint pains.
Headache, dizziness, rapid and forceful heart palpitation.
Reduced appetite, nausea, abdominal discomfort.
Stuttering and hallucinations.
Serious Adverse Effects
Allergic Reactions: Severe skin reactions, extensive bruising due to allergic destruction of blood platelets (see Glossary).
Porphyria (rare).
Liver toxicity (associated with intravenous abuse of the drug).
Muscle damage (rhabdomyolysis).
Idiosyncratic Reaction: Abnormal patterns of behavior.
Abnormally low red blood cell and white blood cell counts (rare and of questionable causation).
Growth suppression (the medicine is often stopped in the summer).

▷ **Possible Effects on Sexual Function:**   None reported.

Natural Diseases or Disorders That May Be Activated by This Drug
Latent epilepsy.

Possible Effects on Laboratory Tests
Blood platelet counts: decreased (rare).
White and red blood cell counts: decreased (rare).

CAUTION
1. This drug should be used ONLY AFTER a careful assessment by a qualified specialist is made. True attention deficit disorder requires careful assessment to differentiate it from behavior problems arising from family tensions or other conditions which do not require Ritalin therapy.
2. Careful dosage adjustments on an individual basis are mandatory.
3. Paradoxical reactions (see Glossary) can occur, causing aggravation of initial symptoms for which this drug was prescribed.

Precautions for Use
By Infants and Children: Safety and effectiveness for those under 6 years of age not established. If this drug is not beneficial in managing an attention deficit disorder after a trial of one month, it should be stopped. During long-term use, monitor the child for normal growth and development.
By Those over 60 Years of Age: Started with small doses. May be increased risk of nervousness, agitation, insomnia, high blood pressure, angina or disturbance of heart rhythm.

▷ **Advisability of Use During Pregnancy**
Pregnancy Category: B. See Pregnancy Code at the back of this book.
  Animal studies: No birth defects found in mouse studies.
  Human studies: Adequate studies of pregnant women are not available.
  Use this drug only if clearly needed. Ask physician for guidance.

Advisability of Use if Breast-Feeding
  Presence of this drug in breast milk: Unknown.
  Avoid drug or refrain from nursing.

Habit-Forming Potential: This drug can produce tolerance and cause serious psychological dependence (see Glossary), a potentially dangerous characteristic of amphetaminelike drugs (see Drug Classes).

Effects of Overdosage: Headache, vomiting, agitation, tremors, muscle twitching, dry mouth, sweating, fever, confusion, hallucinations, seizures, coma.

Possible Effects of Long-Term Use: Suppression of growth (in weight and/or height) has been reported in children during long-term use of this drug. Many patients are taken off the medicine during summer school vacations.

Suggested Periodic Examinations While Taking This Drug (at physician's discretion)
  Complete blood cell counts, blood pressure measurements.

▷ **While Taking This Drug, Observe the Following**
Foods: Avoid foods rich in tyramine (see Glossary); this drug in combination with tyramine may cause an excessive rise in blood pressure.
Beverages: Avoid beverages prepared from meat or meat extracts. This drug may be taken with milk.
▷ *Alcohol:* Avoid beer, Chianti wines and vermouth (may have high tyramine contents).
Tobacco Smoking: No interactions expected.
▷ *Other Drugs*
  Methylphenidate may *increase* the effects of
  • tricyclic antidepressants, and enhance their toxic effects (see Drug Classes).
  Methylphenidate may *decrease* the effects of
  • guanethidine (Ismelin), and impair its ability to lower blood pressure.
  Methylphenidate *taken concurrently* with
  • anticonvulsants may cause a significant change in the pattern of epileptic seizures; dosage adjustments may be necessary for proper control.
  • monoamine oxidase (MAO) type A inhibitor drugs (see Drug Class Section) may cause a significant rise in blood pressure. Avoid the concurrent use of these drugs.

- morphine may be used to great therapeutic benefit to increase alertness, especially if high doses of morphine must be used.
- tricyclic antidepressants (TCAs) may result in undesirable increases in blood pressure.

▷ *Driving, Hazardous Activities:* This drug may cause dizziness or drowsiness. Restrict activities as necessary.

Aviation Note: The use of this drug *is a disqualification* for piloting. Consult a designated Aviation Medical Examiner.

Exposure to Sun: No restrictions.

Discontinuation: If it has been necessary to use this drug for an extended period of time, do not discontinue it abruptly. Careful supervision is necessary during withdrawal to prevent severe depression and erratic behavior.

METHYLPREDNISOLONE (meth il pred NIS oh lohn)

Introduced: 1957   **Prescription:** USA: Yes; Canada: Yes   **Available as Generic:** USA: Yes; Canada: Yes   **Class:** Cortisonelike drugs   **Controlled Drug:** USA: No; Canada: No

Brand Names: A-Methapred, Depmedalone-40, Depmedalone-80, Depo-Medrol, Enpak Refill, Mar-Pred 40, Medrol, ✦Medrol Acne Lotion, Medrol Enpak, ✦Medrol Veriderm Cream, Meprolone, ✦Neo-Medrol Acne Lotion, ✦Neo-Medrol Veriderm, Solu-Medrol

BENEFITS versus RISKS	
Possible Benefits	*Possible Risks*
EFFECTIVE RELIEF OF SYMPTOMS IN A WIDE VARIETY OF INFLAMMATORY AND ALLERGIC DISORDERS EFFECTIVE IMMUNOSUPPRESSION in selected benign and malignant disorders	Use exceeding 2 weeks is associated with many adverse effects: ALTERED MOOD AND PERSONALITY CATARACTS, GLAUCOMA HYPERTENSION OSTEOPOROSIS ASEPTIC BONE NECROSIS INCREASED SUSCEPTIBILITY TO INFECTIONS (See Possible Adverse Effects and Possible Effects of Long-Term Use)

▷ **Principal Uses**

As a Single Drug Product: Uses currently included in FDA approved labeling: (1) Treats a wide variety of allergic and inflammatory conditions. Used most commonly in the management of serious skin disorders, asthma, regional enteritis, multiple sclerosis, lupus erythematosus, ulcerative colitis and all types of major rheumatic disorders including bursitis, tendonitis and most forms of arthritis; (2) helps treat low platelet counts of unknown cause (idiopathic thrombocytopenic purpura); (3) shock due to adrenal gland insufficiency–Addisonian shock); (4) adjunctive role in anaphylactic shock.

Other (unlabeled) generally accepted uses: (1) Treatment of refractory anemia; (2) therapy of chronic obstructive pulmonary disease; (3) combination treatment of acute nonlymphoblastic leukemia; (4) combination therapy of severe vomiting caused by chemotherapy; (5) helps prevent rejection of transplanted organs; (6) combination therapy of pneumocystis carinii pneumonia in AIDS patients; (7) helps treat bone cysts in children; (8) has a role in croup; (9) can help symptoms in Still's disease; (10) used by intramuscular injection to treat polymalgia rheumatica; (11) used to help control cancer pain—especially where inflammation is involved.

How This Drug Works: Anti-inflammatory effect is due to its ability to block normal defensive functions of certain white blood cells. Immunosuppressant effect is attributed to a reduced production of lymphocytes and antibodies.

Available Dosage Forms and Strengths

Injection, solution — 1 gram, 40 mg, 125 mg and 500 mg per vial
Injection, suspension — 40 mg and 80 mg per ml
Ointment — 0.25% and 1%
Retention enema — 40 mg/bottle
Tablets — 2 mg, 4 mg, 8 mg, 16 mg, 24 mg, 32 mg

▷ **Usual Adult Dosage Range:**   Four to 48 mg daily as a single dose or in divided doses. This dose is adjusted depending on the condition being treated and the individual response. **Note: Actual dosage and administration schedule must be determined by the physician for each patient individually.**

Conditions Requiring Dosing Adjustments

Liver function: Specific dosage adjustments in liver compromise are not defined. It is a rare cause of liver changes (hepatomegaly).

Kidney function: This drug can worsen existing kidney compromise. A benefit to risk decision must be made regarding the use of methylprednisolone in these patients.

Obesity: The amount of time this medicine stays in the body has been extended in obese patients. Dosing should be calculated based on ideal body weight.

▷ **Dosing Instructions:**   The tablet may be crushed and taken with or following food to prevent stomach irritation, preferably in the morning.

Usual Duration of Use: For acute disorders: 4 to 10 days. For chronic disorders: according to individual requirements. Duration of use should not exceed the time necessary to obtain adequate symptomatic relief in acute self-limiting conditions, or the time required to stabilize a chronic condition and permit gradual withdrawal. Because of its intermediate duration of action, this drug is appropriate for alternate-day administration. Consult your physician on a regular basis.

▷ **This Drug Should Not Be Taken If**

• you have had an allergic reaction to any dosage form of it previously.
• you have active peptic ulcer disease.
• you have had recent bowel surgery where an anastamosis was performed.
• you have a premature infant and consideration is being given to using the injection form (contains benzyl alcohol).
• you have an active eye infection caused by the herpes simplex virus.
• you have active tuberculosis.

▷ **Inform Your Physician Before Taking This Drug If**
- you have had an adverse reaction to any cortisonelike drug in the past.
- you have a history of peptic ulcer disease, thrombophlebitis or tuberculosis.
- you have any of the following: diabetes, glaucoma, high blood pressure, deficient thyroid function or myasthenia gravis.
- you have been exposed to measles or chickenpox.
- you plan to have surgery of any kind in the near future.
- you have liver compromise.

Possible Side Effects (natural, expected, and unavoidable drug actions)
Increased appetite, weight gain, retention of salt and water, excretion of potassium, increased susceptibility to infection. Suppression of the adrenal gland. Growth retardation with chronic use in children. Increased eye pressure (intraocular).

▷ **Possible Adverse Effects** (unusual, unexpected, and infrequent reactions)
If any of the following develop, consult your physician promptly for guidance.

Mild Adverse Effects
Allergic Reaction: Skin rash.
Headache, dizziness, insomnia.
Easy bruising (ecchymosis).
Acid indigestion, abdominal distention.
Muscle cramping, weakness, and joint pain.
Acne, excessive growth of facial hair.

Serious Adverse Effects
Allergic Reactions: Anaphylaxis.
Mental and emotional disturbances of serious magnitude.
Reactivation of latent tuberculosis, Pneumocystis carinii pneumonia.
Development of peptic ulcer.
Hallucinations.
Seizures.
Decreased ability to heal wounds.
Abnormal heartbeat.
Toxic megacolon.
Liver or kidney compromise.
Blindness, cataracts.
Changes in white blood cell counts.
Cushing's syndrome with chronic use (central obesity, buffalo hump, and moon-shaped face).
Osteoporosis, osteonecrosis.
Hyperglycemia.
Muscle changes (myopathy).
Suppression of the adrenal gland.
Increased blood pressure.
Pancreatitis (rare).
Abnormal heartbeat (arrythmias).
Development of inflammation of the pancreas.
Thrombophlebitis (inflammation of a vein with the formation of blood clot)—

pain or tenderness in thigh or leg, with or without swelling of the foot, ankle, or leg.

Pulmonary embolism (movement of a blood clot to the lung)—sudden shortness of breath, pain in the chest, coughing, bloody sputum.

▷ **Possible Effects on Sexual Function:**   Altered timing and pattern of menstruation.

▷ **Adverse Effects That May Mimic Natural Diseases or Disorders**

Pattern of symptoms and signs resembling Cushing's syndrome.

Natural Diseases or Disorders That May Be Activated by This Drug

Latent diabetes, glaucoma, peptic ulcer disease, tuberculosis.

Possible Effects on Laboratory Tests

Blood amylase and lipase levels: increased (possible pancreatitis).

Glucose tolerance test (GTT): decreased.

Blood potassium level: decreased.

Blood testosterone level: decreased.

CAUTION

1. Best to carry an identification card that says you are taking this drug, if your course of treatment is to exceed 1 week.
2. You have an increased risk of severe infection from viral illnesses such as measles or chickenpox. Try to avoid being exposed, and call your doctor if exposure occurs.
3. Growth and development of children receiving chronic steroids should be carefully followed.
4. Do not stop this drug abruptly after long-term treatment.
5. If vaccination against measles, rabies, smallpox or yellow fever is required, discontinue this drug 72 hours before vaccination and do not resume it for at least 14 days after vaccination.
6. Dermatitis around the mouth may occur. Talk with your doctor if this happens.

Precautions for Use

By Infants and Children: Avoid prolonged use if possible. During long-term use, watch for suppression of normal growth. Intracranial pressure may increase. Long-term use may increase risk for adrenal gland deficiency during stress for as long as 18 months after the drug is stopped.

By Those over 60 Years of Age: Cortisonelike drugs should be used very sparingly after 60 and only when the disorder under treatment is unresponsive to adequate trials of unrelated drugs. Avoid prolonged use of this drug. Continual use (even in small doses) can increase the severity of diabetes, enhance fluid retention, raise blood pressure, weaken resistance to infection, induce stomach ulcer and accelerate the development of cataract and osteoporosis.

▷ **Advisability of Use During Pregnancy**

Pregnancy Category: C. See Pregnancy Code at the back of this book.

Animal studies: Birth defects reported in mice, rats and rabbits.

Human studies: Adequate studies of pregnant women are not available.

Avoid completely during the first 3 months. Limit use during the last 6 months as much as possible. If used, the infant should be examined for possible deficiency of adrenal gland function.

Advisability of Use if Breast-Feeding
Presence of this drug in breast milk: Yes.
Avoid drug or refrain from nursing.

Habit-Forming Potential: Use of this drug to suppress symptoms over an extended period of time may produce a state of functional dependence (see Glossary). In the treatment of asthma and rheumatoid arthritis, the dose should be kept as small as possible and withdrawal should be attempted after periods of reasonable improvement. Such procedures may reduce the degree of "steroid rebound"—the return of symptoms as the drug is withdrawn.

Effects of Overdosage: Fatigue, muscle weakness, stomach irritation, acid indigestion, excessive sweating, facial flushing, fluid retention, swelling of extremities, increased blood pressure.

Possible Effects of Long-Term Use: Increased blood sugar (possible diabetes), increased fat deposits on the trunk of the body ("buffalo hump"), rounding of the face ("moon face"), thinning and fragility of skin, loss of texture and strength of bones (osteoporosis, aseptic necrosis), cataracts, glaucoma, retarded growth and development in children.

Suggested Periodic Examinations While Taking This Drug (at physician's discretion)
Measurements of blood pressure, blood sugar and potassium levels.
Complete eye examinations at regular intervals.
Chest X-ray if history of tuberculosis.
Determination of the rate of development of the growing child to detect retardation of normal growth.
Bone mineral density testing to assess osteoporosis and fracture risk.

▷ **While Taking This Drug, Observe the Following**
Foods: No interactions expected. Ask physician regarding need to restrict salt intake or to eat potassium-rich foods. During long-term use of this drug, it is advisable to eat high-protein diet.
Nutritional Support: During long-term use, take a vitamin supplement. During wound repair, take a zinc supplement.
Beverages: No restrictions. Drink all forms of milk liberally.
▷ *Alcohol:* No interactions expected. Use caution if you are prone to peptic ulcer disease.
Tobacco Smoking: Nicotine increases the blood levels of naturally produced cortisone and related hormones. Heavy smoking may add to the expected actions of this drug and requires close observation for excessive effects.
Marijuana Smoking: May cause additional impairment of immunity.
▷ *Other Drugs*
Methylprednisolone may *decrease* the effects of
• insulin and require higher doses.
• isoniazid (INH, Niconyl, etc.).
• salicylates (aspirin, sodium salicylate, etc.).
Methylprednisolone *taken concurrently* with
• amphotericin B (Fungizone) may result in increased potassium loss.
• carbamazepine (Tegretol) may result decreased methylprednisolone effectiveness.

- cholestyramine (Questran) may decrease the amount of medicine that is absorbed into your body.
- cyclosporine (Sandimmune) can result in increased steroid levels and cyclosporine toxicity.
- loop diuretics such as furosemide (Lasix) or bumetanide (Bumex) may result in increased risk of potassium loss.
- ketoconazole (Nizoral) may increase blood levels of methylprednisolone and result in toxicity (abnormal heart beats or psychiatric reactions).
- NSAIDs may cause increased risk of ulceration of the stomach or intestine.
- oral anticoagulants (warfarin-Coumadin) may either increase or decrease their effectiveness; consult physician regarding the need for prothrombin time testing and dosage adjustment.
- oral hypoglycemic agents (see Drug Classes) or insulin may result in loss of control of blood sugar and require higher doses or more frequent dosing of oral hypoglycemics or insulin in order to control blood sugar.
- primidone (Mysoline) may lead to increased metabolism of methylprednisolone and decreased therapeutic benefit of methylprednisolone.
- rifampin (Rifadin, others) may lead to increased metabolism of methylprednisolone and decreased therapeutic benefit of methylprednisolone.
- thiazide diuretics (see Drug Classes) can result in additive potassium loss.
- theophylline (Theodur) results in variable changes in blood levels. More frequent theophylline blood levels are indicated.
- vaccines (such as flu or pneumococcal) may result in a blunting of the immune response to the vaccine.

The following drugs may **_decrease_** the effects of methylprednisolone
- antacids may reduce its absorption.
- barbiturates (Amytal, Butisol, phenobarbital, etc.).
- phenytoin (Dilantin, etc.).
- rifampin (Rifadin, Rimactane, etc.).

▷ *Driving, Hazardous Activities:* Usually no restrictions. Be alert to the rare occurrence of dizziness.

Aviation Note: The use of this drug **_may be a disqualification_** for piloting. Consult a designated Aviation Medical Examiner.

Exposure to Sun: No restrictions.

Occurrence of Unrelated Illness: This drug may decrease resistance to infection. Tell your doctor if you develop an infection of any kind. It may also reduce your body's ability to respond to stress of acute illness, injury or surgery. Keep your physician fully informed of any significant changes in your state of health.

Discontinuation: After extended use of this drug, do **not** stop it abruptly. Ask your doctor for help regarding gradual withdrawal. For a period of 2 years after discontinuing this drug, it is essential in the event of illness, injury or surgery that you inform attending medical personnel that you have used this drug. The period of impaired response to stress following the use of cortisonelike drugs may last for 1 to 2 years.

METHYSERGIDE (meth i SER jide)

Introduced: 1961   **Prescription:** USA: Yes; Canada: Yes   **Available as**
Generic: USA: No; Canada: No   **Class:** Antimigraine drug   **Controlled**
Drug: USA: No; Canada: No
Brand Name: Sansert

BENEFITS versus RISKS	
Possible Benefits	*Possible Risks*
EFFECTIVE PREVENTION OF MIGRAINE AND CLUSTER HEADACHES	FIBROSIS (SCARRING) INSIDE CHEST AND ABDOMINAL CAVITIES, OF HEART AND LUNG TISSUES, ADJACENT TO MAJOR BLOOD VESSELS AND INTERNAL ORGANS (see Effects of Long-Term Use)
	Aggravation of hypertension, coronary artery disease, and peripheral vascular disease

▷ **Principal Uses**
  As a Single Drug Product: Uses currently included in FDA approved labeling: (1) Prevention of frequent and/or disabling vascular headaches (migraine and cluster neuralgia) that have not responded to other conventional treatment. Other (unlabeled) generally accepted uses: (1) May have a role in therapy of some strokes.

How This Drug Works: By blocking the inflammatory and vasoconstrictor effects of serotonin, this drug prevents blood vessel constriction that initiates vascular headaches.

Available Dosage Forms and Strengths
  Tablets — 2 mg

▷ **Recommended Dosage Ranges** (Actual dosage and administration schedule must be determined by the physician for each patient individually.)
  Infants and Children: Use not recommended.
  12 to 60 Years of Age: 2 to 6 mg daily, in divided doses with meals. A medication-free period of 3 to 4 weeks after every six month course of methysergide must occur.
  Over 60 Years of Age: 2 to 4 mg daily, in divided doses. Use very cautiously, with frequent monitoring for adverse effects.

Conditions Requiring Dosing Adjustments
  Liver function: This drug should not be used in patients with liver compromise.
  Kidney function: This drug should not be used in patients with renal compromise.

▷ **Dosing Instructions:** The tablet may be crushed and taken with food or milk to reduce stomach irritation. Limit continual (uninterrupted) use to 6 months; avoid drug completely for a period of 4 weeks between courses.

Usual Duration of Use: Use on a regular schedule for 3 weeks usually determines effectiveness in preventing recurrence of vascular headache. If significant benefit does not occur during this trial, this drug should be stopped. Long-term use (months to years) requires periodic physician evaluation.

▷ **This Drug Should Not Be Taken If**
- you have had an allergic reaction to it previously.
- you are pregnant.
- you currently have a severe infection.
- you have any of the following conditions:
  - angina pectoris.
  - Buerger's disease.
  - cellulitis of the lower legs.
  - chronic lung disease.
  - connective tissue (collagen) disease.
  - coronary artery disease.
  - hardening of the arteries (arteriosclerosis).
  - heart valve disease.
  - high blood pressure (significant hypertension).
  - kidney disease or significantly impaired kidney function.
  - liver disease or significantly impaired liver function.
  - active peptic ulcer disease.
  - peripheral vascular disease.
  - phlebitis of any kind.
  - Raynaud's disease or phenomenon.

▷ **Inform Your Physician Before Taking This Drug If**
- you have had an adverse reaction to *any other form of ergot*.
- you have a history of peptic ulcer disease.

Possible Side Effects (natural, expected, and unavoidable drug actions)
Fluid retention, weight gain.

▷ **Possible Adverse Effects** (unusual, unexpected, and infrequent reactions)
If any of the following develop, consult your physician promptly for guidance.

Mild Adverse Effects
Allergic Reactions: Skin rashes, flushing of the face, transient loss of scalp hair.
Dizziness, drowsiness, agitation, unsteadiness, altered vision.
Heartburn, nausea, vomiting, diarrhea.
Weight gain.
Transient muscle and joint pains.

Serious Adverse Effects
Idiosyncratic Reactions: Nightmares, hallucinations, acute mental disturbances.
Fibrosis (scar tissue formation) involving the chest and/or abdominal cavities, heart valves, lungs, kidneys, major blood vessels.
Spasm and narrowing of coronary and peripheral arteries: anginal chest pain; cold and painful extremities; leg cramps on walking.
Hemolytic anemia (see Glossary) (rare).
Abnormally low white blood cell counts.
Impaired circulation to the extremities (peripheral ischemia).
Heart attack (myocardial infarction) (very rare).

▷ **Possible Effects on Sexual Function:**   Fibrosis of penile tissues.

▷ **Adverse Effects That May Mimic Natural Diseases or Disorders**
Swelling of the hands, lower legs, feet and ankles (peripheral edema) may suggest heart or kidney dysfunction.

Natural Diseases or Disorders That May Be Activated by This Drug
Latent coronary artery insufficiency (angina), Buerger's disease, Raynaud's disease, peptic ulcer disease.

Possible Effects on Laboratory Tests
Complete blood cell counts: decreased white cells (lymphocytes).
Stomach hydrochloric acid: increased.
Kidney function tests: increased blood urea nitrogen (BUN).

CAUTION
1. Continual use is limited to 6 months. Gradual reduction of dose is advised during the last 2 to 3 weeks of each course to prevent withdrawal headache rebound. Omit drug for a period of 4 to 6 weeks before resuming. This "drug-free" period is mandatory to reduce the risk of developing fibrosis of internal tissues.
2. Promptly report: fatigue, fever, chest pain, difficult breathing, stomach or flank pain, changes in pattern of urination.
3. This drug is useful only for the prevention of recurring vascular headaches; it is not recommended for the treatment of acute attacks of headache. It is ineffective and should not be used for tension headaches.

Precautions for Use
By Infants and Children: Use of this drug is not recommended.
By Those over 60 Years of Age: The age-related changes in blood vessels, circulatory functions and kidney function can make you more susceptible to the serious adverse effects of this drug. See the list of diseases and disorders above that are contraindications to the use this drug. Ask your doctor for help.

▷ **Advisability of Use During Pregnancy**
Pregnancy Category:
X. See Pregnancy Code at the back of this book.
Animal studies: No information available.
Human studies: Adequate studies of pregnant women are not available.
The manufacturer states that this drug is contraindicated during entire pregnancy.

Advisability of Use if Breast-Feeding
Presence of this drug in breast milk: Yes.
Avoid drug or refrain from nursing.

Habit-Forming Potential: None.

Effects of Overdosage: Nausea, vomiting, stomach pain, diarrhea, dizziness, excitement, cold hands and feet.

Possible Effects of Long-Term Use: Formation of scar tissue (fibrosis) inside chest cavity and/or abdominal cavity, on heart valves, in lung tissues, and surrounding major blood vessels and internal organs. This potentially dangerous reaction requires close and continual medical supervision while taking this drug.

Suggested Periodic Examinations While Taking This Drug (at physician's discretion)

Careful examination at regular intervals (6 to 12 months) for scar tissue formation or circulatory complications.

Complete blood cell counts.

Kidney function tests.

▷ **While Taking This Drug, Observe the Following**

Foods: No restrictions other than foods to which you are allergic. Some vascular headaches are due to food allergy.

Beverages: No restrictions.

▷ *Alcohol:* No interactions expected. Observe closely to determine if alcoholic beverages can initiate a migrainelike headache.

Tobacco Smoking: Avoid completely.

▷ *Other Drugs*

Methysergide *taken concurrently* with

• beta blocker drugs (see Drug Classes), may result in hazardous constriction of peripheral arteries; monitor the combined effects of these drugs on circulation in the extremities.

▷ *Driving, Hazardous Activities:* This drug may cause dizziness, drowsiness or impaired vision. Restrict activities as necessary.

Aviation Note: The use of this drug *is a disqualification* for piloting. Consult a designated Aviation Medical Examiner.

Exposure to Sun: No restrictions.

Exposure to Cold: Use caution. Cold environments may increase the occurrence of reduced circulation (blood flow) to the extremities.

Discontinuation: If this drug has been taken for an extended period of time, do not stop it abruptly. Gradual withdrawal (dosage reduction) over 2 to 3 weeks can prevent the development of rebound vascular headaches.

METOCLOPRAMIDE (met oh KLOH pra mide)

Introduced: 1973   **Prescription:** USA: Yes; Canada: Yes   **Available as Generic:** Yes   **Class:** Gastrointestinal drug, antinausea (antiemetic)
Controlled Drug: USA: No; Canada: No

Brand Names: ✦Apo-Metoclop, ✦Clopra, ✦Emex, ✦Maxeran, Maxolon, Octamide, Reclomide, Reglan

BENEFITS versus RISKS	
Possible Benefits	*Possible Risks*
EFFECTIVE STOMACH STIMULANT FOR CORRECTING DELAYED EMPTYING	Sedation and fatigue
	Parkinson-like reactions
	Tardive dyskinesia (rare)
Symptomatic relief in reflux esophagitis	
Relief of nausea and vomiting associated with migraine headache	

▷ **Principal Uses**

As a Single Drug Product: Uses currently included in FDA approved labeling: (1) Helps stomach retention (gastroparesis) associated with diabetes; (2) acid

reflux from the stomach into the esophagus (esophagitis); (3) the nausea
and vomiting associated with migraine headaches; (4) the nausea and vomiting induced by anticancer drugs; (5) helps decrease the time needed to
place a tube in the intestine; (6) used prior to cesarean section to decrease
post-delivery nausea or vomiting.

Other (unlabeled) generally accepted uses: (1) Used as a preparatory drug in
stomach hemorrhage; (2) may help gastrointestinal symptoms in anorexia
nervosa; (3) eases drug-induced slowed functioning of the intestine (ady-
namic ileus); (4) decreases the frequency of accumulations of food in the
stomach (bezoars); (5) can be of benefit in migraine attacks.

How This Drug Works: This drug inhibits relaxation of the stomach muscles
and enhances the stimulation of the parasympathetic nervous system that
is responsible for stomach muscle contractions. This action accelerates
emptying of the stomach into the intestine.

Available Dosage Forms and Strengths

Injection — 5 mg per ml and 10 mg per ml
Solution — 10 mg per ml
Syrup — 5 mg per 5-ml
Tablets — 5 mg, 10 mg

▷ **Usual Adult Dosage Range:**   10 mg taken 30 minutes before breakfast, lunch
and dinner and at bedtime (4 times a day). The total daily dose should not
exceed 0.5 mg per kilogram of body weight. **Note: Actual dosage and administration schedule must be determined by the physician for each
patient individually.**

Conditions Requiring Dosing Adjustments

Liver function: Specific dosage adjustments in liver compromise are not defined. It appears to be safe for use in these patients.

Kidney function: In patients with moderate kidney failure, 75% of the usual dose
can be given at the usual dosing interval. In severe kidney failure, 50% of
the usual dose can be given at the usual dosing interval. A benefit to risk
decision must be made regarding the use of metoclopramide in these patients.

▷ **Dosing Instructions:**   Take tablet or syrup 30 minutes before each meal and at
bedtime. The tablet may be crushed for administration.

Usual Duration of Use: Use on a regular schedule for 5 to 7 days determines
benefit in accelerating stomach emptying and relieving symptoms of heartburn, fullness and belching. Long-term use (months to years) requires physician supervision.

▷ **This Drug Should Not Be Taken If**
- you have had an allergic reaction to it previously.
- you have a seizure disorder of any kind.
- you have active gastrointestinal bleeding.
- you are taking or have taken within the last 14 days a MAO inhibitor (see
Drug Classes).
- you are taking tricyclic antidepressants.
- you have a pheochromocytoma (adrenalin-producing tumor).

▷ **Inform Your Physician Before Taking This Drug If**
- you are allergic or overly sensitive to procaine or procainamide.
- you have impaired liver or kidney function.
- you have Parkinson's disease.
- you have epilepsy.
- you have high blood pressure.
- you have a history of depression.
- you are taking any atropinelike drugs, antipsychotic drugs or opioid analgesics (see Drug Classes Section).

Possible Side Effects (natural, expected, and unavoidable drug actions)
Drowsiness and lethargy, breast tenderness and swelling, milk production.

▷ **Possible Adverse Effects** (unusual, unexpected, and infrequent reactions)
If any of the following develop, consult your physician promptly for guidance.
Mild Adverse Effects
Allergic Reaction: Skin rash. Mild decreases in blood pressure.
Headache, drowsiness, dizziness, restlessness, depression, insomnia.
Dry mouth, nausea, diarrhea, constipation.
Urinary retention or incontinence.
Serious Adverse Effects
Idiosyncratic Reactions: Neuroleptic malignant syndrome (see Glossary), bronchospastic reactions in asthmatics.
Parkinson-like reactions (see Glossary).
Tardive dyskinesia (see Glossary) (rare).
Severe decrease in white blood cells (agranulocytosis) (very rare).
Abnormal heartbeat.
Severe increases in blood pressure (hypertensive crisis).
Drug-induced porphyria.
Abnormal fixed positioning of the eyes (oculogyric crisis).

▷ **Possible Effects on Sexual Function**
Decreased libido, impaired erection, decreased sperm count, sustained painful erection (priapism).
Altered timing and pattern of menstruation, galactorrhea.

Possible Effects on Laboratory Tests
Blood lithium level: increased.
Blood thyroid stimulating hormone (TSH) level: increased.

Precautions for Use
By Infants and Children: Watch for development of Parkinson-like reactions soon after starting therapy. Use of the smallest effective dose can minimize such reactions. For diabetic gastroparesis 0.5 mg per kilogram per day divided into three equal doses given every 8 hours has been used. Children less than 6 years old should NOT receive single doses more than 0.1 mg per kilogram.
By Those over 60 Years of Age: Parkinson-like reactions and tardive dyskinesias are more likely to occur with the use of high doses over an extended period of time. The smallest effective dose should be identified and used only when clearly needed.

▷ **Advisability of Use During Pregnancy**
Pregnancy Category: B. See Pregnancy Code at the back of this book.
Animal studies: No birth defects found due to this drug.
Human studies: Adequate studies of pregnant women are not available.
Use this drug only if clearly needed.

Advisability of Use if Breast-Feeding
Presence of this drug in breast milk: Yes.
Avoid drug or refrain from nursing.

Habit-Forming Potential: None.

Effects of Overdosage: Marked drowsiness, confusion, muscle spasms, jerking movements of head and face, tremors, shuffling gait.

Possible Effects of Long-Term Use: Parkinson-like reactions may appear within several months of use. Tardive dyskinesias usually occur after a year of continual use; they may persist after this drug is discontinued.

Suggested Periodic Examinations While Taking This Drug (at physician's discretion)
During long-term use, observe for the development of fine, wormlike movements on the surface of the tongue; these may be the first indications of an emerging tardive dyskinesia.

▷ **While Taking This Drug, Observe the Following**
Foods: No restrictions.
Beverages: No restrictions. May be taken with milk.
▷   *Alcohol:* Combined effects can result in excessive sedation and marked intoxication. Alcohol is best avoided.
Tobacco Smoking: No interactions expected.
▷   *Other Drugs*
Metoclopramide may *decrease* the effects of
• cimetidine (Tagamet).
• digoxin (slow-dissolving dosage forms), and reduce its effectiveness.
Metoclopramide *taken concurrently* with
• acetaminophen may increase the absorption of this drug. Decreased doses are prudent if chronic acetaminophen use will continue with metoclopramide therapy.
• cyclosporine (Sandimmune) may result in increased cyclosporine levels and toxicity.
• major antipsychotic drugs (phenothiazines, thiothixenes, haloperidol, etc.) may increase the risk of developing Parkinson-like reactions.
• morphine (slow release) may result in faster onset and increased sedation.
• penicillin may result in decreased therapeutic benefits of the antibiotic. Increased doses may be needed.
• quinidine (Quinaglute, others) may result in decreased therapeutic benefits from quinidine. Increased blood level testing and adjustment of dosing to levels is indicated.
The following drugs may *decrease* the effects of metoclopramide
• atropinelike drugs.
• opioid analgesics (see Drug Classes).
▷   *Driving, Hazardous Activities:* This drug may cause drowsiness and dizziness. Restrict activities as necessary.

Aviation Note: The use of this drug *may be a disqualification* for piloting. Consult a designated Aviation Medical Examiner.

Exposure to Sun: No restrictions.

METOLAZONE (me TOHL a zohn)

Introduced: 1974   **Prescription:** USA: Yes; Canada: Yes   **Available as Generic:** USA: No; Canada: No   **Class:** Antihypertensive, diuretic, sulfonamides   **Controlled Drug:** USA: No; Canada: No

Brand Names: Diulo, Microx, Mykrox, Zaroxolyn

BENEFITS versus RISKS	
Possible Benefits	*Possible Risks*
EFFECTIVE, WELL-TOLERATED DIURETIC	Loss of body potassium
POSSIBLY EFFECTIVE IN MILD HYPERTENSION	Increased blood sugar
ENHANCES EFFECTIVENESS OF OTHER ANTIHYPERTENSIVES	Increased blood uric acid
	Rare liver damage, jaundice
	Rare blood cell disorder: abnormally low white blood cell count

Please see thiazide diuretic profile for further information.

METOPROLOL (me TOH proh lohl)

Introduced: 1974   **Prescription:** USA: Yes; Canada: Yes   **Available as Generic:** Yes   **Class:** Antihypertensive, beta-adrenergic blocker   **Controlled Drug:** USA: No; Canada: No

Brand Names: ✦Apo-Metoprolol, ✦Betaloc, ✦Co-Betaloc [CD], Lopressor, Lopressor Slow-release, Lopressor HCT [CD], Lopressor OROS, ✦Novo-Metoprol, ✦Nu-Metop, Toprol, Toprol XL

BENEFITS versus RISKS	
Possible Benefits	*Possible Risks*
EFFECTIVE, WELL-TOLERATED ANTIHYPERTENSIVE in mild to moderate high blood pressure	CONGESTIVE HEART FAILURE in advanced heart disease
MAY HELP REDUCE DEATH FROM HEART ATTACKS	Worsening of angina in coronary heart disease (abrupt withdrawal)
	Masking of low blood sugar (hypoglycemia) in drug-treated diabetes
	Provocation of asthma (with high doses)

▷ **Principal Uses**

As a Single Drug Product: Uses currently included in FDA approved labeling: (1) Treatment of mild to moderately severe high blood pressure. May be used alone or with other antihypertensive drugs, such as diuretics; (2) helps reduce the frequency and severity of angina; (3) used to reduce the risk of a second heart attack.

Other (unlabeled) generally accepted uses: (1) May help reduce symptoms of pathology of the heart muscle (dilated cardiomyopathy); (2) can be a second line drug in treating panic attacks; (3) may decrease operative blood loss and perioperative arrhythmias in elective hysterectomy; (4) used to decrease pressure in the eye (intraocular pressure) in open angle glaucoma.

How This Drug Works: By blocking certain actions of the sympathetic nervous system, this drug
- reduces the rate, the contraction force and ejection pressure of the heart.
- reduces contraction of blood vessel walls, resulting in expansion and consequent lowering of blood pressure.
- prolongs the conduction time of nerve impulses through the heart, of benefit in the management of certain heart rhythm disorders.

Available Dosage Forms and Strengths

Injection — 1 mg per ml
Tablets — 50 mg, 100 mg
Tablets, prolonged-action — 50 mg, 100 mg, 200 mg

▷ **Usual Adult Dosage Range:** Initially, 50 mg once or twice daily (12 hours apart). The dose may be increased gradually at intervals of 7 to 10 days as needed and tolerated, up to 300 mg/day. For maintenance, 100 mg twice/day. The total daily dose should not exceed 450 mg. **Note: Actual dosage and administration schedule must be determined by the physician for each patient individually.**

Conditions Requiring Dosing Adjustments
Liver function: This drug should be used with caution in patients with liver compromise.
Kidney function: The kidneys are minimally involved in the elimination of this drug.

▷ **Dosing Instructions:** The regular tablet may be crushed and taken without regard to eating. Prolonged-action forms should be swallowed whole (not altered). Do not discontinue this drug abruptly.

Usual Duration of Use: Use on a regular schedule for 10 to 14 days determines effectiveness in lowering blood pressure. The long-term use of this drug (months to years) will be determined by your response to an overall treatment program (weight reduction, salt restriction, smoking cessation, etc.). Consult your physician on a regular basis.

Currently a "Drug of Choice"
for initiating treatment of hypertension with a single drug, especially for those subject to bronchial asthma or diabetes.

▷ **This Drug Should Not Be Taken If**
- you have had an allergic reaction to it previously.
- you have congestive heart failure.
- you have had a heart attack and your heart rate is less than 45 beats per minute.
- you have an abnormally slow heart rate or a serious form of heart block.
- you are taking, or have taken within the past 14 days, any monoamine oxidase (MAO) type A inhibitor drug (see Drug Class Section).

▷ **Inform Your Physician Before Taking This Drug If**
  • you have had an adverse reaction to any beta blocker drug in the past (see Drug Classes).
  • you have a history of serious heart disease.
  • you have a history of hay fever (allergic rhinitis), asthma, chronic bronchitis or emphysema. People with bronchial asthma should generally not be given beta blockers. This drug is somewhat selective for the heart, and may be used in asthmatics with great caution.
  • you have a history of overactive thyroid function (hyperthyroidism).
  • you have a history of low blood sugar (hypoglycemia).
  • you have impaired liver or kidney function.
  • you have diabetes or myasthenia gravis.
  • you currently take any form of digitalis, quinidine or reserpine, or any calcium blocker drug (see Drug Class Section).
  • you have a history of poor circulation to the extremities (peripheral vascular disease).
  • you have a history of periodic cramps of your legs (intermittent claudication).
  • you plan to have surgery under general anesthesia in the near future.

Possible Side Effects (natural, expected, and unavoidable drug actions)
  Lethargy and fatigability, cold extremities, slow heart rate, light-headedness in upright position (see Orthostatic Hypotension in Glossary).

▷ **Possible Adverse Effects** (unusual, unexpected, and infrequent reactions)
  If any of the following develop, consult your physician promptly for guidance.
  Mild Adverse Effects
  Allergic Reactions: Skin rash, itching.
  Worsening of psoriasis.
  Headache, fatigue, dizziness, insomnia, abnormal dreams.
  Indigestion, nausea, vomiting, constipation, diarrhea.
  Eye and joint pain.
  Joint and muscle discomfort, fluid retention (edema).
  Serious Adverse Effects
  Mental depression, anxiety.
  Chest pain, shortness of breath, precipitation of congestive heart failure.
  Induction of bronchial asthma (in asthmatic patients).
  Abnormally slow heartbeat (bradycardia).
  Rebound hypertension (if the drug is abruptly stopped).
  Hallucinations.
  Precipitation of myasthenia gravis.
  Carpal tunnel syndrome (rare).
  Low or high blood sugar (hypoglycemia or hyperglycemia).
  Liver compromise (hepatitis) (very rare).

▷ **Possible Effects on Sexual Function:** Decreased libido (4 times more common in men); impaired erection (less common with this drug than with most other beta blockers); Peyronie's disease (see Glossary).

Possible Effects on Laboratory Tests
  Blood HDL cholesterol level: decreased.
  Blood LDL cholesterol level: decreased.

Blood VLDL cholesterol level: increased.
Blood glucose level: increased.
Blood triglyceride levels: increased.

CAUTION
1. ***Do not stop this drug suddenly*** without the knowledge and help of your physician. Carry a note with you that says you take this drug.
2. Ask your doctor or pharmacist before using nasal decongestants usually present in over-the-counter cold preparations and nose drops. These can cause undesirable increases in blood pressure when used with beta blockers.
3. Report the development of any tendency to emotional depression.

Precautions for Use
By Infants and Children: Safety and effectiveness for use by those under 12 years of age have not been established. However, if this drug is used, observe for the development of low blood sugar (hypoglycemia) during periods of reduced food intake.

By Those over 60 Years of Age: Proceed ***cautiously*** with all antihypertensive drugs. Unacceptably high blood pressure should be reduced slowly, avoiding the risks associated with excessively low blood pressure. Therapy is started with small doses, and the blood pressure checked often. Sudden, rapid and excessive reduction of blood pressure can predispose to stroke or heart attack. Watch for dizziness, unsteadiness, tendency to fall, confusion, hallucinations, depression or urinary frequency.

▷ **Advisability of Use During Pregnancy**
Pregnancy Category: C. See Pregnancy Code at the back of this book.
Animal studies: No significant increase in birth defects due to this drug.
Human studies: Adequate studies of pregnant women are not available.
Use this drug only if clearly needed. Ask physician for guidance.

Advisability of Use if Breast-Feeding
Presence of this drug in breast milk: Yes, in large amounts.
Avoid drug or refrain from nursing.

Habit-Forming Potential: None.

Effects of Overdosage: Weakness, slow pulse, low blood pressure, fainting, cold and sweaty skin, congestive heart failure, possible coma and convulsions.

Possible Effects of Long-Term Use: Reduced heart reserve and eventual heart failure in susceptible individuals with advanced heart disease.

Suggested Periodic Examinations While Taking This Drug (at physician's discretion)
Measurements of blood pressure, evaluation of heart function.

▷ **While Taking This Drug, Observe the Following**
Foods: The peak drug concentration and therefore, the peak effect of this drug will increase if it is taken with food. Avoid excessive salt intake.
Beverages: No restrictions. May be taken with milk.
▷ *Alcohol:* Use with caution. Alcohol may exaggerate this drug's ability to lower the blood pressure and may increase its mild sedative effect.

Tobacco Smoking: Nicotine may reduce this drug's benefit in treating high blood pressure. Additionally, high doses of this drug may potentiate the constriction of the bronchial tubes caused by regular smoking.

▷ *Other Drugs*

Metoprolol may *increase* the effects of

- other antihypertensive drugs, and cause excessive lowering of the blood pressure. Dosage adjustments may be necessary.
- reserpine (Ser-Ap-Es, etc.), and cause sedation, depression, slowing of the heart rate and lowering of the blood pressure.
- verapamil (Calan, Isoptin), and cause excessive depression of heart function; monitor this combination closely.

Metoprolol *taken concurrently* with

- amiodarone may result in extremely slow heartbeat and cardiac arrest.
- clonidine (Catapres) requires close monitoring for rebound high blood pressure if clonidine is withdrawn while metoprolol is still being taken.
- fluoxetine (Prozac) may cause metoprolol toxicity.
- fluvoxamine (Luvox) may lead to metoprolol toxicity.
- insulin requires close monitoring to avoid undetected hypoglycemia (see Glossary).
- lidocaine can lead to lidocaine toxicity (cardiac arrest).
- nifedipine (Adalat, Procardia, others) may result in heart failure.
- oral hypoglycemic agents (see Drug Classes) can result in prolonged hypoglycemia if it occurs.
- phenothiazines (see Drug Classes) can result in low blood pressure or toxicity due to the phenothiazine.
- quinidine (Quinaglute, others) can lead to abnormally slow heartbeat and shortness of breath.
- tocainide (Tonocard) may lead to depressed contraction ability of the heart (myocardial contractility).
- venlafaxine (Effexor) may lead to metabolic changes and toxic blood levels of both medicines.

The following drugs may *increase* the effects of metoprolol

- cimetidine (Tagamet).
- diltiazem (Cardizem).
- methimazole (Tapazole).
- MAO inhibitors (see Drug Classes).
- birth control pills (oral contraceptives).
- propylthiouracil (Propacil).

The following drugs may *decrease* the effects of metoprolol

- barbiturates (phenobarbital, etc.).
- indomethacin (Indocin), and possibly other "aspirin substitutes," or NSAIDs may impair metoprolol's antihypertensive effect.
- rifampin (Rifadin, Rimactane).

▷ *Driving, Hazardous Activities:* Use caution until the full extent of drowsiness, lethargy and blood pressure change has been determined.

Aviation Note: The use of this drug *is a disqualification* for piloting. Consult a designated Aviation Medical Examiner.

Exposure to Sun: No restrictions.

Exposure to Heat: Caution advised. Hot environments can lower the blood pressure and exaggerate the effects of this drug.

Exposure to Cold: Caution advised. Cold environments can increase circulatory deficiency in the extremities that may occur with this drug. The elderly should take precautions to prevent hypothermia (see Glossary).

Heavy Exercise or Exertion: It is advisable to avoid exertion that produces light-headedness, excessive fatigue or muscle cramping. The use of this drug may intensify the hypertensive response to isometric exercise.

Occurrence of Unrelated Illness: Fever can lower the blood pressure and require adjustment of dosage. Nausea or vomiting may interrupt the regular dosage schedule. Ask your doctor for help.

Discontinuation: It is advisable to avoid sudden discontinuation of this drug in all situations. If possible, gradual reduction of dose over a period of 1 to 2 weeks is recommended. Ask your physician for specific guidance.

METRONIDAZOLE (me troh NI da zohl)

Introduced: 1960   **Prescription:** USA: Yes; Canada: Yes   **Available as Generic:** Yes   **Class:** Anti-infective   **Controlled Drug:** USA: No; Canada: No

Brand Names: ✦Apo-Metronidazole, Femazole, Flagyl, Flagystatin, Lagyl, Metizol, MetroGel, Metro IV, Metryl, ✦Neo-Tric, ✦Novo-Nidazole, Protostat, SK Metronidazole, ✦Trikacide

---

BENEFITS versus RISKS

Possible Benefits	*Possible Risks*
EFFECTIVE TREATMENT FOR TRICHOMONAS INFECTIONS, AMEBIC DYSENTERY, AND GIARDIASIS, and some anaerobic bacterial infections	Superinfection with yeast organisms Peripheral neuropathy Abnormally low white blood cell count (transient)
Effective local treatment for rosacea	Colitis Aggravation of epilepsy

---

▷ **Principal Uses**

As a Single Drug Product: Uses currently included in FDA approved labeling: (1) Treats Trichomonas infections of the vaginal canal and cervix and of the male urethra; (2) it is also used to treat amebic dysentery and liver abscess, Giardia infections of the intestine and serious infections caused by certain strains of anaerobic bacteria; (3) treats gardnerella infections of the vagina; (4) treatment of rosacea with local application of a gel dosage form; (5) used in therapy of pseudomembranous colitis; (6) has a role in treating bed sores (decubitis ulcers); (7) can help prevent infection (prophylaxis) in gynecologic, appendectomy or colorectal surgery.

Other (unlabeled) generally accepted uses: (1) Combination therapy with gentamicin in treating intra-abdominal infections; (2) combination antibiotic treatment of duodenal ulcers caused by H. pylori; (3) can help treat infections caused by Giardia lamblia; (4) used to help heal the lesions in Crohn's disease.

How This Drug Works: By interacting with DNA, this drug destroys essential components (nucleus) that are needed for life and growth of infecting organisms.

Available Dosage Forms and Strengths

      Capsules — 375 mg

          Gel — 0.75%

      Injection — 500 mg per 100 ml

       Tablets — 250 mg, 500 mg

Vaginal cream — 10%

▷ **Usual Adult Dosage Range:**   Varies with infection to be treated.

For trichomoniasis: One-day course—2 grams as a single dose; or 1 gram for 2 doses 12 hours apart. Seven-day course—250 mg 3 times/day for 7 consecutive days. (The 7-day course is preferred.)

For amebiasis: 500 to 750 mg 3 times/day for 5 to 10 consecutive days.

For giardiasis: 2 grams once/day for 3 days; or 250 to 500 mg 3 times/day for 5 to 7 days.

The total daily dosage should not exceed 4 grams (4000 mg).

Note: Actual dosage and administration schedule must be determined by the physician for each patient individually.

Conditions Requiring Dosing Adjustments

Liver function: The dose should be decreased by one third in mild to moderate liver compromise. It should not be used in severe liver compromise.

Kidney function: In severe kidney failure, 50% of the normal dose can be given at the usual dosing interval. A benefit to risk decision must be made regarding the use of metronidazole in these patients as there is a risk of systemic lupus erythematosus (SLE) from the metabolites of this drug.

▷ **Dosing Instructions:**   The tablet may be crushed and taken with or following food to reduce stomach irritation.

Usual Duration of Use: Use on a regular schedule as outlined is needed to ensure effectiveness. Do not repeat the course of treatment without your physician's approval.

▷ **This Drug Should Not Be Taken If**

- you have had an allergic reaction to it or any the parabens contained in the gel form previously.
- you are pregnant.
- you currently have a bone marrow or blood cell disorder.
- you have any type of central nervous system disorder, including epilepsy.

▷ **Inform Your Physician Before Taking This Drug If**

- you have a history of any type of blood cell disorder, especially one induced by drugs.
- you have a history of seizures or peripheral neuropathy.
- you have impaired liver or kidney function.
- you have a history of alcoholism.
- you are pregnant or breast-feeding.

Possible Side Effects (natural, expected, and unavoidable drug actions)

A sharp, metallic, unpleasant taste.

Dark discoloration of the urine (of no significance).

Superinfection (see Glossary) by yeast organisms in the mouth or vagina.

▷ **Possible Adverse Effects** (unusual, unexpected, and infrequent reactions)

If any of the following develop, consult your physician promptly for guidance.

Mild Adverse Effects
    Allergic Reactions: Skin rash, hives, flushing, itching.
    Headache, dizziness, incoordination, unsteadiness, incontinence.
    Discoloration of urine.
    Loss of appetite, nausea, vomiting, abdominal cramps, diarrhea.
    Irritation of mouth and tongue, possibly due to yeast infection.
Serious Adverse Effects
    Idiosyncratic Reactions: Abnormal behavior; confusion; depression; Herx-
       heimer's reaction—sweating, diarrhea, vomiting, scalding urination, joint
       pain and itching.
    Peripheral neuropathy (see Glossary).
    Abnormally low white blood cell count (transient): fever, sore throat, infec-
       tions (rare).
    Disulfiram-type reaction (nausea, vomiting) if alcoholic beverages are con-
       sumed.
    Seizures (rare).
    Drug-induced pneumonitis (rare).
    Drug-induced porphyria (rare).
    Pseudomembranous colitis.
    Pancreatitis (rare).
    Hemolytic-uremic syndrome (rare).

▷ **Possible Effects on Sexual Function:** Decreased libido; decreased vaginal
    secretions (difficult or painful intercourse).

Possible Delayed Adverse Effects: Studies have shown that this drug can
    cause cancer in mice and possibly in rats. Two researchers concluded that
    the carcinogenic risk is low in doses used to treat episodic vaginitis. Follow
    your physician's instructions exactly. Avoid unnecessary or prolonged use.

▷ **Adverse Effects That May Mimic Natural Diseases or Disorders**
    Behavioral changes may suggest spontaneous psychosis.

Natural Diseases or Disorders That May Be Activated by This Drug
    Latent yeast infections.

Possible Effects on Laboratory Tests
    White blood cell counts: decreased.
    INR (prothrombin time): increased.
    Blood theophylline levels: falsely increased by some methods.

CAUTION
    1. Troublesome and persistent diarrhea can develop. If diarrhea persists for
       more than 24 hours, stop this drug and call your physician.
    2. Stop this drug immediately if you develop any signs of toxic effects on the
       brain or nervous system: Confusion, irritability, dizziness, incoordina-
       tion, unsteady stance or gait, muscle jerking or twitching, numbness or
       weakness in the extremities.

Precautions for Use
    By Infants and Children: Avoid use in those with a history of bone marrow or
       blood cell disorders.
    By Those over 60 Years of Age: Natural changes in the skin may predispose to
       yeast infections in the genital and anal regions. Report the development of
       rashes and itching promptly.

▷ **Advisability of Use During Pregnancy**
  Pregnancy Category: B. See Pregnancy Code at the back of this book.
    Animal studies: No birth defects reported in rat studies. However, this drug is known to cause cancer in mice and possibly in rats.
    Human studies: No increase in birth defects reported in 206 exposures to this drug during the first 3 months. However, information from adequate studies of pregnant women is not available.
    The manufacturer advises against the use of this drug during the first 3 months. Use during the last 6 months is not advised unless it is absolutely essential to the mother's health.

Advisability of Use if Breast-Feeding
  Presence of this drug in breast milk: Yes.
  Avoid drug or refrain from nursing.

Habit-Forming Potential: None.

Effects of Overdosage: Weakness, stomach irritation, nausea, vomiting, confusion, disorientation.

Possible Effects of Long-Term Use: None reported. Avoid long-term use.

Suggested Periodic Examinations While Taking This Drug (at physician's discretion)
  Complete blood cell counts.

▷ **While Taking This Drug, Observe the Following**
  Foods: No restrictions.
  Beverages: No restrictions. May be taken with milk.
▷ *Alcohol:* A disulfiramlike reaction has been reported (see Glossary). It is NOT advisable to drink alcohol while taking metronidazole.
  Tobacco Smoking: No interactions expected.
▷ *Other Drugs*
    Metronidazole may ***increase*** the effects of
    • warfarin (Coumadin, etc.), and cause abnormal bleeding. The INR (prothrombin time) should be monitored closely, especially during the first 10 days of concurrent use.
    Metronidazole ***taken concurrently*** with
    • antacids may decrease absorption of metronidazole.
    • birth control pills (oral contraceptives) may block the effectiveness of contraception and result in pregnancy.
    • cholestyramine (Questran) or other cholesterol lowering resins may decrease metronidazole absorption and lower its therapeutic effect.
    • cotrimoxazole or other sulfa drugs may result in a disulfiram effect.
    • cyclosporine (Sandimmune) can lead to cyclosporine toxicity.
    • disulfiram (Antabuse) may cause severe emotional and behavioral disturbances.
    • lithium (Lithobid, others) can cause lithium toxicity.
    • phenytoin (Dilantin) may result in increased blood levels of phenytoin. More frequent blood level testing is needed, and the phenytoin dose should be adjusted to blood levels.
▷ *Driving, Hazardous Activities:* This drug may cause dizziness or incoordination. Restrict activities as necessary.

Aviation Note: The use of this drug *may be a disqualification* for piloting. Consult a designated Aviation Medical Examiner.
Exposure to Sun: No restrictions.

MEXILETINE (mex IL e teen)

Introduced: 1973   **Prescription:** USA: Yes; Canada: Yes   **Available as**
Generic: No   **Class:** Antiarrhythmic   **Controlled Drug:** USA: No; Canada: No

Brand Name: Mexitil

<table>
<tr><td colspan="2" align="center">BENEFITS versus RISKS</td></tr>
<tr><td align="center">Possible Benefits</td><td align="center">Possible Risks</td></tr>
<tr><td>EFFECTIVE TREATMENT IN
SELECTED HEART RHYTHM
DISORDERS</td><td>NARROW TREATMENT RANGE
FREQUENT ADVERSE EFFECTS
WORSENING OF SOME
ARRHYTHMIAS
Rare seizures, liver injury, and
reduced white blood cell count</td></tr>
</table>

▷ **Principal Uses**
  As a Single Drug Product: Uses currently included in FDA approved labeling: (1)
  Helps correct premature beats that arise in the ventricles (lower heart chambers) which are resistant (refractory) to other agents.
  Other (unlabeled) generally accepted uses: (1) May have a role in reducing symptoms in diabetic nerve damage (neuropathy); (2) has shown some benefit in combination therapy of Wolf-Parkinson-White syndrome.

How This Drug Works: By slowing the transmission of electrical impulses throughout the conduction system of the heart, this drug assists in restoring normal heart rate and rhythm in selected types of arrhythmia.

Available Dosage Forms and Strengths
  Capsules — 150 mg, 200 mg, 250 mg

▷ **Usual Adult Dosage Range:** A loading dose of 400 mg is given, followed by 200 mg every 8 hours. Dose can be increased at intervals of 2 to 3 days, as needed and tolerated in 50 or 100 mg steps to a maximum total daily dose of 1200 mg. Measurement of drug blood levels is advised (when available) to determine the optimal dose and schedule. **Note: Actual dosage and administration schedule must be determined by the physician for each patient individually.**

Conditions Requiring Dosing Adjustments
  Liver function: In liver compromise, the dose should be decreased by one fourth to one third. Blood levels should be obtained at prudent intervals.
  Kidney function: The dose should be decreased and blood levels obtained more frequently in patients with severe kidney failure.

▷ **Dosing Instructions:** The capsule may be opened and taken with food or antacid to reduce stomach irritation. Take at same times each day to obtain uniform results.

Usual Duration of Use: Use on a regular schedule for 1 to 2 weeks determines effectiveness in correcting or preventing responsive rhythm disorders. Long-term use requires physician supervision.

▷ **This Drug Should Not Be Taken If**
- you have had an allergic reaction to it previously.
- you have second-degree or third-degree heart block (determined by electrocardiogram), uncorrected by a pacemaker.

▷ **Inform Your Physician Before Taking This Drug If**
- you have had adverse reactions to other antiarrhythmic drugs in the past.
- you have a history of heart disease of any kind, especially "heart block" or heart failure.
- you have impaired liver function.
- you have Parkinson's disease.
- you are prone to low blood pressure.
- you have a seizure disorder of any kind.
- you take any form of digitalis, a potassium supplement or any diuretic drug that can cause potassium loss (ask physician).

Possible Side Effects (natural, expected, and unavoidable drug actions)
Nervousness, light-headedness.

▷ **Possible Adverse Effects** (unusual, unexpected, and infrequent reactions)
If any of the following develop, consult your physician promptly for guidance.
Mild Adverse Effects
Allergic Reaction: Skin rash.
Headache, dizziness, visual disturbance, fatigue, weakness, tremor.
Loss of appetite, indigestion, nausea, vomiting, constipation, diarrhea, abdominal pain (rare).
Unpleasant taste.
Serious Adverse Effects
Idiosyncratic Reactions: Depression, confusion, amnesia, hallucinations, seizures (all rare).
Drug-induced heart rhythm disorders (rare), shortness of breath, palpitations, chest pain, swelling of feet.
Myelofibrosis (rare).
Seizures.
Ataxia and confusion (up to 50%).
Congestive heart failure and sinus arrest (rare).
Urinary retention.
Liver damage with jaundice (see Glossary).
Abnormally low white blood cell and blood platelet counts (rare): Fever, sore throat, abnormal bleeding or bruising.
Systemic lupus erythematosus (rare).

▷ **Possible Effects on Sexual Function:**   Decreased libido, impotence (rare).

▷ **Adverse Effects That May Mimic Natural Diseases or Disorders**
Liver toxicity may suggest viral hepatitis.

Natural Diseases or Disorders That May Be Activated by This Drug
Latent epilepsy.

Possible Effects on Laboratory Tests

Blood white cell and platelet counts: decreased.

Liver function tests: increased liver enzymes (ALT/GPT, AST/GOT) increased in less than 1% of users.

CAUTION

1. Thorough evaluation of your heart function (including electrocardiograms) is necessary prior to using this drug.
2. Periodic evaluation of your heart function is needed to determine your response to this drug. Some individuals may experience worsening of their heart rhythm disorder and/or deterioration of heart function. Close monitoring of heart rate, rhythm and overall performance is essential.
3. Dosage must be adjusted carefully for each individual. Do not change your dosage without the knowledge and supervision of your physician.
4. Do not take any other antiarrhythmic drug while taking this drug unless you are directed to do so by your physician.
5. Carry a card of personal identification with the notation that you are taking this drug. Inform all attending medical personnel that you are taking this drug, especially if you require surgery of any kind.

Precautions for Use

By Infants and Children: Safety and effectiveness for those under 12 years of age not established. Initial use of this drug requires hospitalization and supervision by a qualified cardiologist.

By Those over 60 Years of Age: Reduced liver function may require reduction in dosage. Observe carefully for light-headedness, dizziness, unsteadiness and tendency to fall.

▷ **Advisability of Use During Pregnancy**

Pregnancy Category: C. See Pregnancy Code at the back of this book.

Animal studies: No birth defects reported in mice, rats or rabbits. However, an increased rate of fetal resorption was found.

Human studies: Adequate studies of pregnant women are not available.

Avoid during first 3 months. Use this drug only if clearly needed. Ask physician for guidance.

Advisability of Use if Breast-Feeding

Presence of this drug in breast milk: Yes.

Avoid drug or refrain from nursing.

Habit-Forming Potential: None.

Effects of Overdosage: Impaired urination, constipation, marked drop in blood pressure, abnormal heart rhythms, congestive heart failure, dizziness, incoordination, seizures.

Possible Effects of Long-Term Use: None reported.

Suggested Periodic Examinations While Taking This Drug (at physician's discretion)

Electrocardiograms, complete blood cell counts, liver function tests, mexiletine blood levels.

▷ **While Taking This Drug, Observe the Following**

Foods: No restrictions. Ask physician regarding need for salt restriction.

Beverages: No restrictions. May be taken with milk.

▷ *Alcohol:* Use caution. Alcohol can increase the blood-pressure-lowering effects of this drug.

Tobacco Smoking: Nicotine can cause irritability of the heart and reduce the effectiveness of this drug. Follow physician's advice regarding smoking.

▷ *Other Drugs*

Mexiletine may ***increase*** the effects of
- antihypertensive drugs, and cause excessive lowering of blood pressure.
- beta blocker drugs (see Drug Classes).
- disopyramide (Norpace).
- theophylline (Theodur, others) leading to theophylline toxicity and seizures.

The following drugs may ***decrease*** the effects of mexiletine
- phenytoin (Dilantin, etc.).
- rifampin (Rifadin, Rimactane).

▷ *Driving, Hazardous Activities:* This drug may cause weakness, dizziness or blurred vision. Restrict activities as necessary.

Aviation Note: The use of this drug ***may be a disqualification*** for piloting. Consult a designated Aviation Medical Examiner.

Exposure to Sun: No restrictions.

Occurrence of Unrelated Illness: Vomiting, diarrhea or dehydration can affect this drug's action adversely. Report such developments promptly.

Discontinuation: This drug should not be stopped abruptly following long-term use. Ask your physician for guidance regarding gradual dose reduction.

MINOXIDIL (min OX i dil)

Introduced: 1972   **Prescription:** USA: Yes; Canada: Yes   **Available as Generic:** Yes   **Class:** Antihypertensive, hair growth stimulant   **Controlled Drug:** USA: No; Canada: No

Brand Names: Alostil, Loniten, Minodyl, Minoximen, Rogaine

Author's note: Rogaine treatment for baldness is now available without a prescription.

BENEFITS versus RISKS

Possible Benefits	*Possible Risks*
POTENT, LONG-ACTING ANTIHYPERTENSIVE	EXCESSIVE BODY HAIR GROWTH SALT AND WATER RETENTION
EFFECTIVE IN CASES OF SEVERE HYPERTENSION, ACCELERATED AND MALIGNANT HYPERTENSION	Excessively rapid heart rate Aggravation of angina Local scalp irritation (topical use)
Moderately effective in treating male-pattern baldness	

▷ **Principal Uses**

As a Single Drug Product: Uses currently included in FDA approved labeling: (1) Treatment of severe high blood pressure that cannot be controlled by conventional therapy; (2) the treatment of female androgenic baldness or male-pattern baldness; (3) effective in patients with high blood pressure and kidney failure.

Other (unlabeled) generally accepted uses: (1) Supportive therapy in hair transplants.

How This Drug Works: (1) Directly relaxes constricted muscles in the walls of small arteries, and permits expansion of the arteries and lowering of blood pressure. (2) The drug may act directly on the hair follicle, and also may increase the size of previously closed small blood vessels in the scalp (improve blood flow) and restore small hair follicles to normal size and activity.

Available Dosage Forms and Strengths

Tablets — 2.5 mg, 10 mg

Topical solution — 2%

▷ **Usual Adult Dosage Range:**   For hypertension: Initially, 5 mg once a day. The dose is then gradually increased as needed and tolerated to 10 mg, 20 mg, then 40 mg per 24 hours, taken in 1 or 2 divided doses daily. The usual maintenance dose is 10 to 40 mg/24 hours. The total daily dosage should not exceed 50 mg. For male-pattern baldness: Apply thinly 1 ml of topical solution to the balding area of the scalp twice daily. The total daily dosage should not exceed 2 ml. **Note: Actual dosage and administration schedule must be determined by the physician for each patient individually.**

Conditions Requiring Dosing Adjustments

Liver function: This drug is metabolized (90%) in the liver. It should be used with caution in patients with liver compromise.

Kidney function: In moderate kidney failure, the dose should be decreased empirically.

▷ **Dosing Instructions:**   For hypertension: Tablets may be crushed and taken with or following food to prevent nausea. Take at the same time each day. For baldness: *The topical solution is for external, local use only; it is not to be swallowed.* Begin application at the center of the bald area; apply thinly to cover the entire area. The scalp and hair must be dry at the time of application. Follow instructions carefully.

Usual Duration of Use: Use on a regular schedule for 3 to 7 days usually determines effectiveness in controlling severe hypertension. Continual use of the topical solution for at least 4 months is necessary to determine its ability to promote hair growth. Long-term use (months to years) of both dosage forms requires physician supervision.

▷ **This Drug Should Not Be Taken If**
- you have had an allergic reaction to it previously.
- you are known to have a pheochromocytoma (an adrenalin-producing tumor).
- you have pulmonary hypertension due to mitral valve stenosis.

▷ **Inform Your Physician Before Taking This Drug If**
- you are pregnant or planning pregnancy.
- you are breast feeding your infant.
- you have had a heart attack.
- you have existing blood vessel disease in your head (cerebrovascular disease).

- you have a history of coronary artery disease or impaired heart function.
- you have a history of stroke or impaired brain circulation.
- you have impaired liver or kidney function.

Possible Side Effects (natural, expected, and unavoidable drug actions)
Increased heart rate, fluid retention with weight gain, excessive hair growth on face, arms, legs, and back (frequent).

▷ **Possible Adverse Effects** (unusual, unexpected, and infrequent reactions)
If any of the following develop, consult your physician promptly for guidance.

Mild Adverse Effects
Allergic Reactions: Skin rash (rare). Localized dermatitis at site of application of topical solution.
Headache, dizziness, fainting (rare).
Nausea, increased thirst.
Hair growth, and changes in hair color.
Weight gain.
Mild increase in liver enzymes.

Serious Adverse Effects
Allergic Reactions: Serious skin rash (Stevens-Johnson syndrome).
Idiosyncratic Reaction: Fluid formation around the heart (pericardial effusion).
Development of angina pectoris; development of high blood pressure in the lung circulation (pulmonary hypertension).
Systemic lupus erythematosus (rare).
Low white blood cells or platelets (rare and transient).

▷ **Possible Effects on Sexual Function:** Male breast tenderness (gynecomastia) (rare). Some data to support this drug balancing male ability to ejaculate and have a healthy sex drive may have been blunted by other drugs which treat high blood pressure.

Natural Diseases or Disorders That May Be Activated by This Drug
Latent coronary artery disease with symptomatic angina.

Possible Effects on Laboratory Tests
Blood HDL cholesterol level: increased.
Blood LDL cholesterol level: decreased.

CAUTION
1. Long-term use for hypertension usually requires the concurrent use of an effective diuretic to counteract salt and water retention.
2. The long-term use of this drug for hypertension may require concurrent use of a beta blocker drug to control excessive acceleration of the heart.
3. Best to avoid combining this drug and guanethidine; the combination can cause severe orthostatic hypotension (see Glossary).
4. Consult your physician regarding the advisability of using a "no salt added" diet.
5. Little of this drug is absorbed into the general circulation when the topical solution is applied to the scalp. However, some systemic effects have been reported. Inform your physician promptly if you experience any unusual symptoms while using the topical solution.

Precautions for Use

By Infants and Children: Dosage schedules should be determined by a qualified pediatrician. In children under 12 years old: starting dose is 0.1 to 0.2 mg per kilogram in a single dose. The dose is then increased as needed and tolerated by 0.1 to 0.2 mg per kilogram per day steps at 3 day intervals. Children over 12 are given the adult dose. Monitor closely for salt and water retention.

By Those over 60 Years of Age: Treatment with small doses and a limit of total daily dose to 75 mg is indicated. Headache, palpitation and rapid heart rate due to this drug are more common in this age group and can mimic acute anxiety states. Observe for dizziness, unsteadiness, fainting and falling.

▷ ### Advisability of Use During Pregnancy

Pregnancy Category: C. See Pregnancy Code at the back of this book.

Animal studies: No birth defects reported in rats or rabbits. However, studies did reveal decreased fertility and increased fetal deaths.

Human studies: Adequate studies of pregnant women are not available.

Avoid during the first 3 months. Use only if clearly needed during the last 6 months.

Advisability of Use if Breast-Feeding

Presence of this drug in breast milk: Yes.

Avoid drug or refrain from nursing.

Habit-Forming Potential: None.

Effects of Overdosage: Headache, dizziness, weakness, nausea, marked low blood pressure, weak and rapid pulse, loss of consciousness.

Possible Effects of Long-Term Use: Excessive growth of body hair occurs in 80% of users after 1 to 2 months of continual treatment for hypertension. Close to 100% of users will experience this effect after 1 year of continual treatment. This may be accompanied by darkening of the skin and coarsening of facial features.

Suggested Periodic Examinations While Taking This Drug (at physician's discretion)

Body weight measurement for insidious gain due to water retention.

Electrocardiographic and echocardiographic heart examinations.

▷ ### While Taking This Drug, Observe the Following

Foods: Avoid excessive salt and heavily salted foods.

Beverages: No restrictions. May be taken with milk.

▷ *Alcohol:* Use with extreme caution. Alcohol can exaggerate the blood-pressure-lowering effects of this drug.

Tobacco Smoking: Best avoided. Nicotine can contribute significantly to the development of angina in susceptible individuals.

▷ *Other Drugs*

Minoxidil may *increase* the effects of

- all other antihypertensive drugs; careful dosage adjustments are mandatory.

Minoxidil *taken concurrently* with

- guanethidine (Ismelin, Esimil) may cause severe orthostatic hypotension; avoid this combination.
- NSAIDs may blunt the therapeutic benefit of minoxidil.
- vitamin E may reverse hair growth.

▷ *Driving, Hazardous Activities:* This drug may cause dizziness and fatigue. Restrict activities as necessary.

Aviation Note: The use of this drug *is a disqualification* for piloting. Consult a designated Aviation Medical Examiner.

Exposure to Sun: No restrictions.

Discontinuation: This drug should not be stopped abruptly. If it is to be discontinued, consult your physician regarding gradual reduction in dosage and appropriate replacement with other drugs for the management of hypertension. Following discontinuation of the topical solution, the pretreatment pattern of baldness may return within 3 to 4 months.

MISOPROSTOL (mi soh PROH stohl)

Introduced: 1987   **Prescription:** USA: Yes; Canada: Yes   **Available as Generic:** USA: No; Canada: No   **Class:** gastrointestinal drug (ulcer preventive)   **Controlled Drug:** USA: No; Canada: No

Brand Name: Arthrotec, Cytotec

BENEFITS versus RISKS	
Possible Benefits	*Possible Risks*
EFFECTIVE PREVENTION OF STOMACH ULCERATION WHILE TAKING ANTI-INFLAMMATORY DRUGS	INCREASED RISK OF ABORTION (if used during pregnancy)
Effective treatment of duodenal ulcer	Diarrhea (transient)
	Neuropathy (rare)

▷ **Principal Uses**

As a Single Drug Product: Uses currently included in FDA approved labeling: (1) Prevents development of stomach ulcers during long-term use of anti-inflammatory drugs as therapy for arthritis and related conditions.

Other (unlabeled) generally accepted uses: (1) Used (in Canada and other countries) for treatment of active duodenal ulcer unrelated to use of anti-inflammatory drugs; (2) has seen some use in inducing abortions; (3) used in combination with cyclosporine or prednisone to decrease transplanted organ rejection; (4) may have a benefit in helping ripen the cervix in preparation for a vaginal delivery.

How This Drug Works: This drug protects the lining of the stomach and duodenum and prevents ulceration due to anti-inflammatory drugs by: (1) replacing tissue prostaglandins that are depleted by anti-inflammatory drugs; (2) inhibiting the secretion of stomach acid; (3) increasing the local production of bicarbonate (to neutralize acids) and of mucus (to protect stomach and duodenal tissues). The combined effects prevent new ulcer formation and promote healing of existing ulcer(s).

Available Dosage Forms and Strengths

Tablets — 100 mcg and 200 mcg

Conditions Requiring Dosing Adjustments

Liver function: Specific dosage adjustments in liver compromise are not defined.

Kidney function: The dose of misoprostol should be decreased if it is used in patients with compromised kidneys, and is not well tolerated.

▷ **Usual Adult Dosage Range**

For prevention of stomach ulcer—200 mcg 4 times daily with food, taken concurrently during the use of any anti-inflammatory drug (see Antiarthritic/Anti-inflammatory Drug Classes).

For treatment of duodenal ulcer—200 mcg 4 times daily for 4 to 8 weeks.

Note: Actual dosage and administration schedule must be determined by the physician for each patient individually.

▷ **Dosing Instructions:**   The tablet may be crushed and taken with each of 3 daily meals; take the last (fourth) dose of the day with food at bedtime.

Usual Duration of Use: For prevention of stomach ulcer, use is recommended for the entire period of anti-inflammatory drug use. For treatment of duodenal ulcer, continual use on a regular schedule for 4 weeks is recommended; if ulcer healing is not complete, a second course of 4 weeks is advised. Long-term use (months to years) requires periodic physician evaluation of response and dosage adjustment.

Possible Advantages of This Drug: Significantly more effective than histamine (H-2)-blocking drugs (cimetidine, famotidine, nizatidine, ranitidine) or sucralfate in preventing the development of stomach ulcers.

▷ **This Drug Should Not Be Taken If**
- you have had an allergic reaction to it previously.
- you are allergic to any type of prostaglandin.
- you are pregnant or breast-feeding.
- you are not able or willing to use effective contraception (oral contraceptives or intrauterine device) while taking this drug.

▷ **Inform Your Physician Before Taking This Drug If**
- you have a history of peptic ulcer disease or Crohn's disease.
- you have inflammatory bowel disease.
- you have impaired kidney function.
- you have a seizure disorder.

Possible Side Effects (natural, expected, and unavoidable drug actions)

Diarrhea (14–40% of users), usually beginning after 13 days of use and subsiding spontaneously after 8 days.

Abortion (miscarriage) of pregnancy (11% of users); this is often incomplete and accompanied by serious uterine bleeding that may require hospitalization and urgent treatment.

▷ **Possible Adverse Effects** (unusual, unexpected, and infrequent reactions)

If any of the following develop, consult your physician promptly for guidance.

Mild Adverse Effects

Allergic Reaction: Skin rash.

Headache, dizziness.

Ringing in the ears.

Passing out (syncope) (rare).

Abdominal pain, indigestion (rare), nausea, vomiting (rare), flatulence, constipation (rare).

Menstrual irregularity (rare), menstrual cramps (rare), heavy menstrual flow (rare), spotting between periods (rare).

Serious Adverse Effects
 Allergic Reactions: Anaphylaxis (rare).
 Postmenopausal vaginal bleeding; this may require further evaluation.
 Anemia and low blood platelets (rare).
 Blood in the urine (rare).
 Bronchospasm (rare).
 Neuropathy (rare).
 Abortion (if taken while pregnant).

▷ **Possible Effects on Sexual Function:**   Reduced libido and impotence reported rarely, but causal relationship not established.

▷ **Natural Diseases or Disorders That May Be Activated by This Drug**
 Latent epilepsy.

Possible Effects on Laboratory Tests
 Mild increase in liver function enzymes.

CAUTION
 1. Do not take this drug if you are pregnant. It can cause abortion.
 2. Do not make this drug available to others who may be pregnant or who may become pregnant.
 3. If this drug is prescribed, it is advisable that you have a negative serum pregnancy test within 2 weeks before starting treatment.
 4. Start taking this drug only on the second or third day of your next normal menstrual period.
 5. Initiate effective contraceptive measures when you begin to take this drug. Discuss the use of oral contraceptives or intrauterine devices with your physician.
 6. Should pregnancy occur while you are taking this drug, stop the drug immediately and inform your physician.

Precautions for Use
 By Infants and Children: Safety and effectiveness for those under 18 years of age not established.
 By Those over 60 Years of Age: This drug is usually well tolerated by this age group. However, some forms of prostaglandins can cause drops in blood pressure; watch for light-headedness or faintness that may indicate low blood pressure. Report any such development to your physician.

▷ **Advisability of Use During Pregnancy**
 Pregnancy Category: X. See Pregnancy Code at the back of this book.
 Animal studies: No birth defects due to this drug found in rat or rabbit studies.
 Human studies: Information from studies of pregnant women confirms that this drug can cause abortion, sometimes incomplete; unpassed products of conception can cause life-threatening complications.
 Avoid this drug completely.

Advisability of Use if Breast-Feeding
 Presence of this drug in breast milk: Unknown.
 Avoid drug or refrain from nursing.

Habit-Forming Potential: None.

Effects of Overdosage: Abdominal pain, diarrhea, fever, drowsiness, weakness, tremor, convulsions, difficult breathing.

Possible Effects of Long-Term Use: Unknown at this time.

Suggested Periodic Examinations While Taking This Drug (at physician's discretion)
   Monitoring for accidental pregnancy.

▷ **While Taking This Drug, Observe the Following**
   Foods: High fat meals may reduce peak blood concentration.
   Beverages: No restrictions. May be taken with milk.
▷ *Alcohol:* No interactions expected. However, alcohol can promote the development of stomach ulcer and reduce the effectiveness of this drug.
   Tobacco Smoking: No interactions expected. However, nicotine is conducive to the development of stomach ulcer. Smoking should be avoided.
▷ *Other Drugs*
   Misoprostol *taken concurrently* with
   • antacids that contain magnesium may increase the risk of diarrhea; avoid this combination. Antacids in general may decrease misoprostol absorption and lessen therapeutic benefit.
   • indomethacin and some other NSAIDs may result in decreased NSAID levels.
▷ *Driving, Hazardous Activities:* This drug may cause dizziness, light-headedness, stomach pain or diarrhea. Restrict activities as necessary.
   Aviation Note: The use of this drug *may be a disqualification* for piloting. Consult a designated Aviation Medical Examiner.
   Exposure to Sun: No restrictions.
   Discontinuation: This drug should be taken as combination therapy while you are taking antiarthritic/anti-inflammatory drugs that can cause stomach ulceration. Call your doctor if you have reason to stop it prematurely.

MOLINDONE (moh LIN dohn)

Introduced: 1971   **Prescription:**   USA: Yes   **Available as Generic:**
No   **Class:**   Strong tranquilizer, antipsychotic   **Controlled Drug:**   USA: No
Brand Name: Moban

BENEFITS versus RISKS	
Possible Benefits	*Possible Risks*
EFFECTIVE TREATMENT OF SOME CASES OF ACUTE AND CHRONIC SCHIZOPHRENIA	NARROW TREATMENT MARGIN SERIOUS TOXIC EFFECTS ON BRAIN:
May be effective in schizophrenia that has not responded to other drugs	Parkinson-like reactions severe restlessness abnormal involuntary movements tardive dyskinesias
	Liver toxicity, jaundice
	Atropinelike side effects

▷ **Principal Uses**
   As a Single Drug Product: Uses currently included in FDA approved labeling: (1) Helps manage acute and chronic schizophrenia to control thought dis-

order, disorientation, hallucinations, perceptual distortions and hostility; (2) may have a small role in helping relieve depression.

Other (unlabeled) generally accepted uses: May be of help in children with conduct disorders.

How This Drug Works: Acts on nerve transmitters (serotonin and dopamine) to restore the activity in the reticular activating system of the brain, and improve distorted patterns of thinking and behavior.

Available Dosage Forms and Strengths
Concentrate — 20 mg per ml
Tablets — 5 mg, 10 mg, 25 mg, 50 mg, 100 mg

▷ **Usual Adult Dosage Range:**   Initially, 50 to 75 mg/day in 3 or 4 divided doses; dose may be increased gradually in 3 days to 100 mg/day as needed and tolerated. For maintenance: mild psychosis—5 to 15 mg, 3 or 4 times/day; moderate psychosis—10 to 25 mg, 3 or 4 times/day; severe psychosis—up to 225 mg/day, in 3 or 4 divided doses. The total daily dosage should not exceed 225 mg. **Note: Actual dosage and administration schedule must be determined by the physician for each patient individually.**

Conditions Requiring Dosing Adjustments
Liver function: Specific dosage adjustments in liver compromise are not defined. It should be used with caution in patients with liver compromise as it is a rare cause of liver toxicity (hepatoxicity).
Kidney function: The kidney is minimally (3%) involved in the elimination of molindone.

▷ **Dosing Instructions:**   The tablet may be crushed and taken with food or milk to reduce stomach irritation. The liquid concentrate may be diluted with water, milk, fruit juice or carbonated beverages.

Usual Duration of Use: Use on a regular schedule for 3 to 6 weeks is usually necessary to determine this drug's effectiveness in controlling the features of schizophrenia. Long-term use (months to years) requires supervision and periodic evaluation by your physician. Consult your physician on a regular basis.

▷ **This Drug Should Not Be Taken If**
• you have had an allergic reaction to it previously.
• you have acute alcoholic intoxication.

▷ **Inform Your Physician Before Taking This Drug If**
• you are taking any drugs that have sedative effects.
• you use alcohol excessively.
• you have any type of seizure disorder.
• you are pregnant or are breast-feeding.
• you have a history of neuroleptic malignant syndrome.
• you have any type of glaucoma.
• you have Parkinson's disease or an enlarged prostate gland.
• you have impaired liver or kidney function.
• you have a history of breast cancer.

Possible Side Effects (natural, expected, and unavoidable drug actions)
Drowsiness, dry mouth, nasal congestion, constipation, impaired urination. Parkinson-like reactions (see Glossary). Orthostatic hypotension, weight gain.

▷ **Possible Adverse Effects** (unusual, unexpected, and infrequent reactions)
  If any of the following develop, consult your physician promptly for guidance.
  Mild Adverse Effects
  Allergic Reaction: Skin rash.
  Headache, dizziness, blurred vision, lethargy, unsteadiness, insomnia, depression, euphoria, ringing in ears.
  Rapid heartbeat, low blood pressure, fainting.
  Loss of appetite, indigestion, nausea.
  Temporary lowering or increase in white blood cells.
  Serious Adverse Effects
  Allergic Reactions: Liver reaction with jaundice (rare, questionable).
  Idiosyncratic Reactions: Neuroleptic malignant syndrome (see Glossary).
  Spasms of face and neck muscles, abnormal involuntary movements of extremities, severe restlessness.
  Development of tardive dyskinesias (see Glossary).
  Lowering of the blood pressure on standing (orthostatic hypotension).
  Lowering of the seizure threshold.
  Muscle damage (rhabdomyolysis) (rare).
  Liver toxicity (rare).

▷ **Possible Effects on Sexual Function**
  Increased libido; male breast enlargement and tenderness; painful and extended erections; female breast enlargement with milk formation.
  Altered timing and pattern of menstruation.

▷ **Adverse Effects That May Mimic Natural Diseases or Disorders**
  Parkinson-like reactions may be mistaken for naturally occurring Parkinson's disease.
  Rare liver reaction may suggest viral hepatitis.

Possible Effects on Laboratory Tests
  Liver function enzymes: increased.
  Blood urea nitrogen: increased.

CAUTION
  1. This drug may alter the pattern of epileptic seizures and require dosage adjustments of anticonvulsant drugs.
  2. Obtain prompt evaluation of any change or disturbance of vision.
  3. There is a very narrow margin between the effective therapeutic dose and the dose that can cause Parkinson-like reactions. Inform your physician promptly if suggestive symptoms develop.

Precautions for Use
  By Infants and Children: Safety and effectiveness for those under 12 years of age not established.
  By Those over 60 Years of Age: Start treatment with small doses. This drug can aggravate an existing prostatism (see Glossary). You may be more susceptible to the development of Parkinson-like reactions or tardive dyskinesia. Report any suggestive symptoms promptly.

▷ **Advisability of Use During Pregnancy**
  Pregnancy Category: C. See Pregnancy Code at the back of this book.
  Animal studies: No birth defects reported in mice, rats or rabbits.

Human studies: Adequate studies of pregnant women are not available.
Because of its inherent toxicity for brain tissue, avoid use during pregnancy if possible.

Advisability of Use if Breast-Feeding
Presence of this drug in breast milk: Unknown.
Avoid drug or refrain from nursing.

Habit-Forming Potential: None.

Effects of Overdosage: Marked drowsiness, weakness, tremor, agitation, impaired stance and gait, stupor progressing to coma, possible seizures.

Possible Effects of Long-Term Use: Development of tardive dyskinesias.

Suggested Periodic Examinations While Taking This Drug (at physician's discretion)
Complete blood cell counts, liver function tests.

▷ **While Taking This Drug, Observe the Following**
Foods: No restrictions.
Beverages: No restrictions. May be taken with milk.
▷ *Alcohol:* Avoid completely. Alcohol can increase the sedative action of this drug and enhance its depressant effects on brain function. Also, this drug can increase the intoxicating effects of alcohol.
Tobacco Smoking: No interactions expected.
▷ *Other Drugs*
Molindone may *increase* the effects of
- all drugs containing atropine or having atropinelike effects (see Drug Class Section).
- all drugs with sedative effects, and cause excessive sedation.

Molindone *taken concurrently* with
- antiepileptic drugs (anticonvulsants) may require close monitoring for changes in seizure patterns and need for dosage adjustments.
- Monoamine oxidase inhibitors (MAO) (see Drug Classes) may result in serious increases in temperature or convulsions. Some patients who do not respond to either medicine may be able to take both at the same time without this effect, but data are limited.

▷ *Driving, Hazardous Activities:* This drug may cause dizziness and drowsiness. Restrict activities as necessary.
Aviation Note: The use of this drug *is a disqualification* for piloting. Consult a designated Aviation Medical Examiner.
Exposure to Sun: No restrictions as far as photosensitivity.
Exposure to Heat: Use caution and avoid excessive heat as much as possible. This drug may impair the regulation of body temperature and increase the risk of heat stroke.
Discontinuation: Do not stop taking this drug suddenly after long-term use. Ask your physician for guidance regarding gradual dosage reduction and withdrawal.

MORPHINE (MOR feen)

Other Name: MS (morphine sulfate)

Introduced: 1806   **Prescription:** USA: Yes; Canada: Yes   **Available as Generic:** Yes   **Class:** Strong analgesic, opioids   **Controlled Drug:** USA: C-II*; Canada: No

Brand Names: Astramorph, Astramorph PF, Duramorph, ✦Epimorph, In-fumorph, ✦Morphine H.P., ✦Morphitec, ✦M.O.S., ✦M.O.S.-S.R., MS Contin, MS-IR, OMS Concentrate, Opium tincture, Oramorph SR, Paregoric, RMS Uniserts, Roxanol, Roxanol 100, Roxanol SR, ✦Statex

---

BENEFITS versus RISKS	
Possible Benefits	*Possible Risks*
EFFECTIVE RELIEF OF MODERATE TO SEVERE PAIN	POTENTIAL FOR HABIT FORMATION (DEPENDENCE)
	Respiratory depression
	Disorientation, hallucinations
	Interference with urination
	Constipation

▷ **Principal Uses**

As a Single Drug Product: Uses currently included in FDA approved labeling: Given by mouth, suppository or injection to relieve moderate to severe pain of: (1)Heart attack, cancer, operations, fluid on the lungs and other causes; (2) it is also used as an adjunct to anesthesia.

Other (unlabeled) generally accepted uses: (1) Therapy of pain in sickle cell crisis; (2) used in patient controlled analgesia pumps to fight pain.

How This Drug Works: Acting primarily as a depressant of certain brain functions, this drug suppresses the perception of pain and calms the emotional response to pain.

Available Dosage Forms and Strengths

Injection — 0.5 mg, 1 mg, 2 mg, 4 mg, 5 mg, 8 mg, 10 mg, 15 mg, 25 mg, 50 mg (all per ml)

Oral Solution — 20 mg per ml; 10 mg, 20 mg, 100 mg per 5-ml

Suppositories — 5 mg, 10 mg, 20 mg, 30 mg

Syrup — 1 mg, 5 mg, 10 mg, 20 mg, 50 mg (all per ml) (50 mg Canada only)

Tablets — 5 mg, 10 mg, 15 mg, 25 mg, 30 mg, 50 mg

Tablets, soluble — 10 mg, 15 mg, 30 mg

Tablets, sustained-release — 15 mg, 30 mg, 60 mg, 100 mg, 200 mg

▷ **Recommended Dosage Ranges** (Actual dosage and administration schedule must be determined by the physician for each patient individually.)

Infants and Children: 0.1 to 0.2 mg/kg of body weight every 4 hours. Single dose should not exceed 15 mg.

12 to 60 Years of Age: By injection—5 to 20 mg every 4 hours.

By mouth (regular solution, syrup and tablets)—10 to 30 mg every 4 hours.

---

*See Schedules of Controlled Drugs at the back of this book.

By mouth (sustained-release forms)—30 mg every 8 to 12 hours.

By suppository—10 to 30 mg every 4 hours.

Over 60 Years of Age: Same as 12 to 60 years of age, using the lower end of the range initially; increase dose cautiously, as needed and tolerated.

Author's note: Previous editions have included as-needed or PRN notations by doses. Current pain treatment theory calls for timed or scheduled dosing. This tends to prevent pain, rather than allowing pain to recur and have to be treated. Some clinicians will use timed dosing immediately after surgery and then revert to as-needed dosing once the most severe period of pain has passed.

Conditions Requiring Dosing Adjustments

Liver function: The dose and frequency **must** be adjusted (decreased) with liver compromise.

Kidney function: The dose and frequency should be adjusted in renal compromise.

▷ **Dosing Instructions:**   The regular tablet may be crushed and taken with or following food to reduce stomach irritation or nausea. The sustained-release tablet should be swallowed whole; do not break it in half, crush it or chew it. The oral liquid may be mixed with fruit juice to improve taste.

Usual Duration of Use: As required to control pain. For short-term, self-limiting conditions, continual use should not exceed 5 to 7 days without interruption and reassessment of need. For the long-term management of severe chronic pain, it is advisable to determine an optimal fixed-dosage schedule.

▷ **This Drug Should Not Be Taken If**
- you have had an allergic reaction to any dosage form of it previously.
- you are having an acute attack of asthma.
- you have acute respiratory depression.

▷ **Inform Your Physician Before Taking This Drug If**
- you are taking, or have taken within the past 14 days, any monoamine oxidase (MAO) type A inhibitor drug (see Drug Class Section).
- you are taking: atropinelike drugs, antihypertensives, metoclopramide (Reglan), zidovudine (AZT).
- you are taking any other drugs that have a sedative effect.
- you have a history of drug abuse or alcoholism.
- you have impaired liver or kidney function.
- you have prostate gland enlargement. (See Prostatism in Glossary.)
- you have a history of asthma, emphysema, epilepsy, gallbladder disease, or inflammatory bowel disease.
- you have a tendency toward constipation.
- you have a history of head injury.
- you have a history of sickle cell anemia.
- you have a history of low blood pressure.
- you plan to have surgery under general anesthesia in the near future.

Possible Side Effects (natural, expected, and unavoidable drug actions)

Drowsiness, light-headedness, weakness, euphoria, dry mouth, urinary retention, constipation.

▷ **Possible Adverse Effects** (unusual, unexpected, and infrequent reactions)

If any of the following develop, consult your physician promptly for guidance.

Mild Adverse Effects
> Allergic Reactions: Skin rash, hives, itching (especially if the intravenous form is injected too quickly).
>
> Headache, dizziness, impaired concentration, sensation of drunkenness, confusion, depression, blurred or double vision.
>
> Miosis or pinpoint pupils.
>
> Facial flushing, sweating, heart palpitation.
>
> Nausea, vomiting.
>
> Spasm of the biliary tract.
>
> Urine retention.

Serious Adverse Effects
> Allergic Reactions: Swelling of throat or vocal cords, spasm of larynx or bronchial tubes.
>
> Hallucinations, psychosis.
>
> Drop in blood pressure, causing severe weakness and fainting.
>
> Disorientation, hallucinations, unstable gait, tremor, muscle twitching.
>
> Drug-induced myasthenia gravis.
>
> Respiratory depression.
>
> Seizures.
>
> Drug-induced porphyria (rare).

▷ **Possible Effects on Sexual Function:**   Reduced libido and/or potency. Amenorrhea and disruption of ovulation.

▷ **Adverse Effects That May Mimic Natural Diseases or Disorders**
Paradoxical behavioral disturbances may suggest psychotic disorder.

Possible Effects on Laboratory Tests
> Blood amylase and lipase levels: increased (natural side effects).
>
> Liver function tests: increased liver enzymes (ALT/GPT, AST/GOT and alkaline phosphatase), increased bilirubin.
>
> Urine screening tests for drug abuse: may be **positive**. (Test results depend upon amount of drug taken and testing method used.)

CAUTION
> 1. If you have asthma, chronic bronchitis or emphysema, excessive use of this drug may cause significant respiratory difficulty, thickening of bronchial secretions and suppression of coughing.
> 2. Taking this drug with atropinelike drugs can increase the risk of urinary retention and reduced intestinal function.
> 3. Do not take this drug following acute head injury.

Precautions for Use
> *By Infants and Children:* Used very cautiously in infants under 2 years of age because of vulnerability to life-threatening respiratory depression. Watch for any indication of paradoxical excitement in this age group.
>
> *By Those over 60 Years of Age:* Small doses and short-term use indicated. There may be increased risk of drowsiness, dizziness, unsteadiness, falling, urinary retention and constipation (often leading to fecal impaction).

▷ **Advisability of Use During Pregnancy**
> *Pregnancy Category:* C. See Pregnancy Code at the back of this book.
>
> Animal studies: Significant skeletal birth defects reported in mouse and hamster studies.

Human studies: Adequate studies of pregnant women are not available. However, no significant increase in birth defects was found in 448 exposures to this drug.

Avoid during the first 3 months. Use sparingly and in small doses during the last 6 months only if clearly needed.

Advisability of Use if Breast-Feeding
Presence of this drug in breast milk: Yes.
Avoid drug or refrain from nursing.

Habit-Forming Potential: This drug can cause psychological and physical dependence (see Glossary).

Effects of Overdosage: Marked drowsiness, dizziness, confusion, restlessness, depressed breathing, tremors, convulsions, stupor progressing to coma.

Possible Effects of Long-Term Use: Psychological and physical dependence, chronic constipation.

Suggested Periodic Examinations While Taking This Drug (at physician's discretion)
None.

▷ **While Taking This Drug, Observe the Following**
Foods: No restrictions.
Beverages: No restrictions. May be taken with milk.
▷ *Alcohol:* Alcohol is best avoided. Opioid analgesics can intensify the intoxicating effects of alcohol, and alcohol can intensify the depressant effects of opioids on brain function, breathing and circulation.
Tobacco Smoking: No interactions expected.
Marijuana Smoking: Increase in drowsiness and pain relief; impairment of mental and physical performance.
▷ *Other Drugs*
Morphine may *increase* the effects of
• other drugs with sedative effects.
• antihypertensives, and cause excessive lowering of blood pressure.
• atropinelike drugs, and increase the risk of constipation and urinary retention.
Morphine may *decrease* the effects of
• metoclopramide (Reglan).
Morphine *taken concurrently* with
• benzodiazepines (see Drug Classes) may result in increased risk of respiratory depression.
• cimetidine (Tagamet) may result in morphine toxicity.
• fluoxetine (Prozac) may antagonize morphine's pain relieving effect.
• hydroxyzine (Vistaril) can increase pain relief, but carries the risk of increased respiratory depression.
• monoamine oxidase (MAO) type A inhibitor drugs (see Drug Classes) may cause the equivalent of an acute narcotic overdose: unconsciousness; severe depression of breathing, heart action and circulation. A variation of this reaction can be excitability, convulsions, high fever and rapid heart action.
• phenothiazines (see Drug Class Section) may cause excessive and prolonged depression of brain functions, breathing and circulation.

- zidovudine (AZT) may increase the toxicity of both drugs; avoid concurrent use.

▷ *Driving, Hazardous Activities:* This drug can impair mental alertness, judgment, reaction time and physical coordination. Avoid hazardous activities.

Aviation Note: The use of this drug *is a disqualification* for piloting. Consult a designated Aviation Medical Examiner.

Exposure to Sun: No restrictions.

Discontinuation: It is advisable to limit this drug to short-term use. Longer-term use requires gradual tapering (decreasing) of doses to minimize possible effects of withdrawal: body aches, fever, sweating, nervousness, trembling, weakness, runny nose, sneezing, rapid heart rate, nausea, vomiting, stomach cramps, diarrhea.

MUPIROCIN (myu PEER oh sin)

Introduced: 1987   **Prescription:** USA: Yes; Canada: Yes   **Available as Generic:** USA: No; Canada: No   **Class:** antibiotic, topical   **Controlled Drug:** USA: No; Canada: No

Brand Names: Bactroban, Bactroban Nasal

BENEFITS versus RISKS	
Possible Benefits	*Possible Risks*
EFFECTIVE TOPICAL TREATMENT OF STAPH AND STREP SKIN INFECTIONS	Skin irritation
EFFECTIVE ERADICATION OF STAPH AUREUS FROM THE NOSE	

▷ **Principal Uses**

As a Single Drug Product: Uses currently included in FDA approved labeling: (1) Used to treat skin infections caused by Staphylococcal and Streptococcal infections such as ecthyma or impetigo; (2) the new intranasal form is specifically formulated to kill Staph aureus bacteria that have colonized the nasal passages. Other (unlabeled) generally accepted uses: (1) Used in burns where resistant Staphylococcus aureus is causing infection; (2) helps prevent opportunistic infections of venous access devices such as intravascular cannulas; (3) treats cellulitis caused by gram positive organisms; (4) has been used in some specific situations in skin surgery to prevent infections; (5) has recently been used to eradicate vaginal Staph infections.

How This Drug Works: This drug binds to a specific enzyme (isoleucyl transfer-RNA synthetase) and stops susceptible bacteria from being able to make critical proteins.

Available Dosage Forms and Strengths

Intranasal form — 2%

Topical ointment — 2%

— 20 mg per gram (Canada)

▷ **Recommended Dosage Ranges (Actual dosage and administration schedule must be determined by the physician for each patient individually.)**
  Infants and Children: Not indicated in infants.
    Children 5 to 15 years old have been given a thin coat of the 2% ointment applied to the infection site 3 times daily for three to five consecutive days.
  16 to 60 Years of Age: The 2% ointment has been applied 3 times daily for 5 to 14 days. Some more involved or extensive infections have been treated for longer periods. If the infection in question has not resolved after the initial course of the ointment, the site should be evaluated by a physician and systemic antibiotics or other treatment considered.
    Intranasal: One half of the ointment from the single-use tube of this new form of mupirocin is applied into one nostril and the other half is applied to the second nostril twice daily in the morning and evening for five consecutive days.
  Over 60 Years of Age: Same as 16 to 60 years of age.

Conditions Requiring Dosing Adjustments
  Liver function: This ointment is not usually systemically absorbed to an appreciable extent. If the ointment is applied to an extensive skin area, metabolism of the active antibiotic does occur in the liver—yet there are no existing guidelines for dosage adjustments.
  Kidney function: A substance in this formulation (polyethylene glycol) may be toxic to the kidneys if the ointment is applied over an extensive burn or wound area.

▷ **Dosing Instructions:**   This medicine should be applied as a thin film or as described by your doctor. Call your doctor if the condition has not improved or worsens during the course of treatment. Do **not** combine this medicine with other ointments or treatments unless your doctor has prescribed this approach.

Usual Duration of Use: Continual use on a regular schedule for several days is usually necessary to determine this drug's effectiveness in treating skin infections. Long-term use (months to years) requires periodic physician evaluation. Consult your physician on a regular basis.

Possible Advantages of This Drug
  Effective topical treatment of skin infections.

▷ **This Drug Should Not Be Taken If**
  • you have had an allergic reaction to any dosage form of it previously.
  • you have extensive burns or open wounds.

▷ **Inform Your Physician Before Taking This Drug If**
  • several days have passed since this medicine has been prescribed and there has been no change or worsening of the wound.
  • pain at the site of the infection increases.
  • you are uncertain of how much mupirocin to apply or how often to apply it.

Possible Side Effects (natural, expected, and unavoidable drug actions)
  Irritation at the site of infection secondary to the polyethylene glycol component.

▷ **Possible Adverse Effects** (unusual, unexpected, and infrequent reactions)
  If any of the following develop, consult your physician promptly for guidance.

Mild Adverse Effects
> Allergic Reactions: Skin rash and irritation at the infection site.
> Soreness, stinging, or pain at the infection site.

Serious Adverse Effects
> Allergic Reactions: Not defined as the medicine is not appreciably absorbed.
> If this medicine is applied to an extensive skin area, polyethylene glycol may be absorbed and cause kidney toxicity.

▷ **Possible Effects on Sexual Function:**   Not reported.

Possible Delayed Adverse Effects: This medicine is indicated for short-term use.

▷ **Adverse Effects That May Mimic Natural Diseases or Disorders**
> None reported.

Natural Diseases or Disorders That May Be Activated by This Drug
> None reported.

Possible Effects on Laboratory Tests
> None reported.

CAUTION
> 1. Do not apply this medicine to an area of skin larger than that your doctor prescribed.

Precautions for Use
> *By Infants and Children:* Safety and effectiveness for use by those under 5 years of age have not been established.
> *By Those over 60 Years of Age:* No special changes needed.

▷ **Advisability of Use During Pregnancy**
> *Pregnancy Category:* B. See Pregnancy Code at the back of this book.
> Animal studies: No fetal problems defined.
> Human studies: Information from adequate studies of pregnant women is not available.

Advisability of Use if Breast-Feeding
> Presence of this drug in breast milk: Unknown.
> Avoid drug or refrain from nursing.

Habit-Forming Potential: None.

Effects of Overdosage: If this medicine is applied to an extensive area of skin, excessive amounts of polyethylene glycol may be absorbed and cause kidney toxicity.

Possible Effects of Long-Term Use: None defined.

Suggested Periodic Examinations While Taking This Drug   (at physician's discretion)
> None.

▷ **While Taking This Drug, Observe the Following**
> *Foods:* No restrictions.
> *Beverages:* No restrictions.

▷ *Alcohol:* No restrictions.
> *Tobacco Smoking:* No interactions expected.

▷ *Other Drugs*
> Mupirocin *taken concurrently* with
> • other medications which are toxic to the kidneys may result in additive kidney toxicity if mupirocin is applied to a large area of skin.

Aviation Note: The use of this drug ***does not appear to be a restriction*** for piloting. Consult a designated Aviation Medical Examiner.
Exposure to Sun: No restrictions.

NABUMETONE (na BYU me tohn)

Introduced: 1984   **Prescription:** USA: Yes   **Available as Generic:** No   **Class:** Nonsteroidal anti-inflammatory drug (NSAID)   **Controlled Drug:** USA: No
Brand Name: Relafen

BENEFITS versus RISKS	
Possible Benefits	*Possible Risks*
EFFECTIVE RELIEF OF MILD TO MODERATE PAIN AND INFLAMMATION ASSOCIATED WITH OSTEOARTHRITIS AND RHEUMATOID ARTHRITIS	Gastrointestinal ulceration (rare) Drug-induced hepatitis (rare) Drug-induced kidney damage (rare) Very rare lung fibrosis Mild fluid retention

Please see the acetic acid nonsteroidal anti-inflammatory drug profile for further information.

NADOLOL (NAY doh lohl)

Introduced: 1976   **Prescription:** USA: Yes; Canada: Yes   **Available as Generic:** Yes   **Class:** Antianginal, antihypertensive, beta blocker   **Controlled Drug:** USA: No; Canada: No
Brand Names: ✤Apo-Nadol, Corgard, Corzide [CD], Syn-Nadol

BENEFITS versus RISKS	
Possible Benefits	*Possible Risks*
EFFECTIVE, WELL-TOLERATED ANTIHYPERTENSIVE for mild to moderate high blood pressure EFFECTIVE ANTIANGINAL DRUG IN CLASSICAL CORONARY ARTERY DISEASE with moderate to severe angina	CONGESTIVE HEART FAILURE in advanced heart disease Provocation of asthma (in predisposed patients) Masking of hypoglycemia in drug-dependent diabetes Worsening of angina following abrupt withdrawal

▷ **Principal Uses**

As a Single Drug Product: Uses currently included in FDA approved labeling: (1) Treats moderate high blood pressure; (2) helps prevent attacks of effort-induced angina. (This drug is contraindicated in Prinzmetal's vasospastic angina.)

Other (unlabeled) generally accepted uses: (1) Helps prevent hemorrhage from bulging veins (esophageal varices) in cirrhosis; (2) may have an adjunctive role in helping prevent and reduce migraine severity; (3) may have a role in helping prevent death after a heart attack (myocardial infarction); (4) may help ease tremor in patients taking lithium; (5) helps decrease risk of ruptured blood vessels in the esophagus (esophageal varices) in patients with cirrhosis.

As a Combination Drug Product [CD]: This drug is available in combination with bendroflumethiazide, a mild diuretic antihypertensive drug. This combination product is more effective and more convenient for long-term use.

How This Drug Works: By blocking certain actions of the sympathetic nervous system, this drug
- reduces the rate and contraction force of the heart, lowering oxygen requirements of the heart muscle, reducing ejection pressure of the blood leaving the heart; consequently reducing the frequency of angina and lowering blood pressure.
- reduces the degree of contraction of blood vessel walls, resulting expansion and consequent lowering of blood pressure.
- prolongs conduction time of nerve impulses through the heart, of benefit in the management of certain heart rhythm disorders.

Available Dosage Forms and Strengths
Tablets — 20 mg, 40 mg, 80 mg, 120 mg, 160 mg

▷ **Usual Adult Dosage Range:**   For hypertension: Initially, 40 mg daily in one dose; this may be increased gradually as needed and tolerated, up to 320 mg/24 hours. The usual maintenance dose is 80 to 320 mg/24 hours. The total daily dosage should not exceed 320 mg. For angina: Initially, 40 mg daily in one dose; increase gradually at intervals of 3 to 7 days up to 240 mg/24 hours. The usual maintenance dose is 80 to 240 mg/24 hours. The total daily dose should not exceed 240 mg. **Note: Actual dosage and administration schedule must be determined by the physician for each patient individually.**

Conditions Requiring Dosing Adjustments
Liver function: The liver is not significantly involved in the elimination of this medication.
Kidney function: In patients with moderate kidney failure, the usual dose should be given every 24 to 36 hours. In patients with severe kidney failure, the dose can be given every 40 to 60 hours.

▷ **Dosing Instructions:**   The tablet may be crushed and taken without regard to eating. Do not stop this drug abruptly.

Usual Duration of Use: Use on a regular schedule for 10 to 14 days determines this drug's effectiveness in lowering blood pressure and preventing angina. The long-term use of this drug (months to years) will be determined by your response to an overall treatment program (weight reduction, salt restriction, smoking cessation, etc.). Consult your physician on a regular basis.

Possible Advantages of This Drug
Does not reduce blood flow to the kidney.
Can be used concurrently with other drugs that may reduce blood flow to the kidney (such as most anti-inflammatory aspirin substitutes).

▷ **This Drug Should Not Be Taken If**
- you have had an allergic reaction to it previously.
- you have congestive heart failure.

- you have an abnormally slow heart rate or a serious form of heart block.
- you are subject to bronchial asthma.
- you are presently experiencing seasonal hay fever.
- you are taking, or have taken within the past 14 days, any monoamine oxidase (MAO) type A inhibitor drug (see Drug Classes).

▷ **Inform Your Physician Before Taking This Drug If**
- you have had an adverse reaction to any beta blocker (see Drug Class Section).
- you have a history of serious heart disease.
- you have a history of hay fever (allergic rhinitis), asthma, chronic bronchitis or emphysema.
- you have a history of overactive thyroid function (hyperthyroidism).
- you have a history of low blood sugar (hypoglycemia).
- you have impaired liver or kidney function.
- you have diabetes or myasthenia gravis.
- you are pregnant or are breast-feeding your infant.
- you have difficulty with blood circulation to the periphery (peripheral vascular disease).
- you are currently taking any form of digitalis, quinidine or reserpine, or any calcium blocker drug (see Drug Class Section).
- you plan to have surgery under general anesthesia in the near future.

Possible Side Effects (natural, expected, and unavoidable drug actions)
Lethargy and fatigability, cold extremities, slow heart rate, light-headedness in upright position (see Orthostatic Hypotension in Glossary).

▷ **Possible Adverse Effects** (unusual, unexpected, and infrequent reactions)
If any of the following develop, consult your physician promptly for guidance.
Mild Adverse Effects
Allergic Reactions: Skin rash, itching, drug fever.
Headache, dizziness, insomnia, vivid dreaming, visual disturbances, ringing in ears, slurred speech, paresthesias.
Hair loss and sweating.
Indigestion, nausea, vomiting, diarrhea, abdominal pain.
Cough.
Increased blood potassium.
Numbness and tingling of extremities.
Serious Adverse Effects
Allergic Reaction: Facial swelling, anaphylaxis.
Chest pain, shortness of breath, precipitation of congestive heart failure.
Intensification of heart block.
Bronchospasm (rare).
Carpal tunnel syndrome (rare).
Induction of bronchial asthma (in asthmatic individuals).
Masking of warning indications of acute hypoglycemia in drug-treated diabetes.
Rare cause of pancreatitis.
Severe slowing of the heart (rare).
May precipitate cramping when walking (intermittent claudication).
Excessively low blood pressure.

▷ **Possible Effects on Sexual Function:**   Decreased libido, impotence (4%), impaired erection (36%).

▷ **Adverse Effects That May Mimic Natural Diseases or Disorders**
Impaired circulation to the extremities may resemble Raynaud's phenomenon.

Natural Diseases or Disorders That May Be Activated by This Drug
Bronchial asthma, Prinzmetal's variant (vasospastic) angina, latent Raynaud's disease, myasthenia gravis (questionable).

Possible Effects on Laboratory Tests
Blood HDL cholesterol level: decreased.
Blood VLDL cholesterol level: increased.
Blood triglyceride levels: increased.

CAUTION
1. ***Do not stop this drug suddenly*** without the knowledge and help of your doctor. Carry a note on your person that you are taking this drug.
2. Ask your physician or pharmacist **before** using nasal decongestants usually present in over-the-counter cold preparations and nose drops. These can cause rapid blood pressure increases when combined with beta blocker drugs.
3. Report the development of any tendency to emotional depression.

Precautions for Use
By Infants and Children: Safety and effectiveness for those under 12 years of age not established. However, if this drug is used, observe for the development of low blood sugar (hypoglycemia) during periods of reduced food intake.
By Those over 60 Years of Age: Unacceptably high blood pressure should be reduced without creating the risks associated with excessively low blood pressure. Small doses, and frequent blood pressure checks needed. Sudden, rapid and excessive reduction of blood pressure can predispose to stroke or heart attack. Watch for dizziness, unsteadiness, tendency to fall, confusion, hallucinations, depression or urinary frequency.

▷ **Advisability of Use During Pregnancy**
Pregnancy Category: C. See Pregnancy Code at the back of this book.
Animal studies: No significant increase in birth defects due to this drug, but embryotoxicity reported in rabbits.
Human studies: Adequate studies of pregnant women are not available.
Avoid use during the first 3 months if possible. Use this drug only if clearly needed. Ask physician for guidance.

Advisability of Use if Breast-Feeding
Presence of this drug in breast milk: Yes, in large amounts.
Avoid drug or refrain from nursing.

Habit-Forming Potential: None.

Effects of Overdosage: Weakness, slow pulse, low blood pressure, fainting, cold and sweaty skin, congestive heart failure, possible coma and convulsions.

Possible Effects of Long-Term Use: Reduced heart reserve and eventual heart failure in susceptible individuals with advanced heart disease.

Suggested Periodic Examinations While Taking This Drug (at physician's discretion)

Measurements of blood pressure, evaluation of heart function.

▷ **While Taking This Drug, Observe the Following**

Foods: No restrictions. Avoid excessive salt intake.

Beverages: No restrictions. May be taken with milk.

▷ *Alcohol:* Use with caution. Alcohol may exaggerate this drug's ability to lower blood pressure and may increase its mild sedative effect.

Tobacco Smoking: Nicotine may reduce this drug's effectiveness in treating high blood pressure and angina. In addition, high doses of this drug may potentiate the constriction of the bronchial tubes caused by regular smoking.

▷ *Other Drugs*

Nadolol may *increase* the effects of

- other antihypertensive drugs, and cause excessive lowering of blood pressure. Dosage adjustments may be necessary.
- reserpine (Ser-Ap-Es, etc.), and cause sedation, depression, slowing of the heart rate and lowering of blood pressure.
- verapamil (Calan, Isoptin) or other calcium channel blockers (see Drug Classes), and cause excessive depression of heart function; monitor this combination closely.

Nadolol may *decrease* the effects of

- ritodrine (Yutopar).
- theophyllines (Aminophyllin, Theo-Dur, etc.), and reduce their effectiveness in treating asthma.

Nadolol *taken concurrently* with

- antacids containing aluminum can block absorption of this medicine and lessen therapeutic nadolol effects.
- amiodarone (Codarone) and cause severe slowing of the heart and potentially stop the heart (cardiac arrest).
- clonidine (Catapres) requires close monitoring for rebound high blood pressure if clonidine is withdrawn while nadolol is still being taken.
- epinephrine can cause serious hypertension, slowing of the heart and should anaphylaxis occur—epinephrine resistance.
- ergot derivatives (see Drug Class) can cause decreased blood flow to the extremities (peripheral ischemia).
- insulin requires close monitoring to avoid undetected hypoglycemia (see Glossary).
- lidocaine can lead to lidocaine toxicity (depressed heart function, cardiac arrest).
- oral hypoglycemic agents (see Drug Class) can cause slowed recovery from any hypoglycemia which may occur.

The following drugs may *decrease* the effects of nadolol

- indomethacin (Indocin), and possibly other "aspirin substitutes," or NSAIDs may impair nadolol's antihypertensive effect.

▷ *Driving, Hazardous Activities:* Use caution until the full extent of drowsiness, lethargy and blood pressure change has been determined.

Aviation Note: The use of this drug *is a disqualification* for piloting. Consult a designated Aviation Medical Examiner.

Exposure to Sun: No restrictions.

Exposure to Heat: Caution advised. Hot environments can lower the blood pressure and exaggerate the effects of this drug.

Exposure to Cold: Caution advised. Cold environments can enhance the circulatory deficiency in the extremities that may occur with this drug. The elderly should take precautions to prevent hypothermia (see Glossary).

Heavy Exercise or Exertion: It is advisable to avoid exertion that produces lightheadedness, excessive fatigue or muscle cramping. The use of this drug may intensify the hypertensive response to isometric exercise.

Occurrence of Unrelated Illness: Fever that accompanies systemic infections can lower blood pressure and require dose decreases. Nausea or vomiting may interrupt the regular dosage schedule. Ask your physician for guidance.

Discontinuation: It is advisable to avoid sudden discontinuation of this drug in all situations. If possible, gradual reduction of dose over a period of 2 to 3 weeks is recommended. Ask your physician for specific guidance.

NAFARELIN (NAF a re lin)

Introduced: 1984   **Prescription:** USA: Yes   **Available as Generic:** USA: No   **Class:** hormones, miscellaneous   **Controlled Drug:** USA: No **Brand Name:** Synarel

BENEFITS versus RISKS	
Possible Benefits	*Possible Risks*
VERY EFFECTIVE TREATMENT OF ENDOMETRIOSIS	Symptoms of estrogen deficiency (during treatment)
	Masculinizing effects (during treatment)
	Loss of bone density
	Lowering of the white blood cell count

▷ **Principal Uses**

As a Single Drug Product: Uses currently included in FDA approved labeling: (1) Treats endometriosis: reduction in the size and activity of endometrial implants within the pelvis; relief of pelvic pain associated with menstruation; (2) also used to treat precocious puberty due to excessive production of gonadotropic hormones.

Other (unlabeled) generally accepted uses: (1) Intranasal dosing helps control abnormal hair growth in women; (2) can be injected below the skin (subcutaneously) to help benign prostatic hyperplasia; (3) may be used before surgery to help decrease size of some tumors (myomas).

How This Drug Works: This drug stimulates the pituitary gland to secrete two additional hormones that regulate production of estrogen by the ovaries. Initially this drug causes an increase in the production of estrogen, but with continued use the high levels of estrogen suppress (via a feed-back mechanism) hormones that stimulate the ovary and thus estrogen production is significantly reduced. The implants of endometrium (from the lining of the uterus) that are attached to the pelvic wall are stimulated by the cyclic rise and fall of estrogen that accompanies menstruation. As a result of suppressing estrogen production, the displaced endometrial tissue (endometriosis) becomes dormant; the conditions responsible for premenstrual and menstrual pain are no longer active.

Available Dosage Forms and Strengths
Nasal solution — 2 mg per ml (10 ml bottle)

▷ **Usual Adult Dosage Range:**   Endometriosis: Pregnancy MUST be excluded prior to starting therapy, then treatment starts with 400 mcg daily. Spray 1 dose of 200 mcg into one nostril in the morning and 1 dose of 200 mcg into the other nostril in the evening, 12 hours apart. Begin treatment between days 2 and 4 of the menstrual cycle.

If regular menstruation persists after 2 months of treatment, the dose may be increased to 800 mcg daily: 1 spray into each nostril (a total of 2 sprays, 400 mcg) in the morning and again in the evening.

Note: Actual dosage and administration schedule must be determined by the physician for each patient individually.

Conditions Requiring Dosing Adjustments
Liver function: The liver plays a minor role in the elimination of this medication.
Kidney function: Specific guidelines are not available for dosing. Decreases may be needed in kidney compromise.

▷ **Dosing Instructions:**   Carefully read and follow the patient instructions provided with this drug. The solution is to be sprayed directly into the nostrils; it is not to be swallowed. Time the start of therapy and daily dosing exactly as directed.

If you need to use a nasal decongestant (spray or drops), the decongestant should not be used for at least 30 minutes after dosing the nafarelin spray; earlier use could impair absorption of nafarelin.

Usual Duration of Use: Use on a regular schedule for 2 to 3 months usually determines effectiveness in relieving endometriosis symptoms. The standard course of treatment is limited to 6 months. After 6 months of treatment, 60% of users are free of symptoms, 32% have mild symptoms, 7% have moderate symptoms and 1% will have severe symptoms. Six months after stopping this drug, of the 60% who obtain complete relief 50% will remain free of symptoms, 33% will have mild symptoms and 17% will have moderate symptoms. If symptoms of endometriosis recur following a 6 month course of treatment and a repeat course is considered, it is advisable to measure bone density before retreatment is started.

Possible Advantages of This Drug
Causes fewer masculinizing effects than danazol.
Less tendency than danazol to increase blood cholesterol levels.
Unlike danazol, this drug does not cause abnormally low HDL cholesterol levels or abnormally high LDL cholesterol levels.

Currently a "Drug of Choice"
for the management of symptoms associated with endometriosis.

▷ **This Drug Should Not Be Taken If**
- you have had an allergic reaction to it previously.
- you are pregnant or breast-feeding.
- you have abnormal vaginal bleeding of unknown cause.

▷ **Inform Your Physician Before Taking This Drug If**
- you have used this drug, danazol or similar drugs previously.
- you are taking any type of estrogen, progesterone or oral contraceptive.
- you are planning pregnancy in the near future.
- you have a family history of osteoporosis.
- you use alcohol or tobacco regularly.
- you have a history of low white blood cells.
- you are using anticonvulsants or cortisonelike drugs.
- you are subject to allergic or infectious rhinitis and use nasal decongestants frequently.

Possible Side Effects (natural, expected, and unavoidable drug actions)

Effects due to reduced estrogen production: hot flashes (90%), headaches, emotional lability, insomnia. Masculinizing effects: acne, muscle aches, fluid retention, increased skin oil, weight gain, excessive hair growth (rare).

▷ **Possible Adverse Effects** (unusual, unexpected, and infrequent reactions)

If any of the following develop, consult your physician promptly for guidance.

Mild Adverse Effects

Allergic Reactions: Skin rash, hives (rare).

Nasal irritation (common).

Vaginal dryness (14–57%)

Depression (rare).

Serious Adverse Effects

Loss of vertebral bone density: at completion of 6 months of treatment, bone density decreases an average of 8.7% and bone mass decreases an average of 4.3%; partial recovery during the post-treatment period restores bone density loss to 4.9% and bone mass loss to 3.3%.

Lowering of the white blood cell count.

Transient prostate enlargement.

Uterine bleeding.

Possible Effects on Sexual Function

Decreased libido (22%), vaginal dryness (14–57%), reduced breast size (10%).

Impotence occurred in most men who had used this drug for prostate problems.

Galactorrhea.

Natural Diseases or Disorders That May Be Activated by This Drug

Worsening of or increased progression of osteoporosis.

Possible Effects on Laboratory Tests

Blood testosterone level: decreased in men with benign enlargement of prostate gland.

Blood progesterone: decreased to less than 4 ng/ml.

Alkaline phosphatase: increased.

Serum estrone: decreased.

CAUTION

1. With continual use of this drug in proper dosage, menstruation will cease. If regular menstruation persists, call your doctor. Dosage adjustment may be necessary.
2. Use this drug consistently on a regular basis. Missed doses can result in breakthrough bleeding and ovulation.

3. It is advisable to avoid pregnancy during the course of treatment. Use a nonhormonal method of birth control; do not use oral contraceptives. Inform your physician promptly if you think you may be pregnant.
4. If you need to use nasal decongestant sprays or drops, delay their use for at least 30 minutes after the intranasal spray of nafarelin.

Precautions for Use

By Infants and Children: Safety and effectiveness for those under 18 years of age not established.

By Those over 60 Years of Age: If used for prostatism, impotence is a common side effect. Depression and hot flashes were also often reported.

▷ ## Advisability of Use During Pregnancy

Pregnancy Category:
X. See Pregnancy Code at the back of this book.
Animal studies: Major fetal abnormalities and increased fetal deaths due to this drug have been demonstrated in rat studies. Human studies: Adequate studies of pregnant women are not available.
Avoid this drug during entire pregnancy.

Advisability of Use if Breast-Feeding

Presence of this drug in breast milk: Unknown.
Avoid drug or refrain from nursing.

Habit-Forming Potential: None.

Effects of Overdosage: No significant effects expected.

Possible Effects of Long-Term Use: Continual use should be limited to 6 months. If repeated courses of treatment are considered, determination of bone density and mass should be made to assess possible bone loss, predisposition to osteoporosis and possible therapy.

Suggested Periodic Examinations While Taking This Drug (at physician's discretion)

Blood cholesterol and triglyceride profiles.
Bone density and mass measurements.

▷ ## While Taking This Drug, Observe the Following

Foods: No restrictions.
Beverages: No restrictions.
▷ *Alcohol:* No interactions expected.
Tobacco Smoking: No interactions expected.
▷ *Other Drugs*
The following drugs will ***decrease*** the effects of nafarelin
• estrogens
• oral contraceptives
▷ *Driving, Hazardous Activities:* No restrictions.
Aviation Note:
The use of this drug ***is not a disqualification*** for piloting. Consult a designated Aviation Medical Examiner for confirmation.
Exposure to Sun: No restrictions.
Discontinuation: Normal ovarian function (ovulation, menstruation, etc.) is usually restored within 4 to 8 weeks after discontinuation of this drug.
Special Storage Instructions: Store in an upright position at room temperature. Protect from light.

NALTREXONE (nahl TREX ohn)

Introduced: 1995   **Prescription:** USA: Yes; Canada: Yes   **Available as Generic:** USA: No; Canada: No   **Class:** Antialcoholism, opioid antagonist **Controlled Drug:** USA: No; Canada: No

Brand Names: Trexan, ReVia

Warning: This medication can cause liver damage if taken in excessive doses. If abdominal pain, white stools, yellowing of the eyes or skin occurs, call your doctor immediately.

BENEFITS versus RISKS

Possible Benefits	*Possible Risks*
CONTROL OF CRAVING FOR ALCOHOL	LIVER DAMAGE IF EXCESSIVE DOSES TAKEN
PART OF AN EFFECTIVE COMBINATION APPROACH TO ALCOHOLISM	
ONCE-DAILY DOSING	

▷ **Principal Uses**

As a Single Drug Product: Uses currently included in FDA approved labeling: (1) Used as part of a comprehensive program to help alcohol dependence; (2) used to treat narcotic addiction.

Other (unlabeled) generally accepted uses: (1) May help women with a specific type of cessation of menstruation (hypothalamic amenorrhea); (2) could have a role in treating Tourette's syndrome.

How This Drug Works: (1) In helping addiction to narcotics, this medicine acts as an antagonist to the effects of opioid medicines and blocks the effects or perceived benefit of the drug to the addicted patient. (2) The exact mechanism of action in alcohol addiction is unknown. It is thought that this drug interferes with the body's own opioids which may be released in response to drinking alcoholic beverages. If the effect of the body's own opioids (endogenous) is blocked, the craving for alcohol is thereby thought to be reduced.

Available Dosage Forms and Strengths

Tablets — 50 mg

▷ **Recommended Dosage Ranges (Actual dosage and administration schedule must be determined by the physician for each patient individually.)**

Infants and Children: Not indicated.

18 to 60 Years of Age: 50 mg daily. The best results are gained when this medicine is used as part of a comprehensive approach to curbing alcohol use.

Over 60 Years of Age: Same as 12 to 60 years of age.

Conditions Requiring Dosing Adjustments

Liver function: This drug is extensively metabolized in the liver and is contraindicated in acute hepatitis or liver failure.

Kidney function: Metabolites of this drug are removed via the kidneys, however, specific guidelines for dosing changes are not available.

▷ **Dosing Instructions:** If there is any question of opioid dependence, a Narcan challenge test must be performed by the physician. Naltrexone is almost completely absorbed after oral dosing. This medicine may be taken with or without food.

Usual Duration of Use:

Continual use on a regular schedule for 12 weeks is usually necessary to determine this drug's effectiveness in treating alcoholism. This drug should be a part of a comprehensive alcohol treatment program. Long-term use (months to years) requires periodic evaluation of response and dosage adjustment. Consult your physician on a regular basis.

Possible Advantages of This Drug

Actually decreases the craving for alcohol.

▷ **This Drug Should Not Be Taken If**

- you have had an allergic reaction to any dosage form of it previously.
- you have liver failure or acute hepatitis.
- you are in opioid withdrawal.
- you are physically dependent on narcotics.

▷ **Inform Your Physician Before Taking This Drug If**

- you have a history of viral hepatitis.
- you are planning surgery or a diagnostic procedure requiring anesthesia.
- you are uncertain of how much naltrexone to take or how often to take it.
- you take other prescription or nonprescription medicines which were not discussed with your doctor when naltrexone was prescribed.

Possible Side Effects (natural, expected, and unavoidable drug actions)

None.

▷ **Possible Adverse Effects** (unusual, unexpected, and infrequent reactions)

If any of the following develop, consult your physician promptly for guidance.

Mild Adverse Effects

Allergic Reactions: Rash.

Oily skin, itching, hair loss.

Nosebleeds.

Joint and muscle pain.

Anorexia, weight loss, fatigue, nervousness.

Sleep disturbances.

Depression.

Serious Adverse Effects

Allergic Reactions: None reported.

Idiosyncratic Reactions: None reported.

Liver toxicity (hepatocellular injury).

Precipitation of acute withdrawal syndrome in patients dependent on narcotics.

Suicidal ideation (rare).

Abnormal platelet function (idiopathic thrombocytopenic purpura) (rare).

▷ **Possible Effects on Sexual Function:**   Delayed ejaculation (less than 10%).

Possible Delayed Adverse Effects: None reported.

▷ **Adverse Effects That May Mimic Natural Diseases or Disorders**

Liver problems may mimic acute hepatitis.

Natural Diseases or Disorders That May Be Activated by This Drug

None.

Possible Effects on Laboratory Tests
Liver function tests: Increased.

CAUTION
1. The therapeutic dose and doses that can cause liver damage are fairly close. Make certain that you understand how much and how often to take this medicine.
2. Self administration of any narcotic drug may be fatal.

Precautions for Use
By Infants and Children: Safety and effectiveness for use by those under 18 years of age have not been established.
By Those over 60 Years of Age: None.

▷ **Advisability of Use During Pregnancy**
Pregnancy Category: C. See Pregnancy Code at the back of this book.
Animal studies: This drug has been shown to be embryocidal in rats and rabbits at roughly 140 times the typical human dose. Human studies: Information from adequate studies of pregnant women is not available. Ask your doctor for help with this benefit to risk decision.

Advisability of Use if Breast-Feeding
Presence of this drug in breast milk: Unknown.
Avoid drug or refrain from nursing.

Habit-Forming Potential: None.

Effects of Overdosage: Human subjects who received over 800 mg daily for a week showed no adverse effects.

Possible Effects of Long-Term Use: None defined.

Suggested Periodic Examinations While Taking This Drug   (at physician's discretion)
Liver function tests.

▷ **While Taking This Drug, Observe the Following**
Foods: No restrictions.
Nutritional Support: Not indicated.
Beverages: No restrictions.
▷ *Alcohol:* Obviously not recommended as this medication is part of a combination approach to help problem drinkers.
Tobacco Smoking: No interactions expected.
Marijuana Smoking: Not to be attempted.
▷ *Other Drugs*
Naltrexone *taken concurrently* with
• narcotic medicines may result in a severe reaction.
• other drugs which are toxic to the liver may result in increased risk of liver toxicity.
• thioridazine (Mellaril) may result in somnolence and lethargy.
▷ *Driving, Hazardous Activities:* This drug may cause fatigue. Restrict activities as necessary.
Aviation Note: Alcoholism *is a disqualification* for piloting. Consult a designated Aviation Medical Examiner.
Exposure to Sun: No restrictions.
Discontinuation: Do not stop this medicine without the knowledge of your doctor.

NAPROXEN (na PROX en)

Introduced: 1974   **Prescription:** USA: No (200 mg) Yes (250 mg); Canada: Yes   **Available as Generic:** Yes   **Class:** Mild analgesic, anti-inflammatory
Controlled Drug: USA: No; Canada: No

Brand Names: Aleve (200 mg nonprescription), Anaprox, Anaprox DS, Apo-Na-pro-NA, ✤Apo-Naproxen, Naprelan, Naprosyn, ✤Naxen, Neo-Prox, ✤Novo-Anaprox, ✤Nu-Naprox, ✤Synflex

BENEFITS versus RISKS	
Possible Benefits	*Possible Risks*
EFFECTIVE RELIEF OF MILD TO MODERATE PAIN AND INFLAMMATION	Gastrointestinal pain, ulceration, bleeding (rare)
	Drug-induced hepatitis with jaundice (rare)
	Rare kidney damage
	Mild fluid retention
	Rare reduced white blood cell counts
	Rare hemolytic anemia

Please see the propionic acid nonsteroidal anti-inflammatory drug profile for further information.

NEDOCROMIL (na DOK ra mil)

Introduced: 1992   **Prescription:** USA: Yes; Canada: Yes   **Available as Generic:** USA: No; Canada: No   **Class:** antiasthmatic, preventive   **Controlled Drug:** USA: No; Canada: No

Brand Names: Tilade

BENEFITS versus RISKS	
Possible Benefits	*Possible Risks*
EFFECTIVE PREVENTION OF RECURRENT ASTHMA	Acute bronchospasm (rare)
Prevention of exercise-induced asthma	Taste disorder

▷ **Principal Uses**

As a Single Drug Product: Uses currently included in FDA approved labeling: (1) Maintenance therapy of mild to moderate bronchial asthma; (2) has a steroid sparing effect which may allow reduction or even elimination of oral steroids; (3) helps manage asthmatic bronchitis.

Other (unlabeled) generally accepted uses: (1) May have a role in helping ease allergic rhinitis; (2) can help vernal conjunctivitis when instilled as an eye drop; (3) may help exercise induced asthma.

How This Drug Works: This drug inhibits the release of inflammatory chemical mediators such as histamine, prostaglandins and leukotrienes which cause bronchial constriction and inflammation seen in acute asthma.

Available Dosage Forms and Strengths
Inhaler — 16.2 gram canister
Solution for inhalation — 2 mg per actuation

▷ **Recommended Dosage Ranges (Actual dosage and administration schedule must be determined by the physician for each patient individually.)**
Infants and Children: Safety and efficacy not established.
12 to 60 Years of Age: Two puffs (inhalations) four times daily to provide a total of 14 mg per day.
Over 60 Years of Age: Same as 12 to 60 years of age.

Conditions Requiring Dosing Adjustments
Liver function: Adjustments in dose in liver compromise are not defined.
Kidney function: Adjustments in dose in kidney compromise are not defined.

▷ **Dosing Instructions:**   Follow the instructions on the leaflet provided in the medication box carefully. Nedocromil use must be continued, even when you are symptom-free.

Usual Duration of Use:
Use on a regular schedule for a week usually determines effectiveness in helping prevent acute asthma. Long-term use (months to years) requires periodic physician evaluation of response and dosage adjustment.

Possible Advantages of This Drug
Usually well tolerated. Rare serious adverse effects.

▷ **This Drug Should Not Be Taken If**
• you have had an allergic reaction to any dosage form of it previously.
• you are having an acute asthma attack.

▷ **Inform Your Physician Before Taking This Drug If**
• you have impaired kidney function.
• you have angina or a heart rhythm disorder.
• you are uncertain of how to take nedocromil, or how often to take it.

Possible Side Effects (natural, expected, and unavoidable drug actions)
Unpleasant taste.
Mild throat irritation or hoarseness. This may be lessened by taking a few swallows of water after each inhalation.

▷ **Possible Adverse Effects** (unusual, unexpected, and infrequent reactions)
If any of the following develop, consult your physician promptly for guidance.
Mild Adverse Effects
Allergic Reactions: Skin rash, hives.
Headache, dizziness (rare).
Unpleasant taste.
Nausea or vomiting (rare).
Cough.
Serious Adverse Effects
Allergic Reactions: Anaphylactoid reaction, allergic pneumonitis (allergic reaction of the lung tissue).
Bronchospasm.

▷ **Possible Effects on Sexual Function:**   None reported.

Possible Delayed Adverse Effects: Pneumonitis (very rare).

Possible Effects on Laboratory Tests

Liver function tests: increased ALT.

CAUTION

1. This drug does **not** act as a bronchodilator and should not be used for immediate relief of acute asthma.
2. If use of this drug has allowed you to stop taking a cortisone-related drug, you may need to resume the cortisone-related drug if you are injured, must stop taking nedocromil, have an infection or need surgery.
3. If severe asthma returns, contact your doctor promptly.
4. If you use a bronchodilator drug by inhalation, it is best to take it about five minutes before inhaling nedocromil.

Precautions for Use

By Infants and Children: Safety and effectiveness for those under 12 years of age not established.

By Those over 60 Years of Age: This drug does not work in therapy of chronic bronchitis or emphysema.

▷ **Advisability of Use During Pregnancy**

Pregnancy Category: B. See Pregnancy Code at the back of this book.

Animal studies: Rat, mice and rabbit studies show no impairment of fertility or harm to the fetus.

Human studies: Adequate studies of pregnant women are not available.

Ask your doctor for guidance.

Advisability of Use if Breast-Feeding

Presence of this drug in breast milk: Unknown.

Avoid drug or refrain from nursing.

Habit-Forming Potential: None.

Effects of Overdosage: Head shaking, tremor and salivation were seen in dogs given high doses.

Suggested Periodic Examinations While Taking This Drug (at physician's discretion)

Sputum analysis and X-ray if pneumonitis suspected.

Liver function tests.

▷ **While Taking This Drug, Observe the Following**

Foods: No restrictions.

Beverages: Avoid all beverages to which you may be allergic.

▷   *Alcohol:* No interaction expected.

Tobacco Smoking: Follow your doctor's advice regarding smoking.

▷   *Other Drugs*

Nedocromil may make it possible to reduce the dose or frequency of use of cortisonelike drugs. Ask your doctor for guidance.

There are no known adverse drug interactions at present.

▷   *Driving, Hazardous Activities:* This drug may cause dizziness. Restrict activities as necessary.

Aviation Note: The use of this drug *may be a disqualification* for piloting. Consult a designated Aviation Medical Examiner.

Exposure to Sun: No restrictions.

Heavy Exercise or Exertion: This drug may enable you to partake in exercise. Ask your doctor for guidance.

Discontinuation: If this drug has made it possible to reduce or stop cortisonelike drugs, and you must stop nedocromil, you may have to resume the cortisonelike drug as well as other measures to control asthma.

NEFAZODONE (na FAZ oh dohn)

Introduced: 1994   **Prescription:** USA: Yes; Canada: Yes   **Available as Generic:** USA: No; Canada: No   **Class:** antidepressant, other   **Controlled Drug:** USA: No; Canada: No
Brand Names: Serzone

BENEFITS versus RISKS	
Possible Benefits	*Possible Risks*
EFFECTIVE TREATMENT OF DEPRESSION	Dizziness
	Mild blood pressure changes on standing
Fewer cardiovascular side effects than older agents	
Minimal anticholinergic side effects	
Decreased sedation	

▷ **Principal Uses**

As a Single Drug Product: Uses currently included in FDA approved labeling: (1) Treatment of major depression.

Other (unlabeled) generally accepted uses: (1) May have a role in pain management.

How This Drug Works: This antidepressant is unique in that it:

1. Blocks the reuptake of a specific nerve transmitting chemical (5-HT).
2. Acts as a 5-HT2 antagonist.

Because of this unique mechanism of action, this drug has fewer cardiovascular and anticholinergic side effects than previously available agents.

Available Dosage Forms and Strengths

Tablets — 100 mg, 150 mg, 200 mg, 250 mg

▷ **Recommended Dosage Ranges (Actual dosage and administration schedule must be determined by the physician for each patient individually.)**

Infants and Children: Not indicated.

18 to 60 Years of Age: The starting dose for this medicine is 200 mg daily. This is given as 100 mg in the morning and 100 mg in the evening. The dose is increased as needed and tolerated in 100 mg increments with at least one week separating any dose increase. The maximum dose is 600 mg daily.

Over 60 Years of Age: Dosing in this population starts with 100 mg daily in two divided doses. The medicine is then increased (however at a slower rate than in younger patients) as needed and tolerated.

Conditions Requiring Dosing Adjustments

Liver function: The dose should be decreased in patients with liver compromise.
Kidney function: No specific dosing changes are presently identified.

▷ **Dosing Instructions:** Food delays the absorption and decreases total absorption, but this effect is not believed to be clinically significant. Water is expected to be the safest liquid to take this medicine with. Grapefruit juice may have an action of some liver enzymes (cytochrome P450) which help remove (metabolize) this medicine. Avoid taking with grapefruit juice until all data are in.

Usual Duration of Use:

Continual use on a regular schedule for four to five weeks is usually necessary to determine this drug's effectiveness in treating depression. Long-term use (months to years) requires periodic evaluation of response and dosage adjustment. See your doctor regularly.

Possible Advantages of This Drug

Two different mechanisms of action.

Decreased side effects versus other available agents.

▷ **This Drug Should Not Be Taken If**

• you have had an allergic reaction to any dosage form of it previously.
• you are taking astemizole or terfenadine.
• you are taking a MAO inhibitor (see Drug Classes).

▷ **Inform Your Physician Before Taking This Drug If**

• you take a triazolobenzodiazepine such as triazolam or alprazolam.
• you have a history of seizure disorder.
• you have a history of heart disease.
• you are uncertain of how much nefazodone to take or how often to take it.
• you take other prescription or nonprescription medicines which were not discussed with your doctor when nefazodone was prescribed.

Possible Side Effects (natural, expected, and unavoidable drug actions)

Dry mouth and constipation.

▷ **Possible Adverse Effects** (unusual, unexpected, and infrequent reactions)

If any of the following develop, consult your physician promptly for guidance.

Mild Adverse Effects

Allergic Reactions: Skin rash.

Dry mouth or blurred vision.

Nausea, ringing in the ears.

Headache, dizziness, and tremor.

Insomnia (rare), confusion, and agitation (rare).

Slowed heart rate.

Serious Adverse Effects

Allergic Reactions: Not defined.

Idiosyncratic Reactions: Not identified.

Lowered blood pressure on standing (postural hypotension).

Activation of mania (one case report).

Seizures (rare).

▷ **Possible Effects on Sexual Function:**   Impotence, absence of orgasm or abnormal ejaculation have all been rarely reported. Priapism has been reported with a structurally similar drug.

Possible Delayed Adverse Effects: None reported.

▷ **Adverse Effects That May Mimic Natural Diseases or Disorders**

None reported.

Natural Diseases or Disorders That May Be Activated by This Drug

None reported.

Possible Effects on Laboratory Tests
Hematocrit: decreased.

CAUTION
1. Risk of suicide is present in depressed patients. Small quantities of this medicine should be dispensed at a time when therapy is started. Appropriate suicide precautions should be taken.
2. This medicine **must not** be taken with MAO inhibitor. 14 days MUST go by once a MAO inhibitor is stopped before nefazodone is started.

Precautions for Use
By Infants and Children: Safety and effectiveness for use by those under 18 years of age have not been established.
By Those over 60 Years of Age: Lower starting doses and more gradual increases in dose are indicated.

▷ **Advisability of Use During Pregnancy**
Pregnancy Category: C. See Pregnancy Code at the back of this book.
Animal studies: Increased rat pup mortality was seen when doses five times the typical human dose were used.
Human studies: Information from adequate studies of pregnant women is not available. Ask your doctor for guidance.

Advisability of Use if Breast-Feeding
Presence of this drug in breast milk: Unknown.
Avoid drug or refrain from nursing.

Habit-Forming Potential: None defined at present, but not expected.

Effects of Overdosage: Nausea, vomiting and somnolence.

Possible Effects of Long-Term Use: None reported.

Suggested Periodic Examinations While Taking This Drug (at physician's discretion)
Periodic checks of heart rate.

▷ **While Taking This Drug, Observe the Following**
Foods: No restrictions.
Beverages: No restrictions.
▷ *Alcohol:* This combination is not recommended.
Tobacco Smoking: No interactions expected.
Marijuana Smoking: Increased somnolence.
▷ *Other Drugs*
Nefazodone may ***increase*** the effects of
- alprazolam (Xanax) and potentially other benzodiazepines (see Drug Classes).
- digoxin (Lanoxin). Increased blood level checks are suggested.
- haloperidol (Haldol).
- triazolam (Halcion).
Nefazodone ***taken concurrently*** with
- acebutolol (Sectral) and perhaps other beta blockers may result in decreased acebutolol levels and increased nefazodone metabolites.
- astemizole (Hismanal) can cause serious heart toxicity.
- clozapine (Clozaril) may result in clozapine toxicity since the P450 system in the liver is involved in removing clozapine from the liver.
- dextromethorphan (cough medicines with DM on the label) may result in

dextromethorphan toxicity since the P450 system in the liver is involved in removing dextromethorphan from the liver.

- MAO inhibitors (see Drug Classes) may cause serious toxicity.
- phenytoin (Dilantin) may result in increased phenytoin levels. More frequent phenytoin blood level checks are needed, and dosing should be adjusted to blood level results.
- terfenadine (Seldane) may cause serious heart rhythm problems.
- tricyclic antidepressants (TCAs see Drug Classes) may result in increased TCA levels and toxicity.

▷ *Driving, Hazardous Activities:* This drug may cause somnolence. Restrict activities as necessary.

Aviation Note: The use of this drug *is a disqualification* for piloting. Consult a designated Aviation Medical Examiner.

Exposure to Sun: Use caution, photosensitivity is possible.

Discontinuation: Do not stop this medication without discussing this with your doctor.

NEOSTIGMINE (nee oh STIG meen)

Introduced: 1931   **Prescription:** USA: Yes; Canada: Yes   **Available as**
Generic: USA: Yes; Canada: Yes   **Class:** Antimyasthenic   **Controlled**
Drug: USA: No; Canada: No
Brand Name: Prostigmin, ♣PMS-Neostigmine, Viaderm-K.C.

BENEFITS versus RISKS	
Possible Benefits	*Possible Risks*
MODERATELY EFFECTIVE TREATMENT OF OCULAR AND MILD FORMS OF MYASTHENIA GRAVIS (symptomatic relief of muscle weakness) Eases postoperative bowel slowing or block (paralytic ileus)	Cholinergic crisis (overdose): excessive salivation, nausea, vomiting, stomach cramps, diarrhea, shortness of breath (asthmalike wheezing), weakness

▷ **Principal Uses**

As a Single Drug Product: Uses currently included in FDA approved labeling: (1) Treats ocular and milder forms of myasthenia gravis by providing temporary relief of muscle weakness and fatigability; (2) reverses depression of bowel function which may occur after surgery; (3) used to ease symptoms of bladder instability.

Other (unlabeled) generally accepted uses: (1) Used to reverse neuromuscular blockade caused by atracurium.

How This Drug Works: This drug inhibits cholinesterase, the enzyme that destroys acetylcholine. This results in higher levels of acetylcholine, the nerve transmitter that facilitates the stimulation of muscular activity. The net effects are increased muscle strength and endurance.

Available Dosage Forms and Strengths

Injection — 0.25, 0.5 and 1.0 mg per ml

Tablets — 15 mg

▷ **Usual Adult Dosage Range:** Initially: 15 mg/3 to 4 hours; adjust dosage as needed and tolerated. Maintenance: up to 300 mg/24 hours; the average dose is 75 to 150 mg/24 hours. **Note: Actual dosage and administration schedule must be determined by the physician for each patient individually.**

Conditions Requiring Dosing Adjustments
Liver function: Neostigmine should be used with caution in patients with compromised livers.
Kidney function: Half of a given dose of neostigmine is eliminated unchanged by the kidney, however, specific guidelines for decreasing doses are not available.

▷ **Dosing Instructions:** The tablet may be crushed and taken with food or milk to reduce the intensity of side effects. Larger portions of the daily maintenance dosage should be timed according to the pattern of fatigue and weakness.

Usual Duration of Use: Use on a regular schedule (with dosage adjustment) for 10 to 14 days determines effectiveness in relieving the symptoms of myasthenia gravis. Long-term use (months to years) requires periodic physician evaluation.

▷ **This Drug Should Not Be Taken If**
- you have had an allergic reaction to it previously.
- you are known to be allergic to bromide compounds.
- you have an obstruction in your urinary tract or intestine.

▷ **Inform Your Physician Before Taking This Drug If**
- you have any type of seizure disorder.
- you are subject to heart rhythm disorders or bronchial asthma.
- you have recurrent urinary tract infections.
- you have prostatism (see Glossary).
- you plan to have surgery under general anesthesia in the near future.

Possible Side Effects (natural, expected, and unavoidable drug actions)
Small pupils, watering of eyes, slow pulse, excessive salivation, nausea, vomiting, stomach cramps, diarrhea, urge to urinate, increased sweating.

▷ **Possible Adverse Effects** (unusual, unexpected, and infrequent reactions)
If any of the following develop, consult your physician promptly for guidance.
Mild Adverse Effects
Allergic Reaction: Skin rash.
Nervousness, anxiety, unsteadiness, muscle cramps or twitching.
Serious Adverse Effects
Confusion, slurred speech, seizures, difficult breathing (asthmatic wheezing).
Increased muscle weakness or paralysis.
Excessive vomiting or diarrhea may induce abnormally low blood potassium levels (hypokalemia). This will accentuate muscle weakness.
Abnormally slow heartbeat (bradycardia) (rare).
Drug-induced porphyria (rare).

▷ **Possible Effects on Sexual Function:** None reported.

▷ **Adverse Effects That May Mimic Natural Diseases or Disorders**
Seizures may suggest the possibility of epilepsy.

Natural Diseases or Disorders That May Be Activated by This Drug
Latent bronchial asthma.

Possible Effects on Laboratory Tests
None reported.

CAUTION

1. Certain drugs can block the action of this drug and reduce its effectiveness in treating myasthenia gravis. (See *Other Drugs* below.) Ask physician before starting any new drug, prescription or over-the-counter.

2. Dosing must be carefully individualized. Variations in response may occur from time to time. Because generalized muscle weakness is a major symptom of both myasthenia crisis (underdosage) and cholinergic crisis (overdosage), it may be difficult to recognize the correct cause. As a rule, weakness that begins within 1 hour after taking this drug probably represents overdosage; weakness that begins 3 or more hours after taking this drug is probably due to underdosage. Observe these time relationships and inform your physician.

3. In long-term therapy, watch for development of resistance to the drug's therapeutic action (loss of effectiveness). Ask your doctor about the advisability of stopping this drug for a few days to see if responsiveness can be restored.

Precautions for Use
By Infants and Children: Dosage and administration schedule must be modified if kidney function is severely impaired.
By Those over 60 Years of Age: The natural decline of kidney function with aging may require smaller doses to prevent accumulation of this drug to toxic levels.

▷ **Advisability of Use During Pregnancy**
Pregnancy Category: C. See Pregnancy Code at the back of this book.
Animal studies: No information available.
Human studies: Adequate studies of pregnant women are not available.
There are no reports of birth defects due to the use of this drug during pregnancy. However, there are reports of significant muscular weakness in 20% of newborn infants whose mothers had taken this drug during pregnancy. Ask your physician for guidance.

Advisability of Use if Breast-Feeding
Presence of this drug in breast milk: Probably not.
Monitor nursing infant closely and discontinue drug or nursing if adverse effects develop.

Habit-Forming Potential: None.

Effects of Overdosage: Generalized muscular weakness, blurred vision, very small pupils, slow heart rate, difficult breathing (wheezing), excessive salivation, nausea, vomiting, stomach cramps, diarrhea, muscle cramps or twitching. This syndrome constitutes the cholinergic crisis.

Possible Effects of Long-Term Use: Development of tolerance (see Glossary) with loss of therapeutic benefit.

Suggested Periodic Examinations While Taking This Drug (at physician's discretion)
Assessment of drug effectiveness and dosage schedule for best results.

▷ **While Taking This Drug, Observe the Following**
Foods: No restrictions.
Beverages: No restrictions. May be taken with milk.
▷ *Alcohol:* Use caution. Weakness and unsteadiness may be accentuated.
Tobacco Smoking: No interactions expected.
▷ *Other Drugs*
The following drugs may *decrease* the effects of neostigmine
- atropine (belladonna).
- clindamycin (Cleocin).
- guanadrel (Hylorel).
- guanethidine (Esimil, Ismelin).
- procainamide (Procan SR, Pronestyl).
- quinidine (Cardioquin, Duraquin, etc.).
- quinine (Quinamm).
Neostigmine *taken concurrently* with
- edrophonium may cause cholinergic crisis in patients with myasthenic weakness.
- hydrocortisone or other corticosteroids (see Drug Classes) can cause decreased neostigmine benefits.
- physostigmine can result in additive adverse effects.
▷ *Driving, Hazardous Activities:* This drug may cause blurred vision, confusion or generalized weakness. Restrict activities as necessary.
Aviation Note: The use of this drug *is a disqualification* for piloting. Consult a designated Aviation Medical Examiner.
Exposure to Sun: No restrictions.
Exposure to Heat: Use caution. This may cause excessive sweating and increased weakness.
Exposure to Environmental Chemicals: Avoid excessive exposure (inhalation, skin contamination) to the insecticides Baygon, Diazinon and Sevin. These can accentuate potential toxicity of this drug.
Discontinuation: Do not stop this drug abruptly without your doctor's knowledge and help.

NIACIN (NI a sin)

Other Names: Nicotinic acid, vitamin B-3

Introduced: 1937   **Prescription:** USA: Tablets and liquid—no; capsules—yes; Canada: No   **Available as Generic:** USA: Yes; Canada: Yes   **Class:** Anticholesterol, vasodilator   **Controlled Drug:** USA: No; Canada: No

Brand Names: ✦Antivert [CD], Endur-Acin, Niac, Niacels, Niacin TR, Niacor, Nia-bid, Niaplus, Nicobid, Nico-400, Nicolar, Nicotinex, ✦Novoniacin, SK-Niacin, Slo-Niacin, Span-Niacin-150, Tega-Span, Tri-B3

```
┌─────────────────────────────────────────────────────────────┐
│                    BENEFITS versus RISKS                       │
│      Possible Benefits              Possible Risks             │
│  EFFECTIVE REDUCTION OF TOTAL   Activation of peptic ulcer     │
│   CHOLESTEROL, LOW-DENSITY      Drug-induced hepatitis         │
│   CHOLESTEROL, AND              Aggravation of diabetes or gout│
│   TRIGLYCERIDES IN TYPES II, III,                              │
│   IV, AND V CHOLESTEROL                                        │
│   DISORDERS                                                    │
│  Specific prevention and treatment of                          │
│   pellagra (niacin-deficiency disease)                         │
└─────────────────────────────────────────────────────────────┘
```

▷ **Principal Uses**

As a *Single Drug Product:* Uses currently included in FDA approved labeling: (1) Certain patterns of abnormally high blood levels of cholesterol and triglycerides; (2) pellagra, a niacin (vitamin B-3) deficiency disorder characterized by dementia, dermatitis and diarrhea; (3) therapy of Hartnup disease.

Other (unlabeled) generally accepted uses: (1) Therapy of certain types of vertigo and tinnitus (ringing in the ears); (2) may help decrease diarrhea in patients with cholera; (3) treatment of Chilblains.

As a *Combination Drug Product* [CD]: In Canada this drug is combined with meclizine to enhance its effectiveness in the treatment of motion sickness and vertigo.

How This Drug Works

It is thought that it may inhibit the initial production of triglycerides and impair the conversion of fatty tissue to cholesterol and triglycerides.

This drug corrects the specific deficiency of vitamin B-3 that is responsible for the symptoms of pellagra.

This drug causes direct dilation of peripheral blood vessels in the skin of the face and neck; for this reason it has been used to increase the blood flow to the inner ear in an attempt to relieve some types of vertigo and ringing in the ears. The effectiveness of this application is questionable.

Available Dosage Forms and Strengths

Capsules, prolonged-action — 125 mg, 250 mg, 300 mg, 400 mg, 500 mg
Oral solution — 50 mg per 5-ml
Tablets — 20 mg, 25 mg, 50 mg, 100 mg, 500 mg
Tablets, prolonged-action — 150 mg, 250 mg, 500 mg, 750 mg

▷ **Usual Adult Dosage Range**

For cholesterol disorders: Initially 100 mg 3 times daily. Dose may be increased in increments of 300 mg daily at intervals of 4 to 7 days as needed and tolerated. The usual maintenance dose is 1 to 2 grams 3 times daily. The total daily dosage should not exceed 6 to 9 grams.

For niacin deficiency: 10 to 20 mg daily.

For treatment of pellagra: 50 mg 3 to 10 times daily.

Note: Actual dosage and administration schedule must be determined by the physician for each patient individually.

Conditions Requiring Dosing Adjustments

Liver function: This drug is metabolized in the liver and is contraindicated in liver disease.

Kidney function: Specific guidelines for adjustment of dosing are not available.

▷ **Dosing Instructions:**   Take with or immediately following meals to prevent stomach irritation. Also take one-half of an adult's aspirin tablet or 1 children's aspirin tablet with each dose of niacin to help prevent facial flushing and itching. Dosage should be increased very slowly over 2 to 3 months as needed. The prolonged-action form of niacin is preferable to improve tolerance. The regular tablet may be crushed for administration, but the prolonged-action capsules and tablets should not be altered.

Usual Duration of Use: Use on a regular schedule for 3 to 5 weeks determines benefit in reducing levels of cholesterol and triglycerides. Long-term use (months to years) requires periodic physician evaluation.

Currently a "Drug of Choice"
for initiating treatment of elevated LDL cholesterol and VLDL triglycerides.

▷ **This Drug Should Not Be Taken If**
  • you have had an allergic reaction to it previously.
  • you have active peptic ulcer disease or inflammatory bowel disease.
  • you have active liver disease.

▷ **Inform Your Physician Before Taking This Drug If**
  • you are prone to low blood pressure.
  • you have a heart rhythm disorder of any kind.
  • you have a history of peptic ulcer disease, inflammatory bowel disease, liver disease, jaundice or gallbladder disease.
  • you have diabetes or gout.

Possible Side Effects (natural, expected, and unavoidable drug actions)
Flushing, itching, tingling, and feeling of warmth, usually in the face and neck. Sensitive individuals may experience orthostatic hypotension (see Glossary).

▷ **Possible Adverse Effects** (unusual, unexpected, and infrequent reactions)
If any of the following develop, consult your physician promptly for guidance.
Mild Adverse Effects
Allergic Reactions: Skin rash, itching, hives.
Headache, dizziness, faintness, impaired vision.
Indigestion, nausea, vomiting, diarrhea.
Flushing and tingling.
Dryness of skin, grayish-black pigmentation of skin folds.
Serious Adverse Effects
Drug-induced hepatitis with jaundice (see Glossary): yellow eyes and skin, dark-colored urine, light-colored stools.
Worsening of diabetes and gout.
Development of heart rhythm disorders.
Myopathy.
Abnormal blood sugar.
Peptic ulcers.

▷ **Possible Effects on Sexual Function:**   None reported.
▷ **Adverse Effects That May Mimic Natural Diseases or Disorders**
Liver reactions may suggest viral hepatitis.

Natural Diseases or Disorders That May Be Activated by This Drug
Latent diabetes, gout, inflammatory bowel disease or peptic ulcer.

Possible Effects on Laboratory Tests

Complete blood cell counts: decreased eosinophils and lymphocytes.

Blood total cholesterol, LDL cholesterol and triglyceride levels: decreased.

Blood HDL cholesterol level: increased.

Blood glucose level: increased.

Glucose tolerance test (GTT): decreased.

Blood uric acid level: increased.

Liver function tests: increased liver enzymes (ALT/GPT, AST/GOT and alkaline phosphatase), increased bilirubin.

Urine sugar tests: inaccurate test results with Benedict's solution.

CAUTION

1. Large doses may cause increases in blood levels of sugar and uric acid. Diabetics or gout patients should monitor their status regularly.
2. Periodic measurements of blood cholesterol and triglyceride levels are essential for monitoring response and determining the need for changes in dosage or medication.
3. Recent reports indicate that the prolonged-action dosage forms of niacin may be more likely to cause liver damage than the rapidly absorbed (crystalline) forms. Ask your doctor which is the most appropriate dosage form and schedule for you.

Precautions for Use

By Infants and Children: Safety and effectiveness for use of large doses by those under 12 years of age have not been established.

By Those over 60 Years of Age: Observe for the possible development of low blood pressure (light-headedness, dizziness, faintness) and heart rhythm disorders.

▷ **Advisability of Use During Pregnancy**

Pregnancy Category: C. See Pregnancy Code at the back of this book.

Animal studies: Significant birth defects due to this drug were found in chicks.

Human studies: Adequate studies of pregnant women are not available.

Use this drug only if clearly needed. Avoid completely during the first 3 months.

Advisability of Use if Breast-Feeding

Presence of this drug in breast milk: Unknown.

Avoid drug or refrain from nursing.

Habit-Forming Potential: None.

Effects of Overdosage: Generalized flushing, nausea, vomiting, stomach cramps, diarrhea, weakness, fainting.

Possible Effects of Long-Term Use: Increased blood levels of sugar and uric acid; liver damage.

Suggested Periodic Examinations While Taking This Drug (at physician's discretion)

Measurements of blood levels of total cholesterol, HDL and LDL cholesterol fractions, triglycerides, sugar and uric acid.

Liver function tests.

▷ **While Taking This Drug, Observe the Following**

Foods: Follow the low-cholesterol diet prescribed by your physician.

Beverages: No restrictions. May be taken with milk.

▷ *Alcohol:* Use with caution. Alcohol used with large doses of this drug may cause excessive lowering of blood pressure. There has been one case report of delirium.

Tobacco Smoking: May increase risk of flushing and dizziness.

▷ *Other Drugs*

Niacin may *increase* the effects of

- some antihypertensive drugs, and cause excessive lowering of blood pressure.

Niacin may *decrease* the effects of

- antidiabetic drugs (insulin and oral hypoglycemic agents; see Drug Classes), by raising the level of blood sugar.
- probenecid (Benemid) and sulfinpyrazone (Anturane), by raising the level of blood uric acid.

Niacin *taken concurrently* with

- Isoniazid (INH) may result in decreased niacin levels and require increased niacin dosing.
- lovastatin and other cholesterol lowering drugs may result in reversible muscle problems (myopathy or rhabdomyolysis).
- nicotine (particularly transdermal) may result in increased risk of flushing and dizziness.

▷ *Driving, Hazardous Activities:* This drug may cause dizziness and faintness. Restrict activities as necessary.

Aviation Note: The use of this drug *may be a disqualification* for piloting. Consult a designated Aviation Medical Examiner.

Exposure to Sun: No restrictions.

Discontinuation: Do not stop this drug without your physician's knowledge and guidance. Abrupt withdrawal may be followed by excessive increase in blood cholesterol and triglyceride levels.

NICARDIPINE (ni KAR de peen)

Introduced: 1984 **Prescription:** USA: Yes **Available as Generic:** USA: No **Class:** Antianginal, antihypertensive, calcium channel blocker **Controlled Drug** USA: No

Brand Name: Cardene, Cardene SR

Controversies In Medicine: Study data indicates that medicines in this class should NOT be used in some patients with extremely compromised hearts. There have also been several FDA hearings held on the calcium channel blocker class. Be certain to ask your doctor about your cardiac output and if the benefits of this medicine outweigh the risks of its use. A recent FDA panel found medicines in this class to be safe and effective. A retrospective chart review yielded data that showed increased risks for nifedipine immediate release forms in those over 71, and cautioned physicians against using the immediate release form for indications other than angina. The immediate release form in question had never been approved for other uses. Most recently, a study of nearly 6,000 patients at Tel Aviv Medical Center found that there was no statistically significant increased risk of death in the patients who took calcium channel blockers versus those who did not.

```
┌─────────────────────────────────────────────────────────────────┐
│                     BENEFITS versus RISKS                         │
│        Possible Benefits              Possible Risks              │
│  EFFECTIVE PREVENTION OF        Increase in angina upon starting  │
│    CLASSICAL ANGINA OF EFFORT     treatment                       │
│  EFFECTIVE TREATMENT OF         Water retention, ankle swelling   │
│    HYPERTENSION                                                   │
└─────────────────────────────────────────────────────────────────┘
```

▷ **Principal Uses**

As a Single Drug Product: Uses currently included in FDA approved labeling: (1) Treats classical angina-of-effort (due to atherosclerotic disease of the coronary arteries) or angina caused by spasm of the coronary arteries; (2) mild to moderate hypertension.

Other (unlabeled) generally accepted uses: (1) Combination therapy in preventing recurrence of stroke; (2) may have a role in helping correct congestive heart failure; (3) can help refractory (not responding to nonsteroidal anti-inflammatory drugs) menstrual pain; (4) may help decrease the frequency and severity of migraine attacks; (5) can halt the progression of atherosclerosis; (6) lowers postoperative hypertension; (7) may prevent vessel spasm in some kinds of vascular surgery; (8) could have a role in some premature labor.

How This Drug Works: By blocking passage of calcium through certain cell walls (which is necessary for the function of nerve and muscle tissue), this drug inhibits the contraction of coronary arteries and peripheral arterioles. As a result of these effects, this drug

• promotes dilation of the coronary arteries (antianginal effect).
• reduces the degree of contraction of peripheral arterial walls, resulting in lowering of blood pressure. This further reduces the workload of the heart during exertion and helps prevent of angina.

Available Dosage Forms and Strengths

Capsules — 20 mg, 30 mg
Injection — 2.5 mg per ml
SR Capsules — 30 mg, 45 mg, 60 mg

▷ **Usual Adult Dosage Range:**   Initially 20 mg 3 times daily, 6 to 8 hours apart. Dose may be increased gradually at 3-day intervals (as needed and tolerated) up to 40 mg 3 times daily. The total daily dosage should not exceed 120 mg. The sustained release form is started at 30 mg twice daily and is increased as needed and tolerated to 60 mg twice daily. **Note: Actual dosage and administration schedule must be determined by the physician for each patient individually.**

Conditions Requiring Dosing Adjustments

Liver function: The dose should be started at 20 mg twice a day. If the dose must be increased, it should be slowly advanced and given twice a day.

Kidney function: In patients with moderate kidney failure, the starting dose should be 20 mg twice daily. If the dose is increased, it should be titrated slowly, and the twice daily dosing interval retained. Nicardipine can cause urine retention, and should be used as a benefit to risk decision in patients with urine outflow problems.

▷ **Dosing Instructions:**   May be taken with or following food to reduce stomach irritation. However, if taken after a high-fat meal, total absorption of this drug may be reduced by 20% to 30%. The capsule should be swallowed whole (not altered).

Usual Duration of Use: Use on a regular schedule for 2 to 4 weeks determines benefit in reducing the frequency and severity of angina or controlling hypertension. For long-term use (months to years), the smallest effective dose should be used. Physician supervision and periodic evaluation are essential.

Possible Advantages of This Drug

Does not impair heart function or cause heart rhythm abnormalities.
Can be used safely with beta blockers, digoxin, diuretics and nitrate.

▷ **This Drug Should Not Be Taken If**
• you have had an allergic reaction to it previously.
• you have advanced aortic stenosis.

▷ **Inform Your Physician Before Taking This Drug If**
• you have had an adverse reaction to any calcium blocker (see Drug Classes).
• you currently take any form of digitalis or a beta blocker drug (see Drug Class Section).
• you are taking any drugs that lower blood pressure.
• you are taking cimetidine (Tagamet) or cyclosporine (Sandimmune).
• you have a history of congestive heart failure, heart attack or stroke.
• you have a history of circulation impairment to the fingers.
• you have Duchenne muscular dystrophy.
• you are subject to disturbances of heart rhythm.
• you have impaired liver or kidney function.

Possible Side Effects (natural, expected, and unavoidable drug actions)

Rapid heart rate, swelling of the feet and ankles, flushing and sensation of warmth.

▷ **Possible Adverse Effects** (unusual, unexpected, and infrequent reactions)

If any of the following develop, consult your physician promptly for guidance.

Mild Adverse Effects

Allergic Reaction: Skin rash (rare).
Headache, dizziness, weakness, nervousness or dream disturbances (rare), ringing in the ears (tinnitus), blurred vision, confusion, increased urination (rare).
Palpitation, shortness of breath (rare).
Indigestion, nausea, vomiting, constipation (all rare).
Joint and muscle pain (rare), cough.
Abnormal growth (hyperplasia) of the gums.

Serious Adverse Effects

Allergic Reactions: None reported.
Increased frequency or severity of angina on initiation of treatment or following an increase in dose.
Difficult urination (rare).
Liver toxicity (rare).
Marked drop in blood pressure with fainting (rare).
Decreased white blood cell counts has been reported with medicines in the same class (agranulocytosis) (very rare).

▷ **Possible Effects on Sexual Function:** Rare impotence (less than 1%).

▷ **Adverse Effects That May Mimic Natural Diseases or Disorders**
Flushing and warmth may resemble menopausal "hot flushes." Increased liver enzymes may resemble infectious hepatitis.

Possible Effects on Laboratory Tests
Liver function tests: elevated (1%).

CAUTION
1. If you are checking your own blood pressure, check it just before each dose and 1 to 2 hours after each dose to obtain an accurate picture of drug effect.
2. Be sure to tell all health care providers who provide care for you that you take this drug. Note the use of this drug on your card of personal identification.
3. You may use nitroglycerin and other nitrate drugs as needed to relieve acute episodes of angina pain. However, if you detect that your angina attacks are becoming more frequent or intense, call your doctor promptly.

Precautions for Use
By Infants and Children: Safety and effectiveness for those under 18 years of age not established.
By Those over 60 Years of Age: Usually well tolerated, however, watch for development of weakness, dizziness, fainting and falling. Take necessary precautions to prevent injury. Report promptly any changes in your pattern of thirst and urination.

▷ **Advisability of Use During Pregnancy**
Pregnancy Category: C. See Pregnancy Code at the back of this book.
Animal studies: Embryo and fetal toxicity reported in small animals, but no birth defects due to this drug.
Human studies: Adequate studies of pregnant women are not available.
Avoid this drug during the first 3 months. Use during the last 6 months only if clearly needed. Ask physician for guidance.

Advisability of Use if Breast-Feeding
Presence of this drug in breast milk: Probably yes.
Avoid drug or refrain from nursing.

Habit-Forming Potential: None.

Effects of Overdosage: Weakness, light-headedness, fainting, fast pulse, low blood pressure, shortness of breath, flushed and warm skin, tremors.

Possible Effects of Long-Term Use: None reported.

Suggested Periodic Examinations While Taking This Drug (at physician's discretion)
Evaluations of heart function, including electrocardiograms; measurements of blood pressure in supine, sitting and standing positions.

▷ **While Taking This Drug, Observe the Following**
Foods: Food decreases the amount of this drug which is absorbed. It is also prudent to avoid excessive salt intake.
Beverages: No restrictions. May be taken with milk.
▷ *Alcohol:* Use with caution until combined effects have been determined. Alcohol may exaggerate the drop in blood pressure experienced by some individuals.

Tobacco Smoking: Nicotine may reduce the effectiveness of this drug. Follow your physician's advice regarding smoking.

Marijuana Smoking: Possible reduced effectiveness of this drug; mild to moderate increase in angina; possible changes in electrocardiogram, confusing interpretation.

▷ **Other Drugs**

Nicardipine may *increase* the effects of

- cyclosporine (Sandimmune), and cause kidney toxicity.

Nicardipine *taken concurrently* with

- amiodarone (Codarone) may result in cardiac arrest.
- beta blocker drugs or digitalis preparations (see Drug Classes Section) may affect heart rate and rhythm adversely. Careful monitoring by your physician is necessary if these drugs are taken concurrently.
- magnesium may cause worsening of neuromuscular blockade and further lowering of blood pressure.
- nonsteroidal anti-inflammatory agents (NSAIDS) (see Drug Classes) may blunt the therapeutic effect of nicardipine.
- phenytoin (Dilantin) may result in phenytoin toxicity or decreased efficacy of Nicardipine.
- rifampin (Rifadin, others) has caused loss of control of blood pressure with some other calcium channel blockers. Caution is advised if these medicines are combined.

The following drugs may *increase* the effects of nicardipine

- cimetidine (Tagamet).

▷ *Driving, Hazardous Activities:* Usually no restrictions. This drug may cause drowsiness or dizziness. Restrict activities as necessary.

Aviation Note: Coronary artery disease and hypertension *are disqualifications* for piloting. Consult a designated Aviation Medical Examiner.

Exposure to Sun: No restrictions.

Exposure to Heat: Caution advised. Hot environments can exaggerate the blood-pressure-lowering effects of this drug. Observe for light-headedness or weakness.

Heavy Exercise or Exertion: This drug may improve your ability to be more active without resulting angina pain. Use caution and avoid excessive exercise that could impair heart function in the absence of warning pain.

Discontinuation: Do not stop this drug abruptly. Ask your doctor about gradual withdrawal. Watch for possible development of rebound angina.

NICOTINE (NIK oh teen)

Introduced: 1992   **Prescription:** USA: Yes for all patches, both nicorettes (2 and 4 mg) are now available without a prescription for those over 18 years of age. **Author's note: Two brands of nicotine patch are now FDA approved for nonprescription use.** Canada: Yes   **Available as Generic:** USA: No; Canada: No   **Class:** Smoking cessation adjunct   **Controlled Drug:** USA: No; Canada: No

Brand Names: Habitrol, Nicoderm, Nicorette, Nicorette DS, Nicotrol, ProStep

BENEFITS versus RISKS	
Possible Benefits	*Possible Risks*
EFFECTIVE REDUCTION OF NICOTINE CRAVING AND WITHDRAWAL EFFECTS when used adjunctively in smoking-cessation treatment programs	Aggravation of existing angina, heart rhythm disorders, hypertension, insulin-dependent diabetes, peptic ulcer, and vascular diseases Increased risk of abortion (if used during pregnancy)

▷ **Principal Uses**

As a Single Drug Product: Uses currently included in FDA approved labeling: Nicotine chewing gum and nicotine transdermal systems are used adjunctively in behavior modification programs to help cigarette smokers who wish to stop smoking.

Other (unlabeled) generally accepted uses: (1) Some European data studying combination gum and patch use appears to show an increased success rate. The technique used the gum to halt "breakthrough" cigarette cravings. The thinking is that the craving resulted from an insufficient nicotine level provided by the patch, and that the gum provided a short term increase which stopped the craving.

How This Drug Works: By providing an alternate source of nicotine (for nicotine-dependent smokers), the appropriate use of these drug products can reduce nicotine craving and lessen smoking withdrawal effects such as irritability, nervousness, headache, fatigue, sleep disturbances, and drowsiness.

Available Dosage Forms and Strengths

Nicotine chewing gum tablets (Newly nonprescription in the United States)
Nicotine (Nicorette—2 mg)
(Nicorette DS— 4 mg) — 2 mg (US, Canada)
— 4 mg (US, Canada).
Nicotine Transdermal Systems — 16-hour Systems (US only): 5 mg, 10 mg, 15 mg
— 24-hour Systems: 7 mg (US, Canada), 11 mg (US), 14 mg (US, Canada), 21 mg (US, Canada) and 22 mg (US)

How to Store

Store nicotine gum at room temperature and protect from light. Store nicotine patches at room temperature and be especially careful to avoid exposing the patches to temperatures greater than 86 degrees F (30 C). Do not store unpouched. Once opened, patches should be used promptly because they may lose their strength.

▷ **Recommended Dosage Ranges (Actual dosage and administration schedule must be determined by the physician for each patient individually.)**

Infants and Children: Avoid use completely in children. Avoid accidental exposure to patches.

12 to 60 Years of Age: For chewing gum tablets: Initially, 1 piece every hour while awake (10 to 12 pieces daily); supplement with 1 additional piece if and when needed to control urge to smoke. Total daily dosage should not exceed 30 pieces (60 mg).

For transdermal systems: Dosage depends upon patient characteristics and product used.

For those weighing 100 pounds or more, smoking 10 or more cigarettes daily, and *without* cardiovascular disease:

Using a 16-hour system (Nicotrol): Initially one 15 mg patch applied for 16 hours daily for 4 to 12 weeks. For those who have abstained from smoking, reduce dose to one 10 mg patch applied for 16 hours daily for the next 2 to 4 weeks; then to one 5 mg patch applied for 16 hours daily for the following 2 to 4 weeks.

Using a 24-hour system: Habitrol, Nicoderm—initially one 21 mg patch applied daily for 4 to 8 weeks. For those who have abstained from smoking, reduce dose to one 14 mg patch daily for the next 2 to 4 weeks; then to one 7 mg patch daily for the following 2 to 4 weeks. ProStep—initially one 22 mg patch applied daily for 4 to 8 weeks. For those who have abstained from smoking, reduce dose to one 11 mg patch daily for 2 to 4 weeks.

For those weighing less than 100 pounds, smoking less than 10 cigarettes daily, or *with* cardiovascular disease:

Using a 24-hour system (Habitrol, Nicoderm): Initially one 14 mg patch applied daily for 4 to 8 weeks. For those who have abstained from smoking, reduce dose to one 7 mg patch daily for the next 2 to 4 weeks. (ProStep): Initially one 11 mg patch applied daily for 4 to 8 weeks.

Over 60 Years of Age: Same as 12 to 60 years of age.

Conditions Requiring Dosing Adjustments
Liver function: Consideration must be given to decreasing the starting dose if the liver is compromised.

Kidney function: Doses are decreased in severe kidney compromise.

▷ **Dosing Instructions:** Carefully follow the manufacturer's directions provided with each product.

For chewing gum: Limit use to one piece of gum at a time. This product is much harder than typical chewing gum. Chew each piece slowly and intermittently for 30 minutes. A tingling of your gum tissue or peppery taste usually indicates release of a sufficient amount of nicotine. Try to gradually reduce the number of pieces chewed each day by using it only when there is an urge to smoke. During participation in a smoking-cessation program, always have the gum available as a defense against smoking.

For transdermal systems: Apply a new patch at the same time each day. Do not alter the patch in any way. Apply the patch to the upper arm or body where the skin is clean, dry, and free of hair, oil, scars and irritation of any kind; alternate sites of application. Press the patch firmly in place for 10 seconds; ensure good contact throughout. Wash your hands when you have finished applying the patch. Replace patches that are dislodged by showering, bathing or swimming.

Usual Duration of Use:
Use on a regular schedule for 2 to 3 months determines effectiveness in achieving lasting cessation of smoking. Nicotine chewing gum should not be used for more than 6 months; transdermal systems should not be used for more than 20 weeks. Long-term use requires periodic physician evaluation of response and dosage adjustment.

Possible Advantages of This Drug
> Provides control and flexibility of gradual nicotine withdrawal for use in supervised smoking-cessation programs.

Currently a "Drug of Choice"
> for people who are motivated to stop smoking but find it difficult to stop abruptly. Since many forms are now available without a prescription, be sure to talk with your doctor or pharmacist about how to most effectively use these medicines.

▷ **This Drug Should Not Be Taken If**
- you have had an allergic reaction to any dosage form of it previously.
- you have severe, uncontrolled or a pattern of worsening angina (physician's discretion).
- you have uncontrolled, life-threatening heart rhythm disorders (physician's discretion).
- you have had a recent heart attack (physician's discretion).

▷ **Inform Your Physician Before Taking This Drug If**
- you have any form of angina (coronary heart disease).
- you have had a heart attack at any time.
- you are subject to heart rhythm disorders.
- you have insulin-dependent diabetes.
- you have hypertension (high blood pressure).
- you have hyperthyroidism (overactive thyroid function).
- you have a pheochromocytoma (adrenalin-producing tumor).
- you have a history of esophagitis or peptic ulcer disease.
- you have a history of Buerger's disease or Raynaud's disorder.
- you currently have any dental problems or skin disorders.
- you have a history of kidney or liver disease.
- you have an increase in cardiovascular effects while you are taking this medicine.
- you have already taken a 3 month course of the patch from another doctor.
- you think you are pregnant or plan to become pregnant.
- you are uncertain of how much or how often to take it.

Possible Side Effects (natural, expected, and unavoidable drug actions)
> For chewing gum: Mouth or throat irritation; injury to teeth or dental repairs.
> For transdermal systems: redness, itching or burning at site of application (mild and transient).

▷ **Possible Adverse Effects** (unusual, unexpected, and infrequent reactions)
> **If any of the following develop, consult your physician promptly for guidance.**
>
> *Mild Adverse Effects*
> Allergic Reactions: Skin rash, hives, itching, local or generalized swellings.
> Headache, light-headedness, dizziness, drowsiness, irritability, nervousness, insomnia, joint pain, muscle aches, abnormal dreams.
> Rapid heartbeat, palpitation, increased sweating.
> Increased or decreased appetite, nausea, dry mouth, indigestion, constipation, or diarrhea.
>
> *Serious Adverse Effects*
> Irregular heart rhythms, chest pain (angina), edema.

See Effects of Overdosage.
Stroke (rare).

▷ **Possible Effects on Sexual Function:**   There is some data questioning an effect on sperm, but a distinct demonstration of an effect is lacking.

Natural Diseases or Disorders That May Be Activated by This Drug
Latent angina, atrial fibrillation, hypertension, peptic ulcer disease, temporomandibular joint (TMJ) disorder (by chewing gum).

Possible Effects on Laboratory Tests
Free fatty acids (FFA blood level): increased.
Blood glucose: increased.
Prothrombin time (INR): decreased.
Urine Screening Test for drug abuse: no effect.

CAUTION
1. For these drug products to be safe and effective, **it is mandatory that all smoking be stopped immediately at the beginning of drug treatment**.
2. Extended use of chewing gum may cause damage to mouth tissues and teeth, may loosen fillings and stick to dentures, and may initiate or aggravate temporomandibular joint dysfunction.
3. Smoking cessation and the use of these drug products can result in increased blood levels of insulin (in insulin-dependent diabetics); dosage reduction of insulin may be necessary to prevent hypoglycemic reactions.
4. If you are taking any of the following drugs, consult your physician regarding the need to reduce their dosage while participating in a smoking-cessation program: aminophylline, oxtriphylline, theophylline, beta blocker drugs, propoxyphene, oxazepam, prazosin, pentazocine, imipramine.
5. If you are taking any of the following drugs, consult your physician regarding the need to increase their dosage while participating in a smoking cessation program: isoproterenol, phenylephrine.
6. Used patches should be folded in half with the adhesive sides sealed together; place them in the original pouch or aluminum foil and dispose of them promptly; keep out of reach of children and animals.
7. Use of antacids such as Tums prior to chewing nicotine gum can increase the amount of nicotine absorbed from the gum.
8. Habitrol patches have only been shown to be effective when they are part of a complete smoking cessation program which includes counseling.

Precautions for Use
By Infants and Children: Safety and effectiveness for those under 12 years of age not established.
By Those over 60 Years of Age: Because of the increased possibility of cardiovascular disorders in this age group, treatment is cautiously started. Watch closely for adverse effects.

▷ **Advisability of Use During Pregnancy**
Pregnancy Category: For nicotine chewing gum: X. For nicotine transdermal systems: D. See Pregnancy Code at the back of this book.
Animal studies: Impaired fertility found in mouse, rat and rabbit studies. Birth defects found in high-dose studies of mice.

Human studies: Adequate studies of pregnant women are not available. However, it is known that cigarette smoking during pregnancy may cause low birth weight, increased risk of abortion, and increased risk of newborn death.

The use of these drug products is not recommended during pregnancy.

Advisability of Use if Breast-Feeding
Presence of this drug in breast milk: Yes.
Avoid drug or refrain from nursing.

Habit-Forming Potential: The prolonged use of these drug products (beyond 3 months) may perpetuate the physical dependence of nicotine-dependent smokers. Patches should have the lowest potential for dependence. Potential exists for abuse of nonprescription forms of this medicine.

Effects of Overdosage: Nausea, vomiting, increased salivation, stomach cramps, diarrhea, headache, dizziness, impaired vision and hearing, weakness, confusion, fainting, difficult breathing, seizures.

Possible Effects of Long-Term Use: Perpetuation of nicotine dependence.

Suggested Periodic Examinations While Taking This Drug (at physician's discretion)
Evaluation of patient's ability to abstain from smoking.
Evaluation of patient's blood pressure and heart function.

▷ **While Taking This Drug, Observe the Following**
Foods: No restrictions.
Beverages: No restrictions.
▷ *Alcohol:* May cause an increase in cardiovascular effects.
Tobacco Smoking: Avoid all forms of tobacco completely.
Marijuana Smoking: Avoid completely.
▷ *Other Drugs*
Nicotine may ***increase*** the effects of
• adenosine.
• niacin (flushing and dizziness).
The following drugs may ***increase*** the effects of nicotine
• antacids such as Tums used prior to chewing nicotine-containing gum may increase the absorption of nicotine from the gum.
• cimetidine (Tagamet).
• lithium.
• ranitidine (Zantac).
Nicotine *taken concurrently* with niacin (Nicobid, others) can cause severe facial flushing.
▷ *Driving, Hazardous Activities:* This drug may cause dizziness or drowsiness. Restrict activities as necessary.
Aviation Note: The use of this drug ***may be a disqualification*** for piloting. Consult a designated Aviation Medical Examiner.
Exposure to Sun: No restrictions.
Exposure to Cold: Use caution until tolerance is determined. Cold environments may enhance the vasospastic action of nicotine.
Heavy Exercise or Exertion: Use caution in patients with angina, coronary artery disease or hypertension.
Discontinuation: As soon as a lasting cessation of smoking has been achieved,

these drugs should be gradually reduced in dosage and then discontinued. Continual use of the chewing gum should not exceed 6 months; continual use of the transdermal systems should not exceed 20 weeks.

NIFEDIPINE (ni FED i peen)

Introduced: 1972   **Prescription:** USA: Yes; Canada: Yes   **Available as Generic:** Yes   **Class:** Antianginal, antihypertensive, calcium channel blocker
Controlled Drug: USA: No; Canada: No
Brand Names: Adalat, Adalat CC, ✦Adalat P.A., ✦Adalat FT, ✦Apo-Nifed, ✦Gen-Nifedipine, ✦Novo-Nifedin, ✦Nu-Nifed, Procardia, Procardia XL
Controversies In Medicine: Study data indicates that medicines in this class should NOT be used in some patients with extremely compromised hearts. There have also been several FDA hearings held on the calcium channel blocker class. Be certain to ask your doctor about your cardiac output and if the benefits of this medicine outweigh the risks of its use. A recent FDA panel found medicines in this class to be safe and effective. A retrospective chart review yielded data that showed increased risks for nifedipine immediate release forms in those over 71, and cautioned physicians against using the immediate release form for indications other than angina. The immediate release form in question had never been approved for other uses. Most recently, a study of nearly 6,000 patients at Tel Aviv Medical Center found that there was no statistically significant increased risk of death in the patients who took calcium channel blockers versus those who did not.

BENEFITS versus RISKS	
Possible Benefits	*Possible Risks*
EFFECTIVE PREVENTION OF BOTH MAJOR TYPES OF ANGINA	Rare increase in angina upon starting treatment
EFFECTIVE TREATMENT OF HYPERTENSION (sustained-release form only)	Rare precipitation of congestive heart failure
	Rare anemia and low white blood cell counts
	Very rare drug-induced hepatitis
	Fainting (rare)

▷ **Principal Uses**

As a Single Drug Product: Uses currently included in FDA approved labeling: (1) Treats angina pectoris due to coronary artery spasm (Prinzmetal's variant angina) that occurs spontaneously and is not associated with exertion; and (2) classical angina-of-effort (due to atherosclerotic disease of the coronary arteries) in people who have not responded to or cannot tolerate the nitrates and beta blocker drugs customarily used to treat this disorder (sustained release form); (2) used to treat mild to moderate hypertension (extended release forms).

Author's note: A recent retrospective chart review has found the immediate release form of this medicine IS NOT recommended for use in treating hypertension, acute myocardial infarction (heart attack), hypertensive crisis and some forms of unstable angina.

Other (unlabeled) generally accepted uses: (1) Treatment of symptoms associated with Raynaud's phenomenon; (2) may stop the progression of atherosclerosis; (3) can have a role in congestive heart failure; (4) therapy of pulmonary hypertension; (5) helps decrease risk of heart attack after coronary artery bypass grafting; (6) could have a role in some neurologically based pain disorders; (7) may have a role in tardive dyskinesia; (8) can help urticaria of unknown cause; (9) therapy of achalasia or esophageal spasm; (10) helps intractable hiccups; (11) helps amaurosis fugax; (12) has a role in helping abnormal reactions to cold (chilblains).

How This Drug Works: By blocking passage of calcium through certain cell walls (which is necessary for the function of nerve and muscle tissue), this drug slows the spread of electrical activity through the heart and inhibits the contraction of coronary arteries and peripheral arterioles. As a result of these combined effects, this drug

- prevents spontaneous spasm of coronary arteries (Prinzmetal's angina).
- reduces the rate and contraction force of the heart during exertion, decreasing oxygen requirements of the heart muscle, and reducing the occurrence of effort-induced angina (classical angina pectoris).
- reduces the degree of contraction of peripheral arterial walls, resulting in their relaxation and consequent lowering of blood pressure. This further reduces the workload of the heart during exertion and helps prevent angina.

Available Dosage Forms and Strengths

Capsules — 5 mg (Canada), 10 mg (US and Canada) and 20 mg (US)

Tablets — 10 mg, 20 mg (Canada)

Tablets, extended-release — 10 mg, 20 mg (Canada), 30 mg, 60 mg, 90 mg (US)

Tablets, sustained-release — 30 mg, 60 mg, 90 mg

▷ **Recommended Dosage Ranges** (Actual dosage and administration schedule must be determined by the physician for each patient individually.)

Infants and Children: Dosage not established.

12 to 60 Years of Age: Extended-release form for high blood pressure: Initially, 30 mg once daily. Dose may be increased gradually at 7- to 14-day intervals (as needed and tolerated) up to 60 mg. Maximum total daily dosage should not exceed 90 mg.

For hypertension: Initially a single 30-mg or 60-mg sustained-release tablet taken once daily. Gradually increased as a single daily dose if needed.

Sublingual: Hypertensive crisis: **the immediate release form of this medicine IS NOT recommended for use in treating hypertension, acute myocardial infarction (heart attack), hypertensive crisis and some forms of unstable angina.**

Over 60 Years of Age: Same as 12 to 60 years of age. **Nifedipine immediate release form in those over 71 has been associated with almost a fourfold increase in risk for all-cause death when compared to ACE inhibitors, beta blockers or other calcium channel blockers.**

Conditions Requiring Dosing Adjustments

Liver function: Specific dosage adjustments in liver compromise are not defined, and the dose should be empirically decreased. This drug is also a rare

cause of liver toxicity (allergic hepatitis), and should be used with caution in patients with compromised livers. It is also a potential cause of portal hypertension, and should not be used in patients with portal hypertension.
Kidney function: In patients with compromised kidneys, nifedipine should be used as a benefit to risk decision as it can lead to kidney toxicity.

▷ **Dosing Instructions:** May be taken with or following food to reduce stomach irritation. The capsule should be swallowed whole (not altered). The sustained-release tablet should be taken whole (not altered).

Usual Duration of Use: Use on a regular schedule for 2 to 4 weeks determines effectiveness in reducing the frequency and severity of angina and in controlling hypertension. For long-term use (months to years), the smallest effective dose should be used. Supervision and periodic physician evaluation are essential.

Possible Advantages of This Drug
The sustained release form of this drug permits effective once-a-day treatment for both angina and hypertension.

▷ **This Drug Should Not Be Taken If**
- you have had an allergic reaction to it previously.
- you have active liver disease.
- you are over 71 and have been prescribed the immediate release form of nifedipine
- you have low blood pressure—systolic pressure below 90.
- you have significant narrowing of your aorta (aortic stenosis). Ask your doctor.

▷ **Inform Your Physician Before Taking This Drug If**
- you have had an adverse response to any calcium blocker.
- you currently take any form of digitalis or a beta blocker drug (see Drug Class Section).
- you are taking any drugs that lower blood pressure.
- you have a history of congestive heart failure, heart attack or stroke.
- you are subject to disturbances of heart rhythm.
- you have cardiomyopathy (nonobstructive) or aortic stenosis.
- you have impaired liver or kidney function.
- you have abnormal circulation to your fingers.
- you have atrial fibrillation.
- you have developed a dermatological condition while taking this medicine.
- you have diabetes or Duchenne muscular dystrophy.
- you have a history of drug-induced liver damage.

Possible Side Effects (natural, expected, and unavoidable drug actions)
Low blood pressure, rapid heart rate, swelling of the feet and ankles, flushing and sensation of warmth, sweating.

▷ **Possible Adverse Effects** (unusual, unexpected, and infrequent reactions)
If any of the following develop, consult your physician promptly for guidance.
Mild Adverse Effects
Allergic Reactions: Skin rash, hives, itching, fever.
Headache, dizziness, weakness, nervousness, blurred vision, eye pain, and swelling around the eyes.

Pedal edema (50%).
Depression (rare).
Abnormal growth of the gums (gingival hyperplasia).
Ringing in the ears (tinnitus).
Sleep disturbances.
Increased or decreased blood potassium.
Bed-wetting (rare).
Palpitation, shortness of breath, wheezing, cough.
Heartburn, nausea, taste disturbances, cramps, diarrhea (rare).
Tremors, muscle cramps.

Serious Adverse Effects

Allergic Reaction: Drug-induced hepatitis (very rare), drug eruptions and erysipelaslike reactions, and exfoliative dermatitis or erythema multiforme.

Idiosyncratic Reactions: Joint stiffness and inflammation.

Increased frequency or severity of angina on initiation of treatment or following an increase in dose.

Abnormal muscle movements (myoclonus) (rare).

Kidney toxicity (rare).

Pulmonary edema (rare).

Bezoars (rare and seen with sustained-release forms).

Acute psychosis (very rare).

Worsening of circulation to the fingers.

Marked drop in blood pressure with fainting.

Low white blood cells, platelets, and hemoglobin (rare).

▷ **Possible Effects on Sexual Function:**   Altered timing and pattern of menstruation; excessive menstrual bleeding.

Tenderness and swelling of the male breast tissue (gynecomastia).

▷ **Adverse Effects That May Mimic Natural Diseases or Disorders**

An allergic rash and swelling of the legs may resemble erysipelas.

Drug-induced hepatitis may suggest viral hepatitis.

Transient increases in liver function tests may suggest infectious hepatitis.

Possible Effects on Laboratory Tests

Bleeding time: increased.

Liver function tests: transient increases.

Blood total cholesterol level: no effect in age group under 60 years old; decreased in those over 60 years old.

Blood HDL cholesterol level: no effect, or increased.

Blood LDL and VLDL cholesterol levels: no effect.

Blood triglyceride levels: no effect, or decreased.

CAUTION

1. Be sure to tell all health care providers you consult that you are taking this drug. Note the use of this drug on your card of personal identification.

2. You may use nitroglycerin and other nitrate drugs as needed to relieve acute episodes of angina pain. However, if you detect that your angina attacks are becoming more frequent or intense, call your doctor.

Precautions for Use

By Infants and Children: Safety and effectiveness for those under 12 years of age not established.

By Those over 60 Years of Age: You may be more susceptible to the development of weakness, dizziness, fainting and falling. Take necessary precautions to prevent injury. Report promptly any changes in your pattern of thirst and urination.

▷ **Advisability of Use During Pregnancy**
Pregnancy Category: C. See Pregnancy Code at the back of this book.
Animal studies: Embryo and fetal deaths reported in mice, rats and rabbits; birth defects reported in rats.
Human studies: Adequate studies of pregnant women are not available.
Avoid this drug during the first 3 months. Use during the last 6 months only if clearly needed. Ask physician for guidance.

Advisability of Use if Breast-Feeding
Presence of this drug in breast milk: Yes.
Avoid drug or refrain from nursing.

Habit-Forming Potential: None.

Effects of Overdosage: Weakness, light-headedness, fainting, fast pulse, low blood pressure, shortness of breath, flushed and warm skin, tremors.

Possible Effects of Long-Term Use: None reported.

Suggested Periodic Examinations While Taking This Drug (at physician's discretion)
Evaluations of heart function, including electrocardiograms; measurements of blood pressure in supine, sitting and standing positions.

▷ **While Taking This Drug, Observe the Following**
Foods: Grapefruit juice may greatly increase the absorption (bioavailability) of nifedipine and result in an exaggerated therapeutic effect. Water is the best liquid to take this medicine with. It is also prudent to avoid excessive salt intake.
Beverages: No restrictions. May be taken with milk.
▷ *Alcohol:* Use with caution. Alcohol may exaggerate the drop in blood pressure experienced by some people.
Tobacco Smoking: Nicotine may reduce the effectiveness of this drug. Follow your physician's advice regarding smoking.
Marijuana Smoking: Possible reduced effectiveness of this drug; mild to moderate increase in angina; possible changes in electrocardiogram, confusing interpretation.
▷ *Other Drugs*
Nifedipine *taken concurrently* with
• amiodarone (Codarone) may cause the heart to stop.
• beta blocker drugs or digitalis preparations (see Drug Classes) may affect heart rate and rhythm adversely. Careful monitoring by your physician is necessary if these drugs are taken concurrently.
• cyclosporine (Sandimmune) can lead to nifedipine toxicity.
• digoxin (Lanoxin) may lead to digoxin toxicity.
• diltiazem may lead to nifedipine toxicity.
• oral hypoglycemic agents (see Drug Classes) or insulin may result in loss of glucose control.
• magnesium can cause additive lowering of the blood pressure.
• phenytoin (Dilantin) can cause phenytoin toxicity.
• rifampin (Rifadin) can decrease nifedipine effectiveness.

- theophylline can reduce the therapeutic benefit of nifedipine and may lead to theophylline toxicity as well.
- vincristine (Oncovin) can cause vincristine toxicity.

The following drug may *increase* the effects of nifedipine
- cimetidine (Tagamet).
- quinidine (Quinaglute, others) can lead to nifedipine toxicity as well as decreased quinidine effectiveness.
- ranitidine (Zantac).

▷ *Driving, Hazardous Activities:* Usually no restrictions. This drug may cause drowsiness or dizziness. Restrict activities as necessary.

Aviation Note: Coronary artery disease *is a disqualification* for piloting. Consult a designated Aviation Medical Examiner.

Exposure to Sun: Caution, rare cases of photoxicity have been reported.

Exposure to Heat: Caution advised. Hot environments can exaggerate the blood-pressure-lowering effects of this drug. Observe for light-headedness or weakness.

Heavy Exercise or Exertion: This drug may improve your ability to be more active without resulting angina pain. Use caution and avoid excessive exercise that could impair heart function in the absence of warning pain.

Discontinuation: Do not stop this drug abruptly. Consult your physician regarding gradual withdrawal. Observe for the possible development of rebound angina.

NITROGLYCERIN (ni troh GLIS er in)

Introduced: 1847   **Prescription:** USA: Yes; Canada: No   **Available as Generic:** Yes   **Class:** Antianginal, nitrates   **Controlled Drug:** USA: No; Canada: No

Brand Names: Deponit, Minitran Transdermal Delivery System, Nitro-Bid, Nitrocap TD, Nitrocine Transdermal, Nitrocine Timecaps, Nitrodisc, Nitro-Dur, Nitro-Dur II, Nitrogard, ✦Nitrogard-SR, Nitroglyn, Nitrol, ✦Nitrol TSAR Kit, Nitrolin, Nitrolingual Spray, Nitrong, ✦Nitrong SR, Nitrospan, ✦Nitrostabilin, Nitrostat, Nitro Transdermal System, NTS Transdermal Patch, Transderm-Nitro, ✦Tridil

BENEFITS versus RISKS	
Possible Benefits	*Possible Risks*
EFFECTIVE RELIEF AND PREVENTION OF ANGINA	Orthostatic hypotension with and without fainting
EFFECTIVE ADJUNCTIVE TREATMENT IN SELECTED CASES OF CONGESTIVE HEART FAILURE	Skin rash (rare)
	Altered hemoglobin with large doses (very rare)
	Low blood platelets (rare)

▷ **Principal Uses**

As a Single Drug Product: Uses currently included in FDA approved labeling: (1) Treatment of symptomatic coronary artery disease. The rapid-action forms are used to relieve acute attacks of anginal pain at their onset. The sustained-action forms are used to prevent the development of angina; (2)

helps improve breathing difficulty caused by heart failure (left ventricle);
(3) intravenous nitroglycerin is used in surgery to control blood pressure;
(4) helps relieve congestive heart failure after heart attacks.

Other (unlabeled) generally accepted uses: (1) May help ease spasms of the
Sphincter of Oddi; (2) topical use may help in impotence; (3) can help reduce the extent of heart damage if given following a heart attack (myocardial infarction); (4) helps relax cocaine-constricted heart arteries; (5) eases
the pain of peripheral neuropathy; may be of help in easing esophageal
problems (achalasia); (6) when the anal sphincter does not work correctly,
this drug can help reduce the muscle pressure and ease constipation; (7)
nitroglycerin in combination with vasopressin may be of use in stopping
bleeding esophageal varices; (8) can help loss of vision that has been caused
by a clot in the retinal artery; (9) if ergot medications (see Drug Class) have
shut down circulation to the extremities, nitroglycerin can open up the circulation; (10) used to delay contractions in order to rotate an abnormally
positioned fetus; (11) may help diabetics with nerve damage (diabetic neuropathy).

How This Drug Works: By direct action on the muscles in blood vessel walls,
this drug relaxes and dilates both arteries and veins. Its beneficial effects in
angina are due to two mechanisms of action: (1) dilation of narrowed coronary arteries; (2) dilation of veins in the general circulation, with consequent reduction of the volume and pressure of blood entering the heart.
The net effects are improved blood supply to the heart muscle and reduced
work load for the heart. Both actions reduce the frequency and severity of
angina.

Available Dosage Forms and Strengths

Canisters, translingual spray — 13.8 grams (200 doses), 0.4 mg per
metered dose

Capsules, prolonged-action — 2.5 mg, 2.6 mg, 6.5 mg, 9 mg

Ointment — 2%

Tablets, buccal — 1 mg, 2 mg, 3 mg

Tablets, prolonged-action — 2.6 mg, 6.5 mg, 9 mg

Tablets, sublingual — 0.15 mg, 0.3 mg, 0.4 mg, 0.6 mg

Transdermal systems — 2.5 mg, 5 mg, 7.5 mg, 10 mg, 15 mg (all per
24 hours)

▷ **Usual Adult Dosage Range:**   According to dosage form:

Sublingual spray—1 metered spray (0.4 mg) under tongue/3 to 5 minutes, up
to 3 doses within 15 minutes, to relieve acute angina. To prevent angina, 1
spray taken 5 to 10 minutes before exertion.

Sublingual tablets—0.15 to 0.6 mg dissolved under tongue at 5-minute intervals to relieve acute angina.

Prolonged-action tablets—2.5 mg at 6 to 8 hour intervals to prevent angina.

Ointment—0.5 inch or 7.5 milligrams applied in a thin, even layer of uniform
size to hairless skin at 3- to 4-hour intervals to prevent angina.

Buccal tablets—1 to 2 mg/4 to 5 hours placed between cheek and gum.

Transdermal patches—5-sq.-cm to 30-sq.-cm patch applied to hairless skin
once/24 hours to prevent angina.

**Author's note: in order to avoid tolerance to the therapeutic effects of
this medicine, a nitrate-free interval of 12 hours daily is recom-**

mended. 24 hour patches are removed after having been applied for 12 hours. Dosing of ointment is interrupted for 12 hours a day. Oral sustained-release formulations are dosed to give a 6- to 12-hour nitrate-free interval. Note: Actual dosage and administration schedule must be determined by the physician for each patient individually.

Conditions Requiring Dosing Adjustments

Liver function: Specific dosage adjustments in liver compromise are not defined.

Kidney function: Specific guidelines for dosing changes are not available. This drug can discolor urine.

▷ **Dosing Instructions:** Dosage forms to be swallowed are best taken when stomach is empty (1 hour before or 2 hours after eating) to obtain maximal blood levels. Tablets should not be crushed for administration. Capsules may be opened, but the contents should not be crushed or chewed before swallowing.

Usual Duration of Use: Use on a regular schedule for 3 to 5 days is often needed to determine effectiveness in preventing and relieving acute anginal attacks. Individual dosage adjustments will be necessary for optimal results. Long-term use (months to years) requires physician supervision.

▷ **This Drug Should Not Be Taken If**
- you have had an allergic reaction to it previously.
- you are severely anemic.
- you have had recent head trauma.
- you have had a heart attack and have an increased heart rate or increased blood pressure.
- you have hyperthyroidism.
- you have increased intraocular pressure.
- you have abnormal growth of the heart muscle in response to vascular disease (hypertrophic cardiomyopathy).
- you have closed-angle glaucoma (inadequately treated).

▷ **Inform Your Physician Before Taking This Drug If**
- you have had an unfavorable response to other nitrate drugs in the past.
- you have low blood pressure.
- you have problems absorbing medicines (malabsorption syndromes) or excessive action of your stomach (gastric hypermotility).
- you have any form of glaucoma.
- you have had recent bleeding in your head.

Possible Side Effects (natural, expected, and unavoidable drug actions)
Flushing of face, headaches (50%), orthostatic hypotension (see Glossary), rapid heart rate, palpitation.

▷ **Possible Adverse Effects** (unusual, unexpected, and infrequent reactions)
If any of the following develop, consult your physician promptly for guidance.
Mild Adverse Effects
Allergic Reaction: Skin rash.
Throbbing headaches (may be severe and persistent), dizziness, fainting.
Nausea, vomiting, taste disorders.
Serious Adverse Effects
Allergic Reactions: Severe skin reactions with peeling.
Idiosyncratic Reaction: Methemoglobinemia (very rare).

Abnormally slow heartbeat (bradycardia) (rare).
Low blood supply to the head (transient ischemic attacks).
Increased intracranial pressure (rare).

▷ **Possible Effects on Sexual Function**
Correction of impotence (1 report following sublingual use).
The preventive use of nitroglycerin prior to sexual activity has been recommended to eliminate or reduce the risk of angina. Consult your physician for guidance.

▷ **Adverse Effects That May Mimic Natural Diseases or Disorders**
Hypotensive spells (sudden drops in blood pressure) due to this drug may be mistaken for late-onset epilepsy.

Possible Effects on Laboratory Tests
Blood platelet count: decreased (very rare).
Bleeding time: prolonged.

CAUTION
1. This drug can provoke migraine headaches in susceptible individuals.
2. Patients with impaired brain circulation (cerebral arteriosclerosis) have increased risk of transient ischemic attacks—periods of temporary speech impairment, paralysis, numbness, etc.
3. Tolerance to long-acting forms of nitrates will happen in most patients after 24 hours of continuous use. A nitrate-free interval of 10 hours usually restores effectiveness.
4. Many over-the-counter (OTC) drug products for allergies, colds and coughs contain drugs that may counteract the desired effects of this drug. Ask your physician or pharmacist for help before using any such medications.

Precautions for Use
By Infants and Children: Limited usefulness and experience in this age group. Dosage schedules not established.
By Those over 60 Years of Age: Begin treatment with small doses and increase dose cautiously as needed and tolerated. You may be more susceptible to the development of flushing, throbbing headache, dizziness, "blackout" spells, fainting and falling.

▷ **Advisability of Use During Pregnancy**
Pregnancy Category: C. See Pregnancy Code at the back of this book.
Animal studies: No information available.
Human studies: Adequate studies of pregnant women are not available.
Use this drug only if clearly needed. Ask physician for guidance.

Advisability of Use if Breast-Feeding
Presence of this drug in breast milk: Unknown.
Watch nursing infant closely and discontinue drug or nursing if adverse effects develop.

Habit-Forming Potential: None.

Effects of Overdosage: Throbbing headache, dizziness, marked flushing, nausea, vomiting, abdominal cramps, confusion, delirium, paralysis, seizures, circulatory collapse.

Possible Effects of Long-Term Use: The development of tolerance (see Glossary) and the temporary loss of effectiveness.

Suggested Periodic Examinations While Taking This Drug (at physician's discretion)
>   Measurements of blood pressure and internal eye pressures.
>   Evaluation of hemoglobin.

▷ **While Taking This Drug, Observe the Following**
>   *Foods:* No restrictions.
>   *Beverages:* No restrictions. May be taken with milk.
▷ *Alcohol:* Avoid alcohol completely. This combination may result in severe lowering of the blood pressure. There is a potential for collapse of the circulation and pumping effectiveness of the heart.
>   *Tobacco Smoking:* Nicotine can reduce the effectiveness of this drug. Follow your physician's advice regarding smoking.
>   *Marijuana Smoking:* Possible reduced effectiveness of this drug; mild to moderate increase in angina; possible changes in the electrocardiogram, confusing interpretation.
▷ *Other Drugs*
>   Nitroglycerin **taken concurrently** with
>   - acetylcysteine (NAC) may reverse tolerance to the intravenous form of this medicine.
>   - antihypertensive drugs may cause excessive lowering of blood pressure. Careful dosage adjustments may be necessary.
>   - diltiazem (Cardizem) can result in abnormally low blood pressure when used with the sustained release form of nitroglycerin.
>   - dihydroergotamine or similar ergot medicines (see drug Classes) may result in ergotamine toxicity.
>   - heparin can result in decreased therapeutic benefit of heparin.
>   - isosorbide dinitrate (Isordil) or mononitrate (Ismo) may result in a decreased nitroglycerin therapeutic benefit.
>   The following drugs may **increase** the effects of nitroglycerin
>   - aspirin, in analgesic doses (500 mg or more).
▷ *Driving, Hazardous Activities:* Usually no restrictions. This drug may cause dizziness or faintness. Restrict activities as necessary.
>   *Aviation Note:* Coronary artery disease **is a disqualification** for piloting. Consult a designated Aviation Medical Examiner.
>   *Exposure to Sun:* No restrictions.
>   *Exposure to Heat:* Hot environments can cause significant lowering of blood pressure.
>   *Exposure to Cold:* Cold environments can increase the need for this drug and limit its effectiveness.
>   *Heavy Exercise or Exertion:* This drug can increase your tolerance for exercise. Use good judgment regarding excessive exertion in the absence of anginal pain.
>   *Discontinuation:* Do not stop this drug abruptly after long-term use. It is advisable to reduce the dose (of the prolonged-action dosage forms) gradually over a period of to 6 weeks. Observe for rebound angina.
>   *Special Storage Instructions:* For sublingual tablets, to prevent loss of strength
>   - keep tablets in the original glass container.
>   - do not transfer tablets to a plastic or metallic container (such as a pillbox).
>   - do not place absorbent cotton, paper (such as the prescription label), or other material inside the container.

- do not store other drugs in the same container.
- close the container tightly immediately after each use.
- store at room temperature.

NIZATIDINE (ni ZA te deen)

Introduced: 1986   **Prescription:** USA: Yes   **Available as Generic:** No   **Class:** H-2 receptor blocker   **Controlled Drug:** USA: No
Brand Name: Axid, Axid AR (nonprescription form)

BENEFITS versus RISKS	
Possible Benefits	*Possible Risks*
EFFECTIVE TREATMENT OF PEPTIC ULCER DISEASE: relief of symptoms, acceleration of healing, and prevention of recurrence in many cases	Drug-induced liver damage (rare) Abnormally low blood platelet count (rare)
CONTROL OF HYPERSECRETORY STOMACH DISORDERS	
Beneficial in treatment of reflux esophagitis	

Please see the histamine (H2) blocking drug profile for more information.

NORFLOXACIN (nor FLOX a sin)

Introduced: 1986   **Prescription:** USA: Yes; Canada: Yes   **Available as Generic:** USA: No; Canada: No   **Class:** Anti-infectives   **Controlled Drug:** USA: No; Canada: No
Brand Name: Noroxin, Noroxin Ophthalmic, Chibroxin

Warning: Some physicians are using the name "Norflox" to identify this drug when issuing orders (for inpatients) or prescriptions (for outpatients). Norflox is not an accepted name for this drug in any setting for any reason. This coinage of an abbreviated name has resulted in serious medication errors—the dispensing of Norflex, the generic drug orphenadrine, a skeletal muscle relaxant. Ask your pharmacist to verify that you are getting the right drug—an anti-infective.

Warning: Reports are being made for some drugs in this class which find tendon rupture as a rare adverse effect. Ask your doctor about limits on strenuous exercise while you are taking this medicine. A rare idiosyncratic reaction has also been reported which presents as mental confusion and disorientation. Use of this medicine after head trauma may be a risk factor. If you have suffered a fall, ask your doctor if a medicine in a different antibiotic class should be substituted. If you are taking this drug and notice a change in your thinking, call your doctor.

BENEFITS versus RISKS	
Possible Benefits	*Possible Risks*
Effective treatment of urinary tract infections	Infrequent nausea, indigestion
	Rare impairment of vision
Effective treatment of bacterial gastroenteritis and gonorrhea	Rare seizure and neurological compromise

▷ **Principal Uses**

As a Single Drug Product: Uses currently included in FDA approved labeling: (1) Treats urinary tract infections (in adults) caused by a wide variety of bacteria sensitive to the action of this drug (including gonorrhea); (2) also used as an ophthalmic solution to treat eye infections and conjunctivitis.

Other (unlabeled) generally accepted uses: (1) Used in a variety of infections where it is effective against the bacteria usually causing the problem such as prostatitis, certain pneumonias and Salmonella; (2) used in gastroenteritis caused by certain bacteria, to prevent traveler's diarrhea.

How This Drug Works: By inhibiting essential enzyme systems of bacterial nucleic acids (DNA), this drug prevents bacterial reproduction (with low doses) and destroys bacteria (with higher doses).

Available Dosage Forms and Strengths

Tablets — 400 mg

Ophthalmic Solution — 3 mg per ml

▷ **Usual Adult Dosage Range:**   Uncomplicated urinary tract infections—400 mg/12 hours for 3 days. Complicated urinary tract infections—400 mg/12 hours for 10 to 21 days. Total daily dosage should not exceed 800 mg. Ophthalmic dosing: 1 to 2 drops to the affected eye four times daily. **Note: Actual dosage and administration schedule must be determined by the physician for each patient individually.**

Conditions Requiring Dosing Adjustments

Liver function: Norfloxacin should be used with caution in patients with compromised livers, and blood levels and liver function tests obtained.

Kidney function: In patients with moderate to severe kidney compromise, the dose should be decreased to 400 mg daily. Since norfloxacin is a rare cause of crystalluria, patients taking the drug should drink adequate quantities of water.

▷ **Dosing Instructions:**   Preferably taken with a full glass of water 1 hour before or 2 hours after eating. Avoid antacids for 2 hours after taking this drug. The tablet may be crushed for administration. Take the full course prescribed.

Usual Duration of Use: Continual use on a regular schedule for 3 to 21 days (depending upon the nature of the infection) is usually necessary to determine this drug's effectiveness in eradicating the infection.

▷ **This Drug Should Not Be Taken If**

• you have had an allergic reaction to any dosage form of it previously.
• you are pregnant or breast-feeding.
• it is prescribed for a child under 18 years of age.

▷ **Inform Your Physician Before Taking This Drug If**

• you are allergic to cinoxacin (Cinobac) or nalidixic acid (NegGram).
• you have a history of psychosis.

- you have a history of intracranial pressure elevation (ask your doctor).
- you have a seizure disorder.
- you have impaired liver or kidney function.

Possible Side Effects (natural, expected, and unavoidable drug actions)
None reported.

▷ **Possible Adverse Effects** (unusual, unexpected, and infrequent reactions)
If any of the following develop, consult your physician promptly for guidance.
Mild Adverse Effects
Allergic Reactions: Skin rash (rare), hives (rare), localized swelling, itching (rare).
Headache (rare), dizziness (rare), mental depression (4 reports), seizures (3 reports).
Drowsiness, mood alterations, nervousness, insomnia, hallucinations (all rare).
Lowering of blood glucose.
Visual disturbances: blurred or double vision, altered color vision, increased sensitivity to light (all rare).
Dry mouth, decreased appetite (rare), nausea (rare), indigestion (rare), vomiting (rare), diarrhea (rare).
Swollen or painful tendons and joints (rare).
Serious Adverse Effects
Allergic Reactions: Exfoliative dermatitis (1 report), anaphylactic reaction (see Glossary).
One medication of this class has had instances of severe neurological compromise reported with use of the drug. Stop the medication immediately and call your doctor if you experience confusion, trouble speaking, or disorientation once taking this drug.
One medicine belonging to this class has been associated with tendon rupture. Ask your doctor for guidance regarding exercise or activity while you are taking this drug.
Lowering of neutrophilic white blood cells (very rare and of questionable causation).
Seizures (rare).
Vaginal discharge.
Kidney toxicity (formation of crystals of the drug in the urine).
Worsening of myasthenia gravis.

▷ **Possible Effects on Sexual Function:**   Vaginitis with discharge has been reported.

Natural Diseases or Disorders That May Be Activated by This Drug
Latent epilepsy.

Possible Effects on Laboratory Tests
Red and white blood cell counts: rarely decreased.
Liver function tests: rarely increased liver enzymes (ALT/GPT, AST/GOT).
Kidney function tests: rarely increased blood creatinine and urea nitrogen (BUN) levels.
Blood sugar: decreased.

CAUTION

1. Crystal formation in the kidney can occur (especially with high doses or prolonged use). This can be prevented by drinking large amounts of water, up to 2 quarts/24 hours.
2. This drug may decrease saliva formation and predispose to formation of dental cavities or gum disease. Consult your dentist if mouth dryness persists.

Precautions for Use

By Infants and Children: Safety for use by those who have not attained complete bone growth not established. This drug can impair normal bone growth and development in test animals. Avoid its use in children until they are 18.

By Those over 60 Years of Age: Impaired kidney function requires dosage reduction. Consult your physician.

▷ **Advisability of Use During Pregnancy**

Pregnancy Category: C. See Pregnancy Code at the back of this book.

Animal studies: Mouse, rat, rabbit and monkey studies reveal no birth defects due to this drug. However, this drug can cause impaired bone development in immature dogs.

Human studies: Adequate studies of pregnant women are not available.

This drug should be avoided during entire pregnancy.

Advisability of Use if Breast-Feeding

Presence of this drug in breast milk: Unknown.

Avoid drug or refrain from nursing.

Habit-Forming Potential: None.

Effects of Overdosage: Nausea, vomiting, diarrhea, seizures.

Possible Effects of Long-Term Use: Crystal formation in kidneys with high doses and inadequate fluid intake.

Suggested Periodic Examinations While Taking This Drug (at physician's discretion)

Liver function tests, urine analysis.

▷ **While Taking This Drug, Observe the Following**

Foods: Avoid taking this drug after eating dairy foods. Take this drug one hour before or two hours after eating dairy foods such as milk or cottage cheese.

Beverages: Caffeine will stay in the body longer than expected. Use care in the number of caffinated beverages (including coffee) that you drink.

▷   *Alcohol:* No interactions expected.

Tobacco Smoking: No interactions expected.

▷   *Other Drugs*

Norfloxacin *taken concurrently* with

- cyclosporine (Sandimmune) may cause toxic effects on the kidney.
- iron salts will decrease the therapeutic benefits of norfloxacin.
- magnesium will decrease the therapeutic benefits of norfloxacin.
- nitrofurantoin (Macrodantin, etc.) may antagonize the antibacterial action of norfloxacin in the urinary tract. Avoid this combination.
- sucralfate (Carafate) will decrease absorption of norfloxacin.
- theophylline (Theodur, others) may lead to theophylline toxicity over time.

- warfarin (Coumadin) will lead to increased risk of bleeding. More frequent INR testing is needed.
- zinc will decrease norfloxacin effectiveness.

The following drug may *increase* the effects of norfloxacin
- probenecid (Benemid).

The following drugs may *decrease* the effects of norfloxacin
- antacids may reduce its absorption.
- calcium supplements.

▷ *Driving, Hazardous Activities:* This drug may cause dizziness or impaired vision. Restrict activities as necessary.

Aviation Note: The use of this drug *may be a disqualification* for piloting. Consult a designated Aviation Medical Examiner.

Exposure to Sun: Sunglasses advised if eyes are overly sensitive to bright light.

Discontinuation: If you experience no adverse effects from this drug, take the full course prescribed for maximal results. Consult your physician when to stop taking this medication.

NORTRIPTYLINE (nor TRIP ti leen)

Introduced: 1963   **Prescription:** USA: Yes; Canada: Yes   **Available as Generic:** USA: Yes; Canada: No   **Class:** Antidepressant   **Controlled Drug:** USA: No; Canada: No

Brand Names: Aventyl, Pamelor

BENEFITS versus RISKS	
Possible Benefits	*Possible Risks*
EFFECTIVE RELIEF OF ENDOGENOUS DEPRESSION Possibly beneficial in other depressive disorders Possibly beneficial in the management of some types of chronic, severe pain	ADVERSE BEHAVIORAL EFFECTS: confusion, disorientation, hallucinations, delusions CONVERSION OF DEPRESSION TO MANIA in manic-depressive (bipolar) disorders Aggravation of schizophrenia Irregular heart rhythms Rare blood cell abnormalities

▷ **Principal Uses**

As a Single Drug Product

Uses currently included in FDA approved labeling (1) Relieves symptoms associated with spontaneous (endogenous) depression. This drug should be used only when a diagnosis of a true, primary depression of significant degree has been established. It should not be used to treat the symptoms of mild and transient (reactive) depression that may be associated with many life situations in the absence of a bona fide affective illness.

Other (unlabeled) generally accepted uses: (1) Used in conjunction with other drugs to manage chronic, severe pain associated with such conditions as cancer, migraine headache, severe arthritis, peripheral neuropathy, AIDS, etc.; (2) helps decrease the frequency of bedwetting; (3) may have a role in helping severe PMS; (4) can help attention deficit hyperactivity disorder (ADHD); (5) may have a role in helping ringing in the ears (tinnitus).

How This Drug Works: It is thought that this drug relieves depression by slowly restoring to normal levels certain constituents of brain tissue (norepinephrine and serotonin) that transmit nerve impulses.

Available Dosage Forms and Strengths

Capsules — 10 mg, 25 mg, 50 mg, 75 mg
Oral solution — 10 mg per 5-ml (alcohol 4%)

▷ **Usual Adult Dosage Range:**   Initially 25 mg 3 or 4 times daily. Dose may be increased cautiously as needed and tolerated by 10 to 25 mg daily at intervals of 1 week. Usual maintenance dose is 50 to 100 mg/24 hours. Total dose should not exceed 150 mg/24 hours. When the optimal requirement is determined, it may be taken at bedtime as one dose. **Note: Actual dosage and administration schedule must be determined by the physician for each patient individually.**

Conditions Requiring Dosing Adjustments

Liver function: Specific dosage adjustments in liver compromise are not defined, however, the patient should be closely followed, and levels obtained. This drug is also a rare cause of hepatoxicity, and should be used with caution in patients with compromised livers.

Kidney function: Specific dosing changes in renal compromise are not usually needed. Nortriptyline can cause a decrease in urine outflow, and should be used as a benefit to risk decision in patients with urine outflow problems.

▷ **Dosing Instructions:**   The capsule may be opened and may be taken without regard to meals.

Usual Duration of Use: Some benefit may be apparent within 1 to 2 weeks, but adequate response may require continual use for 3 months or longer. Long-term use should not exceed 6 months without physician evaluation regarding the need for continuation of the drug.

Possible Advantages of This Drug

Causes less daytime sedation.
Causes fewer atropinelike side effects.
Causes orthostatic hypotension infrequently (see Glossary).

▷ **This Drug Should Not Be Taken If**
- you have had an allergic reaction to it previously.
- you are taking or have taken within the past 14 days any monoamine oxidase (MAO) type A inhibitor drug (see Drug Classes).
- you are recovering from a recent heart attack.
- you have narrow-angle glaucoma.

▷ **Inform Your Physician Before Taking This Drug If**
- you are allergic or sensitive to any other tricyclic antidepressant (see Drug Class Section).
- you have a history of: diabetes, epilepsy, glaucoma, heart disease, prostate gland enlargement or overactive thyroid function.
- you plan to have surgery under general anesthesia in the near future.
- you have a history of bone marrow suppression.
- you have a history of low blood pressure.

Possible Side Effects (natural, expected, and unavoidable drug actions)

Light-headedness, drowsiness, blurred vision, dry mouth, constipation, impaired urination (see Prostatism in Glossary).

▷ **Possible Adverse Effects** (unusual, unexpected, and infrequent reactions)

If any of the following develop, consult your physician promptly for guidance.

Mild Adverse Effects

Allergic Reactions: Skin rash, hives, swelling of face or tongue, drug fever (see Glossary).

Headache, dizziness, memory problems, weakness, fainting, unsteady gait, tremors, blurred vision, hearing toxicity.

Peculiar taste, weight gain, cavities (dental caries), irritation of tongue or mouth, nausea, indigestion.

Fluctuation of blood sugar levels.

Serious Adverse Effects

Allergic Reactions: Hepatitis, with or without jaundice (see Glossary).

Confusion, disorientation, hallucinations, delusions.

Aggravation of paranoid psychoses and schizophrenia; seizures.

Heart palpitation and irregular rhythm.

Bone marrow depression (see Glossary)—fatigue, weakness, fever, sore throat, abnormal bleeding or bruising.

Drug-induced porphyria (rare).

Excessive urination, leading to sodium loss.

Peripheral neuritis (see Glossary)—numbness, tingling, pain, loss of strength in arms and legs.

Parkinson-like disorders (see Glossary)—usually mild and infrequent; more likely to occur in the elderly.

▷ **Possible Effects on Sexual Function:**   Decreased libido, increased libido (antidepressant effect), male impotence (rare), inhibited female orgasm, male and female breast enlargement, milk production, swelling of testicles.

▷ **Adverse Effects That May Mimic Natural Diseases or Disorders**

Liver toxicity may suggest viral hepatitis.

Natural Diseases or Disorders That May Be Activated by This Drug

Latent diabetes, epilepsy, glaucoma, prostatism.

Possible Effects on Laboratory Tests

White blood cell and platelet counts: decreased.

Blood glucose levels: increased and decreased (fluctuations).

Liver function tests: increased liver enzymes (ALT/GPT, AST/GOT and alkaline phosphatase), increased bilirubin.

CAUTION

1. Dose must be individualized. Report for follow-up evaluation and laboratory tests as directed by your physician.
2. It is advisable to withhold this drug if electroconvulsive therapy (ECT, "shock" treatment) is to be used to treat your depression.

Precautions for Use

By Infants and Children: The manufacturer's labeling says that safety and effectiveness for children have not been established.

By Those over 60 Years of Age: Usual dosage is 30 to 50 mg daily in divided doses. During the first 2 weeks of treatment, watch for confusion, agitation, forgetfulness, delusions disorientation and hallucinations. Reduction of dosage or discontinuation may be necessary. Unsteadiness may predispose to falling and injury. This drug can increase the degree of impaired urination associated with prostate gland enlargement (prostatism).

▷ **Advisability of Use During Pregnancy**

Pregnancy Category: D. See Pregnancy Code at the back of this book.

Animal studies: Results are inconclusive.

Human studies: No defects reported in 21 exposures to amitriptyline, a closely related drug. Adequate studies of pregnant women are not available for this drug.

Avoid use of drug during first 3 months. Use during last 6 months only if clearly needed. Ask your physician for guidance.

Advisability of Use if Breast-Feeding

Presence of this drug in breast milk: Yes, in small amounts.

Monitor nursing infant closely and discontinue drug or nursing if adverse effects develop: excessive drowsiness and failure to feed.

Habit-Forming Potential: Psychological or physical dependence is rare and unexpected.

Effects of Overdosage: Confusion, hallucinations, marked drowsiness, heart palpitations, dilated pupils, tremors, stupor, deep sleep, coma, convulsions.

Suggested Periodic Examinations While Taking This Drug (at physician's discretion)

Complete blood cell counts, liver function tests, serial blood pressure readings and electrocardiograms.

▷ **While Taking This Drug, Observe the Following**

Foods: No restrictions. This drug may increase the appetite and cause excessive weight gain.

Beverages: No restrictions. May be taken with milk.

▷ *Alcohol:* Avoid completely. This drug can markedly increase the intoxicating effects of alcohol and accentuate its depressant action on brain function.

Tobacco Smoking: May hasten the elimination of this drug. Higher doses may be necessary.

▷ *Other Drugs*

Nortriptyline may *increase* the effects of
- atropinelike drugs (see Drug Class Section).
- dicoumarol, and increase the risk of bleeding.
- epinephrine (Adrenalin).
- phenytoin (Dilantin) by increasing blood levels.
- warfarin (Coumadin) and require more frequent INR (protime) testing and dosing adjustments based on laboratory results.

Nortriptyline may *decrease* the effects of
- clonidine (Catapres).
- ephedrine (Primatene tablets).
- guanethidine (Ismelin).

Nortriptyline *taken concurrently* with
- activated charcoal will decrease and almost block absorption (useful in overdose situations).
- benzodiazepines (see Drug Classes) may result in additive sedation.
- disulfiram (Antabuse) may cause acute dementia: confusion, disorientation, hallucinations.

- fluconazole (Diflucan) may result in large increases in nortriptyline levels and result in toxic reactions.
- lithium (Lithobid) may pose an increased risk of neurotoxicity in elderly patients.
- monoamine oxidase (MAO) inhibitor drugs may cause high fever, delirium and convulsions (see Drug Class Section).
- nifedipine (Adalat, others) may result in inhibition of nortriptyline's antidepressant effects.
- norepinephrine can cause a serious increase in blood pressure, abnormal heart rhythms and fast heart rate. Avoid the combination.
- phenothiazines (see Drug Class) can result in increased phenothiazine levels and toxicity as well as additive anticholinergic problems.
- thyroid preparations may impair heart rhythm and function. Ask physician for guidance regarding adjustment of thyroid dose.
- venlafaxine (Effexor) may result in nortriptyline or venlafaxine toxicity.

The following drugs may *increase* the effects of nortriptyline
- cimetidine (Tagamet), and cause nortriptyline toxicity.
- fluoxetine (Prozac).
- quinidine (Quinaglute, etc.), and cause nortriptyline toxicity.
- sertraline (Zoloft).

The following drugs may *decrease* the effects of nortriptyline
- ascorbic acid (vitamin C) in high doses.
- barbiturates (see Drug Classes), and reduce its effectiveness.
- carbamazepine (Tegretol).
- conjugated estrogens.
- rifampin (Rifadin).

▷ *Driving, Hazardous Activities:* This drug may impair mental alertness, judgment, physical coordination and reaction time. Avoid hazardous activities.

Aviation Note: The use of this drug *is a disqualification* for piloting. Consult a designated Aviation Medical Examiner.

Exposure to Sun: Use caution. This drug may cause photosensitivity (see Glossary).

Exposure to Heat: This drug can inhibit sweating and impair the body's adaptation to hot environments, increasing the risk of heat stroke. Avoid saunas.

Exposure to Cold: The elderly should use caution and avoid conditions conducive to hypothermia (see Glossary).

Discontinuation: Best to slowly discontinue this drug. Abrupt withdrawal after long-term use can cause headache, malaise and nausea.

OFLOXACIN (oh FLOX a sin)

Introduced: 1984   **Prescription:** USA: Yes   **Available as Generic:** USA: No   **Class:** Anti-infective fluoroquinolone   **Controlled Drug:** USA: No

Brand Name: Floxin, Floxin Uropak, Ocuflox

Warning: Reports are being made for some drugs in this class which find tendon rupture as a rare adverse effect. Ask your doctor about limits on strenuous exercise while you are taking this medicine. A rare idiosyncratic reaction has also been reported which presents as mental confusion and disorientation. Use of this medicine after head trauma may be a risk factor.

If you have suffered a fall, ask your doctor if a medicine in a different antibiotic class should be substituted. If you are taking this drug and notice a change in your thinking, call your doctor.

BENEFITS versus RISKS

Possible Benefits	*Possible Risks*
HIGHLY EFFECTIVE TREATMENT FOR INFECTIONS OF THE LOWER RESPIRATORY TRACT, URINARY TRACT, SKIN, AND SKIN STRUCTURES, due to susceptible organisms	Rare but serious allergic reactions
	Rare seizures and hallucinations or changes in thinking
	Rare reports of tendon rupture with heavy exertion
EFFECTIVE TREATMENT FOR SOME SEXUALLY TRANSMITTED DISEASES	
Effective treatment for some infections of the prostate gland	

▷ **Principal Uses**

As a Single Drug Product: Uses currently included in FDA approved labeling: (1) Treats responsive infections (in adults) of: (1) the lower respiratory tract (lungs and bronchial tubes); (2) the urinary tract (kidneys, bladder, urethra and prostate gland); (3) skin and related tissues; (4) certain sexually transmitted diseases: gonorrheal and chlamydial infections of the urethra and cervix; (5) infections of the eye.

Other (unlabeled) generally accepted uses: (1) May have a role in combination therapy of leprosy; (2) used to treat traveler's diarrhea; (3) treats bone infections in combination with surgery.

How This Drug Works: By interfering with the bacterial enzyme DNA gyrase (required for DNA synthesis and cell reproduction), this drug arrests bacterial growth (in low concentrations) and destroys bacteria (in high concentrations).

Available Dosage Forms and Strengths

Tablets — 200 mg, 300 mg, 400 mg

Ophthalmic solution — 3 mg per ml

▷ **Usual Adult Dosage Range:**   200 mg to 400 mg every 12 hours (for 10 days for lower respiratory infections), depending upon the nature and severity of the infection. The total daily dosage should not exceed 800 mg. **Note: Actual dosage and administration schedule must be determined by the physician for each patient individually.**

Conditions Requiring Dosing Adjustments

Liver function: Dosage adjustments do not appear to be needed.

Kidney function: In patients with moderate kidney failure, the usual dose can be given every 24 hours. In patients with severe failure, one half the usual dose should be given every 24 hours.

▷ **Dosing Instructions:**   Do not take with food. The tablet may be crushed and is preferably taken 1 hour before or 2 hours after eating. Drink fluids liberally during the entire course of treatment. Avoid antacids containing aluminum or magnesium and supplements containing iron or zinc for 2 hours before and after dosing.

Usual Duration of Use: Use on a regular schedule for up to 10 days determines effectiveness in eradicating the infection. The drug should be continued for at least 2 days after all indications of infection have disappeared. Prostate gland infections may require continual treatment for 6 weeks. Long-term use requires periodic physician evaluation of response.

Possible Advantages of This Drug
Very broad spectrum of antibacterial activity.
Capable of establishing effective drug levels throughout the prostate gland.
Effective one-dose treatment for uncomplicated gonorrheal infection of the urethra.
No significant effect on kidney function.
No reports of serious drug-induced colitis.

▷ **This Drug Should Not Be Taken If**
- you have had an allergic reaction to it previously.
- you are allergic to cinoxacin (Cinobac), nalidixic acid (NegGram), ciprofloxacin (Cipro) or norfloxacin (Noroxin).
- you are pregnant or breast-feeding.
- you have a seizure disorder that is not adequately controlled.
- it is prescribed for a person under 18 years of age (as it may cause arthropathy-joint problems, as well as defects in cartilage).

▷ **Inform Your Physician Before Taking This Drug If**
- you have a history of a seizure disorder or a circulatory disorder of the brain.
- you have a history of psychosis or intracranial pressure elevation.
- you have impaired liver or kidney function.
- your work requires heavy manual labor. Several cases of tendon rupture have been reported with fluoroquinolone use. Heavy exercise or work may be contraindicated. Call your doctor immediately if you develop inflammation or pain in a tendon.
- you are taking any form of probenecid or theophylline.

Possible Side Effects (natural, expected, and unavoidable drug actions)
Superinfections (see Glossary): vaginitis.

▷ **Possible Adverse Effects** (unusual, unexpected, and infrequent reactions)
If any of the following develop, consult your physician promptly for guidance.
Mild Adverse Effects
Allergic Reactions: Rash, itching, fever.
Headache, dizziness, weakness, drowsiness, nervousness, joint and muscle pain (rare), insomnia, visual disturbances.
Decreased appetite, altered taste (rare), dry mouth, nausea, vomiting, indigestion (rare), diarrhea.
Serious Adverse Effects
Allergic Reactions: Anaphylactoid reactions (see Glossary).
Idiosyncratic Reactions: Rare extreme confusion and speech problems (aphasia) may be idiosyncratic.
Central nervous system stimulation: restlessness, tremor, confusion, hallucinations, seizures (all very rare).
Intracranial hypertension (rare).
Rare tendon rupture with heavy exertion.
Drug-induced hepatitis (rare).

▷ **Possible Effects on Sexual Function:** Painful menstruation, excessive menstrual bleeding.

▷ **Natural Diseases or Disorders That May Be Activated by This Drug**
Latent epilepsy.

Possible Effects on Laboratory Tests
Complete blood cell counts: rarely decreased lymphocytes; rarely increased eosinophils.
Liver function tests: rarely increased liver enzymes (ALT/GPT, AST/GOT).
Blood creatinine level: rarely increased.
Blood glucose levels: rare fluctuations.

CAUTION
1. Crystal formation in the kidney may occur with high doses and prolonged use. This can be prevented by drinking large amounts of water, up to 2 quarts/24 hours.
2. Drugs of this class may decrease the formation of saliva and predispose to the development of dental cavities or gum disease. Consult your dentist if dry mouth persists.
3. Very rare case reports of aphasia, disorientation and confusion has occurred. Stop the drug and call your doctor immediately if this occurs.
4. Rare reports of tendon rupture with heavy exertion.

Precautions for Use
By Infants and Children: Safety and effectiveness for those under 18 years of age not established. Avoid the use of this drug completely. It can impair normal bone growth and development in immature animals.
By Those over 60 Years of Age: Impaired kidney function will require dosage reduction.
If you are taking theophylline concurrently with this drug, observe closely for possible theophylline accumulation and toxicity.

▷ **Advisability of Use During Pregnancy**
Pregnancy Category: C. See Pregnancy Code at the back of this book.
Animal studies: Mild skeletal defects due to this drug were found in rat studies; toxic effects on the fetus were shown in rat and rabbit studies. This drug can impair normal bone development in immature dogs.
Human studies: Adequate studies of pregnant women are not available. However, the potential for adverse effects on fetal bone development contraindicates the use of this drug during entire pregnancy.

Advisability of Use if Breast-Feeding
Presence of this drug in breast milk: Yes.
Avoid drug or refrain from nursing.

Habit-Forming Potential: None.

Effects of Overdosage: Nausea, vomiting, diarrhea, confusion, hallucinations, seizures.

Possible Effects of Long-Term Use: Superinfections (see Glossary).

Suggested Periodic Examinations While Taking This Drug (at physician's discretion)
Liver function tests, urine analysis.

▷ **While Taking This Drug, Observe the Following**
Foods: No restrictions.
Beverages: Caffeine from any beverages will remain in the body longer than ex-

pected. Take care to limit the total amount of caffeine in your diet (remember sodas and coffee) while taking this medicine. May be taken with milk.

▷ *Alcohol:* No interactions expected.

Tobacco Smoking: No interactions expected.

▷ *Other Drugs*

Ofloxacin may ***increase*** the effects of
- theophylline (Theodur, others), and cause theophylline toxicity.
- warfarin (Coumadin) and lead to bleeding. More frequent INR (protime testing) is needed, and warfarin dosing should be adjusted to laboratory results.

The following drug may ***increase*** the effects of ofloxacin
- probenecid (Benemid).

The following drugs may ***decrease*** the effects of ofloxacin
- antacids containing aluminum or magnesium can reduce the absorption of ofloxacin and lessen its effectiveness.
- calcium supplements.
- iron salts.
- sucralfate (Carafate).
- zinc salts.

▷ *Driving, Hazardous Activities:* This drug may cause drowsiness, dizziness and impaired vision. Restrict activities as necessary.

Aviation Note: The use of this drug ***may be a disqualification*** for piloting. Consult a designated Aviation Medical Examiner.

Exposure to Sun: This drug may cause photosensitivity (see Glossary).

Discontinuation: If you experience no adverse effects from this drug, take the full course prescribed for best results.

OLSALAZINE (ohl SAL a zeen)

Introduced: 1987   **Prescription:** USA: Yes; Canada: Yes   **Available as Generic:** USA: No; Canada: No   **Class:** Bowel anti-inflammatory   **Controlled Drug:** USA: No; Canada: No

Brand Name: Dipentum

BENEFITS versus RISKS	
Possible Benefits	*Possible Risks*
EFFECTIVE SUPPRESSION OF INFLAMMATORY BOWEL DISEASE	RARE BONE MARROW DEPRESSION (see Glossary) Rare drug-induced hepatitis Occasional aggravation of ulcerative colitis

▷ **Principal Uses**

As a Single Drug Product: Uses currently included in FDA approved labeling: Used to maintain remission of chronic ulcerative colitis and proctitis.

Other (unlabeled) generally accepted uses: Has a role in treatment of active ulcerative colitis.

How This Drug Works: This drug suppresses the formation of prostaglandins (and related compounds), tissue substances that induce inflammation, tissue destruction and diarrhea—the main features of ulcerative colitis and proctitis.

Available Dosage Forms and Strengths
Capsules — 250 mg
Tablet (in Canada only) — 500 mg

▷ **Recommended Dosage Ranges** (Actual dosage and administration schedule must be determined by the physician for each patient individually.)
Infants and Children: Dosage not established.
12 to 60 Years of Age: 500 mg twice daily, morning and evening.
Over 60 Years of Age: Same as 12 to 60 years of age.

Conditions Requiring Dosing Adjustments
Liver function: Dosage adjustments do not appear to be needed in liver compromise. This drug rarely causes liver toxicity (granulomatous hepatitis), and should be used with caution in patients with liver problems.
Kidney function: Some of the metabolites of olsalazine are eliminated by the kidneys. There is potential for kidney damage by one of these compounds, and the drug should be used as a benefit to risk in patients with compromised kidneys.

▷ **Dosing Instructions:** The capsule may be opened and taken with food, preferably with breakfast and dinner.

Usual Duration of Use: Use on a regular schedule for 1 to 3 weeks determines effectiveness in controlling the symptoms of ulcerative colitis. Long-term use (months to years) requires physician supervision.

Possible Advantages of This Drug
Does not inhibit sperm production or cause infertility.

▷ **This Drug Should Not Be Taken If**
- you have had an allergic reaction to it previously.
- you have severely impaired kidney function.
- you are allergic to aspirin.

▷ **Inform Your Physician Before Taking This Drug If**
- you are allergic to aspirin (or other salicylates), mesalamine or sulfasalazine.
- you are allergic by nature: history of hay fever, asthma, hives, eczema.
- you have impaired kidney function.
- you have severe liver disease.
- you are currently taking sulfasalazine (Azulfidine).

Possible Side Effects (natural, expected, and unavoidable drug actions)
None.

▷ **Possible Adverse Effects** (unusual, unexpected, and infrequent reactions)
If any of the following develop, consult your physician promptly for guidance.
Mild Adverse Effects
Allergic Reactions: Skin rash, itching (rare).
Headache, drowsiness (rare), depression (rare), dizziness (rare).
Loss of appetite (rare), indigestion, nausea, vomiting (rare), stomach pain, diarrhea.
Paresthesias (rare).

Blurred vision (rare).

Joint aches and pains.

Serious Adverse Effects

Allergic Reactions: Dermatitis, hair loss (rare).

Rare bone marrow depression (see Glossary): fatigue, fever, sore throat, abnormal bleeding or bruising.

Rare drug-induced hepatitis (see Glossary).

Rare pancreatitis.

Rare kidney damage.

Pericarditis (rare).

Spasm of the bronchi of the lung (rare).

▷ **Possible Effects on Sexual Function:** Rare impotence, excessive menstrual flow.

Possible Effects on Laboratory Tests

Complete blood cell counts: decreased red cells, hemoglobin, white cells and platelets; increased eosinophils.

Liver function tests: increased liver enzymes (ALT/GPT, AST/GOT and alkaline phosphatase), increased bilirubin.

Urinalysis: red blood cells and protein present.

CAUTION

1. Report promptly any signs of infection or unusual bleeding or bruising.
2. Report promptly any indications of active or intensified ulcerative colitis: abdominal cramping, bloody diarrhea, fever.

Precautions for Use

By Infants and Children: Safety and effectiveness for those under 12 years of age not established.

By Those over 60 Years of Age: None.

▷ **Advisability of Use During Pregnancy**

Pregnancy Category: C. See Pregnancy Code at the back of this book.

Animal studies: Rat studies reveal toxic effects on the fetus, retarded bone development, and impaired development of internal organs. Human studies: Adequate studies of pregnant women are not available.

Use this drug only if clearly needed. Ask your physician for guidance.

Advisability of Use if Breast-Feeding

Presence of this drug in breast milk: Controversial, has caused diarrhea in some infants.

Avoid drug or refrain from nursing.

Habit-Forming Potential: None.

Effects of Overdosage: Headache, dizziness, nausea, vomiting, abdominal cramping.

Possible Effects of Long-Term Use: Bone marrow depression (impaired production of blood cells).

Suggested Periodic Examinations While Taking This Drug (at physician's discretion)

Complete blood cell counts.

Liver function tests.

Kidney function tests, urinalysis.

▷ **While Taking This Drug, Observe the Following**
  Foods: No restrictions. Follow prescribed diet.
  Beverages: No restrictions. May be taken with milk.
▷ *Alcohol:* No interactions expected.
  Tobacco Smoking: No interactions expected.
▷ *Other Drugs:* Olsalazine **taken concurrently** with
    • varicella vaccine (Varivax) may result in an increased risk of Reye's syndrome. This drug should be avoided for 6 weeks after the vaccine is given.
▷ *Driving, Hazardous Activities:* This drug may cause drowsiness or dizziness. Restrict activities as necessary.
  Aviation Note: The use of this drug **may be a disqualification** for piloting. Consult a designated Aviation Medical Examiner.
  Exposure to Sun: Use caution. This drug can cause photosensitization (see Glossary).

OMEPRAZOLE (oh MEH pra zohl)

Introduced: 1986   **Prescription:** USA: Yes; Canada: Yes   **Available as Generic:** USA: No; Canada: No   **Class:** proton pump inhibitor   **Controlled Drug:** USA: No; Canada: No
Brand Name: Prilosec, ✢Losec

BENEFITS versus RISKS	
Possible Benefits	*Possible Risks*
VERY EFFECTIVE TREATMENT OF CONDITIONS ASSOCIATED WITH EXCESSIVE PRODUCTION OF GASTRIC ACID: Zollinger-Ellison syndrome, mastocytosis, endocrine adenoma VERY EFFECTIVE TREATMENT OF REFLUX ESOPHAGITIS, GASTRIC AND DUODENAL ULCERS EFFECTIVE IN COMBINATION WITH CLARITHROMYCIN in treatment of h. pylori infections	Rare aplastic anemia Rare liver failure

▷ **Principal Uses**
  As a Single Drug Product: Uses currently included in FDA approved labeling: (1) Inhibits stomach acid formation in: acute and chronic gastritis, reflux esophagitis, gastroesophageal reflux disease, Zollinger-Ellison syndrome, mastocytosis, endocrine adenomas and active duodenal ulcer; (2) approved for long-term use in erosive esophagitis; (3) approved for combination (with clarithromycin (Biaxin)) in patients with positive Helicobacter pylori cultures; (4) helps in the short-term treatment of active and benign stomach (gastric) ulcers.
    Other (unlabeled) generally accepted uses: (1) Used to help gastric ulcers; (2) may have a role in severe bleeding of the stomach (hemorrhagic gastritis).
  How This Drug Works: Inhibits a specific enzyme system (proton pump H/K ATPase) in the stomach lining, stopping production of stomach acid and

thereby (1) eliminates a principal cause of the condition under treatment, and (2) creates an environment conducive to healing.

Available Dosage Forms and Strengths

Capsules, delayed-release — 20 mg

▷ **Usual Adult Dosage Range:** Reflux esophagitis: 20 mg once daily for 4 to 8 weeks.

Excessive stomach acid conditions: 60 mg once daily for as long as necessary.

Gastric and duodenal ulcer: 20 mg once daily for 4 to 8 weeks.

In extreme conditions, doses of 120 mg three times a day have been used.

Note: Actual dosage and administration schedule must be determined by the physician for each patient individually.

Conditions Requiring Dosing Adjustments

Liver function: Dosing adjustments not defined, however, patients should be monitored closely.

Kidney function: Dosage adjustments do not appear to be needed.

▷ **Dosing Instructions:** Take immediately before eating, preferably the morning meal. The capsule should be swallowed whole without opening; the contents should not be crushed or chewed. This drug may be taken concurrently with antacids if they are needed to relieve stomach pain.

Usual Duration of Use: Use on a regular schedule for 2 to 3 weeks determines benefit in suppressing stomach acid production. Long-term use (months to years) requires periodic physician evaluation of response.

Possible Advantages of This Drug

Effectively inhibits acid secretion at all times: basal conditions (stomach empty and at rest) and following food, alcohol, smoking or other stimulants. Is more effective than H-2 receptor blocking drugs in treating severe reflux esophagitis and refractory duodenal ulcer.

Currently a "Drug of Choice"

for the short-term treatment of severe reflux esophagitis and for the long-term treatment of Zollinger-Ellison syndrome and erosive esophagitis.

▷ **This Drug Should Not Be Taken If**

• you have had an allergic reaction to it previously.

• you have a currently active bone marrow or blood cell disorder.

▷ **Inform Your Physician Before Taking This Drug If**

• you have a history of liver disease or impaired liver function.

• your history includes any bone marrow or blood cell disorder, especially a drug-induced one.

• you take any anticoagulant medication, or diazepam (Valium) or phenytoin (Dilantin, etc.).

Possible Side Effects (natural, expected, and unavoidable drug actions)

Acid in the stomach actually works to protect from some bacterial infections. Since omeprazole is so effective in decreasing acid, it may increase the likelihood of infection by Campylobacter. This organism causes a gastroenteritis. Symptoms may include mucousy, loose stools and fever. Talk with your doctor if you start to develop these symptoms while taking omeprazole.

▷ **Possible Adverse Effects** (unusual, unexpected, and infrequent reactions)

If any of the following develop, consult your physician promptly for guidance.

Mild Adverse Effects
  Allergic Reactions: Skin rash (rare), itching.
  Headache, dizziness (rare), muscle pain or ringing in the ears (rare), drowsiness, paresthesias, weakness (rare).
  Indigestion, nausea, vomiting (rare), diarrhea, constipation (rare).

Serious Adverse Effects
  Allergic Reactions: Rare allergic kidney damage (interstitial nephritis).
  Rare bone marrow depression (see Glossary): fatigue, weakness, fever, sore throat, infections, abnormal bleeding or bruising.
  Rare liver damage with jaundice (see Glossary).
  Rare urinary tract infection: painful urination, cloudy or bloody urine.
  Rare chest pain or angina.
  Rare half-facial pain.
  Yeast infection (Candida) of the esophagus.
  Rare kidney inflammation (interstitial nephritis).

Possible Effects on Sexual Function
  Drug-induced male breast enlargement and tenderness (gynecomastia) has been rarely reported.

▷ **Adverse Effects That May Mimic Natural Diseases or Disorders**
  Persistent infection or bruising may be bone marrow depression; blood counts advisable.
  Liver reactions may suggest viral hepatitis.

Possible Effects on Laboratory Tests
  Complete blood cell counts: decreased red cells, hemoglobin, white cells and platelets.
  Blood glucose level: decreased.
  Liver function tests: increased liver enzymes (ALT/GPT, AST/GOT and alkaline phosphatase), increased bilirubin.

CAUTION
  1. Take this drug for exactly as long as your doctor told you. Do not extend its use without his guidance.
  2. Report promptly any indications of infection.
  3. Tell your doctor if you plan to take any other medications (prescription or over-the-counter) while taking omeprazole.
  4. Acid in the stomach actually works to protect from some bacterial infections. Since omeprazole is so effective in decreasing acid, it may increase the likelihood of infection by Campylobacter. This organism causes a gastroenteritis. Symptoms may include, mucousy loose stools and fever. Talk with your doctor if you start to develop these symptoms while taking omeprazole.
  5. While this drug effectively treats ulcers, it does not preclude the possibility of cancer of the stomach.

Precautions for Use
  By Infants and Children: Safety and effectiveness for those under 12 years of age not established.
  By Those over 60 Years of Age: Slower elimination of this drug makes it possible to achieve satisfactory response with smaller doses; this reduces the risk of adverse effects. Limit the daily dose to 20 mg if possible.

▷ **Advisability of Use During Pregnancy**
Pregnancy Category:
C. See Pregnancy Code at the back of this book.
Animal studies: No drug-induced birth defects found in rats; drug-induced embryo and fetal toxicity were demonstrated in rats and rabbits.
Human studies: Adequate studies of pregnant women are not available.
Avoid use if possible. Use only if clearly necessary and for the shortest possible time.

Advisability of Use if Breast-Feeding
Presence of this drug in breast milk: Unknown.
Avoid drug or refrain from nursing.

Habit-Forming Potential: None.

Effects of Overdosage: Possible drowsiness, dizziness, lethargy, abdominal pain, nausea.

Possible Effects of Long-Term Use: Some long-term (2 year) studies in rats revealed the development of drug-induced carcinoid tumors in the stomach. To date, long-term use of this drug (more than 5 years) in humans has not revealed any drug-induced tumor potential. Pending more studies of long-term human use, it is advisable to limit the use of this drug to the shortest duration possible.

Suggested Periodic Examinations While Taking This Drug (at physician's discretion)
Complete blood cell counts.

▷ **While Taking This Drug, Observe the Following**
Foods: No restrictions.
Beverages: No restrictions. May be taken with milk.
▷ *Alcohol:* No interactions expected. However, alcohol is best avoided; it stimulates the secretion of stomach acid.
Tobacco Smoking: No interactions expected. However, smoking is best avoided; it may stimulate the secretion of stomach acid.
▷ *Other Drugs*
Omeprazole may *increase* the effects of
• anticoagulants (warfarin, etc.) and increase the risk of bleeding.
• clonazepam (Klonopin) and some other benzodiazepines (see Drug Classes) and lead to benzodiazepine toxicity.
• cyclosporine (Sandimmune) by increasing the level (decreased levels also reported).
• diazepam (Valium) and cause excessive sedation.
• digoxin (Lanoxin) and lead to toxicity.
• phenytoin (Dilantin, etc.) and cause phenytoin toxicity.
• warfarin (Coumadin) and lead to bleeding. More frequent INR (protime) testing is needed. Warfarin doses should be adjusted according to laboratory results.
Omeprazole may *decrease* the effects of
• ampicillin.
• amoxicillin.
• iron preparations.
• ketoconazole (Nizoral).

▷ *Driving, Hazardous Activities:* This drug may cause drowsiness and dizziness. Limit activities as necessary.

Aviation Note: The use of this drug **may be a disqualification** for piloting. Consult a designated Aviation Medical Examiner.

Exposure to Sun: No restrictions.

Discontinuation: The duration of use will vary according to the condition under treatment and individual patient response. Premature discontinuation could result in incomplete healing or prompt recurrence of symptoms.

ONDANSETRON (on DAN sa tron)

Introduced: 1993   **Prescription:** USA: Yes; Canada: Yes   **Available as Generic:** USA: No; Canada: No   **Class:** Antiemetic, 5HT3 antagonist
Controlled Drug: USA: No; Canada: No

Brand Name: Zofran

BENEFITS versus RISKS	
Possible Benefits	*Possible Risks*
EFFECTIVE ORAL TREATMENT AND RELIEF OR PREVENTION OF SEVERE VOMITING which can occur after some types of chemotherapy or radiation treatments	Bronchospasm (rare) Grand mal seizures (rare) Rare liver toxicity Rare heart rate and rhythm changes Rare low potassium

▷ **Principal Uses**

As a Single Drug Product: Uses currently included in FDA approved labeling: (1) Prevention of nausea and vomiting associated with initial and repeat courses of chemotherapy; (2) treatment or prevention of postoperative nausea and vomiting; (3) prevention or treatment of emesis (vomiting) caused by radiation therapy.

Other (unlabeled) generally accepted uses: (1) May have a role in helping patients keep from vomiting medicines used to treat drug overdoses; (2) may have a role in treating schizophrenia.

How This Drug Works: Ondansetron antagonizes 5HT3 receptors. It appears to block vomiting by blocking serotonin (a chemical causing vomiting) at 5HT3 receptors.

Available Dosage Forms and Strengths

Tablets — 4 mg and 8 mg

Intravenous — 2 mg per ml

How To Store

Keep at room temperature. Avoid exposing this medicine to extreme humidity.

▷ **Recommended Dosage Ranges (Actual dosage and administration schedule must be determined by the physician for each patient individually.)**

Infants and Children: Little information is available regarding use in those less than four years old.

4 to 11 Years of Age: Vomiting from chemotherapy: one (four mg) tablet given three times by mouth daily. The method and frequency is the same as for adults.

12 to 60 Years of Age: One 8-mg tablet given three times a day. The first dose should be given 30 minutes before the start of the emetogenic chemotherapy. Subsequent doses should be given 4 hours and 8 hours after the first dose.

Over 60 Years of Age: Same as 12 to 60 years of age.

Conditions Requiring Dosing Adjustments

Liver function: Maximum dose in people with severe liver failure is 8 mg per day.

Kidney function: Studies have not been conducted in patients with impaired kidneys. Decision to use ondansetron in these patients must be made by your physician. Only 5 to 10% of the drug is removed unchanged by the kidneys. Based on this small involvement of the kidneys, no changes are expected to be needed with short-term use.

▷ **Dosing Instructions:**   May be taken on an empty stomach.

Usual Duration of Use:

Since chemotherapy can cause vomiting long after it has been given, continual use on a regular schedule for 3 days is usually necessary.

Possible Advantages of This Drug

Effective oral prevention of severe vomiting caused by some kinds of chemotherapy which have been poorly controlled by earlier agents.

Currently a "Drug of Choice"

for control of vomiting secondary to emetogenic (likely to cause vomiting) cancer chemotherapy.

▷ **This Drug Should Not Be Taken If**

• you have had an allergic reaction to any dosage form of it previously.

▷ **Inform Your Physician Before Taking This Drug If**

• you have a history of liver disease.
• you have a history of kidney disease.
• you have a history of alcoholism.
• you are unsure of how much to take or how often to take ondansetron.

Possible Side Effects (natural, expected, and unavoidable drug actions)
Constipation, sedation.

▷ **Possible Adverse Effects** (unusual, unexpected, and infrequent reactions)
If any of the following develop, consult your physician promptly for guidance.

Mild Adverse Effects
Allergic Reactions: Skin rash (rare).
Headache, sedation, dizziness and light-headedness, constipation, diarrhea, dry mouth.

Serious Adverse Effects
Allergic Reactions: Anaphylaxis (rare).
Rare: Extrapyramidal reactions (abnormal body movements).
Rare seizures.
Bronchospasm (rare).
Angina, tachycardia, arrhythmias (all rare).
Hypokalemia (low potassium) (rare).

▷ **Possible Effects on Sexual Function:**   None reported.

Possible Delayed Adverse Effects: None reported.

▷ **Adverse Effects That May Mimic Natural Diseases or Disorders**

Changes in liver enzymes may mimic hepatitis; however, specific antibodies will not be present. Bronchospasm may mimic asthma.

Natural Diseases or Disorders That May Be Activated by This Drug

Epilepsy, asthma.

Possible Effects on Laboratory Tests

Liver function tests: Transient increases in SGPT, SGOT and bilirubin.

CAUTION

1. Even though you do not feel an urge to vomit, continue ondansetron for the prescribed length of therapy. The vomit-causing effect of cancer chemotherapy or radiation therapy continues after the medicine or radiation has been given.

Precautions for Use

By Infants and Children: Safety and effectiveness for those under 3 years of age not established.

By Those over 60 Years of Age: Same as for general adult population.

▷ **Advisability of Use During Pregnancy**

Pregnancy Category: B. See Pregnancy Code at the back of this book.

Animal studies: Drug and its metabolites pass into the milk. No adverse effects on gestation, postnatal development or reproductive performance has been observed in rats.

Human studies: Adequate studies of pregnant women are not available.

Ask your physician for guidance.

Advisability of Use if Breast-Feeding

Presence of this drug in breast milk: This medicine is excreted in the milk of rats; however, human data is not available. Caution should be used if this medicine is to be used in nursing mothers.

Habit-Forming Potential: None.

Effects of Overdosage: Doses 10 times greater than recommended have not resulted in illness.

Possible Effects of Long-Term Use: Not indicated for long term use.

Suggested Periodic Examinations While Taking This Drug   (at physician's discretion)

Observe for vomiting occurrence and frequency.

▷ **While Taking This Drug, Observe the Following**

Foods: No restrictions.

Beverages: No restrictions.

▷ *Alcohol:* Additive sedation and potential additive urge to vomit if alcohol is taken in large doses. Alcohol abuse which has led to liver problems may limit the total dose which can be given.

Tobacco Smoking: No direct clinical documenting restrictions.

Marijuana Smoking: May induce additive sedation and provide additive antiemetic effects.

▷ *Other Drugs*

The following drugs may *increase* the effects of ondansetron

• allopurinol (Zyloprim).
• cimetidine (Tagamet).
• disulfiram (Antabuse).
• fluconazole (Diflucan).
• isoniazid (Nydrazid).

- macrolide antibiotics (erythromycin, azithromycin and clarithromycin).
- metronidazole (Flagyl).
- monoamine oxidase inhibitor antidepressants (MAO inhibitors—Nardil).

The following drugs may *decrease* the effects of ondansetron

- barbiturates.
- carbamazepine (Tegretol).
- phenylbutazone (Butazolidin, Azolid).
- phenytoin (Dilantin).
- rifampin (Rifadin) and rifabutin (Mycobutin).
- tolbutamide (Orinase).

▷ *Driving, Hazardous Activities:* This drug may cause drowsiness and dizziness. Restrict activities as necessary.

Aviation Note: The use of this drug *may be a disqualification* for piloting. Consult a designated Aviation Medical Examiner.

Exposure to Sun: No restrictions.

Discontinuation: Ondansetron may be stopped after you've completed the prescribed course (usually 3 days) of therapy.

ORAL CONTRACEPTIVES (OR al kon tra SEP tivs)

Other Names: Estrogens/progestins, OCs, Birth control pills

Introduced: 1956 **Prescription:** USA: Yes; Canada: Yes **Available as Generic:** USA: Yes, in some forms; Canada: No **Class:** Female sex hormones **Controlled Drug:** USA: No; Canada: No

Brand Names: Brevicon, Demulen, Desogen, Enovid, Genora, Jenest 28, Levlen, Loestrin, Lo/Ovral, Micronor*, ✚Minestrin 1/20, Min-Ovral, Modicon, NEE, Nelova, Nelova 1/50 M, Nelova 10/11, Norcept-E 1/35, Nordette, Norethin 1/35E, Norethin 1/50M, Norinyl, Norlestrin, Nor-Q.D.*, Ortho Cyclen, Ortho Tri-Cyclen, Ortho-Novum, Ovcon, Ovral, Ovrette*, ✚Synphasic, Tri-Levlen, Tri-Norinyl, Triphasil, Triquilar, Zovia

BENEFITS versus RISKS	
Possible Benefits	*Possible Risks*
HIGHLY EFFECTIVE FOR CONTRACEPTIVE PROTECTION	SERIOUS, LIFE-THREATENING THROMBOEMBOLIC DISORDERS in susceptible individuals
Moderately effective as adjunctive treatment in management of excessive menses and endometriosis	Hypertension
	Fluid retention
	Intensification of migrainelike headaches and fibrocystic breast changes
	Accelerated growth of uterine fibroid tumors
	Drug-induced hepatitis with jaundice
	Benign liver tumors (rare)

*"Mini-Pill" type, contains progestin only.

▷ **Principal Uses**

    As a Single Drug Product: Uses currently included in FDA approved labeling: (1) Prevention of conception. The "Mini-Pill" contains only one component—a progestin. This has been shown to be slightly less effective than the combination of estrogen and progestin in preventing pregnancy; (2) used in cases where women do not make enough hormones (female hypogonadism); (3) helps decrease excessive blood flow at menstruation (menorrhagia); (4) of use in endometriosis as the combination mestranol and norethynodrel.

    Other (unlabeled) generally accepted uses: (1) May be of benefit in abnormal hair growth in women (hirsutism); (2) has a protective effect against osteoporosis.

    As a Combination Drug Product [CD]: Uses currently included in FDA approved labeling: (1) Most oral contraceptives consist of a combination of an estrogen and a progestin. These products are the most effective form of medicinal contraception available; (2) they are sometimes used to treat menstrual irregularity, excessively heavy menstrual flow and endometriosis.

    Other (unlabeled) generally accepted uses: (1) Gestodene has been reported to inhibit certain breast cancer cell lines. Clinical studies are needed; (2) may have a protective effect against osteoporosis; triphasic oral contraceptives can help in the prevention or treatment of menopause symptoms.

How This Drug Works: When estrogen and progestin are taken in sufficient dosage and on a regular basis, the blood and tissue levels of these hormones increase to resemble those that occur during pregnancy. This results in suppression of the two pituitary gland hormones that normally cause ovulation (the formation and release of an egg by the ovary). In addition, these drugs may (1) alter the cervical mucus so that it resists the passage of sperm, and (2) alter the lining of the uterus so that it resists implantation of the egg (if ovulation occurs).

Available Dosage Forms and Strengths

    Tablets — several combinations of synthetic estrogens and progestins in varying strengths; see the package label of the brand prescribed.

▷ **Usual Adult Dosage Range:** Start with the first tablet on the fifth day after the onset of menstruation. Follow with 1 tablet daily (taken at the same time each day) for 21 consecutive days. Resume treatment on the eighth day following the last tablet taken during the preceding cycle. The schedule is to take the drug daily for 3 weeks and to omit it for 1 week. For the Mini-Pill (progestin only), initiate treatment on the first day of menstruation and take 1 tablet daily, every day, throughout the year (no interruption). **Note: Actual dosage and administration schedule must be determined by the physician for each patient individually.**

Conditions Requiring Dosing Adjustments

    Liver function: Should **NOT** be taken if you have liver disease.

    Kidney function: Oral contraceptives are not significantly eliminated by the kidneys.

▷ **Dosing Instructions:** The tablets may be crushed and taken with or after food to reduce stomach upset. To ensure regular (every day) use and uniform blood levels, it is best to take the tablet at the same time daily.

Usual Duration of Use: According to individual needs and circumstances. Long-term use (months to years) requires physician supervision and evaluation every 6 months.

▷ **This Drug Should Not Be Taken If**
- you have had an allergic reaction to any dosage form of it.
- you have a history of thrombophlebitis, embolism, heart attack or stroke.
- you have breast cancer.
- you have active liver disease, seriously impaired liver function or a history of liver tumor.
- you are a heavy smoker.
- you are age 35 and smoke.
- you have diabetes and have developed circulatory disease.
- you have high blood pressure.
- you have not had any periods (amenorrhea).
- you have abnormal and unexplained vaginal bleeding.
- you have sickle cell disease.
- you are pregnant.

▷ **Inform Your Physician Before Taking This Drug If**
- you have had an adverse reaction to any oral contraceptive.
- you have a history of cancer of the breast or reproductive organs.
- you have: fibrocystic breast changes, uterine fibroid tumors, endometriosis, migrainelike headaches, epilepsy, asthma, elevated lipids, prolapse of the mitral valve of the heart, heart disease, high blood pressure, gallbladder disease, diabetes or porphyria.
- you are over 40. This was an age related limit previously, but current thinking says that use of these medicines may occur as a benefit to risk decision.
- you smoke tobacco on a regular basis.
- you plan to have surgery in the near future.

Possible Side Effects (natural, expected, and unavoidable drug actions)
Fluid retention, weight gain, "breakthrough" bleeding (spotting in middle of menstrual cycle), altered menstrual pattern, lack of menstruation (during and following cessation of drug), increased susceptibility to yeast infection of the genital tissues.

▷ **Possible Adverse Effects** (unusual, unexpected, and infrequent reactions)
If any of the following develop, consult your physician promptly for guidance.
Mild Adverse Effects
Allergic Reactions: Skin rash, hives, itching.
Headache, nervous tension, irritability, accentuation of migraine headaches.
Nausea, vomiting, bloating, diarrhea.
Tannish pigmentation of the face.
Reduced tolerance to contact lenses.
Impaired color vision: blue tinge to objects, blue halo around lights.
Serious Adverse Effects
Allergic Reactions: Anaphylaxis, erythema multiforme and nodosum (skin reactions), loss of scalp hair.
Idiosyncratic Reactions: Joint and muscle pains.
Emotional depression, rise in blood pressure (in some people).
Eye changes: optic neuritis, retinal thrombosis, altered curvature of the cornea, cataracts.

Gallbladder disease, benign liver tumors, jaundice, rise in blood sugar.

Erosion of uterine cervix, enlargement of uterine fibroid tumors, cystitislike syndrome.

Abnormal glucose tolerance leading to high blood glucose (hyperglycemia).

Thrombophlebitis (inflammation of a vein with formation of blood clot)—pain or tenderness in thigh or leg, with or without swelling of foot or leg (4 to 11 times greater risk than people not taking these medicines).

Drug-induced porphyria (rare).

Retinopathy (rare).

Pulmonary embolism (movement of blood clot to lung)—sudden shortness of breath, pain in chest, coughing, bloody sputum.

Esophageal ulcers (especially if the medicine is taken lying down with no water).

Stroke (blood clot in brain)—headaches, blackout, sudden weakness or paralysis of any part of the body, severe dizziness, altered vision, slurred speech, inability to speak.

Heart attack (blood clot in coronary artery)—sudden pain in chest, neck, jaw, or arm; weakness; sweating; nausea.

Mesenteric thrombosis—blood clot in abdominal artery.

▷ **Possible Effects on Sexual Function**

Decreased libido (14–50%).

Altered character of menstruation; midcycle spotting.

Breast enlargement and tenderness with milk production.

Absent menstruation and infertility (temporary) after discontinuation of drug.

Possible Delayed Adverse Effects: Estrogens taken during pregnancy can predispose the female child to the later development of cancer of the vagina or cervix following puberty. Non-pregnant use does not increase breast cancer.

▷ **Adverse Effects That May Mimic Natural Diseases or Disorders**

Liver reactions may suggest viral hepatitis.

Natural Diseases or Disorders That May Be Activated by This Drug

Latent hypertension, diabetes mellitus, acute intermittent porphyria, lupus erythematosuslike syndrome.

Possible Effects on Laboratory Tests

Blood lupus erythematosus (LE) cells: positive.

Blood clotting time: decreased.

Blood prothrombin time: decreased.

Blood amylase and lipase levels: increased (very rare pancreatitis).

Blood total cholesterol, HDL cholesterol, LDL and VLDL cholesterol levels: usually no effects; some variability depending upon estrogen and progestin content of preparation used.

Blood triglyceride levels: no effect to increased, depending upon estrogen and progestin content of preparation used.

Blood glucose level: increased.

Blood thyroid stimulating hormone (TSH) level: no effect.

Blood thyroid hormone levels: T_3 and T_4 increased; free T_4 either no effect or decreased.

Liver function tests: increased liver enzymes (ALT/GPT, AST/GOT and alkaline phosphatase), increased bilirubin.

CAUTION

1. Serious adverse effects due to these drugs are a very low risk. However, any unusual development should be reported and evaluated promptly.
2. Studies indicate that women over 30 years of age who smoke and use oral contraceptives are at significantly greater risk of having a serious cardiovascular event than are nonusers.
3. The risk of thromboembolism increases with the amount of estrogen in the product and with the age of the user. Low-estrogen combinations are advised.
4. It is advisable to discontinue these drugs 1 month prior to elective surgery to reduce the risk of postsurgical thromboembolism.
5. Investigate promptly any alteration or disturbance of vision that occurs during the use of these drugs.
6. Investigate promptly the nature of recurrent, persistent or severe headaches that develop while taking these drugs.
7. Observe for significant change of mood. Discontinue this drug if depression develops.
8. Certain commonly used drugs may reduce the effectiveness of oral contraceptives. Some of these are listed in the category of *Other Drugs*.
9. Diarrhea lasting more than a few hours (and occurring during the days the drug is taken) can prevent adequate absorption of these drugs and impair their effectiveness as contraceptives.
10. If two consecutive menstrual periods are missed, ask your doctor if you should get a pregnancy test. Do not continue to use these drugs until you know if you are pregnant.
11. **Many antibiotics may stop the effectiveness of birth control pills** (oral contraceptives). If your doctor prescribes an antibiotic, ask if a different method of birth control is needed.

▷ **Advisability of Use During Pregnancy**

Pregnancy Category: X. See Pregnancy Code at the back of this book.

Animal studies: Genital defects reported in mice and guinea pigs; cleft palate reported in rodents.

Human studies: Information from studies of pregnant women indicates that estrogens can masculinize the female fetus. In addition, limb defects and heart malformations have been reported.

It is now known that estrogens taken during pregnancy can predispose the female child to the development of cancer of the vagina or cervix following puberty.

Avoid these drugs completely during entire pregnancy.

Advisability of Use if Breast-Feeding

Presence of these drugs in breast milk: Yes, in minute amounts.

These drugs may suppress milk formation if started early after delivery.

Breast-feeding is considered to be safe during the use of oral contraceptives.

Habit-Forming Potential: None.

Effects of Overdosage: Headache, drowsiness, nausea, vomiting, fluid retention, abnormal vaginal bleeding, breast enlargement and discomfort.

Possible Effects of Long-Term Use: High blood pressure, gallbladder disease with stones, accelerated growth of uterine fibroid tumors, absent menstruation and impaired fertility after discontinuation of drug.

Suggested Periodic Examinations While Taking This Drug (at physician's discretion)

Regular (every 6 months) evaluation of the breasts and pelvic organs, including Pap smears. Liver function tests as indicated.

▷ **While Taking This Drug, Observe the Following**

Foods: Avoid excessive use of salt if fluid retention occurs.

Beverages: No restrictions. May be taken with milk.

▷ *Alcohol:* No interactions expected.

Tobacco Smoking: Studies indicate that heavy smoking (15 or more cigarettes daily) while taking oral contraceptives significantly increases the risk of heart attack (coronary thrombosis). Heavy smoking should be considered a contraindication to the use of oral contraceptives.

▷ *Other Drugs*

Oral contraceptives may ***increase*** the effects of

- some benzodiazepines (see Drug Classes), and cause excessive sedation.
- cyclosporine (Sandimmune) and cause toxicity.
- metoprolol (Lopressor), and cause excessive beta blocker effects.
- prednisolone and prednisone, and cause excessive cortisonelike effects.
- theophyllines (Theodur, others), and increase the risk of toxic effects.

Oral contraceptives ***taken concurrently*** with

- antibiotics (such as amoxicillin or ampicillin) can seriously impair effectiveness and allow pregnancy to occur.
- antidiabetic drugs may cause unpredictable fluctuations of blood sugar.
- ascorbic acid (vitamin C) may result in increased levels of ethinyl estradiol, and breakthrough bleeding if the vitamin C is stopped.
- tricyclic antidepressants (Elavil, Sinequan, etc.) may enhance their adverse effects and reduce their antidepressant effectiveness.
- troleandomycin (TAO) may increase occurrence of liver toxicity and jaundice.
- warfarin (Coumadin) may cause unpredictable alterations of prothrombin activity. More frequent INR (protime) testing is needed, and warfarin dosing should be adjusted to laboratory test results.

The following drugs may ***decrease*** the effects of oral contraceptives (and impair their effectiveness)

- barbiturates (phenobarbital, etc.; see Drug Class Section).
- carbamazepine (Tegretol).
- griseofulvin (Fulvicin, etc.).
- penicillins (ampicillin, penicillin V).
- phenytoin (Dilantin).
- primidone (Mysoline).
- rifampin (Rifadin, Rimactane).
- tetracyclines (see Drug Classes).

▷ *Driving, Hazardous Activities:* Usually no restrictions. Consult your physician for assessment of individual risk and for guidance regarding specific restrictions.

Aviation Note: Usually no restrictions. However, watch for the rare occurrence of disturbed vision and to restrict activities accordingly. Consult a designated Aviation Medical Examiner.

Exposure to Sun: Use caution. These drugs can cause photosensitivity (see Glossary).

Discontinuation: Do not stop this drug if "breakthrough" bleeding occurs. If spotting or bleeding continues, call your doctor. A higher estrogen pill may be required. Remember: Omitting this drug for only 1 day may allow pregnancy to occur. It is best to avoid pregnancy for 3 to 6 months after stopping these drugs; aborted fetuses from women who became pregnant within 6 months after discontinuation reveal significantly increased chromosome abnormalities.

OXAPROZIN (OX a proh zin)

Introduced: 1992   **Prescription:** USA: Yes   **Available as Generic:** USA: No   **Class:** analgesic, mild; NSAID   **Controlled Drug:** USA: No
Brand Names: Daypro

BENEFITS versus RISKS	
Possible Benefits	*Possible Risks*
EFFECTIVE RELIEF OF MILD TO MODERATE PAIN AND INFLAMMATION	Gastrointestinal pain, ulceration, and bleeding (rare)
ONCE-DAILY DOSING	Rare kidney toxicity
	Rare fluid retention
	Sleep disturbances

Please see the propionic acid nonsteroidal anti-inflammatory drug profile for further information.

OXICAMS
(Nonsteroidal anti-inflammatory drug)

Piroxicam (peer OX i kam)

Introduced: 1978   **Prescription:** USA: Yes; Canada: Yes   **Available as Generic:** Yes   **Class:** Mild analgesic, anti-inflammatory   **Controlled Drug:** USA: No; Canada: No
Brand Names: ✦Apo-Piroxicam, Feldene, ✦Novo-Pirocam, ✦Nu-Pirox

BENEFITS versus RISKS	
Possible Benefits	*Possible Risks*
EFFECTIVE RELIEF OF MILD TO MODERATE PAIN AND INFLAMMATION	Gastrointestinal pain, ulceration, and bleeding
	Drug-induced hepatitis (rare)
	Rare kidney damage
	Mild fluid retention
	Reduced white blood cell and platelet counts

▷ **Principal Uses**

As a Single Drug Product: Uses currently included in FDA approved labeling: (1) Relieves mild to moderately severe pain and inflammation associated with (1) rheumatoid arthritis, (2) osteoarthritis.

Other (unlabeled) generally accepted uses: (1) Treats the morning and evening pain associated with ankylosing spondylitis; (2) helps relieve the pain and inflammation of acute gout; (3) used to treat terminal cancer pain in combination with doxepin; (4) may have a role in easing temporal arteritis.

How This Drug Works: This drug suppresses the formation of prostaglandins (and related compounds), chemicals involved in the production of inflammation and pain.

Available Dosage Forms and Strengths

Capsules — 10 mg and 20 mg
Rectal Suppository — 10 mg and 20 mg

▷ **Usual Adult Dosage Range:**   As antiarthritic: 10 mg twice daily, 12 hours apart; or 20 mg once daily. The total daily dosage should not exceed 40 mg, and then for no more than 5 days. **Note: Actual dosage and administration schedule must be determined by the physician for each patient individually.**

Conditions Requiring Dosing Adjustments

Liver function: This drug should be used with caution and in decreased dose in patients with liver compromise.

Kidney function: Piroxicam should be used with caution in renal compromise and kidney function followed closely. The kidney is a minor path of removal of this medicine.

▷ **Dosing Instructions:**   Take with or following food to prevent stomach irritation. Take with a full glass of water and remain upright (do not lie down) for 30 minutes. The capsule may be opened for administration.

Usual Duration of Use: Use on a regular schedule for 2 weeks usually determines effectiveness in relieving the discomfort of arthritis. Long-term use (months to years) requires physician supervision and periodic evaluation.

▷ **This Drug Should Not Be Taken If**
- you have had an allergic reaction to it previously.
- you are subject to asthma or nasal polyps caused by aspirin.
- you have active peptic ulcer disease or any form of gastrointestinal bleeding.
- you have a bleeding disorder or a blood cell disorder.
- you have active liver disease.
- you have severe impairment of kidney function.

▷ **Inform Your Physician Before Taking This Drug If**
- you are allergic to aspirin or to other aspirin substitutes.
- you have a history of peptic ulcer disease, regional enteritis or ulcerative colitis.
- you have a history of any type of bleeding disorder.
- you have impaired liver or kidney function.
- you develop signs or symptoms of pancreatitis while taking this medicine. (talk with your doctor).
- you have high blood pressure or a history of heart failure.
- you take: acetaminophen, aspirin or other aspirin substitutes, anticoagulants, oral antidiabetic drugs.
- you plan to have surgery of any type in the near future.

Possible Side Effects (natural, expected, and unavoidable drug actions)
Fluid retention (weight gain), prolongation of bleeding time.

▷ **Possible Adverse Effects** (unusual, unexpected, and infrequent reactions)
If any of the following develop, consult your physician promptly for guidance.

Mild Adverse Effects
Allergic Reactions: Skin rash, itching, spontaneous bruising.
Headache, dizziness, hair loss, altered or blurred vision, ringing in the ears, drowsiness, fatigue, paresthesias, inability to concentrate.
Indigestion, nausea, vomiting, abdominal pain, breast pain, diarrhea.

Serious Adverse Effects
Active peptic ulcer, stomach or intestinal bleeding.
Drug-induced liver damage.
Serious skin damage (toxic epidermal necrolysis).
Pancreatitis (rare).
Kidney damage with painful urination, bloody urine, reduced urine formation.
Rare bone marrow depression (see Glossary): fatigue, weakness, fever, sore throat, abnormal bleeding or bruising.
Blood clotting problems.
Esophagitis.
Increased blood potassium.
Decreased sodium (following abnormal urine excretion) (rare).

▷ **Possible Effects on Sexual Function:** None reported.

Possible Delayed Adverse Effects: Mild anemia due to "silent" blood loss from the stomach.

▷ **Adverse Effects That May Mimic Natural Diseases or Disorders**
Liver reaction may suggest viral hepatitis.

Natural Diseases or Disorders That May Be Activated by This Drug
Peptic ulcer disease, ulcerative colitis. This drug may hide symptoms of gout.

Possible Effects on Laboratory Tests
Red blood cell count and hemoglobin level: decreased.
Bleeding time: increased.
Blood uric acid level: increased.
Liver function tests: increased liver enzymes (ALT/GPT, AST/GOT and alkaline phosphatase), increased bilirubin.
Kidney function tests: blood creatinine and urea nitrogen (BUN) levels increased; urine analysis positive for red blood cells, casts and increased protein content (kidney damage).
Fecal occult blood test: positive.

CAUTION
1. The smallest effective dose should always be used.
2. This drug may hide early signs of infection. Tell your doctor if you think you are developing an infection.

Precautions for Use
By Infants and Children: Indications and dose recommendations for those under 12 years of age not established.
By Those over 60 Years of Age: Small doses are advisable until tolerance is deter-

mined. Observe for any indications of liver or kidney toxicity, fluid retention, dizziness, confusion, impaired memory, stomach bleeding or constipation.

▷ **Advisability of Use During Pregnancy**

Pregnancy Category: B. Category D in the last three months of pregnancy. See Pregnancy Code at the back of this book.

Animal studies: No birth defects reported due to this drug.

Human studies: Adequate studies of pregnant women are not available.

The manufacturer does not recommend the use of this drug during pregnancy.

Advisability of Use if Breast-Feeding

Presence of this drug in breast milk: Yes.

Avoid drug or refrain from nursing.

Habit-Forming Potential: None.

Effects of Overdosage: Possible drowsiness, dizziness, ringing in the ears, nausea, vomiting, indigestion.

Possible Effects of Long-Term Use: Development of anemia due to "silent" bleeding from the gastrointestinal tract.

Suggested Periodic Examinations While Taking This Drug (at physician's discretion)

Complete blood cell counts, liver and kidney function tests.

Complete eye examinations if vision is altered in any way.

Hearing examinations if ringing in the ears or hearing loss develops.

▷ **While Taking This Drug, Observe the Following**

Foods: No restrictions.

Beverages: No restrictions. May be taken with milk.

▷ *Alcohol:* Use with caution. Both alcohol and piroxicam can irritate the stomach lining, and can increase the risk of stomach ulceration and/or bleeding.

Tobacco Smoking: No interactions expected.

▷ *Other Drugs*

Piroxicam may ***increase*** the effects of

- acetaminophen (Tylenol, etc.), and increase the risk of kidney damage; avoid prolonged use of this combination.
- anticoagulants (Coumadin, etc.), and increase the risk of bleeding; more frequent INR (prothrombin time) testing is needed and dosing should then be adjusted accordingly.
- lithium (Lithobid, others) can lead to lithium toxicity.
- methotrexate (Mexate) may lead to methotrexate toxicity.

Piroxicam ***taken concurrently*** with the following drugs may increase the risk of bleeding; avoid these combinations:

- aspirin.
- antihypertensives such as thiazides (see drug classes) and others will blunt their therapeutic benefit.
- beta blockers (atenolol and others) can decrease the effectiveness of the beta blocker.
- cholestyramine (Questran).
- dipyridamole (Persantine).
- indomethacin (Indocin).

- sulfinpyrazone (Anturane).
- valproic acid (Depakene).

▷ *Driving, Hazardous Activities:* This drug may cause drowsiness or dizziness. Restrict activities as necessary.

Aviation Note: The use of this drug *may be a disqualification* for piloting. Consult a designated Aviation Medical Examiner.

Exposure to Sun: This drug may cause photosensitivity (see Glossary). Use caution.

OXTRIPHYLLINE (ox TRY fi lin)

Other Names: choline theophyllinate, theophylline cholinate

Introduced: 1965   **Prescription:** USA: Yes; Canada: Yes   **Available as Generic:** Yes   **Class:** Antiasthmatic, bronchodilator, xanthines   **Controlled Drug:** USA: No; Canada: No

Brand Names: ✦Apo-Oxtriphylline, Choledyl, Choledyl Delayed-release, Choledyl SA, ✦Novotriphyl

BENEFITS versus RISKS	
Possible Benefits	*Possible Risks*
EFFECTIVE PREVENTION AND RELIEF OF ACUTE BRONCHIAL ASTHMA	NARROW TREATMENT RANGE FREQUENT STOMACH DISTRESS Gastrointestinal bleeding
MODERATELY EFFECTIVE CONTROL OF CHRONIC, RECURRENT BRONCHIAL ASTHMA	Central nervous system toxicity, seizures Heart rhythm disturbances
Moderately effective symptomatic relief in chronic bronchitis and emphysema	

▷ **Principal Uses**

As a Single Drug Product: Uses currently included in FDA approved labeling: (1) Used to relieve shortness of breath and wheezing characteristic of acute bronchial asthma, and to prevent the recurrence of asthmatic episodes; (2) also useful in relieving the asthmaticlike symptoms that are associated with some types of chronic bronchitis and emphysema.

Other (unlabeled) generally accepted uses: Please see the theophylline profile.

As a Combination Drug Product [CD]: This drug is available in combination with guaifenesin to provide an expectorant effect that thins the mucus secretions in the bronchial tubes.

How This Drug Works: This drug yields 64% free theophylline, the active medicinal component. By inhibiting the enzyme phosphodiesterase, this drug produces an increase in the tissue chemical cyclic AMP. This causes relaxation of the muscles in the bronchial tubes and blood vessels of the lung, resulting in relief of bronchospasm, expanded lung capacity and improved lung circulation.

Available Dosage Forms and Strengths

Oral solution — 100 mg/ 5-ml (20% alcohol)

Syrup — 50 mg/ 5-ml

Tablets — 100 mg, 200 mg (US, Canada) and 300 mg (Canada)

Tablets, delayed-release — 100 mg, 200 mg

Tablets, extended-release — 400 mg, 600 mg

▷ **Recommended Dosage Ranges** (Actual dosage and administration schedule must be determined by the physician for each patient individually.)

Note: All doses of oxtriphylline are to be calculated as theophylline-equivalents; all dosages are the same as in the theophylline profile later in this book. Please see the theophylline profile for further information.

OXYCODONE (ox ee KOH dohn)

Introduced: 1950 **Prescription:** USA: Yes; Canada: Yes **Available as Generic:** USA: Yes; Canada: No **Class:** Analgesic, strong; opioid **Controlled Drug:** USA: C-II*; Canada: No

Brand Names: ✦Endocet [CD], ✦Endodan [CD], ✦Oxycocet [CD], ✦Oxycodan [CD], Percocet [CD], ✦Percocet-Demi [CD], Percodan [CD], Percodan-Demi [CD], Roxicet, Roxicodone, Roxilox, Roxiprin [CD], SK-Oxycodone, ✦Supeudol, Tylox [CD]

BENEFITS versus RISKS	
Possible Benefits	*Possible Risks*
EFFECTIVE RELIEF OF MODERATE TO SEVERE PAIN	POTENTIAL FOR HABIT FORMATION (DEPENDENCE)
	Sedative effects
	Mild allergic reactions (infrequent)
	Nausea, constipation

▷ **Principal Uses**

As a Single Drug Product: Uses currently included in FDA approved labeling: (1) Used in tablet and suppository form (Canada) to relieve moderate to severe pain.

Other (unlabeled) generally accepted uses: None.

As a Combination Drug Product [CD]: Oxycodone is available in combinations with acetaminophen and with aspirin. These milder pain relievers are added to enhance the analgesic effect and to reduce fever when present.

How This Drug Works: Acting primarily as a depressant of certain brain functions, this drug suppresses pain perception and calms the emotional response to pain.

Available Dosage Forms and Strengths

Solution — 5 mg/ 5-ml

Suppositories — 10 mg, 20 mg (Canada)

Tablets — 5 mg, 10 mg (Canada)

Tablets — 2.44 mg, 4.88 mg (in combination drugs)

*See Schedules of Controlled Drugs at the back of this book.

▷ **Usual Adult Dosage Range:** Percodan is given as one tablet (5 mg) every 6 hours. Current pain theory says that pain medicines should be scheduled; for example, given every 4 hours. The outdated "wait until it hurts" method tended to result in suffering. May be increased to 10 mg/ 4 hours if needed for severe pain. The total daily dosage should not exceed 60 mg. **Note: Actual dosage and administration schedule must be determined by the physician for each patient individually.**

Conditions Requiring Dosing Adjustments
Liver function: Dosage adjustments should be empirically made in liver failure.
Kidney function: Dosage adjustment does not appear to be needed. Some combination products contain aspirin which may be contraindicated in kidney failure.

▷ **Dosing Instructions:** The tablet may be crushed and taken with or following food to reduce stomach upset or nausea.

Usual Duration of Use: As required to control pain. Continual use should not exceed 5 to 7 days without interruption and reassessment of need.

▷ **This Drug Should Not Be Taken If**
- you have had an allergic reaction to any dosage form of it previously.
- you are having an acute attack of asthma.
- patients allergic to aspirin should **not** be given Percodan.

▷ **Inform Your Physician Before Taking This Drug If**
- you have had an unfavorable reaction to any narcotic drug in the past.
- you have had a head injury with increased pressure (intracranial) in the head.
- you have a history of drug abuse or alcoholism.
- you have chronic lung disease with impaired breathing.
- you have impaired liver or kidney function.
- you have gallbladder disease, a seizure disorder or an underactive thyroid gland.
- you have difficulty emptying the urinary bladder.
- you are taking any other drugs that have a sedative effect.
- you plan to have surgery under general anesthesia in the near future.

Possible Side Effects (natural, expected, and unavoidable drug actions)
Drowsiness, light-headedness, dry mouth, urinary retention, constipation.

▷ **Possible Adverse Effects** (unusual, unexpected, and infrequent reactions)
If any of the following develop, consult your physician promptly for guidance.
Mild Adverse Effects
Allergic Reactions: Skin rash, hives, itching.
Idiosyncratic Reactions: Skin rash and itching when combined with dairy products (milk or cheese).
Dizziness, impaired concentration, sensation of drunkenness, confusion, depression, blurred or double vision.
Nausea, vomiting.
Serious Adverse Effects
Impaired breathing: use with caution in chronic lung disease.
Abnormal body movements (if the drug is abruptly stopped).

▷ **Possible Effects on Sexual Function:**   Blunted sexual responses.

Possible Effects on Laboratory Tests

Urine screening tests for drug abuse: test result may be falsely **positive**; *confirmatory* test result may be **negative**. (Test results depend upon amount of drug taken and testing method used.)

CAUTION

1. If you have asthma, chronic bronchitis or emphysema, excessive use of this drug may cause significant respiratory difficulty, thickening of bronchial secretions and suppression of coughing.
2. The concurrent use of this drug with atropinelike drugs can increase the risk of urinary retention and reduced intestinal function.
3. Do not take this drug following acute head injury.

Precautions for Use

By Infants and Children: Do not use this drug in children under 2 years of age because of their vulnerability to life-threatening respiratory depression.

By Those over 60 Years of Age: Small starting doses and short-term therapy are indicated. There may be increased susceptibility to the development of drowsiness, dizziness, unsteadiness, falling, urinary retention and constipation (often leading to fecal impaction).

▷ **Advisability of Use During Pregnancy**

Pregnancy Category: C. See Pregnancy Code at the back of this book.

Animal studies: No information available.

Human studies: Adequate studies of pregnant women are not available. Oxycodone taken repeatedly during the last few weeks before delivery may cause withdrawal symptoms in the newborn infant.

Use this drug only if clearly needed and in small, infrequent doses.

Advisability of Use if Breast-Feeding

Presence of this drug in breast milk: Unknown.

Avoid drug or refrain from nursing.

Habit-Forming Potential: Psychological and/or physical dependence can develop.

Effects of Overdosage: Drowsiness, restlessness, agitation, nausea, vomiting, dry mouth, vertigo, weakness, lethargy, stupor, coma, seizures.

Possible Effects of Long-Term Use: Psychological and physical dependence, chronic constipation.

Suggested Periodic Examinations While Taking This Drug (at physician's discretion)

None.

▷ **While Taking This Drug, Observe the Following**

Foods: No restrictions.

Beverages: No restrictions. May be taken with milk.

▷ *Alcohol:* Oxycodone can intensify the intoxicating effects of alcohol, and alcohol can intensify the depressant effects of oxycodone on brain function, breathing and circulation. Combined use is best avoided.

Tobacco Smoking: No interactions expected.

Marijuana Smoking: Increase in drowsiness and pain relief; impairment of mental and physical performance.

▷ *Other Drugs*
> Oxycodone may ***increase*** the effects of
> - other drugs with sedative effects (see Drug Classes for benzodiazepines, tricyclic antidepressants, antihistamines, MAO inhibitors, phenothiazines, and opioid drugs (narcotics)).
> - atropinelike drugs, and increase the risk of constipation and urinary retention.

▷ *Driving, Hazardous Activities:* This drug can impair mental alertness, judgment, reaction time and physical coordination. Avoid hazardous activities accordingly.

Aviation Note: The use of this drug ***is a disqualification*** for piloting. Consult a designated Aviation Medical Examiner.

Exposure to Sun: No restrictions.

Discontinuation: It is best to limit this drug to short-term use. If extended use is needed, discontinuation should be gradual to minimize possible effects of withdrawal.

PAROXETINE (pa ROCKS a teen)

Introduced: 1993   **Prescription:** USA: Yes; Canada: Yes   **Available as Generic:** USA: No; Canada: No   **Class:** antidepressant (other)   **Controlled Drug:** USA: No; Canada: No

Brand Names: Paxil

BENEFITS versus RISKS	
Possible Benefits	*Possible Risks*
EFFECTIVE CONTROL OF DEPRESSION	Withdrawal symptoms
Fewer adverse effects than tricyclic antidepressants	Abnormal ejaculation in males
Helps control obsessive-compulsive disorder and panic disorder	

▷ **Principal Uses**

> *As a Single Drug Product:* Uses currently included in FDA approved labeling: (1) Treatment of depression; (2) helps control obsessive compulsive disorder; (3) helps control panic attacks.
>
> Other (unlabeled) generally accepted uses: (1) Can have a role in diabetic nerve pain (neuropathy); (2) helps long-standing (chronic) daily headaches; (3) can help premature ejaculation.

How This Drug Works: This phenylpiperidine antidepressant inhibits the uptake of a chemical important in mood (serotonin). When more of this chemical is available in the brain, a positive impact on thinking is often realized.

Available Dosage Forms and Strengths

> Capsules — 20 mg, 30 mg

▷ **Recommended Dosage Ranges (Actual dosage and administration schedule must be determined by the physician for each patient individually.)**

Infants and Children: Not indicated.

18 to 60 Years of Age: The usual starting dose is 20 mg, given in the morning. Dose can then be increased as needed and tolerated in 10 mg intervals to a maximum of 50 mg daily.

Over 60 Years of Age: The starting dose in this population is 10 mg daily. The maximum dose is 40 mg daily.

Conditions Requiring Dosing Adjustments

Liver function: Starting dose is 10 mg and the maximum dose is 40 mg daily. Drug levels may be needed.

Kidney function: The starting dose and maximum dose are the same as those used in patients with liver compromise.

▷ **Dosing Instructions:**   The absorption of this medicine is not changed by food.

Usual Duration of Use:

Continual use on a regular schedule for 14 days is usually necessary to determine this drug's effectiveness in treating depression. Long-term use (months to years) requires periodic evaluation of response and dosage adjustment. Consult your physician on a regular basis.

Possible Advantages of This Drug

Fewer side effects than tricyclic antidepressants.

▷ **This Drug Should Not Be Taken If**

• you have had an allergic reaction to any dosage form of it previously.
• you are currently taking, or have taken within the last 14 days a MAO inhibitor (see Drug Classes) medication.

▷ **Inform Your Physician Before Taking This Drug If**

• you are pregnant or are breast feeding.
• you have a history of mania.
• you have a history of seizures.
• you take diuretics or typically drink little water.
• you have a history of liver or kidney disease.
• you take other prescription or nonprescription medicines which were not discussed with your doctor when paroxetine was prescribed.

Possible Side Effects (natural, expected, and unavoidable drug actions)

Lowered blood pressure and fainting upon standing (postural hypotension).

▷ **Possible Adverse Effects** (unusual, unexpected, and infrequent reactions)

If any of the following develop, consult your physician promptly for guidance.

Mild Adverse Effects

Allergic Reactions: Skin rash and itching.
Headache.
Palpitations.
Loss of appetite, taste disorders, or constipation.
Tingling of the hands (paresthesias).
Sweating.
Nervousness, insomnia, sedation.
Dizziness, blurred vision.

Serious Adverse Effects

Allergic Reactions: Not reported.
Idiosyncratic Reactions: None reported.

Abnormal movements or positioning of the mouth or face.

Seizures (rare).

Liver toxicity (rare and of questionable causation).

Abnormal sensation of motion (acathisia) (rare).

▷ **Possible Effects on Sexual Function:**   Galactorrhea. Abnormal ejaculation (12.9%) (mostly delayed), inability to achieve orgasm (10%), impotence or sexual dysfunction (10%), prolonged and painful erection (priapism) (rare).

Possible Delayed Adverse Effects: None reported.

▷ **Adverse Effects That May Mimic Natural Diseases or Disorders**

Increased liver enzymes may mimic early hepatitis.

Natural Diseases or Disorders That May Be Activated by This Drug

None reported.

Possible Effects on Laboratory Tests

Liver function tests: increased.

CAUTION

1. Take this medicine as prescribed and do not stop taking it without talking with your doctor.

Precautions for Use

By Infants and Children: Safety and effectiveness for use by those under 18 years of age have not been established.

By Those over 60 Years of Age: Lower starting and maximum doses are indicated.

▷ **Advisability of Use During Pregnancy**

Pregnancy Category: B. See Pregnancy Code at the back of this book.

Animal studies: Reproduction studies in rabbits or rats using doses of up to 10 times the typical human dose have not revealed any fetal changes.

Human studies: Information from adequate studies of pregnant women is not available.

Ask your doctor for guidance.

Advisability of Use if Breast-Feeding

Presence of this drug in breast milk: Yes, in small amounts.

Ask your doctor for guidance.

Habit-Forming Potential: None, however a withdrawal syndrome characterized by dizziness, confusion, sweating and tremor has been described.

Effects of Overdosage: Confusion, heart rhythm changes, seizures.

Possible Effects of Long-Term Use: Not defined.

Suggested Periodic Examinations While Taking This Drug (at physician's discretion)

Liver function tests.

▷ **While Taking This Drug, Observe the Following**

Foods: No restrictions.

Nutritional Support: Not indicated.

Beverages: No restrictions.

▷ *Alcohol:* The manufacturer recommends avoiding alcohol while taking this medicine.

Tobacco Smoking: No interactions expected.

Marijuana Smoking: Additive sedation.

▷ *Other Drugs*
  Paroxetine may *increase* the effects of
  - benzodiazepines (see Drug Classes).
  - desipramine (and potentially other tricyclic antidepressants; see Drug Classes).
  - haloperidol (Haldol) because paroxetine blocks an enzyme system needed to remove haloperidol.
  - labetalol (Normodyne) and perhaps other beta blockers (see Drug Classes) because paroxetine inhibits an enzyme system needed to remove labetalol.
  - nonsedating antihistamines astemizole and terfenadine because paroxetine may inhibit some liver systems that usually remove paroxetine from the body. This effect has not been documented, but is theoretically possible.

  Paroxetine *taken concurrently* with
  - MAO inhibitors (see Drug Classes) may result in a fatal serotonin syndrome. **Do not** combine these medicines.
  - phenytoin (Dilantin) may result in decreased paroxetine blood levels and lessening of therapeutic benefits. Dose increases may be needed.
  - quinidine (Quinaglute, others) may result in increased paroxetine levels and toxicity. Decreased paroxetine doses may be needed.
  - tryptophan may result in sweating, nausea and dizziness.
  - warfarin (Coumadin) may result in bleeding. More frequent INR (protime) testing is recommended. Warfarin doses should be adjusted based on laboratory results.

  The following drugs may *increase* the effects of paroxetine
  - cimetidine (Tagamet).

▷ *Driving, Hazardous Activities:* This drug may frequently cause sedation. Restrict activities as necessary.
  Aviation Note: The use of this drug *is a disqualification* for piloting. Consult a designated Aviation Medical Examiner.
  Exposure to Sun: No specific restrictions.
  Exposure to Heat: This medicine can cause excessive sweating. If you work or are frequently in a hot environment, be careful to replace enough fluids to avoid dehydration.
  Heavy Exercise or Exertion: Since this medicine may cause excessive sweating, be careful to replace lost fluids.
  Occurrence of Unrelated Illness: Illnesses which cause fevers may be worsened in their ability to cause dehydration.
  Discontinuation: Do not stop this medicine without first talking with your doctor.

PENBUTOLOL (pen BYU toh lohl)

Introduced: 1976   **Prescription:** USA: Yes   **Available as Generic:** No   **Class:** Antihypertensive, beta-adrenergic blocker   **Controlled Drug:** USA: No

Brand Name: Levatol

```
┌─────────────────────────────────────────────────────────────┐
│                    BENEFITS versus RISKS                       │
│      Possible Benefits              Possible Risks             │
│  EFFECTIVE, WELL-TOLERATED      CONGESTIVE HEART FAILURE in     │
│  ANTIHYPERTENSIVE in mild to      advanced heart disease       │
│  moderate high blood pressure   Worsening of angina in coronary│
│                                   heart disease (abrupt withdrawal)│
│                                 Masking of low blood sugar     │
│                                   (hypoglycemia) in drug-treated│
│                                   diabetes                     │
│                                 Provocation of asthma (in asthmatics)│
└─────────────────────────────────────────────────────────────┘
```

▷ **Principal Uses**

As a Single Drug Product: Uses currently included in FDA approved labeling: (1) Treatment of mild to moderate high blood pressure. May be used alone or concurrently with other antihypertensive drugs, such as diuretics.

Other (unlabeled) generally accepted uses: (1) May help curb aggressive behavior; (2) can help decrease the frequency and severity of angina attacks; (3) may help decrease death from heart attack (myocardial infarction); (4) can have a supportive role in panic attacks; (5) a small amount of data supports penbutolol use in glaucoma, but large trials have not been performed as yet.

How This Drug Works: By blocking certain actions of the sympathetic nervous system, this drug
- reduces the rate and contraction force of the heart, lowering ejection pressure of the blood leaving the heart.
- reduces the degree of contraction of blood vessel walls, resulting in their expansion and lower blood pressure.

Available Dosage Forms and Strengths

Tablets — 20 mg

▷ **Usual Adult Dosage Range:**   Initially 20 mg once daily. The dose may be increased gradually by 10 mg/day at intervals of 2 weeks as needed and tolerated up to 80 mg/day. While higher doses have been well tolerated, they have not shown greater efficacy. For maintenance, 20 to 40 mg once daily is usually adequate. The total daily dose should not exceed 80 mg. **Note: Actual dosage and administration schedule must be determined by the physician for each patient individually.**

Conditions Requiring Dosing Adjustments

Liver function: Dosage adjustments should be considered in mild to moderate liver disease; however, specific guidelines are not available.

Kidney function: Penbutolol elimination does not significantly involve the kidneys. No dosing changes are thought to be needed.

▷ **Dosing Instructions:**   The tablet may be crushed and taken without regard to eating. Do not stop this drug abruptly.

Usual Duration of Use: Use on a regular schedule for up to 2 weeks determines the full effect in lowering blood pressure. Long-term use of this drug (months to years) will be determined by the course of your blood pressure over time and your response to an overall treatment program (weight reduction, salt restriction, smoking cessation, etc.).

Possible Advantages of This Drug
Adequate control of blood pressure with a single daily dose.
Causes less slowing of the heart rate than most other beta blocker drugs.

Currently a "Drug of Choice"
for initiating treatment of hypertension with a single drug.

▷ **This Drug Should Not Be Taken If**
- you have had an allergic reaction to it previously.
- you have congestive heart failure.
- you have an abnormally slow heart rate or a serious form of heart block.
- you have abnormal growth of the left side of the heart (left ventricular hypertrophy).
- you are subject to bronchial asthma.

▷ **Inform Your Physician Before Taking This Drug If**
- you have had an adverse reaction to any beta blocker (see Drug Class Section).
- you have a history of serious heart disease.
- you are a diabetic.
- you have a history of hay fever (allergic rhinitis), asthma, chronic bronchitis or emphysema.
- you have a history of overactive thyroid function (hyperthyroidism).
- you have a history of low blood sugar (hypoglycemia).
- you have impaired liver or kidney function.
- you have diabetes or myasthenia gravis.
- you have impaired circulation in the extremities (Raynaud's disorder, claudication pains in legs).
- you take any form of digitalis, quinidine or reserpine, or any calcium blocker drug (see Drug Classes).
- you plan to have surgery under general anesthesia in the near future.

Possible Side Effects (natural, expected, and unavoidable drug actions)
Lethargy and fatigability, cold extremities, slow heart rate, light-headedness in upright position (see Orthostatic Hypotension in Glossary).

▷ **Possible Adverse Effects** (unusual, unexpected, and infrequent reactions)
If any of the following develop, consult your physician promptly for guidance.
Mild Adverse Effects
Allergic Reactions: Skin rash, itching, reversible hair loss.
Headache, dizziness, blurred vision, insomnia, abnormal dreams.
Indigestion, nausea, vomiting, constipation, diarrhea.
Joint and muscle discomfort.
Serious Adverse Effects
Allergic Reactions: Anaphylactoid reaction (see Glossary).
Mental depression, anxiety, disorientation, short-term memory loss, hallucinations.
Carpal tunnel syndrome (rare).
High blood sugar.
Worsening of circulatory problems in those with preexisting conditions such as Raynaud's phenomenon.
Bronchospasm (rare).
Chest pain, shortness of breath, precipitation of congestive heart failure.

Rebound hypertension (if abruptly stopped).
Induction of bronchial asthma (in asthmatic individuals).
Aggravation of myasthenia gravis.
Abnormally low white blood cell and platelet counts: fever, sore throat, abnormal bleeding or bruising.

▷ **Possible Effects on Sexual Function:** Decreased libido and impotence, rare but more common with higher doses; Peyronie's disease (see Glossary).

▷ **Adverse Effects That May Mimic Natural Diseases or Disorders**
Reduced blood flow to extremities may resemble Raynaud's phenomenon (see Glossary).

Natural Diseases or Disorders That May Be Activated by This Drug
Raynaud's disease, intermittent claudication, myasthenia gravis.

Possible Effects on Laboratory Tests
White blood cell and platelet counts: decreased.
Uric acid: increased.
Blood sugar: increased.

CAUTION
1. *Do not stop this drug suddenly* without the knowledge and help of your doctor. Carry a notation on your person that you are taking this drug.
2. Ask your physician or pharmacist **before** using nasal decongestants in over-the-counter cold preparations and nose drops. These can cause sudden increases in blood pressure when taken with beta blockers.
3. Report the development of any tendency to emotional depression.

Precautions for Use
By Infants and Children: Safety and effectiveness for those under 12 years of age not established. However, if this drug is used, observe for the development of low blood sugar (hypoglycemia) during periods of reduced food intake.
By Those over 60 Years of Age: Unacceptably high blood pressure should be reduced without creating the risks associated with excessively low blood pressure. Small starting doses and frequent blood pressure checks are needed. Sudden, rapid and excessive reduction of blood pressure can predispose to stroke or heart attack. Observe for dizziness, unsteadiness, tendency to fall, confusion, hallucinations, depression or urinary frequency.

▷ **Advisability of Use During Pregnancy**
Pregnancy Category: C. See Pregnancy Code at the back of this book.
Animal studies: No birth defects due to this drug found in rat or rabbit studies.
Human studies: Adequate studies of pregnant women are not available.
Use this drug only if clearly needed. Ask physician for guidance.

Advisability of Use if Breast-Feeding
Presence of this drug in breast milk: Unknown.
Avoid drug or refrain from nursing.

Habit-Forming Potential: None.

Effects of Overdosage: Weakness, slow pulse, low blood pressure, fainting, cold and sweaty skin, congestive heart failure, possible coma and convulsions.

Possible Effects of Long-Term Use: Reduced heart reserve and eventual heart failure in susceptible individuals with advanced heart disease.

Suggested Periodic Examinations While Taking This Drug (at physician's discretion)

Measurements of blood pressure, evaluation of heart function.

Complete blood cell counts.

▷ **While Taking This Drug, Observe the Following**

Foods: No restrictions. Avoid excessive salt intake.

Beverages: No restrictions. May be taken with milk.

▷ *Alcohol:* Alcohol may exaggerate this drug's ability to lower the blood pressure and may increase its mild sedative effect.

Tobacco Smoking: Nicotine may reduce this drug's benefit in treating high blood pressure. In addition, high doses of this drug may worsen constriction of the bronchial tubes caused by regular smoking.

▷ *Other Drugs*

Penbutolol may *increase* the effects of

- other antihypertensive drugs, and cause excessive lowering of the blood pressure. Dosage adjustments may be necessary.
- reserpine (Ser-Ap-Es, etc.), and cause sedation, depression, slowing of the heart rate and lowering of the blood pressure. This combination is best avoided.
- verapamil (Calan, Isoptin), and cause excessive depression of heart function; monitor this combination closely.

Penbutolol may *decrease* the effects of

- epinephrine resulting in decreased benefit when used to correct allergic reactions. Slow heartbeat and elevated blood pressure may also occur.

Penbutolol *taken concurrently* with

- amiodarone (Codarone) may result in sinus arrest or symptomatic bradycardia. DO NOT combine these medicines.
- clonidine (Catapres) requires close monitoring for rebound high blood pressure if clonidine is withdrawn while penbutolol is still being taken.
- fluvoxamine (Luvox) may cause very slow heart beat (bradycardia) and excessive lowering of blood pressure.
- insulin or oral hypoglycemic agents requires close monitoring to avoid undetected hypoglycemia (see Glossary).
- venlafaxine (Effexor) may result in increased risk of toxicity from penbutolol.

The following drugs may *increase* the effects of penbutolol

- methimazole (Tapazole).
- birth control pills (oral contraceptives).
- propylthiouracil (Propacil).

The following drugs may *decrease* the effects of penbutolol

- barbiturates (phenobarbital, etc.).
- indomethacin (Indocin), and possibly other "aspirin substitutes," or NSAIDs may impair penbutolol's antihypertensive effect.
- rifampin (Rifadin, Rimactane).

▷ *Driving, Hazardous Activities:* Use caution until the full extent of fatigue, dizziness and blood pressure change have been determined.

Aviation Note: The use of this drug *is a disqualification* for piloting. Consult a designated Aviation Medical Examiner.

Exposure to Sun: No restrictions.

Exposure to Heat: Hot environments can lower the blood pressure and exaggerate the effects of this drug.

Exposure to Cold: Cold environments can worsen the circulatory deficiency in the extremities that may occur with this drug. The elderly should take precautions to prevent hypothermia (see Glossary).

Heavy Exercise or Exertion: Avoid exertion that produces light-headedness, excessive fatigue or muscle cramping. The use of this drug may intensify the hypertensive response to isometric exercise.

Occurrence of Unrelated Illness: Fever can lower the blood pressure and require adjustment of dosage. Nausea or vomiting may interrupt the regular dosage schedule. Ask your physician for guidance.

Discontinuation: It is advisable to avoid sudden discontinuation of this drug in all situations. If possible, gradual reduction of dose over a period of 2 to 3 weeks is recommended. Ask your physician for specific guidance.

PENICILLAMINE (pen i SIL a meen)

Introduced: 1963   **Prescription:** USA: Yes; Canada: Yes   **Available as Generic:** USA: No; Canada: No   **Class:** antiarthritic   **Controlled Drug:** USA: No; Canada: No

Brand Names: Cuprimine, Depen

BENEFITS versus RISKS	
Possible Benefits	*Possible Risks*
EFFECTIVE TREATMENT OF WILSON'S DISEASE (COPPER TOXICITY)	SEVERE ALLERGIC REACTIONS BONE MARROW DEPRESSION Drug-induced damage of lungs, liver, pancreas, and kidneys
Effective treatment of cystinuria and cystine kidney stones	
Partially effective treatment of rheumatoid arthritis and poisoning due to heavy metals: iron, lead, mercury, and zinc	

▷ **Principal Uses**

As a Single Drug Product: Uses currently included in FDA approved labeling: Treatment of (1) Wilson's disease (copper toxicity of brain, cornea, liver and kidneys); (2) severe rheumatoid arthritis that has failed to respond to less hazardous conventional treatment; also helps rheumatoid arthritis which presents with interstitial lung disease; (3) cystinuria and cystine stone formation (excessive amounts of cystine in the urine).

Other (unlabeled) generally accepted uses: (1) Treatment of heavy metal poisoning, especially that due to lead and mercury; (2) may help increase survival in scleroderma; (3) eases progression of systemic sclerosis.

How This Drug Works: In Wilson's disease and heavy metal poisoning—this drug chelates (bonds tightly to) copper, iron, lead, mercury and zinc (in body tissues) to form soluble compounds that are readily extracted and excreted in the urine.

In rheumatoid arthritis—this drug favorably modifies the abnormal immune reactions within joint structures that cause inflammation, swelling, pain and tissue destruction.

In cystinuria—this drug combines with cystine to form a compound that is readily excreted in the urine. The reduction of cystine concentrations prevents the formation of cystine stones in the urinary tract.

Available Dosage Forms and Strengths

Capsules — 125 mg, 250 mg

Tablets — 250 mg

▷ **Recommended Dosage Ranges** (Actual dosage and administration schedule must be determined by the physician for each patient individually.)

Infants and Children: For Wilson's disease: From 6 months to 12 years of age—20 mg/kg of body weight daily, in 4 divided doses.

For rheumatoid arthritis: Initially 3 mg/kg of body weight (up to 250 mg) daily, in 2 divided doses, for 3 months; then 6 mg/kg of body weight (up to 500 mg) daily, in 2 divided doses, for 3 months; as needed and tolerated, gradually increase dose to a maximum of 10 mg/kg of body weight daily, in 3 to 4 divided doses.

For cystinuria: 30 mg/kg of body weight daily, in 4 divided doses.

For lead poisoning: 25 to 40 mg/kg of body weight daily, in 2 to 3 divided doses.

12 to 60 Years of Age: For Wilson's disease: 250 mg 4 times daily.

For rheumatoid arthritis: Initially 125 or 250 mg once daily as a single dose; increase dose gradually, as needed and tolerated, by 125 or 250 mg daily at intervals of 2 to 3 months. The total daily dose should not exceed 1000 mg for small individuals, 1500 mg for large individuals.

For cystinuria and cystine stones: 500 mg 4 times daily.

For heavy metal poisoning (such as lead): 500 mg to 1500 mg daily for 1 to 2 months.

Over 60 Years of Age: Initially 125 mg daily; gradually increase dose, as needed and tolerated, by 125 mg daily at intervals of 2 to 3 months. The total daily dose should not exceed 750 mg.

Conditions Requiring Dosing Adjustments

Liver function: Dosage adjustments do not appear to be needed. This drug is a rare cause of liver toxicity, and should be used with caution in patients with compromised livers.

Kidney function: In patients with moderate to severe kidney failure, the drug should **not** be given. It is also a cause of kidney problems (nephropathy and renal failure), and should be used as a benefit to risk decision in patients with compromised kidneys.

▷ **Dosing Instructions:**   Take this drug on an empty stomach, 1 hour before or 2 hours after eating. The capsule may be opened and the tablet may be crushed for administration.

Usual Duration of Use: Use on a regular schedule for 2 to 3 months determines benefit in relieving the symptoms of Wilson's disease or rheumatoid arthritis. Long-term use (months to years) requires periodic physician evaluation.

▷ **This Drug Should Not Be Taken If**

- you have had an allergic reaction to it previously.
- you are pregnant and using this drug to treat rheumatoid arthritis or cystinuria.

- you currently have a bone marrow or blood cell disorder.
- you are currently taking drugs for malaria, gold therapy or other cytotoxic drugs.
- you have active liver disease.

▷ **Inform Your Physician Before Taking This Drug If**
- you are allergic to any type of penicillin.
- you have a history of drug-induced bone marrow depression.
- you have a history of myasthenia gravis, pancreatitis, peptic ulcer disease or systemic lupus erythematosus.
- you have impaired liver or kidney function.
- you are planning pregnancy.
- you are taking any type of gold or immune-suppressant drugs.
- you are planning surgery or dental procedures in the near future.

Possible Side Effects (natural, expected, and unavoidable drug actions)
Deficiency of pyridoxine (vitamin B_6): optic neuritis (eye pain, blurred vision); peripheral neuritis (pain, numbness, tingling in extremities).

▷ **Possible Adverse Effects** (unusual, unexpected, and infrequent reactions)
If any of the following develop, consult your physician promptly for guidance.

Mild Adverse Effects
Allergic Reactions: Skin rash, hives, itching.
Blurred vision.
Ringing or buzzing in ears.
Loss of appetite, mouth sores, altered taste, nausea, vomiting, stomach pain, diarrhea.

Serious Adverse Effects
Allergic Reactions: Severe dermatitis, fever, joint pain, swollen lymph glands.
Bone marrow depression (see Glossary) (if it occurs, happens after several months of therapy—isolated cases only).
Very, very, rare leukemia (one case of acute lymphoblastic reported).
Bronchiolitis (cough, wheezing, shortness of breath).
Lung toxicity (pulmonary bleeding, Goodpasture's syndrome, or alveolitis).
Abnormal muscle quivering (fasciculation).
Hepatitis with jaundice (see Glossary).
Pancreatitis (fever, severe stomach pain, nausea, vomiting).
Peptic ulcer, stomach or duodenum.
Drug-induced porphyria.
Kidney damage (cloudy/bloody urine, swelling of face, legs, feet).
Protein in the urine.
Myasthenia gravis syndrome (extreme muscle weakness, difficulty breathing, chewing, swallowing, talking; double vision).
Systemic lupus erythematosus (SLE) syndrome (skin rash, skin blisters, fever, fatigue, chest pain, joint pain).

▷ **Possible Effects on Sexual Function:** Swelling and tenderness of male breast tissue.

Possible Delayed Adverse Effects: None reported.

▷ **Adverse Effects That May Mimic Natural Diseases or Disorders**
Drug-induced hepatitis may suggest viral hepatitis.
Myasthenia gravis syndrome.
Systemic lupus erythematosus (SLE) syndrome.

Natural Diseases or Disorders That May Be Activated by This Drug
Peptic ulcer, hemolytic anemia.

Possible Effects on Laboratory Tests
Complete blood cell counts: decreased red cells, hemoglobin, white cells and platelets; increased eosinophils.
Blood LE cells: positive.
Liver function tests: increased liver enzymes (ALT/GPT, AST/GOT and alkaline phosphatase), increased bilirubin.
Kidney function tests: increased blood urea nitrogen (BUN) and creatinine levels; increased urine protein content.
Partial Thromboplastin Time (PTT): Decreased.
Urine copper: increased.

CAUTION
1. Ask your doctor if you need pyridoxine (vitamin B_6) to prevent optic neuritis and peripheral neuritis. The recommended amount is 25 mg daily.
2. Comply fully with your physician's request for periodic laboratory tests: blood counts, liver and kidney function tests.
3. Report promptly any indications of bone marrow depression: unusual fatigue or weakness, fever or sore throat, abnormal bleeding or bruising.
4. Do not interrupt your regular, continual dosing of this drug; even brief periods of interruption may cause significant allergic reactions following resumption of treatment. If dosing is interrupted for any reason, it should be resumed with small doses and gradually increased until the previous full dosage is restored.
5. If you are to have surgery, reduce the dose of this drug to 250 mg daily until your wound is fully healed. This drug can impair or delay wound healing.

Precautions for Use
By Infants and Children: Safety and effectiveness for those under 6 months of age not established.
By Those over 60 Years of Age: May have increased levels of bone marrow depression while using this drug. Report promptly any indication of unusual fatigability, infection, bruising or bleeding.

▷ **Advisability of Use During Pregnancy**
Pregnancy Category: D. See Pregnancy Code at the back of this book.
Animal studies: Rat studies reveal drug-induced cleft palates and skeletal defects.
Human studies: Adequate studies of pregnant women are not available. Birth defects have been reported in infants born to mothers with rheumatoid arthritis or cystinuria who took this drug during pregnancy.
If you have rheumatoid arthritis, do not use this drug. If you have cystinuria, avoid this drug if possible. If you have Wilson's disease, limit the daily dose to 1000 mg; if cesarean section is planned, limit the daily dose to 250 mg during the last 6 weeks of pregnancy and following delivery until wound healing is complete.

Advisability of Use if Breast-Feeding
Presence of this drug in breast milk: Unknown.
Avoid drug or refrain from nursing.

Habit-Forming Potential: None.

Effects of Overdosage: Nausea, vomiting, diarrhea, stomach pain.

Possible Effects of Long-Term Use: Increased risk of bone marrow depression, liver or kidney damage.

Suggested Periodic Examinations While Taking This Drug (at physician's discretion)

Complete blood cell counts every 2 weeks during the first 6 months of treatment; then monthly thereafter.

Urinalysis every 2 weeks during the first 6 months of treatment; then monthly thereafter.

Liver and kidney function tests every 6 months during the first 18 months of treatment.

▷ **While Taking This Drug, Observe the Following**

Foods: Follow the diet prescribed by your physician.

Nutritional Support: Recommended daily supplement of pyridoxine (vitamin B_6)—25 mg.

Beverages: Do not take this drug with milk.

▷ *Alcohol:* No interactions expected.

Tobacco Smoking: No interactions expected.

▷ *Other Drugs*

Penicillamine may *decrease* the effects of
- digoxin (Lanoxin).

The following drugs may *increase* the effects of penicillamine
- chloroquine (Aralen).
- indomethacin (Indocin) and perhaps other NSAIDs.

The following drugs may *decrease* the effects of penicillamine
- all antacids containing aluminum and/or magnesium.
- iron preparations.
- probenecid (Benemid).
- sucralfate (Carafate).

Penicillamine *taken concurrently with*
- birth control pills (oral contraceptives) can result in breast swelling and tenderness.
- gold (Auranofin) may result in increased bone marrow depression and rashes.
- heparin may result in decreased therapeutic benefit.

▷ *Driving, Hazardous Activities:* No restrictions.

Aviation Note: The use of this drug *may be a disqualification* for piloting. Consult a designated Aviation Medical Examiner.

Exposure to Sun: No restrictions.

Discontinuation: To be determined by your physician. Do not stop this drug without your physician's knowledge and guidance.

PENICILLIN V (pen i SIL in VEE)

Introduced: 1953   **Prescription:** USA: Yes; Canada: Yes   **Available as Generic:** USA: Yes; Canada: Yes   **Class:** Antibiotic, penicillins   **Controlled Drug:** USA: No; Canada: No

Brand Names: ✦Apo-Pen-VK, Beepen VK, Betapen-VK, Ledercillin VK, ✦Nadopen-V, ✦Novopen-VK, ✦Nu-Pen-VK, Penapar VK, Pen-V, ✦Pen-Vee, Pen-Vee K, Pfizerpen VK, ✦PVF, ✦PVF K, Robicillin VK, SK-Penicillin VK, Uticillin VK, V-Cillin K, ✦VC-K 500, Veetids

---

BENEFITS versus RISKS

Possible Benefits	*Possible Risks*
EFFECTIVE TREATMENT OF INFECTIONS due to susceptible microorganisms	ALLERGIC REACTIONS, mild to severe Superinfections (yeast) Drug-induced colitis

---

▷ **Principal Uses**

As a Single Drug Product: Uses currently included in FDA approved labeling: (1) Used to treat responsive infections of the upper and lower respiratory tract, the middle ear and the skin; (2) helps prevent rheumatic fever and bacterial endocarditis in people with valvular heart disease.

Other (unlabeled) generally accepted uses: (1) Combination therapy of animal bite wounds; (2) treatment of stage one Lyme disease in children; (3) therapy of Lyme disease involving the central nervous system; (4) can have a role in treating dental abscesses.

How This Drug Works: This drug destroys susceptible infecting bacteria by interfering with their ability to produce new protective cell walls as they multiply and grow.

Available Dosage Forms and Strengths

Oral solution — 125 mg, 250 mg per 5-ml

Tablets — 125 mg, 250 mg, 500 mg

▷ **Usual Adult Dosage Range:** Dosage is based upon sensitivity testing of the bacteria causing the infection, the severity of the infection and response of the patient. Depending upon the specific infection, the dosage range is 125 to 500 mg/6 to 8 hours. For the prevention of bacterial endocarditis: 2 grams (2000 mg) taken 1 hour before the procedure, followed by 1 gram 6 hours later. The total daily dosage should not exceed 7 grams (7000 mg). **Note: Actual dosage and administration schedule must be determined by the physician for each patient individually.**

Conditions Requiring Dosing Adjustments

Liver function: Dosage adjustments do not appear to be needed.

Kidney function: In patients with renal compromise, no more than 250 mg should be given every 6 hours.

▷ **Dosing Instructions:** The tablet may be crushed and taken on an empty stomach or with food or milk. Absorption may be slightly faster if taken when stomach is empty.

Usual Duration of Use: For all streptococcal infections—not less than 10 consecutive days (without interruption) to reduce the possibility of developing rheumatic fever or glomerulonephritis. For all other infections—as long as necessary to eradicate the infection. Talk with your doctor before stopping therapy if you feel you must stop this medicine. Incomplete treatment may lead to serious resistance and aggressive infections requiring combination therapy.

▷ **This Drug Should Not Be Taken If**
- you have had an allergic reaction to any dosage form of it previously.
- you are certain you are allergic to **any** form of penicillin.

▷ **Inform Your Physician Before Taking This Drug If**
- you suspect you may be allergic to penicillin or you have a history of a previous "reaction" of any type to penicillin.
- you are allergic to any cephalosporin antibiotic (Ancef, Anspor, Ceclor, Ceporan, Ceporex, Kafocin, Keflex, Keflin, Kefzol, Loridine, Ultracef, Velosef; see Drug Classes).
- you are allergic by nature (hay fever, asthma, hives, eczema).

Possible Side Effects (natural, expected, and unavoidable drug actions)
Superinfections (see Glossary), often due to yeast organisms.

▷ **Possible Adverse Effects** (unusual, unexpected, and infrequent reactions)
If any of the following develop, consult your physician promptly for guidance.
Mild Adverse Effects
Allergic Reactions: Skin rashes, hives, itching.
Irritations of mouth and tongue, "black tongue," nausea, vomiting, mild diarrhea, dizziness (rare).
Serious Adverse Effects
Allergic Reactions: Anaphylactic reaction (see Glossary), severe skin reactions, drug fever, swollen painful joints, sore throat, abnormal bleeding or bruising.
Severe skin reactions (Stevens-Johnson syndrome, bullous pemphigoid).
Rare drug-induced colitis.
Rare hemolytic anemia.
Drug-induced periarteritis nodosa (rare).
Rare drug-induced meningitis.
Rare drug-induced porphyria.
Rare abnormal liver function.

▷ **Possible Effects on Sexual Function:**   None reported.

Possible Effects on Laboratory Tests
Complete blood counts: decreased red cells, hemoglobin, white cells and platelets; increased eosinophils (allergic reaction).
Prothrombin time: occasionally increased.
Liver function tests: increased aspartate aminotransferase (AST/GOT) and bilirubin.

CAUTION
1. Take the exact dose and the full course prescribed.
2. If this drug must be used concurrently with antibiotics like erythromycin or tetracycline, give the penicillin first.

Precautions for Use
By Infants and Children: Observe the allergic child closely for evidence of a developing allergy to penicillin. This drug may cause diarrhea, which sometimes necessitates discontinuation.

By Those over 60 Years of Age: Natural changes in the skin may predispose to prolonged itching reactions in the genital and anal regions. Report such reactions promptly.

▷ **Advisability of Use During Pregnancy**
Pregnancy Category: B. See Pregnancy Code at the back of this book.
Animal studies: Birth defects of the limbs reported in mice. (Not confirmed in other studies.)
Human studies: Adequate studies of pregnant women indicate no increased risk of birth defects in 3546 pregnancies exposed to penicillin derivatives.
This drug is considered safe for use during any period of pregnancy.

Advisability of Use if Breast-Feeding
Presence of this drug in breast milk: Yes.
The nursing infant may be sensitized to penicillin and be at risk for developing diarrhea or yeast infections.
Avoid drug if possible or refrain from nursing.

Habit-Forming Potential: None.

Effects of Overdosage: Possible nausea, vomiting and/or diarrhea.

Possible Effects of Long-Term Use: Superinfections, often due to yeast organisms.

Suggested Periodic Examinations While Taking This Drug (at physician's discretion)
Complete blood cell counts, kidney function tests.

▷ **While Taking This Drug, Observe the Following**
Foods: No restrictions.
Beverages: No restrictions. May be taken with milk.
▷ *Alcohol:* No interactions expected.
Tobacco Smoking: No interactions expected.
▷ *Other Drugs*
Penicillamine *taken concurrently with*
• aminoglycoside antibiotics (see Drug Classes) may blunt or inactivate the aminoglycoside and decrease the therapeutic benefit it would otherwise confer.
• probenecid (Benemid) will increase and sustain blood levels. This interaction is often used to therapeutic advantage.
Penicillin V may *decrease* the effects of
• birth control pills (oral contraceptives), and impair their effectiveness in preventing pregnancy.
The following drugs may *decrease* the effects of penicillin V
• antacids may reduce the absorption of penicillin V.
• chloramphenicol (Chloromycetin).
• erythromycin (Erythrocin, E-Mycin, etc.).
• tetracyclines (Achromycin, Declomycin, Minocin, etc.). (See Drug Class Section.)
▷ *Driving, Hazardous Activities:* Usually no restrictions. Be alert to the rare occurrence of dizziness and/or nausea, and restrict activities accordingly.
Aviation Note: The use of this drug *may be a disqualification* for piloting. Consult a designated Aviation Medical Examiner.
Exposure to Sun: No restrictions.

Special Storage Instructions: Oral solutions should be refrigerated.

Observe the Following Expiration Times: Do not take the oral solution of this drug if older than 7 days when kept at room temperature or 14 days when kept refrigerated.

PENTAZOCINE (pen TAZ oh seen)

Introduced: 1967   **Prescription:** USA: Yes; Canada: Yes   **Available as Generic:** USA: No; Canada: No   **Class:** Analgesic, strong   **Controlled Drug:** USA: C-IV*; Canada: No

Brand Names: Talacen [CD], Talwin, Talwin Compound [CD], ✦Talwin Compound-50 [CD], Talwin Nx [CD]

BENEFITS versus RISKS

Possible Benefits	*Possible Risks*
EFFECTIVE RELIEF OF MODERATE TO SEVERE PAIN	POTENTIAL FOR HABIT FORMATION (DEPENDENCE) Respiratory depression Sedative effects Mental and behavioral disturbances Low blood pressure, fainting Nausea, constipation

---

▷ **Principal Uses**

As a Single Drug Product: Uses currently included in FDA approved labeling: (1) Relieves acute or chronic pain of moderate to severe degree from any cause. Other (unlabeled) generally accepted uses: None.

As a Combination Drug Product [CD]: Pentazocine is available in combinations with acetaminophen and with aspirin. These milder pain relievers are added to enhance the analgesic effect and to reduce fever when present. In the United States the tablet form of pentazocine also contains naloxone (Talwin Nx), a narcotic antagonist that renders the drug ineffective if abused.

How This Drug Works: Acting primarily as a depressant of certain brain functions, this drug suppresses the perception of pain and calms the emotional response to pain.

Available Dosage Forms and Strengths

Injection — 30 mg per ml
Tablets — 50 mg (Canada)
Tablets — 50 mg with 0.5 mg of naloxone (USA)

▷ **Usual Adult Dosage Range:** Oral dosing: 50 mg every 3 to 4 hours. May be increased to 100 mg every 4 hours for severe pain. The total daily dosage should not exceed 600 mg. Many clinicians now use timed or scheduled dosing of pain medicines (analgesics) particularly early in acute pain as this tends to prevent pain rather than treat it. Others revert to as-needed dosing once the acute pain is controlled. **Note: Actual dosage and administra-**

*See Schedules of Controlled Drugs at the back of this book.

tion schedule must be determined by the physician for each patient individually.

Conditions Requiring Dosing Adjustments

Liver function: Doses should be decreased or the time between doses lengthened, otherwise increased adverse effects may occur.

Kidney function: For moderate to severe kidney failure, the dose should be reduced by 25–50%.

▷ **Dosing Instructions:** The tablet may be crushed and taken with or following food to reduce stomach irritation or nausea.

Usual Duration of Use: As required to control pain. Continual use should not exceed 5 to 7 days without interruption and reassessment of need.

▷ **This Drug Should Not Be Taken If**
- you have had an allergic reaction to any dosage form of it previously.
- you are having an acute attack of asthma.
- you have increased intracranial pressure or brain damage.

▷ **Inform Your Physician Before Taking This Drug If**
- you have had an unfavorable reaction to any narcotic drug in the past.
- you have a history of drug abuse or alcoholism.
- you have chronic lung disease with impaired breathing.
- you have impaired liver or kidney function.
- you have a history of confusion or hallucinations.
- you have gallbladder disease, a seizure disorder or an underactive thyroid gland.
- you have difficulty emptying the urinary bladder.
- you are taking any other drugs that have a sedative effect.
- you plan to have surgery under general anesthesia in the near future.

Possible Side Effects (natural, expected, and unavoidable drug actions)
Drowsiness, light-headedness, weakness, urinary retention, constipation.

▷ **Possible Adverse Effects** (unusual, unexpected, and infrequent reactions)
If any of the following develop, consult your physician promptly for guidance.

Mild Adverse Effects
Allergic Reactions: Skin rash, hives, itching, swelling of face.
Headache, dizziness, impaired concentration, sensation of drunkenness, blurred or double vision, flushing, sweating.
Increased or decreased blood pressure.
Drug fever (rare).
Nausea, vomiting, indigestion, diarrhea.

Serious Adverse Effects
Marked drop in blood pressure, possible fainting.
Impaired breathing (respiratory depression): use with caution in chronic lung disease.
Mental and behavioral disturbances, hallucinations, psychosis.
Drug-induced seizure (rare).
Drug-induced porphyria (rare).
Toxic epidermal necrolysis (rare).
Fibrous muscle replacement (with injection form) (rare).
Rare kidney problems.

Fixed positioning of the eyes (oculogyric crisis) (rare).

Bone marrow depression (see Glossary) of a mild and reversible nature (rare).

Aggravation of prostatism (see Glossary).

▷ **Possible Effects on Sexual Function:**   Blunting of sexual response.

Natural Diseases or Disorders That May Be Activated by This Drug

Porphyria (see Glossary).

Possible Effects on Laboratory Tests

White blood cell count: rarely decreased.

Blood amylase and lipase levels: increased (natural side effects).

CAUTION

1. Use of this drug with atropinelike drugs may increase the risk of urinary retention and reduced intestinal function.
2. Do not take this drug following acute head injury.

Precautions for Use

By Infants and Children: Safety and effectiveness for those under 12 years of age not established.

By Those over 60 Years of Age: Use small doses initially and increase dosage as needed and tolerated. Limit use to short-term treatment only. There may be increased susceptibility to development of drowsiness, dizziness, unsteadiness, falling, urinary retention and constipation.

▷ **Advisability of Use During Pregnancy**

Pregnancy Category: C (B or D in high dose at term or extended use). See Pregnancy Code at the back of this book.

Animal studies: Significant birth defects reported in hamsters.

Human studies: Adequate studies of pregnant women are not available. Pentazocine taken repeatedly during the last few weeks before delivery may cause withdrawal symptoms in the newborn infant.

Avoid this drug during the first 3 months. Use only if clearly needed and in small, infrequent doses during the last 6 months.

Advisability of Use if Breast-Feeding

Presence of this drug in breast milk: Expected.

Avoid drug or refrain from nursing.

Habit-Forming Potential: Psychological and/or physical dependence can develop.

Effects of Overdosage: Anxiety, disturbed thoughts, hallucinations, progressive drowsiness, stupor, depressed breathing.

Possible Effects of Long-Term Use: Psychological and physical dependence, chronic constipation.

Suggested Periodic Examinations While Taking This Drug (at physician's discretion)

Complete blood cell counts, if used for an extended period of time.

▷ **While Taking This Drug, Observe the Following**

Foods: No restrictions.

Beverages: No restrictions. May be taken with milk.

▷   *Alcohol:* Pentazocine can intensify the intoxicating effects of alcohol, and alcohol can intensify the depressant effects of pentazocine on brain function, breathing and circulation. Best to avoid combination.

Tobacco Smoking: Heavy smoking may reduce the effectiveness of pentazocine and make larger doses necessary.

Marijuana Smoking: Increase in drowsiness and pain relief; impairment of mental and physical performance.

▷ *Other Drugs*

Pentazocine may ***increase*** the effects of
- other drugs with sedative effects (see Drug Classes on benzodiazepines, phenothiazines and opioids).
- atropinelike drugs, and increase the risk of constipation and urinary retention.
- cyclosporine (Sandimmune) and cause toxicity.
- MAO inhibitors (see Drug Classes) may result in muscle rigidity.

▷ *Driving, Hazardous Activities:* This drug can impair mental alertness, judgment, reaction time and physical coordination. Avoid hazardous activities accordingly.

Aviation Note: The use of this drug ***is a disqualification*** for piloting. Consult a designated Aviation Medical Examiner.

Exposure to Sun: No restrictions.

Discontinuation: It is advisable to limit this drug to short-term use. If it is necessary to use it for extended periods of time, discontinuation should be gradual to minimize possible effects of withdrawal.

PENTOXIFYLLINE (pen tox I fi leen)

Other Name: Oxpentifylline

Introduced: 1972   **Prescription:** USA: Yes; Canada: Yes   **Available as Generic:** No   **Class:** Blood flow agent, xanthines   **Controlled Drug:** USA: No; Canada: No

Brand Name: Trental

BENEFITS versus RISKS	
Possible Benefits	*Possible Risks*
IMPROVED BLOOD FLOW IN PERIPHERAL ARTERIAL DISEASE	Reduced blood pressure, angina, abnormal heart rhythms
REDUCTION OF INTERMITTENT CLAUDICATION PAIN	Rare low blood counts and aplastic anemia
	Indigestion, nausea, vomiting
	Dizziness, flushing

▷ **Principal Uses**

As a Single Drug Product: Uses currently included in FDA approved labeling: (1) Adjunctive treatment in the management of peripheral obstructive arterial disease to improve arterial blood flow and reduce frequency and severity of muscle pain due to intermittent claudication.

Other (unlabeled) generally accepted uses: (1) Decreases hemodialysis shunt clots (thrombosis); (2) may have a role in treating impotence which is caused by blood vessel problems (vascular impotence); (3) can increase the motility of sperm; (4) helps decrease interleukin 6 and tumor necrosis factor in patients with cerebral malaria; (5) has had variable results in AIDS patients in attempting to halt weight loss which may be caused by tumor necrosis factor; (6) may ease skin tightening in some cases; (7) has been used to relieve symptoms of septic shock; (8) has been used to help heal refractory ulcers in diabetics; (9) can help decrease insulin requirements in diabetics.

How This Drug Works: Improves blood flow and increases oxygen supply to working muscles by way of three mechanisms: (1) reduction of blood viscosity due to decreased levels of fibrinogen in the blood; (2) increased flexibility of the red blood cells (carrying oxygen) due to an increase in cyclic AMP (enzyme) within red blood cells; this permits easier passage through the small blood vessels of the microcirculation; and (3) prevention of red blood cell and platelet aggregation.

Inhibits interleukin-6 and tumor necrosis factor.

Available Dosage Forms and Strengths

Tablets, prolonged-action — 400 mg

▷ **Usual Adult Dosage Range:** 400 mg 3 times/day. If adverse nervous system or gastrointestinal effects occur, reduce the dose to 400 mg twice/day. **Note: Actual dosage and administration schedule must be determined by the physician for each patient individually.**

Conditions Requiring Dosing Adjustments

Liver function: Dosing changes do not appear to be needed in liver compromise.
Kidney function: The dose should be empirically decreased in patients with compromised kidneys.

▷ **Dosing Instructions:** Take with or following food to reduce stomach irritation. Swallow the tablet whole without breaking, crushing or chewing.

Usual Duration of Use: Use on a regular schedule for 2 to 4 weeks determines effectiveness in preventing or delaying the pains of intermittent claudication associated with walking. Treatment for a minimum of 3 months is recommended to determine full effectiveness. Long-term use (months to years) requires physician supervision and periodic evaluation.

Possible Advantages of This Drug

Reduces blood viscosity and thereby improves blood flow through small vessels.

Increases supply of oxygen to working muscles.

▷ **This Drug Should Not Be Taken If**
- you have had an allergic reaction to it previously.

▷ **Inform Your Physician Before Taking This Drug If**
- you are allergic to other xanthine drugs: caffeine, theophylline, theobromine.
- you have impaired kidney function.
- you have low blood pressure, impaired brain circulation or coronary artery disease.
- you are a diabetic.
- you smoke tobacco.
- you are taking any antihypertensive drugs.

Possible Side Effects (natural, expected, and unavoidable drug actions)

Usually none with recommended doses.

▷ **Possible Adverse Effects** (unusual, unexpected, and infrequent reactions)
If any of the following develop, consult your physician promptly for guidance.
Mild Adverse Effects
Allergic Reaction: Skin rash.
Headache (rare), blurred vision and scotoma (rare), dizziness (rare), tremor.
May worsen glucose control in diabetics.
Nosebleeds (rare).
Flu-like syndrome (rare). Indigestion, nausea, vomiting (rare).
Serious Adverse Effects
Development of angina or heart rhythm disorders in the presence of coronary artery disease.
Liver toxicity (rare).
Rare low platelets, white blood cells, or all cells (rare).
Rare auditory hallucinations.
Retinal bleeding (rare).

▷ **Possible Effects on Sexual Function**
May help reverse impotence caused by circulatory problems.

Possible Effects on Laboratory Tests
Complete blood cell counts: rarely decreased red cells, hemoglobin, white cells and platelets.

CAUTION
Use this drug with caution in the presence of impaired circulation within the brain (cerebral arteriosclerosis) or coronary artery disease. If any related symptoms develop, consult your physician for prompt evaluation.

Precautions for Use
By Infants and Children: Safety and effectiveness for those under 18 years of age not established. Use by this age group is not anticipated.
By Those over 60 Years of Age: You may be more susceptible to the adverse effects listed. Observe closely for any indications of dizziness or chest pain and report these promptly.

▷ **Advisability of Use During Pregnancy**
Pregnancy Category: C. See Pregnancy Code at the back of this book.
Animal studies: Increased fetal resorptions reported in rats, but no birth defects found in rats or rabbits.
Human studies: Adequate studies of pregnant women are not available.
Avoid use during the first 3 months. Use otherwise only if clearly needed.

Advisability of Use if Breast-Feeding
Presence of this drug in breast milk: Yes.
Avoid drug or refrain from nursing.

Habit-Forming Potential: None.

Effects of Overdosage: Drowsiness, flushing, faintness, excitement, seizures.

Possible Effects of Long-Term Use: None reported.

Suggested Periodic Examinations While Taking This Drug (at physician's discretion)
Blood pressure measurements, evaluation of heart status.

▷ **While Taking This Drug, Observe the Following**
  Foods: No restrictions.
  Beverages: No restrictions. May be taken with milk.
▷ *Alcohol:* Alcohol may increase the blood-pressure-lowering effect of this drug.
  Tobacco Smoking: Nicotine constricts arteries and will impair the effectiveness
    of this drug significantly. Avoid all use of tobacco.
▷ *Other Drugs*
    Pentoxifylline may *increase* the effects of
    • antihypertensive drugs, and cause excessive lowering of blood pressure.
    • warfarin (Coumadin, etc.), and increase the possibility of unwanted bleed-
      ing; monitor INR (prothrombin times) more frequently. Dosing should be
      adjusted to laboratory values.
    Pentoxifylline *taken concurrently* with
    • cimetidine (Tagamet), nizatidine(Axid), famotidine (Pepcid) or ranitidine
      (Zantac) may result in pentoxifylline toxicity (increases drug absorption).
    • theophylline (Theodur, others) may result in theophylline toxicity.
▷ *Driving, Hazardous Activities:* This drug may cause drowsiness or dizziness. Re-
    strict activities as necessary.
  Aviation Note: The use of this drug *may be a disqualification* for piloting. Con-
    sult a designated Aviation Medical Examiner.
  Exposure to Sun: No restrictions.

PERGOLIDE (PER go lide)

Introduced: 1980   **Prescription:** USA: Yes   **Available as Generic:**
USA: No   **Class:** Antiparkinsonism, ergot derivative   **Controlled Drug:**
USA: No
Brand Name: Permax

BENEFITS versus RISKS	
Possible Benefits	*Possible Risks*
ADDITIVE RELIEF OF SYMPTOMS OF PARKINSON'S DISEASE when used concurrently with levodopa/carbidopa PERMITS A REDUCTION IN SINEMET DOSAGE	ABNORMAL INVOLUNTARY MOVEMENTS HALLUCINATIONS INITIAL FALL IN BLOOD PRESSURE/ORTHOSTATIC HYPOTENSION Premature heart contractions (ventricular)

▷ **Principal Uses**
  As a Single Drug Product: Uses currently included in FDA approved labeling: (1)
    As an adjunct to levodopa/carbidopa treatment of Parkinson's disease for
    people who experience intolerable abnormal movements (dyskinesia) and/
    or increasing "on-off" episodes due to levodopa. The addition of pergolide
    (1) permits reduction of the daily dose of levodopa with consequent lessen-
    ing of dyskinesia and erratic drug response, and (2) provides additional
    relief of parkinsonian symptoms.
  Other (unlabeled) generally accepted uses: (1) May have a role in helping re-

duce drug craving in cocaine withdrawal; (2) helps in some conditions where excess prolactin is made; (3) may be of use in acromegaly.

How This Drug Works: By directly stimulating part of the brain (dopamine receptor sites in the corpus striatum), this drug helps to compensate for the deficiency of dopamine that is responsible for the rigidity, tremor and sluggish movement characteristic of Parkinson's disease.

Available Dosage Forms and Strengths

Tablets — 0.05 mg, 0.25 mg, 1 mg

▷ **Usual Adult Dosage Range**

Parkinson's (in conjunction with levodopa plus carbidopa): initially 0.05 mg daily for the first 2 days; gradually increase the daily dose by 0.1 mg or 0.15 mg every third day over the next 12 days. If needed and tolerated, the daily dose may be increased further by 0.25 mg every third day until an optimal response is achieved. The total daily dosage should be divided into 3 equal portions and given at 6 to 8 hour intervals. The usual maintenance dose is 3 mg/24 hours; do not exceed 5 mg/24 hours.

During the gradual introduction of pergolide, the concurrent dose of levodopa/carbidopa (Sinemet) may be cautiously decreased in accord with your physician's instructions.

Note: Actual dosage and administration schedule must be determined by the physician for each patient individually.

Conditions Requiring Dosing Adjustments

Liver function: Specific guidelines for liver compromise are not available. It should be used with caution.

Kidney function: Consideration should be given to empiric decreases in dosage.

▷ **Dosing Instructions:**   The tablet may be crushed and taken with food or milk to reduce stomach irritation.

Usual Duration of Use: Use on a regular schedule for 4 to 6 weeks determines effectiveness in controlling the symptoms of Parkinson's disease and permitting reduction of levodopa/carbidopa dosage. Long-term use (months to years) requires periodic physician evaluation of response.

Possible Advantages of This Drug: It may provide a more effective and uniform control of parkinsonian symptoms and a reduction of some adverse effects of long-term levodopa therapy.

▷ **This Drug Should Not Be Taken If**

• you have had an allergic reaction to it previously.
• you have had a serious adverse effect from any ergot preparation.
• you have severe coronary artery disease or peripheral vascular disease.

▷ **Inform Your Physician Before Taking This Drug If**

• you have constitutionally low blood pressure.
• you are pregnant or breast-feeding your infant.
• you are taking any antihypertensive drugs or antipsychotic drugs (see Drug Classes).
• you have any degree of coronary artery disease, especially angina or a history of heart attack.
• you have any type of heart rhythm disorder.
• you have impaired liver or kidney function.
• you have a seizure disorder.

Possible Side Effects (natural, expected, and unavoidable drug actions)
> Weakness; chest pain—possibly anginal; peripheral edema; orthostatic hypotension (see Glossary).

▷ **Possible Adverse Effects** (unusual, unexpected, and infrequent reactions)
> **If any of the following develop, consult your physician promptly for guidance.**

Mild Adverse Effects
> Allergic Reactions: Skin rash, facial swelling (rare).
> Headache, dizziness, hallucinations, confusion, drowsiness, insomnia, anxiety, double vision (rare).
> Nasal congestion, shortness of breath, palpitation (rare), fainting (rare).
> Altered taste (rare), loss of appetite, dry mouth, indigestion, nausea, vomiting, constipation, diarrhea.

Serious Adverse Effects
> Allergic Reactions: None reported.
> Idiosyncratic Reactions: Flu-like symptoms.
> Abnormal involuntary movements (dyskinesia) (frequent), psychotic behavior (rare).
> Hallucinations (accounted for 7.8% of patient withdrawals from therapy; 13.8% occurrence).
> Abnormal heartbeat (ventricular arrhythmias).
> Anemia (rare).
> Paranoid delusions.

▷ **Possible Effects on Sexual Function:**   Infrequent reports of altered libido (both increased and decreased), impotence, breast pain, priapism (see Glossary).

▷ **Adverse Effects That May Mimic Natural Diseases or Disorders**
> Effects on mental function and behavior may resemble psychotic disorders.

▷ **Natural Diseases or Disorders That May Be Activated by This Drug**
> Coronary artery disease with anginal syndrome, heart rhythm disorders, Raynaud's syndrome (see Glossary), seizure disorders.

Possible Effects on Laboratory Tests
> Blood prolactin level: decreased (marked reduction).

CAUTION
> 1. May cause abnormal movements (dyskinesias) and intensify existing dyskinesias. Watch carefully for the development of tremors, twitching or abnormal, involuntary movements of any kind. Report these promptly.
> 2. Low starting doses help prevent the possibility of excessive drop in blood pressure. See dosage routine outlined above.
> 3. Inform your physician promptly if you become pregnant or plan pregnancy. This drug has been reported (rarely) to cause abortion and birth defects.

Precautions for Use
> *By Infants and Children:* This drug is not utilized by this age group.
> *By Those over 60 Years of Age:* Small initial doses are mandatory. Watch closely for any tendency to light-headedness or faintness, especially on arising from a lying or sitting position. You may be more susceptible to the development of impaired thinking, confusion, agitation, nightmares or hallucinations.

▷ **Advisability of Use During Pregnancy**

Pregnancy Category: B. See Pregnancy Code at the back of this book.

Animal studies: No birth defects due to this drug were found in mouse or rabbit studies.

Human studies: Adequate studies of pregnant women are not available. However, there are four reports of birth defects associated with the use of this drug and infrequent reports of abortion. Causal relationships have not been established, but prudence advises against the use of this drug during pregnancy. Consult your physician for guidance.

Advisability of Use if Breast-Feeding

Presence of this drug in breast milk: Unknown.

Avoid drug or refrain from nursing.

Habit-Forming Potential: None.

Effects of Overdosage: Nausea, vomiting, palpitations, low blood pressure, agitation, severe involuntary movements, hallucinations, seizures.

Possible Effects of Long-Term Use: Increased risk of developing dyskinesias.

Suggested Periodic Examinations While Taking This Drug (at physician's discretion)

Regular evaluation of drug response, heart function and blood pressure status.

▷ **While Taking This Drug, Observe the Following**

Foods: No restrictions.

Beverages: No restrictions. May be taken with milk.

▷ *Alcohol:* Alcohol can exaggerate the blood-pressure-lowering and sedative effects of this drug.

Tobacco Smoking: No interactions expected.

▷ *Other Drugs*

Pergolide ***taken concurrently*** with

• antihypertensive drugs (and other drugs that can lower blood pressure) requires careful monitoring for excessive drops in pressure. Dosage adjustments may be necessary.

The following drugs may ***decrease*** the effects of pergolide and diminish its effectiveness

• chlorprothixene (Taractan).
• haloperidol (Haldol).
• metoclopramide (Reglan).
• phenothiazines (see Drug Class Section).
• thiothixene (Navane).

▷ *Driving, Hazardous Activities:* This drug may cause dizziness, drowsiness, impaired coordination or fainting. Restrict activities as necessary.

Aviation Note: The use of this drug ***is a disqualification*** for piloting. Consult a designated Aviation Medical Examiner.

Exposure to Sun: No restrictions.

Exposure to Heat: Use caution until the combined effects have been determined. Hot environments can cause lowering of blood pressure.

Discontinuation: Do not stop this drug abruptly. Sudden withdrawal can cause confusion, paranoid thinking and severe hallucinations. Consult your physician regarding a schedule for gradual withdrawal.

PERPHENAZINE (per FEN a zeen)

Introduced: 1957   **Prescription:** USA: Yes; Canada: Yes   **Available as Generic:** USA: Yes; Canada: Yes   **Class:** tranquilizer, major; phenothiazines
Controlled Drug: USA: No; Canada: No

Brand Names: ✦Apo-Perphenazine, ✦PMS-Perphenazine, ✦Elavil Plus [CD], ✦Entrafon, Etrafon [CD], Etrafon-A [CD], Etrafon Forte [CD], ✦Phenazine, ✦PMS-Levazine, ✦PMS-Perphenazine, Triavil [CD], Trilafon

BENEFITS versus RISKS	
Possible Benefits	*Possible Risks*
EFFECTIVE CONTROL OF ACUTE MENTAL DISORDERS	SERIOUS TOXIC EFFECTS ON BRAIN with long-term use
Beneficial effects on thinking, mood, and behavior	Liver damage with jaundice (infrequent)
Relief of anxiety and tension	Rare blood cell disorders: hemolytic
Moderately effective control of nausea and vomiting	anemia, abnormally low white blood cell and platelet counts

▷ **Principal Uses**

As a Single Drug Product: Uses currently included in FDA approved labeling: (1) Used to treat acute and chronic psychotic disorders such as agitated depression, schizophrenia and similar states of mental dysfunction; (2) may be used as a tranquilizer to help agitated and disruptive behavior in the absence of true psychosis; (3) sometimes used to treat severe nausea and vomiting.

Other (unlabeled) generally accepted uses: (1) Can ease tremors caused by tricyclic antidepressants.

As a Combination Drug Product [CD]: Available combined with amitriptyline, an effective antidepressant. In some cases of severe agitated depression, the combination of a specific antipsychotic drug and a specific antidepressant drug will be more effective than either drug used alone.

How This Drug Works: By inhibiting dopamine, this drug acts to correct an imbalance of nerve impulse transmissions thought to be responsible for mental disorders.

Available Dosage Forms and Strengths

Concentrate — 16 mg/ 5-ml

Injection — 5 mg per ml

Tablets — 2 mg, 4 mg, 8 mg, 16 mg

Tablets, prolonged-action — 8 mg

▷ **Usual Adult Dosage Range:** Psychotic symptoms (patients not in the hospital) Initially 4 to 8 mg 3 times daily. Dose may be increased by 4 mg at 3- to 4-day intervals as needed and tolerated. The total daily dosage should not exceed 64 mg. **Note: Actual dosage and administration schedule must be determined by the physician for each patient individually.**

Conditions Requiring Dosing Adjustments

Liver function: The dose should be empirically decreased in patients with liver compromise. Perphenazine is contraindicated in patients with moderate to severe liver compromise.

Kidney function: The kidney is minimally involved in the elimination of this drug.

▷ **Dosing Instructions:**   May be taken with or following meals to reduce stomach irritation. The regular tablets may be crushed for administration; the prolonged-action tablets should be taken whole, not broken, crushed or chewed.

Usual Duration of Use: Use on a regular schedule for several weeks determines this drug's effectiveness in controlling psychotic disorders. If it is not significantly beneficial within 6 weeks, it should be stopped. Long-term use (months to years) requires periodic physician evaluation of response, and consideration of continued need.

▷ **This Drug Should Not Be Taken If**
- you are allergic to any of the drugs bearing the brand names listed.
- you have active liver disease.
- you have brain damage in the subcortical area.
- you have cancer of the breast.
- you have a current blood cell or bone marrow disorder.

▷ **Inform Your Physician Before Taking This Drug If**
- you are allergic or abnormally sensitive to any phenothiazine (see Drug Classes).
- you have impaired liver or kidney function.
- you have any type of seizure disorder.
- you have diabetes, glaucoma or heart disease.
- you have a history of lupus erythematosus.
- you are pregnant or are breast feeding your child.
- you have an allergy to sulfites.
- you have a history of neuroleptic malignant syndrome.
- you are taking any drug with sedative effects.
- you plan to have surgery under general or spinal anesthesia soon.

Possible Side Effects (natural, expected, and unavoidable drug actions)
Drowsiness (usually during the first 2 weeks), orthostatic hypotension (see Glossary), blurred vision, dry mouth, nasal congestion, constipation, impaired urination.
Pink or purple coloration of urine, of no significance.

▷ **Possible Adverse Effects** (unusual, unexpected, and infrequent reactions)
If any of the following develop, consult your physician promptly for guidance.
Mild Adverse Effects
Allergic Reactions: Skin rash, hives, low-grade fever.
Lowering of body temperature, especially in the elderly (see Hypothermia in Glossary).
Increased appetite and weight gain.
Dizziness, weakness, agitation, insomnia, impaired day and night vision.
Chronic constipation, fecal impaction.
Serious Adverse Effects
Allergic Reactions: Hepatitis with jaundice (see Glossary), severe skin reactions (systemic lupus erythematosus [SLE], Stevens-Johnson syndrome), anaphylactic reaction (see Glossary).

Idiosyncratic Reactions: Neuroleptic malignant syndrome (see Glossary).
Depression; disorientation; seizures; deposits in cornea, lens, and retina.
Rapid heart rate, heart rhythm disorders.
Blood cell disorders: hemolytic anemia, reduced white blood cell and blood platelet counts (rare).
Drug-induced porphyria.
Nervous system reactions: Parkinson-like disorders (see Glossary), severe restlessness, muscle spasms involving the face and neck, tardive dyskinesia (see Glossary).

▷ **Possible Effects on Sexual Function**
Altered timing and pattern of menstruation.
Female breast enlargement with milk production.
Male breast enlargement and tenderness.
Painful and extended duration of erection (priapism).
Inhibited ejaculation.
False positive pregnancy test results.

▷ **Adverse Effects That May Mimic Natural Diseases or Disorders**
Nervous system reactions may suggest true Parkinson's disease.
Liver reactions may suggest viral hepatitis.
Reactions resembling systemic lupus erythematosus can occur.

Natural Diseases or Disorders That May Be Activated by This Drug
Latent epilepsy, glaucoma, diabetes mellitus, prostatism (see Glossary).

Possible Effects on Laboratory Tests
White blood cell counts: decreased.
Blood bilirubin level: increased (jaundice—see Glossary).
Blood glucose level: increased.
Glucose tolerance test (GTT): decreased in 35% of those taking this drug.

CAUTION
1. Many over-the-counter medications (see OTC Drugs in Glossary) for allergies, colds and coughs contain drugs that can interact unfavorably with this drug. Ask your physician or pharmacist for help **before** using any such medications.
2. Antacids that contain aluminum and/or magnesium can prevent the absorption of this drug and reduce its effectiveness.
3. Obtain prompt evaluation of any change or disturbance of vision.

Precautions for Use
By Infants and Children: Use of this drug is not recommended in children under 12 years of age. Do not use this drug in the presence of symptoms suggestive of Reye syndrome (see Glossary). Children with acute infectious diseases (flulike infections, chicken pox, measles, etc.) are more prone to develop spasms of the face, back and extremities if this drug is used to control nausea or vomiting.
By Those over 60 Years of Age: Small starting doses are advisable. Increased susceptibility to development of drowsiness, lethargy, constipation, lowering of body temperature (hypothermia) and orthostatic hypotension (see Glossary). This drug can enhance existing prostatism (see Glossary). You may also be more susceptible to the development of Parkinson-like reactions and/or tardive dyskinesia (see discussion of these terms in Glossary).

These reactions must be recognized early since they may become unresponsive to treatment and irreversible.

▷ **Advisability of Use During Pregnancy**
Pregnancy Category: C. See Pregnancy Code at the back of this book.
Animal studies: Cleft palate reported in mouse and rat studies.
Human studies: No increase in birth defects reported in 166 exposures. Information from adequate studies of pregnant women is not available.
Avoid drug during the first 3 months; avoid during the last month because of possible effects on the newborn infant.

Advisability of Use if Breast-Feeding
Presence of this drug in breast milk: Yes, in minute amounts.
Monitor nursing infant closely and discontinue drug or nursing if adverse effects develop.

Habit-Forming Potential: None.

Effects of Overdosage: Marked drowsiness, weakness, tremor, agitation, unsteadiness, deep sleep, coma, convulsions.

Possible Effects of Long-Term Use: Opacities in the cornea or lens of the eye, pigmentation of the retina.
Tardive dyskinesia (see Glossary).

Suggested Periodic Examinations While Taking This Drug (at physician's discretion)
Complete blood cell counts, especially between the fourth and tenth weeks of treatment.
Liver function tests, electrocardiograms.
Complete eye examinations—eye structures and vision.
Careful inspection of the tongue for early evidence of fine, involuntary, wavelike movements that could indicate the beginning of tardive dyskinesia.

▷ **While Taking This Drug, Observe the Following**
Foods: No restrictions.
Nutritional Support: A riboflavin (vitamin B-2) supplement should be taken with long-term use.
Beverages: No restrictions. May be taken with milk.
▷ *Alcohol:* Avoid completely. Alcohol can increase the sedative action of phenothiazines and accentuate their depressant effects on brain function and blood pressure. Phenothiazines can increase the intoxicating effects of alcohol.
Tobacco Smoking: Possible reduction of drowsiness from drug.
Marijuana Smoking: Moderate increase in drowsiness; accentuation of orthostatic hypotension; increased risk of precipitating latent psychoses, confusing the interpretation of mental status and drug responses.
▷ *Other Drugs*
Perphenazine may ***increase*** the effects of
• all sedative drugs, especially meperidine (Demerol), and cause excessive sedation.
• all atropinelike drugs, and cause nervous system toxicity.
Perphenazine may ***decrease*** the effects of
• guanethidine (Ismelin, Esimil), and reduce its effectiveness in lowering blood pressure.

- oral hypoglycemic drugs (see Drug Classes) and cause loss of glucose control.

Perphenazine *taken concurrently* with

- ascorbic acid may blunt the therapeutic effect of perphenazine.
- lithium (Lithobid, Lithotabs) may impair the effectiveness of lithium and cause nervous system toxicity.
- Monoamine oxidase inhibitor drugs (MAO) (see drug Classes) may result in increased extrapyramidal reactions.

The following drugs may *decrease* the effects of perphenazine

- antacids containing aluminum and/or magnesium.
- barbiturates (see Drug Class Section).
- benztropine (Cogentin).
- disulfiram (Antabuse).
- trihexyphenidyl (Artane).

▷ *Driving, Hazardous Activities:* This drug can impair mental alertness, judgment and physical coordination. Avoid hazardous activities.

Aviation Note: The use of this drug *is a disqualification* for piloting. Consult a designated Aviation Medical Examiner.

Exposure to Sun: Use caution. Some phenothiazines can cause photosensitivity (see Glossary).

Exposure to Heat: Use caution and avoid excessive heat as much as possible. This drug may impair the regulation of body temperature and increase the risk of heat stroke.

Exposure to Cold: Use caution and dress warmly. This drug can increase the risk of hypothermia in the elderly.

Discontinuation: After a period of long-term use, do not stop this drug suddenly. Gradual withdrawal over 2 to 3 weeks under physician supervision is recommended. Do not discontinue this drug without your physician's knowledge and approval. The relapse rate of schizophrenia after discontinuation is 50–60%.

PHENELZINE (FEN el zeen)

Introduced: 1961   **Prescription:** USA: Yes; Canada: Yes   **Available as**
Generic: No   **Class:** Antidepressant, MAO type A inhibitor   **Controlled**
Drug: USA: No; Canada: No

Brand Name: Nardil

BENEFITS versus RISKS	
Possible Benefits	*Possible Risks*
EFFECTIVE RELIEF OF REACTIVE, NEUROTIC, ATYPICAL DEPRESSIONS with associated anxiety or phobia	DANGEROUS INTERACTIONS WITH MANY DRUGS AND FOODS CONDUCIVE TO HYPERTENSIVE CRISIS
Beneficial in some depressions that are not responsive to other treatments	DISORDERED HEART RATE AND RHYTHM
	Drug-induced hepatitis (rare)
	Mental changes: agitation, confusion, impaired memory, hypomania

▷ **Principal Uses**

As a Single Drug Product: Uses currently included in FDA approved labeling: (1) Used to treat severe situational (reactive or neurotic) depression, atypical depression, and (though less effective) severe endogenous depression. Because of the supervision required during its use and its potential for serious adverse effects, this drug is usually reserved to treat depressions that have not responded satisfactorily to other antidepressant therapy.

Other (unlabeled) generally accepted uses: (1) Helps control binge eating in bulimia; (2) may be useful in treating chronic headache patients who also suffer from depression or anxiety; (3) a long-term study found phenelzine beneficial in treating social phobia; (4) rare use in intractable narcolepsy; (5) may be of benefit in post-traumatic stress disorder.

How This Drug Works: By blocking an enzyme (monoamine oxidase type A) in brain tissue, this drug produces an increase of nerve impulse transmitters that maintain normal mood and emotional stability.

Available Dosage Forms and Strengths

Tablets — 15 mg

▷ **Usual Adult Dosage Range:**   Initially, 15 mg 3 times/day (or 1 milligram per kilogram divided into three equal doses and given three times daily); increased rapidly up to 60 mg/day, as needed and tolerated, until improvement is apparent. For maintenance, reduce dose gradually over several weeks to the smallest dose that will maintain improvement; this may be as low as 15 mg daily or every other day. The total daily dosage should not exceed 90 mg. **Note: Actual dose and dosing schedule must be individually determined by the physician.**

Conditions Requiring Dosing Adjustments

Liver function: Phenelzine is contraindicated in patients with increased liver function tests or history of liver compromise.

Kidney function: No specific dosing changes are indicated in renal compromise.

▷ **Dosing Instructions:**   The tablet may be crushed and taken on an empty stomach or with food. Do not take this drug in the late evening; it can interfere with sleep.

▷ **Usual Duration of Use:**   Use on a regular schedule for 3 to 4 weeks usually determines effectiveness in relieving depression. Once the optimal maintenance dose has been determined, it may be continued indefinitely. Long-term use (months to years) requires physician supervision.

▷ **This Drug Should Not Be Taken If**

- you have had an allergic reaction to it previously.
- you have advanced heart disease.
- you take meperidene (Demerol).
- you have active liver disease or impaired liver function.
- you have an adrenalin-producing tumor (pheochromocytoma).
- you are taking caffeine containing drinks.
- you are taking any of the following drugs: another MAO type A inhibitor, a tricyclic antidepressant, carbamazepine (see Drug Classes).

▷ **Inform Your Physician Before Taking This Drug If**

- you have high blood pressure.
- you have had a stroke, or you have impaired circulation to the brain.
- you have coronary heart disease.
- you have frequent or severe headaches.

- you have diabetes, epilepsy, schizophrenia or an overactive thyroid gland (hyperthyroidism).
- you are pregnant or are breast-feeding.
- you have impaired kidney function.
- you plan to have surgery under general or spinal anesthesia in the near future.

Possible Side Effects (natural, expected, and unavoidable drug actions)

Insomnia if taken in the evening.

Orthostatic hypotension (see Glossary).

Fluid retention (swelling of feet and ankles).

▷ **Possible Adverse Effects** (unusual, unexpected, and infrequent reactions)

If any of the following develop, consult your physician promptly for guidance.

Mild Adverse Effects

Allergic Reaction: Skin rash.

Headache, dizziness, drowsiness, weakness, agitation, confusion, impaired memory, tremors, muscle twitching, blurred vision, impaired red–green color vision (may be a first sign of toxic amblyopia).

Dry mouth, increased appetite, indigestion, constipation.

Serious Adverse Effects

Drug-induced hepatitis with jaundice (see Glossary).

Hypertensive crisis: rapid and extreme rise in blood pressure, severe throbbing headache, palpitation, nausea, vomiting, sweating, risk of brain hemorrhage.

Peripheral neuropathy (may be secondary to pyridoxine or vitamin B6 deficiency).

Seizures (rare).

Parkinson-like syndrome (rare). Manic episodes.

Drug-induced porphyria (rare).

Neuroleptic malignant syndrome (rare).

Eye toxicity (toxic amblyopia).

Disturbances of heart rate and rhythm.

Low white blood cell count (rare).

▷ **Possible Effects on Sexual Function**

Decreased libido (30% of males, 28% of females).

Impaired erection (50%), painful and extended erection (priapism) (rare), inhibited ejaculation (60%).

Inhibited orgasm (30% of males, 35% of females).

▷ **Adverse Effects That May Mimic Natural Diseases or Disorders**

Drug-induced hepatitis may suggest viral hepatitis.

Natural Diseases or Disorders That May Be Activated by This Drug

Latent epilepsy, schizophrenia.

This drug may convert depression into the manic phase of a manic-depressive disorder.

Possible Effects on Laboratory Tests

White blood cell counts: decreased.

Blood glucose level: increased.

Liver function tests: increased liver enzymes (ALT/GPT and AST/GOT), increased bilirubin.

Systemic lupus erythematosus cells: positive.

CAUTION

1. The lowest effective dose should be identified and not exceeded.
2. The development of a severe headache or palpitation may indicate a dangerous elevation of blood pressure. Stop this drug immediately and call your doctor.
3. This drug may suppress anginal pain that would normally serve as a warning of excessive demand on the heart.
4. May increase the possibility of hypoglycemic reactions if used concurrently with insulin or oral antidiabetic drugs (sulfonylureas; see Drug Class Section). It may also delay recovery from hypoglycemia.
5. This drug can alter the threshold for convulsions in anyone with epilepsy or a seizure disorder. Dose decreases of anticonvulsant drugs may be needed.
6. This drug should be discontinued 2 weeks before elective surgery under general or spinal anesthesia. Consult your surgeon or anesthesiologist.
7. Many over-the-counter drug products contain ingredients that can cause serious interactions if taken with this drug. Avoid use of: cold and sinus medications, nasal decongestants, hay fever preparations, asthma inhalants, appetite and weight control products, "pep" pills. Ask your physician or pharmacist about their safe use with this drug.
8. It is advisable to carry a card of personal identification with the notation that you are taking this drug. Notify all medical personnel that may attend you that you are taking this drug.

Precautions for Use

By Infants and Children: Safety and effectiveness for those under 16 years of age not established.

By Those over 60 Years of Age: This drug is not recommended for use by anyone over 60. However, if poor response to other treatment justifies consideration of a trial of this drug, it should not be used in patients with high blood pressure, hardening of the arteries, impaired circulation within the brain, or coronary artery disease. This drug will intensify existing prostatism (see Glossary). Fluid retention is more prominent in this age group.

▷ Advisability of Use During Pregnancy

Pregnancy Category: C. See Pregnancy Code at the back of this book.

Animal studies: No information available.

Human studies: Adequate studies of pregnant women are not available. Birth defects have been reported with the use of this drug.

Avoid this drug completely if possible. Ask your physician for guidance.

Advisability of Use if Breast-Feeding

Presence of this drug in breast milk: Probably yes.

Avoid drug or refrain from nursing.

Habit-Forming Potential: None.

Effects of Overdosage: Overstimulation, agitation, anxiety, restlessness, insomnia, confusion, delirium, hallucinations, seizures, high fever, circulatory collapse, coma.

Possible Effects of Long-Term Use: The conversion of mental depression into a state of hypomania: excessive mental and physical activity, excitement, agitation, loud and rapid talking, delusional thinking.

Suggested Periodic Examinations While Taking This Drug (at physician's discretion)

Blood pressure measurements in lying, sitting and standing positions.

Complete blood cell counts, liver function tests.

▷ **While Taking This Drug, Observe the Following**

Foods: **All tyramine-rich foods should be avoided completely.** See Tyramine in the Glossary for a complete list of foods and beverages to avoid while taking this drug. A pyridoxine deficiency (vitamin B-6) may develop and require supplementation (symptoms of peripheral neuropathy would result if this vitamin is not replaced).

Beverages: Limit coffee, tea and cola beverages to one serving daily. See Tyramine in Glossary.

▷ *Alcohol:* Alcohol can increase the depressant effects of this drug on brain function.

Tobacco Smoking: No interactions expected.

▷ *Other Drugs*

Phenelzine may *increase* the effects of

- amphetamine and related drugs.
- appetite suppressants.
- all drugs with stimulant effects on the nervous system, and cause excessive rise in blood pressure.
- all drugs with sedative effects, and cause excessive sedation.
- insulin.
- sulfonylureas (see Drug Classes) or other oral hypoglycemic agents.

Phenelzine *taken concurrently* with

- antihistamines (see Drug Classes) can worsen the anticholinergic side effects of antihistamines.
- buspirone (Buspar) may result in undesirable increases in blood pressure.
- carbamazepine (Tegretol) may cause severe toxic reactions.
- dextromethorphan (nonprescription cough medicine with a "DM") and cause severe toxic reactions.
- dopamine (Intropin) may cause severe toxic reactions.
- fluoxetine (Prozac) has resulted in fatal reactions with another MAO inhibitor (tranylcypromine). This combination is to be avoided.
- fluvoxamine (Luvox) or other serotonin reuptake inhibitors may result in neuroleptic malignant syndrome and other serious reactions. This combination is not recommended.
- levodopa (Dopar, Sinemet) may cause a dangerous rise in blood pressure.
- meperidine (Demerol) may cause high fever, seizures and coma. These drugs are NOT to be combined.
- methyldopa (Aldomet) may cause a dangerous rise in blood pressure.
- methylphenidate (Ritalin) may cause severe headache, weakness and numbness in the extremities.
- nadolol (Corgard) and metoprolol (Lopressor) or other beta blockers (see Drug Classes) may result in significant decreases in heart rate.
- nefazodone (Serzone) may result in serious adverse effects. DO NOT combine these drugs.

- paroxetine (Paxil) may result in serious adverse effects. DO NOT combine these drugs.
- phenothiazines (see Drug Classes) or other antipsychotics may cause exaggeration of the central nervous system and depression of breathing effects.
- phenylephrine (various) may result in serious increases in blood pressure. DO NOT combine.
- phenylpropanolamine (various) may result in serious increases in blood pressure. DO NOT combine.
- propoxyphene (Darvon) may result in coma, heart problems or severe increases in temperature. DO NOT combine.
- pseudoephedrine (various) may result in serious adverse effects. DO NOT combine these drugs.
- sertraline (Zoloft) may result in muscle rigidity, CNS toxicity and chills. DO NOT combine these medicines.
- tryptophan (L-Tryptophan) can cause toxic reactions.
- tricyclic antidepressants (see Drug Classes) may cause severe toxic reactions including high fever, delirium, tremor, seizures and coma.
- venlafaxine (Effexor) may result in serious adverse reactions. DO NOT combine these medicines.

Note: Consult your physician before taking *any other drugs* while taking phenelzine.

▷ *Driving, Hazardous Activities:* This drug may cause dizziness, drowsiness and blurred vision. Restrict activities as necessary.

Aviation Note: The use of this drug *is a disqualification* for piloting. Consult a designated Aviation Medical Examiner.

Exposure to Sun: No restrictions.

Occurrence of Unrelated Illness: Because of the very serious and life-threatening interactions that can occur between this drug and many others, you **must** tell each physician and dentist you consult that you are taking this drug.

Discontinuation: If this drug is not effective after 4 weeks of continual use, it should be stopped. If it is effective, continue to take it in proper dosage until advised to stop. Do not stop it abruptly. If another antidepressant is to be tried, a drug-free waiting period of 14 days must pass between stopping this drug and starting the new one. Avoid tyramine-rich foods and other interacting drugs during this 14-day period.

PHENOBARBITAL (fee noh BAR bi tawl)

Other Name: Phenobarbitone

Introduced: 1912   **Prescription:**   USA: Yes; Canada: Yes   **Available as Generic:** Yes   **Class:**   Sedative, anticonvulsant, barbiturates   **Controlled Drug:** USA:C-IV***

Brand Names: Alubelap [CD], Aminodrox-Forte, Antispasmodic[CD], Azpan, Barbidonna [CD], Barbidonna Elixir [CD], Barbita, Belap, Belladenal [CD], Belladenal-S [CD], ✦Belladenal Spacetabs [CD], ✦Bellergal [CD], Bellergal-S [CD], ✦Bellergal Spacetabs [CD], Bronchotabs [CD], Bronkolixir

---

*See Schedules of Controlled Drugs at the back of this book.

[CD], ♣Cafergot-PB, Chardonna-2 [CD], Daricon PB, ♣Diclophen [CD], Dilantin w/Phenobarbital [CD], Donphen, Donna-Sed, Donnatal [CD], Ergobel [CD], Eskabarb, Eskaphen B [CD], Floramine, ♣Gardenal, Hybephen [CD], Hypnaldyne [CD], Isuprel compound [CD], Kinesed [CD], Luminal, Mudrane GG Elixir & Tablets [CD], Mudrane Tablets [CD], Neospect, Novalene, ♣Neuro-Spasex [CD], ♣Neuro-Trasentin [CD], ♣Neuro-Trasentin Forte [CD], Phedral [CD], ♣Phenaphen Capsules [CD], ♣Phenaphen No. 2, 3, 4 [CD], Phenergan w/Codeine [CD], Phyldrox, Quadrinal [CD], Relaxadron, SBP [CD], Scodonnar [CD], Sedacord [CD], SK-Phenobarbital, Solfoton, Spasquid [CD], Spazcaps, Tedral Preparations [CD], T.E.P. [CD], Thalfed [CD], Theocardone, Theocord [CD], Theolixer, Vitaphen

---

BENEFITS versus RISKS

Possible Benefits	*Possible Risks*
EFFECTIVE CONTROL OF TONIC-CLONIC SEIZURES AND ALL TYPES OF PARTIAL SEIZURES	POTENTIAL FOR DEPENDENCE LIFE-THREATENING TOXICITY WITH OVERDOSAGE
EFFECTIVE CONTROL OF FEBRILE SEIZURES OF CHILDHOOD	Drug-induced hepatitis Rare drug-induced decreased kidney function
Effective relief of anxiety and nervous tension	Rare blood cell disorders: abnormally low red cell, white cell, and platelet counts

---

▷ **Principal Uses**

As a Single Drug Product: Uses currently included in FDA approved labeling: (1) Used as a mild sedative; (2) as an anticonvulsant to control grand mal epilepsy and all types of partial seizures. It is also used to control febrile seizures of childhood; (3) used as a sedative, however, newer agents carry fewer drug interactions and effects on sleep cycles. Other (unlabeled) generally accepted uses: (1) May be helpful in detoxification of sedative-hypnotic addiction; (2) can help control seizures found in cerebral malaria; (3) eases neonatal seizures; (4) may have a role in pain syndromes.

As a Combination Drug Product [CD]: This drug is available in many combinations with derivatives of belladonna, an antispasmodic commonly used to treat functional disorders of the gastrointestinal tract. It is also available in combination with bronchodilators for the treatment of asthma, and with ergotamine for the treatment of headaches.

How This Drug Works: By impeding the transfer of sodium and potassium across cell membranes, this drug selectively blocks the transmission of nerve impulses. This could serve to produce a sedative effect and to suppress the spread of nerve impulses that are responsible for epileptic seizures.

Available Dosage Forms and Strengths

Capsules — 16 mg
Elixir — 15 mg, 20 mg per 5-ml
Tablets — 8 mg, 16 mg, 32 mg, 65 mg, 100 mg

▷ **Usual Adult Dosage Range:** As sedative—15 to 30 mg 2 to 3 times/day. As hypnotic: 100 to 200 mg at bedtime. As anticonvulsant—60 to 250 mg given as a single dose at bedtime. Some clinicians give 2 to 3 milligrams per kilogram in order to achieve and maintain a blood level between 15 to 40 micrograms per milliliter. **Note: Actual dose and dosing schedule must be determined by the physician for each patient individually.**

Conditions Requiring Dosing Adjustments

Liver function: It should be used with caution, in decreased doses and blood levels obtained more frequently in patients with liver compromise.

Kidney function: This drug should be used with caution and in decreased dose in patients with compromised kidneys. Blood levels should be obtained at prudent intervals. One researcher suggests that patients with severe kidney failure (creatinine clearance less than 10 ml per minute) can be given typical doses, but only every 12 to 16 hours.

▷ **Dosing Instructions:**   Regular tablets may be crushed and capsules opened and taken with or after food to reduce stomach irritation. Prolonged-action dosage forms should be swallowed whole without alteration.

Usual Duration of Use: Use on a regular schedule for 3 to 5 days determines effectiveness in relieving anxiety and tension, and for 4 to 6 weeks to determine its ability to control seizures. If used to treat anxiety-tension states, its use should not exceed 4 weeks without reappraisal of continued need. Long-term use for seizure control (months to years) requires physician supervision and periodic evaluation.

▷ **This Drug Should Not Be Taken If**
- you have had an allergic reaction to it previously.
- you have severe liver impairment.
- you are subject to acute intermittent porphyria (see Glossary).
- you have respiratory disease that makes it difficult to breathe.

▷ **Inform Your Physician Before Taking This Drug If**
- you are allergic or overly sensitive to any barbiturate (see Drug Class Section).
- you are pregnant or planning pregnancy.
- you have a history of alcohol or drug abuse.
- you are taking any drugs with sedative effects.
- you have a history of depression.
- you have any type of seizure disorder.
- you have myasthenia gravis.
- you have impaired liver, kidney or thyroid gland function.
- you plan to have surgery under general anesthesia in the near future.

Possible Side Effects (natural, expected, and unavoidable drug actions)

Drowsiness, impaired concentration, mental and physical sluggishness.

▷ **Possible Adverse Effects** (unusual, unexpected, and infrequent reactions)
If any of the following develop, consult your physician promptly for guidance.

Mild Adverse Effects

Allergic Reactions: Skin rashes, hives, localized swellings of face, drug fever (see Glossary).

Dizziness, unsteadiness, impaired vision, double vision.

Nausea, vomiting, diarrhea.

Abnormal growth of the gums.

Shoulder-hand syndrome: pain and stiffness in the shoulder, pain and swelling in the hand.

Serious Adverse Effects

Allergic Reactions: Drug-induced hepatitis with jaundice (see Glossary), severe skin disorders (Stevens-Johnson syndrome or toxic epidermal necrolysis).

Osteoporosis (possible with long-term use).

Idiosyncratic Reactions: Paradoxical excitement and delirium (instead of sedation).

Drug-induced myasthenia gravis.

Respiratory depression (dose-related).

Mental depression, abnormal involuntary movements.

Blood cell disorders: deficiencies of all blood cell types causing fatigue, weakness, fever, sore throat, abnormal bleeding or bruising.

Blood clotting disorders in neonates.

Kidney disease (rare).

Optic neuropathy (rare).

Drug-induced seizures.

Low blood calcium.

▷ **Possible Effects on Sexual Function**

Decreased libido and/or impotence (occasional).

Decreased effectiveness of oral contraceptives taken concurrently (71%).

▷ **Adverse Effects That May Mimic Natural Diseases or Disorders**

Liver reactions may suggest viral hepatitis.

Natural Diseases or Disorders That May Be Activated by This Drug

Acute intermittent and/or cutaneous porphyria, systemic lupus erythematosus.

Possible Effects on Laboratory Tests

Complete blood cell counts: decreased red cells, hemoglobin, white cells and platelets.

Blood lupus erythematosus (LE) cells: positive.

Prothrombin time: decreased (when taken concurrently with warfarin).

Blood calcium level: decreased (with long-term use).

Blood thyroxine (T_4) level: decreased.

Liver function tests: increased liver enzymes (ALT/GPT, AST/GOT and alkaline phosphatase), increased bilirubin.

Urine sugar tests: no effect with TesTape; false low results with Clinistix and Diastix.

Urine screening tests for drug abuse: may be **positive**. (Test results depend upon amount of drug taken and testing method used.)

CAUTION

1. Accurate diagnosis and classification of the seizure pattern are essential for correct selection of the most appropriate drug for therapy.
2. Emotional stress or physical trauma (including surgery) may require increased anticonvulsant dosage to control seizures.
3. Prolonged-action dosage forms of this drug are not appropriate for the treatment of seizures and should not be used.

Precautions for Use

By Infants and Children: This drug should not be given to the hyperkinetic child. Observe for possible paradoxical stimulation and hyperactivity; this can occur in 10% to 40% of children. Changes associated with puberty characteristically slow the metabolism of this drug and permit its gradual accumulation. Blood levels of this drug in young adolescents should be monitored every 3 months to detect rising concentrations and early toxicity.

By Those over 60 Years of Age: It is advisable to avoid all barbiturates in the elderly. If use of this drug is attempted, small starting doses are indicated. Watch for confusion, delirium, agitation and excitement. Do not use this drug concurrently with other drugs for mental disorders. This drug is conducive to the development of hypothermia (see Glossary).

▷ **Advisability of Use During Pregnancy**
Pregnancy Category: D. See Pregnancy Code at the back of this book.
Animal studies: Conflicting reports of cleft palate and skeletal defects in mouse, rat and rabbit studies.
Human studies: Information from studies of pregnant women indicates no increase in birth defects in 8037 exposures to this drug. However, it is reported that barbiturates can cause fetal damage when taken during pregnancy.
Avoid use of drug during entire pregnancy if possible. If it is clearly needed to control seizures, the mother should receive vitamin K prior to delivery and the infant should receive it at birth.

Advisability of Use if Breast-Feeding
Presence of this drug in breast milk: Yes, in small amounts.
Monitor nursing infant closely and discontinue drug or nursing if adverse effects develop.

Habit-Forming Potential: Psychological and physical dependence can occur with prolonged use of excessive doses—300 to 700 mg/day for 1 to 2 months. Dependence is not likely to occur with usual sedative or anticonvulsant doses.

Effects of Overdosage: Behavior similar to alcoholic intoxication—confusion, slurred speech, physical incoordination, staggering gait, drowsiness, stupor leading to coma.

Possible Effects of Long-Term Use: Psychological and/or physical dependence; syndrome of chronic intoxication—headache, depression, impaired vision, dizziness, slurred speech, incoordination. Megaloblastic anemia due to folic acid deficiency. Rickets or osteomalacia due to deficiencies of vitamin D and calcium.

Suggested Periodic Examinations While Taking This Drug (at physician's discretion)
When used to control seizures, blood phenobarbital levels are needed.
Time to sample blood for phenobarbital level: Just before next dose.
Recommended therapeutic range: For adults—15–40 mcg/ml; for children—15–30 mcg/ml.
Complete blood cell counts, liver function tests.
During long-term use: blood levels of folic acid, vitamin B-12, calcium and phosphorus; densitometry (DEXA) studies for demineralization of bone.

▷ **While Taking This Drug, Observe the Following**
Foods: No restrictions. Eat liberally of foods rich in folic acid—fortified breakfast cereals, liver, legumes, green leafy vegetables.
Beverages: No restrictions. May be taken with milk or fruit juices.

▷ *Alcohol:* Avoid completely. Alcohol can increase greatly the sedative and depressant actions of this drug on brain functions.

Tobacco Smoking: May enhance the sedative effects of this drug and increase drowsiness.

Marijuana Smoking: Increased drowsiness, unsteadiness; significantly impaired mental and physical performance.

▷ *Other Drugs*

Phenobarbital may *increase* the effects of
- all other drugs with sedative effects, and cause excessive sedation.

Phenobarbital may *decrease* the effects of
- anticoagulants (Coumadin, etc.), and require dosage adjustments based on more frequent INR (protime) testing.
- certain beta blockers (Inderal, Lopressor), and reduce their effectiveness.
- cortisonelike drugs.
- cyclosporine (Sandimmune).
- diltiazem (Cardizem).
- disopyramide (Norpace).
- doxycycline (Vibramycin).
- felodipine (Plendil).
- griseofulvin (Fulvicin, etc.).
- metoprolol (Lopressor, others).
- nimodipine (Nimotop).
- oral contraceptives, and reduce their effectiveness in preventing pregnancy.
- quinidine (Quinaglute, etc.), and reduce its effectiveness.
- propranolol (Inderal).
- theophyllines (Aminophyllin, Theo-Dur, etc.), and reduce their antiasthmatic effectiveness.
- tricyclic antidepressants (see Drug Classes).
- verapamil (Calan) and reduce its effectiveness.
- warfarin (Coumadin) and increase risk of clots.

Phenobarbital *taken concurrently* with
- chloramphenicol (Chloromycetin) may result in decreased chloramphenicol benefits and phenobarbital toxicity. These drugs are NOT to be combined.
- colestipol (Colestid) and other cholesterol lowering resins may bind phenobarbital and limit absorption.
- influenza vaccine may cause phenobarbital toxicity.
- itraconazole (and perhaps other antifungals) may decrease the anti-fungal effect of itraconazole.
- phenytoin (Dilantin) may alter phenytoin blood levels: a high phenobarbital level will increase the phenytoin level; a low phenobarbital level will decrease the phenytoin level. Periodic determination of blood levels of both drugs is advised.
- primidone (Mysoline) may lead to phenobarbital toxicity.

The following drugs may *increase* the effects of phenobarbital
- ascorbic acid (vitamin C).
- felbamate (Felbatol).
- valproic acid (Depakene).

▷ *Driving, Hazardous Activities:* This drug may cause drowsiness and may impair mental alertness, judgment, physical coordination and reaction time. Restrict activities as necessary.

Aviation Note: The use of this drug ***is a disqualification*** for piloting. Consult a designated Aviation Medical Examiner.

Exposure to Sun: Use caution. This drug may cause photosensitivity.

Exposure to Cold: Observe the elderly for possible hypothermia (see Glossary) while taking this drug.

Discontinuation: If used as an anticonvulsant, this drug must not be stopped abruptly. Sudden withdrawal can precipitate status epilepticus (repetitive seizures). Gradual reduction in dosage should be made over a period of 3 months. Total drug withdrawal may be attempted after a period of 3 to 5 years without a seizure. However, seizures are likely to recur in 40% of adults and in 20–30% of children.

PHENYTOIN (FEN i toh in)

Other Name: Diphenylhydantoin

Introduced: 1938   **Prescription:** USA: Yes; Canada: Yes   **Available as Generic:** USA: Yes; Canada: Yes   **Class:** Anticonvulsant, hydantoins, pain syndrome modifier   **Controlled Drug:** USA: No; Canada: No

Brand Names: Dilantin, Dilantin w/Phenobarbital [CD], Di-Phen, Diphenylan, Ekko JR, Ekko Three, ✦Mebroin [CD], ✦Phelantin

BENEFITS versus RISKS	
Possible Benefits	*Possible Risks*
EFFECTIVE CONTROL OF TONIC-CLONIC (GRAND MAL), PSYCHOMOTOR (TEMPORAL LOBE), MYOCLONIC, AND FOCAL SEIZURES	VERY NARROW TREATMENT MARGIN POSSIBLE BIRTH DEFECTS Overgrowth of gums Excessive hair growth Rare blood cell disorders: impaired production of all blood cells Drug-induced hepatitis Drug-induced nephritis

▷ **Principal Uses**

As a Single Drug Product: Uses currently included in FDA approved labeling: (1) As an antiepileptic drug to control grand mal, psychomotor, myoclonic and focal seizures. It can also be used to control seizures following brain surgery.

Other (unlabeled) generally accepted uses: (1) Used to initiate treatment of trigeminal neuralgia; it is sometimes effective in relieving the severe facial pain of this disorder; (2) used in chronic pain syndromes; (3) may have a role (as an applied powder) in helping heal wounds.

As a Combination Drug Product [CD]: This drug is available in combination with phenobarbital, another effective anticonvulsant. Some seizure disorders require the combined actions of these two drugs for effective control.

How This Drug Works: By promoting the loss of sodium from nerve fibers, this drug lowers and stabilizes their excitability and thereby inhibits the repetitious spread of electrical impulses along nerve pathways. This action may prevent seizures altogether, or it may reduce their frequency and severity.

Available Dosage Forms and Strengths
Capsules (extended) — 30 mg, 100 mg
Capsules (prompt) — 30 mg, 100 mg
Injection — 50 mg per ml
Oral suspension — 30 mg, 125 mg per 5-ml
Tablets, chewable — 50 mg

▷ **Usual Adult Dosage Range:**   Seizures: Initially (prompt or extended form): 100 mg 3 times/day. Dose may be increased cautiously by 100 mg/week as needed and tolerated. Once the optimal maintenance dose has been identified, the total daily dose may be taken as a single dose every 24 hours if Dilantin capsules are used. No other formulation is approved for once-a-day use. The total daily dosage should not exceed 600 mg. **Note: Actual dosage and administration schedule must be determined by the physician for each patient individually.**

Conditions Requiring Dosing Adjustments
Liver function: The maintenance dose should be decreased based on blood levels.
Kidney function: The dose or dosing interval must be decreased in moderate kidney failure.
Obesity: The way this medicine is distributed (volume of distribution) changes with increasing body fat. Loading doses must be calculated based on ideal body weight. The product of 1.33 times actual weight divided by the ideal weight is then added to the original number to decide the final loading dose.

▷ **Dosing Instructions:**   May be taken with or after food to reduce stomach irritation. The capsule may be opened and the tablet may be crushed for administration.

Usual Duration of Use: Use on a regular schedule for 2 to 3 weeks usually determines benefit in reducing frequency and severity of seizures. Optimal control will require careful dosage adjustments over a period of several months. Long-term use (months to years) requires ongoing physician supervision.

▷ **This Drug Should Not Be Taken If**
• you have had an allergic reaction to this drug or to other hydantoin drugs previously.
• you have sinus bradycardia or serious heart block.

▷ **Inform Your Physician Before Taking This Drug If**
• you are taking any other drugs at this time.
• you have a history of liver disease or impaired liver function.
• you have low blood pressure, diabetes or any type of heart disease.
• you are pregnant or are planning pregnancy.
• you plan to have surgery under general anesthesia in the near future.

Possible Side Effects (natural, expected, and unavoidable drug actions)
Mild fatigue, sluggishness, and drowsiness (in sensitive individuals).
Pink to red to brown coloration of urine (of no significance).

▷ **Possible Adverse Effects** (unusual, unexpected, and infrequent reactions)
   If any of the following develop, consult your physician promptly for guidance.

Mild Adverse Effects

Allergic Reactions: Skin rashes, hives, drug fever (see Glossary).

Headache, dizziness, nervousness, insomnia, muscle twitching.

Nausea, vomiting, constipation.

Bed-wetting.

Abnormal eye movements.

Low blood calcium (and potential osteoporosis) and elevated blood sugar.

Overgrowth of gum tissues (most common in children).

Excessive growth of body hair (most common in young girls).

Serious Adverse Effects

Allergic Reactions: Drug-induced hepatitis, with or without jaundice (see Glossary). Drug-induced nephritis, with acute kidney failure. Severe skin reactions (toxic epidermal necrolysis [TEN], Stevens-Johnson syndrome, or erythema multiforme). Myocarditis, generalized enlargement of lymph glands (pseudolymphoma).

Idiosyncratic Reaction: Hemolytic anemia (see Glossary).

Acute psychotic episodes (rare).

Blood clotting disorders in infants of mothers maintained on phenytoin (rare).

Bone marrow depression (see Glossary): fatigue, weakness, fever, sore throat, abnormal bleeding or bruising.

Drug-induced periarteritis nodosa.

Drug-induced seizures.

Drug-induced low thyroid function.

Drug-induced myasthenia gravis.

Tardive dyskinesia (very rare).

Abnormal IgA (increased risk of respiratory infections).

Peripheral nerve damage (neuropathy).

Drug-induced porphyria (rare).

Serious heart rhythm problems (with rapid intravenous use).

Mental confusion, unsteadiness, double vision, jerky eye movements, slurred speech.

Myopathy (rare).

Joint pain and swelling.

Elevated blood sugar, due to inhibition of insulin release.

▷ **Possible Effects on Sexual Function**

Decreased libido and/or impotence (occasional).

Swelling and tenderness of male breast tissue (gynecomastia) (rare).

Peyronie's disease (see Glossary).

Decreased effectiveness of oral contraceptives taken concurrently.

▷ **Adverse Effects That May Mimic Natural Diseases or Disorders**

Drug-induced hepatitis may suggest viral hepatitis.

Skin reactions may resemble lupus erythematosus.

Natural Diseases or Disorders That May Be Activated by This Drug

Latent diabetes, porphyria, systemic lupus erythematosus, low bone mineral density predisposing to osteoporosis.

Possible Effects on Laboratory Tests

Complete blood cell counts: decreased red cells, hemoglobin, white cells and platelets; increased eosinophils (allergic reaction).

Blood lupus erythematosus (LE) cells: positive.

Prothrombin time: increased (when taken concurrently with warfarin).

Blood calcium level: decreased.

Blood total cholesterol, LDL and VLDL cholesterol levels: no effects.

Blood HDL cholesterol level: increased.

Blood triglyceride levels: no effect.

Blood glucose level: increased.

Blood thyroid hormone levels: T_3, T_4 and free T_4 increased.

Liver function tests: increased liver enzymes (ALT/GPT, AST/GOT and alkaline phosphatase), increased bilirubin.

CAUTION

1. Some brand name capsules of this drug have a significantly longer duration of action than generic name capsules of the same strength. To assure a correct dosing schedule, it is necessary to distinguish between "prompt" action and "extended" action capsules. Do not substitute one for the other without your physician's knowledge and guidance.
2. When used for the treatment of epilepsy, *this drug must not be stopped abruptly.*
3. Periodic measurements of blood levels of this drug are essential in determining appropriate dosage. (See Therapeutic Drug Monitoring Section.)
4. Regularity of drug use is essential for successful management of seizure disorders. Take this drug at the same time each day.
5. Shake the suspension form of this drug thoroughly before measuring the dose. Use a standard measuring device to assure that the dose is based upon a 5-ml teaspoon.
6. Side effects and mild adverse effects are usually most apparent during the first several days of treatment, and often subside with continued use.
7. It may be necessary to take folic acid to prevent anemia while taking this drug. Consult your physician regarding this.
8. This medicine has an unusual pathway for removal that can fill up (become saturated) and stop working. What this means is that a small change in dose can give a huge change in blood levels. Make certain you know exactly how much phenytoin your doctor wants you to take.
9. It is advisable to carry a card of personal identification with a notation that you are taking this drug.

Precautions for Use

By Infants and Children: Elimination of this drug varies widely with age. Periodic measurement of blood levels is essential for all ages. Some children will require more than one dose daily for good control. Observe for early indications of drug toxicity: jerky eye movements, unsteadiness in stance and gait, slurred speech, abnormal involuntary movements of the extremities and odd behavior.

By Those over 60 Years of Age: You may be more sensitive to all of the actions of this drug and require smaller doses. Observe closely for any indications of early toxicity: drowsiness, fatigue, confusion, unsteadiness, disturbances of vision, slurred speech, muscle twitching.

▷ **Advisability of Use During Pregnancy**

Pregnancy Category: D. See Pregnancy Code at the back of this book.

Animal studies: Cleft lip and palate, skeletal and visceral defects in mice; skeletal and visceral defects in rats.

Human studies: Available information is conflicting. Some studies suggest a small but significant increase in the occurrence of birth defects associated with the use of phenytoin during pregnancy. The incidence of birth defects in children of epileptics not taking anticonvulsant drugs is 3.2%; the incidence with the use of anticonvulsant drugs during pregnancy increases to 6.4%. The "fetal hydantoin syndrome" in the newborn infant exposed to phenytoin during pregnancy consists of birth defects of the skull, face and limbs, deficient growth and development, and subnormal intelligence and performance. Other effects on the infant include reduction in blood clotting factors that predispose it to severe bruising and hemorrhage.

Discuss with your physician the advantages and possible disadvantages of using this drug during pregnancy. It is advisable to use the smallest maintenance dose that will control seizures. In addition, you should be given vitamin K during the last month of pregnancy to prevent a deficiency of blood clotting factors in the fetus.

Advisability of Use if Breast-Feeding

Presence of this drug in breast milk: Yes, in trace amounts.

Monitor nursing infant closely and discontinue drug or nursing if adverse effects develop.

Habit-Forming Potential: None.

Effects of Overdosage: Drowsiness, jerky eye movements, hand tremor, unsteadiness, slurred speech, hallucinations, delusions, nausea, vomiting, stupor progressing to coma.

Possible Effects of Long-Term Use: Low blood calcium resulting in rickets or osteomalacia; megaloblastic anemia; peripheral neuropathy (see Glossary); schizophreniclike psychosis. Lymphosarcoma, malignant lymphoma and leukemia have been associated with long-term use; a cause-and-effect relationship (see Glossary) has not been established.

Suggested Periodic Examinations While Taking This Drug (at physician's discretion)

Monitoring of blood phenytoin levels to guide dosage.

Time to sample blood for phenytoin level: Just before next dose.

Recommended therapeutic range: 10 to 20 ng/ml.

Complete blood cell counts, liver function tests.

Measurements of the following blood levels: glucose, calcium, phosphorus, folic acid, vitamin B-12.

Bone mineral density testing to check risk for osteoporosis and fracture.

▷ **While Taking This Drug, Observe the Following**

Foods: No restrictions.

Nutritional Support: Supplements of folic acid, calcium, vitamin D and vitamin K may be necessary.

Beverages: No restrictions. May be taken with milk.

▷   *Alcohol:* Use extreme caution. Alcohol (in large quantities or with continual use) may reduce this drug's effectiveness in preventing seizures.

Tobacco Smoking: No interactions expected.

▷ *Other Drugs*

Phenytoin may **decrease** the effects of
- acetaminophen.
- conjugated estrogens (Premarin).
- cortisonelike drugs (see Drug Class Section).
- cyclosporine (Sandimmune).
- disopyramide (Norpace).
- doxycycline (Vibramycin, etc.).
- itraconazole (Sporanox).
- levodopa (Larodopa, Sinemet).
- levothyroxine.
- meperidine (Demerol).
- methadone (Dolophine).
- mexiletine (Mexitil).
- miconazole (Monistat, Micatin, others).
- oral contraceptives (birth control pills).
- oral hypoglycemic agents (see Drug Class).
- paroxetine (Paxil).
- quinidine (Quinaglute, etc.).

Phenytoin **taken concurrently** with
- oral anticoagulants (Coumadin, etc.) can either increase or decrease the anticoagulant effect; monitor this combination very closely with serial prothrombin testing.
- carbamazepine (Tegretol) may result in increased or decreased levels of phenytoin.
- chlordiazepoxide (Librium) (and perhaps other benzodiazepines) may increase or decrease phenytoin levels. Levels should be obtained more frequently if these drugs are combined.
- ciprofloxacin (Cipro) may increase or decrease phenytoin levels.
- dopamine will result in very low blood pressure.
- ketorolac (Toradol) may result in seizures. DO NOT combine these medicines.
- primidone (Mysoline) may alter primidone actions and enhance its toxicity.
- theophyllines (Aminophyllin, Theo-Dur, etc.) may cause a decrease in the effectiveness of both drugs.
- valproic acid (Depakene) may result in altered phenytoin or valproic acid levels. Increased blood level testing of both medicines is needed if these medicines are to be combined.
- warfarin (Coumadin) may result in an initial increased risk of bleeding and a subsequent decrease in anticoagulation. More frequent INR testing is needed. Warfarin doses should be adjusted to laboratory results.

The following drugs may **increase** the effects of phenytoin
- amiodarone (Codarone).
- chloramphenicol (Chloromycetin).
- chlorpheniramine.
- cimetidine (Tagamet).
- cotrimoxazole (Bactrim).
- diltiazem (Cardizem).

- disulfiram (Antabuse).
- felbamate (Felbatol).
- fluconazole (Diflucan).
- fluvoxamine (Luvox).
- fluoxetine (Prozac).
- ibuprofen and perhaps other NSAIDs.
- isoniazid (INH, Niconyl, etc.).
- nifedipine (Adalat).
- omeprazole (Prilosec).
- phenacemide (Phenurone).
- sulfonamides (see Drug Class Section).
- tricyclic antidepressants (see drug Classes).
- trimethoprim (Proloprim, Trimpex).
- valproic acid (Depakene).

The following drugs may *decrease* the effects of phenytoin

- bleomycin.
- carmustine.
- cisplatin.
- diazoxide.
- folic acid.
- methotrexate (Mexate).
- rifampin (Rifadin).
- vinblastine.

▷ *Driving, Hazardous Activities:* This drug may impair mental alertness, vision and coordination. Restrict activities as necessary.

Aviation Note: The use of this drug *is a disqualification* for piloting. Consult a designated Aviation Medical Examiner.

Exposure to Sun: Use caution. This drug may cause photosensitivity (see Glossary).

Occurrence of Unrelated Illness: Intercurrent infections may slow the elimination of this drug and increase the risk of toxicity due to higher blood levels.

Discontinuation: This drug must not be discontinued abruptly. Sudden withdrawal can precipitate severe and repeated seizures. If this drug is to be discontinued, gradual reduction in dosage should be made over a period of 3 months. Total drug withdrawal may be attempted after a period of 3 to 4 years without a seizure. However, seizures are likely to recur in 40% of adults and in 20–30% of children.

PILOCARPINE (pi loh KAR peen)

Introduced: 1875   **Prescription:** USA: Yes; Canada: No   **Available as Generic:** Yes   **Class:** Antiglaucoma   **Controlled Drug:** USA: No; Canada: No

Brand Names: Adsorbocarpine, Akarpine, Almocarpine, E-Pilo Preparations [CD], I-Pilopine, Isopto Carpine, ♣Minims, ♣Miocarpine, Ocusert Pilo-20,-40, PE Preparations [CD], Pilagan, Pilocar, Pilopine HS, Piloptic-1,-2, Pilosyst 20/40, Salagen, ♣Spersacarpine

```
┌─────────────────────────────────────────────────────────────────┐
│                    BENEFITS versus RISKS                          │
│        Possible Benefits                   Possible Risks         │
│   EFFECTIVE REDUCTION OF           Mild side effects with systemic│
│     INTERNAL EYE PRESSURE FOR        absorption                   │
│     CONTROL OF ACUTE AND           Minor eye discomfort           │
│     CHRONIC GLAUCOMA               Altered vision                 │
└─────────────────────────────────────────────────────────────────┘
```

▷ **Principal Uses**
    As a Single Drug Product: Uses currently included in FDA approved labeling: (1) Used exclusively for the management of all types of glaucoma. Selection of the appropriate dosage form and strength must be carefully individualized; (2) can help in dry mouth (xerostomia).
    Other (unlabeled) generally accepted uses: (1) Treatment of Adie's syndrome; (2) can help before laser surgery in order to prevent excessive increases in eye (intraocular) pressure after surgery.
    As a Combination Drug Product [CD]: This drug is combined with epinephrine (in eye drop solutions) to utilize the actions of both drugs in lowering internal eye pressure. The opposite effects of these two drugs on the size of the pupil (pilocarpine constricts, epinephrine dilates) provides a balance that prevents excessive constriction or dilation.

How This Drug Works: By directly stimulating constriction of the pupil, this drug enlarges the outflow canal in the anterior chamber of the eye and promotes the drainage of excess fluid (aqueous humor), thus lowering the internal eye pressure.

Available Dosage Forms and Strengths
    Eye drop solutions — 0.25%, 0.5%, 1%, 2%, 3%, 4%, 5%, 6%, 8% and 10%
    Gel — 4%
    Ocuserts — 20 mcg and 40 mcg
    Tablet — 5 mg

▷ **Usual Adult Dosage Range:** For open-angle glaucoma—eye drop solutions: 1 drop of a 1% to 2% solution 3 to 4 times daily. Eye gel: apply 0.5 inch strip of gel into the eye once daily at bedtime. Ocusert: insert one into affected eye and replace every 7 days with a new one. **Note: Actual dose and dosing schedule must be determined by the physician for each patient individually.**

Conditions Requiring Dosing Adjustments
    Liver function: The specific elimination of this drug is unclear.
    Kidney function: The elimination of this drug has yet to be defined.

▷ **Dosing Instructions:** To avoid excessive absorption into the body, press finger against inner corner of the eye (to close off the tear duct) during and for 2 minutes following instillation of the eye drop. Place the gel and the Ocusert in the eye at bedtime.

Usual Duration of Use: Use on a regular schedule for 1 to 2 weeks usually determines this drug's effectiveness in controlling internal eye pressure. Long-term use (months to years) requires physician supervision.

▷ **This Drug Should Not Be Taken If**
- you have had an allergic reaction to it previously.
- you have acute iritis.
- you have active bronchial asthma.

▷ **Inform Your Physician Before Taking This Drug If**
- you have a history of bronchial asthma.
- you have a history of acute iritis.
- you have significant heart disease.
- you have chronic obstructive pulmonary disease.
- you have gallstones.

Possible Side Effects (natural, expected, and unavoidable drug actions)
Temporary impairment of vision, usually lasting 2 to 3 hours following instillation of drops.

▷ **Possible Adverse Effects** (unusual, unexpected, and infrequent reactions)
If any of the following develop, consult your physician promptly for guidance.
Mild Adverse Effects
Allergic Reactions: Itching of the eyes, eyelid itching and/or swelling.
Headache, heart palpitation, tremors.
Sweating, nausea.
Serious Adverse Effects
Provocation of acute asthma in susceptible individuals.
Atrioventricular block (abnormal heart conduction).
Retinal detachment (rare).
Mental status changes (rare).

▷ **Possible Effects on Sexual Function:**   None reported.

Possible Effects on Laboratory Tests
Red blood cell and white blood cell counts: increased.

Precautions for Use
By Those over 60 Years of Age: Maintain personal cleanliness to prevent eye infections. Report promptly any indication of possible infection involving the eyes.

▷ **Advisability of Use During Pregnancy**
Pregnancy Category: C. See Pregnancy Code at the back of this book.
Animal studies: Significant birth defects due to this drug reported in rats.
Human studies: Adequate studies of pregnant women are not available.
Limit use to the smallest effective dose. Minimize systemic absorption (see Dosing Instructions).

Advisability of Use if Breast-Feeding
Presence of this drug in breast milk: May be present in small amounts.
Monitor nursing infant closely and discontinue drug or nursing if adverse effects develop.

Habit-Forming Potential: None.

Effects of Overdosage: Flushing of face, increased flow of saliva, sweating. If solution is swallowed: nausea, vomiting, diarrhea, profuse sweating, rapid pulse, difficult breathing, loss of consciousness.

Possible Effects of Long-Term Use: Development of tolerance (see Glossary), temporary loss of effectiveness.

Suggested Periodic Examinations While Taking This Drug (at physician's discretion)

Measurement of internal eye pressure on a regular basis.

Examination of eyes for development of cataracts.

▷ **While Taking This Drug, Observe the Following**

Foods: No restrictions.

Beverages: No restrictions.

▷ *Alcohol:* Use caution. If this drug is absorbed, it may prolong the effect of alcohol on the brain.

Tobacco Smoking: No interactions expected.

Marijuana Smoking: Sustained additional decrease in internal eye pressure.

▷ *Other Drugs*

The following drugs may *decrease* the effects of pilocarpine

• atropine and drugs with atropinelike actions (see Drug Classes).

Pilocarpine *taken concurrently* with

• epinephrine will result in increased myopia.

• timolol can produce additive effects in treating glaucoma.

▷ *Driving, Hazardous Activities:* This drug may impair your ability to focus your vision properly. Restrict activities as necessary.

Aviation Note: The use of this drug *may be a disqualification* for piloting. Consult a designated Aviation Medical Examiner.

Exposure to Sun: This medicine may make you very sensitive to the sun. Wear sunglasses.

Discontinuation: Do not stop regular use of this drug without consulting your physician. Periodic discontinuation and temporary substitution of another drug may be necessary to preserve its effectiveness in treating glaucoma.

PINDOLOL (PIN doh lohl)

Introduced: 1972   **Prescription:** USA: Yes; Canada: Yes   **Available as Generic:** Yes   **Class:** Antihypertensive, beta-adrenergic blocker   **Controlled Drug:** USA: No; Canada: No

Brand Names: ✤Apo-Pindol, ✤Novo-Pindol, ✤Nu-Pindol, ✤Syn-Pindolol, ✤Viskazide [CD], Visken

BENEFITS versus RISKS	
Possible Benefits	*Possible Risks*
EFFECTIVE, WELL-TOLERATED ANTIHYPERTENSIVE in mild to moderate high blood pressure	CONGESTIVE HEART FAILURE in advanced heart disease
	Worsening of angina in coronary heart disease (abrupt withdrawal)
	Masking of low blood sugar (hypoglycemia) in drug-treated diabetes
	Provocation of asthma (with high doses)

▷ **Principal Uses**

As a Single Drug Product: Uses currently included in FDA approved labeling: (1) The treatment of mild to moderate high blood pressure. May be used alone or concurrently with other antihypertensive drugs, such as diuretics.

Other (unlabeled) generally accepted uses: (1) May be of benefit in helping control aggressive behavior; (2) can help prevent migraine headaches; (3) combination therapy with digoxin may be effective in limiting some abnormal heart rhythms (atrial fibrillation); (4) can be of benefit in some kinds of anxiety; (5) decreases sympathetic output in hyperthyroidism.

As a Combination Drug Product [CD]: This drug is available in combination with hydrochlorothiazide (in Canada). The addition of a thiazide diuretic to this beta blocker drug enhances its effectiveness as an antihypertensive.

How This Drug Works: By blocking certain actions of the sympathetic nervous system, this drug

- reduces the rate and contraction force of the heart, thus lowering the ejection pressure of the blood leaving the heart.
- reduces the degree of contraction of blood vessel walls, resulting in their relaxation and consequent lowering of blood pressure.

Available Dosage Forms and Strengths

Tablets — 5 mg, 10 mg, 15 mg (Canada)

▷ **Usual Adult Dosage Range:** Hypertension: Initially, 5 mg twice daily (12 hours apart). The dose may be increased gradually by 10 mg/day at intervals of 3 to 4 weeks as needed and tolerated up to 60 mg/day. For maintenance, 5 to 10 mg 2 or 3 times/day is often effective. The total daily dose should not exceed 60 mg. **Note: Actual dosage and administration schedule must be determined by the physician for each patient individually.**

Conditions Requiring Dosing Adjustments

Liver function: The dose should be empirically decreased in patients with severe liver compromise and in those with combined liver and kidney compromise.

Kidney function: The dose should be decreased if urine output is significantly decreased.

▷ **Dosing Instructions:** The tablet may be crushed and taken without regard to eating. Do not stop this drug abruptly.

Usual Duration of Use: Use on a regular schedule for 2 to 3 weeks usually determines effectiveness in lowering blood pressure. The long-term use of this drug (months to years) will be determined by the course of your blood pressure over time and your response to an overall treatment program (weight reduction, salt restriction, smoking cessation, etc.). Consult your physician on a regular basis.

Possible Advantages of This Drug: Causes less slowing of the heart rate than most other beta blocker drugs.

Currently a "Drug of Choice"

for initiating treatment of hypertension with a single drug.

▷ **This Drug Should Not Be Taken If**

- you have bronchial asthma.
- you have had an allergic reaction to it previously.
- you have congestive heart failure.

- you have an abnormally slow heart rate or a serious form of heart block.
- you are taking, or have taken within the past 14 days, any monoamine oxidase (MAO) type A inhibitor drug (see Drug Classes).

▷ **Inform Your Physician Before Taking This Drug If**
- you have had an adverse reaction to any beta blocker in the past (see Drug Classes).
- you have a history of serious heart disease.
- you have a history of hay fever (allergic rhinitis), asthma, chronic bronchitis or emphysema.
- you have a history of overactive thyroid function (hyperthyroidism).
- you have a history of low blood sugar (hypoglycemia) or diabetes.
- you have impaired liver or kidney function.
- you have diabetes or myasthenia gravis.
- you currently take any form of digitalis, quinidine or reserpine, or any calcium blocker drug (see Drug Class Section).
- you have bad circulation to your legs or arms (peripheral vascular disease).
- you plan to have surgery under general anesthesia in the near future.

Possible Side Effects (natural, expected, and unavoidable drug actions)
Lethargy and fatigability, cold extremities, slow heart rate, light-headedness in upright position (see Orthostatic Hypotension in Glossary).

▷ **Possible Adverse Effects** (unusual, unexpected, and infrequent reactions)
If any of the following develop, consult your physician promptly for guidance.
Mild Adverse Effects
Allergic Reactions: Skin rash, itching.
Headache, dizziness, insomnia, abnormal dreams, fainting.
Indigestion, nausea, vomiting, constipation, diarrhea.
Joint and muscle discomfort, fluid retention (edema).
Serious Adverse Effects
Mental depression, anxiety.
Chest pain, shortness of breath, precipitation of congestive heart failure.
Induction of bronchial asthma (in asthmatic individuals).
Abnormally slow heartbeat.
Congestive heart failure (rare).
Drug-induced systemic lupus erythematosus (rare).
Drug-induced myasthenia gravis.
Worsening of poor circulation to the arms or legs (intermittent claudication).
Depression.
Carpal tunnel syndrome (reported with other beta-blockers).
Low blood glucose.

▷ **Possible Effects on Sexual Function:** Decreased libido (2%), impaired erection (up to 2%).

Possible Effects on Laboratory Tests
Blood lupus erythematosus (LE) cells: positive (one case of drug-induced LE).
Blood total cholesterol level: decreased (with long-term use).
Blood HDL cholesterol level: increased.
Blood LDL and VLDL cholesterol levels: no effects.
Blood triglyceride levels: no effects.
Glucose tolerance test (GTT): decreased.

Liver function tests: slightly increased liver enzymes (ALT/GPT and AST/GOT) in 7% of drug users.

CAUTION
1. ***Do not stop this drug suddenly*** without the knowledge and help of your doctor. Carry a notation on your person that you are taking this drug.
2. Ask your doctor or pharmacist before using nasal decongestants usually present in over-the-counter cold preparations and nose drops. These can cause sudden increases in blood pressure when taken concurrently with beta blocker drugs.
3. Report the development of any tendency to emotional depression.

Precautions for Use
By Infants and Children: Safety and effectiveness for those under 12 years of age not established. However, if this drug is used, observe for the development of low blood sugar (hypoglycemia) during periods of reduced food intake.

By Those over 60 Years of Age: Unacceptably high blood pressure should be reduced without creating the risks associated with excessively low blood pressure. Small starting doses, and frequent blood pressure checks are indicated. Sudden, rapid and excessive reduction of blood pressure can predispose to stroke or heart attack. Watch for dizziness, unsteadiness, tendency to fall, confusion, hallucinations, depression or urinary frequency.

▷ Advisability of Use During Pregnancy
Pregnancy Category: B. See Pregnancy Code at the back of this book.
Animal studies: No significant increase in birth defects due to this drug.
Human studies: Adequate studies of pregnant women are not available.
Use this drug only if clearly needed. Ask physician for guidance.

Advisability of Use if Breast-Feeding
Presence of this drug in breast milk: Yes.
Avoid drug or refrain from nursing.

Habit-Forming Potential: None.

Effects of Overdosage: Weakness, slow pulse, low blood pressure, fainting, cold and sweaty skin, congestive heart failure, possible coma and convulsions.

Possible Effects of Long-Term Use: Reduced heart reserve and eventual heart failure in susceptible individuals with advanced heart disease.

Suggested Periodic Examinations While Taking This Drug (at physician's discretion)
Measurements of blood pressure, evaluation of heart function.

▷ While Taking This Drug, Observe the Following
Foods: No restrictions. Avoid excessive salt intake.
Beverages: No restrictions. May be taken with milk.
▷ *Alcohol:* Use with caution. Alcohol may exaggerate this drug's ability to lower the blood pressure and may increase its mild sedative effect.
Tobacco Smoking: Nicotine may reduce this drug's effectiveness in treating high blood pressure. In addition, high doses of this drug may worsen constriction of the bronchial tubes caused by regular smoking.

▷   *Other Drugs*

Pindolol may *increase* the effects of
- other antihypertensive drugs, and cause excessive lowering of the blood pressure. Dosage adjustments may be necessary.
- reserpine (Ser-Ap-Es, etc.), and cause sedation, depression, slowing of the heart rate and lowering of the blood pressure.
- verapamil (Calan, Isoptin), and cause excessive depression of heart function; monitor this combination closely.

Pindolol *taken concurrently* with
- amiodarone (Codarone) may cause extremely slow heart beats and risk sinus arrest.
- clonidine (Catapres) requires close monitoring for rebound high blood pressure if clonidine is withdrawn while pindolol is still being taken.
- epinephrine (various) will result in a large increase in blood pressure and reflex increase in heart rate (tachycardia).
- fluoxetine (Prozac) may result in increased risk of pindolol toxicity.
- fluvoxamine (Luvox) may result in increased risk of pindolol toxicity.
- insulin requires close monitoring to avoid undetected hypoglycemia (see Glossary).
- oral hypoglycemic agents (see Drug Classes) can result in slowed recovery from low blood sugar.
- phenylpropanolamine (various) may result in severe increases in blood pressure. Avoid this combination.
- venlafaxine (Effexor) may result in beta blocker or venlafaxine toxicity. Avoid this combination if possible, or use decreased doses of both medicines.

The following drugs may *increase* the effects of pindolol
- cimetidine (Tagamet).
- methimazole (Tapazole).
- oral contraceptives.
- propylthiouracil (Propacil).

The following drugs may *decrease* the effects of pindolol
- barbiturates (phenobarbital, etc.).
- indomethacin (Indocin), and possibly other "aspirin substitutes," or NSAIDs may impair pindolol's antihypertensive effect.
- rifampin (Rifadin, Rimactane).
- theophylline (Theodur, others).

▷   *Driving, Hazardous Activities:* Use caution until the full extent of fatigue, dizziness and blood pressure change have been determined.

Aviation Note: The use of this drug *is a disqualification* for piloting. Consult a designated Aviation Medical Examiner.

Exposure to Sun: No restrictions.

Exposure to Heat: Caution advised. Hot environments can lower the blood pressure and exaggerate the effects of this drug.

Exposure to Cold: Caution advised. Cold environments can enhance the circulatory deficiency in the extremities that may occur with this drug. The elderly should take precautions to prevent hypothermia (see Glossary).

Heavy Exercise or Exertion: It is advisable to avoid exertion that produces lightheadedness, excessive fatigue or muscle cramping. The use of this drug may intensify the hypertensive response to isometric exercise.

Occurrence of Unrelated Illness: Fever can lower the blood pressure and require adjustment of dosage. Nausea or vomiting may interrupt regular doses. Ask your doctor for help.

Discontinuation: It is advisable to avoid sudden discontinuation of this drug in all situations. If possible, gradual reduction of dose over a period of 2 to 3 weeks is recommended. Ask your physician for specific guidance.

PIRBUTEROL (peer BYU ter ohl)

Introduced: 1983   **Prescription:** USA: Yes   **Available as Generic:** No   **Class:** Antiasthmatic, bronchodilator   **Controlled Drug:** USA: No
Brand Name: Maxair

BENEFITS versus RISKS	
Possible Benefits	*Possible Risks*
VERY EFFECTIVE RELIEF OF BRONCHOSPASM	Increased blood pressure
	Nervousness
	Fine hand tremor
	Irregular heart rhythm (with excessive use)

▷ **Principal Uses**

As a Single Drug Product: Uses currently included in FDA approved labeling: (1) Relieves acute attacks of bronchial asthma; (2) reduces the frequency and severity of chronic, recurrent asthmatic attacks (prevention); (3) relieves reversible bronchospasm associated with chronic bronchitis, bronchiectasis and emphysema.

Other (unlabeled) generally accepted uses: May help congestive heart failure.

How This Drug Works: By increasing the production of cyclic AMP, this drug relaxes constricted bronchial muscles to relieve asthmatic wheezing.

Available Dosage Forms and Strengths

Aerosol — 200 mcg per actuation (in canisters of 300 inhalations)

▷ **Usual Adult Dosage Range:** Inhaler—2 inhalations (400 mcg) every 4 to 6 hours. **Do not exceed** 12 inhalations (2400 mcg)/24 hours. Oral dosing: 10 to 15 milligrams three to four times a day. Maximum dose is 60 mg daily. **Note: Actual dosage and administration schedule must be determined by the physician for each patient individually.**

Conditions Requiring Dosing Adjustments

Liver function: It should be used with caution in patients with liver compromise who use it frequently. Guidelines for dosage adjustments are not available.

Kidney function: The kidneys do not appear to play a role in the elimination of this drug.

▷ **Dosing Instructions:** Carefully follow the "Patient's Instructions for Use" provided with the inhaler. Do not overuse.

Usual Duration of Use: According to individual requirements. Do not use beyond the time necessary to terminate episodes of asthma.

Possible Advantages of This Drug

Has a more rapid onset of action and a longer duration of effect than most other drugs of this class.

▷ **This Drug Should Not Be Taken If**
- you have had an allergic reaction to it previously.
- you currently have an irregular heart rhythm.
- you are taking, or have taken within the past 2 weeks, any monoamine oxidase (MAO) type A inhibitor drug (see Drug Classes).

▷ **Inform Your Physician Before Taking This Drug If**
- you have any type of heart or circulatory disorder, especially high blood pressure, coronary heart disease or heart rhythm abnormality.
- you have diabetes or an excessively active thyroid gland (hyperthyroidism).
- you have any type of seizure disorder.
- you are taking any form of digitalis or any stimulant drug.

Possible Side Effects (natural, expected, and unavoidable drug actions)

Aerosol—dryness or irritation of mouth or throat, altered taste.

▷ **Possible Adverse Effects** (unusual, unexpected, and infrequent reactions)

If any of the following develop, consult your physician promptly for guidance.

Mild Adverse Effects

Allergic Reactions: Skin rash, itching (rare).

Headache (rare), dizziness (rare), nervousness, fine tremor of hands.

Palpitations (rare), rapid heart rate, chest pain (rare), cough (rare).

Nausea, diarrhea, taste disorders (all rare).

Serious Adverse Effects

Irregular heart rhythm, increased blood pressure.

▷ **Possible Effects on Sexual Function:**   None reported.

Natural Diseases or Disorders That May Be Activated By This Drug

Latent coronary artery disease, diabetes, epilepsy or high blood pressure.

Possible Effects on Laboratory Tests

None reported.

CAUTION

1. Combined use of this drug by inhalation with beclomethasone aerosol (Beclovent, Vanceril) may increase the risk of toxicity due to fluorocarbon propellants. Advisable to use pirbuterol aerosol 20 to 30 minutes **before** beclomethasone aerosol. This will reduce the risk of toxicity and help beclomethasone reach the lung.

2. Excessive or prolonged use of this drug by inhalation can reduce its effectiveness and cause serious heart rhythm disturbances, including cardiac arrest.

Precautions for Use

By Infants and Children: Safety and effectiveness of use in children under 12 years of age have not been established.

By Those over 60 Years of Age: Avoid excessive and continual use. If acute asthma is not relieved promptly, other drugs will have to be tried. Observe for the development of nervousness, palpitations, irregular heart rhythm and muscle tremors.

▷ **Advisability of Use During Pregnancy**

Pregnancy Category: C. See Pregnancy Code at the back of this book.

Animal studies: High-dose studies in rabbits revealed abortion and increased fetal deaths. Studies in rats and rabbits found no drug associated birth defects.

Human studies: Adequate studies of pregnant women are not available.

Avoid use during first 3 months if possible.

Advisability of Use if Breast-Feeding

Presence of this drug in breast milk: Unknown.

Avoid drug or refrain from nursing.

Habit-Forming Potential: None.

Effects of Overdosage: Nervousness, palpitation, rapid heart rate, sweating, headache, tremor, vomiting, chest pain.

Possible Effects of Long-Term Use: Loss of effectiveness.

Suggested Periodic Examinations While Taking This Drug (at physician's discretion)

Blood pressure measurements, evaluation of heart status.

▷ **While Taking This Drug, Observe the Following**

Foods: No restrictions.

Beverages: Avoid excessive use of caffeine-containing beverages—coffee, tea, cola, chocolate.

▷ *Alcohol:* No interactions expected.

Tobacco Smoking: No interactions expected.

▷ *Other Drugs*

Pirbuterol *taken concurrently* with

• albuterol (Proventil, Ventolin) may result in adverse effects on the heart.

• monoamine oxidase (MAO) type A inhibitor drugs may cause excessive increase in blood pressure and undesirable heart stimulation.

• phenothiazines (see Drug Classes) may result in blunting of the therapeutic effects of pirbuterol.

▷ *Driving, Hazardous Activities:* Use caution if excessive nervousness or dizziness occurs.

Aviation Note: The use of this drug *is a disqualification* for piloting. Consult a designated Aviation Medical Examiner.

Exposure to Sun: No restrictions.

Heavy Exercise or Exertion: Use caution. Excessive exercise can induce asthma in sensitive individuals.

PIROXICAM (peer OX i kam)

Introduced: 1978   **Prescription:** USA: Yes; Canada: Yes   **Available as Generic:** Yes   **Class:** analgesic, mild; NSAID   **Controlled Drug:** USA: No; Canada: No

Brand Names: ✦Apo-Piroxicam, Feldene, ✦Novopirocam, Nu-Pirox

BENEFITS versus RISKS	
Possible Benefits	*Possible Risks*
EFFECTIVE RELIEF OF MILD TO MODERATE PAIN AND INFLAMMATION	Gastrointestinal pain, ulceration, bleeding Drug-induced hepatitis (rare) Rare kidney damage Mild fluid retention Reduced white blood cell and platelet counts

Please see the oxicam nonsteroidal anti-inflammatory drug profile for further information.

PRAVASTATIN (pra vah STA tin)

Introduced: 1986 **Prescription:** USA: Yes; Canada: Yes **Available as Generic:** USA: No; Canada: No **Class:** anticholesterol **Controlled Drug:** USA: No; Canada: No

Brand Name: Pravachol

BENEFITS versus RISKS	
Possible Benefits	*Possible Risks*
EFFECTIVE REDUCTION OF TOTAL BLOOD CHOLESTEROL AND LDL CHOLESTEROL EFFECTIVE REDUCTION IN THE NUMBER OF FIRST-TIME HEART ATTACKS REDUCTION IN THE NUMBER OF PATIENT DEATHS	Drug-induced hepatitis (without jaundice) (rare) Drug-induced myositis (muscle inflammation) (rare)

▷ **Principal Uses**

As a Single Drug Product: Uses currently included in FDA approved labeling: (1) Treatment of abnormally high total blood cholesterol levels (in individuals with Types IIa and IIb hypercholesterolemia) due to increased fractions of low-density lipoprotein (LDL) cholesterol. It is used in conjunction with a cholesterol-lowering diet. It should not be used until an adequate trial of nondrug methods for lowering cholesterol has proved to be ineffective;(2) the FDA has cleared this medicine to help prevent a first heart attack and reduce death from cardiovascular disease in people with increased blood cholesterol levels who are at risk of a first heart attack. Other (unlabeled) generally accepted uses: (1) Familial hypercholesterolemia; (2) appears to have a role in slowing the progression and in some cases making small reversals in coronary artery disease.

How This Drug Works: This drug blocks the liver enzyme that starts production of cholesterol. Its principal action is the reduction of low-density lipoproteins (LDL), the fraction of total blood cholesterol that is thought to increase the risk of coronary heart disease. This drug may also increase the level of high-density lipoproteins (HDL), the cholesterol fraction that is thought to reduce the risk of heart disease.

Available Dosage Forms and Strengths

Tablets — 10 mg, 20 mg (Canada) and 20 mg (United States).

▷ **Recommended Dosage Ranges** (Actual dosage and administration schedule must be determined by the physician for each patient individually.)

Infants and Children: Under 2 years of age—do not use this drug.

2 to 18 years of age—dosage not established.

18 to 60 Years of Age: Initially 10 to 20 mg daily, taken at bedtime. Maintenance dosage is 10 to 20 mg daily; and is adjusted as needed and tolerated at intervals of 4 weeks.

Over 60 Years of Age: Starting dose in those with kidney or liver compromise is 10 mg daily.

Conditions Requiring Dosing Adjustments

Liver function: This drug should be used with caution in patients with liver compromise, and the starting dose decreased to 10 mg per day. Pravastatin is contraindicated in acute liver disease.

Kidney function: Patients with significant renal compromise can be given a starting dose of 10 mg per day. Pravastatin should be used with caution in renal compromise.

▷ **Dosing Instructions:** The tablet may be crushed and can be taken without regard to eating. Preferably taken at bedtime. (The highest rates of cholesterol production occur between midnight and 5 a.m.)

Usual Duration of Use: Use on a regular schedule for 4 to 6 weeks usually determines effectiveness in reducing blood levels of total and LDL cholesterol. Long-term use (months to years) requires periodic physician evaluation.

Possible Advantages of This Drug: Recent studies indicate that drugs of this class (HMG-CoA reductase inhibitors) are more effective and better tolerated than other drugs currently available for reducing total and LDL cholesterol. Its long-term effects are yet to be determined. See Cholesterol Disorders in Section Two.

▷ **This Drug Should Not Be Taken If**
- you have had an allergic reaction to it previously.
- you have active liver disease.
- you are pregnant or breast-feeding your infant.

▷ **Inform Your Physician Before Taking This Drug If**
- you have previously taken any other drugs in this class: lovastatin (Mevacor), simvastatin (Zocor).
- you have a history of liver disease or impaired liver function.
- you are not using any method of birth control, or you are planning pregnancy.
- you regularly consume substantial amounts of alcohol.
- you have kidney disease.
- you have cataracts or impaired vision.
- you develop any kind of unexplained muscle weakness, pain or tenderness.
- you have any type of chronic muscular disorder.
- you plan to have major surgery in the near future.

Possible Side Effects (natural, expected, and unavoidable drug actions)
Development of abnormal liver function tests without associated symptoms.

▷ **Possible Adverse Effects** (unusual, unexpected, and infrequent reactions)
If any of the following develop, consult your physician promptly for guidance.
Mild Adverse Effects
Allergic Reactions: Skin rash, itching (rare).
Headache (rare), dizziness (rare).
Flu-like syndrome, cough (occasional).
Indigestion (rare), stomach pain (rare), nausea, excessive gas, constipation, diarrhea (rare).
Muscle cramps and/or pain (rare).
Serious Adverse Effects
Marked and persistent abnormal liver function tests with focal hepatitis (without jaundice) (rare).
Acute myositis (muscle pain and tenderness), rare during long-term use.
Rhabdomyolysis (rare).
Low white blood cells (leukopenia) (rare).
Neuropathy (rare).

▷ **Possible Effects on Sexual Function:**   None reported.

Possible Delayed Adverse Effects: None reported to date.

Natural Diseases or Disorders That May Be Activated by This Drug
Latent liver disease.

Possible Effects on Laboratory Tests
Blood alanine aminotransferase (ALT) enzyme level: increased (with higher doses of drug).
Blood total cholesterol, LDL cholesterol and triglyceride levels: decreased.
Blood HDL cholesterol level: increased.

CAUTION
1. If pregnancy occurs while taking this drug, discontinue it immediately and consult your physician.
2. Report promptly any development of muscle pain or tenderness, especially if accompanied by fever or malaise.
3. Report promptly the development of altered or impaired vision so that appropriate evaluation can be made.
4. If CPK levels become markedly elevated, this medicine should be stopped.

Precautions for Use
By Infants and Children: Safety and effectiveness for those under 18 years of age not established.
By Those over 60 Years of Age: Inform your physician regarding any personal or family history of cataracts. Comply with all recommendations regarding periodic eye examinations. Report promptly any alterations in vision.

▷ **Advisability of Use During Pregnancy**
Pregnancy Category: X. See Pregnancy Code at the back of this book.
Animal studies: Mouse and rat studies reveal skeletal birth defects due to a closely related drug of this class.

Human studies: Adequate studies of pregnant women are not available. This drug should be avoided during entire pregnancy.

Advisability of Use if Breast-Feeding
Presence of this drug in breast milk: Yes, in small amounts.
Avoid drug or refrain from nursing.

Habit-Forming Potential: None.

Effects of Overdosage: Increased indigestion, stomach distress, nausea, diarrhea.

Possible Effects of Long-Term Use: Abnormal liver function with focal hepatitis.

Suggested Periodic Examinations While Taking This Drug (at physician's discretion)
Blood cholesterol studies: total cholesterol, HDL and LDL fractions.
Liver function tests before treatment, every 6 weeks during the first 3 months of use, every 8 weeks for the rest of the first year, and at 6-month intervals thereafter.
Complete eye examination at beginning of treatment and at any time that significant change in vision occurs. Ask your physician for guidance.

▷ **While Taking This Drug, Observe the Following**
Foods: Follow a standard low-cholesterol diet.
Beverages: No restrictions. May be taken with milk.
▷ *Alcohol:* No interactions expected. Use sparingly.
Tobacco Smoking: No interactions expected.
▷ *Other Drugs*
Pravastatin *taken concurrently* with
• clofibrate (Atromid-S) has been associated with muscle damage (rhabdomyolysis).
• cyclosporine (Sandimmune) increases the risk for myopathy.
• gemfibrozil (Lopid) may alter the absorption and excretion of pravastatin; these drugs should not be taken concurrently.
• warfarin (Coumadin) can increase the risk of bleeding. More frequent INR (Protime) testing is indicated. Ongoing warfarin doses should be based on laboratory results.
The following drug may *decrease* the effects of pravastatin
• cholestyramine (Questran), may reduce absorption of pravastatin; take pravastatin 1 hour before or 4 hours after cholestyramine.
▷ *Driving, Hazardous Activities:* This drug may cause dizziness. Restrict activities as necessary.
Aviation Note: The use of this drug *may be a disqualification* for piloting. Consult a designated Aviation Medical Examiner.
Exposure to Sun: No restrictions.
Discontinuation: Do not stop this drug without your doctor's knowledge and help. There may be a significant increase in blood cholesterol levels following discontinuation of this drug.

PRAZOSIN (PRA zoh sin)

Introduced: 1970   **Prescription:** USA: Yes; Canada: Yes   **Available as Generic:** Yes   **Class:** Antihypertensive   **Controlled Drug:** USA: No; Canada: No

Brand Names: ✦Apo-Prazo, Minipress, Minizide [CD], ✦Novo-Prazin, ✦Nu-Prazo

---

BENEFITS versus RISKS

Possible Benefits	*Possible Risks*
EFFECTIVE INITIAL THERAPY FOR MILD TO MODERATE HYPERTENSION	"First dose" drop in blood pressure with fainting
EFFECTIVE ANTIHYPERTENSIVE IN MODERATE TO SEVERE HYPERTENSION	Cause of paroxysmal tachycardia
EFFECTIVE CONTROL OF HYPERTENSION IN PHEOCHROMOCYTOMA	
Effective in presence of impaired kidney function	

▷ **Principal Uses**

As a Single Drug Product: Uses currently included in FDA approved labeling: (1) Used to start treatment in mild to moderate hypertension. Also used in conjunction with other drugs, to treat moderate to severe hypertension.

Other (unlabeled) generally accepted uses: (1) Combination therapy of congestive heart failure; (2) helps control high blood pressure in a rare tumor (pheochromocytoma); (3) may have an adjunctive role in controlling urine outflow problems caused by prostatic obstruction; (4) may help relieve the symptoms of Raynaud's phenomenon; (5) can ease symptoms of angina; (6) has a role in reducing benign prostatic hyperplasia.

As a Combination Drug Product [CD]: This drug is available in combination with polythiazide, a diuretic of the thiazide class of drugs. By utilizing two different methods of drug action, this combination product is more effective and more convenient for long-term use.

How This Drug Works: By blocking certain actions of the sympathetic nervous system, this drug causes direct relaxation and expansion of blood vessel walls, thus lowering the pressure of the blood within the vessels.

Available Dosage Forms and Strengths

Capsules — 1 mg, 2 mg, 5 mg

▷ **Usual Adult Dosage Range:**   Hypertension: A "test dose" of 1 mg is given to determine the patient's response within the first 2 hours. Patients at risk for first-dose excessive lowering in blood pressure include those with pheochromocytoma and those who have recently suffered a stroke (cerebral vascular accident). If tolerated satisfactorily, dose is increased cautiously up to 15 mg/24 hours in 2 or 3 divided doses. The total daily dosage should not exceed 20 mg. Benign prostatic hyperplasia (BPH): Starting dose is 0.5 mg to one milligram twice a day. This dose is increased (titrated) as needed and tolerated to 2 mgs twice daily. **Note: Actual dose and dosing schedule must be determined by the physician for each patient individually.**

Conditions Requiring Dosing Adjustments

Liver function: It should be used with caution and in lower doses in patients with liver compromise. The drug is 97% protein bound. Dose adjustments and more frequent blood pressure checks are needed.

Kidney function: Patients with kidney failure may have adequate response to smaller doses.

▷ **Dosing Instructions:**   May be taken without regard to food. The capsule may be opened for administration.

Usual Duration of Use: Use on a regular schedule for 4 to 6 weeks usually determines effectiveness in controlling hypertension. Long-term use (months to years) requires supervision and periodic physician evaluation.

Possible Advantages of This Drug

Effective initial treatment of hypertension.

Does not alter blood cholesterol, potassium or sugar levels.

▷ **This Drug Should Not Be Taken If**
- you have had an allergic reaction to it previously.
- you are experiencing mental depression.
- you have angina (active coronary artery disease) and you are not taking a beta-blocking drug. (Consult your physician.)

▷ **Inform Your Physician Before Taking This Drug If**
- you have experienced orthostatic hypotension (see Glossary) when using other antihypertensive drugs.
- you have a history of mental depression.
- you have impaired circulation to the brain, or a history of stroke (you may be more sensitive to this medicine).
- you have coronary artery disease.
- you have active liver disease or impaired liver function.
- you plan to have surgery under general anesthesia in the near future.

Possible Side Effects (natural, expected, and unavoidable drug actions)

Orthostatic hypotension, drowsiness, salt and water retention, dry mouth, nasal congestion, constipation.

▷ **Possible Adverse Effects** (unusual, unexpected, and infrequent reactions)

If any of the following develop, consult your physician promptly for guidance.

Mild Adverse Effects

Allergic Reactions: Skin rash, itching.

Headache, dizziness, fatigue, weakness, nervousness, sweating, numbness and tingling, blurred vision, reddened eyes, ringing in the ears.

Edema and weight gain (rare).

Nosebleeds.

Palpitation, rapid heart rate, shortness of breath.

Nausea, vomiting, diarrhea, abdominal pain, constipation.

Urinary frequency or incontinence (bed-wetting or enuresis also) (rare).

Serious Adverse Effects

Mental depression, sleep disturbance.

Paroxysmal tachycardia (heart rates of 120 to 160).

Slowing of the heart peak and passing out (syncope) (rare).

▷ **Possible Effects on Sexual Function**
Decreased libido (14%); impotence (less than 1%).
Retrograde ejaculation. Priapism (see Glossary).

Natural Diseases or Disorders That May Be Activated by This Drug
Latent coronary artery insufficiency.

Possible Effects on Laboratory Tests
Blood total cholesterol level: no effect in some; decreased in others.
Blood HDL cholesterol level: no effect in some; increased in others.
Blood LDL cholesterol level: no effect.
Blood VLDL cholesterol level: no effect in some; decreased in others.
Blood triglyceride levels: no effect in some; decreased in others.
Blood glucose level: increased.
Liver function tests: increased (rarely).
Glucose tolerance test (GTT): decreased.
Blood thyroid stimulating hormone (TSH) level: increased.
Blood thyroxine (T_4) level: increased.

CAUTION
1. Observe for the possible "first dose" response of precipitous drop in blood pressure, with or without fainting; this usually occurs within 30 to 90 minutes. Limit initial doses to 1 mg taken at bedtime for the first 3 days; remain supine after taking these trial doses.

Precautions for Use
By Infants and Children: Safety and effectiveness for use by those under 12 years of age have not been established.
By Those over 60 Years of Age: Begin treatment with no more than 1 mg/day for the first 3 days. Subsequent increases in dose must be very gradual and carefully supervised by your physician. The occurrence of orthostatic hypotension can cause unexpected falls and injury; sit or lie down promptly if you feel light-headed or dizzy. Report any indications of dizziness or chest pain promptly.

▷ **Advisability of Use During Pregnancy**
Pregnancy Category: C. See Pregnancy Code at the back of this book.
Animal studies: No birth defects found.
Human studies: Adequate studies of pregnant women are not available.
Use this drug only if clearly needed. Ask your physician for guidance.

Advisability of Use if Breast-Feeding
Presence of this drug in breast milk: Yes, in small amounts.
Monitor nursing infant closely and discontinue drug or nursing if adverse effects develop.

Habit-Forming Potential: None.

Effects of Overdosage: Orthostatic hypotension, headache, generalized flushing, rapid heart rate, extreme weakness, irregular heart rhythm, circulatory collapse.

Possible Effects of Long-Term Use: None reported.

Suggested Periodic Examinations While Taking This Drug (at physician's discretion)
Measurements of blood pressure in lying, sitting and standing positions.
Measurements of body weight to detect fluid retention.

▷ **While Taking This Drug, Observe the Following**

Foods: No restrictions. Avoid excessive salt intake.

Beverages: No restrictions. May be taken with milk.

▷ *Alcohol:* Use with extreme caution. Alcohol can exaggerate the blood-pressure-lowering actions of this drug and cause excessive reduction.

Tobacco Smoking: Nicotine can worsen this drug's ability to intensify coronary insufficiency in susceptible individuals. All forms of tobacco should be avoided.

▷ *Other Drugs*

The following drugs may **increase** the effects of prazosin

- other antihypertensive medications (this is often used to help patients).
- beta-adrenergic-blocking drugs (see Drug Classes); severity and duration of the "first dose" hypotensive response may be increased.
- verapamil (Calan) may increase the blood level of prazosin and require dose reduction.

Prazocin **taken concurrently** with

- NSAIDs (see Drug Classes) may result in blunting of the blood-pressure-lowering benefit of prazocin.

▷ *Driving, Hazardous Activities:* This drug may cause dizziness or drowsiness. Restrict activities as necessary.

Aviation Note: The use of this drug **is a disqualification** for piloting. Consult a designated Aviation Medical Examiner.

Exposure to Sun: No restrictions.

Exposure to Cold: Use caution until combined effect has been determined. Cold environments may increase this drug's ability to cause coronary insufficiency (angina) in susceptible individuals.

Heavy Exercise or Exertion: Excessive exertion can augment this drug's ability to induce angina.

Discontinuation: If you are taking this drug as part of your treatment program for congestive heart failure, do not stop it abruptly. Ask your physician for guidance.

PREDNISOLONE (pred NIS oh lohn)

Introduced: 1955 **Prescription:** USA: Yes; Canada: Yes   **Available as Generic:** USA: Yes; Canada: Yes   **Class:** Cortisonelike drugs   **Controlled Drug:** USA: No; Canada: No

Brand Names: ✦Ak-Cide [CD], A & D with prednisolone [CD], ✦Ak-Pred, ✦Ak-Tate, Blephamide, Cortalone, Delta-Cortef, Duapred, Econopred Ophthalmic, Fernisolone-P, Hydelta-TBA, Hydeltrasol, ✦Inflamase, ✦Inflamase Forte, Isopto Cetapred [CD], Key-Pred, Meticortelone, Menti-Derm, Metimyd [CD], Metreton, ✦Minims Prednisolone, Mydrapred, Niscort, Nor-Pred, ✦Nova-Pred, ✦Novoprednisolone, Ophtho-Tate, Optimyd [CD], Otobione [CD], Pediapred, Pediaject, Polypred, Predcor, ✦Pred Forte, Pred-G [CD], ✦Pred Mild, Prelone, PSP-IV, Savacort, Sterane, TBA Pred, ✦Vasocidin [CD]

```
┌─────────────────────────────────────────────────────────────────┐
│                     BENEFITS versus RISKS                         │
│        Possible Benefits              Possible Risks              │
│   EFFECTIVE RELIEF OF            Use exceeding 2 weeks is associated│
│      SYMPTOMS IN A WIDE VARIETY     with many possible adverse effects:│
│      OF INFLAMMATORY AND            ALTERED MOOD AND               │
│      ALLERGIC DISORDERS               PERSONALITY                 │
│   EFFECTIVE                         CATARACTS, GLAUCOMA            │
│      IMMUNOSUPPRESSION in           HYPERTENSION                   │
│      selected benign and malignant  OSTEOPOROSIS                  │
│      disorders                      ASEPTIC BONE NECROSIS          │
│   Prevention of rejection in organ  INCREASED SUSCEPTIBILITY TO    │
│      transplantation                  INFECTIONS                  │
└─────────────────────────────────────────────────────────────────┘
```

▷ **Principal Uses**

As a Single Drug Product: Uses currently included in FDA approved labeling: (1) Used in the treatment of a wide variety of allergic and inflammatory conditions. It is used most commonly in the management of serious skin disorders, asthma, regional enteritis, ulcerative colitis and all types of major rheumatic disorders including bursitis, tendonitis, most forms of arthritis and inflammatory eye conditions; (2) used as part of combination therapy in lymphoma; (3) used in some kinds of adrenal insufficiencies; (4) used to help tuberculosis patients who also have inflammation around the heart without fluid buildup; (5) eases symptoms in ulcerative colitis.

Other (unlabeled) generally accepted uses: (1) Used as part of combination therapy in acute leukemias (lymphoblastic, lymphocytic and myelogenous); (2) may have a role in combination therapy of breast cancer; (3) can help relieve the muscle pain of familial Mediterranean Fever; (4) part of a combination therapy in treating abnormal liver tumors (hemangiomas); (5) can help subfertile men decrease seminal antibodies and become fertile; (6) helps people who have drug-induced lowering of white blood cells recover; (7) treats anaphylactic reactions of unknown cause; (8) treats thrombocytopenic purpura of unknown cause; (9) eases symptoms in myasthenia gravis; (10) can help reflex sympathetic dystrophy.

How This Drug Works: Not fully established. It is thought that this drug's anti-inflammatory effect is due to its ability to inhibit the normal defensive functions of certain white blood cells. Its immunosuppressant effect is attributed to a reduced production of lymphocytes and antibodies.

Available Dosage Forms and Strengths

Eye ointment — 0.6%

Eye suspension — 0.5%, 1%

Oral liquid — 6.7 mg per 5 ml

Syrup — 15 mg per 5-ml

Tablets — 5 mg

▷ **Usual Adult Dosage Range:**   5 to 60 mg daily as a single dose or in divided doses (some patients are put on alternate day schedules). Once an adequate response is achieved, the dose should be decreased to the lowest effective dose. Ophthalmic drops: one to two drops is instilled in to the eye sac (conjunctival sac) every three to 12 hours. Dosing may be increased to every hour in severe cases. **Note: Actual dosage and administration schedule must be determined by the physician for each patient individually.**

Conditions Requiring Dosing Adjustments

Liver function: Dosing adjustments do not appear to be needed in liver compromise.

Kidney function: Dosing adjustments in renal compromise do not appear to be needed. This drug can cause proteinuria, and may be a benefit to risk use in patients with kidney compromise (nephropathy) which causes them to lose protein.

▷ **Dosing Instructions:**   The tablet may be crushed and taken with or following food to prevent stomach irritation, preferably in the morning.

Usual Duration of Use: For acute disorders: 4 to 10 days. For chronic disorders: according to individual requirements. The duration of use should not exceed the time needed to obtain adequate symptomatic relief in acute self-limiting conditions; or the time required to stabilize a chronic condition and permit gradual withdrawal. Because of its intermediate duration of action, this drug is appropriate for alternate day administration. Consult your physician on a regular basis.

Note: The information categories provided in this Profile are appropriate for prednisolone. For specific information that is normally found in those categories that have been omitted from this Profile, the reader is referred to the Drug Profile of prednisone, which follows. Prednisolone is a derivative of prednisone; all significant actions and effects are shared by both drugs.

PREDNISONE (PRED ni sohn)

Introduced: 1955   **Prescription:** USA: Yes; Canada: Yes   **Available as Generic:** USA: Yes; Canada: Yes   **Class:** Cortisonelike drugs   **Controlled Drug:** USA: No; Canada: No

Brand Names: ✦Apo-Prednisone, Aspred-C [CD], Deltasone, Liquid Pred, Meticorten, ✦Metreton [CD], ✦Novoprednisone, Orasone, Panasol-S, Paracort, Prednicen-M, Prednisone Intensol, SK-Prednisone, Sterapred, Sterapred-DS, ✦Winpred

BENEFITS versus RISKS	
Possible Benefits	*Possible Risks*
EFFECTIVE RELIEF OF SYMPTOMS IN A WIDE VARIETY OF INFLAMMATORY AND ALLERGIC DISORDERS	Use exceeding 2 weeks is associated with many possible adverse effects:
EFFECTIVE IMMUNOSUPPRESSION in selected benign and malignant disorders	ALTERED MOOD AND PERSONALITY CATARACTS, GLAUCOMA HYPERTENSION OSTEOPOROSIS ASEPTIC BONE NECROSIS
Prevention of rejection in organ transplantation	INCREASED SUSCEPTIBILITY TO INFECTIONS

▷ **Principal Uses**

As a Single Drug Product: Uses currently included in FDA approved labeling: Treats a wide variety of allergic and inflammatory conditions. It is used most commonly in the management of serious skin disorders, asthma, gout, lupus erythematosus, regional enteritis, ulcerative colitis, nephrotic syndrome and all types of major rheumatic disorders including bursitis, tendonitis and most forms of arthritis; (2) used as part of combination therapy of lymphoma; (3) helps address adrenal insufficiency; (4) used as part of combination therapy of several kinds of leukemia; (5) used in kidney transplant patients; (6) helps patients recover from symptoms of multiple sclerosis.

Other (unlabeled) generally accepted uses: (1) Used in combination therapy of acute (lymphoblastic, lymphocytic and myelogenous) leukemias; (2) combination therapy of breast cancer; (3) may be helpful in therapy of familial Mediterranean fever; (4) used with other medications to treat liver tumors (hemangiomas); (5) may help subfertile men decrease seminal antibodies and become fertile; (6) helps prevent early lung deterioration in children with AIDS; (7) eases symptoms in alcoholics who have hepatitis and encephalopathy; (8) used in some chronic pain syndromes.

How This Drug Works: It is thought that this drug's anti-inflammatory effect is due to its ability to inhibit the normal defensive functions of certain white blood cells. Its immunosuppressant effect is attributed to a reduced production of lymphocytes and antibodies.

Available Dosage Forms and Strengths

Oral solution — 5 mg per 5-ml

Syrup — 5 mg per 5-ml (alcohol 5%)

Tablets — 1 mg, 2.5 mg, 5 mg, 10 mg, 20 mg, 25 mg, 50 mg

▷ **Usual Adult Dosage Range:**   5 to 60 mg daily as a single dose or in divided doses. In myasthenia gravis, patients not responding to 100 mg will not respond to higher doses. Once the initial inflammation has been overcome, the dose should be gradually lowered to the lowest dose that is effective for the condition being treated. **Note: Actual dosage and administration schedule must be determined by the physician for each patient individually.**

Conditions Requiring Dosing Adjustments

Liver function: Dosing adjustments do not appear to be needed in liver compromise.

Kidney function: Dosing adjustments in renal compromise do not appear to be needed. This drug is a possible cause of proteinuria. Its use is a benefit to risk decision in patients who have protein-losing renal compromise (nephropathy).

▷ **Dosing Instructions:**   The tablet may be crushed and taken with or following food to prevent stomach irritation, preferably in the morning.

Usual Duration of Use: For acute disorders: 4 to 10 days. For chronic disorders: according to individual requirements. The duration of use should not exceed the time necessary to obtain adequate symptomatic relief in acute self-limiting conditions; or the time required to stabilize a chronic condition and permit gradual withdrawal. Because of its intermediate duration of action, this drug is appropriate for alternate day administration. Consult your physician on a regular basis.

▷ **This Drug Should Not Be Taken If**
- you have had an allergic reaction to any dosage form of it previously.
- you have active peptic ulcer disease.
- you have an active herpes simplex virus eye infection.
- you have active tuberculosis.
- you have a fungal infection in a large area inside your body (systemic fungal infection).

▷ **Inform Your Physician Before Taking This Drug If**
- you have had an adverse reaction to any cortisonelike drug.
- you have a history of peptic ulcer disease, thrombophlebitis or tuberculosis.
- you have: diabetes, kidney failure, glaucoma, high blood pressure, deficient thyroid function or myasthenia gravis.
- you have osteoporosis.
- you have been exposed to any viral illness such as measles or chickenpox. (cases may be severe if you are taking this medicine.
- you are prone to depression.
- you have diverticulitis.
- you plan to have surgery of any kind in the near future.

Possible Side Effects (natural, expected, and unavoidable drug actions)

Increased appetite, weight gain, retention of salt and water, excretion of potassium, increased susceptibility to infection.

▷ **Possible Adverse Effects** (unusual, unexpected, and infrequent reactions)

If any of the following develop, consult your physician promptly for guidance.

Mild Adverse Effects

Allergic Reaction: Skin rash.

Headache, dizziness, insomnia.

Acid indigestion, abdominal distention.

Patchy blue areas on the great toe (blue toe syndrome).

Muscle cramping and weakness.

Elevated intracranial pressure (pseudotumor cerebri).

Acne, excessive growth of facial hair.

Serious Adverse Effects

Mental and emotional disturbances of serious magnitude.

Reactivation of latent tuberculosis.

Development of peptic ulcer.

Increased blood pressure.

Development of inflammation of the pancreas.

Thrombophlebitis (inflammation of a vein with the formation of blood clot)— pain or tenderness in thigh or leg, with or without swelling of the foot, ankle, or leg.

Seizures (rare).

Increased intraocular (inner eye) pressure.

Kaposi's sarcoma (rare).

Necrosis of bone.

Superinfections.

Increased blood sugar.
Drug-induced porphyria.
Pulmonary embolism (movement of a blood clot to the lung)—sudden shortness of breath, pain in the chest, coughing, bloody sputum.
Low blood platelets (rare).

▷ **Possible Effects on Sexual Function**
Altered timing and pattern of menstruation.
Correction of male infertility when due to autoantibodies that suppress sperm activity.

▷ **Adverse Effects That May Mimic Natural Diseases or Disorders**
Pattern of symptoms and signs resembling Cushing's syndrome.

Natural Diseases or Disorders That May Be Activated by This Drug
Latent diabetes, glaucoma, peptic ulcer disease, tuberculosis.

Possible Effects on Laboratory Tests
Complete blood cell counts: decreased eosinophils, lymphocytes and platelets.
Blood amylase level: increased (possible pancreatitis).
Blood total cholesterol and HDL cholesterol levels: increased.
Blood LDL cholesterol level: no effect.
Blood triglyceride levels: no significant effect.
Blood glucose level: increased.
Glucose tolerance test (GTT): decreased.
Blood potassium level: decreased.
Blood testosterone level: decreased.
Blood thyroid hormone (T_3): decreased.
Blood uric acid level: increased.
Urine sugar tests: no effect with TesTape; false low result with Clinistix and Diastix.
Fecal occult blood test: positive (if gastrointestinal bleeding).

CAUTION
1. If therapy is to exceed one week, it is advisable to carry a card of personal identification with a notation that you are taking this drug.
2. Do not stop this drug abruptly after long-term use.
3. If vaccination against measles, rabies, smallpox or yellow fever is required, discontinue this drug 72 hours before vaccination and do not resume it for at least 14 days after vaccination.

Precautions for Use
By Infants and Children: Avoid prolonged use if possible. During long-term use, observe for suppression of normal growth and the possibility of increased intracranial pressure. Following long-term use, the child may be at risk for adrenal gland deficiency during stress for as long as 18 months after cessation of this drug.
By Those over 60 Years of Age: Cortisonelike drugs should only be used when the disorder under treatment is unresponsive to adequate trials of unrelated drugs. Avoid the prolonged use of this drug. Continual use (even in small doses) can increase severity of diabetes, enhance fluid retention, raise blood pressure, weaken resistance to infection, induce stomach ulcer and accelerate development of cataract and osteoporosis.

▷ **Advisability of Use During Pregnancy**

Pregnancy Category: B or C. See Pregnancy Code at the back of this book.
Animal studies: Birth defects reported in mice, rats and rabbits.
Human studies: Adequate studies of pregnant women are not available.
Avoid completely during the first 3 months. Limit use during the last 6 months as much as possible. If used, examine infant for possible deficiency of adrenal gland function.

Advisability of Use if Breast-Feeding

Presence of this drug in breast milk: Yes.
Avoid drug or refrain from nursing.

Habit-Forming Potential: Long-term use of this drug may produce a state of functional dependence (see Glossary). In therapy of asthma and rheumatoid arthritis, it is advisable to keep the dose as small as possible and to attempt drug withdrawal after periods of reasonable improvement. Such procedures may reduce the degree of "steroid rebound"—the return of symptoms as the drug is withdrawn.

Effects of Overdosage: Fatigue, muscle weakness, stomach irritation, acid indigestion, excessive sweating, facial flushing, fluid retention, swelling of extremities, increased blood pressure.

Possible Effects of Long-Term Use: Increased blood sugar (possible diabetes), increased fat deposits on the trunk of the body ("buffalo hump"), rounding of the face ("moon face"), thinning and fragility of skin, loss of texture and strength of bones (osteoporosis, aseptic necrosis), cataracts, glaucoma, retarded growth and development in children.

Suggested Periodic Examinations While Taking This Drug (at physician's discretion)

Measurements of blood pressure, blood sugar and potassium levels.
Complete eye examinations at regular intervals.
Chest X-ray if history of tuberculosis.
Determination of the rate of development of the growing child to detect retardation of normal growth.

▷ **While Taking This Drug, Observe the Following**

Foods: No interactions expected. Ask physician regarding need to restrict salt intake or to eat potassium-rich foods. During long-term use of this drug, it is advisable to eat a high-protein diet.

Nutritional Support: During long-term use, take a vitamin D supplement. During wound repair, take a zinc supplement. Potassium loss may need to be replaced.

Beverages: No restrictions. Drink all forms of milk liberally.

▷ *Alcohol:* No interactions expected. Use caution if you are prone to peptic ulcers.

Tobacco Smoking: Nicotine increases the blood levels of naturally produced cortisone and related hormones. Heavy smoking may add to the expected actions of this drug and requires close observation for excessive effects.

Marijuana Smoking: May cause additional impairment of immunity.

▷ *Other Drugs*

Prednisone may **decrease** the effects of
• isoniazid (INH, Niconyl, etc.).
• salicylates (aspirin, sodium salicylate, etc.).

Prednisone *taken concurrently* with

- amphotericin B (Fungizone) may result in additive potassium loss.
- birth control pills (oral contraceptives) will prolong the prednisone effect.
- cyclosporine (Sandimmune) can cause increased cyclosporine levels and increased prednisone levels. Dose decreases may be needed for both drugs.
- foscarnet (Foscavir) may result in additive potassium loss.
- ketoconazole (Nizoral) will lessen the therapeutic benefit of ketoconazole.
- loop diuretics (furosemide (Lasix), bumetanide (Bumex)) may have their effects blunted.
- NSAIDs may result in additive stomach and intestinal irritation.
- oral hypoglycemic agents (see Drug Class) or insulin may result in loss of glucose control.
- oral anticoagulants may either increase or decrease their effectiveness; consult physician regarding the need for prothrombin time testing and dosage adjustment.
- pneumococcal or smallpox vaccine will blunt the response to the vaccine.
- thiazide diuretics (see Drug Class) or loop diuretics may result in additive potassium loss.
- theophylline (Theodur, others) may result in variable responses to this medicine. Increased frequency of theophylline levels are recommended.
- vaccines may result in blunted response to the vaccine and decreased preventive benefits.

The following drugs may *decrease* the effects of prednisone

- antacids may reduce its absorption.
- barbiturates (Amytal, Butisol, phenobarbital, etc.).
- carbamazepine (Tegretol).
- phenytoin (Dilantin, etc.).
- primidone (Mysoline).
- rifampin (Rifadin, Rimactane, etc.).

▷ *Driving, Hazardous Activities:* Usually no restrictions. Be alert to the rare occurrence of dizziness.

Aviation Note: The use of this drug *may be a disqualification* for piloting. Consult a designated Aviation Medical Examiner.

Exposure to Sun: No restrictions.

Occurrence of Unrelated Illness: This drug may decrease natural resistance to infection. Tell your doctor if you develop an infection of any kind. It may also reduce your body's ability to respond to the stress of acute illness, injury or surgery. Keep your doctor informed of any significant changes in your state of health.

Discontinuation: After long-term use, do not stop it abruptly. Ask physician for guidance regarding gradual withdrawal. For a period of 2 years after discontinuing this drug, it is essential in the event of illness, injury or surgery that you tell attending medical personnel that you have used this drug in the past. The period of impaired response to stress following the use of cortisonelike drugs may last for 1 to 2 years.

PRIMIDONE (PRI mi dohn)

Introduced: 1953   **Prescription:** USA: Yes; Canada: Yes   **Available as**
Generic: USA: Yes; Canada: Yes   **Class:** Anticonvulsant   **Controlled**
Drug: USA: No; Canada: No

Brand Names: ✢Apo-Primidone, Myidone, Mysoline, ♣PMS-Primidone

BENEFITS versus RISKS	
Possible Benefits	*Possible Risks*
EFFECTIVE CONTROL OF TONIC-CLONIC (GRAND MAL) AND ALL TYPES OF PARTIAL SEIZURES	Allergic skin reactions Rare blood cell disorders: megaloblastic anemia, deficient white blood cells and platelets

▷ **Principal Uses**

As a Single Drug Product: Uses currently included in FDA approved labeling: (1) This drug is used exclusively to control generalized grand mal seizures and all types of partial seizures. It can be used to supplement the anticonvulsant action of phenytoin.

Other (unlabeled) generally accepted uses: (1) May have a minor role in helping in therapy of orthostatic tremor; (2) can help ringing in the ears.

How This Drug Works: Reduces and stabilizes the excitability of nerve fibers and inhibits the repetitive spread of electrical impulses along nerve pathways. This action may prevent seizures altogether, or it may reduce their frequency and severity. (Part of this drug's action is attributable to phenobarbital, one of its conversion products in the body.)

Available Dosage Forms and Strengths

Oral suspensions — 250 mg per 5-ml

Tablets — 50 mg, 250 mg

▷ **Usual Adult Dosage Range:** Initially, 100 mg/24 hours as a single dose at bedtime for 3 days; 100 to 125 mg twice a day for days 4 through 6, 100 to 125 mg three times a day for days 7 through 9, and an ongoing (maintenance) dose of 250 mg 3 or 4 times a day, 6 to 8 hours apart. Total daily dosage should not exceed 2000 mg. **Note: Actual dosage and administration schedule must be determined by the physician for each patient individually.**

Conditions Requiring Dosing Adjustments

Liver function: The dose **must** be decreased, and blood levels obtained more frequently in patients with liver compromise.

Kidney function: In patients with mild to moderate kidney failure, the usual dose can be given every eight hours. Patients with moderate to severe kidney failure can be given the usual dose every 8–12 hours. Patients with severe kidney failure should be given the usual dose every 12–24 hours. Primidone should be used with caution in renal compromise as it can be a cause of crystalluria.

▷ **Dosing Instructions:** The tablet may be crushed and taken with or following food to reduce stomach irritation. Shake the suspension well before measuring the dose.

Usual Duration of Use: Use on a regular schedule for 2 to 4 weeks usually determines effectiveness in reducing the frequency and severity of seizures. Long-term use (months to years) requires physician supervision.

▷ **This Drug Should Not Be Taken If**
- you have had an allergic reaction to it previously.
- you are allergic to phenobarbital.
- you have a history of porphyria.

▷ **Inform Your Physician Before Taking This Drug If**
- you have had an allergic or idiosyncratic reaction to any barbiturate drug in the past.
- you have a family history of intermittent porphyria.
- you have impaired liver, kidney or thyroid gland function.
- you have asthma, emphysema or myasthenia gravis.
- you are pregnant or planning pregnancy.
- you plan to have surgery under general anesthesia in the near future.

Possible Side Effects (natural, expected, and unavoidable drug actions)
Drowsiness, impaired concentration, mental and physical sluggishness.

▷ **Possible Adverse Effects** (unusual, unexpected, and infrequent reactions)
If any of the following develop, consult your physician promptly for guidance.
Mild Adverse Effects
Allergic Reactions: Skin rashes, hives, localized swellings."Hangover" effect, dizziness, unsteadiness, impaired vision, double vision, fatigue, emotional disturbances.
Low blood pressure, faintness.
Shoulder pain, joint pain.
Nausea, vomiting, thirst, increased urine volume.
Serious Adverse Effects
Allergic Reaction: Swelling of lymph glands.
Idiosyncratic Reactions: Paradoxical anxiety, seizures, agitation, restlessness, rage.
Visual hallucinations (rare).
Drug-induced porphyria (rare).
Drug-induced systemic lupus erythematosus (rare).
Drug-induced low thyroid gland function (hypothyroidism).
Blood cell disorders: megaloblastic anemia due to folic acid depletion; deficient production of white blood cells and blood platelets.
Drug induced kidney problems (crystalluria) (rare).
Auditory hallucinations (rare).

▷ **Possible Effects on Sexual Function**
Decreased libido and/or impotence.
Decreased effectiveness of oral contraceptives taken concurrently.

▷ **Adverse Effects That May Mimic Natural Diseases or Disorders**
Allergic swelling of lymph glands may suggest a naturally occurring lymphoma.

Natural Diseases or Disorders That May Be Activated by This Drug
Acute intermittent and/or cutaneous porphyria (see Glossary).
Systemic lupus erythematosus.

Possible Effects on Laboratory Tests

Complete blood cell counts: decreased red cells, hemoglobin, white cells and platelets; increased eosinophils.

Blood lupus erythematosus (LE) cells: positive.

Prothrombin time: decreased (when taken concurrently with warfarin).

Urine screening tests for drug abuse: may be **positive** for phenobarbital (a normal derivative of this drug). (Test results depend upon amount of drug taken and testing method used.)

CAUTION

1. This drug must not be stopped abruptly.
2. The wide variation of this drug's action from person to person requires careful individualization of dosage schedules.
3. Regularity of drug use is essential for the successful management of seizure disorders. Take your medication at the same time each day.
4. Side effects and mild adverse effects are usually most apparent during the first several weeks of treatment and often subside with continued use.
5. It may be necessary to take folic acid to prevent anemia while taking this drug. Consult your physician.
6. It is advisable to carry a card of personal identification with a notation that you are taking this drug.

Precautions for Use

By Infants and Children: This drug should be used with caution in the hyperkinetic (overactive) child. Observe for possible paradoxical hyperactivity. Changes associated with puberty characteristically slow the metabolism of phenobarbital and permit its gradual accumulation. Measurements of blood levels in young adolescents can detect rising concentrations of this drug that could lead to toxicity. (See Therapeutic Drug Monitoring in Section One.)

By Those over 60 Years of Age: It is advisable to avoid all barbiturates in the elderly. If use of this drug is attempted, small starting doses are indicated. Watch for confusion, delirium, agitation or paradoxical excitement. This drug may be conducive to hypothermia (see Glossary).

▷ Advisability of Use During Pregnancy

Pregnancy Category: D. See Pregnancy Code at the back of this book.

Animal studies: Birth defects due to this drug reported in mice.

Human studies: Adequate studies of pregnant women are not available. However, recent reports suggest a possible association between the use of this drug during the first 3 months of pregnancy and the development of birth defects in the fetus. Discuss with your physician the advantages and possible disadvantages of using this drug during pregnancy. If it is used, determine the smallest maintenance dose that will prevent seizures.

The newborn infants of mothers who take this drug during pregnancy may develop abnormal bleeding or bruising due to the deficiency of certain blood clotting factors in the blood. Consult your physician regarding the need to take vitamin K during the last month of pregnancy.

Advisability of Use if Breast-Feeding

Presence of this drug in breast milk: Yes.

Monitor nursing infant closely and discontinue drug or nursing if adverse effects develop.

Habit-Forming Potential: None.

Effects of Overdosage: Drowsiness, jerky eye movements, blurred vision, staggering gait, incoordination, slurred speech, stupor progressing to coma.

Possible Effects of Long-Term Use: Enlargement of lymph glands; enlargement of thyroid gland. Megaloblastic anemia due to folic acid deficiency. Reduced blood levels of calcium and phosphorus, leading to rickets in children and loss of bone texture (osteomalacia) in adults.

Suggested Periodic Examinations While Taking This Drug (at physician's discretion)
Complete blood cell counts. Measurements of blood levels of calcium and phosphorus. Evaluation of lymph and thyroid glands. Skeletal X-ray examinations for bone demineralization during long-term use.

▷ **While Taking This Drug, Observe the Following**
Foods: No restrictions.
Nutritional Support: Consult your physician regarding the need for supplements of calcium, vitamin D, folic acid and vitamin K.
Beverages: No restrictions. May be taken with milk or fruit juice.
▷ *Alcohol:* Avoid completely. Alcohol can increase greatly the sedative and depressant effects of this drug on brain function.
Tobacco Smoking: May enhance the sedative effects of this drug and increase drowsiness.
▷ *Other Drugs*
Note: 15% of primidone is converted to phenobarbital in the body. See the Drug Profile of Phenobarbital for possible interactions with other drugs.
▷ *Driving, Hazardous Activities:* This drug may cause drowsiness and dizziness; it can also impair mental alertness, vision and physical coordination. Restrict activities as necessary.
Aviation Note: The use of this drug *is a disqualification* for piloting. Consult a designated Aviation Medical Examiner.
Exposure to Sun: No restrictions.
Occurrence of Unrelated Illness: Notify your physician of any illness or injury that prevents the use of this drug according to your regular dosage schedule.
Discontinuation: Do not stop this drug without your physician's knowledge and approval. Sudden withdrawal of any anticonvulsant drug can cause severe and repeated seizures.

PROBENECID (proh BEN e sid)

Introduced: 1951   **Prescription:** USA: Yes; Canada: No   **Available as Generic:** USA: Yes; Canada: No   **Class:** Antigout   **Controlled Drug:** USA: No; Canada: No

Brand Names: ✦Ampicin PRB [CD], Benemid, ✦Benuryl, Colabid [CD], Col-Benemid [CD], Polycillin-PRB [CD], Probalan, Probampacin [CD], Proben-C [CD], ✦Pro-Biosan 500 Kit [CD], SK-Probenecid

---

BENEFITS versus RISKS

Possible Benefits	*Possible Risks*
EFFECTIVE LONG-TERM PREVENTION OF ACUTE ATTACKS OF GOUT	Formation of uric acid kidney stones
	Bone marrow depression (aplastic anemia) (rare)
Useful adjunct to penicillin therapy (to achieve high blood and tissue levels of penicillin)	Drug-induced liver and kidney damage (both rare)

▷ **Principal Uses**

As a Single Drug Product: Uses currently included in FDA approved labeling: (1) Used in helping maintain penicillin levels in therapy of gonorrhea; (2) helps decrease elevated uric acid levels caused by thiazide diuretics; (3) helps prevent gout.

Other (unlabeled) generally accepted uses: (1) May have a role in preventing kidney toxicity in cisplatin chemotherapy; (2) adjunctive use in maintaining effective antibiotic levels in treatment of syphilis; (3) helps decrease uric acid in gout patients.

As a Combination Drug Product [CD]: This drug is available in combination with colchicine, a drug often used for the treatment of acute gout. Each drug works in a different way; when used in combination they provide both relief of the acute gout and some measure of protection from recurrence of acute attacks.

How This Drug Works: Works in the kidney (tubular systems) to increase uric acid excretion in the urine, this drug reduces the levels of uric acid in the blood and body tissues. It also works in the kidney to decrease the amount of penicillin excreted in the urine, and prolongs the presence of penicillin in the blood and helps achieve higher concentrations in body tissues.

Available Dosage Forms and Strengths

Tablets — 500 mg

▷ **Usual Adult Dosage Range:**   Antigout: Initially, 250 mg twice/day for 1 week; then 500 mg twice/day. Adjunct to penicillin therapy: 500 mg 4 times/day. **Note: Actual dosage and administration schedule must be determined by the physician for each patient individually.**

Conditions Requiring Dosing Adjustments

Liver function: Specific guidelines for dosage adjustment in liver compromise are not available. It should be used with caution.

Kidney function: Patients with kidney failure (creatinine clearance less than 30 ml per minute) should **not** be given this drug as the effectiveness is questionable. Those with moderate kidney failure may still benefit from this medicine, and dose increases (as needed and tolerated) in 500 mg steps up to 2,000 mg a day in equally divided doses may be required.

▷ **Dosing Instructions:**   The tablet may be crushed and taken with or following food to reduce stomach irritation. Drink 2.5 to 3 quarts of liquids daily.

Usual Duration of Use: Use on a regular schedule for several months usually determines effectiveness in preventing acute attacks of gout. Long-term use (months to years) requires supervision and periodic evaluation by your physician.

▷ **This Drug Should Not Be Taken If**
- you have had an allergic reaction to it previously.
- you have active liver disease.
- you have acute kidney failure.
- you have an active blood cell or bone marrow disorder.
- you are experiencing an attack of acute gout at the present time.

▷ **Inform Your Physician Before Taking This Drug If**
- you have a history of kidney disease or kidney stones.
- you have a history of liver disease or impaired liver function.
- you have a history of peptic ulcer disease.
- you have a history of a blood cell or bone marrow disorder.
- you are taking any drug product that contains aspirin or aspirinlike drugs.

Possible Side Effects (natural, expected, and unavoidable drug actions)
Development of kidney stones (composed of uric acid); this is preventable. Consult your physician regarding the use of sodium bicarbonate (or other urine alkalizer) to prevent stone formation.

▷ **Possible Adverse Effects** (unusual, unexpected, and infrequent reactions)
If any of the following develop, consult your physician promptly for guidance.
Mild Adverse Effects
Allergic Reactions: Skin rash, itching, drug fever (see Glossary).
Headache, dizziness, flushing of face.
Reduced appetite, sore gums, nausea, vomiting.
Serious Adverse Effects
Allergic Reaction: Anaphylactic reaction (see Glossary).
Idiosyncratic Reaction: Hemolytic anemia (see Glossary).
Bone marrow depression (see Glossary): fatigue, weakness, fever, sore throat, abnormal bleeding or bruising (isolated cases).
Drug-induced liver damage with jaundice (see Glossary).
Drug-induced porphyria (rare).
Fluid in the retina (retinal edema) (rare).
Drug-induced kidney damage: marked fluid retention, reduced urine formation.

▷ **Possible Effects on Sexual Function:**   None reported.

▷ **Adverse Effects That May Mimic Natural Diseases or Disorders**
Liver reactions may suggest viral hepatitis.
Kidney reactions may suggest nephrosis.

Possible Effects on Laboratory Tests
Complete blood cell counts: decreased red cells, hemoglobin, white cells and platelets.
Prothrombin time: increased (when taken concurrently with warfarin).
Blood glucose level: decreased.
Blood urea nitrogen (BUN) level: increased (kidney damage).
Blood uric acid level: decreased.
Liver function tests: increased liver enzymes (ALT/GPT, AST/GOT and alkaline phosphatase), increased bilirubin.
Urine sugar tests: false positive with Benedict's solution and Clinitest.

CAUTION
1. This drug should not be started until 2 to 3 weeks after an acute attack of gout has subsided.
2. This drug may increase the frequency of acute attacks of gout during the first few months of treatment. Concurrent use of colchicine is advised to prevent acute attacks.
3. Aspirin (and aspirin-containing drug products) can reduce the effectiveness of this drug. Use acetaminophen or a nonaspirin analgesic for pain relief as needed.

Precautions for Use

By Infants and Children: Safety and effectiveness for those under 2 years of age not established.

By Those over 60 Years of Age: The natural decline in kidney function that occurs after 60 may require adjustment of your dosage. You may be more susceptible to the serious adverse effects of this drug. Report any unusual symptoms promptly for evaluation.

▷ **Advisability of Use During Pregnancy**

Pregnancy Category: B. See Pregnancy Code at the back of this book.
Animal studies: No information available.
Human studies: Adequate studies of pregnant women are not available.
This drug has been used during pregnancy with no reports of birth defects or adverse effects on the fetus. Ask your physician for guidance.

Advisability of Use if Breast-Feeding

Presence of this drug in breast milk: Unknown.
Avoid drug or refrain from nursing.

Habit-Forming Potential: None.

Effects of Overdosage: Stomach irritation, nausea, vomiting, nervous agitation, delirium, seizures, coma.

Possible Effects of Long-Term Use: Formation of kidney stones. Kidney damage in sensitive individuals.

Suggested Periodic Examinations While Taking This Drug (at physician's discretion)

Complete blood cell counts, measurements of blood uric acid, liver and kidney function tests.

▷ **While Taking This Drug, Observe the Following**

Foods: Follow physician's advice regarding the need for a low-purine diet.
Beverages: A large intake of coffee, tea or cola beverages may reduce the effectiveness of treatment.

▷ *Alcohol:* No interactions expected. However, large amounts of alcohol can raise the blood uric acid level and reduce the effectiveness of treatment.

Tobacco Smoking: No interactions expected.

▷ *Other Drugs*

Probenecid may *increase* the effects of
• acyclovir (Zovirax) and result in toxicity unless doses are reduced.
• clofibrate (Atromid S).
• dyphylline (Neothylline).
• ketoprofen and perhaps other NSAIDs (see Drug Classes).

- methotrexate (Mexate), and increase its toxicity.
- midazolam (Versed) and increase the CNS depression.
- oral hypoglycemic agents (see Drug Class).
- thiopental (Pentothal), and prolong its anesthetic effect.
- zalcitabine (Hivid).
- zidovudine (Retrovir) and increase toxicity risk.

Probenecid *taken concurrently* with

- allopurinol (Zyloprim) may result in extended allopurinol half life.
- penicillins (see Drug Classes) may cause a threefold to fivefold increase in penicillin blood levels, greatly increasing the effectiveness of each penicillin dose.
- cephalosporins (see Drug Classes) may cause a doubling of antibiotic levels. Caution must be used to avoid toxicity.
- dapsone may cause up to a 50% increased dapsone level and result in toxicity unless dapsone doses are decreased.
- rifampin (Rifadin, others) may result in increased blood levels of rifampin.

The following drugs may *decrease* the effects of probenecid

- aspirin and other salicylates may reduce its effectiveness in promoting the excretion of uric acid.
- bismuth subsalicylate (Pepto-Bismol, others).

▷ *Driving, Hazardous Activities:* This drug may cause dizziness. Restrict activities as necessary.

Aviation Note: The use of this drug *may be a disqualification* for piloting. Consult a designated Aviation Medical Examiner.

Exposure to Sun: No restrictions.

Discontinuation: Do not stop this drug without consulting your physician.

PROBUCOL (PROH byu kohl)

Introduced: 1971 **Prescription:** USA: Yes; Canada: Yes **Available as Generic:** USA: No; Canada: No **Class:** Anticholesterol **Controlled Drug:** USA: No; Canada: No

Brand Name: Lorelco

Author's note: Hoechst Marion Roussel has discontinued distribution of this drug in the United States. It will only be available until current supplies are used up.

PROCAINAMIDE (proh KAYN a mide)

Introduced: 1950 **Prescription:** USA: Yes; Canada: Yes **Available as Generic:** USA: Yes; Canada: No **Class:** Antiarrhythmic **Controlled Drug:** USA: No; Canada: No

Brand Names: ✦Apo-Procainamide, Procamide SR, Procanbid, Procan SR, Promine, Pronestyl, Pronestyl-SR, Rhythmin

```
┌─────────────────────────────────────────────────────────────────────┐
│                        BENEFITS versus RISKS                          │
│       Possible Benefits                   Possible Risks              │
│   EFFECTIVE TREATMENT OF          NARROW TREATMENT RANGE              │
│     SELECTED HEART RHYTHM         INDUCTION OF SYSTEMIC LUPUS         │
│     DISORDERS                       ERYTHEMATOSUS SYNDROME            │
│                                   Provocation of abnormal heart       │
│                                     rhythms                           │
│                                   Blood cell disorders: insufficient  │
│                                     white blood cells and platelets   │
└─────────────────────────────────────────────────────────────────────┘
```

▷ **Principal Uses**

As a Single Drug Product: Uses currently included in FDA approved labeling: (1) Used to abolish and prevent the recurrence of premature beats arising in the ventricles (lower chambers) of the heart.

Other (unlabeled) generally accepted uses: (1) Used to treat and prevent atrial fibrillation, atrial flutter and abnormally rapid heart rates (tachycardia) that originate in the atria or the ventricles; (2) helps treat myotonia and improve breathing in myotonic dystrophy.

How This Drug Works: By slowing the activity of the pacemaker and delaying the transmission of electrical impulses through the conduction system and muscle of the heart, this drug assists in restoring normal heart rate and rhythm.

Available Dosage Forms and Strengths

Capsules — 250 mg, 375 mg, 500 mg

Injections — 100 mg per ml and 500 mg per ml

Tablets — 250 mg, 375 mg, 500 mg

Tablets, prolonged-action — 250 mg, 500 mg, 750 mg, 1000 mg

▷ **Usual Adult Dosage Range:**   Dose varies according to indication for use. Starting dose is usually 50 mg per kilogram per day of the immediate release form. This calculated dose is then divided into equal doses and is given every 3, 4 or 6 hours. The ongoing daily dose should be adjusted to individual patient response and blood levels. People over 50 years old may get an acceptable clinical response and blood level from a lower dose. The sustained release form is usually started in younger patients who do not have kidney problems at 50 mg per kilogram per day. This calculated dose is divided into equal doses and is given every 6 to 12 hours depending on patient response and blood levels. **Note: Actual dosage and administration schedule must be determined by the physician for each patient individually.**

Conditions Requiring Dosing Adjustments

Liver function: This drug should be used with caution in patients with liver compromise, and blood levels appropriately obtained. Lower ongoing doses are generally used. Procainamide should be used as a benefit to risk in patients with compromised livers as it may be more likely to cause liver problems in this patient population.

Kidney function: Patients with moderate to severe kidney failure can be given the usual doses every 6–12 hours. Patients with severe kidney failure can be given the usual dose every 8–24 hours. The drug should be used with caution in renal compromise, and appropriate blood levels obtained.

▷ **Dosing Instructions:**　Preferably taken on an empty stomach, 1 hour before or 2 hours after eating. However, it may be taken with or following food to reduce stomach irritation. The regular capsules may be opened and the regular tablets may be crushed for administration; however, the prolonged-action tablets should be swallowed whole without alteration.

Usual Duration of Use:　Use on a regular schedule for 24 to 48 hours usually determines effectiveness in correcting or preventing responsive rhythm disorders. Long-term use requires supervision and periodic evaluation by your physician.

▷ **This Drug Should Not Be Taken If**
- you have had an allergic reaction to it previously.
- you have systemic lupus erythematosus.
- you have second-degree or third-degree heart block (determined by electrocardiogram).
- you have myasthenia gravis.

▷ **Inform Your Physician Before Taking This Drug If**
- you are allergic to procaine (Novocain) or to other local anesthetics of the "-cain" drug class, such as those commonly used for glaucoma testing and for dental procedures.
- you have had any adverse reactions to other antiarrhythmic drugs.
- you have a history of heart disease of any kind, especially "heart block."
- you have a history of low blood pressure.
- you have a history of lupus erythematosus.
- you have a history of abnormally low blood platelet counts.
- you have impaired liver or kidney function.
- you have myasthenia gravis.
- you have an enlarged prostate gland.
- you are taking any form of digitalis or any diuretic drug that can cause excessive loss of body potassium (ask physician).
- you plan to have surgery under general anesthesia in the near future.

Possible Side Effects (natural, expected, and unavoidable drug actions)
Drop in blood pressure in susceptible individuals.

▷ **Possible Adverse Effects** (unusual, unexpected, and infrequent reactions)
If any of the following develop, consult your physician promptly for guidance.
Mild Adverse Effects
Allergic Reactions: Skin rash, hives, itching, drug fever (see Glossary).
Weakness, light-headedness.
Loss of appetite, bitter taste, indigestion, nausea, vomiting, diarrhea.
Serious Adverse Effects
Allergic Reactions: Systemic lupus-erythematosus-like syndrome: fever, skin eruptions, joint and muscle pains, pleurisy. (This is reported to occur in at least 20% of users.)
Idiosyncratic Reactions: Mental depression, hallucinations, psychotic behavior, hemolytic anemia (see Glossary).
Severe drop in blood pressure, fainting.
Drug-induced pancreatitis (rare).
Drug-induced liver toxicity.
Myopathy.

Drug-induced myasthenia gravis.

Pericardial effusions (rare).

Asthmalike breathing difficulties.

Induction of new heart rhythm disturbances.

Inability to empty urinary bladder, prostatism (see Glossary).

Peripheral neuropathy.

Anticholinergic syndrome (rare).

Blood cell disorders: abnormally low white blood cell count, causing fever, sore throat, infections; abnormally low blood platelet count, causing abnormal bleeding or bruising (rare).

▷ **Possible Effects on Sexual Function:**   None reported.

▷ **Adverse Effects That May Mimic Natural Diseases or Disorders**

Rare liver reaction may suggest viral hepatitis.

Natural Diseases or Disorders That May Be Activated by This Drug

Systemic lupus erythematosus, myasthenia gravis.

Possible Effects on Laboratory Tests

Complete blood cell counts: decreased red cells, hemoglobin, white cells and platelets; increased eosinophils.

Blood lupus erythematosus (LE) cells: positive.

Blood antinuclear antibodies (ANA): positive (in 50–80% of those using drug after 3 to 6 months).

Liver function tests: increased liver enzymes (ALT/GPT, AST/GOT and alkaline phosphatase), increased bilirubin.

Urine screening tests for drug abuse: **initial** test result may be falsely *positive*; **confirmatory** test result will be *negative*. (Test results depend upon amount of drug taken and testing method used.)

CAUTION

1. Thorough evaluation of your heart function (including electrocardiograms) is necessary prior to using this drug.
2. Periodic evaluation of your heart function is necessary to determine your response to this drug. Some individuals may experience worsening of their heart rhythm disorder and/or deterioration of heart function. Close monitoring of heart rate, rhythm and overall performance is essential.
3. Dosage must be adjusted carefully for each individual. Do not change your dosage without the knowledge and supervision of your physician.
4. Do not take any other antiarrhythmic drug while taking this drug unless directed to do so by your physician.

Precautions for Use

By Infants and Children: Blood cell counts should be monitored for loss of white blood cells.

By Those over 60 Years of Age: Reduced kidney function may require reduction in dosage. Observe carefully for light-headedness, dizziness, unsteadiness and tendency to fall.

▷ **Advisability of Use During Pregnancy**

Pregnancy Category: C. See Pregnancy Code at the back of this book.

Animal studies: No information available.

Human studies: Adequate studies of pregnant women are not available.

Use this drug only if clearly needed.

Advisability of Use if Breast-Feeding
    Presence of this drug in breast milk: Yes.
    Avoid drug or refrain from nursing.

Habit-Forming Potential: None.

Effects of Overdosage: Loss of appetite, nausea, vomiting, weakness, faintness, irregular heart rhythm, stupor, circulatory collapse, heart arrest.

Possible Effects of Long-Term Use: Lupus-erythematosus-like syndrome (see above).

Suggested Periodic Examinations While Taking This Drug (at physician's discretion)
    Complete blood cell counts.
    Blood tests for the development of lupus erythematosus (LE) cells and antinuclear antibodies.
    Electrocardiograms to monitor the full effect of this drug on the mechanisms that influence heart rate and rhythm.

▷ **While Taking This Drug, Observe the Following**
    Foods: No restrictions.
    Beverages: Avoid excessive intake of coffee, tea and cola beverages. Avoid iced drinks. May be taken with milk.
▷   *Alcohol:* Use caution. Alcohol can increase the blood-pressure-lowering effects of this drug.
    Tobacco Smoking: Nicotine can cause irritability of the heart and reduce the effectiveness of this drug. Follow physician's advice regarding smoking.
▷   *Other Drugs*
        Procainamide may *increase* the effects of
        • antihypertensive drugs, and cause excessive lowering of blood pressure.
        The following drugs may *increase* the effects of procainamide
        • amiodarone (Codarone).
        • cimetidine (Tagamet).
        • quinidine (Quinaglute).
        • propranolol (Inderal).
        • ranitidine (Zantac).
        • trimethoprim (Proloprim, Bactrim)
▷   *Driving, Hazardous Activities:* This drug may cause dizziness or weakness. Restrict activities as necessary.
    Aviation Note: The use of this drug *may be a disqualification* for piloting. Consult a designated Aviation Medical Examiner.
    Exposure to Sun: No restrictions.
    Exposure to Heat: Use caution. Hot environments are conducive to lower blood pressure.
    Occurrence of Unrelated Illness: Vomiting, diarrhea or dehydration can affect this drug's action adversely. Report such developments promptly.
    Discontinuation: This drug should not be stopped abruptly after long-term use. Ask your physician for guidance regarding gradual dose reduction.

PROCHLORPERAZINE (proh klor PER a zeen)

Introduced: 1956   **Prescription:** USA: Yes; Canada: Yes   **Available as Generic:** USA: Yes; Canada: Yes   **Class:** antipsychotic, antiemetic, phenothiazines   **Controlled Drug:** USA: No; Canada: No

Brand Names: ✤Combid [CD], Compazine, Eskatrol, ✤PMS-prochlorperazine, Pro-Iso, ✤Stemetil, Ultrazine [CD]

BENEFITS versus RISKS

Possible Benefits	*Possible Risks*
EFFECTIVE CONTROL OF ACUTE MENTAL DISORDERS, NAUSEA, AND VOMITING Relief of anxiety and nervous tension	SERIOUS TOXIC EFFECTS ON BRAIN with long-term use Liver damage with jaundice (infrequent) Rare blood cell disorders: abnormally low white cell and platelet counts

---

▷ **Principal Uses**

As a Single Drug Product: Uses currently included in FDA approved labeling: (1) Relieves severe nausea and vomiting; (2) sometimes used to treat schizophrenia; (3) helps prevent motion sickness.

Other (unlabeled) generally accepted uses: (1) Sometimes used to increase the effects of anesthesia; (2) may be of use in Meniere's disease.

How This Drug Works: By inhibiting the action of dopamine, this drug acts to correct an imbalance of nerve impulse transmissions that is thought to be responsible for certain mental disorders. By blocking the action of dopamine in the chemoreceptor trigger zone of the brain, this drug prevents stimulation of the vomiting center.

Available Dosage Forms and Strengths

Capsules, prolonged-action — 10 mg, 15 mg, 30 mg

Injection — 5 mg per ml

Suppositories — 2.5 mg, 5 mg, 25 mg

Syrup — 5 mg per 5-ml

Tablets — 5 mg, 10 mg, 25 mg

▷ **Usual Adult Dosage Range:** Initially, 5 mg of the immediate release form every 6 to 8 hours. If needed and tolerated, dose may be increased by 5 mg at intervals of 3 to 4 days. Usual range is 50 to 75 mg daily. The total daily dosage should not exceed 150 mg. Nausea and vomiting: 5 to 10 milligrams three or four times daily. The sustained release form can be taken as 15 milligrams when you wake up in the morning or 10 mgs of the sustained release form every 12 hours **Note: Actual dose and dosing schedule must be determined by the physician for each patient individually.**

Conditions Requiring Dosing Adjustments

Liver function: This drug should be used with caution in patients with liver compromise. Specific guidelines for dosage adjustment are not available.

Kidney function: Specific guidelines for adjustment of dosages are not available.

▷ **Dosing Instructions:** The tablets may be crushed and taken with or following food to reduce stomach irritation. Prolonged-action capsules should be swallowed whole without alteration.

Duration of Use: Use on a regular schedule for 12 to 24 hours usually determines effectiveness in controlling nausea and vomiting. If used for severe anxiety-tension states or acute psychotic behavior, a trial of several weeks is usually necessary to determine effectiveness. If not significantly beneficial within 6 weeks, it should be stopped. Consult your physician on a regular basis.

▷ **This Drug Should Not Be Taken If**
- you have had an allergic reaction to it previously.
- you have active liver disease.
- you have extremely low blood pressure.
- you have cancer of the breast.
- you have had it prescribed for a child who is less than two years old or who weighs less than 20 pounds.
- you have a current blood cell or bone marrow disorder.

▷ **Inform Your Physician Before Taking This Drug If**
- you are allergic or abnormally sensitive to any phenothiazine drug (see Drug Class Section).
- you have impaired liver or kidney function.
- you have any type of seizure disorder.
- you have bone marrow depression or history of blood diseases.
- you have diabetes, glaucoma or heart disease.
- you have prostate trouble (prostatic hypertrophy).
- you are pregnant.
- you have had neuroleptic malignant syndrome.
- you have a history of lupus erythematosus.
- you are taking any drug with sedative effects.
- you plan to have surgery under general or spinal anesthesia in the near future.

Possible Side Effects (natural, expected, and unavoidable drug actions)
Drowsiness (usually during the first 2 weeks), orthostatic hypotension (see Glossary), blurred vision, dry mouth, nasal congestion, constipation, impaired urination.
Pink or purple coloration of urine, of no significance.

▷ **Possible Adverse Effects** (unusual, unexpected, and infrequent reactions)
If any of the following develop, consult your physician promptly for guidance.
Mild Adverse Effects
Allergic Reactions: Skin rash, hives, low-grade fever.
Lowering of body temperature, especially in the elderly (see Hypothermia in Glossary).
Increased appetite and weight gain.
Increased blood pressure.
Dizziness, weakness, agitation, insomnia, impaired day and night vision.
Chronic constipation, fecal impaction, incontinence.
Serious Adverse Effects
Allergic Reactions: Hepatitis with jaundice (see Glossary), usually between second and fourth week; high fever; asthma; anaphylactic reaction (see Glossary).

Idiosyncratic Reactions: Toxic dermatitis, Stevens-Johnson syndrome. Neuroleptic malignant syndrome (see Glossary).
Liver toxicity (rare).
Abnormal eye positioning (oculogyric crisis).
Depression, disorientation, seizures.
Abnormally high blood pressure (rare).
Disturbances of heart rhythm, rapid heart rate (rare).
Bone marrow depression (see Glossary): fever, sore throat, abnormal bleeding or bruising.
Drug-induced porphyria (rare).
Parkinson-like disorders (see Glossary); muscle spasms of face, jaw, neck, back, extremities; extreme restlessness; slowed movements, muscle rigidity, tremors; tardive dyskinesias (see Glossary).

▷ **Possible Effects on Sexual Function**
Altered timing and pattern of menstruation.
Female breast enlargement with milk production.
Male breast enlargement and tenderness (gynecomastia).
Inhibited ejaculation; priapism (see Glossary).
Causes false positive pregnancy test result.

▷ **Adverse Effects That May Mimic Natural Diseases or Disorders**
Nervous system reactions may suggest Parkinson's disease.
Liver reactions may suggest viral hepatitis.
Reactions resembling systemic lupus erythematosus can occur.

Natural Diseases or Disorders That May Be Activated by This Drug
Latent epilepsy, glaucoma, diabetes mellitus, prostatism (see Glossary).

Possible Effects on Laboratory Tests
White blood cell count: decreased.
Liver function tests: increased liver enzymes (ALT/GPT, AST/GOT and alkaline phosphatase), increased bilirubin.

CAUTION
1. Many over-the-counter medications (see OTC Drugs in Glossary) for allergies, colds and coughs contain drugs that can interact unfavorably with this drug. Ask your doctor or pharmacist for help before using any such medications.
2. Antacids that contain aluminum and/or magnesium can prevent the absorption of this drug and reduce its effectiveness.
3. Obtain prompt evaluation of any change or disturbance of vision.

Precautions for Use
By Infants and Children: Do not use this drug in infants under 2 years of age, or in children of any age with symptoms suggestive of Reye syndrome (see Glossary). Children with acute illnesses ("flulike" infections, measles, chicken pox, etc.) are very susceptible to adverse effects when this drug is given to control nausea and vomiting.
By Those over 60 Years of Age: Small starting doses are advisable. You may be more susceptible to drowsiness, lethargy, constipation, lowering of body temperature (hypothermia) and orthostatic hypotension (see Glossary). This drug can worsen existing prostatism (see Glossary). You may also be more susceptible to the development of Parkinson-like reactions and/or tardive dyskinesia (see discussion of these terms in Glossary). These reactions

must be recognized early since they may become unresponsive to treatment and irreversible.

▷ **Advisability of Use During Pregnancy**

Pregnancy Category: C. See Pregnancy Code at the back of this book.

Animal studies: Cleft palate reported in mouse and rat studies.

Human studies: No increase in birth defects reported in 2023 exposures. Information from adequate studies of pregnant women is not available.

Limit use to small and infrequent doses. Avoid drug during the last month because of possible effects on the newborn infant.

Advisability of Use if Breast-Feeding

Presence of this drug in breast milk: Yes, in small amounts.

Monitor nursing infant closely and discontinue drug or nursing if adverse effects develop.

Habit-Forming Potential: None, but has been used in combination with pentazocine as a heroin substitute by drug abusers.

Effects of Overdosage: Marked drowsiness, weakness, tremor, agitation, unsteadiness, deep sleep, coma, convulsions.

Possible Effects of Long-Term Use: Tardive dyskinesias. Eye changes: opacities in cornea or lens, retinal pigmentation.

Suggested Periodic Examinations While Taking This Drug (at physician's discretion)

Complete blood cell counts, especially between the fourth and tenth weeks of treatment.

Liver function tests, electrocardiograms.

Complete eye examinations—eye structures and vision.

Careful inspection of the tongue for early evidence of fine, involuntary, wavelike movements that could indicate the beginning of tardive dyskinesia.

▷ **While Taking This Drug, Observe the Following**

Foods: No restrictions.

Nutritional Support: A riboflavin (vitamin B-2) supplement should be taken with long-term use.

Beverages: No restrictions. May be taken with milk.

▷ *Alcohol:* Avoid completely. Alcohol can increase the sedative action of phenothiazines and accentuate their depressant effects on brain function and blood pressure. Phenothiazines can increase the intoxicating effects of alcohol.

Tobacco Smoking: Possible reduction of drowsiness from drug.

Marijuana Smoking: Moderate increase in drowsiness; accentuation of orthostatic hypotension; increased risk of precipitating latent psychoses, confusing the interpretation of mental status and drug responses.

▷ *Other Drugs*

Prochlorperazine may *increase* the effects of

• all sedative drugs, especially meperidine (Demerol), and cause excessive sedation.

• all atropinelike drugs, and cause nervous system toxicity.

Prochlorperazine may *decrease* the effects of

• guanethidine (Ismelin, Esimil), and reduce its effectiveness in lowering blood pressure.

Prochlorperazine *taken concurrently* with

- oral hypoglycemic (see Drug Classes) agents may blunt their therapeutic benefit.
- MAO inhibitors (see Drug Classes) may result in increased risk of abnormal body movements (extrapyramidal reactions).
- propranolol (Inderal) may cause increased effects of both drugs; monitor drug effects closely and adjust dosages as necessary.

The following drugs may *decrease* the effects of prochlorperazine

- antacids containing aluminum and/or magnesium.
- benztropine (Cogentin).
- trihexyphenidyl (Artane).

▷ *Driving, Hazardous Activities:* This drug can impair mental alertness, judgment and physical coordination. Avoid hazardous activities.

Aviation Note: The use of this drug *is a disqualification* for piloting. Consult a designated Aviation Medical Examiner.

Exposure to Sun: Use caution until sensitivity has been determined. Some phenothiazines can cause photosensitivity (see Glossary).

Exposure to Heat: Use caution and avoid excessive heat as much as possible. This drug may impair the regulation of body temperature and increase the risk of heat stroke.

Exposure to Cold: Use caution and dress warmly. This drug can increase the risk of hypothermia in the elderly.

Discontinuation: After long-term use, do not stop this drug suddenly. Gradual withdrawal over 2 to 3 weeks under physician supervision is recommended.

PROPIONIC ACIDS
(Nonsteroidal anti-inflammatory drugs)

Ibuprofen (i BYU proh fen)   **Fenoprofen** (FEN oh proh fen)   **Flurbiprofen** (flur BI proh fen)   **Ketoprofen** (kee toh PROH fen)   **Naproxen** (na PROX in) **Oxaprozin** (OX a proh zin)

Introduced: 1974, 1976, 1977, 1973, 1974, 1992 respectively   **Prescription:** USA: Varies; Canada: Yes   **Available as Generic:**   Yes: ibuprofen, fenoprofen, flurbiprofen, ketoprofen and naproxen   **Class:** analgesic, mild; NSAID **Controlled Drug:** USA: No; Canada: No

Brand Names: Ibuprofen:, Aches-N-Pain, Actiprofen, Advil, ✦Amersol, ✦Apo-Ibuprofen, Arthritis Foundation Pain Reliever/Fever Reducer, Bayer Select, Children's Advil, Children's Motrin, Children's Motrin Drops (nonprescription), Children's Motrin Suspension (nonprescription), CoAdvil [CD], Dimetapp Sinus [CD], Dologesic, Dristan Sinus, Excedrin IB, Genpril, Guildprofen, Haltran, Ibuprohm, Ibu, Junior Strength Motrin Caplets (nonprescription), Medipren, Medi-Profen, Midol IB, Motrin, Motrin IB, ✦Novo-Profen, Nuprin, PediaProfen, Prpfen-IB, Rufen, Superior Pain Medicine, Supreme Pain Medicine, Tab-Profen, Fenoprofen:, Nalfon, Flurbiprofen:, Ansaid, ✦Apo-Flurbiprofen, ✦Froben, ✦Froben-SR, Ocufen, Ketoprofen:, Actron (12.5 mg nonprescription), ✦Apo-Keto, ✦Apo-Keto E, Orudis, Orudis E-50, Orudis E-100, Orudis KT, Orudis SR, Oruvail, Oruvail

ER, ✦Oruvail SR, ✦Rhodis, ✦Rhodis EC, ✦Rhodis EC suppository, Naproxen:, Aleve (nonprescription), Anaprox, Anaprox DS, ✦Apo-Naproxen, Naprelan, Naprosyn, ✦Naxen, Neo-Prox, ✦Novo-Naprox, ✦Nu-Naprox, ✦Synflex, Oxaprozin:, Daypro

---

BENEFITS versus RISKS

Possible Benefits	*Possible Risks*
EFFECTIVE RELIEF OF MILD TO MODERATE PAIN AND INFLAMMATION	Gastrointestinal pain, ulceration, bleeding (rare)
EFFECTIVE RELIEF OF FEVER	Rare kidney damage
	Rare fluid retention
	Rare bone marrow depression (except oxaprozin)
	Rare liver toxicity (naproxen, ketoprofen, and flurbiprofen)

▷ **Principal Uses**

As a Single Drug Product: Uses currently included in FDA approved labeling: (1) All of the 6 agents in this class treat rheumatoid and osteoarthritis; (2) naproxen is useful in: bursitis, gout, dysmenorrhea (ketoprofen and ibuprofen are also approved for use in primary dysmenorrhea), pain, juvenile rheumatoid arthritis and tendonitis; (3) fenoprofen is the only agent approved to treat tennis elbow.

Other (unlabeled) generally accepted uses: (1) Naproxen has been used to treat migraine and colds caused by rhinoviruses; (2) oxaprozin is useful in gout and tendonitis; (3) ketoprofen may have a role in temporal arteritis; (4) flurbiprofen has some support for therapy of periodontal disease and miosis inhibition; (5) fenoprofen has been used successfully in therapy of migraine; (6) ibuprofen treats interleukin 2 toxicity, chronic urticaria and can decrease IUD associated bleeding. All of the agents have been used for a variety of pains and fever.

How These Drugs Work: It is thought that these drugs reduces the tissue concentrations of prostaglandins (and related compounds), chemicals involved in the production of inflammation and pain.

Available Dosage Forms and Strengths

Ibuprofen:

Caplets — 200 mg
Chewable tablets — 50 mg, 100 mg
Oral suspension — 100 mg per 5-ml
Tablets — 40 mg, 200 mg, 300 mg, 400 mg, 600 mg, 800 mg

Fenoprofen:

Capsules — 200 mg, 300 mg, 600 mg
Tablets — 600 mg

Flurbiprofen:

Ophthalmic drops — 0.03%
Tablets — 50 mg, 100 mg

Ketoprofen:

Capsules — 50 mg, 75 mg, 100 mg, 150 mg
Suppositories — 100 mg (in Canada)

Tablets (nonprescription) — 12.5 mg
Enteric tablets — 50 mg (in Canada)
Naproxen:
Caplet — 220 mg
Oral suspension — 125 mg per 5 ml
Rectal suppository — 500 mg (Canada)
Tablets — 125 mg, 250 mg, 275 mg, 375 mg, 500 mg, 550 mg
Tablets, controlled release — 375 mg, 500 mg
Oxaprozin:
Caplet — 600 mg

▷ **Usual Adult Dosage Range:**   Ibuprofen: 200 to 800 mg 3 or 4 times/day. Total daily dosage should not exceed 3200 mg.

Fenoprofen: 300 to 600 mg three or four times daily. Daily maximum is 3200 mg.

Flurbiprofen: 100 to 300 mg daily in 2 to 4 divided doses. The lowest effective dose should be used. Daily maximum is 300 mg.

Ketoprofen: 75 mg three times daily or 50 mg four times daily. Usual daily dose is 100 to 300 mg divided into 3 or 4 doses. Daily maximum is 300 mg.

Naproxen: Gout: 750 mg initially, then 250 mg every 8 hours until attack is relieved. Arthritis: 250, 375 or 500 mg twice daily 12 hours apart.

The new sustained release form (Naprelan) offers an intestinal protective drug absorption system (IPDAS) and once daily (two tablets once daily) dosing. Menstrual pain: 500 mg initially, then 250 mg every 6 to 8 hours as needed. Maximum dose for pain is 1375 mg.

Oxaprozin: 1200 mg as a single daily dose in the morning. Daily maximum is 1800 mg (or 26 mg per kilogram in patients with normal liver and kidney function).

Author's note: Medicines in this class with available nonprescription forms usually have lower daily maximum doses. For example: Children's Motrin: Approved for nonprescription use as temporary relief of minor aches and pains or reduction of fever in children 2 years of age and older.

Less than 11 kg and under 2 years old: consult your doctor; 2 to 3 years old and 11–15.9 kg: 100 mg every 6 to 8 hours. Up to 4 doses may be given a day. Use should NOT go on for longer than 3 days. Please consult individual package labels or ask your pharmacist or doctor for dosing advice.

Note: Actual dose and dosing schedule must be determined by the physician for each patient individually.

Conditions Requiring Dosing Adjustments

Liver function: All of these drugs are metabolized in the liver and are used with caution, and consideration is given to lower doses in patients with liver compromise.

Kidney function: These drugs share the risks common to most nonsteroidal antiinflammatory drugs (NSAIDs). Some patients with kidney compromise are dependent on prostaglandins for kidney function. A benefit to risk decision must be made regarding the use of NSAIDS in these patients.

▷ **Dosing Instructions:**   Take either on an empty stomach or with food or milk to prevent stomach irritation. Take with a full glass of water and remain upright (do not lie down) for 30 minutes. The tablets may be crushed and the capsules opened for administration except for ketoprofen tablets which should not be crushed or altered.

Usual Duration of Use: Use on a regular schedule for 1 to 2 weeks usually determines effectiveness. Peak oxaprozin effect may take 6 weeks. Long-term use requires supervision and periodic evaluation by the physician.

▷ **These Drugs Should Not Be Taken If**
- you have had an allergic reaction to them previously.
- you are subject to asthma or nasal polyps caused by aspirin.
- you have a bleeding disorder or a blood cell disorder.
- flurbiprofen ophthalmic drops should NOT be used in people with herpes simplex keratitis.
- you have severe impairment of kidney function (some cases).

▷ **Inform Your Physician Before Taking These Drugs If**
- you are allergic to aspirin or to other aspirin substitutes.
- you have active peptic ulcer disease or any form of gastrointestinal bleeding.
- you have a history of peptic ulcer disease or any type of bleeding disorder.
- you have impaired liver or kidney function.
- you have high blood pressure or a history of heart failure.
- you are taking any of the following: acetaminophen, aspirin or other aspirin substitutes or anticoagulants.

Possible Side Effects (natural, expected, and unavoidable drug actions)
Fluid retention (weight gain); pink, red, purple, or rust coloration of urine (ibuprofen only). Ringing in the ears.

▷ **Possible Adverse Effects** (unusual, unexpected, and infrequent reactions)
If any of the following develop, consult your physician promptly for guidance.
Mild Adverse Effects
Allergic Reactions: Skin rash, hives, itching.
Headache, dizziness, altered or blurred vision, ringing in the ears, depression.
Stinging or burning of the eyes with ophthalmic flurbiprofen drops.
Sleep disturbances (oxaprozin—up to 3%).
Mouth sores, indigestion, nausea, vomiting, constipation, diarrhea.
Palpitations (fenoprofen—rare).
Serious Adverse Effects
Allergic Reactions: Anaphylaxis (see Glossary), severe skin reactions (rare), lung inflammation (naproxen—pneumonitis) (rare).
Idiosyncratic Reactions: Ibuprofen and naproxen—drug-induced meningitis with fever and coma (rare).
Active peptic ulcer, with or without bleeding.
Inflammation of the colon (rare).
Porphyria (some drugs in this class) (rare).
Pancreatitis (one case with naproxen) (very rare).
Some medicines in this class may cause Parkinson-like symptoms in susceptible patients.
Inflammation of the esophagus (more probable if patients lie down soon after taking these medicines).

One case of naproxen-associated recurrence of lupus erythematosus.

Liver damage with jaundice (see Glossary).

Kidney damage with painful urination, bloody urine, reduced urine formation.

Rare bone marrow depression (see Glossary)—fatigue, weakness, fever, sore throat, abnormal bleeding or bruising.

▷ **Possible Effects on Sexual Function**

Altered timing and pattern of menstruation (ibuprofen, ketoprofen and naproxen), and excessive menstrual bleeding (ibuprofen and ketoprofen); Male breast enlargement and tenderness (ibuprofen) (rare). Naproxen may rarely inhibit ejaculation. Ketoprofen may rarely decrease libido.

Possible Delayed Adverse Effects: Mild anemia due to "silent" blood loss from the stomach (less than that caused by aspirin).

▷ **Adverse Effects That May Mimic Natural Diseases or Disorders**

Liver reaction may suggest viral hepatitis.

Natural Diseases or Disorders That May Be Activated by These Drugs

Peptic ulcer disease, ulcerative colitis.

Possible Effects on Laboratory Tests

Complete blood cell counts: decreased red cells, hemoglobin, white cells and platelets.

Blood cholesterol level: increased.

Blood lithium level: increased.

Blood uric acid level: increased.

Liver function tests: increased liver enzymes (ALT/GPT, AST/GOT and alkaline phosphatase), increased bilirubin.

Kidney function tests: increased blood creatinine and urea nitrogen (BUN) levels.

Fecal occult blood test: positive.

CAUTION

1. Dosage should always be limited to the smallest amount that produces reasonable improvement.
2. These drugs may mask early indications of infection. Inform your physician if you think you are developing an infection of any kind.

Precautions for Use

By Infants and Children: Safety and effectiveness for those under 12 years of age not established.

By Those over 60 Years of Age: Small doses are advisable until tolerance is determined. Watch for signs of liver or kidney toxicity, fluid retention, dizziness, confusion, impaired memory, stomach bleeding or constipation.

▷ **Advisability of Use During Pregnancy**

Pregnancy Category: B for ibuprofen, fenoprofen, flurbiprofen, ketoprofen and naproxen. C for oxaprozin. Ibuprofen and fenoprofen are FDA category D if used in the last three months (trimester) of pregnancy. The manufacturers of ketoprofen and flurbiprofen say that both medicines should be avoided in late pregnancy. See Pregnancy Code at the back of this book.

Animal studies: No birth defects reported in rats or rabbits.

Human studies: Adequate studies of pregnant women are not available.

Avoid these drugs during the last 3 months. Use during the first 6 months only if clearly needed. Ask physician for guidance.

Advisability of Use if Breast-Feeding
Presence of these drugs in breast milk: Yes, or expected.
Avoid drugs or refrain from nursing.

Habit-Forming Potential: None.

Effects of Overdosage: Drowsiness, dizziness, ringing in the ears, nausea, vomiting, diarrhea, confusion, unsteadiness, stupor progressing to coma.

Possible Effects of Long-Term Use: Fluid retention.

Suggested Periodic Examinations While Taking These Drugs (at physician's discretion)
Complete blood cell counts, liver and kidney function tests, complete eye examinations if vision is altered in any way.

▷ **While Taking These Drugs, Observe the Following**
Foods: No restrictions.
Beverages: No restrictions. May be taken with milk.
▷ *Alcohol:* Use with caution. The irritant action of alcohol on the stomach lining, added to the irritant action of these drugs, can increase the risk of stomach ulceration and/or bleeding.
Tobacco Smoking: No interactions expected.
▷ *Other Drugs*
These medicines may ***increase*** the effects of
- acetaminophen (Tylenol, etc.), and increase the risk of kidney damage; avoid prolonged use of this combination.
- anticoagulants (Coumadin, etc.), and increase the risk of bleeding. More frequent INR (prothrombin time) tests are needed and ongoing doses should be adjusted to the laboratory test results.
- enoxaparin (Lovenox) if NSAIDs have been used before hip replacement surgery and enoxaparin is used after surgery.
- lithium (Lithobid, others) by causing toxic lithium levels.
- methotrexate (Mexate, others) and result in major methotrexate toxicity with possible anemia, hemorrhage and blood infections.
These medicines may ***decrease*** the effects of
- diuretics (see Drug Classes) such as hydrochlorothiazide (Esidrix) and furosemide (Lasix).
- beta blockers (see Drug Classes) such as carteolol (Cartrol).
These medicines ***taken concurrently*** with the following drugs may increase the risk of bleeding; avoid these combinations:
- aspirin.
- dipyridamole (Persantine).
- enoxaparin (Lovenox).
- indomethacin (Indocin).
- sulfinpyrazone (Anturane).
- valproic acid (Depakene).
- warfarin (Coumadin).
▷ *Driving, Hazardous Activities:* These drugs may cause drowsiness or dizziness. Restrict activities as necessary.
Aviation Note: The use of these drugs ***may be a disqualification*** for piloting. Consult a designated Aviation Medical Examiner.

Exposure to Sun: Use caution until sensitivity is determined. Ibuprofen, keto-profen, flurbiprofen and naproxen cause photosensitivity (see Glossary).

PROPRANOLOL (proh PRAN oh lohl)

Introduced: 1966   **Prescription:** USA: Yes; Canada: Yes   **Available as Generic:** Yes   **Class:** Antianginal, antiarrhythmic, antihypertensive, antimigraine drug, beta blocker   **Controlled Drug:** USA: No; Canada: No

Brand Names: ✦Apo-Propranolol, ✦Detensol, Inderal, Inderal-LA, Inderide [CD], Inderide LA [CD], Ipran, ✦Novo-Pranol, ✦PMS Propranolol

BENEFITS versus RISKS	
Possible Benefits	*Possible Risks*
EFFECTIVE, WELL-TOLERATED AS: ANTIANGINAL DRUG in effort-induced angina; ANTIARRHYTHMIC DRUG in certain heart rhythm disorders; ANTIHYPERTENSIVE DRUG in mild to moderate hypertension EFFECTIVE PREVENTION OF MIGRAINE HEADACHES Effective adjunct in the prevention of recurrent heart attack and in the management of pheochromocytoma	CONGESTIVE HEART FAILURE in advanced heart disease Worsening of angina in coronary heart disease (if drug is abruptly withdrawn) Masking of low blood sugar (hypoglycemia) in drug-treated diabetes Provocation of asthma Rare depression Rare blood cell disorders: low white cell and platelet counts

▷ **Principal Uses**

As a Single Drug Product: Uses currently included in FDA approved labeling: (1) Used to treat several serious cardiovascular disorders: classical effort-induced angina, certain types of heart rhythm disturbance and high blood pressure. It is also beneficial in preventing the recurrence of heart attacks (myocardial infarction); (2) used to reduce the frequency and severity of migraine headaches.

Other (unlabeled) generally accepted uses: (1) Control of physical signs of anxiety and nervous tension (as in stage fright); (2) helps control familial tremors and symptoms seen with markedly overactive thyroid function (thyrotoxicosis); (3) decreases abnormal abdominal fluid accumulation (ascites) in people with cirrhosis of the liver; (4) may have a role in combination therapy with metronidazole in resistant giardia infections; (5) helps control headaches caused by cyclosporine (Sandimmune); (6) may be useful in certain kinds of pain, especially after amputations; (7) can help control panic attacks; (8) useful in helping decrease bleeding in patients with esophageal varices and liver cirrhosis; (9) helps fight symptoms in narcotic withdrawal cases.

As a Combination Drug Product [CD]: This drug is available in combination with hydrochlorothiazide for the treatment of hypertension. This combination product includes two drugs with different mechanisms of action; it is intended to provide greater effectiveness and convenience for long-term use.

How This Drug Works: By blocking certain actions of the sympathetic nervous system, this drug
- reduces rate and contraction force of the heart, lowering the ejection pressure of the blood leaving the heart and reducing the oxygen requirement for heart function.
- reduces the degree of contraction of blood vessel walls, resulting in their expansion and consequent lowering of blood pressure.
- prolongs the conduction time of nerve impulses through the heart, of benefit in the management of certain heart rhythm disorders.

Available Dosage Forms and Strengths

Capsules, prolonged-action — 60 mg, 80 mg, 120 mg, 160 mg

Concentrate — 80 mg/ml

Injection — 1 mg per ml

Oral solution — 4 mg/ml and 8 mg/ml

Tablets — 10 mg, 20 mg, 40 mg, 60 mg, 80 mg, 90 mg, 120 mg

▷ **Usual Adult Dosage Range:**   Varies with indication.

Antianginal: Initially, 10 mg 3 or 4 times/day; increase dose gradually every 3 to 7 days as needed and tolerated. The total daily dosage should not exceed 400 mg.

Antiarrhythmic: 10 to 30 mg 3 or 4 times/day as needed and tolerated.

Antihypertensive: Initially, 40 mg twice/day; increase dose gradually as needed and tolerated. The total daily dosage should not exceed 640 mg.

Migraine headache prevention: Initially, 20 mg 4 times/day; increase dose gradually as needed and tolerated. The total daily dosage should not exceed 480 mg. Long acting formulations offer the advantage of once daily dosing for many patients. **Note: Actual dosage and administration schedule must be determined by the physician for each patient individually.**

Conditions Requiring Dosing Adjustments

Liver function: This drug should be used with caution in patients with liver compromise, however, specific guidelines for adjustment of dosages are not available. In general, lower starting doses and slower increases as needed and tolerated are indicated.

Kidney function: Used with caution in people with combined kidney and liver compromise. Dose adjustments are not needed in people with compromised kidneys.

▷ **Dosing Instructions:**   Preferably taken 1 hour before eating to maximize absorption. The tablet may be crushed for administration; to prevent harmless possible numbing effect, mix with soft food and swallow promptly. The prolonged-action capsules should be swallowed whole without alteration. Do not stop this drug abruptly.

Usual Duration of Use: Use on a regular schedule for 10 to 14 days usually determines effectiveness in preventing angina, controlling heart rhythm disorders and lowering blood pressure. Maximal effectiveness may require continual use for 6 to 8 weeks. The long-term use of this drug (months to years) will be determined by the course of your symptoms over time and your response to the overall treatment program (weight reduction, salt restriction, smoking cessation, etc.). Consult your physician on a regular basis.

▷ **This Drug Should Not Be Taken If**
- you have bronchial asthma
- you have had an allergic reaction to it previously.
- you have Prinzmetal's variant angina (coronary artery spasm).
- you have congestive heart failure.
- you have Raynaud's disease.
- you have an abnormally slow heart rate or a serious form of heart block.
- you are taking, or have taken within the past 14 days, any monoamine oxidase (MAO) type A inhibitor drug (see Drug Classes).

▷ **Inform Your Physician Before Taking This Drug If**
- you have had an adverse reaction to any beta blocker drug in the past (see Drug Classes).
- you have a history of serious heart disease.
- you have a history of hay fever (allergic rhinitis), asthma, chronic bronchitis or emphysema.
- you have a history of overactive thyroid function (hyperthyroidism).
- you have a history of low blood sugar (hypoglycemia).
- you have impaired liver or kidney function.
- you are allergic to bee stings.
- you have diabetes or myasthenia gravis.
- you are currently taking any form of digitalis, quinidine or reserpine, or any calcium blocker drug (see Drug Classes).
- you plan to have surgery under general anesthesia in the near future.

Possible Side Effects (natural, expected, and unavoidable drug actions)
Lethargy and fatigability, cold extremities, slow heart rate, light-headedness in upright position (see orthostatic hypotension in Glossary).

▷ **Possible Adverse Effects** (unusual, unexpected, and infrequent reactions)
If any of the following develop, consult your physician promptly for guidance.

Mild Adverse Effects
Allergic Reactions: Skin rash, temporary loss of hair, drug fever (see Glossary).
Joint pain.
Headache, dizziness, insomnia, vivid dreams.
Indigestion, taste disorder, nausea, vomiting, diarrhea.
Weight gain.

Serious Adverse Effects
Allergic Reactions: Anaphylaxis.
Idiosyncratic Reactions: Acute behavioral disturbances: disorientation, confusion, hallucinations, amnesia.
Paradoxical hypertension.
Mental depression, anxiety.
Chest pain, shortness of breath, precipitation of congestive heart failure.
Peripheral neuropathy (rare).
Hyperthyroidism (rare).
Drug-induced systemic lupus erythematosus (rare).
Drug-induced myasthenia gravis (rare).
Drug-induced porphyria (rare).
Kidney problems (interstitial nephritis) (rare).

Induction of bronchial asthma (in asthmatic individuals).

May precipitate problems walking (intermittent claudication).

Rare blood cell disorders: abnormally low white blood cell count, causing fever and sore throat; abnormally low blood platelet count, causing abnormal bleeding or bruising.

Carpal tunnel syndrome (rare).

▷ **Possible Effects on Sexual Function**

Decreased libido; impaired erection (28%); impotence (15%).

This drug has been found to have the highest incidence of libido reduction and erectile impairment of all beta blocker drugs. Male infertility (inhibited sperm motility); Peyronie's disease (see Glossary).

▷ **Adverse Effects That May Mimic Natural Diseases or Disorders**

Reduced blood flow to extremities may resemble Raynaud's phenomenon (see Glossary).

Natural Diseases or Disorders That May Be Activated by This Drug

Prinzmetal's variant angina, Raynaud's disease, intermittent claudication, myasthenia gravis (questionable).

Possible Effects on Laboratory Tests

White blood cell count: occasionally decreased.

Blood platelet count: increased or decreased.

Bleeding time: increased.

Blood total cholesterol level: no effect in some; increased in others.

Blood HDL cholesterol level: no effect in some; decreased in others.

Blood LDL cholesterol level: no effect in some; increased and decreased in others.

Blood VLDL cholesterol level: no effect in some; increased in others.

Blood triglyceride levels: no effect in some; increased in others.

Blood glucose level: no effect in some; increased and decreased in others.

Glucose tolerance test (GTT): decreased.

Blood thyroid hormone levels: T_3—no effect in some, decreased in others; T_4—increased; free T_4—increased.

Blood uric acid level: no effect in some; increased in others.

Liver function tests: increased liver enzymes (ALT/GPT, AST/GOT and alkaline phosphatase); effects probably not due to liver damage.

CAUTION

1. ***Do not stop this drug suddenly*** without the knowledge and help of your doctor. Carry a notation on your person that you are taking this drug.

2. Ask your physician or pharmacist before using nasal decongestants usually present in over-the-counter cold preparations and nose drops. These can cause sudden increases in blood pressure when taken concurrently with beta blocker drugs.

3. Report the development of any tendency to emotional depression.

Precautions for Use

By Infants and Children: Safety and effectiveness for those under 12 years of age not established. However, if this drug is used, observe for the development of low blood sugar (hypoglycemia) during periods of reduced food intake.

By Those over 60 Years of Age: Unacceptably high blood pressure should be reduced without creating the risks associated with excessively low blood pressure. Therapy is started with small doses, and blood pressure checked frequently. Sudden, rapid and excessive reduction of blood pressure can predispose to stroke or heart attack. Observe for dizziness, unsteadiness, tendency to fall, confusion, hallucinations, depression or urinary frequency.

▷ **Advisability of Use During Pregnancy**
Pregnancy Category: C. See Pregnancy Code at the back of this book.
    Animal studies: No significant increase in birth defects due to this drug. Some toxic effects on embryo reported.
    Human studies: Adequate studies of pregnant women are not available.
    Avoid use of drug during the first 3 months if possible. Use this drug only if clearly needed. Ask your physician for guidance.

Advisability of Use if Breast-Feeding
    Presence of this drug in breast milk: Yes.
    Monitor nursing infant closely and discontinue drug or nursing if adverse effects develop.

Habit-Forming Potential: None.

Effects of Overdosage: Weakness, slow pulse, low blood pressure, fainting, cold and sweaty skin, congestive heart failure, possible coma and convulsions.

Possible Effects of Long-Term Use: Reduced heart reserve and eventual heart failure in susceptible patients with advanced heart disease.

Suggested Periodic Examinations While Taking This Drug (at physician's discretion)
    Complete blood cell counts.
    Measurements of blood pressure, evaluation of heart function.
    Liver function tests.

▷ **While Taking This Drug, Observe the Following**
Foods: No restrictions. Avoid excessive salt intake.
Beverages: No restrictions. May be taken with milk.
▷ *Alcohol:* Use with caution. Alcohol may exaggerate this drug's ability to lower the blood pressure and may increase its mild sedative effect.
Tobacco Smoking: Nicotine may reduce this drug's effectiveness in treating angina, heart rhythm disorders and high blood pressure. Smoking increases the rate of elimination of this drug and decreases its blood levels, especially in younger individuals. In addition, high doses of this drug may worsen the constriction of the bronchial tubes caused by regular smoking.
▷ *Other Drugs*
    Propranolol may ***increase*** the effects of
    • other antihypertensive drugs, and cause excessive lowering of blood pressure. Dosage adjustments may be necessary.
    • lidocaine (Xylocaine, etc.).
    • reserpine (Ser-Ap-Es, etc.), and cause sedation, depression, slowing of the heart rate and lowering of the blood pressure.
    • verapamil (Calan, Isoptin), and cause excessive depression of heart function; monitor this combination closely.
    • warfarin (Coumadin) and increase bleeding risk. More frequent INR testing (protimes) are needed. Warfarin dosing should be adjusted to laboratory results.

Propranolol may *decrease* the effects of
- albuterol (Proventil).
- theophyllines (Aminophyllin, Theo-Dur, etc.), and reduce their antiasthmatic effectiveness.

Propranolol *taken concurrently* with
- amiodarone (Codaraone) may result in abnormal heart rhythms and low pulse. These agents should not be combined.
- clonidine (Catapres) requires close monitoring for rebound high blood pressure if clonidine is withdrawn while propranolol is still being taken.
- digoxin can result in severe slowing of the heart (bradycardia).
- epinephrine (Adrenalin, etc.) may cause marked rise in blood pressure and slowing of the heart rate.
- fluoxetine (Prozac) may increase the risk of slow heart beat and sedation.
- fluvoxamine (Luvox) may increase the risk of slow heart beat and sedation.
- insulin requires close monitoring to avoid undetected hypoglycemia (see Glossary).
- oral hypoglycemic agents (see Drug Class) and cause slow recovery from any low blood sugar which may occur.
- quinidine (Quinaglute) can increase adverse effects without increased therapeutic benefits.
- venlafaxine (Effexor) may result in increased risk of propranolol toxicity.
- X-ray contrast media such as diatrizoate results in up to an eight fold increased risk of severe allergic (anaphylactoid) drug reactions.

The following drugs may *increase* the effects of propranolol
- chlorpromazine (Thorazine, etc.).
- cimetidine (Tagamet).
- diltiazem (Cardizem).
- disopyramide (Norpace).
- furosemide or other diuretics.
- methimazole (Tapazole).
- nicardipine (Cardene).
- propylthiouracil (Propacil).

The following drugs may *decrease* the effects of propranolol
- antacids.
- barbiturates (phenobarbital, etc.).
- indomethacin (Indocin), and possibly other "aspirin substitutes" or NSAIDs may impair propranolol's antihypertensive effect.
- rifampin (Rifadin, Rimactane).

▷ *Driving, Hazardous Activities:* Use caution until the full extent of drowsiness, lethargy and blood pressure change have been determined.

Aviation Note: The use of this drug *may be a disqualification* for piloting. Consult a designated Aviation Medical Examiner.

Exposure to Sun: No restrictions.

Exposure to Heat: Caution advised. Hot environments can lower blood pressure and exaggerate the effects of this drug.

Exposure to Cold: Caution advised. Cold environments can enhance the circulatory deficiency in the extremities that may occur with this drug. The elderly should take precautions to prevent hypothermia (see Glossary).

Heavy Exercise or Exertion: It is advisable to avoid exertion that produces light-headedness, excessive fatigue or muscle cramping. The use of this drug may intensify the hypertensive response to isometric exercise.

Occurrence of Unrelated Illness: Fever can lower blood pressure and require adjustment of dosage. Nausea or vomiting may interrupt the regular dosage schedule. Ask your physician for guidance.

Discontinuation: It is advisable to avoid sudden discontinuation of this drug in all situations; this is especially true in the presence of coronary artery disease. If possible, gradual reduction of dose over a period of 2 to 3 weeks is recommended. Ask your physician for specific guidance.

PROTRIPTYLINE (proh TRIP ti leen)

Introduced: 1966   **Prescription:** USA: Yes; Canada: Yes   **Available as Generic:** USA: No; Canada: No   **Class:** Antidepressant   **Controlled Drug:** USA: No; Canada: No

Brand Names: ✦Triptil, Vivactil

BENEFITS versus RISKS	
Possible Benefits	*Possible Risks*
EFFECTIVE RELIEF OF MAJOR ENDOGENOUS DEPRESSIONS	ADVERSE BEHAVIORAL EFFECTS: confusion, disorientation, hallucinations, delusions
HELPS MANAGE OTHER DEPRESSIVE DISORDERS	CONVERSION OF DEPRESSION TO MANIA in manic-depressive (bipolar) disorders
Possibly beneficial in the management of attention deficit disorder and of narcolepsy/cataplexy syndrome	Aggravation of schizophrenia
	Irregular heart rhythms
	Rare blood cell abnormalities

▷ **Principal Uses**

As a Single Drug Product: Uses currently included in FDA approved labeling: (1) Relieves symptoms associated with major spontaneous (endogenous) depression, depressed bipolar disorder and mixed bipolar disorder.

Other (unlabeled) generally accepted uses: (1) Treatment of sleep disorders such as apnea, hypersomnia and impaired morning arousal, (2) may have a role in treating glaucoma; (3) used in combination with methylphenidate or amphetamines in narcolepsy

How This Drug Works: It is thought that this drug relieves depression by slowly restoring to normal levels certain constituents of brain tissue (norepinephrine and serotonin) that transmit nerve impulses.

Available Dosage Forms and Strengths

Tablets — 5 mg, 10 mg

▷ **Recommended Dosage Ranges** (Actual dosage and administration schedule must be determined by the physician for each patient individually.)

Infants and Children: Dosage not established.

12 to 60 Years of Age: For depression: Initially 5 to 10 mg, 3 or 4 times daily. The dose is increased cautiously as needed and tolerated by 5 mg daily at intervals of 1 week. The usual maintenance dose is 15 to 40 mg a day, divided into 3 or 4 doses. The total daily dose should not exceed 60 mg.

Over 60 Years of Age: Initially 5 mg, 2 or 3 times daily to evaluate tolerance. Increase dose cautiously as needed and tolerated by 5 mg daily at intervals of 1 week. Doses above 20 mg daily require careful monitoring of heart function and blood pressure. The total daily dose should not exceed 40 mg.

Conditions Requiring Dosing Adjustments

Liver function: The dose should be empirically decreased, and blood levels obtained at appropriate intervals. Protriptyline is a rare cause of hepatotoxicity.

Kidney function: The kidney plays a minor role in the elimination of this drug.

▷ **Dosing Instructions:**   The tablet may be crushed and taken without regard to meals.

For those individuals who experience a stimulating effect from this drug: (1) Necessary dosage increases should be made in the morning; (2) the last daily dose should be taken in the afternoon (3 to 4 p.m.) to avoid insomnia and disturbed dreaming.

Usual Duration of Use: Some benefit may be apparent within 1 to 2 weeks, but adequate response may require continual use for 3 months or longer. Long-term use should not exceed 6 months without evaluation regarding the need for continuation of the drug. Consult your physician on a regular basis.

Possible Advantages of This Drug

Causes less daytime sedation than some other agents.

Causes orthostatic hypotension less frequently (see Glossary).

▷ **This Drug Should Not Be Taken If**
- you have had an allergic reaction to it previously.
- you are taking or have taken within the past 14 days any monoamine oxidase (MAO) type A inhibitor drug (see Drug Classes).
- you are recovering from a recent heart attack.
- you have narrow-angle glaucoma.

▷ **Inform Your Physician Before Taking This Drug If**
- you are allergic or sensitive to any other tricyclic antidepressant (see Drug Classes).
- you have a history of any of the following: diabetes, epilepsy, glaucoma, heart disease, prostate gland enlargement or overactive thyroid function.
- you have a history of psychosis.
- you work outside, particularly in hot weather.
- you plan to have surgery under general anesthesia in the near future.

Possible Side Effects (natural, expected, and unavoidable drug actions)

Light-headedness, blurred vision, dry mouth, constipation, impaired urination (see prostatism in Glossary).

▷ **Possible Adverse Effects** (unusual, unexpected, and infrequent reactions)

If any of the following develop, consult your physician promptly for guidance.

Mild Adverse Effects

Allergic Reactions: Skin rash, hives, swelling of face or tongue, drug fever (see Glossary).

Cavities (dental caries).

Blurred vision.

Ringing in the ears.

Headache, dizziness, weakness, fainting, unsteady gait, tremors.

Peculiar taste, irritation of tongue or mouth, nausea, indigestion.

Fluctuation of blood sugar levels.

Serious Adverse Effects

Allergic Reactions: Hepatitis, with or without jaundice (see Glossary).

Confusion, disorientation, hallucinations, delusions.

Aggravation of paranoid psychoses and schizophrenia; seizures.

Heart palpitation and irregular rhythm.

Bone marrow depression (see Glossary)—fatigue, weakness, fever, sore throat, abnormal bleeding or bruising.

Severe lowering of blood pressure on standing (orthostatic hypotension).

Peripheral neuritis (see Glossary)—numbness, tingling, pain, loss of strength in arms and legs (rare).

Parkinson-like disorders (see Glossary)—usually mild and infrequent; more likely to occur in the elderly.

▷ **Possible Effects on Sexual Function:** Decreased libido, increased libido (antidepressant effect), male impotence, inhibited female orgasm, male and female breast enlargement, milk production, swelling of testicles.

▷ **Adverse Effects That May Mimic Natural Diseases or Disorders**

Liver toxicity may suggest viral hepatitis.

Natural Diseases or Disorders That May Be Activated by This Drug

Latent diabetes, epilepsy, glaucoma, prostatism.

Possible Effects on Laboratory Tests

White blood cell and platelet counts: decreased.

Blood glucose levels: increased and decreased (fluctuations).

Liver function tests: increased liver enzymes (ALT/GPT, AST/GOT and alkaline phosphatase), increased bilirubin.

CAUTION

1. Dosage must be adjusted for each person individually. Report for follow-up evaluation and laboratory tests as directed by your physician.
2. It is advisable to withhold this drug if electroconvulsive therapy (ECT, "shock" treatment) is to be used to treat your depression.

Precautions for Use

By Infants and Children: Safety and effectiveness for those under 6 years of age not established. This drug may be used to relieve symptoms of attention deficit disorder, with or without hyperactivity, in selected children over 6 years of age.

By Those over 60 Years of Age: Usual dosage is 15 to 30 mg daily in divided doses. During the first 2 weeks of treatment, observe for the development of confusion, agitation, forgetfulness, disorientation, delusions and hallucinations. Reduction of dosage or discontinuation may be necessary. Unsteadiness may predispose to falling and injury. This drug can increase the degree of impaired urination associated with prostate gland enlargement (prostatism).

▷ **Advisability of Use During Pregnancy**

Pregnancy Category: C. See Pregnancy Code at the back of this book.

Animal studies: No birth defects found in mouse, rat and rabbit studies.

Human studies: No defects reported in 21 exposures to amitriptyline, a closely related drug. Adequate studies of pregnant women are not available. Avoid use of drug during first 3 months. Use during last 6 months only if clearly needed. Ask your physician for guidance.

Advisability of Use if Breast-Feeding

Presence of this drug in breast milk: Yes, in small amounts.

Monitor nursing infant closely and discontinue drug or nursing if adverse effects develop: excessive drowsiness and failure to feed.

Habit-Forming Potential: Psychological or physical dependence is rare and unexpected.

Effects of Overdosage: Confusion, hallucinations, marked drowsiness, heart palpitations, dilated pupils, tremors, stupor, deep sleep, coma, convulsions.

Suggested Periodic Examinations While Taking This Drug (at physician's discretion)

Complete blood cell counts, liver function tests, serial blood pressure readings and electrocardiograms.

▷ **While Taking This Drug, Observe the Following**

Foods: No restrictions. This drug may increase the appetite and cause excessive weight gain.

Beverages: No restrictions. May be taken with milk.

▷ *Alcohol:* Avoid completely. This drug can markedly increase the intoxicating effects of alcohol and accentuate its depressant action on brain function.

Tobacco Smoking: May hasten the elimination of this drug. Higher doses may be necessary.

▷ *Other Drugs*

Protriptyline may ***increase*** the effects of

- atropinelike drugs (see Drug Class Section).
- dicoumarol, and increase the risk of bleeding.
- epinephrine (Adrenalin).
- norepinephrine.
- phenytoin (Dilantin) and lead to toxicity.
- pseudoephedrine and cause high blood pressure and arrhythmias.

Protriptyline may ***decrease*** the effects of

- clonidine (Catapres), and cause loss of blood pressure control; do not use these drugs concurrently.
- guanethidine (Ismelin).

Protriptyline ***taken concurrently*** with

- carbamazepine (Tegretol) may result in increased carbamazepine levels (toxicity risk) and decreased protryptyline levels (loss of therapeutic benefit).
- disulfiram (Antabuse) may cause acute dementia: confusion, disorientation, hallucinations.
- monoamine oxidase (MAO) inhibitor drugs may cause high fever, delirium and convulsions (see Drug Classes).
- thyroid preparations (see Drug Classes) may impair heart rhythm and function. Ask physician for guidance regarding adjustment of thyroid dose.
- venlafaxine (Effexor) may result in increased protriptyline levels and toxicity.

- warfarin (Coumadin) may result in prolonged anticoagulation. Increased INR testing (prothrombin times) is needed.

The following drugs may *increase* the effects of protriptyline
- cimetidine (Tagamet).
- conjugated estrogens (Premarin).
- fluoxetine (Prozac).
- lithium (Lithobid, etc.).
- methylphenidate (Ritalin).
- oral contraceptives.
- quinidine (Quinaglute, others).
- ranitidine (Zantac).
- sertraline (Zoloft).

The following drugs may *decrease* the effects of protriptyline
- barbiturates (see Drug Classes), and reduce its effectiveness.

▷ *Driving, Hazardous Activities:* This drug may impair mental alertness, judgment, physical coordination and reaction time. Avoid hazardous activities.

Aviation Note: The use of this drug *is a disqualification* for piloting. Consult a designated Aviation Medical Examiner.

Exposure to Sun: Use caution. This drug may cause photosensitivity (see Glossary).

Exposure to Heat: This drug can inhibit sweating and impair the body's adaptation to hot environments, increasing the risk of heat stroke. Avoid saunas.

Exposure to Cold: The elderly should use caution and avoid conditions conducive to hypothermia (see Glossary).

Discontinuation: It is advisable to discontinue this drug gradually. Abrupt withdrawal after long-term use can cause headache, malaise and nausea.

PYRAZINAMIDE (peer a ZIN a mide)

Introduced: 1968   **Prescription:** USA: Yes; Canada: Yes   **Available as Generic:** USA: Yes; Canada: No   **Class:** Anti-infective, antituberculosis drug
Controlled Drug: USA: No; Canada: No

Brand Names: ✦PMS Pyrazinamide, Rifiter, ✦Tebrazid

BENEFITS versus RISKS	
Possible Benefits	*Possible Risks*
EFFECTIVE ADJUNCTIVE TREATMENT OF TUBERCULOSIS	DRUG-INDUCED HEPATITIS (rare) Activation of gouty arthritis and porphyria Rare decreased platelets and hemoglobin

▷ **Principal Uses**

As a Single Drug Product: Uses currently included in FDA approved labeling: (1) Treatment of active tuberculosis, in combination with other antitubercular drugs

Other (unlabeled) generally accepted uses: (1) Combination therapy of Mycobacterium xenopi infections; (2) combination therapy of resistant tuberculosis; (2) combination treatment of tuberculosis in AIDS patients.

As a Combination Drug Product [CD]:
> This medicine is combined with two other antituberculosis (isoniazid and rifampin) medicines in order to attack tuberculosis with combination treatment with a single dosage form

How This Drug Works: This drug is ideal for killing tuberculosis organisms which are in acid environments such as in some kinds of white blood (macrophages) cells.

Available Dosage Forms and Strengths
> Tablets — 500 mg

▷ **Recommended Dosage Ranges** (Actual dosage and administration schedule must be determined by the physician for each patient individually.)

Infants and Children: 7.5 to 15 mg/kg of body weight, twice daily; or 15 to 30 mg/kg of body weight, once daily.
> Total daily dosage should not exceed 1.5 grams.

12 to 60 Years of Age: For tuberculosis—15 to 30 mg per kilogram (up to a maximum of 2,000 mg) daily. Some patients do better with twice weekly dosing: 50 to 70 milligram (mg) per kilogram (up to 4,000 mg).

Author's note: Because of the current resistant tuberculosis problem, most clinicians start all patients on a four antituberculosis medicine regimen until laboratory culture results are available.

Over 60 Years of Age: Same as 12 to 60 years of age.

Conditions Requiring Dosing Adjustments

Liver function: It should be used with caution and in decreased doses in patients with liver compromise. Contraindicated in patients with severe liver dysfunction.

Kidney function: In patients with end stage renal failure, the dose **must** be adjusted. One researcher recommends: 60 milligrams per kilogram twice weekly. The dose of pyrazinamide should be given at least 24 hours before any given dialysis session. Patients should be closely monitored.

▷ **Dosing Instructions:**   The tablet may be crushed and taken with or following food to reduce stomach irritation. Take the full course prescribed. This drug should be taken concurrently with other antitubercular drugs to prevent the development of drug-resistant strains of tuberculosis bacteria.

Usual Duration of Use: Use on a regular schedule for 2 months usually determines effectiveness in controlling active tuberculosis. Long-term use of antitubercular drugs (6 months) requires periodic physician evaluation.

Possible Advantages of This Drug
> May reduce the period of drug treatment from 9 to 6 months in responsive infections.

▷ **This Drug Should Not Be Taken If**
- you have had an allergic reaction to it previously.
- you have permanent liver damage with impaired function.
- you have active gout.
- you have active peptic ulcer disease.

▷ **Inform Your Physician Before Taking This Drug If**
- you have had an allergic reaction to: ethionamide, isoniazid, niacin (nicotinic acid).
- you have a history of liver disease.

- you have a history of peptic ulcer or porphyria.
- you tried to take medicines for tuberculosis before, but did not complete the prescribed therapy.
- you have gout or diabetes.
- you have impaired kidney function.

Possible Side Effects (natural, expected, and unavoidable drug actions)
Increased blood uric acid levels.

▷ **Possible Adverse Effects** (unusual, unexpected, and infrequent reactions)
If any of the following develop, consult your physician promptly for guidance.
Mild Adverse Effects
Allergic Reactions: Skin rash, itching, fever.
Loss of appetite, nausea, vomiting.
Increased uric acid.
Joint pain.
Acne (rare).
Serious Adverse Effects
Idiosyncratic Reactions: Rare sideroblastic anemia.
Decreased blood platelets (rare).
Seizures (rare).
Pellagra.
Drug-induced porphyria (rare).
Kidney problems (interstitial nephritis).
Drug-induced hepatitis, with and without jaundice (see Glossary).
Gouty arthritis, due to increased blood uric acid levels.

▷ **Possible Effects on Sexual Function:**   None reported.

▷ **Adverse Effects That May Mimic Natural Diseases or Disorders**
Drug-induced hepatitis may suggest viral hepatitis.

Natural Diseases or Disorders That May Be Activated by This Drug
Gout, peptic ulcer, porphyria.

Possible Effects on Laboratory Tests
Complete blood cell counts: decreased red cells, hemoglobin and platelets.
INR (prothrombin time): increased.
Blood uric acid level: increased.
Liver function tests: increased liver enzymes (ALT/GPT, AST/GOT and alkaline phosphatase), increased bilirubin.
Urine ketone tests: false positive test result with Acetest and Ketostix.

CAUTION
1. When this drug is used alone, tuberculosis bacteria rapidly develop resistance to it. To be effective, this drug must be used in combination with other effective antitubercular drugs, such as isoniazid and rifampin.
2. This drug may interfere with control of diabetes.

Precautions for Use
By Infants and Children: Safety and effectiveness for those under 12 years of age not established. The rare occurrence of drug-related seizure has been reported in a 2 year old child.
By Those over 60 Years of Age: No specific information available.

▷ **Advisability of Use During Pregnancy**
  Pregnancy Category:
    C. See Pregnancy Code at the back of this book.
    Animal studies: No information available.
    Human studies: Adequate studies of pregnant women are not available.
    Use this drug only if clearly needed. Ask your physician for guidance.

  Advisability of Use if Breast-Feeding
    Presence of this drug in breast milk: Yes.
    Avoid drug or refrain from nursing.

  Habit-Forming Potential: None.

  Effects of Overdosage: Nausea, vomiting, malaise.

  Possible Effects of Long-Term Use: Liver damage.

  Suggested Periodic Examinations While Taking This Drug (at physician's discretion)
    Complete blood cell counts.
    Liver function tests.
    Uric acid blood levels.

▷ **While Taking This Drug, Observe the Following**
    Foods: No restrictions.
    Beverages: No restrictions. May be taken with milk.
▷ *Alcohol:* Use sparingly to minimize liver toxicity.
    Tobacco Smoking: No interactions expected.
▷ *Other Drugs*
    Pyrazinamide may *decrease* the effects of
    • allopurinol (Zyloprim).
    • BCG vaccine.
    • cyclosporine (Sandimmune).
    • probenecid (Benemid).
    • sulfinpyrazone (Anturane).
▷ *Driving, Hazardous Activities:* No restrictions.
    Aviation Note: The use of this drug is probably *not a disqualification* for piloting. Consult a designated Aviation Medical Examiner.
    Exposure to Sun: Use caution. This drug may cause photosensitivity (see Glossary).
    Discontinuation: If tolerated, this drug is usually taken for a minimum of 2 months. Do not stop it without your physician's knowledge and guidance.

PYRIDOSTIGMINE (peer id oh STIG meen)

Introduced: 1962   **Prescription:** USA: Yes; Canada: No   **Available as Generic:** USA: No; Canada: No   **Class:** Antimyasthenic   **Controlled Drug:** USA: No; Canada: No

Brand Names: ✦Anaplex SR, Mestinon, Mestinon-SR, Mestinon Timespan, Regonol

BENEFITS versus RISKS	
Possible Benefits	*Possible Risks*
MODERATELY EFFECTIVE TREATMENT OF OCULAR AND MILD FORMS OF MYASTHENIA GRAVIS (symptomatic relief of muscle weakness)	Cholinergic crisis (overdose): excessive salivation, nausea, vomiting, stomach cramps, diarrhea, shortness of breath (asthmalike wheezing), excessive weakness

▷ **Principal Uses**

As a Single Drug Product: Uses currently included in FDA approved labeling: (1) Used to treat the ocular and milder forms of myasthenia gravis by providing temporary relief of muscle weakness and fatigability. It is most useful in long-term treatment when there is little or no difficulty in swallowing; (2) used to reverse muscle relaxants.

Other (unlabeled) generally accepted uses: (1) Used as part of combination therapy in chronic pain; (2) may help in combination therapy of Huntington's chorea and Lambert-Eaton syndrome; (3) adjunctive use with scopolamine to prevent side effects of scopolamine in treating motion sickness; (4) used in war zones to treat the effects of nerve gas; (5) may have a role in treating nonepidemic parotitis; (6) can have a role in chronic pain (causalgia or thalamic pain) .

How This Drug Works: This drug inhibits cholinesterase, the enzyme that destroys acetylcholine. This results in higher levels of acetylcholine, the nerve transmitter that facilitates the stimulation of muscular activity. The net effects are increased muscle strength and endurance.

Available Dosage Forms and Strengths

Syrup — 60 mg per 5-ml (5% alcohol)

Tablets — 30 mg, 60 mg

Tablets, prolonged-action — 180 mg

▷ **Usual Adult Dosage Range:**   Myasthenia gravis: Initially: One to six normal release tablets spaced throughout the day when maximum strength is needed. Maintenance varies with the severity of the disease: One to three extended release tablets taken every 6 hours. Some patients may need to supplement the extended release tablets with the 30 mg immediate release tablets or the syrup in order to best control symptoms. Nerve gas or agent protection: 30 mg every 8 hours when the threat of a nerve agent attack is present. **Note: Actual dosage and administration schedule must be determined by the physician for each patient individually.**

Conditions Requiring Dosing Adjustments

Liver function: No dosing changes are defined in liver compromise.

Kidney function: This drug is primarily eliminated in the urine, however, specific guidelines for dosage adjustments in renal compromise are not available.

▷ **Dosing Instructions:**   Take with food or milk to reduce the intensity of Side Effects. Larger portions of the daily maintenance dosage should be timed according to the pattern of fatigue and weakness. The syrup will permit a finer adjustment of dosage. The regular tablet may be crushed for administration. The prolonged-action tablet should be taken whole (not altered).

Usual Duration of Use: Use on a regular schedule (with dosage adjustment) for 10 to 14 days usually determines effectiveness in relieving the symptoms of myasthenia gravis. Long-term use (months to years) requires periodic physician evaluation.

▷ **This Drug Should Not Be Taken If**
- you are known to be allergic to bromide compounds.
- you have a urinary obstruction or mechanical intestinal obstruction.

▷ **Inform Your Physician Before Taking This Drug If**
- you are subject to heart rhythm disorders or bronchial asthma.
- you are sensitive to bromides.
- you have recurrent urinary tract infections.
- you have prostatism (see Glossary).
- you plan to have surgery under general anesthesia in the near future.

Possible Side Effects (natural, expected, and unavoidable drug actions)
Small pupils, watering of eyes, slow pulse, excessive salivation, nausea, vomiting, stomach cramps, diarrhea, urge to urinate, increased sweating, increased bronchial secretions.

▷ **Possible Adverse Effects** (unusual, unexpected, and infrequent reactions)
If any of the following develop, consult your physician promptly for guidance.
Mild Adverse Effects
Allergic Reaction: Skin rash.
Nervousness, anxiety, unsteadiness, muscle cramps or twitching.
Loss of scalp hair (alopecia), sweating.
Change in the pupil of the eye (miosis).
Serious Adverse Effects
Confusion, slurred speech, seizures, difficult breathing (asthmatic wheezing).
Increased muscle weakness or paralysis.
Psychosis (rare).
Excessive vomiting or diarrhea may induce abnormally low blood potassium levels (hypokalemia). This will accentuate muscle weakness.

▷ **Possible Effects on Sexual Function:**   None reported.

▷ **Adverse Effects That May Mimic Natural Diseases or Disorders**
Seizures may suggest the possibility of epilepsy.

Natural Diseases or Disorders That May Be Activated by This Drug
Latent bronchial asthma.

Possible Effects on Laboratory Tests
None reported.

CAUTION
1. Some drugs block the action of this drug and reduce its effectiveness in treating myasthenia gravis. (See *Other Drugs* below.) Ask your doctor before starting any new drug, prescription or over-the-counter.
2. Dosing must be carefully individualized. Variations in response may occur from time to time. Because generalized muscle weakness is a major symptom of both myasthenia crisis (underdosage) and cholinergic crisis (overdosage), it may be difficult to recognize the correct cause. As a rule, weakness that begins within 1 hour after taking this drug probably represents overdosage; weakness that begins 3 or more hours after taking this

drug is probably due to underdosage. Observe these time relationships and inform your physician.

3. During long-term use of this drug, watch for development of resistance to the drug's therapeutic action (loss of effectiveness). Ask your doctor if the drug should be stopped for a few days to see if responsiveness can be restored.

Precautions for Use

By Infants and Children: The syrup form of this drug permits greater precision of dosage adjustment and ease of administration in this age group. Neonates have received 5 mg every 4 to 6 hours. Since this is often self limiting in neonates, the medicine can frequently be tapered and stopped.

By Those over 60 Years of Age: The natural decline of kidney function with aging may require smaller doses to prevent accumulation of this drug to toxic levels.

▷ **Advisability of Use During Pregnancy**

Pregnancy Category: C. See Pregnancy Code at the back of this book.

Animal studies: No information available.

Human studies: Adequate studies of pregnant women are not available.

There are no reports of birth defects due to the use of this drug during pregnancy. However, there are reports of significant muscular weakness in newborn infants whose mothers had taken this drug during pregnancy. Ask your physician for guidance.

Advisability of Use if Breast-Feeding

Presence of this drug in breast milk: Yes as roughly 0.01% of the mother's dose.

Monitor nursing infant closely and discontinue drug or nursing if adverse effects develop.

Habit-Forming Potential: None.

Effects of Overdosage: Generalized muscular weakness, blurred vision, very small pupils, slow heart rate, difficult breathing (wheezing), excessive salivation, nausea, vomiting, stomach cramps, diarrhea, muscle cramps or twitching. This syndrome constitutes the cholinergic crisis.

Possible Effects of Long-Term Use: Development of tolerance (see Glossary) with loss of therapeutic effectiveness.

Suggested Periodic Examinations While Taking This Drug (at physician's discretion)

Assessment of drug effectiveness and dosage schedule for optimal therapeutic results.

▷ **While Taking This Drug, Observe the Following**

Foods: No restrictions.

Beverages: No restrictions. May be taken with milk.

▷ *Alcohol:* Use caution until the combined effects are determined. Weakness and unsteadiness may be accentuated.

Tobacco Smoking: No interactions expected.

▷ *Other Drugs*

Protriptyline *taken concurrently* with

• disopyramide (Norpace) may help the decreased sweating, difficulty urinating and other anticholinergic effects.

The following drugs may **decrease** the effects of pyridostigmine
- atropine (belladonna).
- clindamycin (Cleocin).
- guanadrel (Hylorel).
- guanethidine (Esimil, Ismelin).
- procainamide (Procan SR, Pronestyl).
- quinidine (Cardioquin, Duraquin, etc.).
- quinine (Quinamm).
- steroids (see Drug Classes).

▷ *Driving, Hazardous Activities:* This drug may cause blurred vision, confusion or generalized weakness. Restrict activities as necessary.

Aviation Note: The use of this drug *is a disqualification* for piloting. Consult a designated Aviation Medical Examiner.

Exposure to Sun: No restrictions.

Exposure to Heat: Use caution. This may cause excessive sweating and increased weakness.

Exposure to Environmental Chemicals: Avoid excessive exposure (inhalation, skin contamination) to the insecticides Baygon, Diazinon and Sevin. These can worsen potential drug toxicity.

Discontinuation: Do not stop this drug abruptly without your doctor's knowledge and guidance.

QUAZEPAM (KWAH zee pam)

Introduced: 1982 **Prescription:** USA: Yes **Available as Generic:**
USA: No **Class:** Hypnotic, benzodiazepines **Controlled Drug:** USA:
C-IV*

Brand Name: Doral, Dormalin

BENEFITS versus RISKS	
Possible Benefits	*Possible Risks*
EFFECTIVE HYPNOTIC during 4 weeks of continual use	Habit-forming potential with long-term use
NO SUPPRESSION OF REM (RAPID EYE MOVEMENT) SLEEP	Minor impairment of mental functions ("hangover" effect)
NO REM SLEEP REBOUND after discontinuation	
Wide margin of safety with therapeutic doses	

▷ **Principal Uses**
As a Single Drug Product: Uses currently included in FDA approved labeling: (1) Short-term treatment of insomnia consisting of difficulty in falling asleep, frequent nighttime awakenings, and/or early morning awakenings; (2) preoperative use (given the night before surgery) as a hypnotic.
Other (unlabeled) generally accepted uses: None.

*See Schedules of Controlled Drugs at the back of this book.

How This Drug Works: This drug selectively affects the benzodiazepine receptors in the brain (BZ-1 receptors) that are associated primarily with sleep mechanisms. Other benzodiazepine hypnotics affect both BZ-1 and BZ-2 receptors, the latter being associated with awareness, memory and judgment; this could account for the "morning-after" impairment of memory and mental functioning caused by shorter-acting benzodiazepine hypnotics (notably triazolam and temazepam), but not by quazepam.

Available Dosage Forms and Strengths
Tablets — 7.5 mg, 15 mg

▷ **Recommended Dosage Ranges** (Actual dosage and administration schedule must be determined by the physician for each patient individually.)
Infants and Children: Up to 18 years of age—use not recommended.
18 to 60 Years of Age: Initially 15 mg at bedtime; on the third night, decrease to 7.5 mg, evaluate effectiveness; adjust further dosage as needed and tolerated.
Over 60 Years of Age: Same as 18 to 60 years of age. Usual maintenance dose is 7.5 mg, once daily at bedtime; use higher doses with caution.

Conditions Requiring Dosing Adjustments
Liver function: The dose **must** be decreased in patients with liver compromise.
Kidney function: Quazepam should be used with caution in renal compromise.

▷ **Dosing Instructions:**   The tablet may be crushed and taken on an empty stomach or with food or milk. Do not stop this drug abruptly if taken for more than 4 weeks.

Usual Duration of Use: Use for 3 nights usually determines this drug's effectiveness in relieving insomnia. If possible, this drug should be used for periods of 3 to 5 nights intermittently, repeated as needed with appropriate dosage adjustment. Avoid uninterrupted and prolonged use. The duration of use should not exceed 2 weeks without reappraisal of continued need.

Possible Advantages of This Drug
Effective the first night of use.
Maintains effectiveness on continual use for 4 weeks.
No effects on rapid-eye-movement (REM) sleep.
Minimal "hangover" effect on day after use.
Less likely to cause "next-morning" amnesia, cognitive impairment or mental dysfunction.
No daytime anxiety (drug-withdrawal effect).
No rebound insomnia when drug is discontinued.
No blood cell or liver toxicity.

▷ **This Drug Should Not Be Taken If**
• you have had an allergic reaction to it previously.
• you are pregnant.
• you have sleep apnea (periods where breathing stops while you sleep).
• you have acute narrow-angle glaucoma.

▷ **Inform Your Physician Before Taking This Drug If**
• you are allergic to any benzodiazepine (see Drug Classes).
• you have a history of alcoholism or drug abuse.
• you are planning pregnancy.
• you have impaired liver or kidney function.

- you have a history of serious depression or mental disorder.
- you are taking other drugs with sedative effects.
- you have: asthma, emphysema, epilepsy, myasthenia gravis.

Possible Side Effects (natural, expected, and unavoidable drug actions)
Mild "hangover" effects on arising: drowsiness, lethargy.

▷ **Possible Adverse Effects** (unusual, unexpected, and infrequent reactions)
If any of the following develop, consult your physician promptly for guidance.
Mild Adverse Effects
Allergic Reactions: Skin rash, itching (rare).
Headache, dizziness (rare), fatigue (rare), unsteadiness, blurred vision (rare).
Dry mouth, nausea, vomiting, indigestion, constipation, diarrhea (all rare).
Problems in moving and coordination (ataxia).
Serious Adverse Effects
Idiosyncratic Reactions: Nervousness, talkativeness, irritability, apprehension, euphoria, excitement, hallucinations (rare paradoxical reactions that may occur with any benzodiazepine).
Withdrawal symptoms.

▷ **Possible Effects on Sexual Function:** Decreased libido, impotence (rare and questionable).

Possible Effects on Laboratory Tests
Urine screening tests for drug abuse: may be **positive**. (Test results depend upon amount of drug taken and testing method used.)

CAUTION
1. Do not stop taking this drug abruptly if it has been taken continually for more than 4 weeks.
2. Some over-the-counter drug products that contain antihistamines (allergy and cold preparations, sleep aids) can cause excessive sedation.
3. Regular nightly use of any hypnotic drug should be avoided.
4. This drug is changed by the liver into long-acting forms that can persist in the body for 24 hours or more. With continual use of this drug daily, these active drug forms may accumulate and produce increasing sedation. If you experience a "hangover" effect, avoid hazardous activities (driving, etc.) and the use of alcohol.

Precautions for Use
By Infants and Children: Safety and effectiveness for those under 18 years of age not established.
By Those over 60 Years of Age: It is advisable to use smaller doses at longer intervals. Watch for lethargy, indifference, fatigue, weakness, unsteadiness, disturbing dreams, nightmares and paradoxical reactions of excitement, agitation, anger, hostility and rage. Because this is a long-acting benzodiazepine, it may cause residual sluggishness and unsteadiness with increased risk of falling during the day following bedtime use. This drug may also increase the number of periods of sleep apnea in this age group.

▷ **Advisability of Use During Pregnancy**
Pregnancy Category: X. See Pregnancy Code at the back of this book.
Animal studies: No significant birth defects reported in mouse and rabbit studies.

Human studies: Adequate studies of pregnant women are not available.

Several studies indicate an increased risk of birth defects if drugs of this class (benzodiazepines) are used during the first 3 months.

Frequent use in late pregnancy can cause the "floppy infant" syndrome in the newborn: weakness, lethargy, unresponsiveness, depressed breathing, low body temperature.

Avoid use during entire pregnancy.

Advisability of Use if Breast-Feeding

Presence of this drug in breast milk: Yes.

Avoid drug or refrain from nursing.

Habit-Forming Potential: This drug can produce psychological and/or physical dependence (see Glossary) if used in large doses for an extended period of time. Avoid continual use.

Effects of Overdosage: Marked drowsiness, weakness, feeling of drunkenness, staggering gait, tremor, stupor progressing to deep sleep or coma.

Possible Effects of Long-Term Use: Psychological and/or physical dependence.

Suggested Periodic Examinations While Taking This Drug (at physician's discretion)

None.

▷ **While Taking This Drug, Observe the Following**

Foods: No restrictions.

Beverages: Avoid excessive intake of caffeine-containing beverages (coffee, tea, cola) within 4 hours of taking this drug. May be taken with milk.

▷ *Alcohol:* It is advisable to avoid alcohol completely.

Tobacco Smoking: Heavy smoking may reduce the hypnotic action of this drug.

Marijuana Smoking: Increased sedation and significant impairment of intellectual and physical performance.

▷ *Other Drugs*

Quazepam may ***increase*** the effects of
- digoxin (Lanoxin), and cause digoxin toxicity.
- phenytoin (Dilantin), and cause phenytoin toxicity.

Quazepam may ***decrease*** the effects of
- levodopa (Sinemet, etc.), and reduce its effectiveness in treating Parkinson's disease.

The following drugs may ***increase*** the effects of quazepam
- any drug with central nervous system (CNS) depressant action (see Drug Classes for benzodiazepines, opioids, tricyclic antidepressants and phenothiazines among others).
- cimetidine (Tagamet).
- clindamycin (Cleocin) may enhance neuromuscular blockade.
- disulfiram (Antabuse).
- isoniazid (INH, Rifamate, etc.).
- MAO inhibitors (see Drug Classes).
- omeprazole (Prilosec) by inhibiting (removal) metabolism of quazepam.
- oral contraceptives.
- valproic acid (Depakene).

The following drugs may *decrease* the effects of quazepam
- rifampin (Rimactane, etc.).
- theophylline (aminophylline, Theo-Dur, etc.).

▷ *Driving, Hazardous Activities:* This drug may impair mental alertness, judgment, physical coordination and reaction time. Avoid hazardous activities accordingly.

Aviation Note: The use of this drug *is a disqualification* for piloting. Consult a designated Aviation Medical Examiner.

Exposure to Sun: No restrictions.

Exposure to Heat: Use caution until the effect of excessive perspiration is determined. Because of reduced urine volume, this drug may accumulate in the body and produce effects of overdosage.

Discontinuation: Do **not** stop this drug abruptly if this drug has been taken for over 4 weeks without interruption. Dosage should be tapered gradually to prevent a withdrawal syndrome that could include depression, confusion, hallucinations, tremor, seizures, muscle cramping, sweating and vomiting.

QUINACRINE (KWIN a kreen)

Other Name: Mepacrine

Introduced: 1967   **Prescription:** USA: Yes; Canada: No   **Available as Generic:** USA: No; Canada: No   **Class:** Anti-infective   **Controlled Drug:** USA: No; Canada: No

Brand Name: Atabrine

BENEFITS versus RISKS	
Possible Benefits	*Possible Risks*
HIGHLY EFFECTIVE TREATMENT FOR GIARDIASIS	Infrequent adverse behavioral effects: irritability, mood changes, hallucinations, psychotic thinking
Effective treatment for mild to moderate discoid lupus erythematosus	Yellow discoloration of skin
	Rare hepatitis
	Rare corneal and retinal changes, hepatitis, aplastic anemia with high dose and/or long-term use

Author's note: This medicine is derived from a natural source which is no longer available to the manufacturer. While a secondary source is being attempted to be identified, several years has gone by without success. This profile will be suspended to make room for other medicines which are currently available.

QUINAPRIL (KWIN a pril)

Introduced: 1984   **Prescription:** USA: Yes   **Available as Generic:** No   **Class:** Antihypertensive, ACE inhibitor   **Controlled Drug:** USA: No

Brand Name: Accupril

BENEFITS versus RISKS	
Possible Benefits	*Possible Risks*
EFFECTIVE CONTROL OF MILD TO MODERATE HIGH BLOOD PRESSURE	Low blood pressure (rare)
	Low white blood cell counts (rare)
	Allergic swelling of face, tongue, throat, vocal cords (very rare)

▷ **Principal Uses**

As a Single Drug Product: Uses currently included in FDA approved labeling: (1) Treats mild to moderate high blood pressure, either alone or combined with a thiazide diuretic; (2) treats symptoms of congestive heart failure.

Other (unlabeled) generally accepted uses: (1) Improves survival in patients with congestive heart failure; (2) may improve survival in patients with atherosclerosis; (3) other medicines from this class have helped decrease the number of deaths and the severity of ongoing heart compromise.

How This Drug Works: By blocking certain enzyme systems (angiotensin-converting enzyme, ACE) that influence arterial function, this drug helps relax arterial walls and lowers resistance to blood flow that causes high blood pressure. This, in turn, reduces the work load of the heart and improves its performance.

Available Dosage Forms and Strengths

Tablets — 5 mg, 10 mg, 20 mg, 40 mg

▷ **Recommended Dosage Ranges** (Actual dosage and administration schedule must be determined by the physician for each patient individually.)

Infants and Children: Dosage not established.

12 to 60 Years of Age: Initially 10 mg once daily for those not taking a diuretic; 5 mg once daily for those taking a diuretic. Usual maintenance dose is 20 to 40 mg/day taken in a single dose. If once-a-day dosing does not give stable control of blood pressure over a 24 hour period, divide the dose equally into morning and evening doses. The total daily dosage should not exceed 80 mg.

Over 60 Years of Age: Same as 12 to 60 years of age, if kidney function is normal. If kidney function is significantly impaired, reduce dose by 50%. The total daily dose should not exceed 40 mg.

Conditions Requiring Dosing Adjustments

Liver function: Decreases in dose are not needed.

Kidney function: Patients with mild kidney failure can be given 10 mg daily. Those with moderate kidney failure should be given 5 mg daily. In severe kidney failure, 2.5 mg per day may be given. If needed and tolerated, dose increases should only be made every two weeks.

▷ **Dosing Instructions:**   The tablet may be crushed and taken on an empty stomach or with food, at same time each day.

Usual Duration of Use: Use on a regular schedule for 2 to 3 weeks usually determines effectiveness in controlling high blood pressure. The proper treatment of high blood pressure usually requires the long-term use of effective medications. Consult your physician on a regular basis.

Possible Advantages of This Drug
Usually controls blood pressure effectively with one daily dose.
Relatively low incidence of adverse effects.
No adverse influence on asthma, cholesterol blood levels or diabetes.
Sudden withdrawal does not result in a rapid increase in blood pressure.

▷ **This Drug Should Not Be Taken If**
- you have had an allergic reaction to it previously.
- you are pregnant (last 6 months).
- you have experienced swelling of the face (angioedema) from this or other ACE inhibitors.
- you have an abnormally high level of blood potassium.

▷ **Inform Your Physician Before Taking This Drug If**
- you have had an allergic reaction (or other adverse effect) on using any other ACE inhibitor drug (see Drug Classes).
- you currently have a blood cell or bone marrow disorder.
- you are planning pregnancy or are breast feeding your infant.
- you have a history of kidney disease or impaired kidney function.
- you have severe liver disease.
- you are immunosuppressed or are taking an immunosuppressant medicine.
- you are taking potassium supplements or have an elevated blood potassium.
- you have a low white blood cell count.
- you have scleroderma or systemic lupus erythematosus.
- you have cerebral artery disease.
- you have any form of heart disease.
- you are taking any of the following drugs: other antihypertensives, diuretics, nitrates or potassium supplements.
- you plan to have surgery under general anesthesia in the near future.

Possible Side Effects (natural, expected, and unavoidable drug actions)
Dizziness, orthostatic hypotension (rare) (see Glossary), fainting (rare), increased blood potassium level (rare).

▷ **Possible Adverse Effects** (unusual, unexpected, and infrequent reactions)
If any of the following develop, consult your physician promptly for guidance.

Mild Adverse Effects
Allergic Reactions: Skin rash, itching (rare).
Headache, fatigue, drowsiness (rare), numbness and tingling (rare), weakness (rare).
Taste disorders (rare).
Cough (rare), chest pain, muscle pain, palpitation (rare).
Indigestion, nausea/vomiting (rare), constipation (rare).

Serious Adverse Effects
Allergic Reactions: Swelling (angioedema) of face, tongue, and/or vocal cords (rare); can be life-threatening.
Impairment of kidney function (rare).
Blood cell problems have occurred with other ACE inhibitors, and caution should be used here.

Low blood pressure and fainting.
Increased blood potassium.

▷ **Possible Effects on Sexual Function:**   Swelling and tenderness of male breast tissue (gynecomastia).

Possible Effects on Laboratory Tests
Complete blood cell counts: decreased white cells and platelets.
Blood potassium level: increased.
Liver function tests: increased liver enzymes (ALT/GPT, AST/GOT and alkaline phosphatase).
Kidney function tests: increased blood urea nitrogen (BUN) and creatinine.

CAUTION
1. Ask your doctor if other antihypertensive drugs (especially diuretics) should be stopped for 1 week before starting this drug.
2. **Inform your physician immediately if you become pregnant.** This drug should not be taken beyond the first 3 months of pregnancy.
3. **Report promptly** any indications of infection (fever, sore throat), and any indications of water retention (weight gain, puffiness, swollen feet or ankles).
4. Do not use a salt substitute without your physician's knowledge and approval. (Many salt substitutes contain potassium.)
5. Blood cell counts and urine analyses should be checked **before** starting this drug.

Precautions for Use
By Infants and Children: Safety and effectiveness for those in this age group not established.
By Those over 60 Years of Age: Small starting doses are indicated. Sudden and excessive lowering of blood pressure can predispose to stroke or heart attack in those with impaired brain circulation or coronary artery heart disease.

▷ **Advisability of Use During Pregnancy**
Pregnancy Category: C during the first three months (trimester). D in the last six months of pregnancy. See Pregnancy Codes at the back of this book.
Animal studies: No information available.
Human studies: The use of ACE inhibitor drugs during the last 6 months of pregnancy is known to possibly cause very serious injury and possible death to the fetus; skull and limb malformations, lung defects, and kidney failure have been reported in over 50 cases worldwide.
Avoid this drug completely during the last 6 months. During the first 3 months of pregnancy, use this drug only if clearly needed. Ask your physician for guidance.

Advisability of Use if Breast-Feeding
Presence of this drug in breast milk: Unknown.
Avoid drug or refrain from nursing.

Habit-Forming Potential: None.

Effects of Overdosage: Excessive drop in blood pressure, light-headedness, dizziness, fainting.

Possible Effects of Long-Term Use: Gradual increase in blood potassium level.

Suggested Periodic Examinations While Taking This Drug (at physician's discretion)

Before starting drug: Complete blood cell counts; urine analysis with measurement of protein content; blood potassium level.

During use of drug: Blood cell counts; measurements of blood potassium.

▷ **While Taking This Drug, Observe the Following**

Foods: Consult physician regarding salt intake.

Nutritional Support:

Do not take potassium supplements unless directed by your physician.

Beverages: No restrictions. May be taken with milk.

▷ *Alcohol:* Use caution until combined effect has been determined. Alcohol may enhance the blood-pressure-lowering effect of this drug.

Tobacco Smoking: No interactions expected.

▷ *Other Drugs*

Quinapril *taken concurrently* with

- aspirin or other NSAIDs (see Drug Class) may block prostaglandin synthesis and blunt the therapeutic benefit of quinapril.
- cyclosporine (Sandimmune) may cause increased kidney toxicity.
- furosemide (Lasix) or bumetanide (Bumex) may cause decreased blood pressure on standing (postural hypotension).
- lithium (Lithobid, others) can cause increased lithium blood levels and toxicity; monitor lithium blood levels and adjust dosage as necessary.
- potassium preparations (K-Lyte, Slow-K, etc.) may cause increased blood levels of potassium with risk of serious heart rhythm disturbances.
- potassium-sparing diuretics: amiloride (Moduretic), spironolactone (Aldactazide), triamterene (Dyazide) may cause increased blood levels of potassium with risk of serious heart rhythm disturbances.

▷ *Driving, Hazardous Activities:* Usually no restrictions. Be aware of possible drops in blood pressure with resultant dizziness or faintness.

Aviation Note: The use of this drug *may be a disqualification* for piloting. Consult a designated Aviation Medical Examiner.

Exposure to Sun: Caution advised. A similar drug of this class can cause photosensitivity.

Exposure to Heat: Caution advised. Avoid excessive perspiring with resultant loss of body water and drop in blood pressure.

Occurrence of Unrelated Illness: Report promptly any disorder that causes nausea, vomiting or diarrhea. Fluid and chemical imbalances must be corrected as soon as possible.

Discontinuation: This drug may be stopped abruptly without causing a sudden increase in blood pressure. However, you should consult your physician regarding withdrawal of this drug for any reason.

QUINIDINE (KWIN i deen)

Introduced: 1918   **Prescription:** USA: Yes; Canada: No   **Available as Generic:** Yes   **Class:** Antiarrhythmic   **Controlled Drug:** USA: No; Canada: No

Brand Names: ✦Apo-Quinidine, ✦Biquin Durules, Cardioquin, Cin-Quin, Dura-quin, ✦Natisedine, ✦Novoquinidine, Quinaglute Dura-Tabs, ✦Quinate, Quinatime, Quinidex Extentabs, ✦Quinobarb [CD]*, Quinora, Quin-Release, SK-Quinidine sulfate

---

BENEFITS versus RISKS

Possible Benefits	*Possible Risks*
EFFECTIVE TREATMENT OF SELECTED HEART RHYTHM DISORDERS	NARROW TREATMENT RANGE FREQUENT ADVERSE EFFECTS NUMEROUS ALLERGIC AND IDIOSYNCRATIC REACTIONS Dose-related toxicity Provocation of abnormal heart rhythms Abnormally low blood platelet count (rare) Hemolytic anemia (rare) Kidney and liver toxicity (rare)

▷ **Principal Uses**

As a Single Drug Product: Uses currently included in FDA approved labeling: (1) Helps control the following types of abnormal heart rhythm: atrial fibrillation and flutter, paroxysmal atrial tachycardia, paroxysmal ventricular tachycardia, premature atrial and ventricular contractions; (2) intravenous treatment of malaria in people who can not take medicine by mouth.

Other (unlabeled) generally accepted uses: None.

As a Combination Drug Product [CD]: (1) This drug is available (in Canada) in combination with a barbiturate, a mild sedative that is added to allay the anxiety and nervous tension that often accompany heart rhythm disorders.

How This Drug Works: By slowing the activity of the pacemaker and delaying transmission of electrical impulses through the conduction system and muscle of the heart, this drug assists in restoring normal heart rate and rhythm.

Available Dosage Forms and Strengths

Capsules — 200 mg, 300 mg
Injections — 80 mg, 200 mg per ml
Tablets — 100 mg, 200 mg, 275 mg, 300 mg
Tablets, prolonged-action — 250 mg, 300 mg, 324 mg, 330 mg

▷ **Usual Adult Dosage Range:** Dose varies with indication—premature atrial or ventricular contractions: 200 to 400 mg every 4 to 6 hours.

Paroxysmal atrial tachycardia: 400 to 600 mg/2 to 3 hours until paroxysm is terminated.

Atrial flutter: digitalize first; then individualize dosage schedule as appropriate.

Atrial fibrillation: digitalize first; then try 200 mg/2 to 3 hours for 5 to 8 doses; increase dose daily until normal rhythm is restored or toxic effects develop.

Maintenance schedule: 200 to 300 mg 3 or 4 times/day. The total daily dosage should not exceed 4000 mg.

---

*Quinobarb contains phenylethylbarbiturate, a sedative of the barbiturate class.

Note: Actual dosage and administration schedule must be determined by the physician for each patient individually.

Conditions Requiring Dosing Adjustments

Liver function: This drug is extensively metabolized in the liver. Blood levels should be obtained to guide dosing. A larger loading dose and a 50% decreased maintenance dose may be indicated.

Kidney function: Blood levels should be obtained, and used to guide dosing. Quinidine should be used with caution in renal compromise.

▷ **Dosing Instructions:** Preferably taken on an empty stomach to achieve high blood levels rapidly. However, it may be taken with or following food to reduce stomach irritation. The regular tablets may be crushed and the capsules opened for administration. The prolonged-action forms should be swallowed whole without alteration.

Usual Duration of Use: Use on a regular schedule for 2 to 4 days usually determines effectiveness in correcting or preventing responsive abnormal rhythms. Long-term use (months to years) requires physician supervision and periodic evaluation.

▷ **This Drug Should Not Be Taken If**
- you have had an allergic or idiosyncratic reaction to it previously.
- you currently have an acute infection of any kind.
- you have taken too much digoxin (digoxin toxicity).
- you have myasthenia gravis.
- you have abnormal heart rhythms caused by an escape mechanism (ask your specialist).

▷ **Inform Your Physician Before Taking This Drug If**
- you have coronary artery disease or myasthenia gravis.
- you have a history of excessive thyroid function (hyperthyroidism).
- you usually have a very low blood pressure.
- you have had a deficiency of blood platelets in the past from any cause.
- you are now taking, or have taken recently, any digitalis preparation (digitoxin, digoxin, etc.).
- you plan to have surgery under general anesthesia in the near future.
- you have acute rheumatic fever or subacute bacterial endocarditis (SBE).

Possible Side Effects (natural, expected, and unavoidable drug actions)

Drop in blood pressure, may be marked in some patients.

▷ **Possible Adverse Effects** (unusual, unexpected, and infrequent reactions)

If any of the following develop, consult your physician promptly for guidance.

Mild Adverse Effects

Allergic Reactions: Skin rash, hives, itching, drug fever (rare).

Dose-related toxicity (cinchonism): blurred vision, ringing in the ears, loss of hearing, dizziness.

Joint pain.

Irritation of the esophagus (esophagitis).

Nausea, vomiting, diarrhea.

Serious Adverse Effects

Allergic Reactions: Severe skin reactions, hemolytic anemia (see Glossary), joint and muscle pains, anaphylactic reaction (see Glossary), reduced blood platelet count, drug-induced hepatitis (see Glossary).

Idiosyncratic Reactions: Skin rash, rapid heart rate, acute delirium and combative behavior, difficult breathing.

Psychosis (rare).

Drug-induced myasthenia gravis (rare).

Swelling of the lymph glands in the inguinal area (lymphadenopathy).

Kidney toxicity (rare).

Systemic lupus erythematosus (SLE) (rare).

Carpal tunnel syndrome (very rare).

Very low blood pressure, fainting (syncope).

Heart conduction abnormalities.

Optic neuritis, impaired vision.

Abnormally low white blood cell count: fever, sore throat, infections.

▷ **Possible Effects on Sexual Function:**   None reported.

▷ **Adverse Effects That May Mimic Natural Diseases or Disorders**

Drug-induced hepatitis may suggest viral hepatitis.

Natural Diseases or Disorders That May Be Activated by This Drug

Systemic lupus erythematosus, myasthenia gravis, psoriasis (in sensitive individuals).

Possible Effects on Laboratory Tests

Complete blood cell counts: decreased red cells, hemoglobin, white cells and platelets; increased eosinophils (allergic reaction); marked increase of white blood cells in association with "quinidine fever" (very rare).

Antinuclear antibodies (ANA): positive.

Prothrombin time: increased (when taken concurrently with warfarin).

Liver function tests: increased liver enzymes (ALT/GPT, AST/GOT and alkaline phosphatase), increased bilirubin.

CAUTION

1. Wide variation in response from person to person. Dosage adjustments must be based upon individual reaction. Notify your physician of any events that you suspect may be drug related.
2. It is advisable to carry a card of personal identification that includes a notation that you are taking this drug.

Precautions for Use

By Infants and Children: A test for drug idiosyncrasy should be made before starting treatment with this drug. If there is no beneficial response after 3 days of adequate dosage, this drug should be discontinued.

By Those over 60 Years of Age: Small doses are mandatory until your individual response has been determined. Observe for the development of light-headedness, dizziness, weakness or sense of impending faint. Use caution to prevent falls.

▷ **Advisability of Use During Pregnancy**

Pregnancy Category: C. See Pregnancy Code at the back of this book.

Animal studies: No information available.

Human studies: Adequate studies of pregnant women are not available. No birth defects have been reported following use of this drug during pregnancy.

Use this drug only if clearly needed.

Advisability of Use if Breast-Feeding

Presence of this drug in breast milk: Yes.

Avoid drug or refrain from nursing.

Habit-Forming Potential: None.

Effects of Overdosage: Nausea, vomiting, ringing in the ears, headache, jerky eye movements, double vision, altered color vision, confusion, delirium, hot skin, seizures, coma.

Possible Effects of Long-Term Use: None reported.

Suggested Periodic Examinations While Taking This Drug (at physician's discretion)
Complete blood cell counts, electrocardiograms, blood levels.

▷ **While Taking This Drug, Observe the Following**
   Foods: No restrictions.
   Beverages: No restrictions. May be taken with milk.
▷   *Alcohol:* Use caution. Alcohol may enhance the blood-pressure-lowering effects of this drug.
   Tobacco Smoking: Nicotine can increase irritability of the heart and aggravate rhythm disorders. Avoid all forms of tobacco.
▷   *Other Drugs*
   Quinapril *taken concurrently* with
   • aspirin may prolong the bleeding time.
   • beta blockers may result in additive and undesirable beta blockade. Lower starting doses may be needed for both medicines.
   • codeine may blunt the effectiveness of codeine.
   • tricyclic antidepressants (see Drug Classes) may result in antidepressant toxicity.
   • venlafaxine (Effexor) may result in venlafaxine toxicity.
   Quinidine may *increase* the effects of
   • anticoagulants (Coumadin, etc.), and increase the risk of bleeding. More frequent INR (protime) testing is needed.
   • digitoxin and digoxin (Lanoxin), and cause digitalis toxicity.
   • disopyramide (Norpace).
   • tricyclic antidepressants (doxepin).
   • warfarin (Coumadin) and result in bleeding. More frequent testing of INR (protime) is needed.
   The following drugs may *increase* the effects of quinidine
   • amiodarone (Codarone).
   • cimetidine (Tagamet).
   • ketoconazole (Nizoral).
   • verapamil (Verelan).
   The following drugs may *decrease* the effects of quinidine
   • barbiturates (phenobarbital, etc.).
   • phenytoin (Dilantin).
   • rifampin (Rifadin, Rimactane).
   • sucralfate (Carafate).
▷   *Driving, Hazardous Activities:* This drug may cause dizziness and alter vision. Restrict activities as necessary.
   Aviation Note: The use of this drug *may be a disqualification* for piloting. Consult a designated Aviation Medical Examiner.
   Exposure to Sun: Use caution. This drug may cause photosensitivity (See Glossary).

RAMIPRIL (ra MI pril)

Introduced: 1985   **Prescription:** USA: Yes   **Available as Generic:**
No   **Class:** Antihypertensive, ACE inhibitor   **Controlled Drug:** USA: No
Brand Name: Altace

BENEFITS versus RISKS	
Possible Benefits	*Possible Risks*
EFFECTIVE CONTROL OF MILD TO SEVERE HIGH BLOOD PRESSURE	Low blood pressure
	Allergic swelling of face, tongue, or vocal cords (rare)

▷ **Principal Uses**

As a Single Drug Product

Uses currently included in FDA approved labeling: (1) Treats all degrees of high blood pressure, alone or concurrently with thiazide-type diuretics. Mild to moderate high blood pressure usually responds to low doses; severe high blood pressure may require higher doses, with greater risk of serious adverse effects; (2) helps decrease the size of the left ventricle and control blood pressure in people with left ventricular hypertrophy; (3) helps control blood pressure caused by abnormalities (stenosis) in the renal artery; (4) used in patients with atherosclerosis to help prevent heart attacks, angina and need for surgery; (5) used after heart attacks to help prevent death, a second heart attack and undesirable compromises from the first heart attack.

Other (unlabeled) generally accepted uses: (1) Helps improve survival in patients with congestive heart failure.

How This Drug Works: By blocking enzyme systems that influence arterial function, this drug helps relax arterial walls and lower resistance to blood flow that causes high blood pressure. This, in turn, reduces the work load of the heart and improves its performance.

Available Dosage Forms and Strengths

Capsules — 1.25 mg, 2.5 mg, 5 mg, 10 mg

▷ **Usual Adult Dosage Range:**   Initially 2.5 mg once daily for 2 to 4 weeks. Usual maintenance dose is 2.5 to 20 mg/day in a single dose or in 2 divided doses. If taking diuretics: Either discontinue the diuretic for 3 days before initiating this drug, or begin treatment with 1.25 mg of this drug. Total daily dose should not exceed 5 mg if kidney function is significantly impaired. **Note: Actual dosage and administration schedule must be determined by the physician for each patient individually.**

Conditions Requiring Dosing Adjustments

Liver function: Patients should be followed closely if they have compromised livers. No specific dosage recommendations are available.

Kidney function: Patients with moderate kidney failure or creatinine values of greater than 2.5, a dose of 1.25 mg of ramipril can be used daily.

▷ **Dosing Instructions:**   Take on an empty stomach or with food, at same time each day. The capsule may be opened for administration.

Usual Duration of Use: Use on a regular schedule for 2 to 4 weeks usually determines effectiveness in controlling high blood pressure. The proper treatment of high blood pressure usually requires the long-term use of effective medications. Consult your physician on a regular basis.

▷ **This Drug Should Not Be Taken If**
- you have had an allergic reaction to it previously.
- you are pregnant (last 6 months).
- you have a history of angioedema (a serious allergic reaction) from any cause.
- you have active liver disease.
- you have an abnormally high level of blood potassium.

▷ **Inform Your Physician Before Taking This Drug If**
- you have had an unfavorable reaction to angiotensin-converting enzyme (ACE) inhibitor drugs previously: captopril (Capoten), enalapril (Vasotec), lisinopril (Prinivil, Zestril), others (see Drug Classes).
- you are pregnant (first 3 months), planning pregnancy, or breast-feeding.
- you have impaired liver or kidney function.
- you have scleroderma or systemic lupus erythematosus.
- you have any form of heart disease.
- you have diabetes.
- you take: other antihypertensives, diuretics, nitrates or potassium supplements.
- you have abnormal kidney circulation (ask your doctor).
- you take immunosuppressant therapy or have an autoimmune disease.
- you have an abnormally elevated blood potassium level or take a potassium sparing diuretic.
- you have a condition which causes increased temperature.
- you have had low white blood cell counts.
- you plan to have surgery under general anesthesia in the near future.

Possible Side Effects (natural, expected, and unavoidable drug actions)
Dizziness, light-headedness (rare).

▷ **Possible Adverse Effects** (unusual, unexpected, and infrequent reactions)
If any of the following develop, consult your physician promptly for guidance.
Mild Adverse Effects
Allergic Reactions: Skin rash, itching.
Headache, fatigue (rare), drowsiness, nervousness, numbness and tingling, insomnia.
Chest pain, palpitation, drug-induced cough.
Indigestion, stomach pain, nausea (rare), vomiting, diarrhea.
Excessive sweating, joint and muscle aches.
Serious Adverse Effects
Allergic Reactions: Swelling (angioedema) of face, tongue, and/or vocal cords: can be life-threatening (rare).
Profound lowering of the blood pressure.
Liver toxicity (rare).
Increased blood potassium.
Pancreatitis (reported with other ACE inhibitors) (rare).
Abnormally decreased blood sodium.

▷ **Possible Effects on Sexual Function:**   Rare reports of impotence (0.4%). Swelling and tenderness of male breast tissue (gynecomastia) (rare).

Possible Effects on Laboratory Tests

Complete blood cell counts: decreased red cells and hemoglobin (0.4% using this drug alone; 1.5% using this drug and a diuretic); decreased white cells, increased eosinophils (both rare).

Blood potassium level: increased (1%).

Liver function tests: increased liver enzymes (ALT/GPT, AST/GOT and alkaline phosphatase), increased bilirubin.

Kidney function tests: increased blood urea nitrogen (BUN) (0.5% using this drug alone; 3% using this drug and a diuretic); increased creatinine (1.2% using this drug alone; 1.5% using this drug and a diuretic).

Increased erythrocyte sedimentation rate.

Uric acid: increased.

Blood sodium level: decreased.

CAUTION

1. Ask your doctor if other antihypertensive drugs (especially diuretics) should be stopped for 1 week before starting this drug.
2. **Report promptly** any indications of infection (fever, sore throat), and any indications of water retention (weight gain, puffiness, swollen feet or ankles).
3. Do not use a salt substitute without your physician's knowledge and approval. (Many salt substitutes contain potassium.)
4. It is advisable to obtain blood cell counts and urine analyses **before** starting this drug.
5. **Notify your physician immediately if pregnancy occurs.** This drug should not be taken beyond the first 3 months of pregnancy.

Precautions for Use

By Infants and Children: Safety and effectiveness for use by those in this age group have not been established.

By Those over 60 Years of Age: Small doses are advisable until tolerance has been determined. Sudden and excessive lowering of blood pressure can predispose to stroke or heart attack in those with impaired brain circulation or coronary artery heart disease.

▷ Advisability of Use During Pregnancy

Pregnancy Category: C during the first three months. D during the last six months. See Pregnancy Code at the back of this book.

Animal studies: Fetal kidney defects found in rat studies; retarded growth found in mouse studies.

Human studies: Adequate studies of pregnant women are not available. However, drugs of this class taken during the last 6 months of pregnancy have been reported to cause serious fetal defects: skull and facial malformations, limb deformities, lung defects and kidney failure (over 50 cases reported worldwide).

Avoid this drug completely during the last 6 months. During the first 3 months of pregnancy, use this drug only if clearly needed. Ask your physician for guidance.

Advisability of Use if Breast-Feeding

Presence of this drug in breast milk: Yes.

Avoid drug or refrain from nursing.

Habit-Forming Potential: None.

Effects of Overdosage: Excessive drop in blood pressure—light-headedness, dizziness, fainting.

Possible Effects of Long-Term Use: Gradual increase in blood potassium level.

Suggested Periodic Examinations While Taking This Drug (at physician's discretion)

Before starting drug: Complete blood cell counts; urine analysis with measurement of protein content; blood potassium level.

During use of drug: Blood cell counts; measurements of blood potassium.

▷ **While Taking This Drug, Observe the Following**

Foods: Consult physician regarding salt intake.

*Nutritional Support: **Do not take*** potassium supplements unless directed by your physician.

Beverages: No restrictions. May be taken with milk.

▷ *Alcohol:* Use caution until combined effect has been determined. Alcohol may enhance the blood-pressure-lowering effect of this drug.

Tobacco Smoking: No interactions expected.

▷ *Other Drugs*

Ramipril ***taken concurrently*** with

- aspirin or other NSAIDs (see Drug Classes) may blunt the blood pressure lowering response.
- cyclosporine (Sandimmune) may pose increased risk of kidney toxicity.
- lithium (Lithane, Lithotab, etc.) may cause increased blood lithium levels and symptoms of lithium toxicity. Monitor lithium levels closely.
- loop diuretics such as furosemide (Lasix) or bumetanide (Bumex) may cause severe postural hypotension (see Glossary).
- phenothiazines (see Drug Classes) have been reported to cause hypotension with other ACE inhibitors. Caution is advised.
- potassium preparations (K-Lyte, Slow-K, etc.) may cause increased blood levels of potassium with risk of serious heart rhythm disturbances.
- potassium-sparing diuretics: amiloride (Moduretic), spironolactone (Aldactazide), triamterene (Dyazide) may cause increased blood levels of potassium with risk of serious heart rhythm disturbances.

▷ *Driving, Hazardous Activities:* Usually no restrictions. Be aware of possible drops in blood pressure with resultant dizziness or faintness.

Aviation Note: The use of this drug ***may be a disqualification*** for piloting. Consult a designated Aviation Medical Examiner.

Exposure to Sun: Caution advised. A similar drug of this class can cause photosensitivity.

Exposure to Heat: Caution advised. Avoid excessive perspiring with resultant loss of body water and drop in blood pressure.

Occurrence of Unrelated Illness: Nausea, vomiting or diarrhea may cause fluid and chemical imbalances that must be corrected as soon as possible.

RANITIDINE (ra NI te deen)

Introduced: 1981   **Prescription:** USA: Yes; Canada: Yes   **Available as Generic:** Yes   **Class:** H-2 receptor blocker   **Controlled Drug:** USA: No; Canada: No

Brand Name: Zantac, Zantac 75 (nonprescription form), ♣Zantac-C, ♣Apo-Ranitidine, ♣Novo-Ranitidine, ♣Nu-Ranit

Warning: The brand names Zantac and Xanax are similar and can be mistaken for each other; this can lead to serious medication errors. These names represent very different drugs. Zantac is the generic drug ranitidine; it is used to treat peptic ulcer disease. Xanax is the generic drug alprazolam; it is a mild tranquilizer. Verify that you are taking the correct drug.

BENEFITS versus RISKS	
Possible Benefits	**Possible Risks**
EFFECTIVE TREATMENT OF PEPTIC ULCER DISEASE: relief of symptoms, acceleration of healing, prevention of recurrence	Drug-induced hepatitis (rare)
	Confusion (in severely ill elderly patients)
CONTROL OF HYPERSECRETORY STOMACH DISORDERS	Rare blood cell disorders
	Rare pancreatitis
Beneficial in treatment of reflux esophagitis	Rare liver toxicity

Author's note: ALL of the four available H2 receptor blocking drugs are now available without prescription.

Please see the new histamine (H2) blocking drug profile for further information.

RIFABUTIN (RIF a byu tin)

Introduced: 1993   **Prescription:** USA: Yes; Canada: No   **Available as Generic:** USA: No; Canada: No   **Class:** antimycobacterial agent (antitubercular)   **Controlled Drug:** USA: No; Canada: No

Brand Name: Mycobutin

Warning: Rifabutin prophylaxis must not be given to people with active tuberculosis.

BENEFITS versus RISKS	
Possible Benefits	**Possible Risks**
PREVENTION OF DISSEMINATED MYCOBACTERIUM AVIUM COMPLEX (MAC) IN PEOPLE WITH ADVANCED HIV INFECTION	NEUTROPENIA
	Rare low white blood cell counts
	Rare low platelet counts

▷ **Principal Uses**

As a Single Drug Product: Uses currently included in FDA approved labeling: (1) Prevention of disseminated Mycobacterium avium complex (MAC) in patients with advanced HIV infection; (2) combination treatment of MAI infection.

Other (unlabeled) generally accepted use: None.

How This Drug Works: Rifabutin inhibits DNA-dependent RNA polymerase (an enzyme critical to cells that are dividing) in E. coli. The exact mechanism of action of rifabutin in Mycobacterium avium or Mycobacterium intracellulare is not known.

Available Dosage Forms and Strengths

Rifabutin (Mycobutin) capsules — 150 mg

How To Store

Keep at room temperature and avoid exposure to excessive humidity.

▷ **Recommended Dosage Ranges (Actual dosage and administration schedule must be determined by the physician for each patient individually.)**

Infants and Children: Safety and effectiveness of rifabutin in MAC prophylaxis has not clearly been established. Safety data comes from a trial of 22 children who were HIV positive:

Infants one year of age—18.5 mg/kg/day.

Children 2–10 years—8.6 mg/kg/day.

Adolescents 14 years—4.0 mg/kg/day.

14 to 60 Years of Age: 300 mg once a day. People who are prone to nausea and vomiting may take 150 mg 2 times a day with food.

Over 60 Years of Age: Same as 12 to 60 years of age.

Conditions Requiring Dosing Adjustments

Liver function: At present, clear adjustments of dose in hepatic compromise are not defined, but the drug should be used with caution.

Kidney function: Elimination of rifabutin may actually be increased in people with compromised kidneys, yet the clinical effect is as yet unknown.

▷ **Dosing Instructions:** May be taken with food if you are prone to nausea and vomiting. May be mixed with foods such as applesauce for use in children.

Usual Duration of Use:

Use on a regular schedule indefinitely is usually needed to assure this drug's effectiveness in prophylaxis of disseminated MAC. Long-term use (months to years) requires periodic physician evaluation of response.

If rifabutin is being used as a part of combination therapy of a Mycobacterium avium intracellulare infection, the ideal duration of treatment has not been identified, but treatment is usually ongoing.

Possible Advantages of This Drug

Oral treatment of very resistant organisms.

Currently a "Drug of Choice"

for prophylaxis (prevention) of disseminated MAC.

▷ **This Drug Should Not Be Taken If**

- you have had an allergic reaction to any dosage form of it previously.
- you have active tuberculosis (combination therapy with several medications is indicated).

▷ **Inform Your Physician Before Taking This Drug If**

- you are pregnant or plan to become pregnant.
- you are taking an oral contraceptive (a nonhormonal alternative method is advised).

- you have a history of blood disorders.
- you are taking an anticoagulant such as coumadin.
- you take other prescription or nonprescription medicines which were not discussed with your doctor when this medicine was prescribed.
- you are uncertain of how much to take or how often to take rifabutin.

Possible Side Effects (natural, expected, and unavoidable drug actions)

This medication may color saliva, urine, feces, sputum, perspiration, tears, and skin a brown-orange color. Soft contact lenses may become permanently stained by rifabutin or its metabolites.

Emergence of resistant Mycobacterium tuberculosis.

▷ **Possible Adverse Effects** (unusual, unexpected, and infrequent reactions)

If any of the following develop, consult your physician promptly for guidance.

Mild Adverse Effects

Allergic Reactions: Skin rash, fever.

Change in taste perceptions; headache; loss of appetite; gastrointestinal upset; nausea, vomiting, and diarrhea; muscle aches, joint pains, and a flu-like syndrome.

Taste disorders.

Serious Adverse Effects

Very rare confusion and aphasia and seizures; chest pain with dyspnea (trouble breathing); nonspecific T wave changes (a change in the way the heart beats).

Neutropenia (rare).

Rare leukopenia, anemia, and lowered blood platelets (thrombocytopenia).

▷ **Possible Effects on Sexual Function:**   Potential alteration of pattern and timing of menstruation.

Decreased effectiveness of oral contraceptives taken together with this drug.

▷ **Adverse Effects That May Mimic Natural Diseases or Disorders**

Liver reactions similar to viral hepatitis.

Possible Effects on Laboratory Tests

Complete blood cell counts: neutropenia (decreases in a specific kind of white blood cells), thrombocytopenia (decreased platelets), anemia, leukopenia (decreased white blood cells).

Coagulation (clotting tests), decreased prothrombin time (when taken at the same time as coumadin).

Liver enzymes (alkaline phosphatase, SGOT and SGPT) can be increased.

CAUTION

1. The effectiveness of oral contraceptives may be decreased.
2. May hasten the development of resistant Mycobacterium tuberculosis if used as monotherapy (as a single drug).
3. Urine, feces, saliva, sputum, sweat, tears and skin may be colored brown-orange with rifabutin and some of its metabolites. Soft contact lenses may be permanently stained.

Precautions for Use

By Infants and Children: Safety and effectiveness for use in children has not been established.

By Those over 60 Years of Age: Specific precautions have not yet been developed, however since the drug is similar to rifampin, those over 60 may be more sensitive to the adverse effects of rifabutin.

▷ **Advisability of Use During Pregnancy**
  Pregnancy Category: B. See Pregnancy Code at the back of this book.
    Animal studies: At doses equal to 8 times the usual human dose, rifabutin
      caused an increase in skeletal variants in rats. Doses of 16 times the usual
      human dose caused maternotoxicity and fetal skeletal anomalies in rabbits.
    Human studies: Adequate studies of pregnant women are not available.
    Ask your physician for guidance.

Advisability of Use if Breast-Feeding
    Presence of this drug in breast milk: It is not known whether rifabutin is
      excreted in breast milk.
    A decision should be made to avoid drug or refrain from nursing.

Habit-Forming Potential: None.

Effects of Overdosage: No information is currently available on overdosage in
    humans.

Suggested Periodic Examinations While Taking This Drug (at physician's
    discretion)
    This medication may cause neutropenia and thrombocytopenia, therefore,
      white blood cell counts and platelet counts should be checked. Liver func-
      tion tests should also be obtained periodically.

▷ **While Taking This Drug, Observe the Following**
  Foods: No restrictions.
  Beverages: No restrictions.
▷ *Alcohol:* Potential exists for additive liver toxicity. It is best to avoid alcohol.
  Tobacco Smoking: No interactions expected.
  Marijuana Smoking: May be an additive cause of rashes and seizures in people
    with existing seizure disorders. Avoid marijuana completely.

▷ *Other Drugs*
    Rifabutin may *decrease* the effects of
    • antianxiety agents such as diazepam and perhaps other benzodiazepines
      (see Drug Classes).
    • anticoagulants such as warfarin (Coumadin).
    • anticonvulsant drugs such as phenytoin (Dilantin).
    • barbiturates (see Drug Classes).
    • BCG live attenuated vaccine.
    • beta blockers such as metoprolol, propranolol (see Drug Classes).
    • chloramphenicol (Chloromycetin).
    • clofibrate (Atromid-S).
    • cortisonelike drugs (see Drug Class Section).
    • cyclosporine (Sandimmune).
    • dapsone.
    • digitalis preparations (Lanoxin, others).
    • disopyramide (Norpace).
    • ketoconazole (Nizoral).
    • mexilitine (Mexitil).
    • narcotics such as methadone (see Drug Classes—Opioids).
    • oral contraceptives.
    • oral hypoglycemic agents (sulfonylureas such as tolbutamide) (see Drug
      Classes).
    • quinidine (Quinaglute, others).
    • theophylline (Theodur, others).

- verapamil (Verelan).
- zidovudine (AZT) (the therapeutic effect will be lessened by a decreased drug level).

Rifabutin *taken concurrently* with

- anticoagulants such as warfarin (Coumadin) will result in a decreased anticoagulant effect (the INR (protime) will decrease). More frequent INR testing is needed. Warfarin dosing should then be adjusted to INR results.
- fluconazole (Diflucan) may result in increased rifabutin concentrations.
- trimetrexate (Neutrexan) may result in lowered trimetrexate levels and decreased therapeutic benefit from trimetrexate.

▷ *Driving, Hazardous Activities:* This drug may rarely be associated with confusion and seizures. Restrict activities as necessary.

Aviation Note: The use of this drug *may be a disqualification* for piloting. Consult a designated Aviation Medical Examiner.

Exposure to Sun: No restrictions.

Discontinuation: Do not stop or interrupt taking this medication without asking your doctor.

RIFAMPIN (ri FAM pin)

Other Name:	Rifampicin

Introduced: 1967	**Prescription:** USA: Yes; Canada: Yes	**Available as Generic:** No	**Class:** Antibiotic, rifamycins	**Controlled Drug:** USA: No; Canada: No

Brand Names: Rifadin, Rifadin IV, Rifamate [CD], Rifater [CD], Rimactane, Rimactane/INH Dual Pack [CD], ♣Rofact

BENEFITS versus RISKS	
Possible Benefits	*Possible Risks*
EFFECTIVE TREATMENT OF TUBERCULOSIS in combination with other drugs	DRUG-INDUCED HEPATITIS
	DRUG-INDUCED NEPHRITIS
EFFECTIVE PREVENTION OF MENINGITIS by the elimination of meningococcus from the throat of carriers	Rare blood cell disorder: abnormally low blood platelet count
	Rare coagulation defects
	Rare colitis (pseudomembranous)

▷ **Principal Uses**

As a Single Drug Product: Uses currently included in FDA approved labeling: (1) Treats active tuberculosis. It is usually given concurrently with other antitubercular drugs to enhance its effectiveness. It is also used to eliminate the meningitis germ (meningococcus) from the throats of healthy carriers so it cannot be spread to others; (2) treats tuberculosis in coal workers with good outcomes when combined with other antitubercular drugs; (3) used to prevent tuberculosis in people exposed to patients with active disease.

Other (unlabeled) generally accepted uses: (1) Second line agent in combination with doxycycline in treatment of brucellosis; (2) has a place in preventing Haemophilus influenzae infections in people exposed to patients with active disease; (3) combination therapy of lepromatous leprosy; (4) used in combination with cotrimoxazole to eliminate methicillin resistant staphylococcus aureus (MRSA) from people who carry the bacteria.

As a Combination Drug Product [CD]: This drug is available in combination with isoniazid, another antitubercular drug that delays the development of drug-resistant strains of the tuberculosis germ.

How This Drug Works: This drug prevents the growth and multiplication of susceptible tuberculosis organisms by blocking specific enzyme systems that are involved in the formation of essential proteins.

Available Dosage Forms and Strengths

Capsules — 150 mg, 300 mg

▷ **Usual Adult Dosage Range:** For tuberculosis: 10 mg per kilogram per day, up to 600 mg once/day. For meningococcus carriers: 600 mg once/day for 4 days. The total daily dosage should not exceed 600 mg. **Note: Actual dosage and administration schedule must be determined by the physician for each patient individually.**

Conditions Requiring Dosing Adjustments

Liver function: This drug can cause liver damage, and patients should be followed closely. In severe failure, the dose should be limited to 6 to 8 mg per kg twice a week.

Kidney function: For patients with a creatinine clearance (see Glossary) of 10 to 50 ml per minute, one researcher suggests that 50 to 100% of the usual dose should be given.

▷ **Dosing Instructions:** Preferably taken with 8 ounces of water on an empty stomach (1 hour before or 2 hours after eating). However, it may be taken with food if necessary to reduce stomach irritation. The capsule may be opened and the contents mixed with applesauce or jelly for administration.

Usual Duration of Use: Use on a regular schedule for several months usually determines effectiveness in promoting recovery from tuberculosis. Long-term use (possibly 1 to 2 years) requires ongoing physician supervision and periodic evaluation.

▷ **This Drug Should Not Be Taken If**
  • you have had an allergic reaction to it previously.

▷ **Inform Your Physician Before Taking This Drug If**
  • you are pregnant.
  • you have a history of liver disease or impaired liver function.
  • you have active liver disease.
  • you consume alcohol daily.
  • you are taking an oral contraceptive. (An alternate method of contraception is advised.)
  • you are taking an anticoagulant.

Possible Side Effects (natural, expected, and unavoidable drug actions)

Red, orange, or brown discoloration of tears, sweat, saliva, sputum, urine, or stool. Yellow discoloration of the skin (not jaundice). Note: In the absence of symptoms indicating illness, any discoloration is a harmless drug effect and does not indicate toxicity.

Possible fungal superinfections (see Glossary).

▷ **Possible Adverse Effects** (unusual, unexpected, and infrequent reactions)
  If any of the following develop, consult your physician promptly for guidance.

Mild Adverse Effects

Allergic Reactions: Skin rash, hives, itching, drug fever (see Glossary).

Headache, drowsiness, dizziness, blurred vision, impaired hearing, vague numbness and tingling.

Joint and muscle pain.

Loss of appetite, heartburn, nausea, vomiting, abdominal cramps, diarrhea.

Serious Adverse Effects

Skin problems (Stevens-Johnson syndrome or toxic epidermal necrolysis [TEN]).

Flu-like syndrome: fever, chills, headache, dizziness, musculoskeletal pain, difficult breathing.

Drug-induced liver damage, with or without jaundice.

Drug-induced kidney damage: impaired urine production, bloody or cloudy urine.

Drug-induced porphyria (rare).

Excessively low blood platelet count: abnormal bleeding or bruising (rare).

Blood clotting problems (disseminated intravascular coagulopathy) (rare).

Hemolytic anemia (rare).

Suppression of the adrenal gland (rare).

Pseudomembranous colitis (rare).

Gallstones (rare).

Pancreatitis (rare).

▷ **Possible Effects on Sexual Function**

Altered timing and pattern of menstruation.

Decreased effectiveness of oral contraceptives taken concurrently.

▷ **Adverse Effects That May Mimic Natural Diseases or Disorders**

Liver reactions may suggest viral hepatitis.

Kidney reactions may suggest an infectious nephritis.

Possible Effects on Laboratory Tests

Complete blood cell counts: decreased red cells, hemoglobin, white cells and platelets; increased eosinophils (allergic reaction).

Prothrombin time: increased (when taken concurrently with warfarin).

Liver function tests: increased liver enzymes (ALT/GPT, AST/GOT and alkaline phosphatase), increased bilirubin.

CAUTION

1. This drug may permanently discolor soft contact lenses.
2. This drug may reduce the effectiveness of oral contraceptives; unplanned pregnancy could occur; an alternate method of contraception is advised.
3. When this drug is used alone in the treatment of tuberculosis, resistance can develop rapidly. This drug should only be used in conjunction with other antitubercular drugs.
4. To ensure the best possible response to treatment, take the full course of medication prescribed; this may be for several months or years.

Precautions for Use

By Infants and Children: Monitor closely for possible liver toxicity or deficiency of blood platelets.

By Those over 60 Years of Age: Natural changes in body composition and function make you more susceptible to the adverse effects of this drug. Report promptly any indications of possible drug toxicity.

▷ **Advisability of Use During Pregnancy**
  Pregnancy Category: C. See Pregnancy Code at the back of this book.
  Animal studies: Cleft palate and spinal defects reported in rodent studies.
  Human studies: Adequate studies of pregnant women are not available.
  If possible, avoid use of drug during the first 3 months.

Advisability of Use if Breast-Feeding
  Presence of this drug in breast milk: Yes.
  Avoid drug or refrain from nursing.

Habit-Forming Potential: None.

Effects of Overdosage: Nausea, vomiting, drowsiness, unconsciousness, severe liver damage, jaundice.

Possible Effects of Long-Term Use: Superinfections, fungal overgrowth of mouth or tongue.

Suggested Periodic Examinations While Taking This Drug (at physician's discretion)
  Complete blood cell counts, liver and kidney function tests.
  Hearing acuity tests if hearing loss is suspected.

▷ **While Taking This Drug, Observe the Following**
  Foods: No restrictions.
  Beverages: No restrictions.
▷ *Alcohol:* It is best to avoid alcohol completely to reduce the risk of liver toxicity.
  Tobacco Smoking: No interactions expected.
▷ *Other Drugs*
  Rifabutin *taken concurrently* with
  • halothane anesthesia may result in serious liver damage.
  Rifampin may *decrease* the effects of
  • antianxiety agents such as diazepam and perhaps other benzodiazepines (see Drug Classes).
  • anticoagulants such as warfarin (Coumadin).
  • anticonvulsant drugs such as phenytoin (Dilantin).
  • barbiturates (see Drug Classes).
  • BCG live attenuated vaccine.
  • beta blockers such as metoprolol, propranolol (see Drug Classes).
  • some calcium channel blockers (see Drug Classes).
  • chloramphenicol (Chloromycetin).
  • clofibrate (Atromid-S).
  • cortisonelike drugs (see Drug Class Section).
  • cyclosporine (Sandimmune).
  • dapsone.
  • digitalis preparations (Lanoxin, others).
  • disopyramide (Norpace).
  • enalapril (Vasotec).
  • fluconazole (Diflucan).
  • itraconazole (Sporanox).
  • ketoconazole (Nizoral).
  • methadone (Dolophine).
  • mexilitine (Mexitil).
  • narcotics such as methadone (see Drug Classes—Opioids).
  • nifedipine (Adalat).

- oral contraceptives.
- oral hypoglycemic agents (sulfonylureas such as tolbutamide) (see Drug Classes).
- phenytoin (Dilantin).
- progestins.
- quinidine (Quinaglute, others).
- tricyclic antidepressants (see Drug Classes).
- theophylline (Theodur, others).
- verapamil (Verelan).
- warfarin (Coumadin). Increased INR testing is needed.
- zidovudine (AZT) (the therapeutic effect will be lessened by a decreased drug level).

The following drugs may *decrease* the effects of rifampin

- aminosalicylic acid (PAS), and reduce its antitubercular effectiveness.

▷ *Driving, Hazardous Activities:* This drug may cause dizziness, drowsiness, impaired vision and impaired hearing. Restrict activities as necessary.

Aviation Note: The use of this drug *may be a disqualification* for piloting. Consult a designated Aviation Medical Examiner.

Exposure to Sun: No restrictions.

Discontinuation: It is advisable not to interrupt or stop this drug without consulting your physician. Intermittent administration can increase the possibility of developing allergic reactions.

RISPERIDONE (ris peer i dohn)

Introduced: 1993   **Prescription:** USA: Yes; Canada: Yes   **Available as Generic:** USA: No; Canada: No   **Class:** Antipsychotic agent   **Controlled Drug:** USA: No; Canada: No

Brand Names: Risperdal

BENEFITS versus RISKS	
Possible Benefits	*Possible Risks*
TREATMENT OF SCHIZOPHRENIA REFRACTORY TO OTHER AGENTS	Change in heart function (rare)
	Involuntary movement disorder (rare)
DECREASED SIDE EFFECTS COMPARED TO OTHER AVAILABLE DRUGS	Neuroleptic malignant syndrome (rare)
EFFECTIVE TREATMENT OF CERTAIN PSYCHOTIC DISORDERS	

▷ **Principal Uses**

As a Single Drug Product: Uses currently included in FDA approved labeling: (1) Management of the effects (manifestations) of psychotic disorders such as chronic schizophrenia.

Other (unlabeled) generally accepted uses: (1) Treatment of acute schizophrenia; (2) treatment of aggression; (3) treatment of Tourette's syndrome; (4) can have a role in helping behavioral problems in people with mental retardation.

How This Drug Works: This medication acts to balance two nerve transmitters (dopamine and serotonin) and by doing so, helps restore more normal thinking and mood.

Available Dosage Forms and Strengths
>   Oral solution — 1 mg per ml
>   Tablets — 1 mg, 2 mg, 3 mg, 4 mg

▷ **Recommended Dosage Ranges (Actual dosage and administration schedule must be determined by the physician for each patient individually.)**

Infants and Children: Safety and efficacy for those less than 18 years of age are not established.

18 to 60 Years of Age: Usual starting dose is 1 mg taken twice daily. Dosage may be increased as needed and tolerated by 1 mg on the second and third day for a total of 3 mg twice daily by the third day. If further dose changes are needed, they should be made at 1 week intervals. Doses greater than 6 mg per day are not recommended.

Over 60 Years of Age: Therapy is started with 0.5 mg twice daily. The dose is increased if needed and tolerated by 0.5 mg twice daily. Doses greater than 1.5 mg daily are achieved by small increases made at one week intervals. Careful attention must be paid to blood pressure and development of adverse effects.

Conditions Requiring Dosing Adjustments

Liver function: The starting dose must be decreased and adjusted as for those over 60 years old. Additionally there may be an increased amount of the active drug that results from each dose (increased free fraction), and as such a greater than expected effect may be seen.

Kidney function: The starting dose must be decreased and adjusted as for those over 60 years old.

▷ **Dosing Instructions:**   The tablet may be crushed, and medication effect is not changed by food.

Usual Duration of Use:
Use on a regular schedule for 1 to 2 weeks usually determines effectiveness in helping control chronic schizophrenia. If long-term use is attempted, the lowest effective dose should be used. Periodic physician evaluation of response and dosage adjustment is required.

Possible Advantages of This Drug
Treatment of schizophrenia refractory to other therapy.

▷ **This Drug Should Not Be Taken If**
- you have had an allergic reaction to any dosage form of it previously.
- you have had neuroleptic malignant syndrome (ask your doctor).

▷ **Inform Your Physician Before Taking This Drug If**
- you have a history of breast cancer.
- you have liver or kidney compromise.
- you are pregnant or plan to become pregnant.
- you are breast feeding your infant.
- you have had tardive dyskinesia in the past.
- you have a history of Parkinson's disease.
- you have a history of seizures.
- you have a history of heart rhythm disturbances.
- you are uncertain of your risperidone dose or how often to take it.

Possible Side Effects (natural, expected, and unavoidable drug actions)
Increased prolactin levels may result in male and female breast tenderness and swelling.

▷ **Possible Adverse Effects** (unusual, unexpected, and infrequent reactions)
If any of the following develop, consult your physician promptly for guidance.

Mild Adverse Effects
Allergic Reactions: Skin rash.
Somnolence (3% to 41% of high-dose patients).
Difficulty in concentrating/fatigue (rare).
Increased dreaming (rare).
Weight gain.
Constipation.
Palpitations (rare).
Orthostatic hypotension (see Glossary) (rare).
Increased urination (rare).

Serious Adverse Effects
Allergic Reactions: Anaphylactoid reactions.
Abnormal heart function (prolonged QT interval) (rare).
Tardive dyskinesia (see Glossary) (rare).
Neuroleptic malignant syndrome (rare).
Low sodium (rare).
Rare seizures.
Lowered white blood cells (very rare).
Low platelets (rare).
Abnormally low blood pressure on standing (orthostatic hypotension) (rare).
Abnormal liver function (rare).

▷ **Possible Effects on Sexual Function:**   Diminished sexual desire (1%). Delayed or absent orgasm (1%). Erectile dysfunction including priapism (up to 1%), male or female breast tenderness or swelling (1%). Dry vagina or menstrual changes (menorrhagia—1%). Ejaculation failure (rare).

Possible Delayed Adverse Effects: Swelling and tenderness of male and female breast tissue.

Natural Diseases or Disorders That May Be Activated by This Drug
Some human cancers depend on prolactin for growth, and since risperidone increases prolactin, it should be used with caution in people with previously diagnosed breast cancer.

Possible Effects on Laboratory Tests
Liver function tests: increased SGPT, SGOT and LDH.
Complete blood counts: decreased platelets, white blood cells and hemoglobin.
Prolactin: increased.

CAUTION
1. Should be used with great caution, if at all in patients with cancer.
2. Call your doctor promptly if you have an increased tendency to infection or abnormal bleeding or bruising while taking this drug.
3. Used with great caution, if at all in patients with seizure history.

Precautions for Use

By Infants and Children: Safety and effectiveness for those under 18 years of age not established.

By Those over 60 Years of Age: The starting dose of 0.5 mg twice daily is used in patients who are elderly or debilitated and slower increases in dose as needed and tolerated are indicated. Great care should be taken in those with heart disease. You may be more likely to experience postural hypotension (see Glossary) and problems with motor skills. Those with prostate problems may have increased risk of urine retention.

▷ **Advisability of Use During Pregnancy**

Pregnancy Category: C. See Pregnancy Code at the back of this book.

Animal studies: Increased rat pup death during the first few days of lactation.

Human studies: Adequate studies of pregnant women are not available. One case report of lack of formation of the corpus callosum of the brain in a fetus exposed to this drug while in the uterus.

Ask your doctor for guidance.

Advisability of Use if Breast-Feeding

Presence of this drug in breast milk: Yes.

Avoid drug or refrain from nursing.

Habit-Forming Potential: None.

Effects of Overdosage: Drowsiness, hypotension, tachycardia, low sodium and potassium, ECG changes (prolonged QT interval), and seizure.

Suggested Periodic Examinations While Taking This Drug (at physician's discretion)

Liver function tests.

Electrolytes (sodium and potassium).

ECG.

Prolactin level.

▷ **While Taking This Drug, Observe the Following**

Foods: No restrictions.

Beverages: No restrictions.

▷ *Alcohol:* Patients should avoid alcohol while taking risperidone.

Tobacco Smoking: No interactions expected.

Marijuana Smoking: Increased somnolence.

▷ *Other Drugs*

Risperidone may **decrease** the effects of

• levodopa (Sinemet, others).

Risperidone **taken concurrently** with

• carbamazepine (Tegretol) will decrease the drug level and perhaps the therapeutic effect of risperidone.

• other centrally acting medicines may result in increased central effects.

• clozapine (Clozaril) may decrease the therapeutic effects of risperidone.

▷ *Driving, Hazardous Activities:* This drug may cause drowsiness and difficulty concentrating. Restrict activities as necessary.

Aviation Note: The use of this drug **is a disqualification** for piloting. Consult a designated Aviation Medical Examiner.

Exposure to Sun: Use caution. May cause photosensitivity.

Discontinuation: Consult your doctor before stopping this medication.

SALMETEROL (sal ME ter ohl)

Introduced: 1994   **Prescription:** USA: Yes; Canada: Not available in Canada   **Available as Generic:** USA: No   **Class:** bronchodilator   **Controlled Drug:** USA:No

Brand Names: Serevent, Aeromax

BENEFITS versus RISKS

Possible Benefits	*Possible Risks*
LONG-ACTING RELIEF OF BRONCHIAL ASTHMA PREVENTION OF NOCTURNAL ASTHMA SYMPTOMS	Rapid heart rate (tachycardia)

▷ **Principal Uses**

As a Single Drug Product: Uses currently included in FDA approved labeling: (1) Treatment and prevention of bronchospasm in asthma; (2) prevention of nocturnal asthma; (3) prevention of exercise-induced bronchospasm.

Other (unlabeled) generally accepted uses: (1) May have a role in chronic obstructive pulmonary disease (COPD).

How This Drug Works: This drug acts at specific sites (beta-2) in the lung and results in opening of the airways (bronchodilation), decreased airway reactivity and increased movement of mucous. It also appears to block release of chemicals from certain (mast) cells which worsen asthma.

Available Dosage Forms and Strengths

Inhaler — 13 gram canister which gives 21 mcg of salmeterol per use.

▷ **Recommended Dosage Ranges (Actual dosage and administration schedule must be determined by the physician for each patient individually.)**

Infants and Children: Safety and efficacy in those less than 12 years of age not established.

12 to 60 Years of Age: For prevention of asthma: Two inhalations (42 mcg) twice daily in the morning and evening. Doses should be given 12 hours apart.

For prevention of exercised induced asthma: Two inhalations at least 30 to 60 minutes **before** exercise. Additional doses of salmeterol should **not** be given for 12 hours.

Over 60 Years of Age: Same as 12 to 60 years of age.

Conditions Requiring Dosing Adjustments

Liver function: Used with caution as the drug may accumulate in liver failure.

Kidney function: Salmeterol has not been studied in kidney failure patients.

▷ **Dosing Instructions:** Follow written instructions on the inhaler closely. Has not been studied for use with a spacer or similar device. Should be shaken well before using.

Usual Duration of Use:

Use on a regular schedule for 4 to 6 weeks usually determines effectiveness in preventing asthma attacks. Long-term use (months to years) requires periodic physician evaluation of response and dosage adjustment.

Possible Advantages of This Drug

Longer acting beta-two agent than medications previously available.

▷ **This Drug Should Not Be Taken If**

- you have had an allergic reaction to any dosage form of it previously.
- you currently have an irregular heart rhythm.
- you are taking, or have taken within the past 2 weeks, any monoamine oxidase (MAO) type A inhibitor.

▷ **Inform Your Physician Before Taking This Drug If**

- your breathing does not improve after administration of this drug.
- you have an overactive thyroid (hyperthyroidism).
- you have diabetes.
- you have a history of heart problems.
- you have abnormally high blood pressure.
- you are uncertain of how much salmeterol to take or how often to take it.

Possible Side Effects (natural, expected, and unavoidable drug actions)

Dryness or irritation of the mouth or throat, altered taste. Nervousness or palpitations.

Tachyphylaxis.

▷ **Possible Adverse Effects** (unusual, unexpected, and infrequent reactions)

If any of the following develop, consult your physician promptly for guidance.

Mild Adverse Effects

Allergic Reactions: Skin rash and urticaria.

Rhinitis and laryngitis.

Nervousness and fatigue.

Headache, tremor, dizziness, and nervousness.

Serious Adverse Effects

Allergic Reactions: Not defined.

Rapid heart rate (tachycardia) and palpitations.

Paradoxical bronchospasm.

Respiratory arrest (rare).

▷ **Possible Effects on Sexual Function:** Dysmenorrhea.

Possible Delayed Adverse Effects: None defined at present.

▷ **Adverse Effects That May Mimic Natural Diseases or Disorders**

Rapid heart rate may mimic heart disease.

Bronchospasm may mimic asthma.

Natural Diseases or Disorders That May Be Activated by This Drug

Latent coronary artery disease. Diabetes or high blood pressure.

Possible Effects on Laboratory Tests

Blood cholesterol profile: may be increased.

Blood glucose level: increased.

CAUTION

1. Use of this drug by inhalation with beclomethasone aerosol (Beclovent, Vanceril) may increase the risk of fluorocarbon propellant toxicity. Use salmeterol aerosol 20 to 30 minutes **before** beclomethasone aerosol to reduce toxicity and enhance penetration of beclomethasone into the lungs.

2. Serious heart rhythm problems or cardiac arrest can result from excessive and prolonged use.
3. Call your doctor if you begin to have symptoms more frequently than usual, or if you begin to increase your use of the immediate bronchodilator which was prescribed for you.

Precautions for Use

By Infants and Children: Safety and effectiveness for those under 12 years of age not established.

By Those over 60 Years of Age: Avoid increased use. If asthma is not controlled as it has been in the past, call your doctor.

▷ **Advisability of Use During Pregnancy**

Pregnancy Category: C. See Pregnancy Code at the back of this book.

Animal studies: Rabbit studies have revealed cleft palate, limb and paw flexures and delayed bone formation.

Human studies: Adequate studies of pregnant women are not available.

Ask your doctor for guidance.

Advisability of Use if Breast-Feeding

Presence of this drug in breast milk: Yes, but extent not defined.

Avoid drug or refrain from nursing.

Habit-Forming Potential: None.

Effects of Overdosage: Exaggeration of pharmacologic effects: tachycardia and/or arrhythmia, muscle cramps, cardiac arrest and death.

Suggested Periodic Examinations While Taking This Drug   (at physician's discretion)

Blood pressure checks, evaluations of heart (cardiac) status.

▷ **While Taking This Drug, Observe the Following**

Foods: No restrictions.

Beverages: Avoid excessive caffeine as in coffee, tea, cola and chocolate.

▷   *Alcohol:* No interactions expected.

Tobacco Smoking: No interactions expected.

Salmeterol *taken concurrently* with

• monoamine oxidase (MAO) type A inhibitor drugs can cause extreme increases in blood pressure and heart stimulation.

The following drugs may *increase* the effects of salmeterol

• tricyclic antidepressants.
• methylzanthines such as caffeine or theophylline.

▷   *Driving, Hazardous Activities:* This drug may cause nervousness or dizziness. Restrict activities as necessary.

Aviation Note: The use of this drug *is a disqualification* for piloting. Consult a designated Aviation Medical Examiner.

Exposure to Sun: No restrictions.

Heavy Exercise or Exertion: Use caution. May stress protective effects of this drug.

SELEGILINE (se LEDGE i leen)

Other Name: Deprenyl

Introduced: 1981   **Prescription:** USA: Yes   **Available as Generic:** USA: No   **Class:** Antiparkinsonism, monoamine oxidase (MAO) type B inhibitor   **Controlled Drug:** USA: No

Brand Name: Eldepryl

<table>
<tr><th colspan="2">BENEFITS versus RISKS</th></tr>
<tr><th>Possible Benefits</th><th>Possible Risks</th></tr>
<tr>
<td>EFFECTIVE INITIAL TREATMENT OF PARKINSON'S DISEASE when started at the onset of symptoms
ADDITIVE RELIEF OF SYMPTOMS OF PARKINSON'S DISEASE when used concurrently with levodopa/carbidopa
PERMITS UP TO 30% REDUCTION IN SINEMET DOSAGE</td>
<td>ABNORMAL INVOLUNTARY MOVEMENTS
HALLUCINATIONS
INITIAL FALL IN BLOOD PRESSURE/ORTHOSTATIC HYPOTENSION</td>
</tr>
</table>

▷ **Principal Uses**

As a Single Drug Product: Uses currently included in FDA approved labeling: (1) Used to start drug treatment of very early Parkinson's disease (soon after onset of symptoms), thus delaying the use of levodopa/carbidopa. It is also used as an adjunct to levodopa/carbidopa treatment of Parkinson's disease for those individuals who experience intolerable abnormal movements (dyskinesia) and/or increasing "on-off" episodes due to loss of effectiveness of levodopa. The addition of selegiline (1) permits reduction of the daily dose of levodopa (by 25% to 30%) with consequent lessening of dyskinesia and erratic drug response, and (2) provides additional relief of parkinsonian symptoms.

Other (unlabeled) generally accepted uses: (1) Some improvement in Alzheimer's disease in patients treated with this drug.

How This Drug Works: By (1) inhibiting monoamine oxidase type B, the enzyme that inactivates dopamine in the brain, and by (2) slowing the restorage of released dopamine at nerve terminals, this drug helps to correct the deficiency of dopamine that is responsible for the rigidity, tremor and sluggish movement characteristic of Parkinson's disease.

Available Dosage Forms and Strengths

Capsules — 5 mg

Tablets — 5 mg

Author's note: the capsule form of this medicine will eventually replace the tablet form, and is an astute attempt by the company to help avoid confusion with other white tablets or counterfeit copies of Eldepryl.

▷ **Usual Adult Dosage Range**

Parkinsonism: 5 mg once or twice daily. The usual maintenance dose is 5 mg after breakfast and 5 mg after lunch. A total daily dose of 10 mg is adequate to achieve optimal benefit from this drug. Higher doses do not result in further improvement and are not advised.

During the gradual introduction of selegiline, the concurrent dose of levodopa/carbidopa (Sinemet) may be cautiously decreased in accord with your physician's instructions. Concurrent Sinemet dosage should be reduced by 10% to 20% when selegiline is started. **Note: Actual dosage and administration schedule must be determined by the physician for each patient individually.**

Conditions Requiring Dosing Adjustments

Liver function: This drug is extensively metabolized in the liver. Patients with liver compromise should be followed closely.

Kidney function: The kidney does not have a major role in the elimination of this medication. It can cause prostatic hypertrophy, and should be used with caution in patients with urine outflow problems.

▷ **Dosing Instructions:**   The tablet may be crushed and taken with food or milk to reduce stomach irritation.

Usual Duration of Use: Use on a regular schedule for 4 to 6 weeks usually determines effectiveness in controlling the symptoms of Parkinson's disease and permitting reduction of levodopa/carbidopa dosage. Long-term use (months to years) requires periodic physician evaluation of response and dosage adjustment.

Possible Advantages of This Drug

It may provide a more effective and uniform control of parkinsonian symptoms and a significant reduction of some adverse effects associated with long-term levodopa therapy. Fifty to 60% of users show improvement.

It does not lose its effectiveness with long-term use.

It does not require avoidance of foods containing tyramine, as is necessary with monoamine oxidase (MAO) type A inhibitors.

It causes no life-threatening or irreversible adverse effects.

▷ **This Drug Should Not Be Taken If**

- you have had an allergic reaction to it previously.
- you have Huntington's disease, hereditary (essential) tremor or tardive dyskinesia (see Glossary).
- you are pregnant or breast-feeding.
- you take meperidine (Demerol).

▷ **Inform Your Physician Before Taking This Drug If**

- you have constitutionally low blood pressure.
- you have peptic ulcer disease.
- you are taking levodopa.
- you have a history of heart rhythm disorder.
- you are taking any antihypertensive drugs or antipsychotic drugs (see Drug Classes).

Possible Side Effects (natural, expected, and unavoidable drug actions)

Weakness (rare), orthostatic hypotension (see Glossary) (rare), dry mouth (rare), insomnia (rare).

▷ **Possible Adverse Effects** (unusual, unexpected, and infrequent reactions)

If any of the following develop, consult your physician promptly for guidance.

Mild Adverse Effects

Headache (rare), dizziness, blurred vision (rare), agitation.

Palpitations (rare), fainting (rare).
Altered taste (rare), nausea and vomiting, stomach pain, anorexia (common).
Sleep disorders.
Serious Adverse Effects
Dyskinesias: abnormal involuntary movements.
Confusion and hallucinations, depression (rare), psychosis (rare), vivid dreams (rare).
Aggravation of peptic ulcer (rare), gastrointestinal bleeding (rare).
Growth of the prostate (rare).

▷ **Possible Effects on Sexual Function:** Transient decreases in penile sensation and anorgasmia have rarely been reported if doses exceed 10 mg per day. Increased libido may occur.

▷ **Adverse Effects That May Mimic Natural Diseases or Disorders**
Effects on mental function and behavior may resemble psychotic disorders.

▷ **Natural Diseases or Disorders That May Be Activated by This Drug**
Peptic ulcer disease.

Possible Effects on Laboratory Tests
None reported.

CAUTION
1. This drug can initiate dyskinesias and can intensify existing dyskinesias. Watch carefully for the development of tremors, twitching or abnormal, involuntary movements of any kind. Report these promptly.
2. This drug potentiates the effects of levodopa. When this drug is added to current levodopa treatment, adverse effects of levodopa may develop or be intensified. The dose of levodopa must be reduced by 10% to 20% when treatment with selegiline begins.
3. Tell your doctor promptly if you become pregnant or plan pregnancy. The manufacturer does not recommend the use of this drug during pregnancy.

Precautions for Use
By Infants and Children: This drug is not utilized by this age group.
By Those over 60 Years of Age: This drug is well tolerated by the elderly. Observe closely for any tendency to light-headedness or faintness, especially on arising from a lying or sitting position.

▷ **Advisability of Use During Pregnancy**
Pregnancy Category: C. See Pregnancy Code at the back of this book.
Animal studies: No birth defects due to this drug were found in rat studies.
Human studies: Adequate studies of pregnant women are not available. The manufacturer advises that this drug should not be taken during pregnancy.

Advisability of Use if Breast-Feeding
Presence of this drug in breast milk: Unknown.
Avoid drug or refrain from nursing.

Habit-Forming Potential: None.

Effects of Overdosage: Nausea, vomiting, palpitations, low blood pressure, agitation, severe involuntary movements, hallucinations.

Possible Effects of Long-Term Use: None reported.

Suggested Periodic Examinations While Taking This Drug (at physician's discretion)

Regular evaluation of drug response, heart function and blood pressure status.

▷ **While Taking This Drug, Observe the Following**

Foods: Caution should be used regarding tyramine containing foods, although the reaction with this drug may not be as severe as that seen with other MAO inhibitors.

Beverages: No restrictions. May be taken with milk.

▷ *Alcohol:* Use caution until the combined effects have been determined. Alcohol may exaggerate the blood-pressure-lowering and sedative effects of this drug.

Tobacco Smoking: No interactions expected.

▷ *Other Drugs*

Selegiline *taken concurrently* with

- albuterol (Ventolin, others) may result in increased adverse vascular effects.
- amphetamine (Dexedrine) can cause a severe increase in blood pressure.
- antidepressants (see Drug Classes) such as amitriptyline (Elavil) may cause neurotoxic reactions such as seizures.
- antihypertensive drugs (and other drugs that can lower blood pressure) require careful monitoring for excessive drops in pressure. Dosage adjustments may be necessary.
- benzodiazepines (see Drug Classes) may result in increased central nervous system depression.
- buspirone (Buspar) may result in increases in blood pressure.
- dextromethorphan (various) a cough suppressant used in many nonprescription cough medicines has been reported to cause toxicity with low blood pressure, spasms, high fevers and some deaths. These medicines should not be combined.
- ephedrine (various) can result in severe increases in temperature.
- fluoxetine (Prozac) may cause serotonin toxicity syndrome.
- fluvoxamine (Luvox) may result in extreme agitation, rigidity, excessive temperatures and coma. DO NOT combine these medicines.
- lithium (Lithobid) may increase risk of the serotonin toxicity syndrome.
- meperidine (Demerol) may cause a life-threatening reaction of unknown cause; avoid this combination.
- oral hypoglycemic agents (see Drug Classes) may cause very low blood sugars.
- paroxetine (Paxil) may result in central nervous system toxicity.
- phenothiazines (see Drug Classes) may result in increased occurrence of movement disorders.
- phenylpropanolamine (various) can cause severe increases in temperature and blood pressure. DO NOT combine.
- pseudoephedrine (various) can cause severe increases in temperature and blood pressure. DO NOT combine.
- sertraline (Zoloft) may result in central nervous system toxicity.
- tryptophan may cause a fatal serotonin syndrome.

- venlafaxine (Effexor) can result in central and autonomic nervous system toxicity.

The following drugs may *decrease* the effects of selegiline and diminish its effectiveness

- chlorprothixene (Taractan).
- haloperidol (Haldol).
- metoclopramide (Reglan).
- phenothiazines (see Drug Classes).
- reserpine (Ser-Ap-Es, etc.), in high doses.
- thiothixene (Navane).

▷ *Driving, Hazardous Activities:* This drug may cause dizziness, drowsiness, impaired coordination or fainting. Restrict activities as necessary.

Aviation Note: The use of this drug *is a disqualification* for piloting. Consult a designated Aviation Medical Examiner.

Exposure to Sun: Use caution, photosensitivity has been reported.

Exposure to Heat: Use caution until the combined effects have been determined. Hot environments can cause lowering of blood pressure.

Discontinuation: Do not stop this drug abruptly. Sudden withdrawal can cause prompt increase in parkinsonian symptoms and deterioration of control. Consult your physician regarding a schedule for gradual withdrawal and concurrent adjustment of Sinemet or other appropriate drugs.

SERTRALINE (SER tra leen)

Introduced: 1986   **Prescription:** USA: Yes   **Available as Generic:** USA: No   **Class:** Antidepressant   **Controlled Drug:** USA: No
Brand Name: Zoloft

BENEFITS versus RISKS	
Possible Benefits	*Possible Risks*
EFFECTIVE TREATMENT OF MAJOR DEPRESSIVE DISORDERS	Male sexual dysfunction
	Seizures (very rare)
Possibly effective in relieving the symptoms of obsessive-compulsive disorder	

▷ **Principal Uses**

As a Single Drug Product: Uses currently included in FDA approved labeling: (1) Treats major forms of depression that have not responded well to other therapies. This drug should be used only when a diagnosis of a true, primary depression of significant degree has been established.

Other (unlabeled) generally accepted uses: (1) May have a role in treating obesity. Rat studies have shown a decrease in eating that depends on the dose that is taken. Studies in humans are being conducted; (2) treatment of obsessive-compulsive disorder.

How This Drug Works: This drug relieves depression by slowly restoring to normal levels a specific constituent of brain tissue (serotonin) that transmits nerve impulses.

Available Dosage Forms and Strengths
Tablets — 50 mg, 100 mg

▷ **Recommended Dosage Ranges** (Actual dosage and administration schedule must be determined by the physician for each patient individually.)
Infants and Children: Dosage not established.
12 to 60 Years of Age: Initially 50 mg once daily, taken in the morning or evening. The dose is then gradually increased, as needed and tolerated, in increments of 50 mg at intervals of 1 week. The total daily dosage should not exceed 200 mg.
Over 60 Years of Age: Same as 12 to 60 years of age. Adjust dosage as appropriate for impaired liver or kidney function.

Conditions Requiring Dosing Adjustments
Liver function: This drug is a rare cause of liver damage. Patients should be followed closely, and less frequent or lower doses should be used.
Kidney function: The role of the kidneys in the elimination of this drug is unknown.

▷ **Dosing Instructions:** The tablet may be crushed and is best taken with food to enhance absorption, but may be taken at any time with or without food.

Usual Duration of Use: Use on a regular schedule for 4 to 8 weeks usually determines (1) this drug's effectiveness in relieving depression; (2) the pattern of both favorable and unfavorable drug effects. Long-term use (months to years) requires periodic physician evaluation of response and dosage adjustment.

Possible Advantages of This Drug
Does not cause weight gain, a common side effect of tricyclic antidepressants.
Less likely to cause dry mouth, constipation, urinary retention, orthostatic hypotension (see Glossary) and heart rhythm disturbances than tricyclic antidepressants.
Does not cause Parkinson-like reactions.

▷ **This Drug Should Not Be Taken If**
• you have had an allergic reaction to it previously.
• you are currently taking or have taken within the past 14 days any monoamine oxidase (MAO) type A inhibitor drug (see Drug Classes Section).

▷ **Inform Your Physician Before Taking This Drug If**
• you have experienced any adverse effects from antidepressant drugs.
• you have impaired liver or kidney function.
• you have Parkinson's disease.
• you have had a recent heart attack.
• you have a seizure disorder.
• you are pregnant or plan pregnancy while taking this drug.

Possible Side Effects (natural, expected, and unavoidable drug actions)
Decreased appetite, weight loss (average 1 to 2 pounds).

▷ **Possible Adverse Effects** (unusual, unexpected, and infrequent reactions)
If any of the following develop, consult your physician promptly for guidance.
Mild Adverse Effects
Allergic Reactions: Skin rash (rare), itching.
Headache, nervousness, insomnia, drowsiness, fatigue, tremor, dizziness, im-

paired concentration (rare), abnormal vision, numbness and tingling (rare), confusion (rare), hallucinations (rare).

Chest pain and increased blood pressure (rare).

Paresthesias (rare).

Dry mouth, altered taste (rare), indigestion, nausea, vomiting, diarrhea, tongue ulceration (rare).

Serious Adverse Effects

Allergic Reactions: Dermatitis (various forms) (rare).

Drug-induced seizures (rare).

Hemorrhage into the anterior chamber of the eye.

Anemia (rare).

Increased blood cholesterol (hypercholesterolemia) (occasional).

Low blood sugar.

Bronchospasm (occasional).

Low blood sodium (rare case reports of SIADH) (may also occur with other SSRIs).

▷ **Possible Effects on Sexual Function:** Male sexual dysfunction: delayed ejaculation (15.5%); female sexual dysfunction: inhibited orgasm (1.7%).

Swelling and tenderness of male and female breast tissue. Infrequent dysmenorrhea, intermenstrual bleeding or atrophic vaginitis.

Natural Diseases or Disorders That May Be Activated by This Drug

Latent epilepsy.

Possible Effects on Laboratory Tests

Blood total cholesterol and triglyceride levels: increased (occasional).

Blood uric acid levels: decreased.

Hemoglobin or hematocrit: decreased (rare).

Liver function tests: increased liver enzymes (ALT/GPT, AST/GOT and alkaline phosphatase).

Blood sodium: decreased (with rare SIADH).

CAUTION

1. If any type of skin reaction develops (rash, hives, etc.), discontinue this drug and inform your physician promptly.
2. If dryness of the mouth develops and persists for more than 2 weeks, consult your dentist for guidance.
3. Ask your doctor or pharmacist before taking any other prescription or over-the-counter drug while taking this drug.
4. If you are advised to take any monoamine oxidase (MAO) type A inhibitor drug (see Drug Classes), allow an interval of 5 weeks after discontinuing this drug before starting the MAO inhibitor.
5. It is advisable to withhold this drug if electroconvulsive therapy (ECT, "shock" treatment) is to be used to treat your depression.

Precautions for Use

By Infants and Children: Safety and effectiveness for those under 12 years of age not established.

By Those over 60 Years of Age: The lowest effective dose should be used for maintenance treatment and adjusted as needed for reduced kidney function.

▷ **Advisability of Use During Pregnancy**

Pregnancy Category: B. See Pregnancy Code at the back of this book.

Animal studies: Delayed bone development due to this drug found in rat and rabbit studies.

Human studies: Adequate studies of pregnant women are not available. Use this drug only if clearly needed. Ask your physician for guidance.

Advisability of Use if Breast-Feeding
Presence of this drug in breast milk: Unknown.
Avoid drug or refrain from nursing.

Habit-Forming Potential: None.

Effects of Overdosage: Agitation, restlessness, excitement, nausea, vomiting, seizures.

Possible Effects of Long-Term Use: None reported.

Suggested Periodic Examinations While Taking This Drug (at physician's discretion)
None.

▷ **While Taking This Drug, Observe the Following**
Foods: May increase peak blood level.
Beverages: No restrictions. May be taken with milk.
▷ *Alcohol:* Avoid completely.
Tobacco Smoking: No interactions expected.
▷ *Other Drugs*
Sertraline may *increase* the effects of
- diazepam (Valium) and perhaps other benzodiazepines (see Drug Classes).
- tolbutamide (Orinase).
- warfarin (Coumadin) and related oral anticoagulants. More frequent INR (protime) testing is needed. Ongoing warfarin doses should be based on INR results.

Sertraline *taken concurrently* with
- antidiabetic drugs (insulin, oral hypoglycemics) (see Drug Classes) may increase the risk of hypoglycemic reactions; monitor blood and urine sugar levels carefully.
- monoamine oxidase (MAO) type A inhibitor drugs may cause confusion, agitation, high fever, seizures and dangerous elevations of blood pressure. Avoid the concurrent use of these drugs.
▷ *Driving, Hazardous Activities:* This drug may cause drowsiness, dizziness, impaired judgment and altered vision. Restrict activities as necessary.
Aviation Note: The use of this drug *is a disqualification* for piloting. Consult a designated Aviation Medical Examiner.
Exposure to Sun: Use caution. This drug may (rarely) cause photosensitivity (see Glossary).
Discontinuation: The slow elimination of this drug from the body makes it unlikely that any withdrawal effects will result from abrupt discontinuation. However, call your doctor if you plan to stop this drug for any reason.

SIMVASTATIN (sim vah STA tin)

Introduced: 1986   **Prescription:** USA: Yes; Canada: Yes   **Available as Generic:** USA: No; Canada: No   **Class:** anticholesterol   **Controlled Drug:** USA: No; Canada: No

Brand Name: Zocor

BENEFITS versus RISKS	
Possible Benefits	*Possible Risks*
EFFECTIVE REDUCTION OF TOTAL BLOOD CHOLESTEROL AND LDL CHOLESTEROL	Drug-induced hepatitis without jaundice (rare) Drug-induced myositis (rare)

▷ **Principal Uses**

As a Single Drug Product: Uses currently included in FDA approved labeling: (1) Used in patients with elevated cholesterol to reduce death from heart disease (42% in one study) and decrease the number of nonfatal heart attacks; (2) treatment of abnormally high total blood cholesterol levels (in individuals with Types IIa and IIb hypercholesterolemia) due to increased fractions of low-density lipoprotein (LDL) cholesterol. It is used in conjunction with a cholesterol-lowering diet. It should not be used until an adequate trial of nondrug methods for lowering cholesterol has proved to be ineffective; (3) stops the progression and decreases the number of deaths in patients with coronary artery disease.

Other (unlabeled) generally accepted uses: (1) may help reduce lipid disorders that occur in kidney (nephrotic syndrome) problems; (2) can have a role as part of combination therapy in preventing gallstones.

How This Drug Works: This drug blocks the liver enzyme that starts production of cholesterol. It reduces low-density lipoproteins (LDL), the fraction of total blood cholesterol that is thought to increase the risk of coronary heart disease. This drug may also increase the level of high-density lipoproteins (HDL), the cholesterol fraction that reduces the risk of heart disease.

Available Dosage Forms and Strengths

Tablets — 5 mg, 10 mg, 20 mg, 40 mg

▷ **Recommended Dosage Ranges** (Actual dosage and administration schedule must be determined by the physician for each patient individually.)

Infants and Children: Under 2 years of age—do not use this drug.

2 to 20 years of age—dosage not established.

20 to 60 Years of Age: Initially 5 to 10 mg daily, taken at bedtime. The dose is increased as needed to reach desired goals (such as decreased LDL-C reduction of 20%). More aggressive goals may require the 10 mg starting dose. The drug is then increased as needed and tolerated by increments of 5 to 10 mg at intervals of 4 weeks. The total daily dose should not exceed 40 mg.

Over 60 Years of Age:

Initially 5 mg daily. Increase dose as needed and tolerated by increments of 5 mg at intervals of 4 weeks. The total daily dose should not exceed 20 mg.

Conditions Requiring Dosing Adjustments

Liver function: This drug achieves a high concentration in the liver, and is subsequently eliminated in the bile. It can be a rare cause of liver damage, and patients should be followed closely.

Kidney function: In severe kidney failure, the dose should be started at 5 mg, and the patient closely followed.

▷ **Dosing Instructions:**   The tablet may be crushed and taken without regard to eating. Preferably taken at bedtime. (The highest rates of cholesterol production occur between midnight and 5 a.m.).

Usual Duration of Use: Use on a regular schedule for 4 to 6 weeks usually determines effectiveness in reducing blood levels of total and LDL cholesterol. Long-term use (months to years) requires periodic physician evaluation of response and dosage adjustment. Consult your physician on a regular basis.

Possible Advantages of This Drug: Recent studies indicate that drugs of this class (HMG-CoA reductase inhibitors) are more effective and better tolerated than other drugs currently available for reducing total and LDL cholesterol. Its long-term effects are yet to be determined.

▷ **This Drug Should Not Be Taken If**
  • you have had an allergic reaction to it previously.
  • you have active liver disease.
  • you are pregnant or breast-feeding your infant.

▷ **Inform Your Physician Before Taking This Drug If**
  • you have previously taken any other drugs in this class: lovastatin (Mevacor), pravastatin (Pravachol).
  • you have a history of liver disease or impaired liver function.
  • you are not using any method of birth control, or you are planning pregnancy.
  • you regularly consume substantial amounts of alcohol.
  • you have cataracts or impaired vision.
  • you have any type of chronic muscular disorder.
  • you develop muscle pain, weakness or soreness which is unexplained while taking this medicine.
  • you plan to have major surgery in the near future.

Possible Side Effects (natural, expected, and unavoidable drug actions)
  Development of abnormal liver function tests without associated symptoms.

▷ **Possible Adverse Effects** (unusual, unexpected, and infrequent reactions)
  If any of the following develop, consult your physician promptly for guidance.
  Mild Adverse Effects
  Allergic reactions: Rash.
  Headache.
  Indigestion (rare), nausea (rare), excessive gas (rare), constipation, diarrhea (rare).
  Lowering of the blood pressure.
  Insomnia (occasional).
  Serious Adverse Effects
  Marked and persistent abnormal liver function tests with focal hepatitis (without jaundice) (rare).
  Acute myositis (muscle pain and tenderness) occurred rarely during long-term use.
  Rhabdomyolysis (rare).
  Potential for cataracts (based on animal data, not reported in humans).
  Depression (rare).
  Protein in the urine (rare).
  Lichen planus skin rash (rare).

▷ **Possible Effects on Sexual Function:**   None reported.

Possible Delayed Adverse Effects: None reported to date. Doses 15 to 33 times the human dose given to rats caused an increase in liver cancers.

Natural Diseases or Disorders That May Be Activated by This Drug
Latent liver disease.

Possible Effects on Laboratory Tests
Blood alanine aminotransferase (ALT) enzyme level: increased (with higher doses of drug).
Blood total cholesterol, LDL cholesterol and triglyceride levels: decreased.
Blood HDL cholesterol level: increased.

CAUTION
1. If pregnancy occurs while taking this drug, stop it immediately and consult your physician.
2. Report promptly any development of muscle pain or tenderness, especially if accompanied by fever or weakness (malaise).
3. Report promptly the development of altered or impaired vision so that appropriate evaluation can be made.

Precautions for Use
By Infants and Children: Safety and effectiveness for those under 20 years of age not established.
By Those over 60 Years of Age: Inform your physician regarding any personal or family history of cataracts. Comply with all recommendations regarding periodic eye examinations. Report promptly any alterations in vision.

▷ **Advisability of Use During Pregnancy**
Pregnancy Category: X. See Pregnancy Code at the back of this book.
Animal studies: Mouse and rat studies reveal skeletal birth defects due to a closely related drug of this class.
Human studies: Adequate studies of pregnant women are not available.
This drug should be avoided during entire pregnancy.

Advisability of Use if Breast-Feeding
Presence of this drug in breast milk: Unknown.
Avoid drug or refrain from nursing.

Habit-Forming Potential: None.

Effects of Overdosage: Increased indigestion, stomach distress, nausea, diarrhea.

Possible Effects of Long-Term Use: Abnormal liver function with focal hepatitis.

Suggested Periodic Examinations While Taking This Drug (at physician's discretion)
Blood cholesterol studies: total cholesterol, HDL and LDL fractions.
Liver function tests before treatment, every 6 weeks during the first 3 months of use, every 8 weeks for the rest of the first year, and at 6-month intervals thereafter.
Complete eye examination at beginning of treatment and at any time that significant change in vision occurs. Ask your physician for guidance.

▷ **While Taking This Drug, Observe the Following**
Foods: Follow a standard low-cholesterol diet.
Beverages: No restrictions. May be taken with milk.
▷   *Alcohol:* No interactions expected. Use sparingly.

Tobacco Smoking: No interactions expected.

▷ *Other Drugs*

astatin may *increase* the effects of
- digoxin (Lanoxin).
- warfarin (Coumadin); more frequent testing of INR (prothrombin time) will be needed.

Simvastatin *taken concurrently* with
- clofibrate (Atromid-S) or other fibrate compounds may result in increased risk of serious muscle toxicity.
- gemfibrozil (Lopid) may alter the absorption and excretion of simvastatin; these drugs should not be taken concurrently.
- cyclosporine (Sandimmune) can result in kidney failure and myopathy.
- niacin may cause an increased frequency of muscle problems (myopathy) when combined with a related medicine (lovastatin). Caution is advised.

The following drug may *decrease* the effects of simvastatin
- cholestyramine (Questran) may reduce absorption of simvastatin; take simvastatin 1 hour before or 4 hours after cholestyramine.

▷ *Driving, Hazardous Activities:* No restrictions.

Aviation Note: No restrictions.

Exposure to Sun: No restrictions.

Discontinuation: Do not stop this drug without your physician's knowledge and guidance. There may be significant increase in blood cholesterol levels following discontinuation of this drug.

SPIRONOLACTONE (speer on oh LAK tohn)

Introduced: 1959   **Prescription:** USA: Yes; Canada: Yes   **Available as Generic:** USA: Yes   **Class:** Diuretic   **Controlled Drug:** USA: No; Canada: No

Brand Names: Alatone, Aldactazide [CD], Aldactone, ✦Apo-Spirozide, ✦Novospiroton, ✦Novospirozine [CD], ✦Sincomen, Spironazide

BENEFITS versus RISKS	
Possible Benefits	*Possible Risks*
EFFECTIVE PREVENTION OF POTASSIUM LOSS when used adjunctively with other diuretics	ABNORMALLY HIGH BLOOD POTASSIUM LEVEL with excessive use
EFFECTIVE DIURETIC IN REFRACTORY CASES OF FLUID RETENTION when used adjunctively with other diuretics	Enlargement of male breast tissue Masculinization effects in women: excessive hair growth, deepening of the voice Rare hepatitis

▷ **Principal Uses**

As a Single Drug Product: Uses currently included in FDA approved labeling: (1) Used to manage congestive heart failure and disorders of the liver and kidney that are accompanied by excessive fluid retention (edema); (2) it is also used in conjunction with other measures to treat high blood pressure where it is advisable to prevent loss of potassium from the body; (3) used to decrease fluid in patients who have failed glucocorticoid treatment and have nephrotic syndrome.

Other (unlabeled) generally accepted uses: (1) May have an adjunctive role in treating acne; (2) can help treat lung problems (bronchopulmonary dysplasia) and slow the disease process; (3) can help precocious puberty in females; (4) eases fluid buildup in premenstrual syndrome; (5) may help women with excessive facial hair growth (hirsutism).

As a Combination Drug Product [CD]: This drug is available in combination with hydrochlorothiazide, a different kind of diuretic that promotes the loss of potassium from the body. Spironolactone is used in this combination to counteract the potassium-wasting effect of the thiazide diuretic.

How This Drug Works: By inhibiting the action of aldosterone (an adrenal gland hormone), this drug prevents the reabsorption of sodium and the excretion of potassium by the kidney. Thus the drug promotes the excretion of sodium (and water with it) and the retention of potassium.

Available Dosage Forms and Strengths
Tablets — 25 mg, 50 mg, 100 mg

▷ **Usual Adult Dosage Range:** For edema: Initially, 100 mg per day in one dose or divided into several doses. The dose is then adjusted according to individual response. The usual maintenance dose is 50 to 200 mg/day, divided into 2 to 4 doses. If response is not adequate after 5 days, a second fluid medicine (diuretic) is added. **Note: Actual dosage and administration schedule must be determined by the physician for each patient individually.**

Conditions Requiring Dosing Adjustments
Liver function: This drug can be a rare cause of liver damage, and patients should be followed closely.
Kidney function: In patients with mild kidney failure, the drug can be given every 12 hours in the usual dose. In moderate kidney failure, spironolactone can be given every 12 to 24 hours in the usual dose. In severe kidney failure, this drug should **not** be given. Spironolactone is contraindicated in acute renal failure and in severe chronic renal compromise.

▷ **Dosing Instructions:** The tablet may be crushed and taken with or following meals to promote absorption of the drug and to reduce stomach irritation.

Usual Duration of Use: Use on a regular schedule for 5 to 10 days usually determines effectiveness in clearing edema, and for 2 to 3 weeks to determine its effect on hypertension. Long-term use (months to years) requires physician supervision and periodic evaluation.

▷ **This Drug Should Not Be Taken If**
• you have had an allergic reaction to it previously.
• you have severely impaired liver or kidney function.
• your kidneys are not making any urine.
• your blood potassium is excessively high (hyperkalemia).
• your creatinine is greater than 2.5 mg/dl.

▷ **Inform Your Physician Before Taking This Drug If**
• you have a history of liver or kidney disease.
• you have diabetes.
• you take: an anticoagulant, antihypertensives, a digitalis preparation, another diuretic, lithium or a potassium preparation.
• you plan to have surgery under general anesthesia in the near future.

Possible Side Effects (natural, expected, and unavoidable drug actions)
   Abnormally high blood potassium levels (42%), abnormally low blood sodium levels (12%), dehydration (17%).

▷ **Possible Adverse Effects** (unusual, unexpected, and infrequent reactions)
   **If any of the following develop, consult your physician promptly for
   guidance.**
   Mild Adverse Effects
   Allergic Reactions: Skin rash, hives, itching, drug fever (see Glossary).
   Headache, dizziness, unsteadiness, weakness, drowsiness, lethargy, confu-
   sion.
   Dry mouth, nausea, vomiting, diarrhea.
   Serious Adverse Effects
   Allergic Reaction: Abnormally low blood platelet count (rare).
   Symptomatic potassium excess: confusion, numbness and tingling in lips and
   extremities, fatigue, weakness, shortness of breath, slow heart rate, low
   blood pressure.
   Masculine pattern of hair growth and deepening of the voice in women.
   Stomach ulceration with bleeding (rare).
   Possible association with decreased white blood cell counts.
   Disruption in the acid–base balance of the body (hyperchloremic or hyper-
   kalemic metabolic acidosis).
   Liver toxicity (hepatitis) (rare).
   Porphyria (rare).
   Decreased platelet counts (rare).
   Systemic lupus-erythematosus-like syndrome (rare).
   Thinning of the bones (rare).

▷ **Possible Effects on Sexual Function**
   Decreased libido (close to 100%); impaired erection or impotence (30%).
   Male breast enlargement and tenderness (gynecomastia) (increases with
   higher doses).
   Female breast enlargement (100% with high doses); altered timing and pattern of menstruation; postmenopausal bleeding. Decreased vaginal secretion.

Possible Effects on Laboratory Tests
   White blood cell count: decreased (one report only).
   Blood platelet count: decreased.
   Prothrombin time: decreased.
   Blood potassium level: increased.
   Blood uric acid level: no effect in some; increased and decreased in others.

CAUTION
   1. Do not take potassium supplements or increase your intake of potas-
      sium-rich foods while taking this drug.
   2. Do not stop this drug abruptly unless abnormally high blood levels of
      potassium develop.
   3. Ordinary doses of aspirin (600 mg) may reverse the diuretic effect of this
      drug. Observe response to this drug combination.
   4. Avoid the excessive use of salt substitutes that contain potassium; these
      are a potential cause of potassium excess.

Precautions for Use

By Infants and Children: Limit the continual use of this drug in children to 1 month. Observe closely for indications of potassium accumulation.

By Those over 60 Years of Age: The natural decline in kidney function may predispose to potassium retention in the body. Watch for indications of potassium excess: slow heart rate, irregular heart rhythms, low blood pressure, confusion, drowsiness. The excessive use of diuretics can cause harmful loss of body water (dehydration), increased viscosity of the blood and an increased tendency of the blood to clot, predisposing to stroke, heart attack or thrombophlebitis.

▷ **Advisability of Use During Pregnancy**

Pregnancy Category: B. See Pregnancy Code at the back of this book.

Animal studies: This drug causes feminization of male rat fetuses.

Human studies: Adequate studies of pregnant women are not available.

This drug should not be used during pregnancy unless a very serious complication of pregnancy occurs for which this drug is significantly beneficial.

Advisability of Use if Breast-Feeding

Presence of this drug in breast milk: A metabolic end product (canrenone) is present.

Avoid drug or refrain from nursing.

Habit-Forming Potential: None.

Effects of Overdosage: Thirst, drowsiness, fatigue, weakness, nausea, vomiting, confusion, irregular heart rhythm, low blood pressure.

Possible Effects of Long-Term Use: Potassium accumulation to abnormally high blood levels. Male breast enlargement.

Suggested Periodic Examinations While Taking This Drug (at physician's discretion)

Measurements of blood sodium, potassium and chloride levels.

Kidney function tests.

▷ **While Taking This Drug, Observe the Following**

Foods: No restrictions. Avoid excessive restriction of salt.

Beverages: No restrictions. May be taken with milk.

▷ *Alcohol:* Use with caution. Alcohol may enhance the drowsiness and the blood-pressure-lowering effect of this drug.

Tobacco Smoking: No interactions expected.

▷ *Other Drugs*

Spironolactone may *increase* the effects of
- digoxin (Lanoxin).

Spironolactone may *decrease* the effects of
- anticoagulants (Coumadin, etc.). Increased frequency of INR (protime) testing is needed.

Spironolactone *taken concurrently* with
- captopril (Capoten) or other ACE inhibitors (see Drug Classes) may cause excessively high blood potassium levels.
- cyclosporine (Sandimmune) may result in very elevated potassium levels.
- digitoxin (Crystodigin) may cause either increased or decreased digitoxin effects (unpredictable).

- lithium (Lithobid, others) may cause accumulation of lithium to toxic levels.
- potassium preparations may cause excessively high blood potassium levels. The following drugs may **decrease** the effects of spironolactone
- aspirin or other NSAIDs (see Drug Classes) may reduce its diuretic effectiveness.

▷ *Driving, Hazardous Activities:* This drug may cause dizziness and drowsiness. Restrict activities as necessary.

Aviation Note: The use of this drug **may be a disqualification** for piloting. Consult a designated Aviation Medical Examiner.

Exposure to Sun: No restrictions.

Discontinuation: With high dosage or prolonged use, it is advisable to withdraw this drug gradually. Ask your physician for guidance.

STAVUDINE (STAV u dine)

Other Names: d4T

Introduced: June 1994   **Prescription:** USA: Yes; Canada: Yes   **Available as Generic:** USA: No; Canada: No   **Class:** anti-AIDS drug   **Controlled Drug:** USA:No

Brand Name: Zerit

BENEFITS versus RISKS	
Possible Benefits	*Possible Risks*
INCREASED CD4 COUNTS IN ADULTS WITH ADVANCED HIV THERAPEUTIC OPTION FOR THOSE INTOLERANT OF AZIDOTHYMIDINE (AZT) OR DIDANOSINE	PERIPHERAL NEUROPATHY Rare pancreatitis (rare)

▷ **Principal Uses**

As a Single Drug Product: Uses currently included in FDA approved labeling: (1) Treatment of advanced HIV in adults who have failed or are intolerant of AZT or didanosine. Other (unlabeled) generally accepted uses: (1) The drug has been used in a small number of children; (2) approval pending for initial use in HIV positive patients; (3) combination therapy may offer a durable increase in CD4 count and decrease in viral load. Many clinicians are now advocates of combination therapy.

How This Drug Works: This drug inhibits HIV reproduction (replication) by: (1) Inhibiting an HIV enzyme (reverse transcriptase) which blocks the ability of the virus to make nuclear material; (2) inhibiting an enzyme (DNA polymerase gamma and beta) which blocks the ability to make DNA in the mitochondria.

Available Dosage Forms and Strengths

Capsules — 15 mg, 20 mg, 30 mg, 40 mg

▷ **Recommended Dosage Ranges (Actual dosage and administration schedule must be determined by the physician for each patient individually.)**

Infants and Children: Safety and efficacy not established.

18 to 60 Years of Age: Patients who weigh 60 kg (132 pounds) or more should be given 40 mg twice daily. Patients who weigh less than 60 kg should be given 30 mg twice daily.

In those who have had to stop this medicine because of peripheral neuropathy (with complete resolution of symptoms):

20 mg twice daily for patients who weigh 60 kg or more.

15 mg twice daily for those who weigh less than 60 kg.

Over 65 Years of Age: This drug has **not** been studied in those over 65.

Conditions Requiring Dosing Adjustments

Liver function: Liver involvement in elimination has not been studied in humans.

Kidney function: Patients with mild kidney compromise (creatinine clearance greater than 50 ml/min) failure may be given the usual weight-adjusted dose for adults. Those with mild to moderate kidney failure (creatinine clearance 26 to 50) should be given one half of the usual weight adjusted dose every 12 hours.

Those with severe kidney compromise (creatinine clearance 10 to 25 ml/min) should be given one half the usual weight adjusted dose every 24 hours.

▷ **Dosing Instructions:** This drug may be taken without regard to food.

Usual Duration of Use:

Use on a regular schedule for several months usually determines effectiveness in slowing AIDS progression and increasing CD4 counts. Long-term use (months to years) requires periodic physician evaluation of response and dosage adjustment. The response as measured by increased CD4 count and decreased viral burden has been durable over several years in many patients.

Possible Advantages of This Drug

More favorable side-effect profile than other nucleoside analogs.

Increased CD4 count over time (may not be sustained).

Favorable profile for combination therapy.

▷ **This Drug Should Not Be Taken If**

- you have had an allergic reaction to any dosage form of it previously.

▷ **Inform Your Physician Before Taking This Drug If**

- you have had peripheral neuropathy caused by other drugs before.
- you have kidney or liver compromise.
- you have had pancreatitis.
- your bone marrow is depressed.
- you have vitamin B12 deficiency or folic acid deficiency.
- you are uncertain of how much stavudine to take or how often to take it.

▷ **Possible Adverse Effects** (unusual, unexpected, and infrequent reactions)

If any of the following develop, consult your physician promptly for guidance.

Mild Adverse Effects

Allergic Reactions: Skin rash.

Nausea and vomiting.

Abdominal pain.

Serious Adverse Effects

Allergic Reactions: Anaphylactoid reactions (rare).

Peripheral neuropathy (15–21%).

Pancreatitis (rare).

Liver toxicity (rare).

Low white blood cell and platelet counts (rare).

▷ **Possible Effects on Sexual Function:**   Rare impotence.

Possible Delayed Adverse Effects: Unknown.

▷ **Adverse Effects That May Mimic Natural Diseases or Disorders**

Increased liver function tests may mimic hepatitis.

Possible Effects on Laboratory Tests

Liver function tests: increased.

Amylase: increased.

Complete blood counts: decreased platelets and white blood cells.

CAUTION

1. Stavudine has **not** been shown to decrease the risk of giving (transmission) HIV to others through sexual contact or blood contamination.
2. Promptly report the development of stomach pain and vomiting; this could indicate pancreatitis.
3. Report development of pain, numbness, tingling or burning in the hands or feet as this may be peripheral neuropathy.

Precautions for Use

By Infants and Children: Safety and effectiveness for those under 18 years of age not established.

By Those over 65 Years of Age: The drug has not been studied in this age group.

▷ **Advisability of Use During Pregnancy**

Pregnancy Category: C. See Pregnancy Code at the back of this book.

Animal studies: Clinical doses in rats have not revealed teratogenicity, however, doses of 399 times those used in humans have resulted in skeletal problems. Increased early rat death has also occurred at 399 times the human dose.

Human studies: Adequate studies of pregnant women are not available.

Ask your doctor for guidance.

Advisability of Use if Breast-Feeding

Presence of this drug in breast milk: Yes.

Refrain from nursing if you are taking this drug.

Habit-Forming Potential: None.

Effects of Overdosage: Adults treated with 12 to 24 times the recommended daily dose revealed no acute toxicity.

Possible Effects of Long-Term Use: Peripheral neuropathy and hepatic toxicity.

Suggested Periodic Examinations While Taking This Drug   (at physician's discretion)

Liver function tests, amylase and complete blood counts.

CD4 or viral load measurement.

▷ **While Taking This Drug, Observe the Following**

Foods: No restrictions.

Beverages: No restrictions.

▷   *Alcohol:* No interactions expected.

Tobacco Smoking: No interactions expected.

▷   *Other Drugs*

Spironolactone *taken concurrently* with

- other drugs such as metronidazole (Flagyl) which can cause peripheral neuropathy should be avoided if possible.

Stavudine may *increase* the effects of

- didanosine (Videx) at specific drug concentration ratios.
- zidovudine (AZT) at specific drug concentration ratios.

Stavudine may *decrease* the effects of

- didanosine (Videx) at specific drug concentration ratios.
- zidovudine (AZT) at specific drug concentration ratios (may only be a phosphorylated intermediate and not of clinical significance).

▷   *Driving, Hazardous Activities:* This drug may cause dizziness. Restrict activities as necessary.

Aviation Note: The use of this drug *may be a disqualification* for piloting. Consult a designated Aviation Medical Examiner.

Exposure to Sun: No restrictions.

Discontinuation: Do not stop this drug without your doctor's knowledge and guidance.

STRONTIUM-89 (STRON tee um)

Introduced: 1993   **Prescription:** USA: Yes; Canada: Yes   **Available as Generic:** USA: No; Canada: No   **Class:** Systemic radionuclide, pain syndrome modifier   **Controlled Drug:** USA: No; Canada: No

Brand Names: Metastron

BENEFITS versus RISKS	
Possible Benefits	*Possible Risks*
EFFECTIVE RELIEF OF PRIMARY OR METASTATIC BONE CANCER PAIN	BONE MARROW TOXICITY (decreased white blood cells and platelets) Transient increase in bone pain

▷ **Principal Uses**

As a Single Drug Product: Uses currently included in FDA approved labeling: (1) Used to treat metastatic bone cancer pain.

Other (unlabeled) generally accepted uses: None at present.

How This Drug Works: This radiopharmaceutical is selectively taken up by areas of bone cancer. Once it accumulates in cancerous areas, it emits radiation directly at the site of the cancer.

Available Dosage Forms and Strengths

Injection — 10.9 to 22.6 mg of strontium in a total of 1 ml of water.

▷ **Recommended Dosage Ranges (Actual dosage and administration schedule must be determined by the physician for each patient individually.)**

Infants and Children: Safety and efficacy for those less than 18 years old not established.

18 to 60 Years of Age: A dose of 4 mCi (148 MBq) is given intravenously over 1 to 2 minutes. The dose may also be calculated using 40 to 60 mcCI/kg. The dose may be repeated at 90 day intervals, if needed.

Over 60 Years of Age: Same as 18 to 60 years of age.

Conditions Requiring Dosing Adjustments

Liver function: Dosing changes in liver compromise do not appear to be needed.

Kidney function: This agent is primarily removed by the kidneys, however, decreases in doses are not presently defined.

▷ **Dosing Instructions:**   You may eat and drink as you normally would. During the first week after injection, Strontium-89 will be present in the blood and the urine. A normal toilet should be used in preference to a urinal.

Usual Duration of Use:

Use of previously prescribed pain medicine will be expected for 7 to 20 days after the injection. A maximum of 20 days after injection has been needed to determine peak effectiveness in controlling bone cancer pain. The dose may be repeated (if blood tests are acceptable) 90 days after the prior dose was given. Consult your physician on a regular basis.

Possible Advantages of This Drug

Effective control of bone cancer pain without the risks or compromise of narcotics.

▷ **This Drug Should Not Be Taken If**

• you have had an allergic reaction to any dosage form of it previously.
• you have cancer which does **not** involve the bone.

▷ **Inform Your Physician Before Taking This Drug If**

• you have a history of low platelets or white blood cell counts.
• you take other drugs which may lower white cells or platelets.
• you do not understand how to appropriately dispose of your urine or vomit.

Possible Side Effects (natural, expected, and unavoidable drug actions)

May cause a calciumlike flushing when it is injected.
May cause a transient (up to 72 hours) increase in bone pain.

▷ **Possible Adverse Effects** (unusual, unexpected, and infrequent reactions)

If any of the following develop, consult your physician promptly for guidance.

Mild Adverse Effects

Allergic Reactions: Chills and fever.
Mild calciumlike flushing on injection.
Transient (up to 72 hours) increase in bone pain.

Serious Adverse Effects

Allergic Reactions: None defined.
Bone marrow toxicity: low white blood cell counts and low platelets.
Very rare bacterial infection of the blood (septicemia) following drug-induced decreases in white blood cells.

▷ **Possible Effects on Sexual Function:**   None reported.

Possible Delayed Adverse Effects: Lowering of white blood cells (recovery in up to six months) and blood platelets (lowest count 12 to 16 weeks after therapy).

Natural Diseases or Disorders That May Be Activated by This Drug
Aplastic anemia.

Possible Effects on Laboratory Tests
White blood cell counts: decreased.
Platelet counts: decreased.

CAUTION
1. Promptly report any signs of infection (lethargy, temperature, sore throat).
2. It may take up to 20 days for this agent to work. Narcotics will need to be continued.
3. Your blood and urine will contain radioactive Strontium for 7 days after injection. Ask you doctor for help on appropriate disposal.
4. This drug is a potential carcinogen.
5. Promptly report any abnormal bleeding or bruising.

Precautions for Use
By Infants and Children: Safety and effectiveness for those under 18 years of age not established.
By Those over 60 Years of Age: Specific changes not presently needed.

▷ **Advisability of Use During Pregnancy**
Pregnancy Category: D. See Pregnancy Code at the back of this book.
Animal studies: Adequate studies evaluating potential to cause birth defects have not been performed.
Human studies: Adequate studies of pregnant women are not available.
This drug may cause fetal harm. Ask your doctor for advice.

Advisability of Use if Breast-Feeding
Presence of this drug in breast milk: This drug acts like calcium and is expected to be present in breast milk.
Avoid drug or refrain from nursing.

Habit-Forming Potential: None.

Effects of Overdosage: May result in acute radiation syndrome with initial nausea and vomiting followed by depressed white cells, platelets and tendency to infections. Careful dosage calculations are indicated as this drug emits beta radiation.

Possible Effects of Long-Term Use: Not indicated for long-term use.

Suggested Periodic Examinations While Taking This Drug (at physician's discretion)
Complete blood counts should be tested once every other week during therapy.

▷ **While Taking This Drug, Observe the Following**
Foods: No restrictions.
Beverages: No restrictions.
▷ *Alcohol:* No interactions expected.
Tobacco Smoking: No interactions expected.
Marijuana Smoking: No interactions expected.

▷ *Other Drugs*
    Strontium-89 *taken concurrently* with
      • medications which lower white blood cells or platelets may result in severe decreases.
▷ *Driving, Hazardous Activities:* This drug may cause a transient increase in bone pain. Restrict activities as necessary.
    Aviation Note: The use of this drug *may be a disqualification* for piloting. Consult a designated Aviation Medical Examiner.
    Exposure to Sun: No restrictions.
    Discontinuation: Dosing may be repeated if blood counts are acceptable.

SUCRALFATE (soo KRAL fayt)

Introduced: 1978   **Prescription:** USA: Yes; Canada: Yes   **Available as Generic:** No   **Class:** Antiulcer, gastrointestinal drug   **Controlled Drug:** USA: No; Canada: No
Brand Names: Carafate, ✦Sulcrate

BENEFITS versus RISKS	
Possible Benefits	*Possible Risks*
EFFECTIVE TREATMENT IN DUODENAL ULCER DISEASE	Constipation
No serious adverse effects	Skin rash, hives, itching
No significant drug interactions	Rare aluminum toxicity in kidney compromise

▷ **Principal Uses**
    As a Single Drug Product: Uses currently included in FDA approved labeling: (1) Treats and prevents recurrence of duodenal ulcer disease in adults and children. It is effective when used alone, but may be used in with antacids for pain relief.
    Other (unlabeled) generally accepted uses: (1) May be useful in treating gastric ulcers in people who can not tolerate other treatment; (2) can reduce the frequency of diarrhea caused by radiation therapy; (3) may have a role as a douche in promoting healing of vaginal ulcerations that are resistant to other measures; (4) can ease the pain and spasms associated with tonsillectomy.

How This Drug Works: This drug promotes ulcer healing in several ways: (1) formation of a protective coating over the ulcer and ulcer margins, preventing further damage; (2) inhibition of the digestive action of pepsin; (3) the stimulation of active healing (tissue repair).

Available Dosage Forms and Strengths
    Tablets — 0.5 gram and 1 gram
    Suspension — 1 gram per 10 ml

▷ **Usual Adult Dosage Range:** 1 gram 4 times/day. **Note: Actual dosage and administration schedule must be determined by the physician for each patient individually.**

Conditions Requiring Dosing Adjustments
    Liver function: Sucralfate is not absorbed.
    Kidney function: Sucralfate is not absorbed.

▷ **Dosing Instructions:** Take with water on an empty stomach at least 1 hour before or 2 hours after each meal and at bedtime. Swallow the tablets whole; do not alter or chew. Take the full course prescribed.

Usual Duration of Use: Use on a regular schedule for 6 to 8 weeks is usually needed for peak effect in promoting the healing of ulcers. Use beyond 8 weeks must be determined by your physician.

▷ **This Drug Should Not Be Taken If**
  • you have had an allergic reaction to it previously.

▷ **Inform Your Physician Before Taking This Drug If**
  • you have chronic constipation.
  • you have chronic kidney failure.
  • you are taking any other drugs at this time.

Possible Side Effects (natural, expected, and unavoidable drug actions)
  Constipation.

▷ **Possible Adverse Effects** (unusual, unexpected, and infrequent reactions)
  If any of the following develop, consult your physician promptly for guidance.
  Mild Adverse Effects
  Allergic Reactions: Skin rash, hives, itching.
  Dizziness, light-headedness, drowsiness (uncommon).
  Dry mouth, indigestion, nausea, cramping, diarrhea.
  Serious Adverse Effects
  Increased risk of aluminum toxicity (seizures, jerks, and encephalopathy) with patients in end-stage kidney failure.
  Bezoar (a clumping of food) formation in the esophagus or proximal stomach

▷ **Possible Effects on Sexual Function:** None reported.

Possible Effects on Laboratory Tests
  None reported.

CAUTION
  1. If antacids are needed to relieve ulcer pain, do not take them within half an hour before or 2 hours after the dose of sucralfate.
  2. This drug may impair the absorption of other drugs if they are taken close together. It is advisable to avoid taking any other drugs within 2 hours of taking sucralfate. This applies especially to cimetidine (Tagamet), phenytoin (Dilantin) and tetracyclines.

▷ **Advisability of Use During Pregnancy**
  Pregnancy Category: B. See Pregnancy Code at the back of this book.
  Animal studies: No birth defects reported in mouse, rat and rabbit studies.
  Human studies: Adequate studies of pregnant women are not available.
  It should be used only if clearly needed. Ask your physician for guidance.

Advisability of Use if Breast-Feeding
  Presence of this drug in breast milk: Unknown.
  Watch nursing infant closely and stop drug or nursing if adverse effects develop.

Habit-Forming Potential: None.

Effects of Overdosage: Nausea, stomach cramping, possible diarrhea.

Possible Effects of Long-Term Use: Deficiencies of vitamins A, D, E and K due to impaired absorption from the intestine.

Suggested Periodic Examinations While Taking This Drug (at physician's discretion)
None required.

▷ **While Taking This Drug, Observe the Following**
Foods: No restrictions. Follow diet prescribed by your physician.
Beverages: No restrictions. This drug is preferably taken with water.
▷ *Alcohol:* No interactions with drug expected. However, alcohol is best avoided because of its irritant effect on the stomach.
Tobacco Smoking: Nicotine can delay ulcer healing and reduce the effectiveness of this drug. Avoid all forms of tobacco.
▷ *Other Drugs*
Sucralfate may **decrease** the effects of
  • cimetidine (Tagamet).
  • ciprofloxacin (Cipro).
  • digoxin (Lanoxin).
  • enoxacin (Penetrex).
  • fleroxacin (Megalone).
  • ketoconazole (Nizoral).
  • lomefloxacin (Maxaquin).
  • norfloxacin (Noroxin).
  • ofloxacin (Floxin).
  • phenytoin (Dilantin, etc.).
  • quinidine (Quinaglute).
  • tetracycline (Achromycin, Tetracyn, etc.).
  • warfarin (Coumadin, etc.), and reduce its anticoagulant effect. Increased frequency of INR testing (protime) is needed.
▷ *Driving, Hazardous Activities:* This drug may cause dizziness or drowsiness. Restrict activities as necessary.
Aviation Note: The use of this drug **may be a disqualification** for piloting. Consult a designated Aviation Medical Examiner.
Exposure to Sun: No restrictions.

SULFAMETHOXAZOLE (sul fa meth OX a zohl)

Introduced: 1961   **Prescription:** USA: Yes; Canada: Yes   **Available as Generic:** Yes   **Class:** Anti-infective, sulfonamides   **Controlled Drug:** USA: No; Canada: No

Brand Names: ✦Apo-Sulfamethoxazole, ✦Apo-Sulfatrim [CD], ✦Apo-Sulfatrim DS [CD], Azo Gantanol [CD], Bactrim [CD], Bactrim DS [CD], Bethaprim [CD], Comoxol [CD], Cotrim [CD], Gantanol, ✦Novo-Trimel [CD], ✦Novo-Trimel DS [CD], ✦Nu-Cotrimox, ✦Protrin [CD], ✦Protrin DF [CD], ✦Roubac [CD], Septra [CD], Septra DS [CD], Sulfatrim [CD], ✦Uro Gantanol [CD], Uroplus DS [CD], Uroplus SS [CD], Vagitrol

BENEFITS versus RISKS	
Possible Benefits	*Possible Risks*
EFFECTIVE ANTIMICROBIAL ACTION against susceptible bacteria and protozoa Effective adjunctive prevention and treatment of Pneumocystis carinii pneumonia (AIDS-related)	Allergic reactions: mild to severe skin reactions, anaphylaxis, myocarditis Rare blood cell disorders: aplastic anemia, hemolytic anemia, abnormally low white cell and platelet counts Low blood sugar Drug-induced liver damage Drug-induced kidney damage

▷ **Principal Uses**

As a Single Drug Product: Uses currently included in FDA approved labeling: (1) Used to treat a variety of bacterial and protozoal infections: chancroid, cystitis and other infections of the urinary tract. **Should not be used to treat group A Streptococcal infections.**

Other (unlabeled) generally accepted uses: (1) Chlamydia infections; (2) combination therapy of resistant Mycobacterium kansaii infections.

As a Combination Drug Product [CD]: This drug is available in combination with phenazopyridine, an analgesic that relieves discomfort associated with acute urethral infections. This drug is also available in combination with another antibacterial drug—trimethoprim; in some countries this combination is given the generic name co-trimoxazole. This combination is quite effective in the treatment of certain types of middle ear infection, bronchitis, pneumonia and certain infections of the intestinal tract and urinary tract. It is now used as primary prevention and treatment for Pneumocystis carinii pneumonia associated with AIDS.

How This Drug Works: This drug prevents the growth and multiplication of susceptible bacteria by interfering with their formation of folic acid, an essential nutrient.

Available Dosage Forms and Strengths

Oral suspension — 500 mg per 5-ml

Tablets — 500 mg, 1 gram

▷ **Usual Adult Dosage Range:**   Initially, 2 grams; then 1 gram every 8 to 12 hours, depending upon the severity of the infection. The total daily dosage should not exceed 3 grams. **Note: Actual dosage and administration schedule must be determined by the physician for each patient individually.**

Conditions Requiring Dosing Adjustments

Liver function: Patients with compromised livers should be followed closely; however, specific guidelines for decreasing doses are not defined.

Kidney function: The dose should be decreased in patients with compromised kidneys. In moderate failure, 50% of the usual dose can be given at the normal time.

▷ **Dosing Instructions:**   The tablet may be crushed and is preferably taken on an empty stomach, 1 hour before or 2 hours after eating. However, it may be taken with or following food to reduce stomach irritation. Be certain to drink liberal amounts of water while taking this medicine if you are not restricted from doing so.

Usual Duration of Use: Use on a regular schedule for 4 to 7 days usually determines effectiveness in controlling responsive infections. Treatment should be continued until the patient is free of symptoms for 48 hours. Limit treatment to no more than 14 days if possible.

Currently a "Drug of Choice"
(when combined with trimethoprim) for preventing pneumonia (due to Pneumocystis carinii) in patients with AIDS.

▷ **This Drug Should Not Be Taken If**
- you are allergic to **any** sulfonamide drug (see Drug Classes).
- you are in the last month of pregnancy.
- you are breast-feeding your infant.

▷ **Inform Your Physician Before Taking This Drug If**
- you are allergic to any sulfonamide derivative: acetazolamide, thiazide diuretics, sulfonylurea antidiabetics (see Drug Classes).
- you are allergic by nature: history of hay fever, asthma, hives, eczema.
- you have impaired liver or kidney function.
- you have a personal or family history of porphyria.
- you have had a drug-induced blood cell or bone marrow disorder.
- you have a G6PD deficiency in your red blood cells (ask your doctor).
- you currently take any oral anticoagulant, antidiabetic drug or phenytoin.
- you plan to have surgery under pentothal anesthesia while taking this drug.

Possible Side Effects (natural, expected, and unavoidable drug actions)
Brownish coloration of the urine, of no significance.
Superinfections, bacterial or fungal (see Glossary).

▷ **Possible Adverse Effects** (unusual, unexpected, and infrequent reactions)
If any of the following develop, consult your physician promptly for guidance.
Mild Adverse Effects
Allergic Reactions: Skin rashes, hives, itching, localized swellings, reddened eyes.
Myopia (occasional).
Headache, dizziness, unsteadiness, ringing in the ears.
Loss of appetite, irritation of the mouth and tongue, nausea, vomiting, abdominal pain, diarrhea.
Serious Adverse Effects
Allergic Reactions: Drug fever (see Glossary), swollen glands, painful joints, anaphylaxis (see Glossary). Allergic reaction in the heart muscle (myocarditis), allergic pneumonitis, allergic hepatitis. Severe skin reactions.
Idiosyncratic Reaction: Hemolytic anemia (see Glossary).
Bone marrow depression (see Glossary): fatigue, weakness, fever, sore throat, abnormal bleeding or bruising.
Pancreatitis.
Kidney damage: bloody or cloudy urine, reduced urine volume.
Psychotic reactions, hallucinations, seizures, hearing loss, peripheral neuropathy (see Glossary).
Severe hypoglycemia (rare).
Methemoglobinemia (rare).
Drug-induced lupus erythematosus (rare).
Problems in blood clotting (hypoprothrombinemia) (rare).

▷ **Possible Effects on Sexual Function:** None reported.

▷ **Adverse Effects That May Mimic Natural Diseases or Disorders**
Liver reactions may suggest viral hepatitis.
Lung reactions may suggest an infectious pneumonia.

Natural Diseases or Disorders That May Be Activated by This Drug
Goiter, acute intermittent porphyria, polyarteritis nodosa, systemic lupus erythematosus (questionable).

Possible Effects on Laboratory Tests
Complete blood cell counts: decreased red cells, hemoglobin, white cells and platelets; increased eosinophils (allergic reaction).
Prothrombin time: increased (when taken concurrently with warfarin).
Liver function tests: increased liver enzymes (ALT/GPT, AST/GOT and alkaline phosphatase), increased bilirubin.

CAUTION
1. A large intake of water (up to 2 quarts daily) is necessary to ensure an adequate volume of urine.
2. Shake liquid dosage forms thoroughly before measuring each dose.

Precautions for Use
By Infants and Children: This drug should not be used in infants under 2 months of age.
By Those over 60 Years of Age: Small doses taken at longer intervals often achieve adequate blood and tissue drug levels. Observe for the development of reduced urine volume, fever, sore throat, abnormal bleeding or bruising or skin irritation with itching, particularly in the anal or genital regions.

▷ **Advisability of Use During Pregnancy**
Pregnancy Category: C, however, the drug **SHOULD NOT BE TAKEN (**is contraindicated) near the time of the birth of the baby. See Pregnancy Code at the back of this book.
Animal studies: Cleft palate and skeletal birth defects reported in mice and rats.
Human studies: No increase in birth defects reported in 4584 exposures to various sulfonamides during pregnancy.
Avoid use of drug during the last month of pregnancy because of possible adverse effects on the newborn infant.

Advisability of Use if Breast-Feeding
Presence of this drug in breast milk: Yes.
Avoid drug or refrain from nursing.

Habit-Forming Potential: None.

Effects of Overdosage: Headache, dizziness, nausea, vomiting, abdominal cramping, toxic fever, coma, jaundice, kidney failure.

Possible Effects of Long-Term Use: Superinfections, bacterial or fungal. Development of goiter, with or without hypothyroidism. Excessive loss of vitamin C via urine.

Suggested Periodic Examinations While Taking This Drug (at physician's discretion)
Complete blood cell counts, weekly for the first 8 weeks.
Urine analysis weekly.
Liver and kidney function tests.

▷ **While Taking This Drug, Observe the Following**
Foods: No restrictions.
Beverages: No restrictions. May be taken with milk.
▷ *Alcohol:* Use caution. Sulfonamide drugs can increase the intoxicating effects of alcohol.
Tobacco Smoking: No interactions expected.
▷ *Other Drugs*
Sulfamethoxazole may *increase* the effects of
- amantadine (Symmetrel) and cause abnormal heart rhythms and CNS stimulation (confusion, disorientation).
- anticoagulants (Coumadin, etc.), and increase the risk of bleeding.
- methotrexate (Mexate) and cause severe blood toxicity.
- sulfonylureas (see Drug Classes) or other oral hypoglycemic agents, and increase the risk of excessively low blood sugar (hypoglycemia).
- warfarin (Coumadin) and result in bleeding.
- zidovudine (AZT) and result in zidovudine toxicity.
Sulfamethoxazole may *decrease* the effects of
- birth control pills (oral contraceptives).
- cyclosporine (Sandimmune), and reduce its immunosuppressive effect.
- penicillins (see Drug Classes).
▷ *Driving, Hazardous Activities:* This drug may cause dizziness. Restrict activities as necessary.
Aviation Note: The use of this drug *may be a disqualification* for piloting. Consult a designated Aviation Medical Examiner.
Exposure to Sun: Use caution. Some sulfonamide drugs can cause photosensitivity (see Glossary).

SULFASALAZINE (sul fa SAL a zeen)

Introduced: 1949   **Prescription:** USA: Yes; Canada: Yes   **Available as Generic:** USA: Yes; Canada: No   **Class:** Bowel anti-inflammatory, sulfonamides   **Controlled Drug:** USA: No; Canada: No

Brand Names: Azaline, Azulfidine, Azulfidine EN-tabs, ✦PMS Sulfasalazine, ✦PMS Sulfasalazine E.C., ✦Salazopyrin, ✦Salazopyrin EN, ✦SAS-Enema, ✦SAS Enteric-500, SAS-500

BENEFITS versus RISKS	
Possible Benefits	*Possible Risks*
EFFECTIVE SUPPRESSION OF INFLAMMATORY BOWEL DISEASE	Allergic reactions: mild to severe skin reactions
SYMPTOMATIC RELIEF IN TREATMENT OF REGIONAL ENTERITIS AND ULCERATIVE COLITIS	Rare blood cell disorders: aplastic anemia, hemolytic anemia, abnormally low white cell and platelet counts
	Drug-induced liver damage
	Drug-induced kidney damage
	Rare seizures

▷ **Principal Uses**

   As a Single Drug Product: Uses currently included in FDA approved labeling: (1) Treats inflammatory disease of the lower intestinal tract: regional enteritis (Crohn's disease) and ulcerative colitis. It is usually taken by mouth, but may also be used in retention enemas.

   Other (unlabeled) generally accepted uses: (1) Short-term use in therapy of ankylosing spondylitis; (2) treatment of mild to moderate psoriasis; (3) may help juvenile rheumatoid arthritis.

How This Drug Works: Possible method of this drug's action is an anti-inflammatory action that suppresses the formation of prostaglandins (and related compounds), tissue substances that induce inflammation, tissue destruction and diarrhea.

Available Dosage Forms and Strengths

   Oral suspension — 250 mg per 5-ml
   Tablets — 500 mg
   Tablets, enteric-coated — 500 mg

▷ **Usual Adult Dosage Range:**   Ulcerative colitis: Initially, 1 to 2 grams every 6 to 8 hours until symptoms are adequately controlled. For maintenance, 500 mg/6 hours. The total daily dosage should not exceed 12 grams. If diarrhea happens, the dose is often decreased to the earlier dose which worked and did not cause diarrhea. Rheumatoid arthritis: One researcher used 0.5 mg a day to start and then increased the dose by 0.5 grams a day steps at one week intervals. **Note: Actual dosage and administration schedule must be determined by the physician for each patient individually.**

Conditions Requiring Dosing Adjustments

   Liver function: It can be a cause of liver damage, and patients should be followed closely.

   Kidney function: Empiric decreases in doses should be considered. It should be used with caution in kidney compromise.

▷ **Dosing Instructions:**   Preferably taken with 8 ounces of water on an empty stomach, 1 hour before or 2 hours after eating. However, it may be taken with or following food to reduce stomach irritation. Intervals between doses (day and night) should be no longer than 8 hours. The regular tablet may be crushed for administration; the enteric-coated tablet should be swallowed whole without alteration.

Usual Duration of Use: Use on a regular schedule for 1 to 3 weeks usually determines effectiveness in controlling the symptoms of regional enteritis or ulcerative colitis. Long-term use (months to years) requires physician supervision.

▷ **This Drug Should Not Be Taken If**

   • you are allergic to *any* sulfonamide drug (see Drug Classes), or to aspirin (or other salicylates).
   • you are in the last month of pregnancy.
   • it has been prescribed for an infant less than 2 years old.
   • you have a urinary or intestinal obstruction or porphyria.
   • you are breast-feeding.

▷ **Inform Your Physician Before Taking This Drug If**
  • you are allergic to any sulfonamide: acetazolamide, thiazide diuretics or sulfonylurea antidiabetics (see Drug Classes).
  • you are allergic by nature: history of hay fever, asthma, hives, eczema.
  • you have asthma.
  • you have impaired liver or kidney function.
  • you have a G6PD deficiency.
  • you have a personal or family history of porphyria.
  • you have had a drug-induced blood cell or bone marrow disorder.
  • you currently take any oral anticoagulant, antidiabetic drug or phenytoin.
  • you plan to have surgery under pentothal anesthesia soon.

Possible Side Effects (natural, expected, and unavoidable drug actions)
  Brownish coloration of the urine, of no significance.
  Superinfections, bacterial or fungal (see Glossary).

▷ **Possible Adverse Effects** (unusual, unexpected, and infrequent reactions)
  If any of the following develop, consult your physician promptly for guidance.
  Mild Adverse Effects
  Allergic Reactions: Skin rashes, hives, itching.
  Headache, dizziness.
  Discoloration of contact lenses.
  Ringing in the ears.
  Loss of appetite, irritation of the mouth and tongue, nausea, vomiting, abdominal pain, diarrhea.
  Skin pigmentation.
  Taste disorders.
  Serious Adverse Effects
  Allergic Reactions: Drug fever (see Glossary), swollen glands, painful joints, anaphylaxis (see Glossary). Allergic pneumonitis, allergic hepatitis. Severe skin reactions (Stevens-Johnson syndrome or toxic epidermal necrolysis).
  Idiosyncratic Reaction: Hemolytic anemia (see Glossary).
  Bone marrow depression (see Glossary): fatigue, weakness, fever, sore throat, abnormal bleeding or bruising.
  Pancreatitis.
  Folic acid deficiency.
  Lupus erythematosus (drug-induced) (rare).
  Kidney damage: bloody or cloudy urine, reduced urine volume.
  Peripheral neuropathy (see Glossary).
  Myopathy (rare).
  Inflammation of the tissue around the heart (pericarditis).

▷ **Possible Effects on Sexual Function:**   Decreased production of sperm, reversible infertility.

▷ **Adverse Effects That May Mimic Natural Diseases or Disorders**
  Liver reactions may suggest viral hepatitis.
  Lung reactions may suggest an infectious pneumonia.

Natural Diseases or Disorders That May Be Activated by This Drug
  Goiter, acute intermittent porphyria.

Possible Effects on Laboratory Tests
  Complete blood cell counts: decreased red cells, hemoglobin, white cells and platelets; increased eosinophils (allergic reaction).

Liver function tests: increased liver enzymes (ALT/GPT, AST/GOT and alkaline phosphatase), increased bilirubin.

Sperm count: decreased; abnormal sperm common; effects reversible on discontinuation of drug.

CAUTION

1. A large intake of water (up to 2 quarts daily) is necessary to ensure an adequate volume of urine.
2. Shake liquid dosage forms thoroughly before measuring each dose.

Precautions for Use

By Infants and Children: Safety and effectiveness for those under 2 years of age are not established.

By Those over 60 Years of Age: Observe for the development of reduced urine volume, fever, sore throat, abnormal bleeding or bruising or skin irritation with itching, particularly in the anal or genital regions.

▷ **Advisability of Use During Pregnancy**

Pregnancy Category: B, however, this drug should **not** be used near the time of the birth of the baby. See Pregnancy Code at the back of this book.

Animal studies: Cleft palate and skeletal birth defects due to sulfonamides reported in mice and rats.

Human studies: No increase in birth defects reported in 4584 exposures to various sulfonamides during pregnancy.

Avoid use of drug during the last month of pregnancy because of possible adverse effects on the newborn infant.

Advisability of Use if Breast-Feeding

Presence of this drug in breast milk: Yes.

Avoid drug or refrain from nursing.

Habit-Forming Potential: None.

Effects of Overdosage: Headache, dizziness, nausea, vomiting, abdominal cramping, toxic fever, coma, jaundice, kidney failure.

Possible Effects of Long-Term Use: Development of goiter, with or without hypothyroidism. An orange-yellow discoloration of the skin has been reported. This is not jaundice.

Suggested Periodic Examinations While Taking This Drug (at physician's discretion)

Complete blood cell counts, weekly for the first 8 weeks.

Urine analysis weekly.

Liver and kidney function tests.

▷ **While Taking This Drug, Observe the Following**

Foods: No restrictions. Follow prescribed diet.

Beverages: No restrictions. May be taken with milk.

▷ *Alcohol:* Use caution. Sulfonamide drugs can increase the intoxicating effects of alcohol.

Tobacco Smoking: No interactions expected.

▷ *Other Drugs*

Sulfasalazine may ***increase*** the effects of

- anticoagulants (Coumadin, etc.), and increase the risk of bleeding. More frequent INR testing is needed.
- sulfonylureas or other oral hypoglycemic agents (see Drug Classes), and increase the risk of hypoglycemia.

Sulfasalazine may *decrease* the effects of
- digoxin (Lanoxin).

Sulfasalazine *taken concurrently* with
- ampicillin and perhaps other penicillins may result in lower than expected therapeutic benefit from sulfasalazine.
- calcium supplements (gluconate) may result in decreased therapeutic benefit from sulfasalazine.
- iron salts or calcium may decrease sulfasalazine benefits.
- some barbiturates (see Drug Classes) may result in decreased sulfasalazine therapeutic benefits.

▷ *Driving, Hazardous Activities:* This drug may cause dizziness. Restrict activities as necessary.

Aviation Note: The use of this drug *may be a disqualification* for piloting. Consult a designated Aviation Medical Examiner.

Exposure to Sun: Use caution. Some sulfonamide drugs can cause photosensitivity (see Glossary).

SULFISOXAZOLE (sul fi SOX a zohl)

Introduced: 1949   **Prescription:** USA: Yes; Canada: Yes   **Available as Generic:** Yes   **Class:** Anti-infective, sulfonamides   **Controlled Drug:** USA: No; Canada: No

Brand Names: Azo Gantrisin [CD], Azo-Sulfisoxazole, Eryzole [CD], Gantrisin, Gulfasin, Lipo Gantrisin, ✦Novosoxazole, Pediazole [CD], SK-Soxazole, Sulfalar

BENEFITS versus RISKS	
Possible Benefits	*Possible Risks*
EFFECTIVE ANTIMICROBIAL ACTION against susceptible bacteria and protozoa	Allergic reactions: mild to severe skin reactions, anaphylaxis
	Rare blood cell disorders: aplastic anemia, hemolytic anemia, abnormally low white cell and platelet counts
	Drug-induced liver damage
	Drug-induced kidney damage

▷ **Principal Uses**

As a Single Drug Product: Uses currently included in FDA approved labeling: (1) Used to treat a variety of bacterial and protozoal infections: ear infections, malaria, nocardia, toxoplasmosis and trachoma. It is most often used to treat urinary tract infections. Other (unlabeled) generally accepted uses: (1) Treats meningitis caused by Haemophilus influenzae; (2) has a role in chlamydia infections; (3) may help prevent ear infections when used in long-term therapy; (4) can have a role in preventing plague.

As a Combination Drug Product [CD]: This drug is available in combination with phenazopyridine, an analgesic drug that relieves the discomfort associated with acute infections of the urinary bladder and urethra. This combination provides early symptomatic relief while the underlying infection is being eradicated.

How This Drug Works: This drug prevents the growth and multiplication of susceptible bacteria by interfering with their formation of folic acid, an essential nutrient.

Available Dosage Forms and Strengths

Emulsion, prolonged-action — 1 gram per 5-ml

Eye drops — 4%

Eye ointment — 4%

Injection — 400 mg per ml

Pediatric suspension — 500 mg per 5-ml

Syrup — 500 mg per 5-ml

Tablets — 500 mg

▷ **Usual Adult Dosage Range:** Initially, 2 to 4 grams; then 750 to 1500 mg (1.5 grams) every 4 hours, or 1 to 2 grams every 6 hours, depending upon the severity of the infection. The total daily dosage should not exceed 12 grams. **Note: Actual dosage and administration schedule must be determined by the physician for each patient individually.**

Conditions Requiring Dosing Adjustments

Liver function: This drug can be a rare cause of liver damage, and patients should be followed closely.

Kidney function: In patients with mild to moderate kidney failure, sulfasoxazole can be given every 6 hours in the usual dose. In moderate to severe kidney failure, it can be given every 12 to 24 hours in the usual dose. In severe kidney failure, it can be given once a day. Increased elimination of this drug may be seen in patients with alkaline urine. It should be used with caution in renal compromise.

▷ **Dosing Instructions:** Preferably taken with 8 ounces of water on an empty stomach, 1 hour before or 2 hours after eating. However, it may be taken with or following food to reduce stomach irritation. The tablet may be crushed for administration.

Usual Duration of Use: Use on a regular schedule for 7 to 10 days usually determines effectiveness in controlling responsive infections. Treatment should be continued until the patient is free of symptoms for 48 hours. Limit treatment to no more than 14 days if possible.

▷ **This Drug Should Not Be Taken If**
- you are allergic to *any* sulfonamide drug (see Drug Classes).
- you are in the last month of pregnancy.
- you are breast-feeding your infant.
- it has been prescribed for an infant less than 2 months old (unless congenital toxoplasmosis is being treated).

▷ **Inform Your Physician Before Taking This Drug If**
- you are allergic to any sulfonamide: acetazolamide, thiazide diuretics, sulfonylurea antidiabetic drugs (see Drug Classes).
- you are allergic by nature: history of hay fever, asthma, hives, eczema.
- you have impaired liver or kidney function.
- you have a low glucose-6-phosphate dehydrogenase.
- you have a personal or family history of porphyria.

- you have had a drug-induced blood cell or bone marrow disorder.
- you currently take any oral anticoagulant, antidiabetic drug or phenytoin.
- you plan to have surgery under pentothal anesthesia while taking this drug.

Possible Side Effects (natural, expected, and unavoidable drug actions)

Brownish coloration of the urine, of no significance.

Superinfections, bacterial or fungal (see Glossary).

▷ **Possible Adverse Effects** (unusual, unexpected, and infrequent reactions)

If any of the following develop, consult your physician promptly for guidance.

Mild Adverse Effects

Allergic Reactions: Skin rashes, hives, itching, localized swellings, reddened eyes.

Headache, dizziness, unsteadiness, ringing in the ears.

Loss of appetite, irritation of the mouth and tongue, nausea, vomiting, abdominal pain, diarrhea.

Serious Adverse Effects

Allergic Reactions: Drug fever (see Glossary), swollen glands, painful joints, anaphylaxis (see Glossary). Allergic hepatitis. Severe skin reactions.

Idiosyncratic Reaction: Hemolytic anemia (see Glossary).

Bone marrow depression (see Glossary): fatigue, weakness, fever, sore throat, abnormal bleeding or bruising.

Kidney damage: bloody or cloudy urine, reduced urine volume.

Peripheral neuropathy (see Glossary).

Liver damage (rare).

Drug-induced parotitis (rare).

Drug-induced systemic lupus erythematosus (rare).

Drug-induced disulfiram reaction.

▷ **Possible Effects on Sexual Function:**   None reported.

▷ **Adverse Effects That May Mimic Natural Diseases or Disorders**

Liver reactions may suggest viral hepatitis.

Natural Diseases or Disorders That May Be Activated by This Drug

Goiter, acute intermittent porphyria.

Possible Effects on Laboratory Tests

Complete blood cell counts: decreased red cells, hemoglobin, white cells and platelets; increased eosinophils (allergic reaction).

Blood lupus erythematosus (LE) cells: positive.

Blood amylase and lipase levels: increased (pancreatitis).

Liver function tests: increased liver enzymes (ALT/GPT, AST/GOT and alkaline phosphatase), increased bilirubin.

CAUTION

1. A large intake of water (up to 2 quarts daily) is necessary to ensure an adequate volume of urine.
2. Shake liquid dosage forms thoroughly before measuring each dose.

Precautions for Use

By Infants and Children: This drug should not be used in infants under 2 months of age.

By Those over 60 Years of Age: Small doses taken at longer intervals often achieve adequate blood and tissue drug levels. Watch for development of reduced urine volume, fever, sore throat, abnormal bleeding or bruising or skin irritation with itching, particularly in the anal or genital regions.

▷ **Advisability of Use During Pregnancy**
Pregnancy Category: C. See Pregnancy Code at the back of this book.
Animal studies: Cleft palate and skeletal birth defects due to sulfonamides reported in mice and rats.
Human studies: No increase in birth defects reported in 4287 exposures to this drug during pregnancy.
Avoid use of drug during the last three months of pregnancy because of possible adverse effects on the newborn infant.

Advisability of Use if Breast-Feeding
Presence of this drug in breast milk: Yes.
Avoid drug or refrain from nursing.

Habit-Forming Potential: None.

Effects of Overdosage: Headache, dizziness, nausea, vomiting, abdominal cramping, toxic fever, coma, jaundice, kidney failure.

Possible Effects of Long-Term Use: Superinfections, bacterial or fungal. Development of goiter, with or without hypothyroidism. Excessive loss of vitamin C via urine.

Suggested Periodic Examinations While Taking This Drug (at physician's discretion)
Complete blood cell counts, weekly for the first 8 weeks.
Urine analysis weekly.
Liver and kidney function tests.

▷ **While Taking This Drug, Observe the Following**
Foods: No restrictions.
Beverages: No restrictions. May be taken with milk.
▷ *Alcohol:* Use caution. Sulfonamide drugs can increase the intoxicating effects of alcohol.
Tobacco Smoking: No interactions expected.
▷ *Other Drugs*
Sulfisoxazole may *increase* the effects of
• anticoagulants (Coumadin, etc.), and increase the risk of bleeding. More frequent INR testing (protime) is needed. Ongoing warfarin doses should be decided based on laboratory results.
• methotrexate (Mexate), and cause serious blood toxicity.
• sulfonylureas (see Drug Class Section), or other oral hypoglycemic agents and increase the risk of hypoglycemia.
Sulfisoxazole may *decrease* the effects of
• birth control pills (oral contraceptives).
• penicillins (see Drug Classes).
▷ *Driving, Hazardous Activities:* This drug may cause dizziness. Restrict activities as necessary.
Aviation Note: The use of this drug *may be a disqualification* for piloting. Consult a designated Aviation Medical Examiner.
Exposure to Sun: Use caution. Some sulfonamide drugs cause photosensitivity (see Glossary).

SULINDAC (sul IN dak)

Introduced: 1976   **Prescription:** USA: Yes; Canada: Yes   **Available as Generic:** USA: Yes; Canada: Yes   **Class:** analgesic, mild; NSAID   **Controlled Drug:** USA: No; Canada: No
Brand Name: , ✦Apo-Sulin, Clinoril, Novo-Sundac

BENEFITS versus RISKS	
Possible Benefits	*Possible Risks*
EFFECTIVE RELIEF OF MILD TO MODERATE PAIN AND INFLAMMATION	Gastrointestinal pain, ulceration, bleeding (rare) Rare liver damage Rare kidney damage Rare bone marrow depression (aplastic anemia) Rare auditory and visual hallucinations Rare pancreatitis

Please see the acetic acid nonsteroidal anti-inflammatory drug profile for further information.

SUMATRIPTAN (soo ma TRIP tan)

Introduced: 1993   **Prescription:** USA: Yes; Canada: Yes   **Available as Generic:** USA: No; Canada: No   **Class:** Antimigraine drug, serotonin 1 receptor agonist   **Controlled Drug:** USA: No; Canada: No
Brand Name: Imitrex

BENEFITS versus RISKS	
Possible Benefits	*Possible Risks*
RAPID AND EFFECTIVE RELIEF OR PREVENTION OF MIGRAINE GENERALLY WELL TOLERATED Relieves photophobia (light sensitivity) Relieves phonophobia (sound sensitivity) Relieves nausea and vomiting	Fainting (very rare) Rare myocardial infarction (probably secondary to coronary vasospasm) Rare serious atrial and ventricular arrhythmias

▷ **Principal Uses**

 As a Single Drug Product: Uses currently included in FDA approved labeling: (1) Acute treatment of migraine with or without aura in adults.

  Other (unlabeled) generally accepted uses: (1) Treatment of cluster headache; (2) may have a role in post-traumatic headaches.

 How This Drug Works: Sumatriptan acts on blood vessels to cause vasoconstriction (shrinking of the blood vessels). This relieves swelling thought to be the cause of migraine. The drug binds to a receptor arteries such as the basilar artery and in vasculature (blood vessels) associated with the dura mater (part of the lining of the brain).

Available Dosage Forms and Strengths

Sumatriptan succinate (Imitrex) injection

SELFdose system kit which has two syringes with 6 mg in 0.5 ml of liquid in a 1 ml size syringe, a dosing device and instructions.

Unit-of-use syringes with 6 mg in 0.5 ml of liquid in a 1 ml syringe packaged in a carton containing two syringes.

6 mg single-dose vials with 0.5 ml of liquid in a 2 ml vial. These vials are packaged in cartons of 5 vials.

All of the liquid in these products should be a colorless to pale yellow, clear solution. Particles or precipitates should never be present.

Tablets — 25 mg

How To Store

Keep out of reach of children. Store at room temperature in a room where the temperature will not exceed 86 degrees. Keep away from heat and light.

▷ **Recommended Dosage Ranges (Actual dosage and administration schedule must be determined by the physician for each patient individually.)**

Infants and Children: The safety and effectiveness in pediatrics have **not** been determined.

18 to 60 Years of Age: Subcutaneous: Maximum adult dose is 6 mg. The dose should be given as soon as possible after the symptoms of acute migraine are recognized. Controlled clinical trials have failed to demonstrate a benefit of repeat injections if the initial injection is unsuccessful. If symptoms return, a second 6 mg injection may be given 12 hours after the first injection was given. If side effects occur, use the lowest dose in the approved dosage range that is effective for you.

Oral: 25 milligrams taken as soon as headache pain start. If the symptoms are not improved after two hours, a second 25 mg may be taken. Maximum single oral dose is 100 mg, but there is presently no evidence that doses this large provide greater relief of symptoms.

Over 65 Years of Age: Safety and effectiveness **not** evaluated in this age group. Since declines in renal and hepatic function and coronary artery disease are more common in those over 65, the possibility of an increase in side effects would be expected.

Conditions Requiring Dosing Adjustments

Liver function: The effect of liver impairment on sumatriptan has not been specifically studied, and dosage or interval adjustments have not been established.

Kidney function: Presently, there are no determined requirements for dosage adjustment in renal compromise.

▷ **Dosing Instructions:** This drug must be given subcutaneously, **not intravenously**. Intravenous injection must be avoided because of its potential to cause coronary vasospasm (constriction of the blood vessels which supply the heart). This medicine should be colorless to pale yellow and clear. Be certain to check the medicine before injecting it. Particles should never be present. There is extensive information on self-injection available from your doctor or pharmacist. The first dose is usually given in the doctor's office. The tablet form may take more than an hour to work. The tablet form may be taken with food.

Usual Duration of Use: The maximum dose is two 6-mg doses (injections) in 24 hours. This medication relieves existing migraines, and will not change the frequency or number of attacks. Recurring use of this medicine will be needed. If your migraines increase in frequency or severity, consult your doctor. If this medicine is not effective in helping your migraine, consult your doctor.

Possible Advantages of This Drug
Effective subcutaneous treatment of acute nonbasilar nonhemiplegic migraine. Better side effect profile and treatment of migraine-associated nausea and vomiting and phono- and photophobia than other currently available agents.

Currently a "Drug of Choice"
for nonbasilar nonhemiplegic migraine.

▷ **This Drug Should Not Be Taken If**
- you have had an allergic reaction to any dosage form of it previously.
- you are unfamiliar with the subcutaneous route. Particular care must be taken to avoid intravenous use because this may lead to coronary vasospasm (constriction of the blood vessels that supply the heart).
- you have ischemic heart disease with symptoms such as: angina pectoris, silent ischemia or history of MI (myocardial infarction).
- you have Prinzmetal's angina (a specific kind of chest pain).
- you have ischemic heart disease (history of heart attack, documented silent ischemia or angina pectoris).
- you have uncontrolled hypertension (high blood pressure).
- you have basilar or hemiplegic migraine.
- you have taken a MAO inhibitor within the last two weeks.
- you have (within 24 hours) taken an ergotamine preparation.

▷ **Inform Your Physician Before Taking This Drug If**
- you are pregnant or plan to become pregnant.
- you are breast-feeding your infant.
- you have high blood pressure.
- you have chest pain, heart disease or irregular heartbeats.
- you have had a heart attack.
- you have taken or have prescriptions for other migraine medications.
- you have allergies or trouble taking other medication, whether prescription or over the counter.
- you have liver or kidney disease.
- you are uncertain of how much to take or when to take this medicine.
- you do not understand the subcutaneous injection technique.
- you have Raynaud's syndrome.

Possible Side Effects (natural, expected, and unavoidable drug actions)
Excessive thirst and frequent urination. Transient rises in blood pressure.

▷ **Possible Adverse Effects** (unusual, unexpected, and infrequent reactions)
If any of the following develop, consult your physician promptly for guidance.
Mild Adverse Effects
Allergic Reactions: Red itching skin, skin rash and tenderness.

Atypical sensations such as tingling (rare with injection, 8% with tablet form).
Confusion and other mental changes or dizziness (rare).
Flushing (rare), tightness in the chest or jaw (infrequent).
Gastroesophageal reflux and diarrhea.
Pain at the injection site; joint pain, weakness, and stiffness (rare).

Serious Adverse Effects
Allergic Reactions: Anaphylactoid reactions.
Syncope (fainting) (rare), CVA (rare), dysphasia (rare), seizure (rare).
Serious changes in heart rate and rhythm (rare).
Raynaud's syndrome (rare), dyspnea (difficulty breathing) (rare).
Kidney stones (renal calculi) (rare).
Prinzmetal's angina (rare).
Heart attack (myocardial infarction) (very rare).
Sudden kidney failure (acute renal failure) (very rare).

▷ **Possible Effects on Sexual Function:** Dysmenorrhea, erection problems (rare).

Possible Delayed Adverse Effects: None identified.

▷ **Adverse Effects That May Mimic Natural Diseases or Disorders**
Changes in heart rate and rhythm may mimic a number of cardiac conditions. Drug induced acute renal failure (ARF) may mimic non-drug induced ARF. Drug induced hypertension may mimic hypertension from other causes.
Urological symptoms may mimic benign prostatic hypertrophy. Sumatriptan can mimic Raynaud's syndrome.

Natural Diseases or Disorders That May Be Activated by This Drug
Hypertension.

Possible Effects on Laboratory Tests
Liver function tests: Rare increases in SGOT and SGPT.

CAUTION
1. Do not use sumatriptan if you are pregnant.
2. Call your doctor if you have any pain or tightness in the chest or throat when you use this medicine.
3. Do not use sumatriptan if you have used an ergotamine containing preparation within the last 24 hours.
4. This medication is **not** to be used intravenously.
5. If you are diagnosed as having ischemic heart disease after sumatriptan has been prescribed for you, do not use the medicine again.

Precautions for Use
By Infants and Children: Safety and effectiveness for those under 18 years of age not established.
By Those over 65 Years of Age: Have not been established.

▷ **Advisability of Use During Pregnancy**
Pregnancy Category: C. See Pregnancy Code at the back of this book.
Animal studies: Sumatriptan has been lethal to rabbit embryos when given in doses that were three fold higher than those produced by a 6 mg dose. Term fetuses from rabbits treated with sumatriptan exhibited an increase in cervicothoracic vascular defects and minor skeletal abnormalities.
Human studies: Adequate studies of pregnant women are not available.
Ask your physician for guidance.

Advisability of Use if Breast-Feeding

Presence of this drug in breast milk: Sumatriptan is excreted in the breast milk of animals, however no human data is available.

Use of this medication in nursing mothers is a benefit to risk decision to be made by a physician.

Habit-Forming Potential: Not clearly defined.

Effects of Overdosage: Patients have received doses of 8 to 12 mg without adverse effects. Healthy volunteers have taken up to 16 mg subcutaneously without serious adverse events. Coronary vasospasm has resulted from intravenous administration of normal doses. Animal data presents: convulsions, tremor, flushing, decreased breathing and activity, cyanosis, ataxia and paralysis.

Possible Effects of Long-Term Use: Not defined.

Suggested Periodic Examinations While Taking This Drug   (at physician's discretion)

Liver function tests, electrocardiogram.

▷ **While Taking This Drug, Observe the Following**

Foods: No restrictions; however, some foods or additives such as monosodium glutamate or chocolate may be a risk factor for migraines. Skipping meals can also be a risk factor for migraines.

Beverages: No restrictions.

▷ *Alcohol:* May cause additive sedation. Alcohol may also be a precipitating factor for migraine.

Tobacco Smoking: No interactions expected.

Marijuana Smoking: May cause additive dizziness, drowsiness and lethargy, may cause additive increases in blood pressure.

▷ *Other Drugs*

Sumatriptan *taken concurrently* with

- ergotamine containing preparations (see Drug Classes) may result in additive vasospasm (prolonged constriction of the blood vessels). These medicines should not be taken within 24 hours of any sumatriptan dose.
- monoamine oxidase inhibitors (MAOIs see Drug Classes) may result in toxic levels of sumatriptan. MAO inhibitors and sumatriptan should never be combines. It is important that 14 days should go by after your last dose of a MAO inhibitor before you take any form of sumatriptan.

▷ *Driving, Hazardous Activities:* This drug may cause dizziness and drowsiness. Restrict activities as necessary.

Aviation Note: The use of this drug *may be a disqualification* for piloting. Consult a designated Aviation Medical Examiner.

Exposure to Sun: No restrictions.

Exposure to Cold: Use caution until tolerance is determined. Cold may enhance sumatriptan vasoconstriction.

Heavy Exercise or Exertion: Strenuous exercise can be a risk factor for migraines in some patients

Special Storage Instructions: Keep this medicine out of reach of children.

Observe the Following Expiration Times: There is an expiration date printed on the treatment package. Throw the medication away if it has expired. The autoinjector may be used again.

TACRINE (TA kreen)

Introduced: 1993   **Prescription:** USA: Yes; Canada: Not available in Canada   **Available as Generic:** USA: No   **Class:** Cholinesterase inhibitor, anti-Alzheimer's drug   **Controlled Drug:** USA:No

Brand Names: Cognex

BENEFITS versus RISKS	
Possible Benefits	*Possible Risks*
IMPROVEMENT OF MEMORY IN MILD TO MODERATE ALZHEIMER'S DISEASE	LIVER TOXICITY Hallucinations

▷ **Principal Uses**

As a Single Drug Product: Uses currently included in FDA approved labeling: (1) Treatment of symptoms of mild to moderate Alzheimer's disease.

Other (unlabeled) generally accepted uses: (1) Significant increases in protective white blood cells (CD4 lymphocytes) occurred when tacrine was used to treat AIDS dementia; (2) some early data indicated a benefit in movement disorders (tardive dyskinesia).

How This Drug Works: Alzheimer's disease is thought to be caused by a loss of nerve cells that make a nerve transmitter (acetylcholine). Tacrine acts to increase levels of neurotransmitter (acetylcholine) in the brain.

Available Dosage Forms and Strengths

Capsules — 10 mg, 20 mg, 30 mg, 40 mg

▷ **Recommended Dosage Ranges (Actual dosage and administration schedule must be determined by the physician for each patient individually.)**

Infants and Children: No data are available on use of this drug in infants and children.

18 to 60 Years of Age: Adult starting dose is 10 mg taken four times a day. The dose can be increased at 6-week intervals if needed. Maximum daily dose is 160 mg.

Over 60 Years of Age: Same as 12 to 60 years of age.

Conditions Requiring Dosing Adjustments

Liver function: Used with great caution or not at all in liver compromise.

Kidney function: Dose decreases in kidney compromise are not presently indicated.

▷ **Dosing Instructions:** Tablet may be crushed and is best taken 1 hour before meals. Food decreases the amount that gets into your body by 30 to 40%.

Usual Duration of Use: Use on a regular schedule for 1 to 4 weeks is usually needed to see clinical improvement in this drug. Dose increases are made at 6-week intervals.

Long-term use (months to years) requires periodic physician evaluation of response and dosage adjustment.

Possible Advantages of This Drug

Improvement of memory and other symptoms of mild to moderate Alzheimer's with fewer side effects of other available agents.

Currently a "Drug of Choice"
for treatment of symptoms of mild to moderate Alzheimer's disease.

▷ **This Drug Should Not Be Taken If**
- you have had an allergic reaction to any dosage form of it previously.
- you have had tacrine-caused hepatoxicity and blood bilirubin levels greater than 3 mg/dl.
- you have bronchial asthma.
- you have a slow heartbeat (bradycardia), an abnormal electrical conduction system in your heart (AV conduction defect) or excessively low blood pressure.
- you have an overly active thyroid (hyperthyroidism).
- you have peptic ulcer disease.
- you have an intestinal or urinary tract obstruction.

▷ **Inform Your Physician Before Taking This Drug If**
- you have a history of seizure disorder.
- you have had liver disease.
- you take a NSAID (see Drug Classes section).
- you take muscle relaxants.
- you have gluacoma (angle closure).

Possible Side Effects (natural, expected, and unavoidable drug actions)
Symptoms of cholinergic excess (abdominal upset).

▷ **Possible Adverse Effects** (unusual, unexpected, and infrequent reactions)
If any of the following develop, consult your physician promptly for guidance.
Mild Adverse Effects
Allergic Reactions: Skin rash.
Increased sweating.
Muscle aches.
Nausea or vomiting, belching and diarrhea, decreased appetite.
Dizziness, confusion, and insomnia.
Serious Adverse Effects
Allergic Reactions: Anaphylactoid reactions.
Liver toxicity (20 to 40%), starts within 6 to 8 weeks after therapy begins.
Agitation, hallucinations (rare).
Purpura (rare).
Excessive urination.
Severe decrease in white blood cells (very rare).
Respiratory compromise (rare).
Slow heart rate (bradycardia) or abnormal rhythm (rare).
Low white blood cell count (rare).

▷ **Possible Effects on Sexual Function:**   Very rare effect in inducing lactation.

Possible Delayed Adverse Effects: Liver toxicity, rash, low white blood cell count.

▷ **Adverse Effects That May Mimic Natural Diseases or Disorders**
Liver toxicity may mimic acute hepatitis.

Natural Diseases or Disorders That May Be Activated by This Drug
May worsen bronchial asthma and precipitate seizures. May exacerbate peptic ulcer disease.

Possible Effects on Laboratory Tests
Liver function tests: increased SGOT, SGPT and CPK.
Complete blood count: decreased white blood cells.

CAUTION
1. This drug should **not** be stopped abruptly as acute deterioration of cognitive abilities may result.
2. Changes in color of stools (light or very black) should be promptly reported to your doctor.
3. This drug does **not** alter the course of Alzheimer's disease. Over time, the benefit of this drug may be lost.
4. The dose **must** be decreased by 40 mg per day if the liver function levels (transaminases) rise to 3 to 5 times the upper normal value.
5. Blood levels achieved by females are 50% higher than those in men. Dose-related side effects may occur sooner (with lower doses) in women than in men. Therapeutic doses may be lower for women than men.

Precautions for Use
By Infants and Children: Safety and effectiveness for those under 18 years of age not established.
By Those over 60 Years of Age: No specific changes are presently indicated.

▷ Advisability of Use During Pregnancy
Pregnancy Category: C. See Pregnancy Code at the back of this book.
Animal studies: Data not available.
Human studies: Adequate studies of pregnant women are not available.
Consult your doctor.

Advisability of Use if Breast-Feeding
Presence of this drug in breast milk: Unknown.
Monitor nursing infant closely and discontinue drug or nursing if adverse effects develop.

Habit-Forming Potential: None.

Effects of Overdosage: May precipitate a cholinergic crisis—severe nausea and vomiting, slow heart beat, low blood pressure, extreme muscle weakness, collapse and convulsions.

Suggested Periodic Examinations While Taking This Drug   (at physician's discretion)
Assessment of mental status: periodically to check benefit of therapy and potential loss of effectiveness as the underlying disease progresses.
Liver function tests: should be checked every 2 weeks for the first 16 weeks of therapy, then monthly for 2 months and then every 3 months thereafter if the same dose is maintained. If the dose is increased, liver function tests should be checked weekly for 7 weeks and then the above schedule should be followed.
Complete blood count: checked periodically or if symptoms of low blood count occur.

▷ While Taking This Drug, Observe the Following
Foods: Best **not** taken with food.
Beverages: No restrictions.
▷ *Alcohol:* Occasional small amounts of alcohol acceptable. Frequent use of alcohol may worsen memory impairment and adversely effect liver enzymes.

Tobacco Smoking: No interactions expected.

Marijuana Smoking: Additive dizziness may occur.

▷ *Other Drugs*

Tacrine may ***increase*** the effects of
- bethanechol (Duvoid, others).
- theophylline (Theo-Dur, others) by doubling the drug level.
- succinylcholine (Anectine, others).

Tacrine may ***decrease*** the effects of
- anticholinergic medications (see Drug Classes).

The following drugs may ***increase*** the effects of tacrine
- cimetidine (Tagamet).

▷ *Driving, Hazardous Activities:* This drug may cause confusion. Restrict activities as necessary.

Aviation Note: The use of this drug ***may be a disqualification*** for piloting. Consult a designated Aviation Medical Examiner.

Exposure to Sun: No restrictions.

Exposure to Heat: Increased sweating may routinely occur with this drug. The combination of increased sweating and hot environments may lead to more rapid dehydration.

Discontinuation: This drug should **not** be abruptly stopped. Some adverse effects are dose related, and may abate if the dose is decreased. Slow withdrawal of the drug is indicated if it is not tolerated and must be stopped.

TAMOXIFEN (ta MOX i fen)

Introduced: 1973   **Prescription:** USA: Yes; Canada: Yes   **Available as Generic:** No   **Class:** Antiestrogen, anticancer   **Controlled Drug:** USA: No; Canada: No

Brand Names: ✦Alpha-Tamoxifen, ✦Apo-Tamox, Nolvadex, ✦Nolvadex-D, ✦Novo-Tamoxifen, ✦Tamofen, ✦Tamone

BENEFITS versus RISKS	
Possible Benefits	*Possible Risks*
EFFECTIVE ADJUNCTIVE TREATMENT IN ADVANCED BREAST CANCER	UTERINE CANCER Severe increase in tumor or bone pain, transient Thrombophlebitis, pulmonary embolism Abnormally high blood calcium levels Eye changes: corneal opacities, retinal injury

▷ **Principal Uses**

As a Single Drug Product: Uses currently included in FDA approved labeling: (1) Used as an alternative to estrogens and androgens (male sex hormones) to treat advanced breast cancer in postmenopausal women; (2) treats advanced breast cancer in men that has spread (metastasized) from a prior site; (3) used to delay the recurrence of breast cancer in women.

Other (unlabeled) generally accepted uses: (1) May have a role in treating cancer of the liver or lung; (2) used to stimulate ovulation in premenopausal women with infertility; (3) used to treat rare desmoid tumors; (4) helps prevent osteoporosis in women in whom the drug is being used to prevent the recurrence of cancer; (4) can help retroperitoneal fibrosis; (5) could have a role in tenderness and swelling of male breast tissue (gynecomastia) of unknown cause (idiopathic); (6) helps lipid (cholesterol) levels.

How This Drug Works: It is thought that by blocking the uptake of estradiol (estrogen), this drug removes or reduces a stimulus to breast cancer cells.

Available Dosage Forms and Strengths
  Tablets — 10 mg, 15.2 mg (in Canada), 20 mg (in Canada) and 30.4 mg (in Canada)

▷ **Usual Adult Dosage Range:**   Breast cancer: 10 to 20 mg two to three times a day for 2 to 5 years. **Note: Actual dosage and administration schedule must be determined by the physician for each patient individually.**

Conditions Requiring Dosing Adjustments
  Liver function: Dose decreases are not defined in patients with compromised livers.
  Kidney function: The kidney plays a minor role in the elimination of this drug, however, tamoxifen should be used with caution in renal compromise.

▷ **Dosing Instructions:**   The tablet may be crushed and taken either on an empty stomach or with food.

Usual Duration of Use: Use on a regular schedule for 4 to 10 weeks usually determines effectiveness in controlling the growth and spread of advanced breast cancer. In the presence of bone involvement, treatment for several months may be required to evaluate effectiveness. Long-term use (months to years) requires physician supervision and periodic evaluation.

▷ **This Drug Should Not Be Taken If**
  • you have had a serious allergic or adverse reaction to it previously.
  • you have active phlebitis.
  • you have a significant deficiency of white blood cells or blood platelets.
  • you are pregnant.

▷ **Inform Your Physician Before Taking This Drug If**
  • you have a history of thrombophlebitis or pulmonary embolism.
  • you have a history of abnormally high blood calcium levels.
  • you have a history of any type of blood cell or bone marrow disorder.
  • you have cataracts or other visual impairment.
  • you have impaired liver function.
  • you plan to have surgery in the near future.

Possible Side Effects (natural, expected, and unavoidable drug actions)
  Hot flashes, fluid retention, weight gain.

▷ **Possible Adverse Effects** (unusual, unexpected, and infrequent reactions)
  If any of the following develop, consult your physician promptly for guidance.
  Mild Adverse Effects
  Allergic Reaction: Skin rash.
  Visual impairment.
  Headache, dizziness, drowsiness, depression, fatigue, confusion.
  Nausea, vomiting, itching in genital area, loss of hair.
  Serious Adverse Effects
  Initial "flare" of severe pain in tumor or involved bone.

Development of thrombophlebitis, risk of pulmonary embolism.

Eye changes: corneal opacities, retinal injury.

Delusions (rare).

Increased uterine cancer risk (increased karyopyknotic index of vaginal epithelium).

Development of abnormally high blood calcium levels.

Transient decreases in white blood cells and blood platelets.

Agranulocytosis (very rare).

Liver toxicity (rare).

▷ **Possible Effects on Sexual Function**

Premenopausal: altered timing and pattern of menstruation.

Postmenopausal: vaginal bleeding. Decreased libido.

Abnormal and painful erections (Priapism).

This drug may be effective in treating the following conditions:
- male infertility due to abnormally low sperm counts.
- male breast enlargement and tenderness.
- chronic female breast pain (mastalgia).

Possible Effects on Laboratory Tests

Complete blood cell counts: decreased red cells, hemoglobin, white cells and platelets.

Blood calcium level: increased.

Blood thyroid hormone levels: T_3, T_4 and free T_4 increased.

Liver function tests: increased liver enzyme (AST/GOT), increased bilirubin (one case report).

Sperm count: increased or decreased.

CAUTION

1. If this drug is used prior to your menopause, it may induce ovulation and predispose to pregnancy. Since this drug should not be used during pregnancy, some method of contraception (other than oral contraceptives) is advised.

2. Do not take any form of estrogen while taking this drug; estrogens can inhibit tamoxifen's effectiveness.

3. Tamoxifen has recently been shown to cause an increased incidence of uterine cancer. Women who have received or who are receiving this drug should have regular gynecologic examinations. Report menstrual irregularity, abnormal vaginal bleeding or vaginal discharge, pelvic pain or pressure promptly to your doctor.

▷ **Advisability of Use During Pregnancy**

Pregnancy Category: D. See Pregnancy Code at the back of this book.

Animal studies: No birth defects due to this drug reported.

Human studies: Adequate studies of pregnant women are not available.

This drug can have estrogenic effects. It should not be used during pregnancy.

Advisability of Use if Breast-Feeding

Presence of this drug in breast milk: Unknown.

Avoid drug or refrain from nursing.

Habit-Forming Potential: None.

Effects of Overdosage: Severe extension of the pharmacologic effects.

Possible Effects of Long-Term Use: Development of abnormally high blood calcium levels.

Suggested Periodic Examinations While Taking This Drug (at physician's discretion)

Complete blood cell counts, measurements of blood calcium levels.

Complete eye examinations if impaired vision occurs.

Women who have been given or who are now receiving tamoxifen **must** have regular gynecologic examinations.

▷ **While Taking This Drug, Observe the Following**

Foods: No restrictions.

Beverages: No restrictions. May be taken with milk.

▷ *Alcohol:* No interactions expected.

Tobacco Smoking: No interactions expected.

Marijuana Smoking: Animal studies show an increased suppression of the immune system. Significance in humans is not known.

▷ *Other Drugs*

The following drugs may *decrease* the effects of tamoxifen

- estrogens.
- oral contraceptives (those that contain estrogens).

Tamoxifen *taken concurrently* with

- allopurinol (Zyloprim) may worsen allopurinol toxicity to the liver.
- cyclosporine (Sandimmune) may increase cyclosporine levels and cause toxicity.
- mitomycin will cause increased risk of hemolytic uremic syndrome.
- pneumococcal and perhaps other vaccines will blunt the vaccine's immune response (benefit).
- warfarin (Coumadin) presents an increased risk of bleeding. Increased frequency of INR testing is needed.

▷ *Driving, Hazardous Activities:* This drug may cause dizziness or drowsiness. Restrict activities as necessary.

Aviation Note: The use of this drug *may be a disqualification* for piloting. Consult a designated Aviation Medical Examiner.

Exposure to Sun: No restrictions.

TERAZOSIN (ter AY zoh sin)

Introduced: 1987   **Prescription:** USA: Yes   **Available as Generic:**
No   **Class:** Antihypertensive   **Controlled Drug:** USA: No
Brand Name: Hytrin

BENEFITS versus RISKS	
Possible Benefits	*Possible Risks*
EFFECTIVE TREATMENT OF MILD TO MODERATE HYPERTENSION when used alone or in combination with other antihypertensive drugs LOWERED LOW-DENSITY LIPOPROTEINS AND TOTAL CHOLESTEROL LOWERED TRIGLYCERIDE LEVELS	"First dose" drop in blood pressure with fainting (very rare) Fluid retention

▷ **Principal Uses**

As a Single Drug Product: Uses currently included in FDA approved labeling: (1) Used to treat mild to moderate hypertension. Also used in combination with other drugs to treat moderate to severe hypertension; (2) treats symptomatic benign prostatic hyperplasia (BPH).

Other (unlabeled) generally accepted uses: (1) Used to help correct symptoms in congestive heart failure; (2) may have a beneficial effect in lowering cholesterol levels.

How This Drug Works: Terazosin blocks some actions of the sympathetic nervous system, causing direct opening of blood vessel walls, lowering blood pressure. In BPH it relaxes the smooth muscle around the bladder neck and prostate allowing opening of the urethra and increased urine flow.

Available Dosage Forms and Strengths

Tablets — 1 mg, 2 mg, 5 mg, 10 mg

▷ **Usual Adult Dosage Range:**   Treatment is started with a "test dose" of 1 mg and the patient's response is observed for 2 hours (some physicians have the patient take the medicine at bedtime). If terazosin is tolerated, dose can be slowly (as needed and tolerated) increased up to 5 mg daily. Maximum daily dosage should not exceed 20 mg. Benign prostatic hyperplasia: 1 milligram is given at bedtime. This dose is gradually increased as needed and tolerated to the desired response. Many patients need 10 mg for 4 to 6 weeks in order to get symptom relief. **Note: Actual dosage and administration schedule must be determined by the physician for each patient individually.**

Conditions Requiring Dosing Adjustments

Liver function: Dose should be decreased in patients with severe liver problems.
Kidney function: Dose changes are not needed in patients with severe kidney failure.

▷ **Dosing Instructions:**   The tablet may be crushed and taken without regard to food. Best taken at bedtime to avoid orthostatic hypotension (see Glossary).

Usual Duration of Use: Use on a regular schedule for 6 to 8 weeks usually determines effectiveness in controlling hypertension. Four to six weeks of scheduled use is needed in benign prostatic hyperplasia (BPH). See your doctor regularly.

Possible Advantages of This Drug

May be used to initiate treatment.
Usually effective with once-a-day dosage.
Rarely causes depression or impotence.
Does not alter blood cholesterol, potassium or sugar.

▷ **This Drug Should Not Be Taken If**

• you have had an allergic reaction to it previously.
• you are experiencing mental depression.
• you have angina (active coronary artery disease) and you are not taking a beta-blocking drug. (See your physician.)

▷ **Inform Your Physician Before Taking This Drug If**

• you have experienced orthostatic hypotension (see Glossary).
• you have a history of mental depression.
• you have impaired circulation to the brain, or a history of stroke.

- your job requires alertness or dexterity in operating heavy machinery (this medicine may cause somnolence or drowsiness).
- you have coronary artery disease.
- you have impaired liver or kidney function.
- surgery under general anesthesia is planned soon.

Possible Side Effects (natural, expected, and unavoidable drug actions)

Orthostatic hypotension (rare), drowsiness, salt and water retention, dry mouth, nasal congestion, constipation.

▷ **Possible Adverse Effects** (unusual, unexpected, and infrequent reactions)

If any of the following develop, consult your physician promptly for guidance.

Mild Adverse Effects

Allergic Reaction: Skin rash.

Headache, dizziness, fatigue, weakness, nervousness, sweating, numbness and tingling, blurred vision (rare).

Weight gain.

Congestion of the nose.

Palpitation, rapid heart rate (rare), shortness of breath.

Nausea, vomiting, diarrhea, abdominal pain.

Serious Adverse Effects

Mental depression (rare).

▷ **Possible Effects on Sexual Function:**   Impotence (1.2%).

Natural Diseases or Disorders That May Be Activated by This Drug

Latent coronary artery insufficiency.

Possible Effects on Laboratory Tests

Blood total cholesterol, LDL and VLDL cholesterol levels: decreased.

Blood HDL cholesterol level: no effect.

Blood triglyceride levels: no effect.

CAUTION

1. A "first dose" precipitous drop in blood pressure, with or without fainting can happen (usually within 30 to 90 minutes). Limit initial doses to 1 mg taken at bedtime (for first 3 days); stay laying down after taking trial doses.
2. Call your doctor if you plan to use over-the-counter remedies for allergic rhinitis or head colds. Serious drug interactions are possible.

Precautions for Use

By Infants and Children: Safety and effectiveness for those under 12 years of age not established.

By Those over 60 Years of Age: Therapy is started with no more than 1 mg/day for the first 3 days. Any dose increases must be very gradual and closely physician supervised. Orthostatic hypotension can cause falls and injury. Sit or lie down promptly if you feel light-headed or dizzy. Report dizziness or chest pain promptly.

▷ **Advisability of Use During Pregnancy**

Pregnancy Category: C. See Pregnancy Code at the back of this book.

Animal studies: No birth defects found in rat or rabbit studies.

Human studies: Adequate studies of pregnant women are not available.

Use this drug only if clearly needed. Ask your physician for guidance.

Advisability of Use if Breast-Feeding
Presence of this drug in breast milk: Unknown.
Watch infant closely and stop drug or nursing if adverse effects start.

Habit-Forming Potential: None.

Effects of Overdosage: Orthostatic hypotension, headache, flushing, fast heart rate, extreme weakness, irregular heart rhythm, circulatory collapse.

Possible Effects of Long-Term Use: None reported.

Suggested Periodic Examinations While Taking This Drug (at physician's discretion)
Measurements of blood pressure in lying, sitting and standing positions.
Measurements of body weight to detect fluid retention.

▷ **While Taking This Drug, Observe the Following**
Foods: No restrictions. Avoid excessive salt intake.
Beverages: No restrictions. May be taken with milk.
▷ *Alcohol:* Alcohol can exaggerate the blood-pressure-lowering actions of this drug and cause excessive reduction. Use with extreme caution.
Tobacco Smoking: Nicotine can intensify this drug's ability to worsen coronary insufficiency. All forms of tobacco should be avoided.
▷ *Other Drugs*
The following drugs may *increase* the effects of terazosin
• beta-adrenergic-blocking drugs (see Drug Classes Section); severity and duration of the "first dose" response may be increased.
• verapamil (Verelan, Calan, others) and cause excessive lowering of blood pressure.
The following drugs may *decrease* the effects of terazosin
• estrogens (see Drug Classes).
• indomethacin (Indocin) and other NSAIDs (see Drug Classes).
▷ *Driving, Hazardous Activities:* This drug may cause dizziness or drowsiness. Restrict activities as necessary.
Aviation Note: The use of this drug *is a disqualification* for piloting. Consult a designated Aviation Medical Examiner.
Exposure to Sun: No restrictions.
Exposure to Cold: Cold environments may increase this drug's ability to cause coronary insufficiency (angina) and hypothermia (see Glossary). Use caution.
Heavy Exercise or Exertion: Excessive exertion can increase likelihood of chest pain. See Angina in Section Two.
Discontinuation: Do not stop this medicine abruptly if it is being used to treat congestive heart failure. Ask your physician for guidance.

TERBUTALINE (ter BYU ta leen)

Introduced: 1974   **Prescription:** USA: Yes; Canada: Yes   **Available as Generic:** No   **Class:** Antiasthmatic, bronchodilator   **Controlled Drug:** USA: No; Canada: No

Brand Names: Brethaire, Brethine, Bricanyl, ✦Bricanyl Spacer

```
┌─────────────────────────────────────────────────────────────────────┐
│                      BENEFITS versus RISKS                            │
│      Possible Benefits                    Possible Risks              │
│  VERY EFFECTIVE RELIEF OF          Increased blood pressure           │
│  BRONCHOSPASM                      Fine hand tremor                   │
│                                    Irregular heart rhythm (with       │
│                                    excessive use)                     │
└─────────────────────────────────────────────────────────────────────┘
```

▷ **Principal Uses**

   As a Single Drug Product: Uses currently included in FDA approved labeling: (1) Relieves acute bronchial asthma and reduces frequency and severity of chronic, recurrent asthmatic attacks; (2) also used to relieve reversible bronchospasm associated with chronic bronchitis and emphysema.

   Other (unlabeled) generally accepted uses: (1) May have a role in helping ease fetal distress in some patients; (2) used to help stop premature labor; (3) can be an alternative to intravenous isoproterenol in therapy of status asthmaticus; (4) has a role in easing sustained and painful erections (priapism); (5) may be used in combination therapy in patients who have wheals and itching of unknown cause (idiopathic urticaria).

How This Drug Works: By stimulating certain sympathetic nerve terminals, this drug acts to dilate those bronchial tubes that are in sustained constriction, thereby increasing the size of the airway and improving the ability to breathe.

Available Dosage Forms and Strengths

   Aerosol — 0.2 mg/actuation and 0.25 mg/actuation (Canada)

   Injection — 1 mg per ml

   Tablets — 2.5 mg, 5 mg

▷ **Usual Adult Dosage Range:**   For the Aerosol: 0.4 mg taken in 2 separate inhalations 1 minute apart; repeat every 4 to 6 hours as needed. Tablets: 2.5 to 5 mg taken every 6 hours. The total daily dosage **should not** exceed 15 mg. **Note: Actual dosage and administration schedule must be determined by the physician for each patient individually.**

Conditions Requiring Dosing Adjustments

   Liver function: This drug is extensively metabolized in the liver, however, guidelines for dosing changes in patients with compromised livers are not available.

   Kidney function: In patients with moderate to severe kidney failure, 50% of the usual dose can be given at the usual time. In severe failure, the drug should not be used.

▷ **Dosing Instructions:**   Tablets may be crushed and taken on empty stomach or with food or milk. For aerosol, follow the written instructions carefully. Do not overuse.

Usual Duration of Use: According to individual requirements. Do not use beyond the time necessary to terminate episodes of asthma.

Possible Advantages of This Drug

   Rapid onset of action.

   Long duration of action.

   Highly effective relief of asthma.

▷ **This Drug Should Not Be Taken If**
- you have had an allergic reaction to any dosage form of it previously.
- you currently have an irregular heart rhythm.
- you are taking, or have taken within the past 2 weeks, any monoamine oxidase (MAO) type A inhibitor drug (see Drug Classes).

▷ **Inform Your Physician Before Taking This Drug If**
- you are overly sensitive to other drugs that stimulate the sympathetic nervous system.
- you are currently using epinephrine (Adrenalin, Primatene Mist, etc.) to relieve asthmatic breathing.
- you have a seizure disorder.
- you have liver or kidney failure.
- you have any type of heart or circulatory disorder, especially high blood pressure or coronary heart disease.
- you have diabetes or an overactive thyroid gland (hyperthyroidism).
- you are taking any form of digitalis or any stimulant drug.

Possible Side Effects (natural, expected, and unavoidable drug actions)
Aerosol: dryness or irritation of mouth or throat, altered taste. Tablet: nervousness, tremor, palpitation.

▷ **Possible Adverse Effects** (unusual, unexpected, and infrequent reactions)
If any of the following develop, consult your physician promptly for guidance.
Mild Adverse Effects
Headache, dizziness, drowsiness, restlessness, insomnia.
Rapid, pounding heartbeat; increased sweating; muscle cramps in arms and legs.
Nausea, heartburn, vomiting.
Increased blood sugar.
Serious Adverse Effects
Rapid or irregular heart rhythm, intensification of angina, increased blood pressure.
Lowered blood calcium or potassium (especially with intravenous use).
Liver toxicity (very rare).
Severe lowering of blood pressure (hypotension).
Increased blood sugar.

▷ **Possible Effects on Sexual Function:**   None reported.

Natural Diseases or Disorders That May Be Activated By This Drug
Latent coronary artery disease, diabetes or high blood pressure.

Possible Effects on Laboratory Tests
Blood total cholesterol and LDL cholesterol levels: no effect.
Blood HDL cholesterol level: increased.
Blood triglyceride levels: no effect.
Blood thyroid hormone levels: T_3 increased; T_4 decreased; free T_4 no effect.
Glucose tolerance test: abnormal test.
Liver function tests: May be elevated.

CAUTION
1. Combination of this drug by aerosol with beclomethasone aerosol (Beclovent, Vanceril) may increase the risk of toxicity due to fluorocarbon propellants. Best to use this aerosol 20 to 30 minutes **before** beclometha-

sone aerosol. This will reduce the risk of toxicity and will help beclomethasone get into the lungs.

2. **Avoid excessive use of aerosol inhalation.** The excessive or prolonged use of this drug by inhalation can reduce its effectiveness and cause serious heart rhythm disturbances, including cardiac arrest.

3. Do not use this drug concurrently with epinephrine. These two drugs may be used alternately if an interval of 4 hours is allowed between doses.

4. If you do not respond to your usually effective dose, ask your physician for guidance. Do not increase the size or frequency of the dose without your physician's approval.

Precautions for Use

By Infants and Children: Safety and effectiveness for those under 12 years of age not established.

By Those over 60 Years of Age: Avoid excessive and continual use. If acute asthma is not relieved promptly, other drugs will be needed. Watch for nervousness, palpitations, irregular heart rhythm and muscle tremors. Use with extreme caution if you have hardening of the arteries, heart disease or high blood pressure.

▷ **Advisability of Use During Pregnancy**

Pregnancy Category: B. See Pregnancy Code at the back of this book.

Animal studies: No significant birth defects reported in mouse and rat studies.

Human studies: Adequate studies of pregnant women are not available.

Use only if clearly needed. Ask your physician for guidance.

Advisability of Use if Breast-Feeding

Presence of this drug in breast milk: Yes.

Monitor nursing infant closely and discontinue drug or nursing if adverse effects develop.

Habit-Forming Potential: None.

Effects of Overdosage: Nervousness, palpitation, rapid heart rate, sweating, headache, tremor, vomiting, chest pain.

Possible Effects of Long-Term Use: Loss of effectiveness. See *CAUTION* category above.

Suggested Periodic Examinations While Taking This Drug (at physician's discretion)

Blood pressure measurements, evaluation of heart status.

▷ **While Taking This Drug, Observe the Following**

Foods: No restrictions.

Beverages: Avoid excessive use of caffeine-containing beverages: coffee, tea, cola, chocolate.

▷ *Alcohol:* No interactions expected.

Tobacco Smoking: No interactions expected.

▷ *Other Drugs*

Terbutaline *taken concurrently* with

- monoamine oxidase (MAO) type A inhibitor drugs may cause excessive increase in blood pressure and undesirable heart stimulation (see Drug Classes).
- theophylline (Theodur, others) may cause decreased theophylline effectiveness.

The following drugs may *decrease* the effects of terbutaline
- beta blocker drugs may impair terbutaline effectiveness (see Drug Classes).

▷ *Driving, Hazardous Activities:* Usually no restrictions. Use caution if excessive nervousness or dizziness occurs.

Aviation Note: The use of this drug *is a disqualification* for piloting. Consult a designated Aviation Medical Examiner.

Exposure to Sun: No restrictions.

Heavy Exercise or Exertion: Use caution. Excessive exercise can induce asthma in some patients.

TERFENADINE (ter FEN a deen)

Introduced: 1977   **Prescription:** USA: Yes; Canada: No   **Available as Generic:** No   **Class:** Antihistamine, nonsedating or minimally sedating
Controlled Drug: USA: No; Canada: No
Brand Names: ✦Contact Allergy Formula, Seldane, Seldane-D

BENEFITS versus RISKS	
Possible Benefits	*Possible Risks*
EFFECTIVE RELIEF OF ALLERGIC RHINITIS AND ALLERGIC SKIN DISORDERS	RARE HEART RHYTHM DISTURBANCES (DRUG INTERACTION EFFECT) Minor digestive disturbances Slight atropinelike effects

▷ **Principal Uses**

As a Single Drug Product: Uses currently included in FDA approved labeling: (1) Provides symptomatic relief in allergic and related disorders: seasonal and perennial allergic rhinitis (hay fever), allergic conjunctivitis and vasomotor rhinitis.

Other (unlabeled) generally accepted uses: (1) Helps relieve hives and localized swellings (angioedema) of allergic origin; (2) can decrease or prevent symptoms of grass pollen-sensitive asthmatic patients; (3) relieves the symptoms of the common cold; (4) helps prevent exercise-induced asthma; (5) can ease the blockage of eustachian tubes seen in otitis media.

How This Drug Works: Antihistamines reduce the intensity of the allergic response by blocking the action of histamine after it has been released from sensitized tissue cells in the eyes, nose and skin.

Available Dosage Forms and Strengths
      Caplet (Canada) — 120 mg
   Extended release tablet — 60 mg
         Suspension — 30 mg per 5-ml (Canada)
         Tablets — 60 mg

▷ **Usual Adult Dosage Range:** For those 12 years old to 60 years old: Use sixty (60) mg every 12 hours as needed. The total daily dosage **should not** exceed 120 mg. **Note: Actual dosage and administration schedule must be determined by the physician for each patient individually.**

Conditions Requiring Dosing Adjustments

Liver function: This drug is extensively metabolized in the liver and it is contraindicated in liver compromise.

Kidney function: Changes in dosing do not appear to be needed in renal compromise.

▷ **Dosing Instructions:**   The tablet may be crushed and taken with food or milk to prevent stomach irritation.

Usual Duration of Use: Use on a regular schedule for 2 to 3 days usually determines effectiveness in relieving the symptoms of allergic rhinitis and dermatosis. It may be necessary to take this drug throughout the entire pollen season, depending upon individual sensitivity. However, antihistamines should not be taken continually (without interruption) for long-term use. Limit their use to periods that require symptomatic relief. Consult your physician on a regular basis.

Possible Advantages of This Drug
Fast onset of action, relief within 1 hour.
No loss of effectiveness with continual use.
Little drowsiness or impaired mental function.

▷ **This Drug Should Not Be Taken If**
• you have had an allergic reaction to any dosage form of it previously.
• you are currently undergoing allergy skin tests.
• you have severely impaired liver function.
• you are taking erythromycin, clarithromycin, azithromycin, ketoconazole, itraconazole or troleandomycin.

▷ **Inform Your Physician Before Taking This Drug If**
• you have had any allergic reactions or unfavorable responses to antihistamines.
• you have a history of heart rhythm disorders.
• you have a history of liver disease.
• you have bronchial asthma.

Possible Side Effects (natural, expected, and unavoidable drug actions)
Dry nose, mouth, or throat.

▷ **Possible Adverse Effects** (unusual, unexpected, and infrequent reactions)
If any of the following develop, consult your physician promptly for guidance.
Mild Adverse Effects
Allergic Reactions: Skin rash, itching.
Headache, nervousness, fatigue.
Increased urination (rare).
Visual disturbances (rare).
Increased appetite, indigestion, nausea, vomiting.
Serious Adverse Effects
Significant heart rhythm disorders (resulting from excessive dosage or interactions with other drugs).
Liver toxicity (rare).
Lowered blood platelets (rare).

▷ **Possible Effects on Sexual Function**
Altered timing and pattern of menstruation.
Female breast enlargement with milk production.

Possible Effects on Laboratory Tests
None reported.

CAUTION
1. Do not exceed recommended doses; high blood levels may cause serious heart rhythm disturbances.
2. Do not take this drug concurrently with any form of erythromycin, ketoconazole (Nizoral), itraconazole or troleandomycin (TAO).
3. Report promptly the development of faintness, dizziness, heart palpitation, or chest pain.
4. Stop this drug 4 days before diagnostic skin testing procedures in order to prevent false negative test results.
5. Lowered blood potassium or magnesium may increase the risk of undesirable cardiovascular effects. Talk with your doctor if you are taking a diuretic or tend to lose a lot of fluid.
6. Do not use this drug if you have active bronchial asthma, bronchitis or pneumonia. It may thicken bronchial mucus and make it more difficult to remove (by absorption or coughing).

Precautions for Use
By Infants and Children: Safety and effectiveness for those under 12 years of age are not established.
By Those over 60 Years of Age: You may be more susceptible to the development of headache and fatigue. Use smaller doses at longer intervals if necessary.

▷ **Advisability of Use During Pregnancy**
Pregnancy Category: C. See Pregnancy Code at the back of this book.
Animal studies: No birth defects due to this drug reported.
Human studies: Adequate studies of pregnant women are not available.
Use this drug only if clearly needed. Ask your physician for guidance.

Advisability of Use if Breast-Feeding
Presence of this drug in breast milk: Expected, but not well studied.
Avoid drug or refrain from nursing.

Habit-Forming Potential: None.

Effects of Overdosage: Possible development of serious heart rhythm disturbances.

Possible Effects of Long-Term Use: None reported.

Suggested Periodic Examinations While Taking This Drug (at physician's discretion)
Electrocardiograms for those with heart disorders.

▷ **While Taking This Drug, Observe the Following**
Foods: No restrictions.
Beverages: Grapefruit juice, especially in large volumes, may lead to increased blood levels and toxicity. May be taken with milk or water.
▷ *Alcohol:* No interactions expected.
Tobacco Smoking: No interactions expected.
▷ *Other Drugs:* Terfenadine **taken concurrently** with
• amiodarone (Codarone) may result in increased risk of adverse cardiovascular effects.
• carbamazepine (Tegretol) may result in carbamazepine toxicity.
• ciprofloxacin (Cipro) may result in increased risk of adverse cardiovascular effects.
• disopyramide (Norpace) may result in increased risk of adverse cardiovascular effects.

- fluoxetine (Prozac) may result in terfenadine toxicity.
- fluvoxamine (Luvox) may result in terfenadine toxicity.
- ketoconazole (Nizoral) may cause increased blood levels of terfenadine resulting in serious heart rhythm disorders.
- itraconazole (Sporanox) may cause increased blood levels of terfenadine resulting in serious heart rhythm disorders.
- macrolide antibiotics (see Drug Classes): erythromycin, azithromycin, clarithromycin, dirithromycin, troleandomycin, others, may cause increased blood levels of terfenadine resulting in serious heart rhythm disorders.
- miconazole (Monistat) may result in increased risk of cardiovascular effects.
- paroxetine (Paxil) may interact with terfenadine and result in terfenadine toxicity.
- quinidine (Quinaglute, others) may result in increased risk of adverse cardiovascular effects.
- sotolol (Betapace) may result in abnormal and serious heart rhythm changes.
- tricyclic antidepressants (see Drug Classes) may result in increased risk of adverse cardiovascular effects.

Hazardous Activities: No restrictions.

Aviation Note: The use of this drug *is probably not a disqualification* for piloting. Consult a designated Aviation Medical Examiner.

Exposure to Sun: Rare cases of photosensitivity have been reported. Use caution.

TETRACYCLINE (te trah SI kleen)

Introduced: 1953   **Prescription:** USA: Yes; Canada: Yes   **Available as Generic:** Yes   **Class:** Antibiotic, tetracyclines   **Controlled Drug:** USA: No; Canada: No

Brand Names: Achromycin, Achromycin V, ✦Acrocidin, ✦Apo-Tetra, Actisite, Aureomycin, Contimycin, Cyclinex, Cyclopar, Lemtrex, ✦Medicycline, Mysteclin-F [CD], ✦Neo-Tetrine, ✦Novo-Tetra, ✦Nor-Tet, ✦Novotetra, ✦Nu-Tetra, Panmycin, Retet, Robitet, SK-Tetracycline, Sumycin, Teline, Tetra-C, Tetracap, Tetra-Con, Tetracyn, Tetralan, Tetram, Tropicycline

BENEFITS versus RISKS	
Possible Benefits	*Possible Risks*
EFFECTIVE TREATMENT OF INFECTIONS due to susceptible bacteria and protozoa	ALLERGIC REACTIONS, mild to severe: ANAPHYLAXIS, DRUG-INDUCED HEPATITIS (rare)
	Drug-induced colitis
	Superinfections (bacterial or fungal)
	Rare blood cell disorders: hemolytic anemia, abnormally low white cell and platelet counts

▷ **Principal Uses**

As a Single Drug Product: Uses currently included in FDA approved labeling: (1) Treats a broad range of infections caused by susceptible bacteria and protozoa (short-term use); and (2) treats severe, resistant pustular acne (long-term use); (3) used in a sustained release form (Actisite) to treat gum disease (periodontitis) in adults.

Other (unlabeled) generally accepted uses: (1) Combination antibiotic treatment of duodenal ulcers caused by H. pylori; (2) used in vaginal and vulval cysts (gartner) and in vaginal hydrocele; (3) topical tetracycline is useful in chronic eye problems (blepharitis); (4) treats cancer (malignant) fluid (pericardial effusion) build-up around the heart; (5) used to treat Stage One Lyme disease; (6) has a role in acne rosacea in decreasing the number of papules or nodules.

As a Combination Drug Product [CD]: This drug is available in combination with amphotericin B, an antifungal antibiotic that is provided to reduce the risk of developing an overgrowth of yeast organisms (superinfection) of the gastrointestinal tract.

How This Drug Works: This drug prevents the growth and multiplication of susceptible bacteria by interfering with their formation of essential proteins.

Available Dosage Forms and Strengths

Capsules — 100 mg, 250 mg, 500 mg

Ointment — 3%

Ointment, ophthalmic — 10 mg per gram

Solution, topical — 2.2 mg per ml

Suspension, ophthalmic — 10 mg per ml

Suspension, oral — 125 mg per 5-ml

Tablets — 250 mg, 500 mg

▷ **Usual Adult Dosage Range:** 250 to 500 milligrams every 6 hours, or 500 to 1000 mg every 12 hours. The total daily dosage should not exceed 4000 mg (4 grams). **Note: Actual dosage and administration schedule must be determined by the physician for each patient individually.**

Conditions Requiring Dosing Adjustments

Liver function: Tetracycline is a cause of hepatoxicity. A benefit to risk decision should be made to use this drug in patients with compromised livers. The maximum daily dose in liver disease is one gram a day.

Kidney function: Patients with mild to moderate kidney failure can be given the usual dose every 8 to 12 hours. Patients with moderate to severe kidney failure can be given the usual dose every 12 to 24 hours. In severe kidney failure (creatinine clearance less than 10 ml/min.), tetracycline should be avoided.

▷ **Dosing Instructions:** The tablet may be crushed and the capsule opened and preferably taken on an empty stomach, 1 hour before or 2 hours after eating. However, to reduce stomach irritation it may be taken with crackers that contain insignificant amounts of iron, calcium, magnesium or zinc. Avoid all dairy products for 2 hours before and after taking this drug. Take at the same time each day, with a full glass of water. Take the full course prescribed.

Usual Duration of Use: The time required to control the acute infection and be free of fever and symptoms for 48 hours. This varies with the nature of the infection. Long-term use (months to years, as for treatment of acne) requires supervision and periodic evaluation. Treatment of Stage One Lyme disease requires longer lengths of therapy (often 3 to 4 weeks). Consult your physician on a regular basis.

Currently a "Drug of Choice"
for the initial treatment of early Lyme disease. (Note: Children under 8 years of age and pregnant/breast-feeding women should use penicillin instead of tetracycline.)

▷ **This Drug Should Not Be Taken If**
   • you are allergic to any tetracycline (see Drug Class Section).
   • you are pregnant or breast-feeding.
   • you have severe liver compromise.

▷ **Inform Your Physician Before Taking This Drug If**
   • it is prescribed for a child under 8 years of age.
   • you have a history of liver or kidney disease.
   • you have systemic lupus erythematosus.
   • you are taking any penicillin drug.
   • you are taking any anticoagulant drug.
   • you plan to have surgery under general anesthesia in the near future.

Possible Side Effects (natural, expected, and unavoidable drug actions)
   Superinfections (see Glossary), often due to yeast organisms. These can occur in the mouth, intestinal tract, rectum, and/or vagina, resulting in rectal and vaginal itching.
   Tooth discoloration (when used in children less than 8 years old).

▷ **Possible Adverse Effects** (unusual, unexpected, and infrequent reactions)
   If any of the following develop, consult your physician promptly for guidance.
   Mild Adverse Effects
   Allergic Reactions: Skin rash, hives, itching of hands and feet, swelling of face or extremities.
   Loss of appetite, stomach irritation, taste disorders, nausea, vomiting, diarrhea.
   Warts (very rare and of questionable causality).
   Irritation of mouth or tongue, "black tongue," sore throat, abdominal cramping or pain.
   Serious Adverse Effects
   Allergic Reactions: Anaphylactic reaction (see Glossary), asthma, fever, swollen joints and lymph glands.
   Serious skin problems (Stevens-Johnson syndrome, Jarisch-Herxheimer reaction).
   Drug-induced hepatitis with jaundice.
   Permanent discoloration and/or malformation of teeth when taken under 8 years of age, including unborn child and infant.
   Impaired vision, increased intracranial pressure.
   Drug-induced colitis.
   Drug-induced myasthenia gravis.
   Worsening of existing systemic lupus erythematosus.

Pancreatitis (rare).

Rare blood cell disorders: hemolytic anemia (see Glossary); abnormally low white blood cell count, causing fever, sore throat, and infections; abnormally low blood platelet count, causing abnormal bleeding or bruising.

Impairment of blood clotting.

Increased intracranial pressure (pseudotumor cerebri).

Kidney problems (rare).

Drug-induced porphyria.

Drug-induced low blood potassium.

Drug-induced esophageal ulcers.

▷ **Possible Effects on Sexual Function:** Decreased effectiveness of oral contraceptives taken concurrently (several case reports of pregnancy). Decreased male fertility.

▷ **Adverse Effects That May Mimic Natural Diseases or Disorders**

Drug-induced hepatitis may suggest viral hepatitis.

Natural Diseases or Disorders That May Be Activated by This Drug

Systemic lupus erythematosus.

Possible Effects on Laboratory Tests

Complete blood cell counts: decreased red cells, hemoglobin, white cells and platelets; increased eosinophils (allergic reaction).

Blood lupus erythematosus (LE) cells: positive.

Blood amylase level: increased (toxic effect in pregnant women).

Liver function tests: increased liver enzymes (ALT/GPT, AST/GOT and alkaline phosphatase), increased bilirubin.

Kidney function tests: increased blood creatinine and urea nitrogen (BUN) levels (kidney damage).

Urine sugar tests: false positive results with Benedict's solution and Clinitest.

CAUTION

1. Antacids, dairy products and preparations containing aluminum, bismuth, calcium, iron, magnesium or zinc can prevent adequate absorption of this drug and reduce its effectiveness significantly.
2. Troublesome and persistent diarrhea can develop. If diarrhea persists for more than 24 hours, stop this drug and call your doctor.
3. If general anesthesia is required while taking this drug, the choice of anesthetic agent must be selected carefully to prevent kidney damage.

Precautions for Use

By Infants and Children: If possible, tetracyclines should not be given to children under 8 years of age because of the risk of permanent discoloration and deformity of the teeth. Rarely, infants may develop increased intracranial pressure within the first 4 days of receiving this drug. Tetracyclines may inhibit normal bone growth and development.

By Those over 60 Years of Age: Dosage must be carefully individualized based on kidney function. Natural skin changes may predispose to severe and prolonged itching reactions in the genital and anal regions.

▷ **Advisability of Use During Pregnancy**

Pregnancy Category: D. See Pregnancy Code at the back of this book.

Animal studies: Tetracycline causes limb defects in rats, rabbits and chickens.

Human studies: Information from studies of pregnant women indicates that this drug can cause impaired development and discoloration of teeth and other developmental defects.

It is advisable to avoid this drug completely during entire pregnancy.

Advisability of Use if Breast-Feeding

Presence of this drug in breast milk: Yes.

Avoid drug or refrain from nursing.

Habit-Forming Potential: None.

Effects of Overdosage: Stomach burning, nausea, vomiting, diarrhea.

Possible Effects of Long-Term Use: Superinfections; rarely, impairment of bone marrow, liver or kidney function.

Suggested Periodic Examinations While Taking This Drug (at physician's discretion)

Complete blood cell counts, liver and kidney function tests.

During extended use, sputum and stool examinations may detect early superinfection due to yeast organisms.

▷ **While Taking This Drug, Observe the Following**

Foods: Avoid cheeses, yogurt, ice cream, iron-fortified cereals and supplements and meats for 2 hours before and after taking this drug. Calcium and iron can combine with this drug and reduce its absorption significantly.

Beverages: Avoid all forms of milk for 2 hours before and after taking this drug.

▷   *Alcohol:* Reduced doxycycline blood levels. Alcohol should be avoided with doxycycline, and perhaps another tetracycline substituted, particularly in those who have drinking problems. Alcohol is also best avoided if you have active liver disease.

Tobacco Smoking: No interactions expected.

▷   *Other Drugs*

Tetracyclines may *increase* the effects of

• oral anticoagulants such as warfarin (Coumadin), and make it necessary to reduce their dosage. Increased INR (protime testing is needed).

• digoxin (Lanoxin), and cause digitalis toxicity.

• lithium (Eskalith, Lithane, etc.), and increase the risk of lithium toxicity.

Tetracyclines may *decrease* the effects of

• birth control pills (oral contraceptives), and impair their effectiveness in preventing pregnancy.

• penicillins (see Drug Classes) and impair their effectiveness in treating infections.

Tetracyclines *taken concurrently* with

• furosemide (Lasix) will tend to increase blood urea nitrogen (BUN).

• isotretinoin (Accutane)may worsen tetracycline induced increased intracranial pressure and cause additive toxicity.

• methoxyflurane anesthesia may impair kidney function.

• theophylline (Theodur) may result in variable changes in drug levels. More frequent theophylline blood levels are needed if these medicines are to be combined.

• warfarin (Coumadin) poses an increased risk of bleeding. INR (prothrombin testing) should be checked more frequently, and doses adjusted if needed.

The following drugs may *decrease* the effects of tetracyclines

• antacids (aluminum and magnesium preparations, sodium bicarbonate, etc.) may reduce drug absorption.

- bismuth subsalicylate (Pepto Bismol, others).
- calcium supplements (various brands).
- cholestyramine (Questran) and other cholesterol lowering resins.
- colestipol (Colestid).
- iron, zinc, magnesium and mineral preparations may reduce drug absorption.
- sucralfate (Carafate).

▷ *Driving, Hazardous Activities:* Usually no restrictions. However, this drug may cause nausea or diarrhea. Restrict activities as necessary.

Aviation Note: The use of this drug **may be a disqualification** for piloting. Consult a designated Aviation Medical Examiner.

Exposure to Sun: Use caution. Some tetracyclines can cause photosensitivity (see Glossary).

THEOPHYLLINE (thee OFF i lin)

Introduced: 1900 **Prescription:** USA: Yes; Canada: Yes **Available as Generic:** Yes **Class:** Antiasthmatic, bronchodilator, xanthines **Controlled Drug:** USA: No; Canada: No

Brand Names: Accurbron, ✦Acet-Am, A.E.A., Aerolate, Aminodrox-Forte, ✦Apo-Oxtriphylline, ✦Aquaphyllim, ✦Asbron [CD], Asmalix, Azpan, Brocomar, Bronchial Gelatin Capsule, Broncomar, Bronkotabs, Bronkaid Tablets [CD], Bronkodyl, Bronkolixir [CD], Bronkotabs [CD], Constant-T, Duraphyl, Elixicon, Elixomin, Elixophyllin, For-Az-Ma [CD], Isuprel Compound [CD], Labid, Lanophyllin, Lixolin, Lodrane, Lodrane CR, Marax [CD], Marax DF [CD], Mudrane GG Elixir [CD], Phedral [CD], Phyllocontin, Physpan, ✦PMS Theophylline, Primatene, ✦Pulmophylline, Quadrinal [CD], Quibron [CD], Quibron-300 [CD], Quibron Plus [CD], Quibron-T Dividose, Quibron-T/SR, Respbid, Slo-bid, Slo-bid Gyrocaps, Slo-Phyllin, Slo-Phyllin GG [CD], Slo-Phyllin Gyrocaps, Somophyllin, Sompphyllin-12, Sustaire, Tedral [CD], Tedral SA [CD], T.E.H. [CD], T.E.P., Thalfed, Theobid Duracaps, ✦Theo-Bronc, Theochron, Theoclear, Theoclear L.A., Theocord, Theo-Dur, Theo-Dur Sprinkle, Theolair, Theolair-SR, Theolate [CD], Theolixir, Theomar [CD], Theomax DF, Theon, Theophyl-SR, Theo-24, Theospan-SR, Theo-SR, Theo-Time, Theovent, Theox, Theozine, Therex [CD], Uni-Dur, ✦Uniphyl, Vitaphen [CD]

BENEFITS versus RISKS	
Possible Benefits	*Possible Risks*
EFFECTIVE PREVENTION AND RELIEF OF ACUTE BRONCHIAL ASTHMA	NARROW TREATMENT RANGE FREQUENT STOMACH DISTRESS
	Gastrointestinal bleeding
MODERATELY EFFECTIVE CONTROL OF CHRONIC, RECURRENT BRONCHIAL ASTHMA	Central nervous system toxicity, seizures
	Heart rhythm disturbances
Moderately effective symptomatic relief in chronic bronchitis and emphysema	

▷ **Principal Uses**

As a Single Drug Product: Uses currently included in FDA approved labeling: (1) Used to relieve shortness of breath and wheezing of acute bronchial asthma, and to prevent the recurrence of asthmatic episodes; (2) It is also useful in relieving the asthmaticlike symptoms that are associated with some types of chronic bronchitis, chronic obstructive pulmonary disease and emphysema.

Other (unlabeled) generally accepted uses: (1) May have a role in combination therapy of cystic fibrosis; (2) can help decrease excessive production of red blood cells in kidney transplant patients; (3) may have a role in helping decrease the risk of sudden infant death syndrome; (4) may have a supportive role with steroids and other agents in helping prevent rejection of transplanted kidneys; (5) can help ease essential tremor; (6) decreases risk of breathing cessation in neonatal apnea; (7) helps in treating SIDS children; (8) may have a role in sleep apnea.

As a Combination Drug Product [CD]: Available in combination with several other drugs that help in overall management of bronchial asthma and related conditions. Ephedrine is added to enhance the bronchodilator effects; guaifenesin is added to provide an expectorant effect that thins mucus in the bronchial tubes; mild sedatives such as phenobarbital are added to allay the anxiety that often accompanies acute attacks of asthma.

How This Drug Works: By inhibiting the enzyme phosphodiesterase, this drug produces an increase in the tissue chemical cyclic AMP. This causes relaxation of the muscles in the bronchial tubes and blood vessels of the lung, resulting in relief of bronchospasm, expanded lung capacity and improved lung circulation.

Available Dosage Forms and Strengths

Capsules —	100 mg, 200 mg, 250 mg, 260 mg
Capsules, prolonged-action —	50 mg, 60 mg, 65 mg, 75 mg, 100 mg, 125 mg, 130 mg, 200 mg, 250 mg, 260 mg, 300 mg
Elixir —	27 mg, 50 mg per 5-ml
Oral solution —	27 mg, 53.3 mg per 5-ml
Oral suspension —	100 mg per 5-ml
Syrup —	27 mg, 50 mg per 5-ml
Tablets —	100 mg, 125 mg, 200 mg, 250 mg, 300 mg
Tablets, prolonged-action —	50 mg, 60 mg, 65 mg, 75 mg, 100 mg, 125 mg, 130 mg, 200 mg, 225 mg, 250 mg, 260 mg, 300 mg, 350 mg, 400 mg, 450 mg, 500 mg, 600 mg

▷ **Recommended Dosage Ranges** (Actual dosage and administration schedule must be determined by the physician for each patient individually.)

Infants and Children: For acute attack of asthma (not currently taking theophylline)—loading dose of 5 to 6 mg/kg of body weight.

For acute attack while currently taking theophylline—a single dose of 2.5 mg/kg of body weight, if no indications of theophylline toxicity. Monitor blood levels of theophylline.

For maintenance during acute attack—dosage is based on age:

Up to 6 months of age—0.07 for each week of age + 1.7 = the mg/kg of body weight, given every 8 hours.

6 months to 1 year of age—0.05 for each week of age + 1.25 = the mg/kg of body weight, given every 6 hours.

1 to 9 years of age—5 mg/kg of body weight, every 6 hours.

9 to 12 years of age—4 mg/kg of body weight, every 6 hours.

12 to 16 years of age—3 mg/kg of body weight, every 6 hours.

For chronic treatment to prevent recurrence of asthma—dosage is based on age:

Initially 16 mg/kg of body weight, in 3 or 4 divided doses at 6 to 8 hour intervals, up to a maximum of 400 mg daily. Increase dose as needed and tolerated by increments of 25% every 2 to 3 days. Limit total daily dosage as follows:

Up to 1 year of age—0.3 for each week of age + 8.0 = the mg/kg of body weight, per day.

1 to 9 years of age—22 mg/kg of body weight, per day.

9 to 12 years of age—20 mg/kg of body weight, per day.

12 to 16 years of age—18 mg/kg of body weight, per day.

16 years of age and over—13 mg/kg of body weight or 900 mg per day, whichever is less.

Note: It is advisable to measure blood levels of theophylline periodically during chronic therapy.

16 to 60 Years of Age: For acute attack of asthma (not currently taking theophylline)—loading dose of 5 to 6 mg/kg of body weight.

For acute attack while currently taking theophylline—a single dose of 2.5 mg/kg of body weight, if no indications of theophylline toxicity. Monitor blood levels of theophylline.

For maintenance during acute attack—for nonsmokers: 3 mg/kg of body weight, every 8 hours; for smokers: 4 mg/kg of body weight, every 6 hours.

For chronic treatment to prevent recurrence of asthma—Initially 6 to 8 mg/kg of body weight, in 3 or 4 divided doses at 6 to 8 hour intervals, up to a maximum of 400 mg daily. Increase dose as needed and tolerated by increments of 25% every 2 to 3 days. The total daily dosage should not exceed 13 mg/kg of body weight or 900 mg, whichever is less.

Prolonged action formulations may allow twice daily dosing with good results.

Over 60 Years of Age: For acute attack—same as 16 to 60 years of age.

For maintenance during acute attack—2 mg/kg of body weight, every 8 hours.

Conditions Requiring Dosing Adjustments

Liver function: The dose **must** be lowered, and blood levels obtained frequently. Doses may need to be decreased by 50 % in some cases.

Kidney function: Levels should be followed closely in severe kidney failure.

▷ **Dosing Instructions:**   May be taken with or following food to reduce stomach irritation. The regular capsules may be opened and the regular tablets may be crushed for administration. The prolonged-action dosage forms should be swallowed whole and not altered. Shake the oral suspension well before measuring each dose. Do not refrigerate any liquid dosage forms of this drug.

Usual Duration of Use: Use on a regular schedule for 48 to 72 hours usually determines effectiveness in controlling the breathing impairment associated with bronchial asthma and chronic lung disease. Long-term use (months to years) requires supervision and periodic physician evaluation.

▷ **This Drug Should Not Be Taken If**
- you have had an allergic reaction to it, or to aminophylline, dyphylline or oxtriphylline.
- you have active peptic ulcer disease.
- you have an uncontrolled seizure disorder.
- you have had a blood level drawn and it is in the "toxic" range.

▷ **Inform Your Physician Before Taking This Drug If**
- you have had an unfavorable reaction to any xanthine (see Drug Class Section).
- you have a seizure disorder of any kind.
- you have a history of peptic ulcer disease.
- you have a history of underactive thyroid (hypothyroidism).
- you have impaired liver or kidney function.
- you take any of the drugs listed in the "Other Drugs" section.
- you have hypertension, heart disease or any type of heart rhythm disorder.

Possible Side Effects (natural, expected, and unavoidable drug actions)
Nervousness, insomnia, rapid heart rate, increased urine volume.

▷ **Possible Adverse Effects** (unusual, unexpected, and infrequent reactions)
If any of the following develop, consult your physician promptly for guidance.

Mild Adverse Effects
Allergic Reactions: Skin rash, hives.
Headache, dizziness, irritability, tremor, fatigue, weakness.
Loss of appetite, nausea, vomiting (may be an early warning of toxicity), abdominal pain, diarrhea, excessive thirst.
Flushing of face.

Serious Adverse Effects
Allergic Reactions: Severe skin rash (Stevens-Johnson syndrome).
Idiosyncratic Reactions: Marked anxiety, confusion, behavioral disturbances.
Central nervous system toxicity: muscle twitching, seizures.
Heart rhythm abnormalities, rapid breathing, low blood pressure.
Gastrointestinal bleeding.
Defects in clotting (coagulation).
Drug-induced abnormal urine production (SIADH) (rare).
Drug-induced porphyria (rare).
Worsening of ulcers.
Liver toxicity.
Serious skin disorder (Stevens-Johnson syndrome).

▷ **Possible Effects on Sexual Function:**   None reported.

Natural Diseases or Disorders That May Be Activated by This Drug
Latent peptic ulcer disease.

Possible Effects on Laboratory Tests
Blood uric acid level: increased.
Fecal occult blood test: positive (large doses may cause stomach bleeding).

CAUTION
1. This drug should not be taken at the same time as other antiasthmatic drugs unless your doctor prescribes the combination. Serious overdose could result.
2. Influenza vaccine may delay the elimination of this drug and cause accumulation to toxic levels.

Precautions for Use

By Infants and Children: Do not exceed recommended doses. Watch for toxicity: irritability, agitation, tremors, lethargy, fever, vomiting, rapid heart rate and breathing, seizures. Blood levels needed during long-term use.

By Those over 60 Years of Age: Small starting doses are indicated. You may be at increased risk for stomach irritation, nausea, vomiting or diarrhea. When used concurrently with coffee (caffeine) or with nasal decongestants, this drug may cause excessive stimulation and a hyperactivity syndrome.

▷ **Advisability of Use During Pregnancy**

Pregnancy Category: C. See Pregnancy Code at the back of this book.

Animal studies: Significant birth defects due to this drug reported in mice.

Human studies: Adequate studies of pregnant women are not available. No increase in birth defects reported in 394 exposures to this drug.

Avoid this drug during the first 3 months. Use it otherwise only if clearly needed. Ask your physician for guidance.

Advisability of Use if Breast-Feeding

Presence of this drug in breast milk: Yes.

Avoid drug or refrain from nursing.

Habit-Forming Potential: None.

Effects of Overdosage: Nausea, vomiting, restlessness, irritability, confusion, delirium, seizures, high fever, weak pulse, coma.

Possible Effects of Long-Term Use: Gastrointestinal irritation.

Suggested Periodic Examinations While Taking This Drug (at physician's discretion)

Periodic testing of blood theophylline levels, especially with high dosage or long-term use. (See Therapeutic Drug Monitoring Section.)

Time to sample blood for theophylline level: 2 hours after regular (standard) dosage forms; 5 hours after sustained-release dosage forms.

Recommended therapeutic range: 10 to 20 mcg/ml.

▷ **While Taking This Drug, Observe the Following**

Foods: No restrictions.

Beverages: Avoid excessive use of caffeine-containing beverages: coffee, tea, cola; this combination could cause nervousness and insomnia.

▷ *Alcohol:* No interactions expected. May have additive effect on stomach irritation.

Tobacco Smoking: May hasten the elimination of this drug and reduce its effectiveness. Higher doses may be necessary to maintain a therapeutic blood level.

Marijuana Smoking: May hasten the elimination of this drug and reduce its effectiveness. Higher doses may be necessary to maintain a therapeutic blood level.

▷ *Other Drugs*

Theophylline may *decrease* the effects of

• lithium (Lithane, Lithobid, etc.), and reduce its effectiveness.

Theophylline *taken concurrently* with

• halothane (anesthesia) may cause heart rhythm abnormalities.

• phenytoin (Dilantin) may cause decreased effects of both drugs. Monitor blood levels and adjust dosages as appropriate.

The following drugs may *increase* the effects of theophylline

• allopurinol (Lopurin, Zyloprim).

• amiodarone (Codarone).

- cimetidine (Tagamet).
- ciprofloxacin (Cipro).
- clarithromycin (Biaxin).
- disulfiram (Antabuse).
- doxycycline and other tetracyclines.
- enoxacin (Penetrex).
- ephedrine.
- erythromycin (E-Mycin, Erythrocin, etc.).
- famotidine (Pepcid).
- fluvoxamine (Luvox).
- furosemide (Lasix).
- imipenem-cilastatin (Primaxin).
- influenza vaccine.
- interferon alpha.
- isoniazid (INH).
- methotrexate (Mexate)
- mexiletine (Mexitil).
- nicotine (Nicorette, Pro-Step, others).
- norfloxacin (Noroxin).
- oral contraceptives.
- pentoxyfylline (Trental).
- ranitidine (Zantac).
- tacrine (Cognex).
- thiabendazole.
- ticlopidine (Ticlid).
- troleandomycin (TAO).
- verapamil (Calan, Verelan).
- viloxazine.

The following drugs may *decrease* the effects of theophylline

- barbiturates (phenobarbital, etc.).
- beta blocker drugs (see Drug Classes).
- carbamazepine (Tegretol).
- isoproterenol.
- primidone (Mysoline).
- rifampin (Rifadin, Rimactane, etc.).
- sulfinpyrazone (Anturane).

▷ *Driving, Hazardous Activities:* This drug may cause dizziness. Restrict activities as necessary.

Aviation Note: The use of this drug *may be a disqualification* for piloting. Consult a designated Aviation Medical Examiner.

Exposure to Sun: No restrictions.

Occurrence of Unrelated Illness: Acute viral respiratory infections may decrease drug elimination. Watch for signs of toxicity. Dosing **must** be changed if this occurs. Fever can decrease the rate of removal (clearance) of this medicine. Increased frequency of blood levels are suggested. Seizure disorders may be worsened by this medicine. It is only used with extreme caution in seizure patients. Theophylline is also only used with extreme caution in active peptic ulcer disease or heart arrhythmias (cardiac, not including slow or bradyarrhythmias).

Discontinuation: Avoid prolonged or unnecessary use of this drug. When your asthma resolves, withdraw this drug gradually over several days.

THIAZIDE DIURETICS

Bendromethiazide (ben droh meh THI a zide)   **Hydrochlorothiazide** (hi droh klor oh THI a zide)   **Hydroflumethiazide** (hi droh flu meh THI a zide)   **Chlorothiazide** (klor oh THI a zide)   **Methyclothiazide** (METH i klo THI a zide) **Trichlormethiazide** (tri klor me THI a zide)   **Chlorthalidone** (KLOR thal i dohn)   **Metolazone** (me TOHL a zohn)

Introduced: 1960, 1959, 1961, 1957, 1959, 1962, 1960, 1974 respectively **Prescription:**   USA: Yes; Canada: Yes   **Available as Generic:**   USA: Yes; Canada: Yes   **Class:**   Antihypertensive, diuretic, thiazides   **Controlled Drug:** USA: No; Canada: No

Brand Names: Bendroflumethiazide: Naturetin, **Hydrochlorothiazide**: Aldactazide [CD], Aldoril-15/25 [CD], Aldoril D30/D50 [CD], ✦Apo-Amilzide,
   ✦Apo-Hydro, ✦Apo-Methazide [CD], ✦Apo-Triazide [CD], Apresazide [CD],
   Apresoline-Esidrix [CD], Capozide [CD], ✦Co-Betaloc [CD], Diaqua, ✦Diuchlor H, Dyazide [CD], Esidrix, Ezide, H-H-R, H.H.R., HydroDIURIL, Hydromal, Hydro-Par, Hydropres [CD], Hydroserpine [CD], Hdroserpine Plus
   [CD], Hydro-T, Hydro-Z-50, Inderide [CD], Inderide LA [CD], ✦Ismelin-Esidrix [CD], Lopressor HCT [CD], Maxzide [CD], Maxzide-25 [CD], M Dopazide [CD], Mictrin, ✦Moduret [CD], Moduretic [CD], ✦Natrimax, ✦Neo-
   Codema, Normozide [CD], ✦Novo-Doparil [CD], ✦Novo-Hydrazide,
   ✦Novo-Spirozine [CD], ✦Novo-Triamzide [CD], Oretic, Oreticyl [CD],
   ✦PMS Dopazide [CD], Prinzide [CD], Ser-Ap-Es [CD], Serpasil-Esidrix
   [CD], SK-Hydrochlorothiazide, Thiuretic, Timolide [CD], Trandate HCT
   [CD], Unipres [CD], ✦Urozide, Vaseretic [CD], ✦Viskazide [CD], Zestoretic
   [CD], Ziac, Zide, **Chlorothiazide:** Aldochlor [CD], Diachlor, Diupres [CD],
   Diurigen, Diuril, SK-Chlorothiazide, ✦Supres [CD], **Hydroflumethiazide:**
   Diucardin, Saluron, **Methyclothiazide:** ✦Duretic, Aquatensen, ✦Duretic,
   Enduron, **Trichlormethiazide**: Diurese, Marazide II, Metahydrin, Naqua,
   Naquival [CD], **Chlorthalidone**: ✦Apo-Chlorthalidone, Combipress [CD],
   Demi-Regroton [CD], Hygroton, ✦Hygroton-Resperpine [CD], Hylidone,
   ✦Novothalidone, Regroton [CD], Thalitone, ✦Uridon, Tenoretic, Metolazone: Diulo, Microx, Mykrox, Zaroxolyn

BENEFITS versus RISKS	
Possible Benefits	*Possible Risks*
EFFECTIVE, WELL-TOLERATED DIURETICS	Loss of body potassium and magnesium (especially with higher doses)
POSSIBLY EFFECTIVE IN MILD HYPERTENSION	Cardiac arrhythmias caused by decreased electrolytes (recently
ENHANCES EFFECTIVENESS OF OTHER ANTIHYPERTENSIVES	studied in chlorthalidone and hydrochlorothiazide)
Beneficial in treatment of diabetes insipidus	Increased blood sugar
	Increased blood uric acid
	Increased blood calcium
	Rare blood cell disorders
	Rare liver toxicity (chlorothiazide or hydrochlorothiazide)

▷ **Principal Uses**

As a Single Drug Product: Uses currently included in FDA approved labeling: (1) Increase the volume of urine (diuresis) to correct fluid retention (edema) seen in congestive heart failure, corticosteroid or estrogen use and certain types of liver and kidney disease; and (2) starting therapy for high blood pressure (hypertension).

Other (unlabeled) generally accepted uses: (1) Prevention of kidney stones that contain calcium; (2) may help decrease the frequency of hip fractures in the elderly; (3) methyclothiazide has been used to help maintain blood calcium levels in Paget's disease; (4) may have a role in helping prevent osteoporosis (by correcting abnormally high elimination of calcium in the urine or hypercalciuria); (5) of use in diabetes insipidus (nephrogenic) in decreasing the urine volume.

As a Combination Drug Product [CD]: Used to treat blood pressure that has not responded to single-drug therapy.

How These Drugs Work: By increasing the elimination of salt and water in the urine, these drugs reduce fluid volume and body sodium. They also relax the walls of smaller arteries and the combined effect of these two actions (reduced blood volume in expanded space) results in lowering of the blood pressure.

Available Dosage Forms and Strengths

Hydrochlorothiazide:
Solution — 50 mg per 5-ml
Solution, intensol — 100 mg per ml
Tablets — 25 mg, 50 mg, 100 mg
Chlorothiazide:
Injection — 500 mg per 20 ml
Oral suspension — 250 mg per 5 ml
Tablets — 250 mg, 500 mg
Methyclothiazide:
Tablets — 2.5 mg, 5 mg
Trichlormethiazide:
Tablets — 2 mg, 4 mg
Chlorthalidone:
Tablets — 25 mg, 50 mg, 100 mg
Metolazone:
Tablets — 0.5 mg, 2.5 mg, 5 mg, 10 mg

▷ **Usual Adult Dosage Range:** Hydrochlorothiazide: As antihypertensive: 50 to 100 mg/day initially; 50 to 200 mg/day for maintenance. As diuretic: 50 to 200 mg/day initially; the smallest effective dose should be determined (**see cautions**). The total daily dose should not exceed 200 mg, however, this maximum may change in light of recent data.

Chlorothiazide: As antihypertensive: 500 to 1000 mg per day to start and 500 to 2000 mg daily as a maintenance dose. As a diuretic: 500 to 2000 mg per day with use of the smallest effective dose. Daily maximum is 2000 mg.

Methyclothiazide: As antihypertensive or diuretic: 2.5 to 5 mg daily are used. Maximum daily diuretic dose is 10 mg. Pediatric dose: 0.05 to 0.2 mg per kg daily.

Trichlormethiazide: As antihypertensive or diuretic: Therapy may be started with 1 to 4 mg twice daily. Usual maintenance dose is 1 to 4 mg once daily.

Chlorthalidone As antihypertensive: 25 to 50 mg daily to start therapy, then 50 to 100 mg for maintenance. As a diuretic: 50 to 100 mg daily, then maintenance with the smallest effective dose **(see cautions).** Daily maximum is 200 mg, however, this may change with recently published data.

Note: Actual dosage and administration schedule must be determined by the physician for each patient individually.

Conditions Requiring Dosing Adjustments

Liver function: Electrolyte balance is critical in liver failure, and these drugs may precipitate encephalopathy. Hydrochlorothiazide and chlorothiazide are also a rare cause of cholestatic jaundice and are used with caution in liver failure.

Kidney function: These drugs can be used with caution in patients with mild kidney failure, and are not effective in patients with moderate failure. Contraindicated in patients severe kidney failure, and can be a rare cause of kidney damage.

▷ **Dosing Instructions:**   The tablets may be crushed and taken with or following meals to reduce stomach irritation. Best taken in the morning to avoid nighttime urination.

Usual Duration of Use: Use on a regular schedule for 2 to 3 weeks determines effectiveness in lowering high blood pressure. Long-term use (months to years) requires periodic physician evaluation.

▷ **These Drugs Should Not Be Taken If**
- you have had an allergic reaction to any dosage form of it previously.
- your kidneys are not making urine.

▷ **Inform Your Physician Before Taking These Drugs If**
- you are allergic to any form of "sulfa" drug.
- you are pregnant or planning pregnancy.
- you have a history of kidney or liver disease.
- you have a history of pancreatitis.
- you have asthma or allergies to other medicines.
- you have had laboratory testing of electrolytes ordered by another physician which your doctor has not seen.
- you develop muscle cramps, weakness or abnormal heart beats while taking one of these medicines.
- you have diabetes, gout or lupus erythematosus.
- you are allergic to the dye tartrazine as some of these medicines contain it.
- you take any form of cortisone, digitalis, oral antidiabetic drug or insulin.
- you plan to have surgery under general anesthesia in the near future.

Possible Side Effects (natural, expected, and unavoidable drug actions)

Light-headedness on arising from sitting or lying position (see Orthostatic Hypotension in Glossary).

Increase in blood sugar level, affecting control of diabetes.

Increase in blood uric acid level, affecting control of gout.

Decrease in blood potassium level, causing muscle weakness and cramping.

Decreased blood magnesium, combined with loss of potassium, may lead to increased risk of sudden cardiac death, especially if high doses are used for extended periods.

▷ **Possible Adverse Effects** (unusual, unexpected, and infrequent reactions)
If any of the following develop, consult your physician promptly for guidance.

Mild Adverse Effects

Allergic Reactions: Skin rashes, hives, drug fever.

Headache, dizziness, blurred or yellow vision.

Reduced appetite, indigestion, nausea, vomiting, diarrhea.

Serious Adverse Effects

Allergic Reactions: Hepatitis with jaundice (see Glossary), anaphylactic reaction (see Glossary), severe skin reactions.

Inflammation of the pancreas—severe abdominal pain.

Bone marrow depression (see Glossary)—fatigue, weakness, fever, sore throat, abnormal bleeding or bruising.

Data from studies of hydrochlorothiazide and chlorthalidone suggest that potassium and magnesium loss associated with higher-dose therapy increases the risk of sudden cardiac death.

Precipitation of acute gout in some patients (because this medicine decreases the elimination of uric acid).

Pancreatitis.

Loss of blood glucose control.

Short-term (less than one year) increase in serum lipids (returns to pretreatment levels in about one year).

▷ **Possible Effects on Sexual Function:** Decreased libido (hydrochlorothiazide, chlorthalidone); impotence (bendroflumethiazide, chlorothiazide, hydrochlorothiazide).

▷ **Adverse Effects That May Mimic Natural Diseases or Disorders**

Liver reaction may suggest viral hepatitis.

Natural Diseases or Disorders That May Be Activated by These Drugs

Diabetes, gout, systemic lupus erythematosus. People with asthma or other drug allergies may be more likely to have allergic reactions.

Possible Effects on Laboratory Tests

Complete blood counts: decreased red cells, hemoglobin, white cells and platelets.

Blood amylase level: increased (possible pancreatitis).

Blood calcium level: increased.

Blood sodium and chloride levels: decreased.

Blood cholesterol and triglyceride levels: increased, short-term.

Blood glucose level: increased.

Glucose tolerance test (GTT): decreased.

Blood lithium level: increased.

Blood potassium and magnesium level: decreased.

Blood urea nitrogen (BUN) level: increased with long-term use.

Blood uric acid level: increased.

Liver function tests (hydrochlorothiazide and chlorothiazide): increased liver enzymes (ALT/GPT, AST/GOT and alkaline phosphatase), increased bilirubin.

CAUTION
1. A recent study found a strong association between higher doses of hydrochlorothiazide and chlorthalidone and combination drugs containing these diuretics and electrolyte loss and sudden cardiac death. This did appear to be a result of magnesium and potassium loss, and may be circumvented by close following of those electrolytes.
2. Take exactly as prescribed. Excessive loss of sodium and potassium can lead to loss of appetite, nausea, fatigue, weakness, confusion and tingling in the extremities.
3. If you take digitalis (digitoxin, digoxin), adequate potassium is critical. Periodic testing and high-potassium foods may be needed to prevent potassium deficiency—a potential cause of digitalis toxicity. (See Table of High Potassium Foods in Section Six.)

Precautions for Use
By Infants and Children: Overdose could cause serious dehydration. Significant potassium loss can occur within the first 2 weeks of drug use.
By Those over 60 Years of Age: Starting doses may be as low as 12.5 mg. Increased risk of impaired thinking, orthostatic hypotension, potassium loss and blood sugar increase. Overdose or extended use can cause excessive loss of body water, thickening (increased viscosity) of blood and increased tendency for the blood to clot—predisposing to stroke, heart attack or thrombophlebitis (vein inflammation with blood clot).

▷ **Advisability of Use During Pregnancy**
Pregnancy Category: Metolazone: B by manufacturer, D by other independent researchers. All other thiazides in this class are D. See Pregnancy Code at the back of this book.
Animal studies: No birth defects found in rat studies.
Human studies: Reports are conflicting and inconclusive. Use of thiazides can cause a variety of maternal complications which may cause adverse fetal effects, including death. They should not be used during pregnancy unless a very serious complication occurs for which this drug is significantly beneficial. Ask physician for guidance.

Advisability of Use if Breast-Feeding
Presence of these drugs in breast milk: Yes.
Avoid drug or refrain from nursing.

Habit-Forming Potential: None.

Effects of Overdosage: Dry mouth, thirst, lethargy, weakness, muscle cramping, nausea, vomiting, drowsiness progressing to stupor or coma.

Possible Effects of Long-Term Use: Impaired balance of water, salt, magnesium and potassium in blood and body tissues. Development of diabetes in predisposed individuals. Pathological changes in parathyroid glands with increased blood calcium levels and decreased blood phosphate levels.

Suggested Periodic Examinations While Taking These Drugs (at physician's discretion)
Complete blood cell counts, measurements of blood levels of sodium, potassium, chloride, sugar and uric acid.
Kidney and liver function tests.

▷ **While Taking These Drugs, Observe the Following**

Foods: Ask your doctor if you need to eat foods rich in potassium. See the Table of High Potassium Foods if needed. Follow physician's advice regarding the use of salt. Magnesium should be routinely checked, and supplemented if these medicines have lowered blood levels.

Beverages: No restrictions. This drug may be taken with milk.

▷ *Alcohol:* Use with caution—alcohol may exaggerate the blood-pressure-lowering effects of this drug and cause orthostatic hypotension.

Tobacco Smoking: No interactions expected. Follow physician's advice.

▷ *Other Drugs*

These drugs may ***increase*** the effects of
- other antihypertensive drugs; dosage adjustments may be necessary to prevent excessive lowering of blood pressure.
- lithium (Lithobid, others), and cause lithium toxicity.

These drugs may ***decrease*** the effects of
- oral antidiabetic drugs (see Drug Classes) (sulfonylureas); dosage adjustments may be necessary for proper control of blood sugar.
- oral anticoagulants such as warfarin (Coumadin) and require dose adjustments. Increased frequency of INR testing is needed.

These drugs ***taken concurrently*** with
- allopurinol (Zyloprim) may decrease kidney function.
- amphotericin B (Fungizone) may result in additive potassium loss. Increased frequency of laboratory testing is needed.
- calcium may result in the Milk-alkali syndrome: with increased calcium, alkalosis and kidney failure.
- carbamazepine (Tegretol) may result in low sodium levels and symptomatic hyponatremia.
- cortisone or other corticosteroid medicines may result in excessive potassium loss with resultant heart rhythm changes and lethargy.
- digitalis preparations (digitoxin, digoxin) requires careful monitoring and dose changes to prevent low potassium levels and serious disturbances of heart rhythm.
- nonsteroidal anti-inflammatory drugs (see Drug Classes) such as sulindac (Clinoril) and naproxen (Naprosyn, Aleve, Anaprox, others) may result in decreased effectiveness of the thiazide.

The following drugs may ***decrease*** the effects of these thiazides
- cholestyramine (Cuemid, Questran) may interfere with its absorption.
- colestipol (Colestid) may interfere with its absorption.

Take cholestyramine and colestipol 1 hour before any oral diuretic.

▷ *Driving, Hazardous Activities:* Use caution until the possible occurrence of orthostatic hypotension, dizziness or impaired vision has been determined.

Aviation Note: The use of this drug ***may be a disqualification*** for piloting. Consult a designated Aviation Medical Examiner.

Exposure to Sun: Use caution until sensitivity has been determined. This drug can cause photosensitivity (see Glossary).

Exposure to Heat: Caution—excessive perspiring could cause additional loss of salt and water from the body.

Heavy Exercise or Exertion: Avoid exertion that produces light-headedness, excessive fatigue or muscle cramping. Isometric exercises can raise blood pressure significantly. Ask doctor for help regarding participation in this form of exercise.

Occurrence of Unrelated Illness: Vomiting or diarrhea can produce a serious imbalance of important body chemistry. Consult your physician for guidance.

Discontinuation: These drugs should not be stopped abruptly following long-term use; sudden discontinuation can cause serious thiazide-withdrawal fluid retention (edema). The dose should be reduced gradually. It may be advisable to discontinue this drug 5 to 7 days before major surgery. Ask your physician, surgeon and/or anesthesiologist for guidance.

THIORIDAZINE (thi oh RID a zeen)

Introduced: 1959   **Prescription:** USA: Yes; Canada: Yes   **Available as Generic:** USA: Yes; Canada: Yes   **Class:** tranquilizer, major; phenothiazines
Controlled Drug: USA: No; Canada: No

Brand Names: ✦Apo-Thioridazine, Mellaril, Mellaril-S, Millazine, ✦Novoridazine, ✦PMS-Thioridazine, SK-Thioridazine

<table>
<tr><td colspan="2" align="center">BENEFITS versus RISKS</td></tr>
<tr><td align="center">Possible Benefits</td><td align="center">Possible Risks</td></tr>
<tr><td>EFFECTIVE CONTROL OF ACUTE MENTAL DISORDERS: beneficial effects on thinking, mood, and behavior
Relief of anxiety, agitation, and tension
Possibly effective in the management of the hyperactivity syndrome in children</td><td>SERIOUS TOXIC EFFECTS ON BRAIN with long-term use
Liver damage with jaundice (infrequent)
Rare blood cell disorder: abnormally low white blood cell count</td></tr>
</table>

▷ **Principal Uses**

As a Single Drug Product: Uses currently included in FDA approved labeling: (1) Helps manage: moderate to marked depression with significant anxiety and nervous tension; agitation, anxiety, depression and exaggerated fears in the elderly; (2) of use in severe behavioral problems in children characterized by hyperexcitability, combativeness, short attention span and rapid swings in mood (temper tantrums).

Other (unlabeled) generally accepted uses: (1) May have a role in treating alcohol withdrawal in patients who can not tolerate benzodiazepines; (2) can be used to treat unexplained infertility; (3) may help control premature ejaculation and nocturnal emissions in men; (4) can help borderline personality disorder; (5) of use in some chronic pain syndromes; (6) may be of use in hypersexuality.

How This Drug Works: By inhibiting the action of dopamine in certain brain centers, this drug acts to correct an imbalance of nerve impulse transmissions that is thought to be responsible for certain mental disorders. May help control premature ejaculation by inhibiting the muscle (longitudinal) that controls the vas deferens.

Available Dosage Forms and Strengths

Concentrate — 30 mg, 100 mg per ml

Oral suspension — 25 mg, 100 mg per 5-ml

Tablets — 10 mg, 15 mg, 25 mg, 50 mg, 100 mg, 150 mg, 200 mg

▷ **Usual Adult Dosage Range:** Initially, 25 to 100 mg 3 times/day. Dose may be increased by 25 to 50 mg at 3 to 4 day intervals as needed and tolerated. Usual dosage range (psychosis) is 200 to 800 mg daily, divided into 2 to 4 doses. The total daily dosage should not exceed 800 mg. **Note: Actual dosage and administration schedule must be determined by the physician for each patient individually.**

Conditions Requiring Dosing Adjustments

Liver function: This drug is extensively metabolized in the liver and should be used with caution in liver compromise, and the patient closely monitored.

Kidney function: Patients with compromised kidneys should be closely followed.

▷ **Dosing Instructions:** The tablets may be crushed and taken with or following meals to reduce stomach irritation.

Usual Duration of Use: Use on a regular schedule for 3 to 4 weeks usually determines effectiveness in controlling psychotic disorders. If not significantly beneficial within 6 weeks, it should be stopped. Long-term use (months to years) requires periodic physician evaluation of response, appropriate dosage adjustment and consideration of continued need.

▷ **This Drug Should Not Be Taken If**

- you are allergic to any of the drugs bearing the brand names listed above.
- you have active liver disease.
- you have cancer of the breast.
- you have a constitutionally low blood pressure.
- you have a current blood cell or bone marrow disorder.

▷ **Inform Your Physician Before Taking This Drug If**

- you are allergic or abnormally sensitive to any phenothiazine (see Drug Classes).
- you have impaired liver or kidney function.
- you have any type of seizure disorder.
- you have diabetes, glaucoma or heart disease.
- you have a history of lupus erythematosus.
- you are taking any drug with sedative effects.
- you plan to have surgery under general or spinal anesthesia in the near future.

Possible Side Effects (natural, expected, and unavoidable drug actions)

Drowsiness (usually during the first 2 weeks), orthostatic hypotension (see Glossary), blurred vision, dry mouth, nasal congestion, constipation, impaired urination.

Pink or purple coloration of urine, of no significance.

▷ **Possible Adverse Effects** (unusual, unexpected, and infrequent reactions)

If any of the following develop, consult your physician promptly for guidance.

Mild Adverse Effects

Allergic Reactions: Skin rash, hives, low-grade fever.

Lowering of body temperature, especially in the elderly (see Hypothermia in Glossary).

Abnormal body hair growth (hirsutism).

Urinary incontinence.

Increased appetite and weight gain.

Inflammation of the parotid gland.

Weakness, agitation, insomnia, impaired day and night vision.

Chronic constipation, fecal impaction.

Serious Adverse Effects

Allergic Reactions: Hepatitis with jaundice (see Glossary), severe skin reactions (Stevens-Johnson syndrome or erythema multiforme).

Idiosyncratic Reactions: Neuroleptic malignant syndrome (see Glossary).

Depression, disorientation, seizures, loss of peripheral vision.

Rapid heart rate, heart rhythm disorders.

Blood cell disorders: reduced white blood cell count (more common in the elderly).

Sudden death syndrome (rare).

Excessive production of urine (SIADH).

Pituitary tumors (rare).

Nervous system reactions: Parkinson-like disorders (see Glossary), severe restlessness, muscle spasms involving the face and neck, tardive dyskinesia (see Glossary).

Retinopathy.

Liver toxicity (cholestatic jaundice).

Abnormally low blood pressure.

▷ **Possible Effects on Sexual Function**

Decreased male and female libido; inhibited ejaculation (49% to 60%); impotence (54%); impaired female orgasm; priapism (see Glossary).

Male breast enlargement and tenderness (gynecomastia).

Female breast enlargement with milk production.

Altered timing and pattern of menstruation.

False positive pregnancy test results.

May help control premature ejaculation and nocturnal emissions.

▷ **Adverse Effects That May Mimic Natural Diseases or Disorders**

Nervous system reactions may suggest true Parkinson's disease.

Liver reactions may suggest viral hepatitis.

Reactions resembling systemic lupus erythematosus can occur.

Natural Diseases or Disorders That May Be Activated by This Drug

Latent epilepsy, glaucoma, diabetes mellitus, prostatism (see Glossary).

Possible Effects on Laboratory Tests

Complete blood cell counts: decreased red cells, hemoglobin, white cells and platelets.

Liver function tests: increased liver enzymes (ALT/GPT, AST/GOT and alkaline phosphatase), increased bilirubin.

Urine pregnancy tests: falsely positive result with Prognosticon.

CAUTION

1. Many over-the-counter medications (see OTC Drugs in Glossary) for allergies, colds and coughs contain drugs that can interact unfavorably with

this drug. Ask your doctor or pharmacist for help **before** using any such medications.

2. Antacids that contain aluminum and/or magnesium can prevent the absorption of this drug and reduce its effectiveness.

3. Obtain prompt evaluation of any change or disturbance of vision.

Precautions for Use

By Infants and Children: NOT recommended in children under 2 years of age. Do not use this drug in the presence of symptoms suggestive of Reye syndrome (see Glossary). Children with acute infectious diseases ("flulike" infections, chicken pox, measles, etc.) are more prone to develop muscular spasms of the face, back and extremities when this drug is given for any reason.

By Those over 60 Years of Age: Small starting doses are advisable. You may be more susceptible to drowsiness, lethargy, constipation, lowering of body temperature (hypothermia) and orthostatic hypotension (see Glossary). This drug can worsen existing prostatism (see Glossary). You may also be more susceptible to Parkinson-like reactions and/or tardive dyskinesia (see discussion of these terms in Glossary). These reactions must be recognized early since they may become unresponsive to treatment and irreversible.

▷ **Advisability of Use During Pregnancy**

Pregnancy Category: C. See Pregnancy Code at the back of this book.

Animal studies: The results of rodent studies are conflicting.

Human studies: No increase in birth defects reported in 23 exposures. Adequate studies of pregnant women are not available.

Avoid drug during the first 3 months. Use it otherwise only if clearly needed. Ask your physician for guidance.

Advisability of Use if Breast-Feeding

Presence of this drug in breast milk: Yes, in minute amounts.

Monitor nursing infant closely and discontinue drug or nursing if adverse effects develop.

Habit-Forming Potential: None.

Effects of Overdosage: Marked drowsiness, weakness, tremor, agitation, unsteadiness, deep sleep, coma, convulsions.

Possible Effects of Long-Term Use: Opacities in the cornea or lens of the eye, pigmentation of the retina. Tardive dyskinesia (see Glossary).

Suggested Periodic Examinations While Taking This Drug (at physician's discretion)

Complete blood cell counts, especially between the fourth and tenth weeks of treatment.

Liver function tests, electrocardiograms.

Complete eye examinations—eye structures and vision.

Careful inspection of the tongue for early evidence of fine, involuntary, wavelike movements that could be the beginning of tardive dyskinesia.

▷ **While Taking This Drug, Observe the Following**

Foods: No restrictions.

Nutritional Support: A riboflavin (vitamin B-2) supplement should be taken with long-term use.

Beverages: No restrictions. May be taken with milk.

▷ *Alcohol:* Avoid completely. Alcohol can increase the sedative action of phenothiazines and accentuate their depressant effects on brain function and blood pressure. Phenothiazines can increase the intoxicating effects of alcohol.

Tobacco Smoking: Possible reduction of drowsiness from drug.

Marijuana Smoking: Moderate increase in drowsiness; accentuation of orthostatic hypotension; increased risk of precipitating latent psychoses, confusing the interpretation of mental status and drug responses.

▷ *Other Drugs*

Thioridazine may ***increase*** the effects of
• all sedative drugs, especially meperidine (Demerol), and cause excessive sedation.
• all atropinelike drugs, and cause nervous system toxicity.

Thioridazine may ***decrease*** the effects of
• bromocriptine (Parlodel).
• guanethidine (Ismelin, Esimil), and reduce its effectiveness in lowering blood pressure.
• oral hypoglycemic agents (see Drug Classes).

Thioridazine ***taken concurrently*** with
• ascorbic acid (vitamin C) may result in decreased thioridazine therapeutic benefits.
• lithium (Lithobid, Lithotabs) may impair the effectiveness of lithium and cause nervous system toxicity.
• phenytoin (Dilantin) may increase or decrease blood levels.

The following drugs may ***decrease*** the effects of thioridazine
• antacids containing aluminum and/or magnesium.
• barbiturates (see Drug Classes).
• benztropine (Cogentin).
• disulfiram (Antabuse).
• trihexyphenidyl (Artane).

▷ *Driving, Hazardous Activities:* This drug can impair mental alertness, judgment and physical coordination. Avoid hazardous activities.

Aviation Note: The use of this drug ***is a disqualification*** for piloting. Consult a designated Aviation Medical Examiner.

Exposure to Sun: Use caution. Some phenothiazines can cause photosensitivity (see Glossary).

Exposure to Heat: Use caution and avoid excessive heat as much as possible. This drug may impair the regulation of body temperature and increase the risk of heat stroke.

Exposure to Cold: Use caution and dress warmly. This drug can increase the risk of hypothermia in the elderly.

Discontinuation: After long-term use, do not stop this drug suddenly. Gradual withdrawal over 2 to 3 weeks under physician supervision is recommended. Do not discontinue this drug without your physician's knowledge and approval.

THIOTHIXENE (thi oh THIX een)

Introduced: 1967   **Prescription:** USA: Yes; Canada: Yes   **Available as
Generic:** USA: Yes; Canada: No   **Class:** tranquilizer, major; thioxanthenes
Controlled Drug: USA: No; Canada: No

Brand Name: Navane

BENEFITS versus RISKS	
Possible Benefits	*Possible Risks*
EFFECTIVE CONTROL OF ACUTE MENTAL DISORDERS: beneficial effects on thinking, mood, and behavior	SERIOUS TOXIC EFFECTS ON BRAIN with long-term use Liver damage with jaundice (rare) Rare blood cell disorder: abnormally low white blood cell count

▷ **Principal Uses**

As a Single Drug Product: Uses currently included in FDA approved labeling: (1) Used to relieve the psychotic thinking and behavior associated with acute psychoses of unknown nature, episodes of mania and paranoia, and acute schizophrenia.

Other (unlabeled) generally accepted uses: (1) Can be of use in significant borderline personality disorder.

How This Drug Works: Present theory is that, by inhibiting the action of dopamine, this drug acts to correct an imbalance of nerve impulse transmissions (at both D1 and D2 receptors) that is thought to be responsible for certain mental disorders.

Available Dosage Forms and Strengths

Capsules — 1 mg, 2 mg, 5 mg, 10 mg, 20 mg
Concentrate — 5 mg per ml
Injections — 2 mg, 5 mg per ml

▷ **Usual Adult Dosage Range:** Initially, 2 to 5 mg 2 or 3 times daily. Dose may be increased by 2 mg at 3 to 4 day intervals as needed and tolerated. Usual dosage range is 20 to 30 mg daily. The total daily dosage should not exceed 60 mg. **Note: Actual dosage and administration schedule must be determined by the physician for each patient individually.**

Conditions Requiring Dosing Adjustments

Liver function: This drug should be used with caution in liver compromise.
Kidney function: Patients with compromised kidneys should be closely followed.

▷ **Dosing Instructions:** The capsules may be opened and taken with or following meals to reduce stomach irritation. The liquid concentrate must be diluted just before administration by adding it to 8 ounces of water, milk, fruit juice or carbonated beverage.

Usual Duration of Use: Use on a regular schedule for several weeks usually determines effectiveness in controlling psychotic disorders. If not beneficial within 6 weeks, it should be stopped. Long-term use (months to years) requires periodic physician evaluation of response, appropriate dosage adjustment and consideration of continued need.

▷ **This Drug Should Not Be Taken If**
- you have had an allergic reaction to it previously.
- you have active liver disease.
- you have cancer of the breast.
- you have a current blood cell or bone marrow disorder.

▷ **Inform Your Physician Before Taking This Drug If**
- you are allergic or abnormally sensitive to other thioxanthene drugs or any phenothiazine drug (see Drug Classes).
- you have impaired liver or kidney function.
- you have any type of seizure disorder.
- you have diabetes, glaucoma or heart disease.
- you have a history of lupus erythematosus.
- you have Parkinson's disease.
- you have had neuroleptic malignant syndrome.
- you are taking any drug with sedative effects.
- you drink alcohol daily.
- you plan to have surgery under general or spinal anesthesia in the near future.

Possible Side Effects (natural, expected, and unavoidable drug actions)
Mild drowsiness (usually during the first 2 weeks), orthostatic hypotension (see Glossary), blurred vision, dry mouth, nasal congestion, constipation, impaired urination.

▷ **Possible Adverse Effects** (unusual, unexpected, and infrequent reactions)
If any of the following develop, consult your physician promptly for guidance.
Mild Adverse Effects
Allergic Reactions: Skin rash, hives, itching.
Lowering of body temperature, especially in the elderly (see Hypothermia in Glossary).
Fluid retention, weight gain.
Dizziness, weakness, agitation, insomnia, impaired vision.
Nausea, vomiting.
Serious Adverse Effects
Allergic Reactions: Rare hepatitis with jaundice (see Glossary), anaphylactic reaction (see Glossary).
Idiosyncratic Reactions: Paradoxical worsening of psychotic symptoms. Development of the neuroleptic malignant syndrome (see Glossary).
Abnormal production of urine and loss of blood sodium (SIADH).
Depression, disorientation, seizures.
Deposits in cornea and lens of the eye.
Abnormal fixed eye positioning (oculogyric crisis).
Drug-induced oculogyric crisis.
Rapid heart rate, heart rhythm disorders.
Systemic lupus erythematosus (rare).
Blood cell disorders: reduced white blood cell count (rare).
Nervous system reactions: Parkinson-like disorders (see Glossary), severe restlessness, muscle spasms involving the face and neck, tardive dyskinesia (see Glossary).
Severe reduction in blood pressure (rare).

▷ **Possible Effects on Sexual Function**

Altered timing and pattern of menstruation.
Impotence (rare).
Priapism and retrograde ejaculation.
Male breast enlargement and tenderness.
Female breast enlargement with milk production.

▷ **Adverse Effects That May Mimic Natural Diseases or Disorders**

Nervous system reactions may suggest true Parkinson's disease or Reye syndrome (see Glossary).
Liver reactions may suggest viral hepatitis.

Natural Diseases or Disorders That May Be Activated by This Drug

Latent epilepsy, glaucoma, prostatism (see Glossary).

Possible Effects on Laboratory Tests

Complete blood cell counts: decreased red cells, hemoglobin, white cells and platelets; increased eosinophils.
Blood glucose level: increased and decreased (fluctuations).
Liver function tests: increased liver enzymes (ALT/GPT, AST/GOT and alkaline phosphatase), increased bilirubin.
Urine pregnancy tests: falsely positive result with some tests.

CAUTION

1. Many over-the-counter medications (see OTC Drugs in Glossary) for allergies, colds and coughs contain drugs that can interact unfavorably with this drug. Ask your doctor or pharmacist for help **before** using any such medications.
2. Antacids that contain aluminum and/or magnesium may prevent the absorption of this drug and reduce its effectiveness.
3. Obtain prompt evaluation of any change or disturbance of vision.

Precautions for Use

By Infants and Children: Use of this drug is not recommended in children under 12 years of age. Do not use this drug in the presence of symptoms suggestive of Reye syndrome (see Glossary). Children with acute infectious diseases ("flulike" infections, chicken pox, measles, etc.) are more prone to develop muscular spasms of the face, back and extremities when this drug is given.

By Those over 60 Years of Age: Small starting doses are advisable. Increased risk of drowsiness, lethargy, constipation, lowering of body temperature (hypothermia) and orthostatic hypotension (see Glossary). This drug can worsen existing prostatism (see Glossary). You may also be more susceptible to the development of Parkinson-like reactions and/or tardive dyskinesia (see discussion of these terms in Glossary). These reactions must be recognized early since they may become unresponsive to treatment and irreversible.

▷ **Advisability of Use During Pregnancy**

Pregnancy Category: C. See Pregnancy Code at the back of this book.
Animal studies: No birth defects reported in rats, rabbits or monkeys.
Human studies: Adequate studies of pregnant women are not available.
Avoid drug during the first 3 months if possible. Avoid during the last month because of possible effects on the newborn infant.

Advisability of Use if Breast-Feeding

Presence of this drug in breast milk: Expected in small amounts, but no data are available.

Avoid drug or refrain from nursing.

Habit-Forming Potential: None.

Effects of Overdosage: Marked drowsiness, weakness, tremor, agitation, unsteadiness, deep sleep, coma, convulsions.

Possible Effects of Long-Term Use: Opacities in the cornea or lens of the eye, pigmentation of the retina. Tardive dyskinesia (see Glossary).

Suggested Periodic Examinations While Taking This Drug (at physician's discretion)

Complete blood cell counts, especially between the fourth and tenth weeks of treatment.

Liver function tests, electrocardiograms.

Complete eye examinations—eye structures and vision.

Careful inspection of the tongue for early evidence of fine, involuntary, wavelike movements that could indicate the beginning of tardive dyskinesia.

▷ **While Taking This Drug, Observe the Following**

Foods: No restrictions.

Beverages: No restrictions. May be taken with milk.

▷ *Alcohol:* Avoid completely. Alcohol can increase the sedative action of thiothixene and accentuate its depressant effects on brain function and blood pressure. Thiothixene can increase the intoxicating effects of alcohol.

Tobacco Smoking: No interactions expected.

Marijuana Smoking: Moderate increase in drowsiness; accentuation of orthostatic hypotension; increased risk of precipitating latent psychoses, confusing the interpretation of mental status and drug responses.

▷ *Other Drugs*

Thiothixene may *increase* the effects of

• all sedative drugs, especially barbiturates and narcotic analgesics, and cause excessive sedation.

• all atropinelike drugs, and cause nervous system toxicity.

Thiothixene may *decrease* the effects of

• guanethidine (Ismelin, Esimil), and reduce its effectiveness in lowering blood pressure.

Thiothixene *taken concurrently* with

• ketorolac (Toradol) may result in hallucinations.

• lithium (Lithobid, others) may result in exaggerated neurotoxicity (rigidity and tremor).

• monoamine oxidase inhibitors (MAO) (see Drug Classes) may result in worsening of the central nervous system and breathing depressive effects of thiothixene.

The following drugs may *decrease* the effects of thiothixene

• antacids containing aluminum and/or magnesium.

• barbiturates (see Drug Class Section).

• benztropine (Cogentin).

• trihexyphenidyl (Artane).

▷ *Driving, Hazardous Activities:* This drug can impair mental alertness, judgment and physical coordination.

Avoid hazardous activities.

Aviation Note: The use of this drug *is a disqualification* for piloting. Consult a designated Aviation Medical Examiner.

Exposure to Sun: Use caution until sensitivity has been determined. This drug can cause photosensitivity (see Glossary).

Exposure to Heat: Use caution and avoid excessive heat as much as possible. This drug may impair the regulation of body temperature and increase the risk of heat stroke.

Exposure to Cold: Use caution and dress warmly. This drug can increase the risk of hypothermia in the elderly.

Discontinuation: After a period of long-term use, do not stop this drug suddenly. Gradual withdrawal over 2 to 3 weeks under physician supervision is recommended. Do not discontinue this drug without your physician's knowledge and approval. The relapse rate of schizophrenia after discontinuation is 50% to 60%.

TICLOPIDINE (ti KLOH pi deen)

Introduced: 1985 **Prescription:** USA: Yes **Available as Generic:** USA: No **Class:** antiplatelet **Controlled Drug:** USA: No **Brand Name:** Ticlid

BENEFITS versus RISKS	
Possible Benefits	*Possible Risks*
SIGNIFICANT REDUCTION IN THE RISK OF STROKE FOR THOSE WITH TRANSIENT ISCHEMIC ATTACK (TIA) OR PREVIOUS STROKE	SIGNIFICANT REDUCTION IN WHITE BLOOD CELL COUNTS (uncommon) Increase of 8–10% in total blood cholesterol level Rare drug-induced hepatitis with jaundice

▷ **Principal Uses**

As a Single Drug Product: Uses currently included in FDA approved labeling: Used in selected individuals (who are intolerant to aspirin) to prevent: (1) Recurrent stroke following initial thrombotic stroke.

Other (unlabeled) generally accepted uses: (1) Used in some patients with peripheral vascular disease and intermittent claudication to prevent blood clots (thrombosis); (2) used in people who have had bypass surgery to help prevent clot formation and keep the graft working; may have a role in slowing the progression of eye problems (retinopathy) in diabetics; (3) combined with other agents to keep patients with angina from having heart attacks; (4) used in combination therapy to help lessen the symptoms of rheumatoid arthritis; (5) may help prevent strokes in patients who have experienced transient ischemic atacks (TIAs); (6) can help patients with kidney failure keep from building up phosphate, urea and creatinine.

How this Drug Works: By inhibiting clumping of blood platelets, this drug prevents the beginning of processes that lead to blood clot formation within atherosclerotic vessels (arterial thrombosis).

Available Dosage Forms and Strengths

Tablets — 250 mg

▷ **Recommended Dosage Ranges (Actual dosage and administration schedule must be determined by the physician for each patient individually.)**
Infants and Children: Dosage not established.
18 to 60 Years of Age: 250 mg twice daily, 12 hours apart, taken with food.
Over 60 Years of Age: Same as 18 to 60 years of age.
Conditions Requiring Dosing Adjustments
Liver function: This drug is contraindicated in patients with severe liver impairment. Doses may need to be decreased in people with compromised livers.
Kidney function: Changes in dosing in kidney compromise patients does not appear to be needed.

▷ **Dosing Instructions:**   The tablet may be crushed and is best taken with meals to enhance absorption and reduce stomach irritation.

Usual Duration of Use: Use on a regular schedule for 6 to 12 months usually determines effectiveness in preventing stroke. Long-term use (months to years) requires periodic physician evaluation of response and dosage adjustment.

Possible Advantages of This Drug
A reduction in risk of initial stroke during first year following TIA (in contrast to aspirin).
A reduction in risk of recurrent stroke during first year following initial stroke.
Effective in both men and women.

▷ **This Drug Should Not Be Taken If**
• you have had an allergic reaction to it previously.
• you currently have a bone marrow, blood cell or bleeding disorder.
• you have active peptic ulcer disease, Crohn's disease or ulcerative colitis.
• you have severely impaired liver function.
• you are taking aspirin, anticoagulants or cortisonelike drugs.

▷ **Inform Your Physician Before Taking This Drug If**
• you have a history of a drug-induced bone marrow depression or blood cell disorder.
• you have gastric or duodenal ulcers.
• you have impaired liver or kidney function.
• you plan to have surgery in the near future; this drug should be discontinued 10 to 14 days prior to surgery.

Possible Side Effects (natural, expected, and unavoidable drug actions)
Spontaneous bruising (purpura) (rare).

▷ **Possible Adverse Effects** (unusual, unexpected, and infrequent reactions)
If any of the following develop, consult your physician promptly for guidance.
Mild Adverse Effects
Allergic Reactions: Rash, itching (rare).
Dizziness (rare), ringing in the ears.
Loss of appetite (rare), indigestion, nausea, vomiting (rare), stomach pain, diarrhea.
Serious Adverse Effects
Allergic Reactions: Drug-induced hepatitis with jaundice (rare). This usually occurs during the first 4 months of treatment (see Jaundice in Glossary).
Idiosyncratic Reactions: Decreased production of white blood cells (neutrophils and granulocytes): fever, sore throat, susceptibility to infection.

Very rare aplastic anemia (see Glossary).
Lupus erythematosus (rare).

▷ **Possible Effects on Sexual Function:**   None reported.

▷ **Adverse Effects That May Mimic Natural Diseases or Disorders**
Drug-induced hepatitis may suggest viral hepatitis.

Possible Effects on Laboratory Tests
Complete blood cell counts: decreased red cells, hemoglobin, white cells and platelets.
Bleeding time: increased.
Total cholesterol and triglyceride levels: increased.
Liver function tests: increased liver enzymes (ALT/GPT, AST/GOT and alkaline phosphatase), increased bilirubin.

CAUTION
1. If significantly low white blood cell counts occurs, it usually begins between 3 weeks and 3 months after treatment starts. White blood cell counts **must** be obtained every 2 weeks from the second week to the end of the third month of drug administration.
2. Report promptly any indications of infection: fever, chills, sore throat, cough, etc.
3. Report promptly any abnormal or unusual bleeding or bruising.
4. Do not take any type of aspirin or anticoagulant drug while taking this drug without your physician's approval.
5. Inform all health care professionals who prescribe medicines for you that you are taking this drug.

Precautions for Use
By Infants and Children: Safety and effectiveness for those under 18 years of age not established.
By Those over 60 Years of Age: You may be more susceptible to bone marrow depression and blood cell decreases. Observe carefully for any tendency to infections or unusual bleeding or bruising. Report such developments promptly.

▷ **Advisability of Use During Pregnancy**
Pregnancy Category: B. See Pregnancy Code at the back of this book.
Animal studies: No drug-induced birth defects found in mouse, rat or rabbit studies.
Human studies: Adequate studies of pregnant women are not available.
Use this drug only if clearly needed. Ask your physician for guidance.

Advisability of Use if Breast-Feeding
Presence of this drug in breast milk: Unknown.
Avoid drug or refrain from nursing.

Habit-Forming Potential: None.

Effects of Overdosage: Abnormal bleeding or bruising, dizziness, nausea, diarrhea.

Possible Effects of Long-Term Use: None reported.

Suggested Periodic Examinations While Taking This Drug (at physician's discretion)
Complete blood cell counts. **See *CAUTION*.**
Liver function tests.

▷ **While Taking This Drug, Observe the Following**
   Foods: High fat meals may increase absorption by 20%.
   Beverages: No restrictions. May be taken with milk.
▷ *Alcohol:* No interactions expected. Avoid if you have active peptic ulcer disease.
   Tobacco Smoking: No interactions expected.
▷ *Other Drugs*
   Ticlopidine may ***increase*** the effects of
   • aspirin.
   • theophylline (theodur, others).
   • warfarin (Coumadin) and also increase the risk of hepatitis. The combination is **not** recommended.
   Ticlodipine may ***decrease*** the effects of
   • cyclosporine (Sandimmune) and decrease effectiveness.
   The following drug may ***increase*** the effects of ticlopidine
   • cimetidine (Tagamet).
   The following drugs may ***decrease*** the effects of ticlopidine
   • antacids decrease absorption of ticlopidine.
▷ *Driving, Hazardous Activities:* This drug may cause dizziness. Restrict activities as necessary.
   Aviation Note: The use of this drug ***may be a disqualification*** for piloting. Consult a designated Aviation Medical Examiner.
   Exposure to Sun: No restrictions.
   Discontinuation: To be determined and guided by your physician.

TIMOLOL (TI moh lohl)

Introduced: 1972   **Prescription:** USA: Yes; Canada: Yes   **Available as Generic:** USA: Yes; Canada: No   **Class:** Antianginal, antiglaucoma, antihypertensive, beta blocker   **Controlled Drug:** USA: No; Canada: No

Brand Names: ✦Apo-Timolol, ✦Apo-Timop, Betimol, Blocadren, ✦Timolide [CD], Timoptic, Timoptic Ocudose, Timoptic-XE

BENEFITS versus RISKS	
Possible Benefits	*Possible Risks*
EFFECTIVE, WELL-TOLERATED AS: ANTIANGINAL DRUG in effort-induced angina; ANTIGLAUCOMA DRUG in open-angle glaucoma; ANTIHYPERTENSIVE DRUG in mild to moderate hypertension EFFECTIVE PREVENTION OF MIGRAINE HEADACHES Effective adjunct in the prevention of recurrent heart attack (myocardial infarction)	CONGESTIVE HEART FAILURE in advanced heart disease Worsening of angina in coronary heart disease (if drug is abruptly withdrawn) Masking of low blood sugar (hypoglycemia) in drug-treated diabetes Provocation of asthma

▷ **Principal Uses**

As a Single Drug Product: Uses currently included in FDA approved labeling: (1) Treats classical effort-induced angina, certain types of heart rhythm disturbance and high blood pressure; (2) helps lower increased internal eye pressure in chronic open-angle glaucoma; (3) beneficial when given within 24 hours and for 28 days thereafter in decreasing the size of the heart damage, decreasing arrhythmias and preventing repeat heart attacks (myocardial infarction) ; (4) used to reduce the frequency and severity of migraine headaches.

Other (unlabeled) generally accepted uses: (1) Has been used in people who are afraid to fly on airplanes (air travel phobia); (2) may be helpful in decreasing the incidence of abnormal heart rhythms that arise in the atria of the heart (atrial fibrillation and flutter); (3) helps prevent abnormally increased intraocular pressure following cataract surgery; (4) can be of use in patients with detached retinas which have not torn.

As a Combination Drug Product [CD]: This drug is available in combination with hydrochlorothiazide for the treatment of hypertension. This combination product includes two drugs with different mechanisms of action; it is intended to provide greater effectiveness and convenience for long-term use.

How This Drug Works: By blocking certain actions of the sympathetic nervous system, this drug
- reduces the rate and contraction force of the heart, lowering the ejection pressure of blood and reducing the amount of oxygen the heart needs to work.
- reduces the degree of contraction of blood vessel walls, resulting in their expansion and consequent lowering of blood pressure.
- prolongs the conduction time of nerve impulses through the heart, of benefit in the management of certain heart rhythm disorders.
- slows formation of fluid (aqueous humor) in the anterior chamber of the eye and improves its drainage from the eye, lowering the internal eye pressure.

Available Dosage Forms and Strengths

Eye solutions — 0.25% and 0.5%
　　Tablets — 5 mg, 10 mg, 20 mg

▷ **Usual Adult Dosage Range:**   Varies with indication.

Antianginal and antihypertensive: Initially, 10 mg 2 times/day; increase dose gradually every 7 days as needed and tolerated. Usual maintenance dose is 10 to 20 mg once a day or divided into two equal doses and given twice daily. The total daily dosage should not exceed 60 mg.

Migraine headache prevention: Initially, 10 mg 2 times/day; increase dose as needed to 10 mg in the morning and 20 mg at night.

Preventing repeat heart attack: 10 mg twice/day.

Antiglaucoma: 1 drop in affected eye every 12 to 24 hours.

Note: Actual dosage and administration schedule must be determined by the physician for each patient individually.

Conditions Requiring Dosing Adjustments

Liver function: Consideration must be given to empirically decreasing the dose in patients with compromised livers.

Kidney function: Patients with kidney compromise should be followed closely, and the dose decreased if the medication appears to be accumulating.

▷ **Dosing Instructions:**   Preferably taken 1 hour before eating to maximize absorption. The tablet may be crushed for administration. Do not stop this drug abruptly.

Usual Duration of Use: Use on a regular schedule for 10 to 14 days usually determines effectiveness in preventing angina, controlling heart rhythm disorders and lowering blood pressure. Peak benefit may require continual use for 6 to 8 weeks. The long-term use of this drug (months to years) will be determined by the course of your symptoms over time and your response to an overall treatment program (weight reduction, salt restriction, smoking cessation, etc.). Consult your physician on a regular basis.

▷ **This Drug Should Not Be Taken If**
  • you have bronchial asthma.
  • you have severe obstructive lung disease.
  • you have had an allergic reaction to it previously.
  • you have Prinzmetal's variant angina (coronary artery spasm).
  • you have congestive heart failure.
  • you have an abnormally slow heart rate or a serious form of heart block.
  • you are taking, or have taken within the past 14 days, any monoamine oxidase (MAO) type A inhibitor drug (see Drug Classes).

▷ **Inform Your Physician Before Taking This Drug If**
  • you have had an adverse reaction to any beta blocker (see Drug Class Section).
  • you have a history of serious heart disease.
  • you have a history of hay fever (allergic rhinitis), asthma, chronic bronchitis or emphysema.
  • you have a history of overactive thyroid function (hyperthyroidism).
  • you have a history of low blood sugar (hypoglycemia).
  • you have impaired liver or kidney function.
  • you have Raynaud's phenomenon.
  • you have diabetes or myasthenia gravis.
  • you currently take any form of digitalis, quinidine or reserpine, or any calcium blocker drug (see Drug Classes).
  • you plan to have surgery under general anesthesia in the near future.

Possible Side Effects (natural, expected, and unavoidable drug actions)
  Lethargy and fatigability, cold extremities, slow heart rate, light-headedness in upright position (see Orthostatic Hypotension in Glossary).

▷ **Possible Adverse Effects** (unusual, unexpected, and infrequent reactions)
  If any of the following develop, consult your physician promptly for guidance.
  Mild Adverse Effects
  Allergic Reactions: Skin rash, itching.
  Loss of hair involving the scalp, eyebrows, and/or eyelashes. This effect can occur with use of the oral tablets or the eyedrops (used to treat glaucoma). Regrowth occurs with discontinuation of this drug.
  Headache, dizziness, visual disturbances, vivid dreams.
  Indigestion, nausea, vomiting, diarrhea.
  Numbness and tingling in extremities, joint pain.

Serious Adverse Effects

Allergic Reactions: Laryngospasm, severe dermatitis.

Idiosyncratic Reactions: Acute behavioral disturbances—depression, hallucinations.

Chest pain, shortness of breath, precipitation of congestive heart failure.

Induction of bronchial asthma (in asthmatic individuals).

Masking of warning signs of impending low blood sugar (hypoglycemia) in drug-treated diabetes.

Drug-induced myasthenia gravis (rare).

Periodic cramping of the leg (intermittent claudication).

Stopping of breathing (respiratory arrest) (rare).

▷ **Possible Effects on Sexual Function**

Decreased libido, impaired erection, impotence.

Note: All of these effects can occur with the use of timolol eye drops at recommended dosage.

▷ **Adverse Effects That May Mimic Natural Diseases or Disorders**

Reduced blood flow to extremities may resemble Raynaud's phenomenon (see Glossary).

Natural Diseases or Disorders That May Be Activated by This Drug

Prinzmetal's variant angina, Raynaud's disease, intermittent claudication, myasthenia gravis (questionable).

Possible Effects on Laboratory Tests

None reported.

CAUTION

1. ***Do not stop this drug suddenly*** without the knowledge and guidance of your doctor. Carry a notation on your person that take this drug.

2. Ask your doctor or pharmacist before using nasal decongestants usually present in over-the-counter cold preparations and nose drops. These can cause sudden increases in blood pressure when taken concurrently with beta blocker drugs.

3. Report the development of any tendency to emotional depression (rare with this drug).

Precautions for Use

By Infants and Children: Safety and effectiveness for those under 12 years of age not established. However, if this drug is used, watch for low blood sugar (hypoglycemia) during periods of reduced food intake.

By Those over 60 Years of Age: Unacceptably high blood pressure should be reduced without creating the risks associated with excessively low blood pressure. Small starting doses, and frequent blood pressure checks are needed. Sudden, rapid and excessive reduction of blood pressure can predispose to stroke or heart attack. Observe for dizziness, unsteadiness, tendency to fall, confusion, hallucinations, depression or urinary frequency.

▷ **Advisability of Use During Pregnancy**

Pregnancy Category: C. See Pregnancy Code at the back of this book.

Animal studies: No significant increase in birth defects due to this drug.

Human studies: Adequate studies of pregnant women are not available.

Avoid use of drug during the first 3 months if possible. Use this drug only if clearly needed. Ask your physician for guidance.

Advisability of Use if Breast-Feeding

Presence of this drug in breast milk: Yes.

Monitor nursing infant closely and discontinue drug or nursing if adverse effects develop.

Habit-Forming Potential: None.

Effects of Overdosage: Weakness, slow pulse, low blood pressure, fainting, cold and sweaty skin, congestive heart failure, possible coma and convulsions.

Possible Effects of Long-Term Use: Reduced heart reserve and eventual heart failure in susceptible individuals with advanced heart disease.

Suggested Periodic Examinations While Taking This Drug (at physician's discretion)

Complete blood cell counts (because of adverse effects of other drugs of this class).

Measurements of blood pressure, evaluation of heart function.

▷ **While Taking This Drug, Observe the Following**

Foods: No restrictions. Avoid excessive salt intake.

Beverages: No restrictions. May be taken with milk.

▷ *Alcohol:* Use with caution. Alcohol may exaggerate this drug's ability to lower the blood pressure and may increase its mild sedative effect.

Tobacco Smoking: Nicotine may reduce this drug's effectiveness in treating angina, heart rhythm disorders and high blood pressure. In addition, high doses of this drug may worsen constriction of the bronchial tubes caused by regular smoking.

▷ *Other Drugs*

Timolol may *increase* the effects of

- other antihypertensive drugs, and cause excessive lowering of blood pressure. Dosage adjustments may be necessary.
- amiodarone (Codarone) and cause cardiac arrest and bradycardia.
- lidocaine (Xylocaine, etc.).
- reserpine (Ser-Ap-Es, etc.), and cause sedation, depression, slowing of the heart rate and lowering of the blood pressure.
- verapamil (Calan, Isoptin), and cause excessive depression of heart function; monitor this combination closely.

Timolol may *decrease* the effects of

- theophyllines (Aminophyllin, Theo-Dur, etc.), and reduce their antiasthmatic effectiveness.

Timolol *taken concurrently* with

- clonidine (Catapres) requires close monitoring for rebound high blood pressure if clonidine is withdrawn while timolol is still being taken.
- epinephrine (Adrenalin, etc.) may cause marked rise in blood pressure and slowing of the heart rate.
- insulin may hide the symptoms of hypoglycemia (see Glossary).
- oral hypoglycemic agents (see Drug Classes) such as acetohexamide (Dymelor) and glipizide (Glucotrol) may result in prolonged low blood sugar.
- venlafaxine (Effexor) may result in increased risk of timolol toxicity.

The following drugs may *increase* the effects of timolol

- chlorpromazine (Thorazine, etc.)

- cimetidine (Tagamet).
- fluoxetine (Prozac).
- fluvoxamine (Luvox).
- methimazole (Tapazole).
- propylthiouracil (Propacil).

The following drugs may *decrease* the effects of timolol
- barbiturates (phenobarbital, etc.).
- indomethacin (Indocin), and possibly other "aspirin substitutes" or NSAIDs may impair timolol's antihypertensive effect.
- rifampin (Rifadin, Rimactane).

▷ *Driving, Hazardous Activities:* Use caution until the full extent of dizziness, lethargy and blood pressure change have been determined.

Aviation Note: The use of this drug *may be a disqualification* for piloting. Consult a designated Aviation Medical Examiner.

Exposure to Sun: No restrictions.

Exposure to Heat: Caution advised. Hot environments can exaggerate the effects of this drug.

Exposure to Cold: Caution advised. Cold environments can worsen circulatory deficiency in the extremities that may occur with this drug. The elderly should take precautions to prevent hypothermia (see Glossary).

Heavy Exercise or Exertion: It is advisable to avoid exertion that produces light-headedness, excessive fatigue or muscle cramping. The use of this drug may intensify the hypertensive response to isometric exercise.

Occurrence of Unrelated Illness: Fever can lower blood pressure and require adjustment of dosage. Nausea or vomiting may interrupt the dosing schedule. Ask your doctor for help.

Discontinuation: It is advisable to avoid sudden discontinuation of this drug in all situations; this is especially true in the presence of coronary artery disease. If possible, gradual reduction of dose over a period of 2 to 3 weeks is recommended. Ask your physician for specific guidance.

TOLBUTAMIDE (tohl BYU ta mide)

Introduced: 1956   **Prescription:** USA: Yes; Canada: Yes   **Available as Generic:** Yes   **Class:** Antidiabetic, sulfonylureas   **Controlled Drug:** USA: No; Canada: No

Brand Names: ✦Apo-Tolbutamide, ✦Mobenol, ✦Novobutamide, Oramide, Orinase, Sk-Tolbutamide

Warning: The brand names Orinase, Ornade and Ornex are similar and can be mistaken for each other; this can lead to serious medication errors. These names represent very different drugs. Orinase is the generic drug tolbutamide; it is used to treat diabetes. Ornade is a combination of chlorpheniramine and phenylpropanolamine; used to treat nasal and sinus congestion. Ornex is a combination of acetaminophen and phenylpropanolamine; used to treat head-colds and sinus pain. Verify that you are taking the correct drug.

```
┌─────────────────────────────────────────────────────────────────┐
│                      BENEFITS versus RISKS                        │
│        Possible Benefits                    Possible Risks        │
│   Assistance in regulating blood sugar   INCREASED RISK OF        │
│     in noninsulin-dependent diabetes        CARDIOVASCULAR DEATH  │
│     (adjunctive to appropriate diet and  HYPOGLYCEMIA, severe and │
│     weight control)                         prolonged             │
│                                           Drug-induced liver damage│
│                                           Rare bone marrow depression│
│                                           Hemolytic anemia        │
└─────────────────────────────────────────────────────────────────┘
```

▷ **Principal Uses**

   As a Single Drug Product: Uses currently included in FDA approved labeling: (1) Helps control mild to moderately severe type II diabetes mellitus (adult, maturity-onset) that does not require insulin, but that cannot be adequately controlled by diet alone. Other (unlabeled) generally accepted uses: (1) Has been used intravenously to help diagnose tumors which secrete insulin.

How This Drug Works: It is thought that this drug (1) stimulates the release of insulin (by a pancreas that is capable of responding to stimulation), and (2) enhances the utilization of insulin by appropriate tissues.

Available Dosage Forms and Strengths

   Tablets — 250 mg, 500 mg

▷ **Usual Adult Dosage Range:**   Initially, 500 mg twice a day. The dose may be increased or decreased every 48 to 72 hours until the minimal amount required for satisfactory control is determined. The usual range is 500 to 2000 mg a day. Three grams (3,000 mgs is the maximum daily dose). **Note: Actual dosage and administration schedule must be determined by the physician for each patient individually.**

Conditions Requiring Dosing Adjustments

   Liver function: Consideration should be given to decreasing the dose in patients with compromised livers. Tolbutamide can be a rare cause of liver damage, and patients should be followed closely.

   Kidney function: Dosing decreases are not needed in kidney compromise.

▷ **Dosing Instructions:**   May be taken with food (morning and evening meals) to reduce stomach irritation. The tablet may be crushed for administration.

Usual Duration of Use: Use on a regular schedule for 5 to 7 days weeks usually determines effectiveness in controlling diabetes. Failure to respond to maximal doses within 1 month constitutes a primary failure. Up to 15% of those who respond initially may develop secondary failure of the drug within the first year. The duration of effective use can only be determined by periodic measurement of the blood sugar. See your physician on a regular basis.

▷ **This Drug Should Not Be Taken If**
   • you have had an allergic reaction to it previously.
   • you have severe impairment of liver or kidney function.
   • you are undergoing major surgery.
   • you have a severe infection.

- you have diabetes complicated by formation of excess acid (acidosis).
- you are pregnant.

▷ **Inform Your Physician Before Taking This Drug If**
- you are allergic to other sulfonylurea drugs or to "sulfa" drugs. (See Drug Classes).
- your diabetes has been unstable or "brittle" in the past.
- you do not know how to recognize or treat hypoglycemia (see Glossary).
- you have an infection and a fever.
- you have a deficiency of G6PD in your red blood cells (ask your doctor).
- you have a history of congestive heart failure, peptic ulcer disease, cirrhosis of the liver, hypothyroidism or porphyria.

Possible Side Effects (natural, expected, and unavoidable drug actions)
If drug dose is excessive or food intake is delayed or inadequate, abnormally low blood sugar (hypoglycemia) will occur.

▷ **Possible Adverse Effects** (unusual, unexpected, and infrequent reactions)
If any of the following develop, consult your physician promptly for guidance.
Mild Adverse Effects
Allergic Reactions: Skin rash, hives, itching, drug fever.
Headache, ringing in the ears, weakness.
Indigestion, heartburn, nausea, vomiting.
Serious Adverse Effects
Allergic Reactions: Hepatitis with jaundice (see Glossary).
Idiosyncratic Reactions: Hemolytic anemia (see Glossary); disulfiramlike reaction with concurrent use of alcohol (see Glossary), infrequent with this drug.
Seizures (rare).
Low blood sodium (SIADH).
Drug-induced porphyria (rare).
Drug-induced urinary tract stones (urolithiasis).
Disulfiramlike reaction.
Bone marrow depression (see Glossary): fatigue, weakness, fever, sore throat, abnormal bleeding or bruising.
Abnormally low thyroid gland function (hypothyroidism).
Increased risk of cardiovascular death versus management by diet or insulin.

▷ **Possible Effects on Sexual Function**
None reported.

▷ **Adverse Effects That May Mimic Natural Diseases or Disorders**
Liver reactions may suggest viral hepatitis.

Natural Diseases or Disorders That May Be Activated by This Drug
Acute intermittent porphyria (see Glossary).

Possible Effects on Laboratory Tests
Complete blood cell counts: decreased red cells, hemoglobin, white cells and platelets.
Blood glucose level: decreased.
Liver function tests: increased liver enzymes (ALT/GPT, AST/GOT and alkaline phosphatase), increased bilirubin.

CAUTION

1. This drug must be regarded as only one part of the total program for the management of your diabetes. It is not a substitute for a properly prescribed diet and regular exercise.
2. Over a period of time (usually several months), this drug may lose its effectiveness in controlling blood sugar levels. Periodic follow-up examinations are necessary to monitor all aspects of response to drug treatment.

Precautions for Use

By Infants and Children: This drug is not effective in type I (juvenile, growth-onset) insulin-dependent diabetes.

By Those over 60 Years of Age: This drug should be used with caution in this age group. Start treatment with 500 mg/day; increase dosage cautiously and monitor closely to prevent hypoglycemic reactions. Repeated episodes of hypoglycemia in the elderly can cause brain damage.

▷ **Advisability of Use During Pregnancy**

Pregnancy Category: C. See Pregnancy Code at the back of this book.

Animal studies: Ocular and bone birth defects reported in rat studies.

Human studies: Adequate studies of pregnant women are not available.

Because uncontrolled blood sugar levels during pregnancy are associated with a higher incidence of birth defects, many experts recommend that insulin (instead of an oral agent) be used as necessary to control diabetes during the entire pregnancy.

Use during pregnancy is not recommended by the manufacturer.

Advisability of Use if Breast-Feeding

Presence of this drug in breast milk: Yes.

Avoid drug or refrain from nursing.

Habit-Forming Potential: None.

Effects of Overdosage: Symptoms of mild to severe hypoglycemia: headache, light-headedness, faintness, nervousness, confusion, tremor, sweating, heart palpitation, weakness, hunger, nausea, vomiting, stupor progressing to coma.

Possible Effects of Long-Term Use: Reduced function of the thyroid gland (hypothyroidism). Reports of increased frequency and severity of heart and blood vessel diseases associated with long-term use of this class of drugs are highly controversial and inconclusive. A direct cause-and-effect relationship (see Glossary) is tenuous. Ask your physician for guidance.

Suggested Periodic Examinations While Taking This Drug (at physician's discretion)

Complete blood cell counts, liver function tests, thyroid function tests, periodic evaluation of heart and circulatory system.

▷ **While Taking This Drug, Observe the Following**

Foods: Follow the diabetic diet prescribed by your physician.

Beverages: As directed in the diabetic diet. May be taken with milk.

▷ *Alcohol:* Use with extreme caution. Alcohol can exaggerate this drug's hypoglycemic effect. This drug infrequently causes a marked intolerance of alcohol resulting in a disulfiramlike reaction (see Glossary): facial flushing, sweating, palpitation.

Tobacco Smoking: Decreased tolbutamide blood levels are found in smokers.

▷ *Other Drugs*

The following drugs may *increase* the effects of tolbutamide
- aspirin, and other salicylates.
- chloramphenicol (Chloromycetin).
- cimetidine (Tagamet).
- clofibrate (Atromid S).
- cotrimoxazole (Bactrim, others).
- fenfluramine (Pondimin).
- fluconazole (Diflucan).
- ketoconazole (Nizoral) .
- itraconazole (Sporanox).
- monoamine oxidase (MAO) type A inhibitors (see Drug Classes).
- phenylbutazone (Butazolidin).
- ranitidine (Zantac).
- sulfonamide drugs (see Drug Classes).
- valproic acid (depakene).

The following drugs may *decrease* the effects of tolbutamide
- beta blocker drugs (see Drug Classes).
- bumetanide (Bumex).
- corticosteroids (see Drug Classes).
- diazoxide (Proglycem).
- ethacrynic acid (Edecrin).
- furosemide (Lasix).
- phenytoin (Dilantin).
- rifampin (Rifadin, Rimactane).
- thiazide diuretics (see Drug Classes).
- thyroid hormones (see Drug Classes).

Tolbutamide *taken concurrently* with
- colestipol (Colestid) can result in decreased colestipol response.
- digoxin may result in increased risk of digoxin toxicity.
- insulin will result in additive lowering of the blood sugar.
- sulfa drugs (see Drug Classes) may result in a greater than expected effect of tolbutamide. Caution against hypoglycemia is advised along with consideration for lower tolbutamide doses while the medicines are combined..

▷ *Driving, Hazardous Activities:* Regulate your dosage schedule, eating schedule and physical activities very carefully to prevent hypoglycemia. Be able to recognize the early symptoms of hypoglycemia so you can avoid hazardous activities and take corrective measures.

Aviation Note: Diabetes *is a disqualification* for piloting. Consult a designated Aviation Medical Examiner.

Exposure to Sun: Use caution. Some drugs of this class can cause photosensitivity (see Glossary).

Occurrence of Unrelated Illness: Acute infections, illnesses causing vomiting or diarrhea, serious injuries and surgical procedures can interfere with diabetic control and may require insulin. If any of these conditions occur, call your doctor promptly.

Discontinuation: Because of the possibility of secondary failure, it is advisable to evaluate the continued benefit of this drug every 6 months.

TOLMETIN (TOHL met in)

Introduced: 1976   **Prescription:** USA: Yes; Canada: Yes   **Available as Generic:** Yes   **Class:** analgesic, mild; NSAID   **Controlled Drug:** USA: No; Canada: No

Brand Names: Tolectin, Tolectin DS, Tolectin 600

BENEFITS versus RISKS	
Possible Benefits	*Possible Risks*
EFFECTIVE RELIEF OF MILD TO MODERATE PAIN AND INFLAMMATION	Increased blood pressure Gastrointestinal pain, ulceration, bleeding (rare) Rare liver damage Rare kidney damage Rare blood cell disorders: hemolytic anemia, abnormally low white blood cell and platelet counts

Please see the new combined acetic acid nonsteroidal anti-inflammatory drug profile for further information.

TRAZODONE (TRAZ oh dohn)

Introduced: 1967   **Prescription:** USA: Yes; Canada: Yes   **Available as Generic:** USA: Yes; Canada: No   **Class:** Antidepressants   **Controlled Drug:** USA: No; Canada: No

Brand Name: Desyrel, ✤Desyrel Dividose, Trialodine

BENEFITS versus RISKS	
Possible Benefits	*Possible Risks*
EFFECTIVE TREATMENT IN ALL TYPES OF DEPRESSIVE ILLNESS	Adverse behavioral effects Potential for causing heart rhythm disorders in people with heart disease

▷ **Principal Uses**

As a Single Drug Product: Uses currently included in FDA approved labeling: (1) Used to provide symptomatic relief in all types of depression, with or without anxiety or agitation.

Other (unlabeled) generally accepted uses: (1) May have a role in reducing the symptoms of agoraphobia; (2) may help drug-induced (such as MAO inhibitors) insomnia; (3) can have a role in combination therapy of some pain syndromes; (4) may be of help in essential tremor; (5) can ease bouts of repetitive screaming.

How This Drug Works: It is thought that this drug increases the availability of the nerve impulse transmitter serotonin within certain brain centers and thereby relieves the symptoms of emotional depression.

Available Dosage Forms and Strengths
   Tablets — 50 mg, 100 mg, 150 mg, 300 mg

▷ **Usual Adult Dosage Range:**   Initially, 50 mg 3 times/day. The dose may be increased by 50 mg daily at intervals of 3 or 4 days as needed and tolerated. The total daily dosage should not exceed 400 mg. **Note: Actual dosage and administration schedule must be determined by the physician for each patient individually.**

Conditions Requiring Dosing Adjustments
   Liver function: Blood levels should be obtained to guide dosing. It can be a rare cause of liver damage, and patients should be followed closely.
   Kidney function: Trazodone metabolites are eliminated by the kidneys, however, dosage adjustment in renal compromise is not defined.

▷ **Dosing Instructions:**   Best taken with food to improve absorption. The tablet may be crushed for administration. If excessive drowsiness or dizziness occurs, it is advisable to take a larger portion of the total daily dose at bedtime and to divide the remaining amount into 2 or 3 smaller doses to be taken during the day.

Usual Duration of Use: Use on a regular schedule for 2 to 4 weeks usually determines effectiveness in relieving the symptoms of depression. Long-term use (weeks to months) requires supervision and periodic evaluation by your physician.

▷ **This Drug Should Not Be Taken If**
   • you have had an allergic reaction to it previously.
   • you are recovering from a recent heart attack (myocardial infarction).
   • you have carcinoid syndrome.
   • you are taking, or have taken within the past 14 days, any monoamine oxidase (MAO) type A inhibitor (see Drug Classes).

▷ **Inform Your Physician Before Taking This Drug If**
   • you have a history of any of the following: alcoholism, epilepsy, heart disease (especially heart rhythm disorders).
   • you have impaired liver or kidney function.
   • you are pregnant or are breast feeding your infant.
   • you are taking any antihypertensive drugs.
   • you plan to have surgery under general anesthesia in the near future.

Possible Side Effects (natural, expected, and unavoidable drug actions)
   Drowsiness, light-headedness, blurred vision, dry mouth, constipation.

▷ **Possible Adverse Effects** (unusual, unexpected, and infrequent reactions)
   If any of the following develop, consult your physician promptly for guidance.
   Mild Adverse Effects
   Allergic Reaction: Skin rash.
   Headache, dizziness, fatigue, impaired concentration, nervousness, tremors.
   Rapid heart rate, palpitations.
   Peculiar taste, constipation, stomach discomfort, nausea, vomiting, diarrhea.
   Weight gain, blurred vision.
   Dry mouth (xerostomia).
   Urinary retention.

Cavities (dental caries).

Muscular aches and pains.

Serious Adverse Effects

Allergic Reactions: Serious skin rashes (erythema multiforme).

Behavioral effects: confusion, anger, hostility, disorientation, impaired memory, delusions, hallucinations, nightmares.

Irregular heart rhythms, low blood pressure, fainting.

Erythema multiforme.

Seizures (rare).

Liver toxicity.

▷ **Possible Effects on Sexual Function**

Decreased male libido; increased female libido.

Inhibited ejaculation, impotence, priapism (see Glossary).

Altered timing and pattern of menstruation.

Possible Effects on Laboratory Tests

Liver enzymes: increased.

CAUTION

1. If you experience a significant degree of mouth dryness while using this drug, consult your dentist regarding the risk of gum erosion or tooth decay. Ask for his guidance in ways to keep the mouth comfortably moist.
2. It is advisable to withhold this drug if electroconvulsive therapy (ECT) is to be used.

Precautions for Use

By Infants and Children: Safety and effectiveness for use by those under 18 years of age have not been established.

By Those over 60 Years of Age: During the first two weeks of treatment, observe for the development of restlessness, agitation, excitement, forgetfulness, confusion or disorientation. Be aware of possible unsteadiness and incoordination that may predispose to falling. This drug may enhance prostatism (see Glossary).

▷ **Advisability of Use During Pregnancy**

Pregnancy Category: C. See Pregnancy Code at the back of this book.

Animal studies: Fetal deaths and birth defects reported.

Human studies: Adequate studies of pregnant women are not available.

Avoid this drug completely during the first 3 months. Use otherwise only if clearly needed. Ask your physician for guidance.

Advisability of Use if Breast-Feeding

Presence of this drug in breast milk: Yes.

Avoid drug or refrain from nursing.

Habit-Forming Potential: None.

Effects of Overdosage: Marked drowsiness, weakness, confusion, tremors, low blood pressure, rapid heart rate, stupor, coma, possible seizures.

Possible Effects of Long-Term Use: None reported.

Suggested Periodic Examinations While Taking This Drug (at physician's discretion)

Complete blood cell counts. (This drug may cause slight reductions in white blood cell counts. This should be monitored closely if infection, sore throat or fever develops.)

Serial blood pressure readings and electrocardiograms.

▷ **While Taking This Drug, Observe the Following**
  Foods: No restrictions.
  Beverages: No restrictions. May be taken with milk.
▷ *Alcohol:* Avoid completely. This drug can increase markedly the intoxicating effects of alcohol and accentuate its depressant action on brain functions.
  Tobacco Smoking: No interactions expected.
▷ *Other Drugs*
  Trazodone may ***increase*** the effects of
  • antihypertensive drugs, and cause excessive lowering of blood pressure; dosage adjustments may be necessary.
  • drugs with sedative effects, and cause excessive sedation.
  • phenytoin (Dilantin), by raising its blood level; observe for phenytoin toxicity.
  Trazodone ***taken concurrently*** with
  • clonidine will lessen the therapeutic effect of clonidine.
  • fluoxetine (Prozac) may result in an increased trazodone level and toxicity.
  • monoamine oxidase inhibitors (MAO) (see Drug Classes) may result in undesirable side effects in some patients, and beneficial therapeutic effects in others.
  • other drugs that cause central nervous system depression (see benzodiazepines, opioids and tranquilizers) may have additive effects.
  • some phenothiazines (see Drug Classes) may result in excessively lowered blood pressure.
  • warfarin (Coumadin) may result in a decreased therapeutic benefit of warfarin. INR (prothrombin times) should be checked three times a week while combined warfarin and trazodone therapy are undertaken.
▷ *Driving, Hazardous Activities:* This drug may cause dizziness or drowsiness. Restrict activities as necessary.
  Aviation Note: The use of this drug ***is a disqualification*** for piloting. Consult a designated Aviation Medical Examiner.
  Exposure to Sun: No restrictions.
  Discontinuation: It is advisable to discontinue this drug gradually. Ask your physician for guidance in dosage reduction over an appropriate period of time.

TRIAMCINOLONE (tri am SIN oh lohn)

Introduced: 1985   **Prescription:** USA: Yes; Canada: Yes   **Available as Generic:** No   **Class:** Antiasthmatic, cortisonelike drugs   **Controlled Drug:** USA: No; Canada: No

Brand Name: Amcort, Aristocort, Aristocort R, Aristoform D, ✦Aristospan, Articulose LA, ✦Aureocort, Azmacort, Cenocort, Cenocort Forte, Flutex, ✦Kenacomb, Kenacort, Kenaject, Kenalog, Kenalog H, Kenalog IN, Kenalone, Mycogen II, Mycomar, Mytrex [CD], Nasacort, Nasacort AQ, Sk-Triamcinolone, TAC-40, TAC-D, Triacet, ✦Triaderm Mild, ✦Triaderm Regular, Triam-A, Triam-Forte, Triamolone 40, Triderm, Tri-Kort, Trilog, Tristoject, ✦Viaderm-K.C.

```
┌─────────────────────────────────────────────────────────────────────┐
│                     BENEFITS versus RISKS                             │
│       Possible Benefits              Possible Risks                   │
│  EFFECTIVE CONTROL OF SEVERE,   Yeast infections of mouth and throat  │
│    CHRONIC BRONCHIAL ASTHMA     Suppression of normal cortisone       │
│  EFFECTIVE SUPPRESSION OF A       production                          │
│    VARIETY OF INFLAMMATORY      Euphoria and psychotic episodes       │
│    DISORDERS                    Cushing's syndrome (moon face,         │
│  POSSIBLE REDUCTION IN            obesity, and buffalo hump)          │
│    SYSTEMIC STEROID USE         Muscle wasting (with long-term use)   │
│  EFFECTIVE TREATMENT OF         Osteoporosis (with long-term use)     │
│    SEASONAL OR PERENNIAL                                              │
│    ALLERGIC RHINITIS IN ADULTS                                        │
│    AND CHILDREN                                                       │
└─────────────────────────────────────────────────────────────────────┘
```

▷ **Principal Uses**

As a Single Drug Product: Uses currently included in FDA approved labeling: (1) In inhaler form used to treat chronic bronchial asthma in people who require cortisonelike drugs for asthma control. This dosage form is better than cortisone taken by mouth (swallowed) or by injection because it works more locally on the respiratory tract and does not require absorption and systemic distribution. This helps prevent the more serious adverse effects that usually result from the long-term use of cortisone taken for systemic effects; (2) the tablet form can be used in a variety of inflammatory disorders; (3) tablet form is used to ease drug reactions; (4) these medicines are also used as part of combination treatment of acute lymphocytic leukemia in children; (5) used in autoimmune hemolytic anemia; (6) The nasal inhaler form helps adults and children with symptoms of seasonal or perennial allergic rhinitis.

Other (unlabeled) generally accepted uses: (1) May have a role in postherpetic nerve pain (neuralgia); (2) corticosteroids may be of use in Pneumocystis carinii pneumonia in extreme cases where conventional therapy has not worked; (3) may help Guillain-Barre syndrome; (4) can help myasthenia gravis; (5) short-term therapy of psoriasis.

How This Drug Works: By increasing the amount of cyclic AMP in appropriate tissues, this drug may thereby increase the concentration of epinephrine, which is an effective bronchodilator and antiasthmatic. Additional benefit is due to the drug's ability to reduce local allergic reaction and inflammation in the lining tissues of the respiratory tract.

Available Dosage Forms and Strengths

Inhalation aerosol — 0.1 mg per metered spray

Tablets — 1 mg, 2 mg, 4 mg, 8 mg

▷ **Recommended Dosage Ranges** (Actual dosage and administration schedule must be determined by the physician for each patient individually.)

Infants and Children: Up to 6 years of age—Dosage not established.

6 to 12 years of age—0.1 to 0.2 mg (1 or 2 metered sprays) 3 or 4 times a day. Adjust dosage as needed and tolerated. Limit total daily dosage to 1.2 mg (12 metered sprays).

12 to 60 Years of Age: Initially 0.2 mg (2 metered sprays) 3 or 4 times a day. For severe asthma—1.2 to 1.6 mg (12 to 16 metered sprays) per day, in divided doses. Adjust dosage as needed and tolerated. It is usually used as 2 inhalations three to four times a day. Results are better when used in this fashion versus on an as needed basis. Limit total daily dose to 1.6 mg (16 metered sprays).

Nasacort AQ and Nasacort may prove effective with a starting dose of 220 mcg per day.

For tablets: 4 to 48 mg daily for inflammatory conditions.

Cream: 0.025% is usually applied to the affected area 2 to 4 times a day.

Over 60 Years of Age: Same as 12 to 60 years of age.

Conditions Requiring Dosing Adjustments

Liver function: This drug is metabolized in the liver. Dosing changes in liver compromise are not defined.

Kidney function: Dosing adjustments do not appear warranted in patients with compromised kidneys.

▷ **Dosing Instructions:** For inhalation form: May be used as needed without regard to eating. Shake the container well before using. Carefully follow the printed patient instructions provided with the unit. Rinse the mouth and throat (gargle) with water thoroughly after each inhalation; do not swallow the rinse water. The Nasacort AQ form is a water based formulation for treatment of allergic rhinitis and does not contain chlorofluorocarbon propellants. For oral tablets: May cause stomach upset, and can be taken with meals or snacks.

Usual Duration of Use: Use on a regular schedule for 1 to 2 weeks usually determines effectiveness in controlling severe, chronic asthma. Long-term use requires the supervision and guidance of the physician.

▷ **This Drug Should Not Be Taken If**
- you have had an allergic reaction to it previously.
- you are having severe acute asthma or status asthmaticus that requires immediate relief.
- you have a form of nonallergic bronchitis with asthmatic features.
- you have a systemic fungal infection.

▷ **Inform Your Physician Before Taking This Drug If**
- you are now taking or have recently taken any cortisone-related drug (including ACTH by injection) for any reason (see Drug Classes).
- you have a history of tuberculosis of the lungs.
- you have chronic bronchitis or bronchiectasis.
- you have diabetes, glaucoma, myasthenia gravis, or peptic ulcer disease.
- you have had unexpected surgery (may delay wound healing).
- you have an underactive thyroid (hypothyroidism).
- you think you may have an active infection of any kind, especially a respiratory infection.
- you are taking any of the following drugs: warfarin, oral antidiabetic drugs, insulin or digoxin

Possible Side Effects (natural, expected, and unavoidable drug actions)

Yeast infections (thrush) of the mouth and throat.

Irritation of mouth, tongue, or throat.

▷ **Possible Adverse Effects** (unusual, unexpected, and infrequent reactions)

If any of the following develop, consult your physician promptly for guidance.

Mild Adverse Effects
 Allergic Reaction: Skin rash.
 Memory loss, weight loss.
 Easy bruising (ecchymosis).
 Swelling of face, hoarseness, voice change, cough.
Serious Adverse Effects
 Allergic Reactions: Rare.
 Bronchospasm, asthmatic wheezing (rare).
 Can be a cause of high blood pressure with long-term use.
 Edema or swelling, especially with kidney or heart vessel disease.
 May cause euphoria, manic-depressive illness, or paranoid states with long-
  term oral use.
 Can cause a syndrome (Cushing's) characterized by: moon face, obesity, and
  poorly controlled high blood pressure.
 Decrease of circulating T lymphocytes.
 Drug-induced seizures.
 Rare electrolyte disturbances.
 Excessive thyroid activity (hyperthyroidism).
 Long-term use can be associated with osteoporosis.
 Long-term oral dosing can result in duodenal ulcer development.
 Cataract formation has occurred with long-term use.
 Muscle wasting can occur with long-term use.
 Pancreatitis (rare).
 Decreased blood potassium.
 Elevated blood sugar.
 Toxic megacolon (rare).
 Toxic psychosis has occurred with other steroids.
▷ **Possible Effects on Sexual Function:** None reported.

Natural Diseases or Disorders That May Be Activated by This Drug
 Latent amebiasis, congestive heart failure, diabetes, glaucoma, hypertension,
  myasthenia gravis, peptic ulcer.
 Cortisone-related drugs (used by inhalation) that produce systemic effects
  can impair immunity and lead to reactivation of "healed" or quiescent tuberculosis of the lungs. Individuals with a history of tuberculosis should be
  observed closely during use of cortisonelike drugs by inhalation.

Possible Effects on Laboratory Tests
 Blood calcium levels: decreased.
 Blood total cholesterol levels: increased.
 Blood glucose levels: increased.
 Blood potassium levels: decreased.
 Blood sodium levels: increased.

CAUTION
 1. This drug does not act primarily as a brochodilator and should not be
  relied upon for the immediate relief of acute asthma.
 2. If you were using any cortisone-related drugs for treatment of your
  asthma **before** transferring to this inhaler drug, it may be necessary to
  resume the former cortisone-related drug if you experience injury or infection of any kind, or if you require surgery. Be sure to notify your attending physician of your prior use of cortisone-related drugs taken either by mouth or by injection.

3. If you experience a return of severe asthma while using this drug, notify your physician immediately so that additional supportive treatment with cortisone-related drugs by mouth or injection can be provided as needed.
4. It is advisable to carry a card of personal identification with a notation (if applicable) that you have used cortisone-related drugs within the past year. During periods of stress it may be necessary to resume cortisone treatment in adequate dosage.
5. An interval of approximately 5 to 10 minutes should separate the inhalation of bronchodilators such as albuterol, epinephrine, pirbuterol, etc. (which should be used first), and the inhalation of this drug. This sequence will permit greater penetration of triamcinolone into the bronchial tubes. The delay between inhalations will also reduce the possibility of adverse effects from the propellants used in the two inhalers.

Precautions for Use
By Infants and Children: Safety and effectiveness for use of the oral inhaler by those under 6 years of age have not been established. To ensure adequate penetration of the drug and to obtain maximal benefit, the use of a spacer device is recommended for inhalation therapy in children.
By Those over 60 Years of Age: Individuals with chronic bronchitis or bronchiectasis should be observed closely for the development of lung infections.

▷ ### Advisability of Use During Pregnancy
Pregnancy Category: C. See Pregnancy Code at the back of this book.
Animal studies: Rat and rabbit studies reveal significant toxic effects on the embryo and fetus and multiple birth defects due to this drug.
Human studies: Adequate studies of pregnant women are not available.
Limit use to very serious illness for which no satisfactory treatment alternatives are available.

Advisability of Use if Breast-Feeding
Presence of this drug in breast milk: Unknown.
Ask your doctor for guidance.

Habit-Forming Potential: With recommended dosage, a state of functional dependence (see Glossary) is not likely to develop.

Effects of Overdosage: Indications of cortisone excess (due to systemic absorption)—fluid retention, flushing of the face, stomach irritation, nervousness.

Possible Effects of Long-Term Use: Significant suppression of normal cortisone production.

Suggested Periodic Examinations While Taking This Drug (at physician's discretion)
Inspection of mouth and throat for evidence of yeast infection.
Assessment of the status of adrenal gland function (cortisone production).
X-ray examination of the lungs of individuals with a prior history of tuberculosis.

▷ ### While Taking This Drug, Observe the Following
Foods: No specific restrictions beyond those advised by your physician.
Beverages: No specific restrictions.
▷ *Alcohol:* No interactions expected.
Tobacco Smoking: No interactions expected. However, smoking can affect the condition under treatment and reduce the effectiveness of this drug. Follow your physician's advice.

▷ *Other Drugs*

The following drugs may *increase* the effects of triamcinolone

- inhalant bronchodilators—albuterol, bitolterol, epinephrine, pirbuterol, etc.
- oral bronchodilators—aminophylline, ephedrine, terbutaline, theophylline, etc.

The following drugs may *decrease* the effects of triamcinolone

- carbamazepine (Tegretol) increases triamcinolone metabolism and may result in decreased effectiveness.
- phenytoin (Dilantin) increases triamcinolone metabolism and may result in decreased effectiveness.
- primidone (Mysoline) increases steroid metabolism and may result in decreased triamcinolone metabolism.
- rifampin (Rifadin).

Triamcinolone *taken concurrently* with

- aspirin may result in blunting of the therapeutic benefits of aspirin.
- cyclosporine (Sandimmune) may result in changes in the blood levels of both medicines.
- oral hypoglycemic agents (see Drug Classes) may result in loss of glucose control.
- thiazide diuretics (see Drug Classes) can result in loss of glucose control.
- vaccines (flu, rabies, others) may result in a less than optimal vaccine response.
- warfarin (Coumadin) can result in variation in the degree of anticoagulation. Increased INR (prothrombin time) testing is indicated.

▷ *Driving, Hazardous Activities:* No restrictions.

Aviation Note: The use of this drug and the disorder for which this drug is prescribed *may be disqualifications* for piloting. Consult a designated Aviation Medical Examiner.

Exposure to Sun: No restrictions.

Occurrence of Unrelated Illness: Acute infections, serious injuries, and surgical procedures can create an urgent need for the administration of additional supportive cortisone-related drugs given by mouth and/or injection. Notify your physician immediately in the event of new illness or injury of any kind.

Discontinuation: If the regular use of this drug has made it possible to reduce or discontinue maintenance doses of cortisonelike drugs by mouth, *do not* discontinue this drug abruptly. If you find it necessary to discontinue this drug for any reason, consult your physician promptly. It may be necessary to resume cortisone preparations and to institute other measures for satisfactory management.

Special Storage Instructions: Store at room temperature. Avoid exposure to temperatures above 120 degrees F (49 degrees C). Do not store or use this inhaler near heat or open flame.

TRIAMTERENE (tri AM ter een)

Introduced: 1964   **Prescription:** USA: Yes; Canada: Yes   **Available as Generic:** Yes   **Class:** Diuretic   **Controlled Drug:** USA: No; Canada: No
Brand Names: ✤Apo-Triazide [CD], Dyazide [CD], Dyrenium, Maxzide [CD], Maxzide-25 [CD], ✤Novo-Triamzide [CD], ✤Nu-Triazide

---

BENEFITS versus RISKS	
Possible Benefits	*Possible Risks*
EFFECTIVE PREVENTION OF POTASSIUM LOSS when used adjunctively with other diuretics	ABNORMALLY HIGH BLOOD POTASSIUM LEVEL with excessive use
EFFECTIVE DIURETIC IN REFRACTORY CASES OF FLUID RETENTION when used adjunctively with other diuretics	Rare blood cell disorders: megaloblastic anemia, abnormally low white blood cell and platelet counts
	Rare kidney stones

▷ **Principal Uses**

As a Single Drug Product: Uses currently included in FDA approved labeling: (1) Used as part of combination therapy of congestive heart failure and disorders of the liver and kidney that are accompanied by excessive fluid retention (edema); (2) used in conjunction with other measures to treat high blood pressure. It is used primarily in situations where it is advisable to prevent loss of potassium from the body.

Other (unlabeled) generally accepted uses: None.

As a Combination Drug Product [CD]: This drug is available in combination with hydrochlorothiazide, a different kind of diuretic that promotes the loss of potassium from the body. Triamterene is used in this combination to counteract the potassium-wasting effect of the thiazide diuretic.

How This Drug Works: By inhibiting the enzyme system that initiates the sodium-potassium exchange process, this drug prevents the reabsorption of sodium and the excretion of potassium by the kidney. Thus the drug promotes the excretion of sodium (and water with it) and the retention of potassium.

Available Dosage Forms and Strengths

Capsules — 50 mg, 100 mg

▷ **Usual Adult Dosage Range:** Hypertension: Initially, 50 to 100 mg twice daily. The dose is then adjusted according to individual response. The usual maintenance dose is 100 to 200 mg/day, divided into 2 doses. The total daily dosage should not exceed 300 mg. **Note: Actual dosage and administration schedule must be determined by the physician for each patient individually.**

Conditions Requiring Dosing Adjustments

Liver function: The dose should be reduced and used with extreme caution in patients with severe liver disease.

Kidney function: Patients with mild to moderate kidney failure may be given the usual dose every 12 hours. In severe or progressive kidney failure, this medication should **not** be used.

▷ **Dosing Instructions:**   May be taken with or following meals to promote absorption of the drug and to reduce stomach irritation. The capsule may be opened for administration. Intermittent or alternate-day use is recommended to minimize the possibility of sodium and potassium imbalance.

Usual Duration of Use: Use on a regular schedule for 3 to 5 days usually determines effectiveness in clearing edema, and for 2 to 3 weeks to determine its effect on hypertension. Long-term use (months to years) requires physician supervision and periodic evaluation.

▷ **This Drug Should Not Be Taken If**
  • you have had an allergic reaction to it previously.
  • you have severely impaired liver or kidney function.
  • your kidney disease is progressive or you have a creatinine greater than 2.5 mg/dl (ask your doctor).
  • your blood potassium level is significantly elevated (ask your doctor).

▷ **Inform Your Physician Before Taking This Drug If**
  • you have a history of liver or kidney disease.
  • you have diabetes or gout.
  • you are taking any of the following: antihypertensives, a digitalis preparation, another diuretic, lithium or a potassium preparation.
  • you have a history of G6PD deficiency (ask your doctor).
  • you have a history of blood cell disorders.
  • you plan to have surgery under general anesthesia in the near future.

Possible Side Effects (natural, expected, and unavoidable drug actions)
  With excessive use: abnormally high blood potassium levels, abnormally low blood sodium levels, dehydration.
  Blue coloration of the urine (of no significance).

▷ **Possible Adverse Effects** (unusual, unexpected, and infrequent reactions)
  If any of the following develop, consult your physician promptly for guidance.
  Mild Adverse Effects
  Allergic Reactions: Skin rash, itching.
  Headache, dizziness, unsteadiness, weakness, drowsiness, lethargy.
  Dry mouth, nausea, vomiting, diarrhea.
  Serious Adverse Effects
  Allergic Reaction: Anaphylactic reaction (see Glossary).
  Symptomatic potassium excess: confusion, numbness and tingling in lips and extremities, fatigue, weakness, shortness of breath, slow heart rate, low blood pressure.
  Rare blood cell disorders: megaloblastic anemia, causing weakness and fatigue; abnormally low white blood cell count, causing infection, fever, or sore throat; abnormally low blood platelet count, causing abnormal bleeding or bruising.
  Abnormal urine production (SIADH).
  Hemolytic anemia (in those with deficiency of G6PD in red cells).
  Rare formation of kidney stones and kidney toxicity.
  Rare liver toxicity.

▷ **Possible Effects on Sexual Function:**   None reported.

Possible Effects on Laboratory Tests

Complete blood cell counts: decreased red cells, hemoglobin, white cells and platelets; increased eosinophils (allergic reaction).

Blood glucose level: increased in diabetics.

Blood lithium level: increased.

Blood potassium level: increased.

Blood uric acid level: increased in 17% of users.

Kidney function tests: increased blood creatinine and urea nitrogen (BUN) levels (kidney damage).

CAUTION

1. Do not take potassium supplements or increase your intake of potassium-rich foods while taking this drug.
2. Patients who take quinidine (Quinaglute, others) may have falsely increased laboratory test results if fluorescent measurement techniques are used.
3. Do not stop this drug abruptly unless abnormally high blood levels of potassium develop.
4. Avoid the liberal use of salt substitutes that contain potassium; these are a potential cause of potassium excess.

Precautions for Use

By Infants and Children: This drug is not recommended for use in children.

By Those over 60 Years of Age: The natural decline in kidney function may predispose to potassium retention in the body. Watch for indications of potassium excess: slow heart rate, irregular heart rhythms, low blood pressure, confusion, drowsiness. Excessive use of diuretics can cause harmful loss of body water (dehydration), increased viscosity of the blood and an increased tendency of the blood to clot, predisposing to stroke, heart attack or thrombophlebitis.

▷ **Advisability of Use During Pregnancy**

Pregnancy Category: B by the manufacturer, D by one researcher. See Pregnancy Code at the back of this book.

Animal studies: No birth defects due to this drug reported.

Human studies: Adequate studies of pregnant women are not available.

This drug should not be used during pregnancy unless a very serious complication of pregnancy occurs for which this drug is significantly beneficial.

Advisability of Use if Breast-Feeding

Presence of this drug in breast milk: Yes.

Avoid drug or refrain from nursing.

Habit-Forming Potential: None.

Effects of Overdosage: Thirst, drowsiness, fatigue, weakness, nausea, vomiting, confusion, irregular heart rhythm, low blood pressure.

Possible Effects of Long-Term Use: Potassium accumulation to abnormally high blood levels.

Suggested Periodic Examinations While Taking This Drug (at physician's discretion)

Complete blood cell counts.

Measurements of blood sodium, potassium and chloride levels.

Kidney function tests.

▷ **While Taking This Drug, Observe the Following**

Foods: Diets high in high potassium foods (see table) may cause problems. Avoid excessive restriction of salt.

Beverages: No restrictions. May be taken with milk.

▷ *Alcohol:* Use with caution. Alcohol may enhance the drowsiness and the blood-pressure-lowering effect of this drug.

Tobacco Smoking: No interactions expected.

▷ *Other Drugs*

Triamterene may *increase* the effects of
- amantadine (Symmetrel).
- digoxin (Lanoxin).

Triamterene *taken concurrently* with
- captopril (Capoten) or other ACE inhibitors may cause excessively high blood potassium levels.
- H2 blockers (see Drug Classes) may decrease the absorption of triamterine and decrease the therapeutic effect of triamterine.
- indomethacin (Indocin) may increase the risk of kidney damage.
- lithium may cause accumulation of lithium to toxic levels.
- NSAIDs (see Drug Classes) may blunt the blood pressure lowering effect of triamterine.
- potassium preparations may cause excessively high blood potassium levels.

▷ *Driving, Hazardous Activities:* This drug may cause dizziness and drowsiness. Restrict activities as necessary.

Aviation Note: The use of this drug *may be a disqualification* for piloting. Consult a designated Aviation Medical Examiner.

Exposure to Sun: Use caution. This drug may cause photosensitivity (see Glossary).

Discontinuation: With high dosage or prolonged use, it is advisable to withdraw this drug gradually. Sudden discontinuation may cause rebound potassium excretion and resultant potassium deficiency. Ask your physician for guidance.

TRICHLORMETHIAZIDE (tri KLOR meth i a zide)

Introduced: 1961   **Prescription:** USA: Yes; Canada: Yes   **Available as Generic:** Yes   **Class:** Thiazide diuretics   **Controlled Drug:** USA: No; Canada: No

Brand Names: Diurese, Marzide II, Metahydrin, Naqua, Naquival

BENEFITS versus RISKS	
Possible Benefits	*Possible Risks*
Effective, well-tolerated diuretic	Loss of body potassium and
Helpful in mild hypertension	magnesium
Increases effectiveness of other	Cardiac risk caused by electrolyte loss
antihypertensives	Increased blood sugar
Helps diabetes insipidus	Rare blood cell disorders
	Rare liver toxicity

Please see the combined thiazide diuretic profile for further information.

TRIFLUOPERAZINE (tri flu oh PER a zeen)

Introduced: 1958   **Prescription:** USA: Yes; Canada: Yes   **Available as Generic:** USA: Yes; Canada: No   **Class:** tranquilizer, major; phenothiazines
Controlled Drug: USA: No; Canada: No

Brand Names: ✤Apo-Trifluoperazine, ✤Novo-Flurazine, ✤Solazine, Stelabid [CD], Stelazine, Suprazine, ✤Terfluzine

---

BENEFITS versus RISKS

Possible Benefits	*Possible Risks*
EFFECTIVE CONTROL OF ACUTE MENTAL DISORDERS: beneficial effects on thinking, mood, and behavior	SERIOUS TOXIC EFFECTS ON BRAIN with long-term use Liver damage with jaundice (infrequent) Rare blood cell disorders: abnormally low red and white blood cell and platelet counts

---

▷ **Principal Uses**

As a Single Drug Product: Uses currently included in FDA approved labeling: (1) Treats psychotic thinking and behavior associated with acute psychoses of unknown nature, mania, paranoid states and acute schizophrenia. It is most effective in those who are withdrawn and apathetic and in those with agitation, delusions and hallucinations; (2) approved for treatment of anxiety disorders, but is not a drug of first choice.

Other (unlabeled) generally accepted uses: (1) May have a role in combination therapy of some kinds of chronic pain; (2) may help in combination therapy of chemotherapy induced nausea or vomiting.

How This Drug Works: Present theory is that by inhibiting the action of dopamine, this drug acts to correct an imbalance of nerve impulse transmissions that is thought to be responsible for certain mental disorders.

Available Dosage Forms and Strengths

Concentrate — 10 mg per ml
Injection — 2 mg per ml
Tablets — 1 mg, 2 mg, 5 mg, 10 mg

▷ **Usual Adult Dosage Range:** Non-psychotic anxiety: Initially, 1 or 2 mg twice daily. The dose may be increased by 1 or 2 mg at 3 to 4 day intervals to a maximum dose of 4 milligrams in patients who are not in the hospital. For psychosis: 2 to 5 mgs twice a day. The dose is then increased every 3 or 4 days as needed and tolerated. Usual dosage range is 15 to 20 mg daily. The total daily dosage should not exceed 40 mg. Some rare cases have required 100 mgs per day. **Note: Actual dosage and administration schedule must be determined by the physician for each patient individually.**

Conditions Requiring Dosing Adjustments

Liver function: This drug should be used with caution in liver compromise.
Kidney function: Patients with compromised kidneys should be closely followed.

▷ **Dosing Instructions:** The tablets may be crushed and taken with or following meals to reduce stomach irritation.

Usual Duration of Use: Use on a regular schedule for several weeks usually determines effectiveness in controlling psychotic disorders. If not significantly beneficial within 6 weeks, it should be stopped. Long-term use (months to years) requires periodic physician evaluation of response, appropriate dosage adjustment and consideration of continued need.

▷ **This Drug Should Not Be Taken If**
  • you are allergic to any of the drugs bearing the brand names listed above.
  • you have active liver disease.
  • you have cancer of the breast.
  • you have a current blood cell or bone marrow disorder.

▷ **Inform Your Physician Before Taking This Drug If**
  • you are allergic or abnormally sensitive to any phenothiazine drug (see Drug Classes).
  • you have impaired liver or kidney function.
  • you have a history of anginal pain (this drug may worsen it).
  • you have any type of seizure disorder.
  • you have diabetes, glaucoma or heart disease.
  • you have a history of lupus erythematosus.
  • you are taking any drug with sedative effects.
  • you have had neuroleptic malignant syndrome (ask your doctor).
  • you plan to have surgery under general or spinal anesthesia in the near future.

Possible Side Effects (natural, expected, and unavoidable drug actions)
  Drowsiness (usually during the first 2 weeks), orthostatic hypotension (see Glossary), blurred vision, dry mouth, nasal congestion, constipation, impaired urination.
  Pink or purple coloration of urine, of no significance.

▷ **Possible Adverse Effects** (unusual, unexpected, and infrequent reactions)
  If any of the following develop, consult your physician promptly for guidance.
  Mild Adverse Effects
  Allergic Reactions: Skin rash, hives, low-grade fever.
  Lowering of body temperature, especially in the elderly (see Hypothermia in Glossary).
  Increased appetite and weight gain.
  Dizziness, weakness, agitation, insomnia, impaired day and night vision.
  Chronic constipation, fecal impaction.
  Serious Adverse Effects
  Allergic Reactions: Hepatitis with jaundice (see Glossary), severe skin reactions, anaphylactic reaction (see Glossary).
  Idiosyncratic Reactions: Neuroleptic malignant syndrome (see Glossary).
  Depression, disorientation, loss of peripheral vision.
  Serious skin disorders (Stevens-Johnson syndrome).
  Drug-induced glaucoma or abnormal eye positioning (oculogyric crisis).
  Seizures.
  Drug-induced porphyrias (rare).
  Drug-induced pituitary tumors (rare).
  Rapid heart rate, heart rhythm disorders.
  Blood cell disorders: significant reduction in all cellular elements of the blood

(reduced counts of red cells, white cells, and blood platelets) (see Bone Marrow Depression in Glossary).

Phenothiazine-induced sudden death syndrome (rare).

Nervous system reactions: Parkinson-like disorders (see Glossary), severe restlessness, muscle spasms involving the face and neck, tardive dyskinesia (see Glossary).

▷ **Possible Effects on Sexual Function**

Altered timing and pattern of menstruation.

Male breast enlargement and tenderness (gynecomastia). Female breast enlargement with milk production.

Spontaneous male orgasm, paradoxical (1 case reported).

Inhibited ejaculation, painful ejaculation, painful and extended erections (priapism) (see Glossary).

Delayed female orgasm.

▷ **Adverse Effects That May Mimic Natural Diseases or Disorders**

Nervous system reactions may suggest true Parkinson's disease.

Liver reactions may suggest viral hepatitis.

Reactions resembling systemic lupus erythematosus may occur.

Natural Diseases or Disorders That May Be Activated by This Drug

Latent epilepsy, glaucoma, diabetes mellitus, prostatism (see Glossary).

Possible Effects on Laboratory Tests

Complete blood cell counts: decreased red cells, hemoglobin, white cells and platelets.

Liver function tests: increased liver enzymes (ALT/GPT, AST/GOT and alkaline phosphatase), increased bilirubin.

Urine pregnancy tests: falsely positive result with some.

CAUTION

1. Many over-the-counter medications (see **OTC Drugs** in Glossary) for allergies, colds and coughs contain drugs that can interact unfavorably with this drug. Ask your doctor or pharmacist for help before using any such medications.
2. Antacids that contain aluminum and/or magnesium may prevent the absorption of this drug and reduce its effectiveness.
3. Obtain prompt evaluation of any change or disturbance of vision.

Precautions for Use

By Infants and Children: Use of this drug is not recommended in children under 6 years of age. Do not use this drug in the presence of symptoms suggestive of Reye syndrome (see Glossary). Children with acute infectious diseases ("flulike" infections, chicken pox, measles, etc.) are more prone to develop muscular spasms of the face, back and extremities when this drug is given.

By Those over 60 Years of Age: Small starting doses are advisable. May be increased risk of: drowsiness, lethargy, constipation, lowering of body temperature (hypothermia) and orthostatic hypotension (see Glossary). This drug may enhance existing prostatism (see Glossary). You may also be more susceptible to the development of Parkinson-like reactions and/or tardive dyskinesia (see discussion of these terms in Glossary). These reactions must be recognized early since they may become unresponsive to treatment and irreversible.

▷ **Advisability of Use During Pregnancy**
Pregnancy Category: C. See Pregnancy Code at the back of this book.
Animal studies: Significant birth defects reported in mouse and rat studies.
Human studies: No increase in birth defects reported in 700 exposures. Adequate studies of pregnant women are not available.
Avoid drug during the first 3 months; avoid during the last month because of possible adverse effects on the newborn infant.

Advisability of Use if Breast-Feeding
Presence of this drug in breast milk: Yes, in minute amounts.
Monitor nursing infant closely and discontinue drug or nursing if adverse effects develop.

Habit-Forming Potential: None.

Effects of Overdosage: Marked drowsiness, weakness, tremor, agitation, unsteadiness, deep sleep, coma, convulsions.

Possible Effects of Long-Term Use: Tardive dyskinesia (see Glossary).

Suggested Periodic Examinations While Taking This Drug (at physician's discretion)
Complete blood cell counts, especially between the fourth and tenth weeks of treatment.
Liver function tests, electrocardiograms.
Complete eye examinations of eye structures and vision.
Careful inspection of the tongue for early evidence of fine, involuntary, wavelike movements that could indicate the beginning of tardive dyskinesia.

▷ **While Taking This Drug, Observe the Following**
Foods: No restrictions.
Nutritional Support: A riboflavin (vitamin B-2) supplement should be taken with long-term use.
Beverages: Caffeine may slightly blunt the calming effect of this medicine. May be taken with milk.
▷ *Alcohol:* Avoid completely. Alcohol can increase the sedative action of phenothiazines and accentuate their depressant effects on brain function and blood pressure. Phenothiazines can increase the intoxicating effects of alcohol.
Tobacco Smoking: Possible reduction of drowsiness from drug.
Marijuana Smoking: Moderate increase in drowsiness; accentuation of orthostatic hypotension; increased risk of precipitating latent psychoses, confusing the interpretation of mental status and drug responses.
▷ *Other Drugs*
Trifluoperazine may *increase* the effects of
• all sedative drugs, especially narcotic analgesics (also see Drug Classes for opioids and benzodiazepines), and cause excessive sedation.
• all atropinelike drugs, and cause nervous system toxicity.
Trifluoperazine may *decrease* the effects of
• guanethidine (Ismelin, Esimil), and reduce its effectiveness in lowering blood pressure.
Trifluoperazine *taken concurrently* with
• ascorbic acid (vitamin C) may result in decreased therapeutic benefits from trifluoperazine.

- lithium (Lithobid, Lithotabs) may impair the effectiveness of lithium and cause nervous system toxicity.
- oral hypoglycemic agents (see drug Classes) will blunt the beneficial effects of the oral hypoglycemic agents.
- monoamine oxidase inhibitors (MAO) (see Drug Classes) may result in an increased risk of extrapyramidal (see Glossary) reactions.

The following drugs may *decrease* the effects of trifluoperazine
- antacids containing aluminum and/or magnesium.
- barbiturates (see Drug Classes).
- benztropine (Cogentin).
- disulfiram (Antabuse).
- trihexyphenidyl (Artane).

▷ *Driving, Hazardous Activities:* This drug can impair mental alertness, judgment and physical coordination. Avoid hazardous activities.

Aviation Note: The use of this drug *is a disqualification* for piloting. Consult a designated Aviation Medical Examiner.

Exposure to Sun: Use caution. Some phenothiazines can cause photosensitivity (see Glossary).

Exposure to Heat: Use caution and avoid excessive heat as much as possible. This drug may impair the regulation of body temperature and increase the risk of heat stroke.

Exposure to Cold: Use caution and dress warmly. This drug can increase the risk of hypothermia in the elderly.

Discontinuation: After a period of long-term use, do not stop this drug suddenly. Gradual withdrawal over 2 to 3 weeks under physician supervision is recommended. Do not discontinue this drug without your physician's knowledge and approval. The relapse rate of schizophrenia after discontinuation is 50–60%.

TRIMETHOPRIM (tri METH oh prim)

Introduced: 1966   **Prescription:** USA: Yes; Canada: Yes   **Available as Generic:** USA: Yes; Canada: No   **Class:** Anti-infective   **Controlled Drug:** USA: No; Canada: No

Brand Names: ✦Apo-Sulfatrim [CD], ✦Apo-Sulfatrim DS [CD], Bactrim [CD], Bactrim DS [CD], Bethaprim [CD], Comoxol [CD], ✦Coptin [CD], Cotrim [CD], ✦Novo-Trimel [CD], ✦NovoTrimel DS [CD], ✦Nu-Cotrimox, Polytrim, Proloprim, ✦Protrin [CD], ✦Protrin DF [CD], ✦Roubac [CD], Septra [CD], Septra DS [CD], SMZ-TMP [CD], Sulfatrim D/S, Trimpex, Uroplus DS [CD], Uroplus SS [CD]

BENEFITS versus RISKS	
Possible Benefits	*Possible Risks*
EFFECTIVE TREATMENT OF INFECTIONS due to susceptible microorganisms	Rare blood cell disorders: megaloblastic anemia, methemoglobinemia, abnormally low white blood cell and platelet counts
Effective adjunctive prevention and treatment of Pneumocystis carinii pneumonia (AIDS-related)	

▷ **Principal Uses**

As a Single Drug Product: Uses currently included in FDA approved labeling: (1) Used to treat certain infections of the urinary tract that are not complicated by the presence of kidney stones or obstructions to the normal flow of urine. It is sometimes used to prevent the recurrence of such infections; (2) treats eye infections caused by sensitive organisms.

Other (unlabeled) generally accepted uses: (1) Used in combination with dapsone to treat pneumocystis carinii pneumonia in AIDS patients; (2) may have a role in combination therapy of resistant acne; (3) prevention (prophylaxis) of urinary tract infections.

As a Combination Drug Product [CD]: This drug is available in combination with sulfamethoxazole; the generic name co-trimoxazole is used in some countries to identify this combination. It is very effective in the treatment of certain urinary tract infections, middle ear infections, chronic bronchitis, acute enteritis and certain types of pneumonia. Now used as primary prevention and treatment of Pneumocystis carinii pneumonia associated with AIDS.

How This Drug Works: This drug prevents the growth and multiplication of susceptible infecting organisms by inactivating the enzyme systems that are necessary for the formation of essential nuclear elements and cell proteins.

Available Dosage Forms and Strengths

Tablets — 100 mg, 200 mg
Tablets — 80 mg combined with 400 mg of sulfamethoxazole
Tablets — 160 mg combined with 800 mg of sulfamethoxazole
Ophthalmic — 1 mg per ml
Oral suspension — 40 mg combined with 200 mg of sulfamethoxazole per 5-ml

▷ **Usual Adult Dosage Range:**   Orally for infections: 100 mg every 12 hours for 10 days. For certain pneumonias, the same dose is given every 6 hours. The total daily dosage should not exceed 640 mg. Ophthalmic: 1 drop in the affected eye every 3 hours (up to 6 doses a day) for 7 to 10 days. **Note: Actual dosage and administration schedule must be determined by the physician for each patient individually.**

Conditions Requiring Dosing Adjustments

Liver function: This drug should be used with caution in patients with both liver and kidney compromise.

Kidney function: Patients with mild kidney compromise can be given the usual dose every 12 hours. Patients with moderate to severe kidney failure (creatinine clearances of 15 to 50 ml/min.) can be given the usual dose every 18 hours. The drug is contraindicated in patients with severe and worsening kidney failure.

▷ **Dosing Instructions:**   The tablet may be crushed and taken without regard to meals. However, it may also be taken with or following food if necessary to reduce stomach irritation.

Usual Duration of Use: Use on a regular schedule for 7 to 14 days usually determines effectiveness in controlling responsive infections. The actual duration of use will depend upon the nature of the infection.

Currently a "Drug of Choice"
  (when combined with sulfamethoxazole) for preventing pneumonia (due to Pneumocystis carinii) in patients with AIDS.

▷ **This Drug Should Not Be Taken If**
  • you have had an allergic reaction to it previously.
  • you have an anemia due to folic acid deficiency (megaloblastic anemia).

▷ **Inform Your Physician Before Taking This Drug If**
  • you have a history of folic acid deficiency.
  • you have impaired liver or kidney function.
  • you are pregnant or breast-feeding.

Possible Side Effects (natural, expected, and unavoidable drug actions)
  None with short-term use.

▷ **Possible Adverse Effects** (unusual, unexpected, and infrequent reactions)
  If any of the following develop, consult your physician promptly for guidance.
  Mild Adverse Effects
  Allergic Reactions: Skin rash, itching, drug fever.
  Headache, abnormal taste, sore mouth or tongue, loss of appetite, nausea, vomiting, abdominal cramping, diarrhea.
  Serious Adverse Effects
  Allergic Reactions: Severe dermatitis with peeling of skin (toxic epidermal necrolysis [TEN]).
  Blood cell disorders: megaloblastic anemia, methemoglobinemia, abnormally low white blood cell and platelet counts (all rare).
  Worsening of hyperkalemia (increased blood potassium).
  Kidney toxicity (rare).
  Liver toxicity (rare).
  Aseptic meningitis (of questionable causal relationship) (extremely rare).

▷ **Possible Effects on Sexual Function:**   None reported.

Possible Effects on Laboratory Tests
  Complete blood cell counts: decreased red cells, hemoglobin, white cells and platelets.
  INR (prothrombin time): increased (when taken concurrently with warfarin).

CAUTION
  1. Certain strains of bacteria that cause urinary tract infections can develop resistance to this drug. If you do not show significant improvement within 10 days, consult your physician.
  2. Comply with your physician's request for periodic blood counts during long-term therapy.

Precautions for Use
  By Infants and Children: Safety and effectiveness for those under 2 months of age not established.
  By Those over 60 Years of Age: The natural decline in liver and kidney function may require smaller doses. If you develop itching reactions in the genital or anal areas, report this promptly.

▷ **Advisability of Use During Pregnancy**
  Pregnancy Category: C. See Pregnancy Code at the back of this book.

Animal studies: Birth defects due to this drug reported in rat and rabbit studies.

Human studies: Adequate studies of pregnant women are not available.

Avoid use of drug during the first 3 months and during the last 2 weeks of pregnancy. Use this drug otherwise only if clearly needed. Ask your physician for guidance.

Advisability of Use if Breast-Feeding

Presence of this drug in breast milk: Yes.

Avoid drug or refrain from nursing.

Habit-Forming Potential: None.

Effects of Overdosage: Headache, dizziness, confusion, depression, nausea, vomiting, bone marrow depression, possible liver toxicity with jaundice.

Possible Effects of Long-Term Use: Impaired production of red and white blood cells and blood platelets.

Suggested Periodic Examinations While Taking This Drug (at physician's discretion)

Complete blood cell counts.

▷ **While Taking This Drug, Observe the Following**

Foods: No restrictions.

Beverages: No restrictions. May be taken with milk.

▷ *Alcohol:* No interactions expected.

Tobacco Smoking: No interactions expected.

▷ *Other Drugs*

Trimethoprim may *increase* the effects of

- amantadine (Symmetrel) and also result in increased levels of trimethoprim resulting in toxicity.
- cyclosporine (Sandimmune) and result in increased kidney toxicity.
- dapsone and result in dapsone or trimethoprim toxicity.
- phenytoin (Dilantin), and cause phenytoin toxicity.
- procainamide (Procan SR) and result in procainamide toxicity.

The following drugs may *decrease* the effects of trimethoprim

- cholestyramine (Questran) and perhaps other cholesterol lowering medicines (see Drug Classes) of the same class will bind trimethoprim and blunt the beneficial effects of trimethoprim by inhibiting absorption.
- rifampin (Rifadin, Rimactane).

▷ *Driving, Hazardous Activities:* No restrictions.

Aviation Note: The use of this drug is probably not a disqualification for piloting. Consult a designated Aviation Medical Examiner.

Exposure to Sun: No restrictions.

VALACYCLOVIR (VALA si klo veer)

Introduced: 1996   **Prescription:** USA: Yes; Canada: Yes   **Available as Generic:** USA: No; Canada: No   **Class:** Antiviral   **Controlled Drug:** USA: No; Canada: No

Brand Names: Valtrex

BENEFITS versus RISKS

Possible Benefits	*Possible Risks*
EFFECTIVE TREATMENT OF HERPES ZOSTER (SHINGLES)	Rare reports of thrombotic thrombocytopenic purpura in some patients with compromised immune systems
EFFECTIVE EPISODIC TREATMENT OF GENITAL HERPES	Nausea

▷ **Principal Uses**
> *As a Single Drug Product:* Uses currently included in FDA approved labeling: (1) To treat Herpes zoster (shingles); (2) used in recurrent genital herpes in patients with intact immune systems.
> Other (unlabeled) generally accepted uses: None at present.

How This Drug Works: This medicine is rapidly converted to acyclovir, and moves into the body to a much greater extent (dose to dose) than acyclovir. It is thought that by blocking the formation of genetic material by the virus, this medicine stops the ability of the virus to multiply and spread.

Available Dosage Forms and Strengths
> Caplets — 500 mg

▷ **Usual Adult Dosage Range (Actual dosage and administration schedule must be determined by the physician for each patient individually):** Herpes zoster (shingles): One gram (1,000 mg) three times a day for seven days. Genital Herpes simplex: This medicine is best started within 24 hours of the onset of symptoms, and is given as 500 mg twice daily for five days.

Conditions Requiring Dosing Adjustments
> *Liver function:* This medicine is not recommended for use in patients with cirrhosis. In moderate to severe cases of liver compromise, this medicine is converted to the active form more slowly, but achieves the same amount of conversion.
> *Kidney function:* Dosing changes MUST be made for patients with compromised kidneys, including the typical age-related decline in kidney function.

▷ **Dosing Instructions:** May be taken without regard to meals.

Usual Duration of Use: Use on a regular schedule for 7 days in Herpes zoster and 5 days in genital herpes has been effective in addressing those conditions.

Possible Advantages of This Drug: Generally well-tolerated antiviral which decreases the length of time patients are in pain from genital herpes.
> Achieves blood levels similar to INTRAVENOUS acyclovir with a medicine taken by mouth (the oral route).
> Patients do not have to take it as may times a day as acyclovir.

▷ **Advisability of Use During Pregnancy**
> *Pregnancy Category:* B. See Pregnancy Code at the back of this book.
> Animal studies: NOT teratogenic in rabbits or rats.
> Human studies: Adequate studies of pregnant women are not available.
> Physicians should call 1–800–722–9292, ext.: 58465 to register their patients.

Advisability of Use if Breast-Feeding
> Presence of this drug in breast milk: Expected.

Given to breast feeding mothers with caution or not at all. Discuss the benefits versus risks with your doctor.

Habit-Forming Potential: None.

Possible Effects of Long-Term Use: None reported.

▷ *Driving, Hazardous Activities:* This drug may cause dizziness or weakness. Restrict activities as necessary.

Discontinuation: Talk with your doctor or pharmacist about how long and how best to take this medicine. **Author's note: further details will be added to this profile as more information about this medicine becomes available.**

VALPROIC ACID (val PROH ik a sid)

Introduced: 1967   **Prescription:** USA: Yes; Canada: Yes   **Available as**
Generic: USA: Yes; Canada: No   **Class:** Anticonvulsant   **Controlled**
Drug: USA: No; Canada: No

Brand Names: Depa, Depakene, Depakote (divalproex sodium), Deproic, ✦Epival

BENEFITS versus RISKS	
Possible Benefits	*Possible Risks*
EFFECTIVE CONTROL OF MULTIPLE SEIZURE TYPES: ABSENCE SEIZURES, TONIC-CLONIC SEIZURES, MYOCLONIC SEIZURES, PSYCHOMOTOR SEIZURES, when used adjunctively with other antiseizure drugs HELPS CONTROL REFRACTORY MIGRAINES DIVALPROEX SODIUM HELPS MANIA	LIVER TOXICITY, infrequent but may be severe Rare reduction of blood platelets and impaired platelet function with risk of bleeding Rare pancreatitis Rare liver toxicity

▷ **Principal Uses**

As a Single Drug Product: Uses currently included in FDA approved labeling: (1) Used to manage the following types of epilepsy: simple and complex absence seizures (petit mal); tonic-clonic seizures (grand mal); myoclonic seizures; complex partial seizures (psychomotor, temporal lobe epilepsy). It is sometimes used adjunctively with other anticonvulsants as needed; (2) used for people who do not respond to medicine once they have a migraine or those who have more than two migraines a month; (2) divalproex sodium (Depakote) was recently approved for use in treating mania.

Other (unlabeled) generally accepted uses: (1) Can help relieve the symptoms of trigeminal neuralgia; (2) can have a role in intractable hiccups; (3) has had some use in patients with epilepsy and hepatic porphyria; (4) may be of help in writer's cramp.

How This Drug Works: It is thought that by increasing the availability of the nerve impulse transmitter gamma-aminobutyric acid (GABA), this drug suppresses the spread of abnormal electrical discharges that cause seizures.

Available Dosage Forms and Strengths

Capsules — 250 mg

Capsules, sprinkle — 125 mg

Syrup — 250 mg per 5-ml

Tablets, enteric-coated — 125 mg, 250 mg, 500 mg

▷ **Usual Adult Dosage Range:**   Starting dose is 15 mg per kg per day. The dose is increased cautiously by 5 to 10 mg/kg/24 hours every 7 days as needed and tolerated. ***The usual daily dose is from 1000 mg to 1600 mg in divided doses.*** The total daily dosage should not exceed 60 mg/kg. Blood levels are used to guide ongoing dosing. **Note: Actual dosage and administration schedule must be determined by the physician for each patient individually.**

Conditions Requiring Dosing Adjustments

Liver function: This medicine SHOULD NOT be given to patients with significant liver compromise or liver disease.

Kidney function: No dosing changes are anticipated in patients with compromised kidneys.

▷ **Dosing Instructions:**   Preferably taken 1 hour before meals. However, it may be taken with or following food if necessary to prevent stomach irritation. The regular capsule should not be opened and the tablet should not be crushed for administration. The sprinkle-capsule may be opened and the contents sprinkled on soft food for administration. Do not administer the syrup in carbonated beverages. It may be diluted in water or milk.

Usual Duration of Use: Use on a regular schedule for 2 weeks usually determines effectiveness in reducing the frequency and severity of seizures. Long-term use (months to years) requires physician supervision and periodic evaluation.

▷ **This Drug Should Not Be Taken If**

- you have had an allergic reaction to it previously.
- you have active liver disease.
- you are pregnant.
- you have an active bleeding disorder.

▷ **Inform Your Physician Before Taking This Drug If**

- you have a history of liver disease or impaired liver function.
- you have a history of any type of bleeding disorder.
- you are pregnant or planning pregnancy.
- you have myasthenia gravis.
- you are taking: anticoagulants; other anticonvulsants; antidepressants, either the tricyclic type or monoamine oxidase (MAO) type A inhibitors (see Drug Classes).
- you plan to have surgery or dental extraction in the near future.

Possible Side Effects (natural, expected, and unavoidable drug actions)

Drowsiness and lethargy.

▷ **Possible Adverse Effects** (unusual, unexpected, and infrequent reactions)

If any of the following develop, consult your physician promptly for guidance.

Mild Adverse Effects
   Allergic Reaction: Skin rash (rare).
   Headache, dizziness, confusion, unsteadiness, tremor (dose-related), slurred speech.
   Nausea, indigestion, stomach cramps, diarrhea.
   Weight gain.
   Bed-wetting at night.
   Temporary loss of scalp hair.

Serious Adverse Effects
   Idiosyncratic Reactions: Bizarre behavior, psychosis, hallucinations.
   Drug-induced hepatitis with jaundice (see Glossary). **Children less than 2 years old have considerably increased risk of fatal hepatotoxicity.**
   Possible Reye's syndrome (see Glossary).
   Increased blood ammonia level.
   Increased blood glucose.
   Drug-induced porphyria (rare).
   Drug-induced lowered function of the thyroid gland (hypothyroidism).
   Decreased selenium levels.
   Reduced formation of blood platelets and impaired function of platelets, with increased risk of abnormal bleeding.
   Drug-induced pancreatitis (rare)
   Reduced formation of red blood cells (rare).
   Increased pressure in the head (pseudotumor cerebri).
   Can cause a Reye's-like syndrome.

▷ **Possible Effects on Sexual Function**
   Altered timing and pattern of menstruation.
   Female breast enlargement with milk production.
   Decreased libido.
   Decreased effectiveness of oral contraceptives taken concurrently (6%).

▷ **Adverse Effects That May Mimic Natural Diseases or Disorders**
   Liver reactions may suggest viral hepatitis.

Possible Effects on Laboratory Tests
   Complete blood cell counts: decreased white cells and platelets.
   Bleeding time: increased.
   INR (prothrombin time): increased.
   Blood amylase level: increased (possible pancreatitis).
   Liver function tests: increased liver enzymes (ALT/GPT, AST/GOT and alkaline phosphatase), increased bilirubin.

CAUTION
1. The capsules and tablets should be swallowed whole without alteration to avoid irritation of the mouth and throat.
2. This drug can impair normal blood clotting mechanisms. In the event of injury, dental extraction, or need for surgery, inform your physician or dentist that you are taking this drug.
3. Because this drug can impair the normal function of blood platelets, it is advisable to avoid aspirin (which has the same effect).
4. Over-the-counter drug products that contain antihistamines (allergy and cold remedies, sleep aids) can enhance sedative effects.

Precautions for Use

By Infants and Children: The concurrent use of aspirin with this drug can cause abnormal bleeding or bruising. Children with mental retardation, organic brain disease or severe seizure disorders may be at increased risk for severe liver toxicity while taking this drug. Observe closely for the development of fever that could indicate the onset of a drug-induced Reye syndrome (see Glossary). Avoid concurrent use of clonazepam (Clonopin); the combined use could result in continuous petit mal episodes.

By Those over 60 Years of Age: Start treatment with small doses and increase dosage cautiously. Observe closely for excessive sedation, confusion or unsteadiness that could predispose to falling and injury.

▷ **Advisability of Use During Pregnancy**

Pregnancy Category: D. See Pregnancy Code at the back of this book.

Animal studies: Palate and skeletal birth defects reported in mouse, rat and rabbit studies.

Human studies: Adequate studies of pregnant women are not available. There have been several reports of birth defects attributed to the use of this drug during early pregnancy.

Consult your physician regarding the advantages and disadvantages of using this drug. If it is used, it is advisable to keep the dose as low as possible.

Advisability of Use if Breast-Feeding

Presence of this drug in breast milk: Yes.

Monitor nursing infant closely and discontinue drug or nursing if adverse effects develop.

Habit-Forming Potential: None.

Effects of Overdosage: Increased drowsiness, weakness, unsteadiness, confusion, stupor progressing to coma.

Possible Effects of Long-Term Use: None reported.

Suggested Periodic Examinations While Taking This Drug (at physician's discretion)

Complete blood cell counts and baseline liver function tests should be done before treatment is started. During treatment, blood counts should be repeated every month and liver function tests repeated every 2 months.

▷ **While Taking This Drug, Observe the Following**

Foods: No restrictions.

Beverages: Do not administer the syrup in carbonated beverages; this could liberate the valproic acid and irritate the mouth and throat. This drug may be taken with milk.

▷ *Alcohol:* Alcohol can increase the sedative effect of this drug. Also, this drug can increase the depressant effects of alcohol on brain function.

Tobacco Smoking: No interactions expected.

▷ *Other Drugs*

Valproic acid may ***increase*** the effects of

- anticoagulants (Coumadin, etc.), and increase the risk of bleeding. Increased frequency of INR testing is needed.
- antidepressants, both monoamine oxidase (MAO) type A inhibitors and tricyclics, and cause toxicity.
- nimodipine (Nimotop) and cause nimodipine toxicity.

- phenobarbital, and cause barbiturate intoxication.
- phenytoin (Dilantin), and cause phenytoin toxicity.

Valproic acid *taken concurrently* with

- antacids (Maalox) will decrease absorption and decrease therapeutic benefit.
- antiplatelet drugs: aspirin, dipyridamole (Persantine), sulfinpyrazone (Anturane) may enhance the inhibition of platelet function and increase the risk of bleeding.
- aspirin can lead to valproic acid toxicity.
- carbamazepine (Tegretol) may have a variable effect on blood levels. More frequent blood level testing is advised
- clonazepam (Klonopin) may result in repeated episodes of absence seizures (absence status).
- cyclosporine (Sandimmune) may increase risk of liver toxicity.
- erythromycin (Ery-Tab, others) may increase the level of valproic acid and result in toxicity. The newer macrolides (azithromycin or clarithromycin) may also cause problems.
- felbamate (Felbatol) can lead to increased valproic acid levels.
- isoniazid (INH) can cause valproic acid or isoniazid toxicity.

▷ *Driving, Hazardous Activities:* This drug may cause drowsiness, dizziness or confusion. Restrict activities as necessary.

Aviation Note: The use of this drug *is a disqualification* for piloting. Consult a designated Aviation Medical Examiner.

Exposure to Sun: Caution. This drug has caused photosensitivity.

Discontinuation: Do not stop this drug suddenly. Abrupt withdrawal can cause repetitive seizures that are difficult to control.

VANCOMYCIN (van koh MI sin)

Introduced: 1974   **Prescription:** USA: Yes; Canada: Yes   **Available as Generic:** USA: Yes; Canada: No   **Class:** Anti-infective   **Controlled Drug:** USA: No; Canada: No

Brand Name: Vancocin, Vancoled, Vancor

Note: Vancomycin is used to treat a variety of serious infections. It is given intravenously to treat some infections and orally to treat others. In the past, the information provided in this Drug Profile was limited to the use of vancomycin taken by mouth. Since resistant organisms have increased intravenous use, the profile has been broadened to help patients understand vancomycin's broadened role in infectious disease.

BENEFITS versus RISKS	
Possible Benefits	*Possible Risks*
HIGHLY EFFECTIVE IN TREATING ANTIBIOTIC-ASSOCIATED PSEUDOMEMBRANOUS COLITIS	Ringing in ears (tinnitus) Loss of hearing

▷ **Principal Uses**

As a Single Drug Product: Uses currently included in FDA approved labeling: Treatment of (1) Oral form is used in antibiotic-associated pseudomembra-

nous colitis caused by *Clostridium difficile*; (2) the oral form is also used in enterocolitis caused by staphylococcal organisms; (3) the intravenous form is used to treat a variety of serious infections such those in heart valves, bones (ostemyelitis), endocarditis and meningitis, including those caused by Methicillin Resistant Staphylococci (MRSA).
Other (unlabeled) generally accepted uses: None.

How This Drug Works: By inhibiting the formation of bacterial cell walls and the production of RNA, this drug destroys susceptible strains of infecting bacteria.

Available Dosage Forms and Strengths
Capsules — 125 mg, 250 mg
Intravenous — 500 mg or one gram per 15 ml
Oral solution — 250 mg per 5-ml teaspoonful and 500 mg per 5-ml

▷ **Recommended Dosage Ranges (Actual dosage and administration schedule must be determined by the physician for each patient individually.)**
Infants and Children: 10 mg/kg of body weight every 6 hours, for 5 to 10 days. The total daily dose should not exceed 2000 mg (2 grams). Repeat course as necessary.
12 to 60 Years of Age: Many clinicians use a 15 mg per kilogram loading dose and then calculate ongoing doses based on individual patient height, weight, kidney function and suspected bacteria (bacterial pathogen). Calculations are made in order to attain a peak blood level of 30–40 mcg/ml and a lowest blood level (trough) of 5 to 10 mcg/ml. Oral dosing for pseudomembranous colitis caused by *C. difficile:* 125 mg by mouth every 6 hours for 10 days.
Over 60 Years of Age: Intravenous dosing: The loading dose is the same as for younger patients. Ongoing doses may be much smaller and may need to be given much less often than in younger patients (such as once a day or once every two days). For oral dosing: Same as 12 to 60 years of age (since the vancomycin in pseudomembranous colitis is not absorbed).

Conditions Requiring Dosing Adjustments
Liver function: The liver is not involved in the elimination of vancomycin.
Kidney function: Oral vancomycin is minimally absorbed. Intravenous vancomycin MUST be given in decreased dose or increased interval in kidney failure. This medicine is also a potential cause of kidney failure, and should only be given if other alternatives are not available. Daily measures of kidney function and more frequent blood levels are indicated if this medicine is used in patients with compromised kidneys.

▷ **Dosing Instructions:**   May be taken with or following food to reduce stomach irritation. Because of this drug's unpleasant taste, it is preferable to swallow the capsule whole without alteration. Use a measuring device to ensure accuracy of dose when taking the oral solution. Observe the expiration date.

Usual Duration of Use: Oral use: use on a regular schedule for 48 to 72 hours usually determines effectiveness in controlling infection in the colon. If response is prompt, limit treatment to 10 days. If symptoms warrant, continue treatment for 14 to 21 days. Consult your physician on a regular basis. For intravenous use, the length of treatment depends on the severity and site of the infection (for example, bone infections may take 6 weeks to cure).

Currently a "Drug of Choice"

for treating metronidazole treatment failures in antibiotic-associated pseudo-membranous colitis caused by *C. difficile*.

▷ **This Drug Should Not Be Taken If**
- you have had an allergic reaction to it previously.

▷ **Inform Your Physician Before Taking This Drug If**
- you have a history of Crohn's disease or ulcerative colitis.
- you have impaired kidney function.
- you are pregnant.
- you have any degree of hearing loss.
- you are taking cholestyramine (Questran) or colestipol (Colestid).

Possible Side Effects (natural, expected, and unavoidable drug actions)
Bitter, unpleasant taste for the oral form.

▷ **Possible Adverse Effects** (unusual, unexpected, and infrequent reactions)
If any of the following develop, consult your physician promptly for guidance.

Mild Adverse Effects
Allergic Reactions: Skin rash (with large doses or prolonged use).
Nausea, vomiting.
Chills.

Serious Adverse Effects
Allergic Reactions: Anaphylaxis. Serious skin rashes (exfoliative dermatitis or Stevens-Johnson syndrome).
Ringing or buzzing in ears, sensation of ear fullness, loss of hearing.
Lowering of white blood cells (reversible, and seen with the intravenous form).
Red-man syndrome (excessive lowering of the blood pressure; sudden rash on the neck, chest, face, and extremities).
Cardiac arrest (rare).
Hearing loss (may be reversible).
Pseudomembranous colitis.
Kidney toxicity (may be dose-dependent).
Thrombophlebitis.

▷ **Possible Effects on Sexual Function:**   None reported.

Natural Diseases or Disorders That May Be Activated by This Drug
Latent hearing loss, kidney failure.

Possible Effects on Laboratory Tests
Serum creatinine : increased (a sign of kidney toxicity).

CAUTION
1. Report promptly the development of fullness, ringing or buzzing in either ear. This may indicate the onset of nerve damage that could lead to hearing loss.
2. Do not take any medication to stop your diarrhea without calling your doctor. The bacterial toxin that causes colitis is eliminated by diarrhea; stopping the elimination could intensify and prolong your illness.
3. Blood levels MUST be used to guide dosing. Keep all appointments for laboratory work.

Precautions for Use

By Infants and Children: This drug is usually well tolerated. Some cases may require doses up to 50 mg/kg of body weight daily.

By Those over 60 Years of Age: You may be more susceptible to drug-induced hearing loss. Use the minimum course of treatment required to cure your colitis or other infection.

▷ **Advisability of Use During Pregnancy**

Pregnancy Category: B. See Pregnancy Code at the back of this book.

Animal studies: Rat and rabbit studies reveal no drug-induced birth defects.

Human studies: Adequate studies of pregnant women are not available.

Use this drug only if clearly needed. Ask your physician for guidance.

Advisability of Use if Breast-Feeding

Presence of this drug in breast milk: Yes.

Avoid drug or refrain from nursing.

Habit-Forming Potential: None.

Effects of Overdosage: Possible nausea, vomiting, ringing in ears.

Possible Effects of Long-Term Use: Hearing loss.

Suggested Periodic Examinations While Taking This Drug (at physician's discretion)

Hearing tests.

▷ **While Taking This Drug, Observe the Following**

Foods: No restrictions.

Beverages: No restrictions. May be taken with milk.

▷ *Alcohol:* No interactions expected. Use sparingly; alcohol may aggravate colitis.

Tobacco Smoking: No interactions expected.

▷ *Other Drugs*

The following drugs may **decrease** the effects of vancomycin

- cholestyramine (Questran).
- colestipol (Colestid).

Vancomycin **taken concurrently** with

- aminoglycoside antibiotics (see Drug Classes) such as gentamicin or tobramycin may cause additive toxicity risk to the ears and kidneys.
- cyclosporine (Sandimmune) may result in increased toxicity risk.
- warfarin (Coumadin) may cause an increased risk of bleeding. Increased INR (protime) testing is needed.

▷ *Driving, Hazardous Activities:* Usually no restrictions.

Aviation Note: The use of this drug **is probably not a disqualification** for piloting. Consult a designated Aviation Medical Examiner.

Exposure to Sun: No restrictions.

Discontinuation: To be determined by your physician.

Special Storage Instructions: Refrigerate the oral solution.

Observe the Following Expiration Times: Provided on your prescription label by your pharmacist.

VARICELLA VIRUS VACCINE (VAHR a cel la)

Introduced: 1995   **Prescription:** USA: Yes; Canada: Yes   **Available as Generic:** USA: No; Canada: No   **Class:** Vaccine   **Controlled Drug:** USA: No; Canada: No

Brand Names: Varivax

BENEFITS versus RISKS	
Possible Benefits	*Possible Risks*
PREVENTION OF VARICELLA (chicken pox)	Rash (infrequent) Soreness at the injection site Anaphylactoid reaction (rare)

▷ **Principal Uses**

As a Single Drug Product: Uses currently included in FDA approved labeling: (1) Prevention of chicken pox.

Other (unlabeled) generally accepted uses: None.

How This Drug Works: By stimulating the immune system, the vaccine prepares the body to fight any exposure to the wild type virus.

Available Dosage Forms and Strengths

vaccine (multi-dose vial): — a single dose vial of vaccine (1500 PFU per dose)

How To Store

This product **must** be kept frozen prior to use.

Author's note: The Center for Disease Control's (CDC) Immunization Practices Committee has recommended that all children 12 to 18 months old should be given varicella vaccine if they have not previously contracted chicken pox. The vaccine is also recommended by the committee for children 19 months to 13 years old. Finally, adults or adolescents who have not had chicken pox and are at risk for exposure should also be given the vaccine.

▷ **Recommended Dosage Ranges (Actual dosage and administration schedule must be determined by the physician for each patient individually.)**

Infants and Children from one to 12 years old: Not indicated in infants. Children 1 year old or older are given 0.5 ml injected under the skin.

12 to 55 Years of Age: Same as the children's dose, providing the patient has not had chicken pox.

Over 55 Years of Age: Not studied.

Conditions Requiring Dosing Adjustments

Liver function: Not a consideration.

Kidney function: Not a consideration.

▷ **Dosing Instructions:** This vaccine is to be injected under the skin. It may be given with measles, mumps and rubella vaccine.

Usual Duration of Benefit: Exposure to chicken pox 5 years after vaccination may result in 20% of patients developing mild disease. More experience is needed before the question of repeat vaccination is answered.

Possible Advantages of This Drug

Prevention of chicken pox.

Currently a "Drug of Choice"
for prevention of chicken pox.

▷ **This Drug Should Not Be Taken If**
- you have had an allergic reaction to any dosage form of it previously.
- you have a history of anaphylactoid reaction to neomycin.
- you have a history of blood diseases, leukemia, or have AIDS.
- you are taking medicines which suppress the immune system.
- you have tuberculosis which has not been treated.
- you are allergic to eggs.
- you are pregnant.
- you have an active infection.

▷ **Inform Your Physician Before Taking This Drug If**
- you are planning pregnancy in the near future.
- you have a condition which may require steroids.
- you take salicylates (aspirin, others) on a regular basis. This should NOT be done for 6 weeks following vaccination as it is a risk for Reye's syndrome.
- you live with someone who has a depressed immune system (such as an AIDS patient). Because this vaccine is a live virus vaccine, you may be infectious to them.

Possible Side Effects (natural, expected, and unavoidable drug actions)
Pain at the injection site, fever.

▷ **Possible Adverse Effects** (unusual, unexpected, and infrequent reactions)
If any of the following develop, consult your physician promptly for guidance.
Mild Adverse Effects
Allergic Reactions: Skin rash.
Varicella-like rash.
Irritability, fatigue, and loss of appetite.
Chills, stiff neck, and joint pain.
Serious Adverse Effects
Allergic Reactions: Anaphylactoid reaction.
Idiosyncratic Reactions: None reported.
Febrile seizures (rare).
Herpes zoster.
Pneumonitis (very rare and of questionable causation).

▷ **Possible Effects on Sexual Function:** None reported.

Possible Delayed Adverse Effects: None reported.

▷ **Adverse Effects That May Mimic Natural Diseases or Disorders**
Rash may resemble chicken pox.

Natural Diseases or Disorders That May Be Activated by This Drug
None reported.

Possible Effects on Laboratory Tests
None reported.

CAUTION
1. **Do not** give aspirin or other salicylates to patients who have recently received the vaccine. The risk of Reye's syndrome is associated with such aspirin use.

Precautions for Use

By Infants and Children: Safety and effectiveness for use by those under 12 months of age have not been established.

By Those over 60 Years of Age: Not studied.

▷ **Advisability of Use During Pregnancy**

Pregnancy Category: C. See Pregnancy Code at the back of this book.

Animal studies: Have not been conducted with this vaccine.

Human studies: Information from adequate studies of pregnant women is not available. The manufacturer says that the vaccine should not be given to pregnant women and pregnancy should be avoided for three months following vaccination.

Advisability of Use if Breast-Feeding

Presence of this drug in breast milk: Expected.

Avoid drug or refrain from nursing.

Habit-Forming Potential: None.

Effects of Overdosage: Not defined.

Possible Effects of Long-Term Use: Not intended for long-term use.

Suggested Periodic Examinations While Taking This Drug (at physician's discretion)

None suggested.

▷ **While Taking This Drug, Observe the Following**

Foods: No restrictions.

Beverages: No restrictions.

▷   *Alcohol:* No interactions expected.

Tobacco Smoking: No interactions expected.

▷   *Other Drugs*

Varicella vaccine ***taken concurrently*** with

- acyclovir (Zovirax) may result in a blunted immune benefit from the vaccine.
- aspirin or any salicylates (various) may result in Reye's syndrome. DO NOT take aspirin for 6 weeks after vaccination.
- corticosteroids (see Drug Classes) may result in extreme reactions.
- immune globulins may result in decreased beneficial response to the vaccine.
- immunosuppressant medicines (such as cyclosporine—Sandimmune) may result in extreme reactions.
- mesalamine (Asacol) may result in risk of Reye's syndrome. DO NOT take salicylates for 6 weeks after vaccination.
- olsalazine (Dipentum) may result in risk of Reye's syndrome. DO NOT take salicylates for 6 weeks after vaccination.

▷   *Driving, Hazardous Activities:* This drug may cause soreness at the injection site. Restrict activities as necessary.

Aviation Note: The use of this drug ***is probably not a disqualification*** for piloting. Consult a designated Aviation Medical Examiner.

Exposure to Sun: No restrictions.

Occurrence of Unrelated Illness: This vaccination should not be given in the presence of any other active infection.

Special Storage Instructions: This vaccine must be stored frozen.

Author's note: There is now a Vaccine Adverse Event Reporting System (VAERS). The toll free number is 1-800–822-7967.

VENLAFAXINE (ven la FAX een)

Introduced: 1993   **Prescription:** USA: Yes   **Available as Generic:**
USA: No   **Class:** Antidepressant   **Controlled Drug:** USA: No
Brand Names: Effexor

BENEFITS versus RISKS	
Possible Benefits	*Possible Risks*
EFFECTIVE TREATMENT OF DEPRESSION	INCREASED BLOOD PRESSURE
BETTER SIDE-EFFECT PROFILE THAN TRICYCLIC ANTIDEPRESSANTS	Seizures (rare)
	Constipation
	Increased heart rate
	Increased serum lipids
RAPID ONSET OF EFFECT	

▷ **Principal Uses**

As a Single Drug Product: Uses currently included in FDA approved labeling: (1) Treatment of depression.

Other (unlabeled) generally accepted uses: (1) May be useful in treatment of obsessive-compulsive disorder.

How This Drug Works: This bicyclic (second generation) antidepressant inhibits the return of (reuptake) of nerve transmitters (serotonin, norepinephrine and dopamine) and helps return normal mood and thinking.

Available Dosage Forms and Strengths

Tablets — 25 mg, 37.5 mg, 50 mg, 75 mg, 100 mg.

▷ **Recommended Dosage Ranges (Actual dosage and administration schedule must be determined by the physician for each patient individually.)**

Infants and Children: Safety and efficacy for those under 18 years of age not established.

18 to 60 Years of Age: For depression: therapy is started with 75 mg per day, given as 25 mg doses 3 times daily.

If needed and tolerated, the dose may be increased at 4 day intervals up to a maximum of 225 mg per day. Some hospitalized patients have been given a maximum of 375 mg per day.

Over 60 Years of Age: Low starting doses and slow increases are indicated. Natural declines in kidney function may lead to drug accumulation at higher doses. This drug may worsen a constipation problem that you already face.

Conditions Requiring Dosing Adjustments

Liver function: The total daily dose must be reduced by 50% in patients with moderate liver compromise. Further dose decreases and individualized dosing is indicated in patients with liver cirrhosis. The drug is changed to an active form in the liver.

Kidney function: Patients with compromised kidneys (creatinine clearance of 10 to 70 ml/min.) should be given 75% of the usual daily dose.

▷ **Dosing Instructions:** Food has no clinically significant effect on venlafaxine absorption.

Usual Duration of Use: Use on a regular schedule for 2 weeks usually determines effectiveness in treating depression. Long-term use (months to years) requires periodic physician evaluation of response and dosage adjustment.

Possible Advantages of This Drug

Effective treatment of depression with fewer side effects than other currently available agents. Starts to have a therapeutic effect more rapidly than other available agents.

▷ **This Drug Should Not Be Taken If**
- you have had an allergic reaction to any dosage form of it previously.
- you are taking a monoamine oxidase inhibitor (see Drug Classes).

▷ **Inform Your Physician Before Taking This Drug If**
- you have a history of high blood pressure.
- you have a history of abnormally increased lipids (hyperlipidemia).
- you have a history of seizures.
- you have a history of hypomania or mania.
- you are uncertain of how much venlafaxine to take or how often to take it.

Possible Side Effects (natural, expected, and unavoidable drug actions)

Constipation and headache.

▷ **Possible Adverse Effects** (unusual, unexpected, and infrequent reactions)

If any of the following develop, consult your physician promptly for guidance.

Mild Adverse Effects

Allergic Reactions. Not characterized.

Palpitations.

Nausea and vomiting.

Dizziness (may disappear without treatment), fatigue, and headache.

Anxiety or insomnia (may stop on its own).

Somnolence.

Blurred vision.

Sweating.

Weight loss, dry mouth.

Small increases in cholesterol (2–3 mg/dl).

Serious Adverse Effects

Allergic Reactions: None reported.

Idiosyncratic Reactions: None reported.

Increased blood pressure.

Seizures (rare).

▷ **Possible Effects on Sexual Function:**   Delayed orgasm, abnormal ejaculation, impotence and erectile failure (all infrequent).

Possible Delayed Adverse Effects: None reported.

▷ **Adverse Effects That May Mimic Natural Diseases or Disorders**

None reported.

Natural Diseases or Disorders That May Be Activated by This Drug

None reported.

Possible Effects on Laboratory Tests

Serum cholesterol: Increased slightly.

CAUTION
1. This drug should **not** be taken with MAO inhibitor (see Glossary) drugs. If you have recently stopped a MAO inhibitor, 14 days should pass before venlafaxine is started.

▷ **Advisability of Use During Pregnancy**

Pregnancy Category: C. See Pregnancy Code at the back of this book.

Animal studies: There was an increase in stillborn rats at 10 times the usual human dose.

Human studies: Adequate studies of pregnant women are not available. Ask your doctor for guidance.

Advisability of Use if Breast-Feeding

Presence of this drug in breast milk: Unknown.

Monitor nursing infant closely and discontinue drug or nursing if adverse effects develop.

Habit-Forming Potential: None.

Effects of Overdosage: Nausea, vomiting, constipation, seizure potential.

Possible Effects of Long-Term Use: None noted.

Suggested Periodic Examinations While Taking This Drug (at physician's discretion)

Blood pressure checks.

▷ **While Taking This Drug, Observe the Following**

Foods: No restrictions.

Nutritional Support: No special support indicated.

Beverages: Since venlafaxine is metabolized in the liver, and grapefruit juice has been shown to inhibit the removal (metabolism) of some other medications, caution is advised. Water may be the best liquid to take this medicine with.

▷   *Alcohol:* May increase somnolence if combined.

Tobacco Smoking: No interactions expected.

Marijuana Smoking: Additive effect on somnolence.

▷   *Other Drugs*

Venlafaxine *taken concurrently* with

- beta blockers (see Drug Classes) may result in larger than expected pharmacological effects from the beta blockers. Because these agents are metabolized in the liver, and venlafaxine may block this metabolism, caution is advised.
- calcium channel blockers (see Drug Classes) may result in toxicity. Because these agents are metabolized in the liver, and venlafaxine may block this metabolism, caution is advised.
- cimetidine (Tagamet) may lead to venlafaxine toxicity.
- drugs with sedative properties will increase those effects.
- MAO inhibitors may lead to undesirable side effects. Do not combine.
- quinidine (Quinaglute, others) may result in venlafaxine toxicity.
- tricyclic antidepressants (see Drug Classes) may result in toxicity. Because these agents are metabolized in the liver, and venlafaxine may block this metabolism, caution is advised.
- warfarin (Coumadin) may result in bleeding. More frequent INR (protime testing) is needed. Ongoing coumadin doses should be adjusted to laboratory results.

▷   *Driving, Hazardous Activities:* This drug may cause somnolence. Restrict activities as necessary.

Aviation Note: The use of this drug *is a disqualification* for piloting. Consult a designated Aviation Medical Examiner.

Exposure to Sun: No restrictions.
Exposure to Heat: No restrictions.
Discontinuation: Talk to your doctor before stopping this medication.

VERAPAMIL (ver AP a mil)

Introduced: 1967   **Prescription:** USA: Yes; Canada: Yes   **Available as Generic:** USA: Yes; Canada: No   **Class:** Antianginal, antiarrhythmic, antihypertensive, calcium channel blocker   **Controlled Drug:** USA: No; Canada: No

Brand Names: ✦Apo-Verap, Calan, Calan SR, Isoptin, Isoptin SR, ✦Novo-Veramil, ✦Nu-Verap, Verelan

> **Controversies in Medicine:** Study data indicates that medicines in this class should NOT be used in some patients with extremely compromised hearts. There have also been several FDA hearings held on the calcium channel blocker class. Be certain to ask your doctor about your cardiac output and if the benefits of this medicine outweigh the risks of its use. A recent FDA panel found medicines in this class to be safe and effective. A retrospective chart review yielded data that showed increased risks for nifedipine immediate release forms in those over 71, and cautioned physicians against using the immediate release form for indications other than angina. The immediate release form in question had never been approved for other uses. Most recently, a study of nearly 6,000 patients at Tel Aviv Medical Center found that there was no statistically significant increased risk of death in the patients who took calcium channel blockers versus those who did not.

BENEFITS versus RISKS

Possible Benefits	*Possible Risks*
EFFECTIVE PREVENTION OF BOTH MAJOR TYPES OF ANGINA	Congestive heart failure
	Low blood pressure (infrequent)
EFFECTIVE CONTROL OF HEART RATE IN CHRONIC ATRIAL FIBRILLATION AND FLUTTER	Heart rhythm disturbance
	Fluid retention (rare)
	Liver damage without jaundice (very rare)
EFFECTIVE PREVENTION OF PAROXYSMAL ATRIAL TACHYCARDIA (PAT)	Swelling of male breast tissue
EFFECTIVE TREATMENT OF HYPERTENSION	

▷ **Principal Uses**

As a Single Drug Product: Uses currently included in FDA approved labeling: Used to treat (1) angina pectoris due to coronary artery spasm (Prinzmetal's variant angina) that occurs spontaneously and is not associated with exertion; (2) classical angina-of-effort (due to atherosclerotic disease of the coronary arteries) in individuals who have not responded to or cannot tolerate the nitrates and beta blocker drugs customarily used to treat this disorder; (3) abnormally rapid heart rate due to chronic atrial fibrillation or flutter; (4) recurrent paroxysmal atrial tachycardia; and (5) primary hypertension.

Other (unlabeled) generally accepted uses: (1) May help prevent abnormal heart rhythms that occur after surgery; (2) can help relieve symptoms and may help reverse hypertrophic cardiomyopathy; (3) may help decrease the severity or occurrence of cluster headaches; (4) used to help control the symptoms of panic attacks; (5) can be of use in post-ischemic acute kidney failure; (6) may stop the progression of abnormal buildup on the inside of blood vessels (atherosclerosis); (7) may help decrease severity and occurrence of nocturnal leg cramps; (8) could have a place in combination therapy of multiple myeloma; (9) can help stuttering; (10) may have a role in Tourette's syndrome.

How This Drug Works: By blocking passage of calcium through certain cell walls (which is necessary for the function of nerve and muscle tissue), this drug slows the spread of electrical activity through the heart and inhibits the contraction of coronary arteries and peripheral arterioles. As a result of these combined effects, this drug
- prevents spontaneous coronary artery spasm (Prinzmetal's type of angina).
- reduces the rate and contraction force of the heart during exertion, thus lowering the oxygen requirement of the heart muscle; this reduces the occurrence of effort-induced angina (classical angina pectoris).
- reduces the degree of contraction of peripheral arterial walls, resulting in their relaxation and consequent lowering of blood pressure. This further reduces the work load of the heart during exertion and contributes to the prevention of angina.
- slows the rate of electrical impulses through the heart and thereby prevents excessively rapid heart action (tachycardia).

Available Dosage Forms and Strengths

Caplets, sustained release — 120 mg, 180 mg, 240 mg
Capsules, sustained release — 360 mg
Injection — 5 mg per 2 ml
Tablets — 40 mg, 80 mg, 120 mg
Tablets, sustained release — 120 mg, 180 mg, 240 mg

▷ **Usual Adult Dosage Range:**   Hypertension: Initially, 80 mg 3 times daily. The dose may be increased gradually at 1 to 7 day intervals as needed and tolerated. The usual maintenance dose is from 240 mg to 360 mg daily in 3 or 4 divided doses. The prolonged-action (sustained release) dosage forms permit once-a-day dosing. The total daily dosage should not exceed 360 mg.

Once-a-day treatment may be initiated with 1 prolonged-action capsule of 120 mg or 1 tablet of 180 mg.

Note: Actual dosage and administration schedule must be determined by the physician for each patient individually.

Conditions Requiring Dosing Adjustments

Liver function: Blood levels should be obtained, and used to guide dosing. In patients with liver compromise, the dose should be decreased to 20–50% of the usual dose and may be given at the usual interval. Verapamil can be a rare cause of liver damage, and patients should be followed closely. Changes in the electrocardiogram may provide an early indication of increasing blood levels.

Kidney function: In severe kidney compromise, the dose should be decreased by 50–75%.

▷ **Dosing Instructions:**   Preferably taken with meals and with food at bedtime. The regular tablet may be crushed for administration. The prolonged-action dosage forms (capsules and tablets) should be swallowed whole and not altered. Verelan capsules may be taken without regard to food intake.

Usual Duration of Use: Use on a regular schedule for 2 to 4 weeks usually determines effectiveness in reducing the frequency and severity of angina. Reduction of elevated blood pressure may be apparent within the first 1 to 2 weeks. For long-term use (months to years), the smallest effective dose should be used. Periodic physician evaluation is needed.

Possible Advantages of This Drug

No adverse effects on blood levels of glucose, potassium or uric acid.

Does not increase blood cholesterol or triglyceride levels.

Does not impair capacity for exercise.

The new 360 mg strength of Verelan allows once daily dosing for those patients who require more than 240 mg daily. The company has noted that there is no increase in side effects when comparing the 240 mg capsules to the new 360 mg ones.

Currently a "Drug of Choice"

for (1) initiating treatment of hypertension with a single drug; (2) treating hypertension in African-Americans.

▷ **This Drug Should Not Be Taken If**

• you have had an allergic reaction to it previously.
• you have active liver disease.
• you have a "sick sinus" syndrome (and do not have an artificial pacemaker).
• you have been told that you have a second-degree or third-degree heart block.
• you have low blood pressure; systolic pressure below 90.
• you have advanced aortic stenosis (ask your doctor).

▷ **Inform Your Physician Before Taking This Drug If**

• you have had an unfavorable response to any calcium blocker.
• you are currently taking any other drugs, especially digitalis or a beta blocker drug (see Drug Class Section).
• you have had a recent stroke or heart attack.
• you have a history of congestive heart failure or heart rhythm disorders.
• you have poor circulation to your extremities, or you have gangrene.
• you have impaired liver or kidney function.
• you have a history of drug-induced liver damage.

Possible Side Effects (natural, expected, and unavoidable drug actions)

Low blood pressure, fluid retention (rare).

▷ **Possible Adverse Effects** (unusual, unexpected, and infrequent reactions)

If any of the following develop, consult your physician promptly for guidance.

Mild Adverse Effects

Allergic Reactions: Skin rash, hives, itching, aching joints.

Headache (rare), dizziness, fatigue (rare).

Nausea (rare), indigestion, constipation.

Abnormal growth of the gums.

Sensation of numbness or coldness in the extremities.

Serious Adverse Effects
Serious disturbances of heart rate and/or rhythm, congestive heart failure (rare).
Drug-induced liver damage without jaundice (very rare).
Antiplatelet effect and extended time to form blood clots.
Ventricular fibrillation (with intravenous use in patients with atrial fibrillation).
Excessive lowering of blood pressure.
Unmasking of parkinsonism (rare).
Low blood sugar.

▷ **Possible Effects on Sexual Function**
Altered timing and pattern of menstruation.
Male breast enlargement and tenderness (gynecomastia).
Impotence (20%).

Possible Effects on Laboratory Tests
Blood total cholesterol and HDL cholesterol levels: no effect in some; decreased in others.
Blood LDL cholesterol level: no effect.
Blood triglyceride levels: no effect.
Glucose tolerance test (GTT): decreased.
Liver function tests: increased liver enzymes (ALT/GPT and AST/GOT), increased bilirubin (one case report).

CAUTION
1. Be sure to inform all physicians and other health care professionals who provide medical care for you that you take this drug. Note the use of this drug on your card of personal identification.
2. You may use nitroglycerin and other nitrate drugs as needed to relieve acute episodes of angina pain. However, if you detect that your angina attacks are becoming more frequent or intense, notify your physician promptly.
3. If this drug is used concurrently with a beta blocker drug, you may develop excessively low blood pressure.
4. This drug may cause swelling of the feet and ankles. This may not be indicative of either heart or kidney dysfunction.

Precautions for Use
By Infants and Children: Safety and effectiveness for those under 12 years of age not established.
By Those over 60 Years of Age: You may be more susceptible to the development of weakness, dizziness, fainting and falling. Take necessary precautions to prevent injury. Report promptly any changes in your pattern of thirst and urination.

▷ **Advisability of Use During Pregnancy**
Pregnancy Category: C. See Pregnancy Code at the back of this book.
Animal studies: Toxic effects on the embryo and retarded growth of the fetus (but no birth defects) reported in rat studies.
Human studies: Adequate studies of pregnant women are not available.
Avoid this drug during the first 3 months. Use during the last 6 months only if clearly needed. Ask your physician for guidance.

Advisability of Use if Breast-Feeding
Presence of this drug in breast milk: Yes.
Discuss the benefits and risks of nursing your infant. While levels are present in the infant, most researchers find them to be below clinically significant levels. Monitor infant for adverse effects.

Habit-Forming Potential: None.

Effects of Overdosage: Flushed and warm skin, sweating, light-headedness, irritability, rapid heart rate, low blood pressure, loss of consciousness.

Possible Effects of Long-Term Use: None reported.

Suggested Periodic Examinations While Taking This Drug (at physician's discretion)
Evaluations of heart function, including electrocardiograms; liver and kidney function tests, with long-term use.

▷ **While Taking This Drug, Observe the Following**
Foods: No restrictions. Avoid excessive salt intake.
Beverages: Caffeine levels will be increased if caffeine-containing beverages are consumed while you are on verapamil. May be taken with milk.
▷   *Alcohol:* Use with caution until combined effects have been determined. Alcohol may exaggerate the drop in blood pressure, and change the elimination of alcohol experienced by some patients.
Tobacco Smoking: Nicotine can reduce the effectiveness of this drug. Avoid all forms of tobacco.
Marijuana Smoking: Possible reduced effectiveness of this drug; mild to moderate increase in angina; possible changes in electrocardiogram, confusing interpretation.
▷   *Other Drugs*
Verapamil may *increase* the effects of
• carbamazepine (Tegretol), and cause carbamazepine toxicity.
• digitoxin and digoxin, and cause digitalis toxicity.
Verapamil *taken concurrently* with
• aspirin may result in bleeding.
• amiodarone (Codarone) may result in cardiac arrest.
• beta blocker drugs (see Drug Class Section) may affect heart rate and rhythm adversely. Careful monitoring by your physician is necessary if these drugs are taken concurrently.
• calcium supplements (various) may blunt the therapeutic benefits of verapamil. Separate calcium and verapamil dosing by two hours.
• cyclosporine (Sandimmune) may result in cyclosporine toxicity and renal compromise.
• dantrolene will cause elevated blood potassium and depression of the heart.
• disopyramide (Norpace) can cause congestive heart failure.
• lithium (Lithobid, others) may result in lithium toxicity and mania.
• NSAIDs (see Drug Classes) may blunt the therapeutic effect of verapamil on blood pressure.
• oral hypoglycemic agents (see Drug Classes) may lead to excessively low blood sugar.
• phenytoin (Dilantin) may result in decreased effectiveness of verapamil.
• quinidine (Quinaglute, others) can result in quinidine toxicity.

- rifampin (Rifadin, others) will decrease the therapeutic benefit of verapamil.
- sulfinpyrazone increases the removal of verapamil and lessens the therapeutic effect.
- terazocin (Hytrin) can lead to excessive decreases in blood pressure.
- theophylline (Theodur, others) can lead to theophylline toxicity.

The following drugs may **increase** the effects of verapamil

- cimetidine (Tagamet) and other H2 blocking (see Drug Classes) drugs .
- tricyclic antidepressants (see Drug Classes).

▷ *Driving, Hazardous Activities:* Usually no restrictions. This drug may cause dizziness. Restrict activities as necessary.

Aviation Note: Coronary artery disease *is a disqualification* for piloting. Consult a designated Aviation Medical Examiner.

Exposure to Sun: Use caution until sensitivity has been determined. This drug may cause photosensitivity (see Glossary).

Exposure to Heat: Caution advised. Hot environments can exaggerate the blood-pressure-lowering effects of this drug. Observe for light-headedness or weakness.

Heavy Exercise or Exertion: This drug may improve your ability to be more active without resulting angina pain. Use caution and avoid excessive exercise that could impair heart function in the absence of warning pain.

Discontinuation: Do not stop this drug abruptly. Consult your physician regarding gradual withdrawal to prevent the development of rebound angina.

WARFARIN (WAR far in)

Introduced: 1941   **Prescription:** USA: Yes; Canada: Yes   **Available as Generic:** USA: No; Canada: No   **Class:** Anticoagulant, coumarins   **Controlled Drug:** USA: No; Canada: No

Brand Names: Coumadin, Sofarin

BENEFITS versus RISKS	
Possible Benefits	*Possible Risks*
EFFECTIVE PREVENTION OF BOTH ARTERIAL AND VENOUS THROMBOSIS	NARROW TREATMENT RANGE Dose-related bleeding Skin and soft tissue hemorrhage with tissue death (rare)
EFFECTIVE PREVENTION OF EMBOLIZATION IN THROMBOEMBOLIC DISORDERS	
HELPS PREVENT RECURRENCE OF HEART ATTACK	
HELPS PREVENT STROKES IN PATIENTS WITH ATRIAL FIBRILLATION	

▷ **Principal Uses**

As a Single Drug Product: Uses currently included in FDA approved labeling: Used in: (1) Acute thrombosis (clot) or thrombophlebitis of the deep veins; (2) acute pulmonary embolism, resulting from blood clots that originate anywhere in the body; (3) atrial fibrillation, to prevent clotting of blood inside the heart that could result in embolization of small clots to any part of the body; (4) acute myocardial infarction (heart attack), to prevent clotting and embolization and therefore a recurrence of heart attack; (5) mitral valve replacement; (6) helps prevent blood clots in the lungs (pulmonary embolism) which may start after hip replacement surgery. Other (unlabeled) generally accepted uses: (1) Helps prevent embolization from the heart in those individuals with artificial heart valves; (2) may help patients with low blood platelets caused by heparin.

How This Drug Works: The coumarin anticoagulants interfere with the production of four essential blood clotting factors by blocking the action of vitamin K. This leads to a deficiency of these clotting factors in circulating blood and inhibits blood clotting mechanisms.

Available Dosage Forms and Strengths

Injection — 5 mg

Tablets — 1 mg, 2 mg, 2.5 mg, 5 mg, 7.5 mg, 10 mg

▷ **Usual Adult Dosage Range:**   Initially, 2 to 5 mg daily for 2 to 3 days. A large loading dose is inappropriate and may be hazardous. For maintenance, the dose is decided based on INR (protime) results and the condition being treated. In many conditions an INR of 2 to 3 is considered therapeutic. **Note: Actual dosage and administration schedule must be determined by the physician for each patient individually.**

Conditions Requiring Dosing Adjustments

Liver function: Blood testing (prothrombin times) should be obtained to guide dosing. It is contraindicated in patients with liver disease.

Kidney function: This drug should be used with caution in renal compromise, however, as warfarin may cause microscopic kidney stones.

▷ **Dosing Instructions:**   The tablet may be crushed and is preferably taken when the stomach is empty, and at the same time each day to ensure uniform results.

Usual Duration of Use: Use on a regular schedule for 3 to 5 days usually determines effectiveness in providing significant anticoagulation. An additional 10 to 14 days is required to determine the optimal maintenance dose for each individual. Long-term use (months to years) requires physician supervision.

▷ **This Drug Should Not Be Taken If**

- you have had an allergic reaction to it previously.
- you have an active peptic ulcer or active ulcerative colitis.
- you are pregnant.
- you have had recent anesthesia (lumbar block) to the spine.
- you have arterial aneurysm.
- you have low blood platelets.
- you have infective pericarditis.
- you have liver disease.
- you have esophageal varices (ask your doctor).
- you have had a recent stroke.

▷ **Inform Your Physician Before Taking This Drug If**

- you are now taking *any other drugs,* either prescription drugs or over-the-counter drug products.

- you are planning pregnancy.
- you have a history of a bleeding disorder.
- you have high blood pressure.
- you have abnormally heavy or prolonged menstrual bleeding.
- you have diabetes.
- you are using an indwelling catheter.
- you have impaired liver or kidney function.
- you plan to have surgery or dental extraction in the near future.

Possible Side Effects (natural, expected, and unavoidable drug actions)

Minor episodes of bleeding may occur even though dosage and prothrombin times are well within the recommended range.

▷ **Possible Adverse Effects** (unusual, unexpected, and infrequent reactions)

If any of the following develop, consult your physician promptly for guidance.

Mild Adverse Effects

Allergic Reactions: Skin rash, hives.

Loss of scalp hair.

Loss of appetite, nausea, vomiting, cramping, diarrhea.

Serious Adverse Effects

Allergic Reaction: Drug fever (see Glossary).

Idiosyncratic Reactions: Bleeding into skin and soft tissues causing gangrene of breast, toes, and localized areas anywhere (rare).

Hereditary warfarin resistance (rare).

Abnormal bleeding from nose, gastrointestinal tract, lungs, urinary tract, or uterus.

Pericardial tamponade.

Hemolytic anemia (rare).

Sudden nerve damage (femoral neuropathy) (rare).

Kidney problems (tubulointerstitial nephritis) (rare).

▷ **Possible Effects on Sexual Function:**   None reported.

▷ **Adverse Effects That May Mimic Natural Diseases or Disorders**

Drug-induced fever may suggest infection.

Natural Diseases or Disorders That May Be Activated by This Drug

Bleeding from "silent" peptic ulcer, intestinal or bladder polyp or tumor.

Possible Effects on Laboratory Tests

Complete blood cell counts: decreased red cells, hemoglobin and white cells.

Bleeding time: increased.

INR (prothrombin time): increased.

Blood uric acid level: increased (in men).

Liver function tests: increased liver enzymes (ALT/GPT, AST/GOT and alkaline phosphatase).

CAUTION

1. Always carry a personal identification card that includes a statement that *you are taking an anticoagulant drug.*
2. While taking this drug, always consult your physician *before* starting any new drug, changing the dosage schedule of any drug or stopping any drug.
3. Data from the Agency For Health Care Policy and Research have shown that expanded use of warfarin could cut in half the 80,000 strokes that occur every year in patients who have atrial fibrillation.

Precautions for Use

By Those over 60 Years of Age: Small starting doses are mandatory. Watch regularly for excessive drug effects: prolonged bleeding from shaving cuts, bleeding gums, bloody urine, rectal bleeding, excessive bruising. Some study data reveals that the beneficial effects of this medicine are not as widely known as needed and are underprescribed in those over 60.

▷ **Advisability of Use During Pregnancy**

Pregnancy Category: D. See Pregnancy Code at the back of this book.

Animal studies: Fetal hemorrhage and death due to this drug reported in mice.

Human studies: Information from studies of pregnant women indicates fetal defects and fetal hemorrhage due to this drug.

The manufacturers state that this drug is contraindicated during entire pregnancy.

Advisability of Use if Breast-Feeding

Presence of this drug in breast milk: Yes.

Avoid drug or refrain from nursing.

Habit-Forming Potential: None.

Effects of Overdosage: Episodes of bleeding from minor surface bleeding (nose, gums, small lacerations) to major internal bleeding: vomiting blood, bloody urine or stool.

Possible Effects of Long-Term Use: None reported.

Suggested Periodic Examinations While Taking This Drug (at physician's discretion)

Regular determinations of prothrombin time are essential to safe dosage and proper control.

Urine analyses for blood.

▷ **While Taking This Drug, Observe the Following**

Foods: A larger intake than usual of foods rich in vitamin K may reduce the effectiveness of this drug and make larger doses necessary. Foods rich in vitamin K include: asparagus, bacon, beef liver, cabbage, cauliflower, fish, green leafy vegetables. Vitamin E may increase risk of bleeding.

Beverages: No restrictions. May be taken with milk.

▷ *Alcohol:* Limit alcohol to one drink daily. Note: Heavy users of alcohol with liver damage may be very sensitive to anticoagulants and require smaller than usual doses.

Tobacco Smoking: Heavy smokers may require relatively larger doses of this drug.

▷ *Other Drugs*

Warfarin may *increase* the effects of
- oral hypoglycemic agents (see Drug Classes).
- phenytoin (Dilantin).

The following drugs may *increase* the effects of warfarin
- acetaminophen (high dose).
- allopurinol (Zyloprim).
- amiodarone (Codarone).
- androgens (see Drug Classes).
- aspirin and some other NSAIDs (see Drug Classes).

- azithromycin (Zithromax).
- bismuth subsalicylate (Pepto Bismol).
- carbamazepine (Tegretol).
- cephalosporins (see Drug Classes).
- chloral hydrate (Noctec).
- chloramphenicol (Chloromycetin).
- cimetidine (Tagamet).
- ciprofloxacin and other quinolone antibiotics (see drug Classes).
- clarithromycin (Biaxin).
- clofibrate (Atromid-S).
- cotrimoxazole (Bactrim).
- dextrothyroxine.
- dirithromycin.
- disulfiram (Antabuse).
- disopyramide (Norpace).
- erythromycin (various).
- felbamate (Felbatol).
- fluconazole (Diflucan).
- fluvoxamine (Luvox).
- gemfibrozil (Lopid).
- glucagon.
- influenza vaccine (Various).
- isoniazid (INH).
- itraconazole (Sporonox).
- ketoconazole (Nizoral).
- metronidazole (Flagyl).
- mesna (Mesnex).
- miconazole (Monistat).
- nonsteroidal anti-inflammatory drugs (see Drug Classes).
- omeprazole (Prilosec).
- pravastatin (Pravachol).
- propranolol (Inderal).
- quinidine (Quinaglute).
- ranitidine (Zantac).
- salicylates (aspirin, etc.).
- sertraline (Zoloft).
- simvastatin (Zocor).
- streptokinase.
- sulfinpyrazone (Anturane).
- sulfonamides (see Drug Classes).
- tamoxifen (Nolvidex).
- tetracyclines (see Drug Classes).
- thyroid hormones (various).
- tricyclic antidepressants (see Drug Classes).
- vancomycin (Vancoled).
- vitamin E.

The following drugs may *decrease* the effects of warfarin
- azathioprine (Imuran).
- barbiturates (see Drug Classes).
- birth control pills (oral contraceptives).

- carbamazepine (Tegretol).
- cholestyramine (Questran).
- estrogens (unclear, but possible).
- ethchlorvynol (Placidyl).
- glutethimide (Doriden).
- griseofulvin (Grispeg).
- phytonadione (vitamin K).
- primidone (Mysoline).
- some penicillins (see Drug Classes).
- spironolactone.
- sucralfate (Carafate).
- rifampin (Rifadin).
- vitamin K.

▷ *Driving, Hazardous Activities:* No restrictions.

Aviation Note: The use of this drug *is a disqualification* for piloting. Consult a designated Aviation Medical Examiner.

Exposure to Sun: No restrictions.

Discontinuation: Do not stop this drug abruptly unless abnormal bleeding occurs. Ask your physician for guidance regarding gradual reduction in dosage over a period of 3 to 4 weeks.

ZALCITABINE (zal SIT a been)

Other Names: Dideoxycytidine, DDC

Introduced: 1987   **Prescription:** USA: Yes   **Available as Generic:** USA: No   **Class:** Antiviral, anti-AIDS drug   **Controlled Drug:** USA: No

Brand Name: HIVID

BENEFITS versus RISKS	
Possible Benefits	*Possible Risks*
DELAYED PROGRESSION OF DISEASE IN HIV-INFECTED PATIENTS WITH AIDS OR AIDS-RELATED COMPLEX	DRUG-INDUCED PERIPHERAL NEURITIS
	Rare drug-induced pancreatitis
	Rare drug-induced esophageal ulcers
	Rare drug-induced cardiomyopathy/congestive heart failure
	Drug-induced arthritis

▷ **Principal Uses**

As a Single Drug Product: Uses currently included in FDA approved labeling: (1) This drug is approved for advanced (CD4 cell count less than or equal to 300 cells per cubic millimeter) HIV infection in adults who do not tolerate zidovudine or have progression of their disease while taking zidovudine. The drug is NOT approved for use in patients with CD4 counts less than 150 cells per cubic millimeter. This drug is not a cure for AIDS, and it does not reduce the risk of transmission of HIV infection to others through sexual contact or contamination of blood.

Other (unlabeled) generally accepted uses: (1)Very recent data suggests that combination treatment with saquinavir (Invirase) decreases death from

AIDS by 70% versus single agent treatment with either medicine alone; (2) may have a role in pediatric AIDS.

How This Drug Works: By interfering with essential HIV enzyme systems, this drug is thought to prevent the growth and reproduction of HIV particles within infected cells, thus limiting the severity and extent of HIV infection.

Available Dosage Forms and Strengths

Zalcitabine (Hivid) tablets — 0.375 mg
— 0.75 mg

▷ **Recommended Dosage Ranges** (Actual dosage and administration schedule must be determined by the physician for each patient individually.)

Infants and Children: Under investigation.

12 to 60 Years of Age: The recommended combination regimen is: One 0.75 mg tablet orally to be taken with 200 mg of zidovudine every eight hours. The total daily dose for both drugs then becomes: 2.25 mg of zalcitabine and 600 mg of zidovudine. The initial dose does not need to be reduced unless the patient weighs less than 30 kg (66 pounds).

Conditions Requiring Dosing Adjustments

Liver function: Liver toxicity may be more likely in people with a prior history of alcohol abuse or liver damage. The patient should be monitored closely, and the dosage reduced or the medication interrupted if toxicity occurs. Patients with liver function enzymes which are more than five times the upper limit of normal should have the drug stopped.

Kidney function: Patients with moderate kidney failure can be given zalcitabine 0.75 mg every 12 hours. In severe kidney failure, the patient can be given 0.75 mg every 24 hours.

▷ **Dosing Instructions:** When combination therapy is being given, dose adjustments must be based on the toxicity profiles for each drug. For example: if the patient experiences peripheral neuropathy, or severe oral ulcers, the zalcitabine dose should be decreased or interrupted. Secondly: if the patient experiences anemia or granulocytopenia, the zidovudine dose should be decreased or interrupted. If the zalcitabine is interrupted or stopped, the zidovudine dose should be changed from 200 mg every 8 hours to 100 mg every 4 hours. Zalcitabine is **not** indicated for use as the only therapy. If zalcitabine is stopped, the physician **must** consider alternative antiretroviral therapy.

The largest peak concentration, the time that it takes for the peak to be achieved, and the amount absorbed are all changed if this drug is taken with food. It is better to take this medication on an empty stomach.

Usual Duration of Use: Use on a regular schedule for several months usually determines effectiveness in slowing the progression of AIDS. Long-term use (months to years) requires periodic physician evaluation of response and dosage adjustment.

Possible Advantages of This Drug

Does not cause serious depression of bone marrow function (production of blood cells).

▷ **This Drug Should Not Be Taken If**
- you have had an allergic reaction to it previously.
- you have had pancreatitis recently.

▷ **Inform Your Physician Before Taking This Drug If**
- you have had allergic reactions to any drugs in the past.
- you are taking any other drugs currently.
- you have a history of pancreatitis or peripheral neuritis.
- you have a history of severe myelosuppression (ask your doctor).
- you have a history of esophageal ulcers.
- you have congestive heart failure or cardiac muscle damage (cardiac myopathy).
- you have a history of alcoholism.
- you have impaired liver or kidney function.

Possible Side Effects (natural, expected, and unavoidable drug actions)
Mild and infrequent decreases in red blood cell, white blood cell, and platelet counts.

▷ **Possible Adverse Effects** (unusual, unexpected, and infrequent reactions)
If any of the following develop, consult your physician promptly for guidance.
Mild Adverse Effects
Allergic Reactions: Skin rash and itching.
Fever, joint pains.
Ringing in the ears.
Mouth sores, nausea, vomiting, diarrhea, stomach pain.
Serious Adverse Effects
Allergic Reactions: Anaphylaxis (rare).
Drug-induced peripheral neuritis (see Glossary), usually occurring after 7 to 18 weeks of treatment. This is more frequent and severe with high doses, and less frequent and mild with low doses.
Drug-induced cardiomyopathy/congestive heart failure (rare).
Drug-induced pancreatitis, usually within the first 6 months of treatment (rare).
Electrolyte changes (lowered phosphorous, sodium, magnesium, or calcium) (rare).
Ototoxicity and hearing loss (rare).
Worsening of preexisting liver disease or hepatotoxicity in patients with a history of alcohol abuse.

▷ **Possible Effects on Sexual Function:**   None reported.

▷ **Adverse Effects That May Mimic Natural Diseases or Disorders**
None reported to date.

Possible Effects on Laboratory Tests
Complete blood cell counts: decreased red cells, white cells and platelets (infrequent and mild).
Blood amylase level: increased (infrequent).
Blood glucose level: increased.
Liver function tests: increased (SGOT, SGPT AND LDH).

CAUTION
1. This drug does not cure HIV infection. Taking it does not reduce the risk of transmitting infection to others through sexual contact or contamination of blood.
2. Report promptly the development of stomach pain with nausea and vom-

iting; this could indicate the onset of pancreatitis. It may be necessary to discontinue this drug.

3. MOST clinicians are advocating combination therapy of this disease.
4. Report promptly the development of pain, numbness, tingling or burning in the hands or feet; this could indicate the onset of peripheral neuritis. It may be necessary to discontinue this drug.
5. It is advisable to avoid all other drugs that are known to cause pancreatitis or peripheral neuritis; ask your physician for guidance.

Precautions for Use

By Infants and Children: Safety and effectiveness for use by this age group have not been established. Children may also be at risk for developing drug-induced pancreatitis and peripheral neuritis; monitor closely for significant symptoms.

By Those over 60 Years of Age: Reduced kidney function may require dosage reduction.

▷ **Advisability of Use During Pregnancy**

Pregnancy Category: C. See Pregnancy Code at the back of this book.

Animal studies: This drug has been shown to be teratogenic in mice at doses of 1365 and 2730 times that achieved at the maximum recommended human dose (MRHD). Increased embryolethality was observed in mice with use of 2730 times the MRHD.

Human studies: Information from adequate studies of pregnant women is not available. The manufacturer recommends that fertile women should not receive zalcitabine unless they are using effective contraception during therapy.

Consult your physician for specific guidance.

Advisability of Use if Breast-Feeding

Presence of this drug in breast milk: Unknown.

Avoid drug or refrain from nursing.

Note: HIV has been found in human breast milk. Breast-feeding may result in transmission of HIV infection to the nursing infant.

Habit-Forming Potential: None.

Effects of Overdosage: Nausea, vomiting, stomach pain, diarrhea, pain in hands and feet.

Possible Effects of Long-Term Use: Peripheral neuritis (see Glossary).

Suggested Periodic Examinations While Taking This Drug (at physician's discretion)

Complete blood cell counts before starting treatment and weekly thereafter until tolerance is established.

Blood amylase levels, fractionated for salivary gland and pancreatic origin.

Triglyceride levels should be tested at baseline (before therapy is started) and periodically.

Assessment of CD4 counts.

Measurement of viral load can be the clearest indication of pending failure and reason to change to other agents.

▷ **While Taking This Drug, Observe the Following**

Foods: No restrictions.

Beverages: No restrictions.

▷ *Alcohol:* No interactions expected.
   Tobacco Smoking: No interactions expected.
▷ *Other Drugs*
   Zalcitabine may ***increase*** the effects of
   • zidovudine (Retrovir), and enhance its antiviral effect against HIV. Serious patient reactions to either of these medicines should be reported to the FDA.
   Zalcitabine ***taken concurrently*** with
   • cimetidine (Tagamet) may result in toxic zalcitabine levels.
   • didanosine (Videx) may result in additive neurotoxicity.
   • metoclopramide (Reglan) may result in lowered blood levels of zalcitabine and reduced therapeutic benefits.
   • other drugs which cause neurotoxicity or pancreatitis are best avoided.
   • probenecid (Benemid) may lead to zalcitabine toxicity.
▷ *Driving, Hazardous Activities:* This drug may cause pain and weakness in the extremities. Restrict activities as necessary.
   Aviation Note: The use of this drug ***is a disqualification*** for piloting. Consult a designated Aviation Medical Examiner.
   Exposure to Sun: No restrictions.
   Discontinuation: Do not stop this drug without your physician's knowledge and guidance.

ZIDOVUDINE (zi DOH vyoo deen)

Other Names: AZT, azidothymidine, Compound S, ZDV

Introduced: 1987   **Prescription:** USA: Yes; Canada: Yes   **Available as Generic:** USA: No; Canada: No   **Class:** Antiviral, anti-AIDS drugs   **Controlled Drug:** USA: No; Canada: No

Brand Name: Retrovir

BENEFITS versus RISKS	
Possible Benefits	*Possible Risks*
DELAYED PROGRESSION OF DISEASE IN HIV-INFECTED PATIENTS	SERIOUS BONE MARROW DEPRESSION
REDUCED INCIDENCE OF INFECTIONS IN TREATING ACTIVE AIDS AND AIDS-RELATED COMPLEX	Brain toxicity
	Lip, mouth, and tongue sores

▷ **Principal Uses**
   As a Single Drug Product: Uses currently included in FDA approved labeling: (1) Used to treat selected patients who have acquired immunodeficiency syndrome (AIDS) or acquired immunodeficiency syndrome-related complex (ARC) caused by human immunodeficiency virus (HIV). This drug is not a cure for AIDS, and it does not reduce the risk of transmission of AIDS infection to others through sexual contact or contamination of blood; (2) recently approved to help prevent transmission of HIV from mother to infant; (3) approved for combination therapy with other agents; (4) approved for

children 3 months or older who have laboratory values that indicate HIV infection or HIV immunosuppression; (5) approved for use in HIV positive patients who are as yet asymptomatic.

Other (unlabeled) generally accepted uses: (1) Used to treat Kaposi's sarcoma; (2) helps remove hairy leukoplakia in the mouth; (3) used to treat heart dysfunction in people with HIV; (4) may prevent HIV in health care workers exposed to the AIDS virus; (5) appears to increase AIDs-related low platelet counts; (6) may have a role in adult T-cell leukemia or lymphoma in combination with interferon alpha.

Author's note: While this drug has historically been used as a single drug to treat AIDS, a medical consensus has developed that limits the use of this drug to combination therapy.

How This Drug Works: By interfering with essential enzyme systems, this drug is thought to prevent the growth and reproduction of HIV particles within tissue cells, thus limiting the severity and extent of HIV infection.

Available Dosage Forms and Strengths

Capsules — 100 mg

Injection — 10 mg per ml

Syrup — 50 mg per 5-ml

▷ **Usual Adult Dosage Range:**   For asymptomatic (CD4 500 or less) HIV infection: 100 mg/4 hours while awake (500 mg/day).

For symptomatic HIV infection: Initially 100 mg every 4 hours, 5 times a day, or 200 mg every 8 hours. This regimen is used unless HIV encephalopathy is present. Some authors recommend a maximum daily dose of 400 to 600 mg.

For prevention of maternal fetal transmission in pregnancy: 100 mg by mouth five times per day until the start of labor. During labor, AZT is given intravenously (2 mg/kg of total body weight), followed by 1 mg/kg/hour (again based on total body weight). This dose is continued until the umbilical cord is clamped. The infant then receives 1.5 mg/kg every 6 hours.

Note: Actual dosage and administration schedule must be determined by the physician for each patient individually.

Author's note: There is controversy present as to the ideal time to start antiretroviral therapy. Some clinicians wait until the CD4 count has declined to 500 or 400 cells. Since it is now known that HIV does *not* have a dormant period, many clinicians are starting therapy once the infection is diagnosed.

Conditions Requiring Dosing Adjustments

Liver function: The dose should be decreased by 50% or the dosing interval should be doubled in patients with significant liver compromise. It can be a rare cause of liver damage, and patients should be followed closely.

Kidney function: Specific guidelines for dosage adjustments in patients with compromised kidneys are not available. It should be used with caution in renal compromise.

▷ **Dosing Instructions:**   Preferably taken on an empty stomach, but may be taken with or following food. Take exactly as prescribed. The capsule may be opened and the contents mixed with food just prior to administration. It is best to take the capsule with at least 120 ml of water.

Usual Duration of Use: Use on a regular schedule for 10 to 12 weeks usually determines effectiveness in improving the course of symptomatic AIDS infection. Long-term use requires periodic physician evaluation of response and dosage adjustment.

▷ **This Drug Should Not Be Taken If**
- you have had a serious allergic reaction to it previously.
- you have a serious degree of uncorrected bone marrow depression.

▷ **Inform Your Physician Before Taking This Drug If**
- you have a history of either folic acid or vitamin B-12 deficiency.
- you have impaired liver or kidney function.
- you take other drugs which can have a bad effect on the bone marrow (are myelosuppressive).

Possible Side Effects (natural, expected, and unavoidable drug actions)
None reported.

▷ **Possible Adverse Effects** (unusual, unexpected, and infrequent reactions)
If any of the following develop, consult your physician promptly for guidance.
Mild Adverse Effects
Allergic Reactions: Skin rash, hives, itching.
Headache, weakness, drowsiness, dizziness, nervousness, insomnia.
Nausea, stomach pain, diarrhea, loss of appetite and vomiting, altered taste, lip sores, swollen mouth or tongue.
Paresthesias.
Muscle aches, fever, sweating.
Serious Adverse Effects
Confusion, loss of speech, twitching, tremors, seizures (representing brain toxicity).
Eye problems (macular edema).
Muscle toxicity (myopathy).
Mania (rare).
Seizures (rare).
Muscle toxicity of the heart (cardiomyopathy).
Bone marrow depression (see Glossary): fatigue, weakness, fever, sore throat, abnormal bleeding or bruising. Anemia occurs most commonly after 4 to 6 weeks of treatment; abnormally low white blood cell counts occur after 6 to 8 weeks of treatment.
Esophageal ulcers (patients should take this medicine with at least 120 ml of water and not lie down for an hour).
Liver toxicity.

▷ **Possible Effects on Sexual Function**
None reported.

Possible Delayed Adverse Effects: Significant anemia and deficient white blood cell counts may develop after this drug has been discontinued. Myopathy.

▷ **Adverse Effects That May Mimic Natural Diseases or Disorders**
Seizures may suggest the possibility of epilepsy.

Possible Effects on Laboratory Tests
Complete blood cell counts: decreased red cells, hemoglobin, white cells and platelets.

CAUTION

1. This drug is not a cure for AIDS or AIDS-related complex. Nor does it protect completely against other infections or complications. Follow your physician's instructions and take all medications exactly as prescribed.
2. This drug does not reduce the risk of transmitting AIDS to others through sexual contact or contamination of the blood. The use of an effective condom is mandatory. Needles for drug administration should not be shared.

Precautions for Use

By Infants and Children: Zidovudine syrup is used in HIV-infected pediatric patients who are greater than 3 months old. The usual dose is 180 mg/square meter.

By Those over 60 Years of Age: Impaired kidney function will require dosage reduction.

▷ **Advisability of Use During Pregnancy**

Pregnancy Category: C. See Pregnancy Code at the back of this book.

Animal studies: Rat studies reveal no birth defects.

Human studies: Adequate studies of pregnant women are not available.

Consult your physician for specific guidance. This medicine has been shown to dramatically reduce the transference of HIV from mother to infant. If the decision is made to use this medicine in pregnancy, cases should be reported to 800–722-9292 ext. 8465.

Advisability of Use if Breast-Feeding

Presence of this drug in breast milk: Unknown.

Avoid drug or refrain from nursing.

Habit-Forming Potential: None.

Effects of Overdosage: Nausea, vomiting, diarrhea, bone marrow depression.

Possible Effects of Long-Term Use: Serious anemia and loss of white blood cells.

Muscle toxicity (myopathy).

Suggested Periodic Examinations While Taking This Drug (at physician's discretion)

Complete blood cell counts before starting treatment and weekly thereafter until tolerance is established. Continual monitoring for bone marrow depression is necessary during entire course of treatment.

Periodic CD4 counts or measurements of viral load are indicators that treatment is failing and demand change of antiretroviral therapy.

▷ **While Taking This Drug, Observe the Following**

Foods: No restrictions.

Beverages: No restrictions. May be taken with milk.

▷ *Alcohol:* No interactions expected.

Tobacco Smoking: No interactions expected.

▷ *Other Drugs*

The following drugs may *increase* the effects of zidovudine and enhance its toxicity

- acetaminophen.
- acyclovir (Zovirax).
- amphotericin B (Fungizone).

- aspirin.
- benzodiazepines (see Drug Class Section).
- cimetidine (Tagamet).
- fluconazole (Diflucan).
- ganciclovir (Cytovene).
- indomethacin.
- interferon beta.
- morphine (various).
- probenecid (Benemid).
- sulfonamides (see Drug Class Section).

Zidovudine *taken concurrently* with
- didanosine may result in increased risk of myelosuppression.
- filgrastim (Neupogen) may help maintain the white blood cell count.
- rifampin (Rifadin) can lead to decreased zidovudine blood levels.
- trimexate may cause additive hematological toxicity.

▷ *Driving, Hazardous Activities:* This drug may cause dizziness or fainting. Restrict activities as necessary.

Aviation Note: The use of this drug *is a disqualification* for piloting. Consult a designated Aviation Medical Examiner.

Exposure to Sun: No restrictions.

Discontinuation: Do not stop this drug without your physician's knowledge and guidance.

ZOLPIDEM (ZOL pi dem)

Introduced: 1993   **Prescription:** USA: Yes   **Available as Generic:**
USA: No   **Class:** Hypnotic, Imidazopyridine   **Controlled Drug:** USA:
C-IV*

Brand Names: Ambien

BENEFITS versus RISKS	
Possible Benefits	*Possible Risks*
GIVES SHORT-TERM RELIEF OF INSOMNIA WITH MINIMAL SLEEP DISRUPTION (REM)	Habit-forming potential with prolonged use Rebound insomnia upon withdrawal

▷ **Principal Uses**

As a Single Drug Product: Uses currently included in FDA approved labeling: (1) Short-term treatment of insomnia in adults.

Other (unlabeled) generally accepted uses: Long-term (more than one year) treatment of insomnia has been accomplished successfully in limited trials.

How This Drug Works: This drug attaches (binds) to a specific receptor (omega-1) and: reduces time it takes to fall asleep, increases total sleep time while producing a pattern and benefit of sleep that is similar to normal sleep patterns.

*See Schedules of Controlled Drugs at the back of this book.

Available Dosage Forms and Strengths
Tablets — 5 mg, 10 mg

▷ **Recommended Dosage Ranges (Actual dosage and administration schedule must be determined by the physician for each patient individually.)**
Infants and Children: Safety and efficacy for those under 18 years of age not established.
18 to 60 Years of Age: Ten mg is given immediately before bedtime. Patients should be reevaluated after taking this drug for ten days.
Over 60 Years of Age: Therapy should be started with 5 mg taken at bedtime. The dose may be cautiously increased to 10 mg at bedtime.

Conditions Requiring Dosing Adjustments
Liver function: The dose should be reduced by 50% in patients with liver compromise.
Kidney function: The half life is doubled in chronic kidney compromise, and the dose must be decreased.

▷ **Dosing Instructions:** The tablet may be crushed and is best taken on an empty stomach. Do **not** stop this drug abruptly if taken for more than 7 days.

Usual Duration of Use: Use on a regular schedule for two nights usually determines effectiveness in treating insomnia. Your physician should assess the benefit of this drug after 10 days.

Possible Advantages of This Drug
Low occurrence of adverse effects.
May produce less of an undesirable effect on normal sleep patterns.

Currently a "Drug of Choice"
for short-term management of insomnia in adults.

▷ **This Drug Should Not Be Taken If**
• you have had an allergic reaction to any dosage form of it previously.

▷ **Inform Your Physician Before Taking This Drug If**
• you have abnormal liver or kidney function.
• you are pregnant or planning pregnancy.
• you have a history of alcoholism or drug abuse.
• you have a serious lung problem (respiratory impairment).
• you have a history of serious depression or mental disorder.
• you are uncertain of how much zolpidem to take or how often to take it.

Possible Side Effects (natural, expected, and unavoidable drug actions)
Drowsiness and blurred vision, "hangover" effects following long-term use.

▷ **Possible Adverse Effects** (unusual, unexpected, and infrequent reactions)
If any of the following develop, consult your physician promptly for guidance.
Mild Adverse Effects
Allergic Reactions: Skin rash.
Drowsiness (rare) and dizziness (rare).
Nausea and diarrhea (rare).
Muscle tremors (infrequent).
Blurred vision (infrequent).
Serious Adverse Effects
Allergic Reactions: Not defined.

Abnormal thoughts or hallucinations (infrequent).

Rare elevation of liver function tests.

Paradoxical aggression, agitation, or suicidal thoughts (rare).

▷ **Possible Effects on Sexual Function:**   None reported.

Possible Effects on Laboratory Tests

Liver function tests: increased SGOT, SGPT and CPK.

CAUTION

1. This drug works quickly. It is best to take it just before bed time.
2. Do **not** drink alcohol while taking this drug.
3. Withdrawal (see Glossary) may occur even if this drug was only taken for a week or two. Ask your doctor for advice before stopping zolpidem.
4. You may experience trouble going to sleep for one or two nights after stopping this drug (rebound insomnia). This effect is usually short-term.
5. Sleep disturbances may be a symptom of underlying psychological problems. Inform your doctor if unusual behaviors or odd thoughts occur.
6. Drugs which depress the central nervous system may produce additive effects with this drug. Ask your doctor or pharmacist **before** combining other prescription or nonprescription drugs with zolpidem.

Precautions for Use

By Infants and Children: Safety and effectiveness for those under 18 years of age not established.

By Those over 60 Years of Age: The starting dose should be decreased to 5 mg. Since this drug works quickly, it is best taken immediately before going to bed. You may be at increased risk for falls if the drug remains in your system in the morning. Watch for lethargy, unsteadiness, nightmares and paradoxical agitation and anger.

▷ **Advisability of Use During Pregnancy**

Pregnancy Category: B. See Pregnancy Code at the back of this book.

Animal studies: In rats, abnormal skull bone formation was reported. In rabbits, abnormal bone formation was found.

Human studies: Adequate studies of pregnant women are not available.

Use during pregnancy **not** advisable. Ask your doctor for guidance.

Advisability of Use if Breast-Feeding

Presence of this drug in breast milk: Yes.

Avoid drug or refrain from nursing.

Habit-Forming Potential: This drug may cause dependence (see Glossary).

Effects of Overdosage: Marked change from lethargy to coma. Cardiovascular and respiratory compromise was also reported. The drug flumazenil may help reverse symptoms.

Possible Effects of Long-Term Use: Psychological and/or physical dependence.

Suggested Periodic Examinations While Taking This Drug   (at physician's discretion)

Liver function tests.

▷ **While Taking This Drug, Observe the Following**

Foods: This drug should **not** be taken with food.

Beverages: Avoid caffeine-containing beverages: coffee, tea, cola.

▷   *Alcohol:* This drug should **not** be combined with alcohol.

Tobacco Smoking: Nicotine is a stimulant and should be avoided.

Marijuana Smoking: May cause additive drowsiness.

▷   *Other Drugs*

Zolpidem may *increase* the effects of

- chlorpromazine (Thorazine).
- narcotics or other CNS depressant drugs (see Drug Classes for opioids, phenothiazines, antihistamines and benzodiazepines).

▷   *Driving, Hazardous Activities:* This drug may cause drowsiness and impair coordination. Restrict activities as necessary.

Aviation Note: The use of this drug *is a disqualification* for piloting. Consult a designated Aviation Medical Examiner.

Discontinuation: This drug should **not** be stopped abruptly even after a week of use. Ask your doctor for help regarding an appropriate withdrawal schedule.

THE LEADING EDGE

This section is designed to help the reader become more fully aware of medications which show promise in novel applications or are FDA approvable. "The Leading Edge" is also intended to bring information about new concepts in medication delivery which show great promise. Finally, a few interesting medications still in early clinical trials may be included as stars on the horizon.

It is impossible to predict which medicines or delivery systems will achieve final FDA approval or will be used in specific drugs, but many of those successful ones will be covered in subsequent editions. Finally, there will be many potential medicines or delivery systems which could be covered in a given year. The author will choose those which in his opinion offer the most potential to the readers of this book.

THALIDOMIDE (thall ID oh myde)

Novel Application

This medicine has a terrible past in that when it was marketed in Europe as a sedative and was given to pregnant women, terrible limb and other birth defects resulted. The interesting news for this drug (Synovir) is that while it MUST NEVER be given to pregnant women, some new uses appear to have great promise. It may have a role in treating canker sores in AIDS patients, systemic lupus erythematosus (SLE) rashes, refractory rheumatoid arthritis, and AIDS wasting syndrome, and halting progression of HIV and erythema nodosum. The mechanism of action is not presently known, but if ongoing studies yield results in concurrence with earlier trials, this medicine may help many diseases and inflammatory conditions. The fact that this medicine should NEVER be used in pregnancy places it in Pregnancy Risk Category X. There are many medicines in wide clinical use that have this designation.

CORTISOL (KOR ti zall)

New Roles Identified for a Biological Substance

Cortisol has long been known as a very strong hormone that is made by the adrenal gland. Blood levels of this hormone are known to be increased in cancer, depression, ulcers, arthritis, and AIDS. Research has begun into anti-cortisols as potential therapeutic agents in all of the aforementioned conditions, especially AIDS.

MIBEFRADIL (mi BEH frah dill)

Star on the Horizon

The documents needed to file for FDA approval will be sent to the FDA for mibefradil. This medicine belongs to the calcium-channel-blocker class but is the first vascular-selective agent. Currently available calcium channel blockers act on L channels, while mibefradil acts preferentially on T channels. What this means is that it appears capable of lowering the blood pressure *without* affecting heart function.

LIPOSOMES (LIP oh soams)

Medication Delivery

Once again liposomes, and the ability to place medications in them, appear to offer greatly improved results (outcomes) from medicines. Three examples include a product called TLC-99 (liposomal doxorubicin) and TLC C-53 (liposomal prostaglandin E1). TLC-99 shows fewer side effects while allowing higher doses to be used and thus a more aggressive attack on metastatic breast cancer. TLC C-53 is used in a life-threatening illness known as adult respiratory distress syndrome or ARDS. A small early clinical trial showed impressive results, and would represent a true advance if larger ongoing studies result in the same benefits. A "Stealth" liposome formulation of doxorubicin (Doxil) has been approved for treatment of Kaposi's sarcoma in AIDS patients.

INTEGRASE (IN ta grace)

Star on the Horizon

Integrase, and research into medicines that can interfere with it, may result in a new class of medicines in the war against AIDS. These drugs act at a different point in the life cycle of the virus than the four nucleoside analogs or the new protease inhibitors that are currently available. Some very early data shows that one flavone has some activity, but further research is needed. Still another point of attack may be found in preventing HIV's ability to enter and infect cells. A new drug known as ALX40–4C appears to block viral entry. A molecule called fusin appears to act as a needed factor (cofactor) for HIV to enter healthy cells. Both of these new approaches used alone or in combination with existing medicines may well turn AIDS into a more survivable, chronic disease.

LIDOCAINE TRANSORAL (LIE dough kane)

FDA Approved

Considering the prevalence of dental cavities (caries), and the reality that most patients receive an injection when a cavity is filled, DentiPatch, a new transoral mucosal delivery system for lidocaine, may help many people. This patch is applied to injection site and works to numb tissues for up to 45 minutes. This will prevent the pain of oral injections or soft tissue procedures.

AMLEXANOX (am LEX I nocks)

FDA Approvable

This will be the first product to be approved for treatment of canker sores. The present approvable status is for the treatment of signs and symptoms of apthous ulcers (canker sores).

MIDODRINE (ME dough drean)

FDA Approvable

Midodrine (ProAmatine) has been found to be FDA approvable to treat orthostatic hypotension (see Glossary). The drug will be the first cardiovascular agent to be approved under the accelerated approval process. This medicine may stop the light-headedness which many patients experience if they stand up suddenly. In some cases, this effect may be related to treatment of hypertension, and midodrine could make a variety of high blood pressure medicines much more tolerable.

CERVICAL CANCER AND LYME DISEASE VACCINE

Star on the Horizon

Research into a Lyme disease vaccine has been conducted using a specific protein called OSP-A. Recently a protein called decorin has been identified, and research is now underway toward development of a vaccine using this protein. Since a virus known as HPV is now known to cause cervical cancer, MedImmune is working to develop a vaccine to protect against HPV types 18 and 16. Once again, it is always better to prevent a disease or condition than to have to treat it.

OLANZAPINE (oh LANZ a peen)

Star on the Horizon

Medicines to help treat psychiatric problems have focused on dopamine receptors to address psychosis for many years. The newest approach looks at serotonin–dopamine antagonism. This profile of strong 5HT2A- and weak D2-blocking ability gives an improved side-effect profile and better patient results. Data on olanzapine (Zyprex), a chemical derivative of clozapine, has been submitted to the FDA for approval. If early data holds, this medicine may represent a major advance in treating mental illness.

AIDS VACCINE (AIDS)

Star on the Horizon
At the recent AIDS conference in Vancouver, information from the University of Nebraska and another center was presented about a P17 AIDS vaccine which shows promise.

ROTAVIRUS VACCINE (ROW ta)

Star on the Horizon
Rotavirus is a significant cause of mortality and morbidity in infants and young children because of dehydrating gastroenteritis. New research involving 1,278 healthy infants showed significant results. Future trials are needed to confirm safety and efficacy, but it appears a final vaccine formulation is not far away.

GENOMICS COLLABORATION (JEAN oh mix)

Star on the Horizon
Schering-Plough, SmithKline Beecham, and Human Genome Sciences have forged an agreement to discover and further develop new (novel) human medicines and therapeutic proteins from the human cDNA database which has been created by Human Genome Sciences. Although specific products have not been yet identified, I believe this collaboration and approach offers some potential fundamental advances in identifying novel ways to treat a variety of human diseases and conditions.

DRUG CLASSES

Throughout the Drug Profiles, reference is made to various drug classes. The reader may be advised to consult Section Four to become familiar with the drugs which belong to a particular class of drugs that share important characteristics in their chemical composition or in their actions within the body. Often it is important to know that *any* drug (or *all* drugs) within a given class can be expected to behave in a particular way. This may be useful in preventing interactions that could reduce the effectiveness of the drugs in use or result in unanticipated and sometimes hazardous adverse effects.

The presentation of each Drug Class consists of the drug class designation followed by an alphabetic listing of the generic names of the drugs that constitute the class. Following each generic name (and enclosed in parentheses) is the widely recognized brand name(s) of that particular drug. In some instances the number of brand names in use is so large that a complete listing is not possible. In such cases, to be certain that you are consulting the correct drug class, call your pharmacist or physician to determine the generic name of the drug that concerns you and consult the master list to see if it is included there. The generic name listings are sufficiently complete to serve the scope of this book.

ACE (Angiotensin-Converting Enzyme) Inhibitors

benazepril (Lotensin)
captopril (Capoten)
enalapril (Vasotec)
fosinopril (Monopril)
lisinopril (Prinivil, Zestril)

moexipril (Univasc)
quinapril (Accupril)
ramipril (Altace)
spirapril (Renormax)

Adrenocortical Steroids (Cortisonelike Drugs)

amcinonide (Cyclocort)
beclomethasone (Beclovent, Vanceril)
betamethasone (Celestone)
budesonide (Rhinocort)
cortisone (Cortone)

dexamethasone (Decadron)
fludrocortisone (Florinef)
flunisolide (AeroBid, Nasarel)
fluorometholone (FML)
fluticasone (Flonase)

halcinonide (Halog)
halobetasol (Ultravate)
hydrocortisone (Cortef)
medrysone (HMS Ophthalmic Suspension)
methylpredisolone (Medrol)
mometasone (Elocon)

paramethasone (Haldrone)
prednisolone (Delta-Cortef)
prednisone (Deltasone)
rimexalone (Vexol)
triamcinolone (Aristocort, Azmacort)

Alpha-Glucosidase Inhibitors

acarbose (Precose)

Amebicides (Anti-Infectives)

chloroquine (Aralen)
emetine
iodoquinol (Yodoxin)

metronidazole (Flagyl)
paromomycin (Humatin)

Aminoglycosides (Anti-Infectives)

kanamycin (Kantrex)
neomycin (Mycifradin, Neobiotic)

paromomycin (Humatin)

Amphetaminelike Drugs

amphetamine
benzphetamine (Didrex)
dextroamphetamine (Dexedrine)
diethylpropion (Tenuate, Tepanil)
methamphetamine (Desoxyn)

methylphenidate (Ritalin)
phendimetrazine (Anorex, Plegine)
phenmetrazine (Preludin)
phentermine (Fastin, Ionamin)
phenylpropanolamine (Dexatrim)

Analgesics, Mild

acetaminophen (Datril, Tylenol)
aspirin
lidocaine/prilocaine cream (Emla)

See also Nonsteroidal Anti-Inflammatory
   Drugs (NSAIDs)

Analgesics, Strong

See Opioid Drugs

Androgens (Male Sex Hormones)

fluoxymesterone (Halotestin)
methyltestosterone (Android, Metandren,

Oreton)
testosterone (Androderm, Depotest, Testone)

Angiotensin Two-Receptor Antagonists

losartan (Cozaar)

Anorexiants (Appetite Suppressants)

dexfenfluramine (Redux)
fenfluramine (Pondimin)

mazindol (Mazanor, Sanorex)
See also Amphetaminelike Drugs

Anti-Acne Drugs

benzoyl peroxide (Epi-Clear, others)
erythromycin (Eryderm)
isotretinoin (Accutane)

tetracycline (Achromycin V)
tretinoin (Retin-A)

Anti-AIDS Drugs (Anti-Retrovirals)

didanosine (DDI, Videx)
indinavir (Crixivan)
lamivudine (3TC, Epivir)
nevirapine (Viramune)
saquinavir (Invirase)

ritonavir (Norvir)
stavudine (Zerit)
zalcitabine (dideoxycytidine, DDC, Hivid)
zidovudine (AZT, Retrovir)

Antialcoholism Drugs

disulfiram (Antabuse)

naltrexone (Trexan, ReVia)

Anti-Alzheimer's Drugs

tacrine (Cognex)

Antianginal Drugs

bepridil (Vascor)
diltiazem (Cardizem)
nicardipine (Cardene)
nifedipine (Adalat, Procardia)

nitrates (see class below)
verapamil (Calan, Isoptin)
See also Beta-Blockers

Antianxiety Drugs (Mild Tranquilizers)

buspirone (Buspar)
chlormezanone (Trancopal)
hydroxyzine (Atarax, Vistaril)

lorazepam (Ativan)
meprobamate (Equanil, Miltown)
See also Benzodiazepines

Antiarrhythmic Drugs (Heart Rhythm Regulators)

acebutolol (Sectral)
amiodarone (Codarone)
digitoxin (Crystodigin)
digoxin (Lanoxin)
disopyramide (Norpace)
flecainide (Tambocor)
mexiletine (Mexitil)

procainamide (Procan SR, Pronestyl)
propafenone (Rythmol)
propranolol (Inderal)
quinidine (Quinaglute, Quinidex, Quinora)
tocainide (Tonocard)
verapamil (Calan, Isoptin)

Antiarthritics

aspirin
azathioprin (Imuran) (rheumatoid only)
chloroquine (Aralen) (rheumatoid only)

penicillamine (Cuprimine)
See also Nonsteroidal Anti-Inflammatory
   Drugs (NSAIDs)

Antiasthmatic Drugs

Bronchodilators

albuterol (Proventil, Ventolin)
aminophylline (Phyllocontin)
bitolterol (Tornalate)
dyphylline (Lufyllin)
ephedrine (Efed II)

epinephrine (Adrenalin, Bronkaid Mist,
   Primatene Mist)
ipratropium
isoetharine (Bronkosol, Dey-Lute)
isoproterenol (Isuprel)

metaproterenol (Alupent, Metaprel)
oxtriphylline (Choledyl)
pirbuterol (Maxair)
salmeterol (Serevent)

terbutaline (Brethaire, Brethine, Bricanyl)
theophylline (Bronkodyl, Elixophyllin,
   Slo-Phyllin, others)

Mast Cell Stabilizing Agents

cromolyn sodium (Gastlrocom, Intal)

nedocromil (Tilade)

Anti-Inflammatory Agents

corticosteroids

Preventive Agents

chromolyn (Intal)

nedocromil (Tilade)

Anti-Attention Deficit Hyperactivity Disorder (ADHD) Drugs

clonidene   methylphenidate (Ritalin)   pemoline

Antibiotics

See specific antibiotic class (Cephalosporins, Penicillins, Tetracyclines, etc.)

Topical, Anti-Infectives

mupirocin (Bactroban)

Anticancer Drugs (Antineoplastics or Chemotherapy)

chlorambucil (Leukeran)
cyclophosphamide (Cytoxan)
flutamide (Eulexin)
hydroxyurea (Hydrea)

mercaptopurine (Purinethol)
methotrexate (Rheumatrex)
tamoxifen (Nolvadex)

Anticholesterol Drugs

See Cholesterol-Reducing Drugs

Anticholinergic Drugs (Atropinelike Drugs)

atropine
belladonna
hyoscyamine
scopolamine
antidepressants, tricyclic (see class below)
antihistamines, some (see class below)

antiparkinsonism drugs, some (see class
   below)
antispasmodics, synthetic, some (see class
   below)
muscle relaxants, some (see class below)

Anticoagulant Drugs

anisindione (Miradon)
dicumarol

warfarin (Coumadin)

Anticonvulsant Drugs (Antiepileptic Drugs)

acetazolamide (Diamox)
carbamazepine (Tegretol)
clonazepam (Klonopin)
clorazepate (Tranxene)

diazepam (Valium)
ethosuximide (Zarontin)
ethotoin (Peganone)
felbamate (Felbatol)

gabapentin (Neurontin)
lamotrigine (Lamictal)
mephenytoin (Mesantoin)
methsuximide (Celontin)
paramethadione (Paradione)
phenacemide (Phenurone)

phenobarbital (Luminal)
phensuximide (Milontin)
phenytoin (Dilantin)
primidone (Mysoline)
trimethadione (Tridione)
valproic acid (Depakene)

Anti-Cystic Fibrosis Agents (Recombinant DNase)

dornase alfa (Pulmozyme)

Antidepressant Drugs

Bicyclic Antidepressants

fluoxetine (Prozac)

venlafaxine (Effexor)

Tricyclic Antidepressants

amitriptyline (Elavil, Endep)
amoxapine (Asendin)
clomipramine (Anafranil)
desipramine (Norpramin, Pertofrane)
doxepin (Adapin, Sinequan)

imipramine (Janimine, Tofranil)
nortriptyline (Aventyl, Pamelor)
protriptyline (Vivactil)
trimipramine (Surmontil)

Tetracyclic Antidepressants

maprotiline (Ludiomil)

Other Antidepressants

bupropion (Wellbutrin)
fluvoxamine (Luvox)
nefazodone (Serzone)
paroxetine (Paxil)

sertraline (Zoloft)
trazodone (Desyrel)
See also Monoamine Oxidase (MAO)
    Inhibitors

Antidiabetic Drugs

Oral

See Alpha-Glucosidase Inhibitors, Biguanides, and Sulfonylureas

Injectable

insulin

Antidiarrheal Drugs

loperamide

Antiemetic Drugs (Anti-Motion Sickness, Antinausea Drugs)

chlorpromazine (Thorazine)
cyclizine (Marezine)
dimenhydrinate (Dramamine)
diphenhydramine (Benadryl)
granisetron (Kytril)
hydroxyzine (Atarax, Vistaril)

meclizine (Antivert, Bonine)
ondansetron (Zofran)
prochlorperazine (Compazine)
promethazine (Phenergan)
scopolamine (Transderm Scop)
trimethobenzamide (Tigan)

Antiepileptic Drugs

See Anticonvulsant Drugs

Antifungal Drugs (Anti-Infectives)

amphotericin B (Fungizone)
fluconazole (Diflucan)
flucytosine (Ancobon)
griseofulvin (Fulvicin, Grifulvin, Grisactin)
itraconazole (Sporanox)

ketoconazole (Nizoral)
lipid-associated amphotericin B (Abelcet)
miconazole (Monistat)
nystatin (Mycostatin)

Anti-Glaucoma Drugs

acetazolamide (Diamox)
betaxolol (Betoptic)
epinephrine (Glaucon)

pilocarpine (Isopto-carpine)
timolol (Timoptic, Betimol)

Anti-Gout Drugs

allopurinol (Zyloprim)
colchicine
diclofenac (Cataflam, Voltaren)
fenoprofen (Nalfon)
ibuprofen (Advil, Motrin, Nuprin, Rufin)
indomethacin (Indocin)
ketoprofen (Orudis)

mefenamic acid (Ponstel)
naproxen (Anaprox, Naprosyn)
oxaprozin (Daypro)
piroxicam (Feldene)
probenecid (Benemid)
sulfinpyrazone (Anturane)
sulindac (Clinoril)

Antihistamines

astemizole (Hismanal)
azatadine (Optimine)
brompheniramine (Dimetane, others)
carbinoxamine (Clistin, Rondec)
cetirizine (Zyrtec)
chlorpheniramine (Chlor-Trimeton, Teldrin)
clemastine (Tavist)
cyclizine (Marezine)
cyproheptadine (Periactin)
dimenhydrinate (Dramamine)
diphenhydramine (Benadryl)

doxylamine (Unisom)
loratadine (Claritin, Claritin Extra)
meclizine (Antivert, Bonine)
orphenadrine (Norflex)
pheniramine (component of Triaminic)
promethazine (Phenergan, others)
pyrilamine (component of Triaminic)
terfenadine (Seldane)
tripelennamine (Pyribenzamine, PBZ)
triprolidine (component of Actifed and
    Sudahist)

Non-Sedating or Minimally Sedating

astemizole (Hismanal)
fexofenadine (Allegra)

loratadine (Claritin)
terfenadine (Seldane)

Antihypertensive Drugs

amlodipine/benazepril (Lotrel)
clonidine (Catapres)
doxazosin (Cardura)
guanabenz (Wytensin)
guanadrel (Hylorel)
guanethidine (Ismelin)
guanfacine (Tenex)

hydralazine (Apresoline)
methyldopa (Aldomet)
minoxidil (Loniten)
prazosin (Minipres)
reserpine (Serpasil)
terazosin (Hytrin)
bisprolol/hydrochlorothiazide (Ziac)

See also ACE Inhibitors, Angiotensin Two-Receptor Antagonists, Beta-Blockers, Calcium Blockers, and Diuretics

Anti-Infective Drugs

See the specific anti-infective drug class:

Amebicides
Aminoglycosides
Antifungal Drugs
Antileprosy Drugs
Antimalarial Drugs
Antituberculosis Drugs
Antiviral Drugs

Cephalosporins
Fluoroquinolones
Macrolide Antibiotics
Penicillins
Sulfonamides
Tetracyclines

Miscellaneous Anti-Infective Drugs

atovaquone (Mepron)
chloramphenicol (Chloromycetin)
clindamycin (Cleocin)
colistin (Coly-Mycin S)
furazolidone (Furoxone)
lincomycin (Lincocin)

nalidixic acid (NegGram)
nitrofurantoin (Furadantin, Macrodantin)
novobiocin (Albamycin)
pentamidine (Pentam-300)
trimethoprim (Proloprim, Trimpex)
vancomycin (Vancocin)

Antileprosy Drugs (Anti-Infectives)

clofazimine (Lamprene)

dapsone

Antimalarial Drugs (Anti-Infectives)

chloroquine (Aralen)
doxycycline (Vibramycin)
hydroxychloraquine (Plaquenil)
mefloquine (Lariam)
primaquine

pyrimethamine (Daraprim)
quinacrine (Atabrine)
quinine
sulfadoxine/pyrimethamine (Fansidar)

Anti-Migraine Drugs

atenolol (Tenormin)
ergotamine (Ergostat)
methysergide (Sansert)
metoprolol (Lopressor)
nadolol (Corgard)

nifedipine (Procardia)
propranolol (Inderal)
sumatriptan (Imitrex)
timolol (Blocadren)
verapamil (Calan, Isoptin)

Anti-Motion Sickness/Antinausea Drugs

See Antiemetic Drugs

Anti-Myasthenics

neostigmine

Anti-Mycobacterial Agents

rifabutin

Anti-Osteoporotics

alendronate
calcitonin

etidronate
miacalcin

Antiparkinsonism Drugs

amantadine (Symmetrel)
benztropine (Cogentin)

bromocriptine (Parlodel)
diphenhydramine (Benadryl)

levodopa (Dopar, Larodopa)
levodopa/bensarazide (Prolopa)
levodopa/carbidopa (Sinemet, Sinemet CR)

pergolide (Permax)
selegiline (Eldepryl)
trihexyphenidyl (Artane)

Antiplatelet Drugs (Platelet Aggregation Inhibitors)

aspirin
dipyridamole (Persantine)

sulfinpyrazone (Anturane)
ticlopidine (Ticlid)

Antipsoriatic Drugs

etretinate

methotrexate

Antipsychotic Drugs (Neuroleptics, Major Tranquilizers)

chlorprothixene (Taractan)
clozapine (Clozaril)
haloperidol (Haldol)
loxapine (Loxitane)
molindone (Moban)

olanzapine (Zyprex)
pimozide (Orap)
risperidone (Risperdal)
thiothixene (Navane)
See also Phenothiazines

Antipyretic Drugs (Fever-Reducing Drugs)

acetaminophen
aspirin

See also Nonsteroidal Anti-Inflammatory
   Drugs (NSAIDs)

Anti-Sickle Cell Anemia Drugs

hydroxyurea (Hydrea)

Antispasmodics, Synthetic

anisotropine (Valpin)
clidinium (Quarzan)
glycopyrrolate (Robinul)
hexocyclium (Tral)
isopropamide (Darbid)

mepenzolate (Cantil)
methantheline (Banthine)
methscopamine (Pamine)
propantheline (Pro-Banthine)
tridihexethyl (Pathilon)

Antituberculosis Drugs

aminosalicylate sodium (Sodium P.A.S.)
capreomycin (Capastat)
cycloserine (Seromycin)
ethambutol (Myambutol)
ethionamide (Trecator-SC)

isoniazid (Laniazid, Nidrazid)
pyrazinamide
rifampin (Rifadin, Rimactane)
rifabutin (Mycobutin)
streptomycin

Antitussive Drugs (Cough Suppressants)

benzonatate (Tessalon)
codeine
dextromethorphan (Hold DM, Suppress)
diphenhydramine (Benylin)

hydrocodone (Hycodan)
hydromorphone (Dilaudid)
promethazine (Phenergan)

Antiviral Drugs (Anti-Infectives)

acyclovir (Zovirax)
amantadine (Symmetrel)

didanosine (Videx)
famciclovir (Famvir)

foscarnet (Foscavir)
ganciclovir (Cytovene)
indinvair (Crixivan)
lamivudine (Epivir)
nevirapine (Viramune)
ribavirin (Virazole)
rimantadine

saquinavir (Invirase)
stavudine (Zerit)
valacyclovir (Valtrex)
vidarabine (Vira A)
zalcitabine (Hivid)
zidovudine (Retrovir)

Appetite Suppressants

See Anorexiants

Atropinelike Drugs

See Anticholinergic Drugs

Barbiturates

amobarbital (Amytal)
aprobarbital (Alurate)
butabarbital (Butisol)
mephobarbital (Mebaral)
metharbital (Gemonil)

pentobarbital (Nembutal)
phenobarbital (Luminal, Solfoton)
secobarbital (Seconal)
talbutal (Lotusate)

Benzodiazepines

alprazolam (Xanax)
bromazepam (Lectopam)
chlordiazepoxide (Libritabs, Librium)
clonazepam (Klonopin)
clorazepate (Tranxene)
diazepam (Valium, Vazepam)
flurazepam (Dalmane)
halazepam (Paxipam)
ketazolam (Loftran)

lorazepam (Ativan)
midazolam (Versed)
nitrazepam (Mogadon)
oxazepam (Serax)
prazepam (Centrax)
quazepam (Doral)
temazepam (Restoril)
triazolam (Halcion)

Beta-Blockers (Beta-Adrenergic-Blocking Drugs)

acebutolol (Sectral)
atenolol (Tenormin)
betaxolol (Kerlone)
bisoprolol (Zebta)
bisoprolol/hydrochlorothiazide (Ziac)
carteolol (Cartrol)
labetalol (Normodyne, Trandate)

metoprolol (Lopressor)
nadolol (Corgard)
penbutolol (Levatol)
pindolol (Visken)
propranolol (Inderal)
timolol (Blocadren)

Biguanides (Oral Antidiabetic Drugs)

metformin (Glucophage)

Blood Flow Agents

pentoxifylline (Trental)

Bowel Anti-Inflammatory Drugs (Inflammatory Bowel Disease Suppressants)

azathioprine (Imuran)
mesalamine (Rowasa, Asacol)
metronidazole (Flagyl)

olsalazine (Dipentum)
sulfasalazine (Azulfidine)

Bronchodilators

See Antiasthmatic Drugs

Calcium Blockers (Calcium-Channel-Blocking Drugs)

amlodipine (Norvasc)
bepridil (Vascor)
nisoldipine (Sular)
diltiazem (Cardizem)
felodipine (Plendil)

isradipine (DynaCirc)
nicardipine (Cardene)
nifedipine (Adalat, Procardia)
nimodipine (Nimotop)
verapamil (Calan, Isoptin)

Cephalosporins (Anti-Infectives)

cefaclor (Ceclor)
cefadroxil (Duricef, Ultracef)
cefamandole (Mandol)
cefazolin (Ancef, Kefzol, Zolicef)
cefixime (Suprax)
cefmetazole (Zefazone)
cefonicid (Monocid)
cefoperazone (Cefobid)
ceforanide (Precef)
cefotaxime (Claforan)
cefotetan (Cefotan)

cefoxitin (Mefoxin)
cefprozil (Cefzil)
ceftazidime (Fortaz, Tazidime, Tazicef)
ceftizoxime (Cefizox)
ceftriaxone (Rocephin)
cefuroxime (Ceftin, Kefurox, Zinacef)
cephalexin (Keflex, Keftab)
cephalothin (Keflin)
cephapirin (Cefadyl)
cephradine (Anspor, Velosef)
moxalactam (Moxam)

Cholesterol-Reducing Drugs

cholestyramine (Cholybar, Questran)
clofibrate (Atromid-S)
colestipol (Colestid)
dextrothyroxine (Choloxin)
fenofibrate (Lipidil)
fluvastatin (Lescol)

gemfibrozil (Lopid)
lovastatin (Mevacor)
niacin (Nicobid, Slo-Niacin, others)
pravastatin (Pravachol)
probucol (Lorelco)
simvastatin (Zocor)

Cortisonelike Drugs

See Adrenocortical Steroids

Cough Suppressants

See Antitussive Drugs

Decongestants

ephedrine (Efedron, Ephedsol)
naphazoline (Naphcon, Vasocon)
oxymetazoline (Afrin, Duration, others)
phenylephrine (Neo-Synephrine, others)
phenylpropanolamine (Propadrine,

Propagest,
  others)
pseudoephedrine (Afrinol, Sudafed, others)
tetrahydrozoline (Tyzine, Visine, others)
xylometazoline (Otrivin)

Digitalis Preparations

deslanoside (Cedilanid-D)
digitoxin (Crystodigin)

digoxin (Lanoxicaps, Lanoxin)

Diuretics

acetazolamide (Diamox)
amiloride (Midamor)
bumetanide (Bumex)
chlorthalidone (Hygroton)
ethacrynic acid (Edecrin)
furosemide (Lasix)

indapamide (Lozol)
metolazone (Diulo, Zaroxolyn)
spironolactone (Aldactone)
triamterene (Dyrenium)
See also Thiazide Diuretics

Ergot Derivatives

bromocriptine (Parlodel)
ergotamine (Bellergal)

methysergide (Sansert)
pergolide (Permax)

Estrogens (Female Sex Hormones)

chlorotrianisene (Tace)
diethylstilbestrol (DES, Stilphostrol)
estradiol (Estrace, Estraderm, others)
estrogens, conjugated (Premarin)
estrogens, esterified (Estratab, Menest)

estrone (Theelin, others)
estropipate (Ogen)
ethinyl estradiol (Estinyl)
quinestrol (Estrovis)

Female Sex Hormones

See Estrogens and Progestins

Fever-Reducing Drugs

See Antipyretic Drugs

Five-Alpha-Reductase Inhibitors

finasteride (Proscar)

Fluoroquinolones (Anti-Infectives)

ciprofloxacin (Cipro)
lomefloxacin (Maxaquin)

norfloxacin (Noroxin)
ofloxacin (Floxin)

Gastrointestinal Drugs

Miscellaneous

metoclopramide (Reglan)

cisapride (Propulsid)

Ulcer Preventatives

misoprostol (Cytotec)

Hair Growth Stimulants

minoxidil (Rogaine)

finasteride (Proscar)

Heart Rhythm Regulators

See Antiarrhythmic Drugs

Hematopoietic Agents

filgrastim (Neupogen)

H-2 Blockers (Histamine [H-2]-Blocking Drugs)

cimetidine (Tagamet)
famotidine (Pepcid)

nizatidine (Axid)
ranitidine (Zantac)

Hormones

Miscellaneous

nafarelin (Synarel)

See also Androgens for male sex hormones; Estrogens and Progestins for female sex hormones

Hypnotic Drugs (Sedatives/Sleep Inducers)

acetylcarbromal (Paxarel)
chloral hydrate (Aquachloral, Noctec)
estazolam (ProSom)
ethchlorvynol (Placidyl)
ethinamate (Valmid)
flurazepam (Dalmane)
glutethimide (Doriden)
methyprylon (Noludar)

paraldehyde (Paral)
propiomazine (Largon)
quazepam (Doral)
temazepam (Restoril)
triazolam (Halcion)
zolpidem (Ambien)
See also Barbiturates

Immunosuppressants

azathioprine (Imuran)
chlorambucil (Leukeran)
cyclophosphamide (Cytoxan)

cyclosporine (Sandimmune)
hydroxychloroquine (Plaquenil)

Macrolide Antibiotics (Anti-Infectives)

azithromycin (Zithromax)
clarithromycin (Biaxin)
dirithromycin (Dynabac)

erythromycin (E-Mycin, Ilosone, Erythrocin,
  E.E.S.)
troleandomycin (Tao)

Male Sex Hormones

See Androgens

Mast Cell Stabilizing Agents

See Antiasthmatic Drugs

Monoamine Oxidase (MAO) Inhibitor Drugs (Type A: Antidepressants)

isocarboxazid (Marplan)
phenelzine (Nardil)

tranylcypromine (Parnate)

Muscle Relaxants (Skeletal Muscle Relaxants)

baclofen (Lioresal)
carisoprodol (Rela, Soma, others)
chlorphenesin carbamate (Maolate)
chlorzoxazone (Paraflex, Parafon Forte)
cyclobenzaprine (Flexeril)
dantrolene (Dantrium)

diazepam (Valium)
meprobamate (Equanil, Miltown, others)
metaxalone (Skelaxin)
methocarbamol (Robaxin, others)
orphenadrine (Norflex, others)

Nitrates

amyl nitrate (Amyl Nitrate Vaporole, others)
erythrityl tetranitrate (Cardilate)
isosorbide dinitrate (Isordil, Sorbitrate, others)
isosorbide mononitrate (Ismo, Imdur)

nitroglycerin (Nitrostat, Nitrolingual, Nitrogard, Nitrong, others)
pentaerythritol tetranitrate (Duotrate, Peritrate)

Nonnucleoside reverse transcriptase inhibitors

nevirapine (Viramune)

Nonsteroidal Anti-Inflammatory Drugs (NSAIDs) (Aspirin Substitutes)

Acetic Acids

diclofenac Potassium (Cataflam)
diclofenac Sodium (Voltaren)
etodolac (Lodine)
indomethacin (Indochron E-R, Indocin, Indocin SR)

ketorolac (Toradol)
nabumetone (Relafen)
sulindac (Clinoril)
tolmetin (Tolectin, Tolectin DS)

Fenamates

meclofenamate (Meclomen)

mefenamic acid (Ponstel)

Oxicams

piroxicam (Feldene)

Propionic Acids

diflunisal (Dolobid)
fenoprofen (Nalfon)
flurbiprofen (Ansaid)
ibuprofen
ketoprofen (Orudis, Orvail)
naproxen (Naprosyn)

naproxen sodium (Aleve, Anaprox, Anaprox DS)
oxaprozin (Daypro)
oxyphenbutazone (Oxalid)
suprofen (Profenal)

Opioid Drugs (Narcotics)

alfentanil (Alfenta)
codeine
fentanyl (Sublimaze, Duragesic)
hydrocodone (Hycodan)
hydromorphone (Dilaudid)
levorphanol (Levo-Dromoran)
meperidine (Demerol)

methadone (Dolophine)
morphine (Astramorph, Duramorph, MS Contin, Roxanol)
oxycodone (Roxicodone)
oxymorphone (Numorphan)
propoxyphene (Darvon)
sufentanil (Sufenta)

Opioid Antagonists

naltrexone (ReVia)

Pain Syndrome Modifiers (also adjuvants)

carbamazepine (Tegretol)
phenytoin (Dilantin)

strontium-89 (Metastron)

Penicillins (Anti-Infectives)

amoxicillin (Amoxil, Larotid, Polymox,
  Trimox, others)
amoxicillin/clavulanate (Augmentin)
ampicillin (Omnipen, Polycillin, Principen,
  Totacillin)
ampicillin/sulbactam (Unasyn)
bacampicillin (Spectrobid)
carbenicillin (Geocillin, Geopen, Pyopen)
cloxacillin (Cloxapen, Tegopen)
dicloxacillin (Dynapen, Pathocil, Veracillin)

methicillin (Staphcillin)
mezlocillin (Mezlin)
nafcillin (Nafcil, Unipen)
oxacillin (Prostaphlin)
penicillin G (Pentids, others)
penicillin V (Pen Vee K, V-Cillin K, Veetids,
  others)
piperacillin (Pipracil)
ticarcillin (Ticar)
ticarcillin/clavulanate (Timentin)

Phenothiazines (Antipsychotic Drugs)

acetophenazine (Tindal)
chlorpromazine (Thorazine)
fluphenazine (Permitil, Prolixin)
mesoridazine (Serentil)
perphenazine (Trilafon)

prochlorperazine (Compazine)
promazine (Sparine)
thioridazine (Mellaril)
trifluoperazine (Stelazine)
triflupromazine (Vesprin)

Progestins (Female Sex Hormones)

ethynodiol
hydroxyprogesterone (Duralutin, Gesterol
  L.A., others)
medroxyprogesterone (Amen, Curretab,
  Prempro, Premphase, Provera)

megestrol (Megace)
norethindrone (Micronor, Norlutate,
  Norlutin)
norgestrel (Ovrette)
progesterone (Gesterol 50, Progestaject)

Proton Pump Inhibitors (H/K ATPase Inhibitors)

lansoprazole (Prevacid)

omeprazole (Prilosec)

Radiopharmaceuticals

strontium-89 (Metastron)

Salicylates

aspirin
choline salicylate (Arthropan)
magnesium salicylate (Doan's, Magan,
  Mobidin)

salsalate (Amigesic, Disalcid, Salsitab)
sodium salicylate
sodium thiosalicylate (Rexolate, Tusal)

Sedatives/Sleep Inducers

See Hypnotic Drugs

Smoking Cessation Adjuncts

nicotine

Sulfonamides (Anti-Infectives)

multiple sulfonamides (Triple Sulfa No. 2)
sulfacytine (Renoquid)
sulfadiazine
sulfamethizole (Thiosulfil)

sulfamethoxazole (Gantanol)
sulfasalazine (Azulfidine)
sulfisoxazole (Gantrisin)

Sulfonylureas (Oral Antidiabetic Drugs)

acetohexamide (Dymelor)
chlorpropamide (Diabinese)
glimepiride (Amaryl)
glipizide (Glucotrol)

glyburide (DiaBeta, Micronase)
tolazamide (Ronase, Tolamide, Tolinase)
tolbutamide (Orinase)

Tetracyclines (Anti-Infectives)

demeclocycline (Declomycin)
doxycycline (Doryx, Doxychel, Vibramycin)
methacycline (Rondomycin)
minocycline (Minocin)

oxytetracycline (Terramycin)
tetracycline (Achromycin V, Panmycin,
   Sumycin)

Thiazide Diuretics

bendroflumethiazide (Naturetin)
benzthiazide (Aquatag, Exna, Marazide)
chlorothiazide (Diuril)
cyclothiazide (Anhydron)
hydrochlorothiazide (Esidrix, Hydrodiuril,

Oretic)
hydroflumethiazide (Diucardin, Saluron)
methyclothiazide (Enduron, Aquatensen)
polythiazide (Renese)
trichlormethiazide (Metahydrin, Naqua)

Thyroid Hormones

levothyroxine (Synthroid)

liothyronine (Cytomel)

Tranquilizers, Major

See Antipsychotic Drugs

Tranquilizers, Minor

See Antianxiety Drugs

Vaccines (Immune Modulators)

influenza vaccine (Fluogen, Flu-Shield,
   Fluzone)

varicella virus vaccine (Varivax)

Vasodilators (Peripheral Vasodilators)

cyclandelate (Cyclospasmol)
ethaverine (Ethaquin, Isovex)
isoxsuprine (Vasodilan)

nylidrin (Arlidin)
papaverine (Cerespan, Pavabid)

Xanthines (Bronchodilators)

aminophylline (Phyllocontin, Truphylline)
dyphylline (Dilor, Lufyllin)
oxtriphylline (Choledyl)

theophylline (Bronkodyl, Slo-Phyllin,
Theolair, others)

A GLOSSARY
OF
DRUG-RELATED TERMS

Glossary

addiction Although there is disagreement among authorities as to how inclusive this designation should be, addiction is generally recognized to be a state of intense dependence (upon a drug) that is characterized by uncontrollable drug-seeking behavior, *tolerance* for the drug's pleasure-giving effects, and *withdrawal* manifestations when the drug is withheld. These features constitute *physical dependence*—a state of physical incorporation of the drug into the fundamental biochemistry of specific brain activities. (See the terms dependence and tolerance for a further account of physical and psychological dependence.)

adverse effect or reaction An abnormal, unexpected, infrequent, and usually unpredictable injurious response to a drug. Used in this restrictive sense, the term *adverse reaction* does *not* include effects of a drug which are normally a part of its pharmacological action, even though such effects may be undesirable and unintended. (See side effect.) Adverse reactions are of three basic types: those due to drug *allergy*, those caused by individual *idiosyncrasy*, and those representing *toxic* effects of drugs on tissue structure and function (see ALLERGY [DRUG], IDIOSYNCRASY, and TOXICITY).

allergy (drug) An abnormal mechanism of drug response that occurs in individuals who produce injurious antibodies* that react with foreign substances—in this instance, a drug. The person who is allergic by nature and has a history of hay fever, asthma, hives, or eczema is more likely to develop drug allergies. Allergic reactions to drugs take many forms: skin eruptions of various kinds, fever, swollen glands, painful joints, jaundice, interference with breathing, acute collapse of circulation, etc. Drug allergies can develop gradually over a long period of time, or they can appear with dramatic suddenness and require life-saving intervention.

alternative delivery system (ADS) A term coined to describe a variety of health care forms other than the traditional fee-for-service model such as HMOs, PPOs, and others.

*Antibodies are special tissue proteins that combine with substances foreign to the body. Protective antibodies destroy bacteria and neutralize toxins. Injurious antibodies, reacting with foreign substances, cause the release of histamine, the principal chemical responsible for allergic reactions.

analgesic A drug that is used primarily to relieve pain. Analgesics are of three basic types: (1) Simple, nonnarcotic analgesics that relieve pain by suppressing the local production of prostaglandins and related substances—examples are acetaminophen, aspirin, and the large group of nonsteroidal anti-inflammatory drugs known as aspirin substitutes (Motrin, Advil, Naprosyn, etc.); (2) narcotic analgesics or opioids ("like opium" derivatives) that relieve pain by suppressing its perception in the brain—examples are morphine, codeine, and hydrocodone (natural derivatives of opium), and meperidine or pentazocine (synthetic drug products); (3) local anesthetics that prevent or relieve pain by rendering sensory nerve endings insensitive to painful stimulation—an example is the urinary tract analgesic phenazopyridine (Pyridium).

anaphylactic (anaphylactoid) reaction A group of symptoms which represent (or resemble) a sometimes overwhelming and dangerous allergic reaction due to extreme hypersensitivity to a drug. Anaphylactic reactions, whether mild, moderate, or severe, often involve several body systems. Mild symptoms consist of itching, hives, nasal congestion, nausea, abdominal cramping, and/or diarrhea. Sometimes these precede more severe symptoms such as choking, shortness of breath, and sudden loss of consciousness (usually referred to as anaphylactic shock).

Characteristic features of anaphylactic reaction must be kept in mind. It can result from a very small dose of drug; it develops suddenly, usually within a few minutes after taking the drug; it can be rapidly progressive and can lead to fatal collapse in a short time if not reversed by appropriate treatment. A developing anaphylactic reaction is a true medical emergency. Any adverse effect that appears within 20 minutes after taking a drug should be considered the early manifestation of a possible anaphylactic reaction. Obtain medical attention immediately! (See allergy [drug], and hypersensitivity.)

antihypertensive A drug used to lower excessively high blood pressure. The term *hypertension* denotes blood pressure above the normal range. It does not refer to excessive nervous or emotional tension. The term *antihypertensive* is sometimes used erroneously as if it had the same meaning as *antianxiety* (or tranquilizing) drug action.

Today there are more than 80 drug products in use for treating hypertension. Those most frequently prescribed for long-term use fall into three major groups:

1. drugs that increase urine production (the diuretics)
2. drugs that relax blood vessel walls
3. drugs that reduce the activity of the sympathetic nervous system

Regardless of their mode of action, all these drugs share an ability to lower the blood pressure. It is important to remember that many other drugs can interact with antihypertensive drugs: some add to their effect and cause excessive reduction in blood pressure; others interfere with their action and reduce their effectiveness. Anyone who is taking medications for hypertension should consult with his or her physician whenever drugs are prescribed for the treatment of other conditions as well.

antipyretic A drug that is used to treat fever because of its ability to lower body temperature that is elevated above the normal. Antipyretics relieve fever through their effects on the temperature-regulating center in the hypothalamus of the brain. Their actions cause dilation of the blood vessels (capillary beds) in the skin, bringing overheated blood to the surface for cooling; in addition, the sweat glands are stimulated to provide copious perspiration that cools the body further through evaporation. An antipyretic drug may also be analgesic (acetaminophen), or analgesic and anti-inflammatory (aspirin).

aplastic anemia A form of bone marrow failure in which the production of all three types of blood cells is seriously impaired (also known as pancytopenia). Aplastic anemia can occur spontaneously from unknown causes, but about one-half of reported cases are induced by certain drugs or chemicals. The offending drug may be difficult to identify; a delay of from one to six months may occur between the use of a causative drug and the detection of anemia. The symptoms reflect the consequences of inadequate supplies of all three blood cell types: deficiency of red blood cells (anemia) results in fatigue, weakness, and pallor; deficiency of white blood cells (leukopenia) predisposes to infections; deficiency of blood platelets (thrombocytopenia) leads to spontaneous bruising and hemorrhage. Treatment is difficult and the outcome unpredictable. Even with the best of care, approximately 50% of cases end fatally.

Although aplastic anemia is a rare consequence of drug treatment (3 in 100,000 users of quinacrine, for example), anyone taking a drug capable of inducing it should have complete blood cell counts periodically if the drug is to be used over an extended period of time. For a listing of causative drugs, see Section Six, Table 5.

bioavailability The measurable characteristics of a drug product (usually a tablet or a capsule) that represent how rapidly the active drug ingredient is absorbed into the bloodstream and to what extent it is absorbed. Two types of measurements—(1) blood levels of the drug at certain time intervals after administration, and (2) the duration of the drug's presence in the blood—indicate how much of the drug is available for biological activity and for how long.

Another method of determining a drug product's bioavailability is to measure (1) the cumulative amount of the drug (or any breakdown product after transformation) that is excreted in the urine, and (2) the rate of drug accumulation in the urine.

The two major factors that govern a drug product's bioavailability are the chemical and physical characteristics (the formulation) of the dosage form given, and the functional state of the digestive system of the individual who takes it. A drug product that disintegrates rapidly in a normally functioning stomach and small intestine produces blood levels of the absorbed drug quite promptly. Such a drug product can be demonstrated to possess good bioavailability.

Specially designed laboratory tests are now available to evaluate a drug product's potential bioavailability when taken by the "average" individual.

bioequivalence It is generally accepted that the ability of a drug product to produce its intended therapeutic effect is directly related to its bioavailability. When a particular drug is marketed by several manufacturers, often in a variety of dosage forms, it is critically important that the drug product selected for use be one that possesses the bioavailability necessary to be therapeutically effective. Substantial variations occur among manufacturers in the formulation of their drug products. Although the principal drug ingredient of products from different firms may be identical chemically, it cannot be assumed that these products possess equal bioavailability and are therefore therapeutically equal.

The bioavailability of any drug product is governed to a large extent by the physical characteristics of its formulation; these in turn determine how rapidly and how completely the drug product disintegrates and releases its active drug component(s) for absorption into the bloodstream. Drug products that contain the same principal drug ingredient but are combined with different inert additives, are coated with different substances, or are enclosed in capsules of different composition may or may not possess the same bioavailability. Those that do are said to be bioequivalent, and can be relied upon to be equally effective in achieving therapeutic results.

If you consider having your prescription filled with the generic equivalent of a brand-name drug product, ask your physician *and* pharmacist for guidance. This decision requires professional judgment in each case. In many treatment situations, reasonable differences in the bioavailability patterns among drug products are acceptable. In some situations, however, because of the serious nature of the illness, or because it is mandatory that blood levels of the drug be maintained within a narrowly defined range, it is essential to use the drug product that has been demonstrated to possess reliable bioavailability.

blood platelets The smallest of the three types of blood cells produced by the bone marrow. Platelets are normally present in very large numbers. Their primary function is to assist the process of normal blood clotting so as to prevent excessive bruising and bleeding in the event of injury. When present in proper numbers and functioning normally, platelets preserve the retaining power of the walls of the smaller blood vessels. By initiating appropriate clotting processes in the blood, platelets seal small points of leakage in the vessel walls, thereby preventing spontaneous bruising or bleeding (that which is unprovoked by trauma).

Certain drugs and chemicals may reduce the number of available blood platelets to abnormally low levels. Some of these drugs act by suppressing platelet formation; other drugs hasten their destruction. When the number of functioning platelets falls below a critical level, blood begins to leak through the thin walls of smaller vessels. The outward evidence of this leakage is the spontaneous appearance of scattered bruises in the skin of the thighs and legs. This is referred to as purpura. Bleeding may occur anywhere in the body, internally as well as superficially into the tissues immediately beneath the skin. See Section Six, Table 5.

bone marrow depression A serious reduction in the ability of the bone marrow to carry on its normal production of blood cells. This can occur as an adverse reaction to the toxic effect of certain drugs and chemicals on bone marrow components. When functioning normally, the bone marrow produces the majority of the body's blood cells. These consist of three types: the red blood cells (erythrocytes), the white blood cells (leukocytes), and the blood platelets (thrombocytes). Each type of cell performs one or more specific functions, all of which are indispensable to the maintenance of life and health.

Drugs that are capable of depressing bone marrow activity can impair the production of all types of blood cells simultaneously or of only one type selectively. Periodic examinations of the blood can reveal significant changes in the structure and number of the blood cells that indicate a possible drug effect on bone marrow activity.

Impairment of the production of red blood cells leads to anemia, a condition of abnormally low red cells and hemoglobin. This causes weakness, loss of energy and stamina, intolerance of cold environments, and shortness of breath on physical exertion. A reduction in the formation of white blood cells can impair the body's immunity and lower its resistance to infection. These changes may result in the development of fever, sore throat, or pneumonia. When the formation of blood platelets is suppressed to abnormally low levels, the blood loses its ability to quickly seal small points of leakage in blood vessel walls. This may lead to episodes of unusual and abnormal spontaneous bruising or to prolonged bleeding in the event of injury.

Any of these symptoms can occur in the presence of bone marrow depression. These symptoms should alert both patient and physician to the need for prompt studies of blood and bone marrow. See Section Six, Table 5.

brand name The registered trade name given to a drug product by its manufacturer. Many drugs are marketed by more than one manufacturer or distributor. Each company adopts a distinctive trade name to distinguish its brand of the generic drug from that of its competitors. Thus a brand name designates a proprietary drug—one that is protected by patent or copyright. Generally, brand names are shorter, easier to pronounce, and more readily remembered than their generic counterparts.

capitation A system where a set amount of money is used to cover the cost of health care for a given person. For instance, a health plan or hospital is paid monthly on a negotiated per-person rate where the plan or hospital provides all health services for the people in the plan.

cause-and-effect relationship A possible causative association between a drug and a biological event—most commonly a side effect or an adverse effect. Knowledge of a drug's full spectrum of effects (wanted and unwanted) is highly desirable when weighing its benefits and risks. However, it is often impossible to establish that a particular drug is the primary agent responsible for an adverse effect. Meticulous consideration must be given to such factors as the time sequence of drug adminis- tration and possible reaction, the use of multiple drugs, possible interactions among these drugs, the effects of the disease under treatment, the physiological and psychological characteristics of the patient, and the influence of unrecognized disorders and malfunctions.

The majority of adverse drug reactions occur sporadically, unpredictably, and infrequently in the general population. A *definite* cause-and-effect relationship be- tween drug and reaction is established when (1) the adverse effect immediately follows administration of the drug; or (2) the adverse effect disappears after the drug is discontinued (dechallenge) and promptly reappears when the drug is used again (rechallenge); or (3) the adverse effects are clearly the expected and predicta- ble toxic consequences of drug overdosage.

In contrast to the obvious "causative" (definite) relationship, there exists a large gray area of "probable," "possible," and "coincidental" associations as- sociated with varying degrees of uncertainty. These classifications often apply to alleged drug reactions that require a relatively long time to develop, are rare, and for which there are no clear-cut means to show a causal mechanism that links drug and reaction. Clarification of cause-and-effect relationships in these uncertain groups requires carefully designed observation over a long period of time, fol- lowed by sophisticated statistical analysis. Occasionally the public is alerted to a newly found "relationship" based upon suggestive but incomplete data. Though early warning is in the public interest, such announcements should make clear whether the presumed relationship is based upon definitive criteria or is simply inferred. It is critical to avoid losing valuable medication use because of poorly designed or reported studies that find their way to the newspaper or television.

The most competent techniques for evaluating cause-and-effect relationships of adverse drug reactions have been devised by the Division of Tissue Reactions to Drugs, a research unit of the Armed Forces Institute of Pathology. Based upon a highly critical examination of all available evidence, the Division's study of 2,800 drug-related deaths yielded the following levels of certainty:

No association	5.0%
Coincidental	14.5%
Possible	33.0%
Probable	30.0%
Causative	17.5%

It is significant that expert evaluation of 2,800 drug-related cases concluded that only 47.5% could be substantiated as definitely or probably causative.

contraindication A condition or disease that precludes the use of a particular drug.

Some contraindications are *absolute*, meaning that the use of the drug would expose the patient to extreme hazard and therefore cannot be justified. Other contraindications are *relative*, meaning that the condition or disease does not entirely bar the use of the drug but requires that special consideration be given to factors that could aggravate existing disease, interfere with current treatment, or produce new injury.

covered lives A term used by health maintenance organizations to indicate how many people have enrolled in their plan. From the HMO's point of view, a minimum number of covered lives is necessary to support a certain number of family practice physicians, a certain number of subspecialists, and so on. Understanding their logic helps explain why some HMOs have one urologist while others have several.

creatinine clearance A measure of how effectively the kidneys are eliminating waste, toxins, and impurities from the body. A low creatinine clearance (such as 20 ml per minute or ml/min) means poorer kidney function; a high creatinine clearance (such as 120 ml/min) means better kidney function. People who have low creatinine clearances often receive lower initial doses and smaller incremental dosages of medicines which are eliminated from the body by the kidneys.

critical or clinical pathway An assortment of coordinated measures taken by a hospital or clinic to organize the care of their patients with specific diseases or conditions. All diagnostic tests, treatments, discharge planning, and other measures are the result of careful study and practice aimed at providing the maximum benefit to all patients in the most cost-effective manner.

dependence A term used to identify the drug-dependent states of *psychological dependence* (or *habituation*) and *physical dependence* (or *addiction*). In addition, a third kind of drug dependence can be included under this term. This might be called *functional dependence*—the need to use a drug continuously in order to sustain a particular body function, the impairment of which causes annoying symptoms of varying degree and significance.

    Psychological dependence is a form of neurotic behavior—an "emotional" dependence. It is an obsession to satisfy a particular desire, be it one of self-gratification or one of escape from some real or imagined distress. Psychological dependence is a very human trait seen often in many socially acceptable patterns and practices such as entertainment, gambling, sports, and collecting. A common form in today's culture is the increasing reliance upon drugs to help in coping with the everyday problems of living: pills for frustration, disappointment, nervous stomach, tension headache, and insomnia. This compulsive drug abuse is characterized by little or no tendency to increase the dose (see TOLERANCE) and no or only minor physical symptoms on withdrawal. Some authorities choose to broaden the definition of addiction to include psychological dependence.

    Physical dependence, which is true addiction, includes two elements: *tolerance* and *withdrawal* manifestations. Addicting drugs provide relief from anguish and pain; they also induce a physiological tolerance that requires increasing dose or repeated use to remain effective. These two features foster continued need for the drug and lead to its becoming a functioning component in the biochemistry of the brain. As this occurs, the drug assumes an "essential" role in ongoing chemical processes. (Thus some authorities prefer the term *chemical dependence*.) Sudden removal of the drug from the system causes a major upheaval in body chemistry and provokes a withdrawal syndrome—the intense mental and physical pain experienced by the addict when intake of the drug is stopped abruptly—that is the hallmark of addiction. It must be noted that true addiction is rare, and fear of addiction, even with potent narcotics, should never stand in the way of effective pain control.

Functional dependence differs significantly from both psychological and physical dependence. It occurs when a drug relieves an annoying or distressing condition and the body function involved becomes increasingly dependent upon the action of the drug to provide a sense of well-being. Drugs that cause functional dependence are used primarily for the relief of symptoms. They do not act on the brain to produce alteration of mood or consciousness as do those drugs with potential for either psychological or physical dependence. The most familiar example of functional dependence is the "laxative habit." Some types of constipation are made worse by the wrong choice of laxative, and natural bowel function fades as the colon becomes more and more dependent upon the laxative drug.

disulfiramlike (Antabuse-like) reaction The symptoms that result from the interaction of alcohol and any drug that is capable of provoking the pattern of response typical of the "Antabuse effect." The interacting drug interrupts the decomposition of alcohol by the liver and permits accumulation of a toxic by-product that enters the bloodstream. When sufficient levels of both alcohol and drug are present in the blood, the reaction occurs. It consists of intense flushing and warming of the face, a severe throbbing headache, shortness of breath, chest pains, nausea, repeated vomiting, sweating, and weakness. If the amount of alcohol ingested has been large enough, the reaction may progress to blurred vision, vertigo, confusion, marked drop in blood pressure, and loss of consciousness. Severe reactions may lead to convulsions and death. The reaction can last from 30 minutes to several hours, depending upon the amount of alcohol in the body. As the symptoms subside, the individual is exhausted and usually sleeps for several hours.

diuretic A drug that alters kidney function to increase the volume of urine. Diuretics use several different mechanisms to increase urine volume, and these, in turn, have different effects on body chemistry. Diuretics are used primarily to (1) remove excess water from the body (as in congestive heart failure and some types of liver and kidney disease) and (2) treat hypertension by promoting the excretion of sodium from the body.

disease management An approach to the prevention and treatment of a specific condition which attempts to identify the frequency of its occurrence in the population, organize available resources, and allocate money to reach the best balance of dollars spent and results achieved.

divided doses The total daily dose of a medicine is split into smaller individual doses over the course of a day.

dosage forms and strengths This information category in the individual Drug Profiles (Section Two) uses several abbreviations to designate measurements of weight and volume. These are:

mcg	=	microgram	= 1,000,000th of a gram (weight)
mg	=	milligram	= 1000th of a gram (weight)
ml	=	milliter	= 1000th of a liter (volume)
gm	=	gram	= 1,000 milligrams (weight)

There are approximately 65 mg in 1 grain.
There are approximately 5 ml in 1 teaspoon.
There are approximately 15 ml in 1 tablespoon.
There are approximately 30 ml in 1 ounce.
1 milliliter of water weighs 1 gram.
There are approximately 454 grams in 1 pound.

drug class A group of drugs that are similar in chemistry, method of action, and use in treatment. Because of their common characteristics, many drugs within a class will produce the same side effects and have similar potential for related adverse reactions and interactions. However, significant variations among members within a drug class can occur. This sometimes allows the physician an important degree of selectivity in choosing a drug if certain beneficial actions are desired or particular side effects are to be minimized. Examples: Antihistamines, phenothiazines, and tetracyclines (see Section Four).

drug, drug product Terms often used interchangeably to designate a medicine (in any of its dosage forms) used in medical practice. Strictly speaking, the term *drug* refers to the single chemical entity that provokes a specific response when placed within a biological system—the "active" ingredient. A *drug product* is the manufactured dosage form—tablet, capsule, elixir, etc.—that contains the active drug intermixed with inactive ingredients to provide for convenient administration.

Drug products that contain only one active ingredient are referred to as single-entity drugs. Drug products with two or more active ingredients are called combination drugs (designated [CD] in the lists of brand names in the Drug Profiles, Section Two).

drug fever The elevation of body temperature that occurs as an unwanted manifestation of drug action. Drugs can induce fever by several mechanisms; these include allergic reactions, drug-induced tissue damage, acceleration of tissue metabolism, constriction of blood vessels in the skin with resulting decrease in loss of body heat, and direct action on the temperature-regulating center in the brain.

The most common form of drug fever is associated with allergic reactions. It may be the only allergic manifestation apparent, or it may be part of a complex of allergic symptoms that can include skin rash, hives, joint swelling and pain, enlarged lymph glands, hemolytic anemia, or hepatitis. The fever usually appears about 7 to 10 days after starting the drug and may vary from low-grade to alarmingly high levels. It may be sustained or intermittent, but it usually persists for as long as the drug is taken. In previously sensitized individuals drug fever may occur within 1 or 2 hours after taking the first dose of medication.

Although many drugs are capable of producing fever, the following are more commonly responsible:

allopurinol	novobiocin
antihistamines	para-aminosalicylic acid
atropinelike drugs	penicillin
barbiturates	pentazocine
coumarin anticoagulants	phenytoin
hydralazine	procainamide
iodides	propylthiouracil
isoniazid	quinidine
methyldopa	rifampin
nadalol	sulfonamides

extension effect An unwanted but predictable drug response that is a logical consequence of mild to moderate overdosage. An extension effect is an exaggeration of the drug's normal pharmacological action; it can be thought of as a mild form of dose-related toxicity (see OVERDOSAGE and TOXICITY).

Example: The continued "hangover" of drowsiness and mental sluggishness that persists after arising in the morning is a common extension effect of a long-acting sleep-inducing drug (hypnotic) taken the night before.

Example: The persistent intestinal cramping and diarrhea that result from too generous a dose of laxative are extension effects of the drug's anticipated action.

FDA approvable A stage in the Food and Drug Administration's review and approval process. A medicine is considered FDA approvable once the panel which reviewed the supporting data submitted to the FDA finds that data acceptable. In general, at this point only final details need to be resolved before the drug becomes FDA approved and is made available for general prescription use.

generic name The official, common, or public name used to designate an active drug entity, whether in pure form or in dosage form. Generic names are coined by committees of officially appointed drug experts and are approved by governmental agencies for national and international use, thus they are nonproprietary. Many drug products are marketed under the generic name of the principal active ingredient and bear no brand name of the manufacturer.

While the total number of prescriptions written in the United States in 1986 increased by 0.6%, prescriptions specifying the *generic name* of the drug increased by 8.6%. Generically written prescriptions now account for 13.5% of all new prescriptions written in the United States. The drugs most commonly prescribed by generic name are listed below, ranked in descending order of the number of new prescriptions issued.

amoxicillin	erythromycin
penicillin VK	hydrochlorothiazide
ampicillin	acetaminophen/codeine
tetracycline	doxycycline
prednisone	phenobarbital

genetic therapy Perhaps the most promising area of therapy in medicine today. Specific healthy genetic material is isolated and inserted into appropriate, but diseased, cells. For example, normal lung genes are given to a person with cystic fibrosis. Still very experimental, it may someday allow people suffering with genetically-based diseases or conditions to receive therapy that changes the effected genes and actually *cure* those conditions.

habituation A form of drug dependence based upon strong psychological gratification. The habitual use of drugs that alter mood or relieve minor discomforts results from a compulsive need to feel pleasure and satisfaction or to escape emotional distress. The abrupt cessation of habituating drugs does not produce the withdrawal syndrome seen in addiction. Thus habituation is a *psychological dependence.* (See dependence for a further account of psychological and physical dependence.)

hemolytic anemia A form of anemia (deficient red blood cells and hemoglobin) resulting from the premature destruction (hemolysis) of red blood cells. Several mechanisms can cause hemolytic anemia; among these is the action of certain drugs and chemicals. Some patients are susceptible to hemolytic anemia because of a genetic deficiency in the makeup of their red blood cells. If such people are given certain antimalarial drugs, sulfa drugs, or numerous other drugs, some of their red cells will disintegrate on contact with the drug. (About 10% of African-Americans have this genetic trait.)

Another type of drug-induced hemolytic anemia is a form of drug allergy. Many drugs in wide use (including quinidine, methyldopa, levodopa, and chlorpromazine) are known to cause hemolytic destruction of red cells as a hypersensitivity (allergic) reaction.

Hemolytic anemia can occur abruptly (with evident symptoms) or silently. The acute form lasts about 7 days and is characterized by fever, pallor, weakness, dark-colored urine, and varying degrees of jaundice (yellow coloration of eyes and skin). When drug-induced hemolytic anemia is mild, involving the destruction of only a small number of red blood cells, there may be no symptoms to indicate its presence. Such episodes are detected only by means of laboratory studies (see IDIOSYNCRASY and ALLERGY [DRUG]).

For listings of causative drugs, see Section Six, Table 5.

hepatitislike reaction Changes in the liver, induced by certain drugs, which resemble those produced by viral hepatitis. The symptoms of drug-induced hepatitis and virus-induced hepatitis are often so similar that the correct cause cannot be established without precise laboratory studies.

Hepatitis due to drugs may be a form of drug allergy (as in reaction to many of the phenothiazines), or it may represent a toxic adverse effect (as in reaction to some of the monoamine oxidase inhibitor drugs). Liver reactions of significance usually result in jaundice and represent serious adverse effects (see JAUNDICE). See Section Six, Table 8.

HMO Abbreviation for Health Maintenance Organization: A health care delivery system that provides a broad spectrum of medical therapies and services by a collective group of practitioners within a common organization.

hypersensitivity A term subject to varying usages for many years. One common use has been to identify the trait of overresponsiveness to drug action, that is, an intolerance to even small doses. Used in this sense, the term indicates that the nature of the response is appropriate but the degree of response is exaggerated.

The term is more widely used today to identify a state of allergy. To have a *hypersensitivity* to a drug is to be *allergic* to it (see ALLERGY [DRUG]).

Some individuals develop cross-hypersensitivity. This means that once a person has developed an allergy to a certain drug, that person will experience an allergic reaction to other drugs that are closely related in chemical composition.

Example: The patient was known to be *hypersensitive* by nature, having a history of seasonal hay fever and asthma since childhood. His *allergy* to tetracycline developed after his third course of treatment. This drug *hypersensitivity* manifested itself as a diffuse, measleslike rash.

hypnotic A drug that is used primarily to induce sleep. There are several classes of drugs that have hypnotic effects: antihistamines, barbiturates, benzodiazepines, and several unrelated compounds. Within the past 15 years the benzodiazepines, because of their relative safety and lower potential for inducing dependence, have largely replaced the barbiturates as the most commonly used hypnotics. The body usually develops a tolerance to the hypnotic effect after several weeks of continual use. To maintain their effectiveness, hypnotics should be used intermittently for short periods of time.

hypoglycemia A condition where the amount of glucose (a sugar) in the blood is below the normal range. Since normal brain function depends upon an adequate supply of glucose, reducing the level of glucose in the blood below a critical point will cause serious impairment of brain activity. The resulting symptoms are characteristic of hypoglycemia. Early indications are headache, a sensation resembling mild drunkenness, and an inability to think clearly. These may be accompanied by hunger. As the level of blood glucose continues to fall, nervousness and confusion develop. Varying degrees of weakness, numbness, trembling, sweating, and rapid heart action follow. If sugar is not provided at this point and the blood glucose level drops further, impaired speech, incoordination, and unconsciousness, with or without convulsions, will follow.

Hypoglycemia in any stage requires prompt recognition and treatment. Because of the potential for injury to the brain, the mechanisms and management of hypoglycemia should be understood by all who use drugs capable of producing it.

hypothermia A state of the body characterized by an unexpected decline of internal body temperature to levels significantly below the norm of 98.6 degrees F or 37 degrees C. By definition, hypothermia means a body temperature of less than 95 degrees F or 35 degrees C. The elderly and debilitated are more prone to develop hypothermia if clothed inadequately and exposed to cool environments. Most episodes are initiated by room temperatures below 65 degrees F or 18.3 degrees C. The condition often develops suddenly, can mimic a stroke, and has a mortality rate of 50%. Some drugs, such as phenothiazines, barbiturates, and benzodiazepines, are conducive to causing hypothermia.

idiosyncrasy An abnormal mechanism of drug response that occurs in people who have a peculiar defect in their body chemistry (often hereditary) which produces an effect totally unrelated to the drug's normal pharmacological action. Idiosyncrasy is not a form of allergy. The actual chemical defects responsible for certain idiosyncratic drug reactions are well understood; others are not.

Example: Approximately 100 million people in the world (including 10% of African-Americans) have an enzyme deficiency in their red blood cells that causes these cells to disintegrate when exposed to drugs such as sulfonamides (Gantrisin, Kynex), nitrofurantoin (Furadantin, Macrodantin), probenecid (Benemid), quinine, and quinidine. As a result of this reaction, these drugs (and others) can cause a significant anemia in susceptible individuals.

Example: Approximately 5% of the population of the United States is susceptible to the development of glaucoma on prolonged use of cortisone-related drugs (see Cortisonelike drug class in Section Four).

immunosuppressive A drug that significantly impairs (suppresses) the functions of the body's immune system. In some cases, immunosuppression is an intended drug effect (cyclosporine to prevent the immune system from rejecting a transplanted kidney). In other instances, it is an unwanted side effect as in the long-term use of cortisonelike drugs (to control asthma) suppressing the immune system sufficiently to permit reactivation of a dormant tuberculosis. Immunosuppressant drugs are being used to treat several chronic disorders that are thought to be autoimmune diseases, notably advanced rheumatoid arthritis, ulcerative colitis, and systemic lupus erythematosus.

interaction An unwanted change in the body's response to a drug that results when a second drug that can alter the action of the first is administered at the same time. Some drug interactions can enhance the effect of either drug, producing an overresponse similar to overdosage. Other interactions may reduce drug effectiveness and cause inadequate response. A third type of interaction can produce a seemingly unrelated toxic response with no associated increase or decrease in the pharmacological actions of the interacting drugs.

Theoretically many drugs can interact with one another, but in reality drug interactions are comparatively infrequent. Many interactions can be anticipated, and the physician can make appropriate adjustments in dosage to prevent or minimize unintended fluctuations in drug response.

jaundice A yellow coloration of the skin (and the white portion of the eyes) that occurs when excessive bile pigments accumulate in the blood as a result of impaired liver function. Jaundice can be produced by several mechanisms. It may occur as a manifestation of a wide variety of diseases, or it may represent an adverse reaction to a particular drug. At times it is difficult to distinguish between disease-induced jaundice and drug-induced jaundice.

Jaundice due to a drug is always a serious adverse effect. Anyone taking a drug that is capable of causing jaundice should watch closely for any significant change in the color of urine or feces. Dark discoloration of the urine and paleness (lack of color) of the stool may be early indications of a developing jaundice. Should either of these symptoms occur, it is advisable to discontinue the drug and notify the prescribing physician promptly. Diagnostic tests are available to clarify the nature of the jaundice. See Section Six, Table 8.

lupus erythematosus (LE) A serious disease of unknown cause that occurs in two forms, one limited to the skin (discoid LE) and the other involving several body systems (systemic LE). Both forms occur predominantly in young women. About 5% of cases of the discoid form convert to the systemic form. Systemic LE is a disorder of the body's immune system which may result in chronic, progressive inflammation and destruction of the connective tissue framework of the skin, blood vessels, joints, brain, heart muscle, lungs, and kidneys. Altered proteins in the blood lead to antibody formation which reacts with certain organ tissues to produce the inflammation and destruction characteristic of the disease. A reduction in the number of white blood cells and blood platelets often occurs. The course of systemic LE is usually quite protracted and unpredictable. While no cure is known, satisfactory management may be achieved in some cases by the judicious use of cortisonelike drugs.

Several drugs are capable of initiating a form of systemic LE quite similar to that which occurs spontaneously. Symptoms may appear as early as 2 weeks or as late as 8 years after starting the responsible drug. The initial symptoms usually consist of low-grade fever, skin rashes of various kinds, aching muscles, and multiple joint pains. Chest pains (pleurisy) are fairly common. Enlargement of the lymph glands occurs less frequently. Symptoms usually subside if the drug is stopped, but laboratory evidence of the reaction may persist for many months.

neuroleptic malignant syndrome (NMS) A rare, serious, sometimes fatal idiosyncratic reaction to the use of neuroleptic (antipsychotic) drugs. The principal features of the reaction are hyperthermia (temperatures of 102 to 104 degrees F), marked muscle rigidity, and coma. Other symptoms include rapid heart rate and breathing, profuse sweating, tremors, and seizures. Two-thirds of reported cases occurred in men, one-third in women. The mortality rate is 15% to 20%.

The following drugs have a potential for inducing this reaction:

amitriptyline + perphenazine (Triavil)	metoclopramide (Reglan, Octamide)
amoxapine (Asendin)	molindone (Moban)
chlorpromazine (Thorazine)	perphenazine (Etrafon, Trilafon)
chlorprothixene (Taractan)	pimozide (Orap)
clomipramine (Anafranil)	prochlorperazine (Compazine)
fluphenazine (Permitil, Prolixin)	thioridazine (Mellaril)
haloperidol (Haldol)	thiothixene (Navane)
imipramine (Tofranil, etc.)	trifluoperazine (Stelazine)
levodopa + carbidopa (Sinemet)	trimeprazine (Temaril)
loxapine (Loxitane)	

orthostatic hypotension A type of low blood pressure that is related to body position or posture (also called postural hypotension). The individual who is subject to orthostatic hypotension may have a normal blood pressure while lying down, but on sitting upright or standing he or she will experience sudden sensations of lightheadedness, dizziness, and a feeling of an impending faint that compels him or her to return quickly to a lying position. These symptoms are manifestations of inadequate blood flow (oxygen supply) to the brain due to a delay in the rise in blood pressure that always occurs as the body adjusts the circulation to the erect position.

Many drugs (especially the stronger antihypertensives) may cause orthostatic hypotension. Individuals who experience this drug effect should report it to their physician so that appropriate dosage adjustment can be made. Failure to correct or to compensate for these sudden drops in blood pressure can lead to severe falls and injury.

The tendency to orthostatic hypotension can be reduced by avoiding sudden standing, prolonged standing, vigorous exercise, and exposure to hot environments. Alcoholic beverages should be used cautiously until their combined effect with the drug in use has been determined.

outcomes research A current concept in health care evaluation that considers the comparative benefits (gauged by a variety of measures) of using a particular medication over another. This may lead to the cheapest drug **not** being the drug of choice, because the outcomes from the therapy do not stand up over time or may be subject to significant treatment failure.

overdosage The meaning of this term should not be limited to the concept of doses that exceed the normal dosage range recommended by the manufacturer. The optimal dose of many drugs (that amount which gives the greatest benefit with least distress) varies greatly from person to person. What may be an average dose for most people will be an overdose for some and an underdose for others. Numerous factors, such as age, body size, nutritional status, and liver and kidney function, have significant influence on dosage requirements. Drugs with narrow safety margins often produce indications of overdosage if something delays the elimination of the customary daily dose. In this instance, overdosage results from accumulation of prescribed daily doses. Massive overdosage—as occurs with accidental ingestion of drugs by children or with suicidal intention by adults—is referred to as poisoning.

over-the-counter (OTC) drugs Drug products that can be purchased without prescription. Many are available in food stores, variety stores, and newsstands as well as in conventional drug stores. Because of the unrestricted availability, many people do not look upon OTC medicines as drugs. But drugs they are! And like the more potent drug products that are sold only on prescription, they are chemicals that are capable of a wide variety of actions on biological systems. Within the last 30 years, many OTC drugs have assumed greater importance because of their ability to interact unfavorably with widely used prescription drugs. Serious problems in drug management can arise when (1) the patient fails to tell the physician of the OTC drug(s) he or she is taking ("because they really aren't drugs") and (2) the physician fails to specify that his or her question about what medicines are being taken currently *includes all OTC drugs.* During any course of treatment, whether medical or surgical, the patient should consult with the physician regarding any OTC drug that he or she wishes to take.

The major classes of OTC drugs for internal use include:

allergy medicines (antihistamines)	laxatives
antacids	menstrual aids
antiworm medicines	motion sickness remedies
aspirin and aspirin combinations	pain relievers
aspirin substitutes	reducing aids
asthma aids	salt substitutes
cold medicines (decongestants)	sedatives and tranquilizers
cough medicines	sleeping pills
diarrhea remedies	stimulants (caffeine)
digestion aids	sugar substitutes (saccharin)
diuretics	tonics
iron preparations	vitamins

paradoxical reaction An unexpected drug response that is not consistent with the known pharmacology of the drug. Such reactions are due to individual sensitivity or variability and can occur in any age group. They are seen more commonly, however, in children and the elderly.

Example: An 80-year-old man was admitted to a nursing home following the death of his wife. He had difficulty adjusting to his new environment and was restless, agitated, and irritable. He was given a trial of the tranquilizer diazepam (Valium) to relax him, starting with small doses. On the second day of medication he became confused and erratic in behavior. The dose of diazepam was increased. On the third day he began to wander aimlessly, talked incessantly in a loud voice, and displayed anger and hostility when attempts were made to help him. Suspecting the possibility of a paradoxical reaction, the diazepam was discontinued. All behavioral disturbances gradually subsided within 3 days.

Parkinson-like disorders (parkinsonism) A group of symptoms that resembles those caused by Parkinson's disease, a chronic disorder of the nervous system also known as shaking palsy. The characteristic features of parkinsonism include a fixed, emotionless facial expression (masklike in appearance); a prominent trembling of the hands, arms, or legs; and stiffness of the extremities that limits movement and produces a rigid posture and gait.

Parkinsonism is a fairly common adverse effect that occurs in about 15% of all patients who take large doses of phenothiazines or use them over an extended period of time. If recognized early, the Parkinson-like features will lessen or disappear with reduced dosage or change in medication. In some instances, however, Parkinson-like changes may become permanent, requiring appropriate medication.

peripheral neuritis (peripheral neuropathy) A group of symptoms that results from injury to nerve tissue in the extremities. A variety of drugs and chemicals are capable of inducing changes in nerve structure or function. The characteristic pattern consists of a sensation of numbness and tingling that usually begins in the fingers and toes and is accompanied by an altered sensation to touch and vague discomfort ranging from aching sensations to burning pain. Severe forms of peripheral neuritis may include loss of muscular strength and coordination.

A relatively common form of peripheral neuritis is that seen with the long-term use of isoniazid in the treatment of tuberculosis. If vitamin B6 (pyridoxine) is not given concurrently with isoniazid, peripheral neuritis may occur in sensitive individuals. Vitamin B6 can be both preventive and curative in this form of drug-induced peripheral neuritis.

Since peripheral neuritis can also occur as a late complication following many viral infections, care must be taken to avoid assigning a cause-and-effect relationship to a drug which is not responsible for the nerve injury (see CAUSE-AND-EFFECT RELATIONSHIP).

See Section Six, Table 10 for further discussion of drug-induced nerve damage.

Peyronie's disease A permanent deformity of the penis caused by the formation of dense fibrous (scarlike) tissue within the system of penile vessels that become engorged with blood during the process of erection. During sexual arousal, this inelastic fibrous tissue causes a painful downward bowing of the penis that hampers or precludes satisfactory intercourse. This condition has been associated with the use of phenytoin (Dilantin, etc.) and with most members of the beta-blocker class of drugs (see drug class, Section Four). See Section Six, Table 11.

pharmacoeconomics The discipline within pharmacology that studies specifically the issues of costs versus benefits, utilizing a variety of measures: material and personnel costs, treatment outcomes, quality of patient life, etc. Study results are used in deciding where and how health care resources should be utilized.

pharmacology The medical science that relates to the development and use of medicinal drugs and their composition and action in animals and man. Used in its broadest sense, pharmacology embraces the related sciences of medicinal chemistry, experimental therapeutics, and toxicology.

Example: The widely used sulfonylurea drugs (Diabinese, Dymelor, Orinase, Tolinase) are effective in the treatment of some forms of diabetes because of the accidental discovery that some of their parent "sulfa" drugs produced hypoglycemia (low blood sugar) during their early therapeutic trials as anti-infectives. Subsequent investigation of the mechanisms of action (*pharmacology*) of these drugs revealed that they are capable of stimulating the pancreas to release more insulin.

Pharmacological studies on another group of "sulfa"-related drugs—the thiazide diuretics—revealed that they could induce the kidney to excrete more water and salt in the urine. This drug action is of great value in treating high blood pressure and heart failure.

photosensitivity A drug-induced change in the skin that results in the development of a rash or exaggerated sunburn on exposure to the sun or ultraviolet lamps. The reaction is confined to uncovered areas of skin, providing a clue to the nature of its cause. See Section Six, Table 2.

porphyria The porphyrias are a group of hereditary disorders characterized by excessive production of porphyrins, essential respiratory pigments of the body. (One porphyrin is a component of hemoglobin, the pigment of red blood cells.) Two forms of porphyria—acute intermittent porphyria and cutaneous porphyria—can be activated by the use of certain drugs. Acute intermittent porphyria involves damage to the nervous system; an acute attack can include fever, rapid heart rate, vomiting, pain in the abdomen and legs, hallucinations, seizures, paralysis, and coma. Some examples include barbiturates, "sulfa" drugs, chlordiazepoxide (Librium), chlorpropamide (Diabinese), methyldopa (Aldomet), and phenytoin (Dilantin). Cutaneous porphyria involves damage to the skin and liver. An episode can include reddening and blistering of the skin, followed by crust formation, scarring, and excessive hair growth; repeated liver damage can lead to cirrhosis. This form of porphyria can be precipitated by chloroquine, estrogen, oral contraceptives, and excessive iron.

priapism The prolonged, painful erection of the penis usually associated with sexual arousal or stimulation. It is caused by obstruction to the outflow (drainage) of blood through the veins at the root of the penis. Erection may persist for 30 minutes to a few hours and then subside spontaneously; or it may persist for up to 30 hours and require surgical drainage of blood from the penis for relief. More than half of the episodes of priapism induced by drugs result in permanent impotence. Sickle cell anemia (or trait) may predispose to priapism; individuals with this disorder should avoid all drugs that may induce priapism.

Drugs reported to induce priapism include the following:

anabolic steroids (male hormonelike drugs: Anadrol, Anavar, Android, Halotestin, Metandren, Oreton, Testred, Winstrol)
chlorpromazine (Thorazine)
cocaine
guanethidine (Ismelin)
haloperidol (Haldol)
heparin
levodopa (Sinemet)
molindone (Moban)
prazosin (Minipress)
prochlorperazine (Compazine)
trazodone (Desyrel)
trifluoperazine (Stelazine)
warfarin (Coumadin)

prostatism This term refers to the difficulties associated with an enlarged prostate. As the prostate enlarges (a natural development in aging men), it constricts the urethra (outflow passage) where it joins the urinary bladder and impedes urination. This causes a reduction in the size and force of the urinary stream, hesitancy in starting the flow of urine, interruption of urination, and incomplete emptying of the bladder. Atropine and drugs with atropinelike effects can impair the bladder's ability to compensate for the obstructing prostate gland, thus intensifying all of the above symptoms.

Raynaud's phenomenon This term refers to intermittent episodes of reduced blood flow into the fingers or toes, with resulting paleness, discomfort, numbness, and tingling. It is due to an exaggerated constriction of the small arteries that supply blood to the digits. Characteristically an attack is precipitated either by emotional stress or exposure to cold. It can occur as part of a systemic disorder (lupus erythematosus, scleroderma), or it can occur without apparent cause (Raynaud's disease). Some widely used drugs, notably beta-adrenergic blockers and products that contain ergotamine, are conducive to the development of Raynaud-like symptoms in predisposed individuals.

Reye (Reye's) syndrome An acute, often fatal, childhood illness characterized by swelling of the brain and toxic degeneration of the liver. It usually develops during recovery from a flu-like infection, measles, or chicken pox. Symptoms include fever, headache, delirium, loss of consciousness, and seizures. It is one of the 10 major causes of death in children ages 1 to 10 years. Evidence to date suggests that the syndrome may be due to the combined effects of viral infection and chemical toxins (possibly drugs) in a genetically predisposed child. Drugs that have been used just prior to the onset of symptoms include acetaminophen, aspirin, antibiotics, and antiemetics (drugs to control nausea and vomiting). Although it has not been definitely established that drugs actually cause Reye syndrome, it is thought that they may contribute to its development or adversely affect its course. Current recommendations are to avoid the use of acetaminophen, aspirin, and antiemetic drugs in children with flu-like infections, chicken pox, or measles.

secondary effect A by-product or complication of drug use which does not occur as part of the drug's primary pharmacological activity. Secondary effects are unwanted consequences and may therefore be classified as adverse effects.

   Example: The reactivation of dormant tuberculosis can be a *secondary effect* of long-term cortisone administration for arthritis. Cortisone and related drugs (see Cortisonelike drug class, Section Four) suppress natural immunity and lower resistance to infection.

   Example: The cramping of leg muscles can be a *secondary effect* of diuretic (urine-producing) drug treatment for high blood pressure. Excessive loss of potassium through increased urination renders the muscle vulnerable to painful spasm during exercise.

side effect A normal, expected, and predictable response to a drug that accompanies the principal (intended) response sought in treatment. Side effects are part of a drug's pharmacological activity and thus are unavoidable. Most side effects are undesirable. The majority cause minor annoyance and inconvenience; some may cause serious problems in managing certain diseases; a few can be hazardous.

   Example: The drug propantheline (Pro-Banthine) is used to treat peptic ulcers because one of the consequences of its pharmacological action is the reduction of acid formation in the stomach (an intended effect). Other consequences can include blurring of near vision, dryness of the mouth, and constipation. These are *side effects.*

superinfection (suprainfection) The development of a second infection that is superimposed upon an initial infection currently under treatment. The superinfection is caused by organisms that are not susceptible to the killing action of the drug(s) used to treat the original (primary) infection. Superinfections usually occur during or immediately following treatment with a broad-spectrum antibiotic—one that is capable of altering the customary balance of bacterial populations in various parts of the body. The disturbance of this balance permits the overgrowth of organisms that normally exist in numbers too small to cause disease. The superinfection may also require treatment, using those drugs that are effective against the offending organism.

Example: Recurrent infections of the kidney and bladder often require repeated courses of treatment with a variety of anti-infective drugs. When these are taken by mouth they can suppress the normally dominant types of bacteria present in the colon and rectum, encouraging the overgrowth of yeast organisms that are capable of causing colitis. When this occurs, colitis is a *superinfection.*

tardive dyskinesia A late-developing, drug-induced disorder of the nervous system characterized by involuntary bizarre movements of the eyelids, jaws, lips, tongue, neck, and fingers. It occurs after long-term treatment with the more potent drugs used in the management of serious mental illness. While it may occur in any age group, it is more common in the middle-aged and the elderly. Older, chronically ill women are particularly susceptible to this adverse drug effect. Once developed, the pattern of uncontrollable chewing, lip puckering, and repetitive tongue protruding (fly-catching movement) appears to be irreversible. No consistently satisfactory treatment or cure is available. To date, there is no way of identifying beforehand the individual who may develop this distressing reaction to drug treatment, and there is no known prevention. Fortunately, the persistent dyskinesia (abnormal movement) is not accompanied by further impairment of mental function or deterioration of intelligence.

tolerance An adaptation by the body that lessens responsiveness to a drug on continuous administration. Body tissues become accustomed to the drug's presence and react to it less vigorously. Tolerance can be beneficial or harmful in treatment.

Examples: Beneficial tolerance occurs when the hay fever sufferer finds that the side effect of drowsiness gradually disappears after 4 or 5 days of continuous use of antihistamines.

Harmful tolerance occurs when the patient with "shingles" (herpes zoster) finds that the usual dose of codeine is no longer sufficient to relieve pain and that the need for increased dosage creates a risk of physical dependence or addiction.

toxicity The capacity of a drug to dangerously impair body functions or to damage body tissues. Most drug toxicity is related to total dosage: the larger the overdose, the greater the toxic effects. Some drugs, however, can produce toxic reactions when used in normal doses. Such adverse effects are not due to allergy or idiosyncrasy; in many instances their mechanisms are not fully understood. Toxic effects due to overdosage are generally a harmful extension of the drug's normal pharmacological actions and—to some extent—are predictable and preventable. Toxic reactions which occur with normal dosage are unrelated to the drug's known pharmacology and for the most part are unpredictable and unexplainable.

tyramine A chemical present in many common foods and beverages that causes no difficulties to body functioning under normal circumstances. The main pharmacological action of tyramine is to raise the blood pressure. Normally, enzymes present in many body tissues neutralize this action of tyramine in the quantities in which it is consumed in the average diet. The principal enzyme responsible for neutralizing the blood-pressure-elevating action of tyramine (and chemicals related to it) is monoamine oxidase (MAO) type A. Monoamine oxidase type A serves an important regulatory function that helps to balance several of the chemical processes in the body that control certain activities of the nervous system. Stabilization of the blood pressure is one of these activities. If the action of monoamine oxidase type A is blocked, chemical substances like tyramine function unopposed, and relatively small amounts can cause alarming and dangerous elevations of blood pressure.

Several drugs in use today are capable of blocking the action of monoamine oxidase type A. These drugs are commonly referred to as monoamine oxidase (MAO) type A inhibitors (see drug class, Section Four). If an individual is taking one of these drugs and his or her diet includes foods or beverages that contain a significant amount of tyramine, he or she may experience a sudden increase in blood pressure. Before this interaction of food and drug was understood, several deaths due to brain hemorrhage occurred in persons taking MAO type A inhibitor drugs as a result of an extreme elevation of blood pressure following a meal of tyramine-rich foods.

It should be noted also that MAO inhibitor drugs can interact with many other drugs and cause serious adverse effects. Consult your physician before taking *any* drug concurrently with one that can inhibit the action of monoamine oxidase type A or B.

Any protein-containing food that has undergone partial decomposition may present a hazard because of its increased tyramine content. The following foods and beverages have been reported to contain varying amounts of tyramine. Unless their tyramine content is known to be insignificant, they should be avoided altogether while taking a MAO type A inhibitor drug. Consult your physician about the advisability of using any of the foods or beverages on these lists if you are taking such drugs.

FOODS

Aged cheeses of all kinds*
Avocado
Banana skins
Bean curd
Bologna
"Bovril" extract
Broad bean pods
Chicken liver (unless fresh and used at
  once)
Chocolate
Figs, canned
Fish, canned
Fish, dried and salted
Herring, pickled
Liver, if not very fresh
"Marmite" extract
Meat extracts
Meat tenderizers
Pepperoni
Raisins
Raspberries

BEVERAGES

Beer (unpasteurized)
Chianti wine
Sherry wine
Vermouth

*Cottage cheese, cream cheese and processed cheese are safe to eat.

Salami
Shrimp paste
Sour cream
Soy sauce
Yeast extracts

NOTE: *Any* high-protein food that is aged or has undergone breakdown by putre-faction probably contains tyramine and could produce a hypertensive crisis in anyone taking MAO type A inhibiting drugs.

viral load or viral burden A term used in reference to AIDS patients to describe the amount of HIV virus present in the body at any given time. The amount of virus relates to the effectiveness of the drug therapy which is being used, and can be a reason to change medication if the load increases.

WHO pain ladder A therapeutic scheme of utilizing increasing strengths of pain medications (analgesics) which include NSAIDs, opiates, and adjuvant drugs to control pain as specified by the World Health Organization. It is *not* an absolute treatment scheme, but should be used to organize the approach to effective analgesia.

TABLES OF DRUG INFORMATION

TABLE 1

Drugs That May Adversely Affect the Fetus and Newborn Infant

Following the confirmation in 1961 that the hypnotic drug thalidomide, taken during early pregnancy, could cause major birth defects, interest and concern regarding medicinal drugs as possible teratogens have greatly intensified. Numerous studies have increased our understanding of how drugs can adversely affect the developing fetus and newborn infant; they have also helped to identify those drugs that appear to have potential for causing significant harm to the unborn and newborn child. It is now recognized that some drugs can cause (or contribute to) malformations, retarded growth, functional disorders and death of the fetus or newborn infant. However, in many instances, it is not possible to clearly separate adverse effects due to the mother's disease or disorder from those that may be induced by the drugs used as therapy. Based upon our current knowledge, it is strongly recommended that only those drugs that confer clear and essential benefits should be used during pregnancy.

Drugs that *probably* cause adverse effects when taken during the *first trimester*

aminopterin	fluorouracil	opioid analgesics*
anticonvulsants*	iodides	progestins*
antithyroid drugs	isotretinoin	quinine
cytarabine	kanamycin	streptomycin
danazol	mercaptopurine	testosterone
diethylstilbestrol	methotrexate	warfarin
etretinate	misoprostol	

Drugs that *possibly* cause adverse effects when taken during the *first trimester*

angiotensin converting enzyme inhibitors*	lithium	piperazine
busulfan	mebendazole	rifampin
chlorambucil	monoamine oxidase inhibitors*	tetracyclines*
estrogens*	oral contraceptives	

Drugs that *probably* cause adverse effects when taken during the *second and third trimesters*

amiodarone	iodides	rifampin
androgens*	kanamycin	streptomycin
angiotensin converting enzyme inhibitors*	lithium	sulfonamides*
antithyroid drugs	nonsteroidal anti-inflammatory drugs*	sulfonylureas*
aspirin		tetracyclines*
benzodiazepines*	opioid analgesics*	thiazide diuretics*
chloramphenicol	phenothiazines*	tricyclic antidepressants*
estrogens*	progestins*	warfarin

Drugs that *possibly* cause adverse effects when taken during the *second and third trimesters*

acetazolamide	ethacrynic acid	hydroxyzine
clemastine	fluoroquinolones*	promethazine
diphenhydramine	haloperidol	

*See Drug Class, Section Four.

TABLE 2

Drugs That May Cause Photosensitivity on Exposure to Sun

Some drugs are capable of sensitizing the skin to the action of ultraviolet light. This can cause uncovered areas of the skin to react with a rash or exaggerated burn on exposure to sun or ultraviolet lamps. If you are taking any of the following drugs, ask your physician for guidance and use caution with regard to sun exposure.

acetazolamide
acetohexamide
alprazolam
amantadine
amiloride
aminobenzoic acid
amiodarone
amitriptyline
amoxapine
barbiturates
bendroflumethiazide
benzocaine
benzoyl peroxide
benzophenones
benzthiazide
captopril
carbamazepine
chlordiazepoxide
chloroquine
chlorothiazide
chlorpromazine
chlorpropamide
chlortetracycline
chlorthalidone
ciprofloxacin
clindamycin
clofazimine
clofibrate
clomipramine
cyproheptadine
dacarbazine
dapsone
demeclocycline
desipramine
desoximetasone
diethylstilbestrol
diflunisal
diltiazem
diphenhydramine
disopyramide

doxepin
doxycycline
enoxacin
estrogen
etretinate
flucytosine
fluorescein
fluorouracil
fluphenazine
furosemide
flutamide
glipizide
glyburide
gold preparations
griseofulvin
haloperidol
hexachlorophene
hydrochlorothiazide
hydroflumethiazide
ibuprofen
imipramine
indomethacin
isotretinoin
ketoprofen
lincomycin
lomefloxacin
maprotiline
mesoridazine
methacycline
methotrexate
methyclothiazide
methyldopa
metolazone
minocycline
minoxidil
nabumetone
nalidixic acid
naproxen
nifedipine
norfloxacin

nortriptyline
ofloxacin
oral contraceptives
oxyphenbutazone
oxytetracycline
para amino benzoic acid
perphenazine
phenobarbital
phenylbutazone
phenylzine
phenytoin
piroxicam
polythiazide
prochlorperazine
promazine
promethazine
protriptyline
pyrazinamide
quinidine
quinine
sulfonamides
sulindac
tetracycline
thiabendazole
thioridazine
thiothixene
tolazamide
tolbutamide
tranylcypromine
trazodone
tretinoin
triamterene
trichlormethiazide
trifluoperazine
trifluopromazine
trimeprazine
trimethoprim
trimipramine
triprolidine
vinblastine

TABLE 3

Drugs That May Adversely Affect Behavior

In addition to producing side effects that can alter mood and disturb emotional stability, some drugs are capable of causing unexpected and unpredictable patterns of ab-

*See Drug Class, Section Four.

normal thinking and behavior. Such responses are relatively infrequent, but the nature and degree of mental disturbance can, at times, be quite alarming and potentially dangerous for both patient and family. It is now well recognized that such paradoxical responses are often of an idiosyncratic nature, and that someone with a history of a serious mental or emotional disorder is more likely to experience bizarre reactions involving disturbed behavior.

It is often difficult to judge whether a particular aberration of thought or behavior is primarily a feature of the disorder under treatment or an effect of one (or more) drugs the patient may be taking at the time. If in doubt, it is advisable to discontinue any drug with potential for such side effects and observe for changes during a drug-free period.

Drugs reported to impair *concentration* and/or *memory*

antihistamines*	isoniazid	primidone
antiparkinsonism drugs*	monoamine oxidase	scopolamine
barbiturates*	inhibitor drugs*	
benzodiazepines*	phenytoin	

Drugs reported to cause *confusion, delirium* or *disorientation*

acetazolamide	cycloserine	metoclopramide
aminophylline	digitalis	narcotic pain relievers
amphotericin B	digitoxin	(analgesics)
antidepressants*	digoxin	NSAIDs
antihistamines*	disulfiram	para-aminosalicylic acid
atropinelike drugs*	diuretics	phenelzine
antipsychotics	ethchlorvynol	phenothiazines*
barbiturates*	ethinamate	phenytoin
benzodiazepines*	fenfluramine	piperazine
bromides	glutethimide	primidone
carbamazepine	H2 receptor antagonists	propranolol
chloroquine	isoniazid	reserpine
cimetidine	levodopa	scopolamine
clonidine	meprobamate	theophylline
cortisonelike drugs*	methyldopa	tricyclic antidepressants

Drugs reported to cause *paranoid thinking*

bromides	diphenhydramine	isoniazid
cortisonelike drugs*	disulfiram	levodopa

Drugs reported to cause *schizophreniclike behavior*

amphetamines*	fenfluramine	phenylpropanolamine
ephedrine	phenmetrazine	

Drugs reported to cause *maniclike behavior*

antidepressants*	levodopa	inhibitor drugs*
cortisonelike drugs*	monoamine oxidase	

Less apparent—but no less important—are the mood-altering *side effects* of some drugs which are prescribed primarily for altogether unrelated conditions, with no intention of modifying emotional status. In keeping with the wide variation of individual response to the primary and intended effects of drugs, it is to be expected that emotional and behavioral secondary effects will also be quite unpredictable and will vary

*See Drug Class, Section Four.

enormously from person to person. However, the following experiences have been seen with sufficient frequency to establish recognizable patterns.

Drugs reported to cause *nervousness* (anxiety and irritability)

amantadine
amphetaminelike drugs*
   (appetite suppressants)
antihistamines*
caffeine
chlorphenesin
cortisonelike drugs*
ephedrine
epinephrine

isoproterenol
levodopa
liothyronine (in excessive
   dosage)
methylphenidate
methysergide
monoamine oxidase
   inhibitor drugs*
nylidrin

oral contraceptives
theophylline
thyroid (in excessive
   dosage)
thyroxine (in excessive
   dosage)

Drugs reported to cause *emotional depression*

amantadine
amphetamine* (on
   withdrawal)
benzodiazepines*
carbamazepine
chloramphenicol
cortisonelike drugs*
cycloserine
digitalis
digitoxin
digoxin
diphenoxylate

estrogens
ethionamide
fenfluramine (on
   withdrawal)
fluphenazine
guanethidine
haloperidol
indomethacin
isoniazid
levodopa
methsuximide
methyldopa

methysergide
metoprolol
oral contraceptives
phenylbutazone
procainamide
progesterones
propranolol
reserpine
sulfonamides*
vitamin D (in excessive
   dosage)

Drugs reported to cause *euphoria*

amantadine
aminophylline
amphetamines
antihistamines* (some)
antispasmodics, synthetic*
aspirin
barbiturates*
benzphetamine
chloral hydrate
clorazepate

codeine
cortisonelike drugs*
diethylpropion
diphenoxylate
ethosuximide
flurazepam
haloperidol
levodopa
meprobamate
methysergide

monoamine oxidase
   inhibitor drugs*
morphine
pargyline
pentazocine
phenmetrazine
propoxyphene
scopolamine
tybamate

Drugs reported to cause *excitement*

acetazolamide
amantadine
amphetaminelike drugs*
antidepressants*
antihistamines*
atropinelike drugs*
barbiturates* (paradoxical
   response)
benzodiazepines*
   (paradoxical response)
cortisonelike drugs
cycloserine

diethylpropion
digitalis
ephedrine
epinephrine
ethinamate (paradoxical
   response)
ethionamide
glutethimide (paradoxical
   response)
isoniazid
isoproterenol
levodopa

meperidine and MAO
   inhibitor drugs*
methyldopa and MAO
   inhibitor drugs*
methyprylon (paradoxical
   response)
nalidixic acid
orphenadrine
quinine
scopolamine

*See Drug Class, Section Four.

TABLE 4

Drugs That May Adversely Affect Vision

Approximately 3.5% of all adverse drug effects involve impairment of vision or eye damage. Some effects, such as blurring of vision or double vision, may occur shortly after starting a drug. These quickly disappear with adjustment of dosage. More subtle and serious effects, such as cataract development or damage to the retina or optic nerve, may not occur until a drug has been in continuous use for an extended period of time. Some of these changes are irreversible. If you are taking a drug that can affect the eye in any way, promptly report any eye discomfort or change in vision so that appropriate evaluation can be made and corrective action taken as soon as possible.

Drugs reported to cause *blurring of vision*

acetazolamide	chlorthalidone	norfloxacin
antiarthritic/anti-inflamm-	ciprofloxacin	oral contraceptives
atory drugs	cortisonelike drugs*	phenytoin
antidepressants*	diethylstilbestrol	sulfonamides*
antihistamines*	etretinate	tetracyclines*
atropinelike drugs*	fenfluramine	thiazide diuretics*

Drugs reported to cause *double vision*

antidepressants*	digitalis	nitrofurantoin
antidiabetic drugs*	digitoxin	norfloxacin
antihistamines*	digoxin	oral contraceptives
aspirin	ethionamide	orphenadrine
barbiturates*	ethosuximide	oxyphenbutazone
benzodiazepines*	etretinate	pentazocine
bromides	guanethidine	phenothiazines*
carbamazepine	hydroxychloroquine	phensuximide
carisoprodol	indomethacin	phenylbutazone
chloroquine	isoniazid	phenytoin
chlorprothixene	levodopa	primidone
ciprofloxacin	mephenesin	propranolol
clomiphene	methocarbamol	quinidine
colchicine	methsuximide	sedatives/sleep inducers*
colistin	morphine	thiothixene
cortisonelike drugs*	nalidixic acid	tranquilizers*

Drugs reported to cause *farsightedness*

ergot	sulfonamides* (possibly)
penicillamine	tolbutamide (possibly)

Drugs reported to cause *nearsightedness*

acetazolamide	ethosuximide	phensuximide
aspirin	methsuximide	spironolactone
carbachol	morphine	sulfonamides*
chlorthalidone	oral contraceptives	tetracyclines*
codeine	penicillamine	thiazide diuretics*
cortisonelike drugs*	phenothiazines*	

Drugs reported to *alter color vision*

acetaminophen	amyl nitrite	atropine
amodiaquine	aspirin	barbiturates*

*See Drug Class, Section Four.

Drugs reported to *alter color vision* (cont.)

belladonna
chloramphenicol
chloroquine
chlorpromazine
chlortetracycline
ciprofloxacin
cortisonelike drugs*
digitalis
digitoxin
digoxin
disulfiram
epinephrine
ergotamine
erythromycin
ethchlorvynol
ethionamide
fluphenazine
furosemide

hydroxychloroquine
indomethacin
isocarboxazid
isoniazid
mephenamic acid
mesoridazine
methysergide
nalidixic acid
norfloxacin
oral contraceptives
oxyphenbutazone
paramethadione
pargyline
penicillamine
pentylenetetrazol
perphenazine
phenacetin
phenylbutazone

primidone
prochlorperazine
promazine
promethazine
quinacrine
quinidine
quinine
reserpine
sodium salicylate
streptomycin
sulfonamides*
thioridazine
tranylcypromine
trifluoperazine
triflupromazine
trimeprazine
trimethadione

Drugs reported to cause *sensitivity to light* (photophobia)

antidiabetic drugs*
atropinelike drugs*
bromides
chloraquine
ciprofloxacin
clomiphene
digitoxin
doxepin
ethambutol

ethionamide
ethosuximide
etretinate
hydroxychloroquine
mephenytoin
methsuximide
monoamine oxidase
   inhibitor drugs*
nalidixic acid

norfloxacin
oral contraceptives
paramethadione
phenothiazines*
quinidine
quinine
tetracyclines*
trimethadione

Drugs reported to cause *halos around lights*

amyl nitrite
chloroquine
cortisonelike drugs*
digitalis
digitoxin

digoxin
hydrochloroquine
nitroglycerin
norfloxacin
oral contraceptives

paramethadione
phenothiazines*
quinacrine
trimethadione

Drugs reported to cause *visual hallucinations*

amantadine
amphetaminelike drugs*
amyl nitrite
antihistamines*
aspirin
atropinelike drugs*
barbiturates*
benzodiazepines*
bromides
carbamazepine
cephalexin
cephaloglycin
chloroquine
cycloserine

digitalis
digoxin
disulfiram
ephedrine
furosemide
griseofulvin
haloperidol
hydroxychloroquine
indomethacin
isosorbide
levodopa
nialamide
oxyphenbutazone
pargyline

pentazocine
phenothiazines*
phenylbutazone
phenytoin
primidone
propranolol
quinine
sedatives/sleep inducers*
sulfonamides*
tetracyclines*
tricyclic antidepressants*
tripelennamine

*See Drug Class, Section Four.

Drugs reported to impair the use of *contact lenses*

brompheniramine	dexbrompheniramine	furosemide
carbinoxamine	dexchlorpheniramine	oral contraceptives
chlorpheniramine	dimethindene	terfenadine
cyclizine	diphenhydramine	tripelennamine
cyproheptadine	diphenpyraline	

Drugs reported to cause *cataracts* or *lens deposits*

allopurinol	methotrimeprazine	thioridazine
busulfan	perphenazine	thiothixene
chlorpromazine	phenmetrazine	trifluoperazine
chlorprothixene	pilocarpine	triflupromazine
cortisonelike drugs*	prochlorperazine	trimeprazine
fluphenazine	promazine	
mesoridazine	promethazine	

TABLE 5

Drugs That May Cause Blood Cell Dysfunction or Damage

All blood cells originate and mature in the bone marrow. They arise from "stem" cells that have the ability to differentiate into specific cell lines that produce fully developed, distinctive blood cell forms: erythrocytes (red blood cells), leukocytes (white blood cells), thrombocytes (blood platelets); the leukocytes include three varieties: granulocytes, monocytes (macrophages), and lymphocytes. Drugs that adversely affect the formation and development of blood cells can (1) act on any stage of cell production; (2) impair the production of one cell line; (3) influence the production of all cell lines.

Through a variety of mechanisms, some medicinal drugs can adversely affect mature cells circulating in the blood stream. Examples can be found in the tables that follow.

Drugs that cause inevitable (dose-dependent) *aplastic anemia* (see Glossary)

actinomycin D	cytarabine	mercaptopurine
azathioprine	doxorubicin	methotrexate
busulphan	epirubicin	mitomycin
carboplatin	etoposide	mitozantrone
carmustine	fluorouracil	plicamycin
chlorambucil	hydroxyurea	procarbazine
cisplatin	lomustine	thioguanine
cyclophosphamide	melphalan	thiotepa

Drugs that may cause idiosyncratic (dose-independent) *aplastic anemia*

amodiaquine	mepacrine	pyrimethamine
benoxaprofen	oxyphenbutazone	sulfonamides*
carbimazole	penicillamine	sulindac
chloramphenicol	phenylbutazone	thiouracils
chlorpromazine	phenytoin	trimethoprim/sulfamethox-
gold	piroxicam	azole
indomethacin	prothiaden	

*See Drug Class, Section Four.

Drugs that may *impair red blood cell production* (only)

azathioprine
carbamazepine
chloramphenicol
chlorpropamide
dapsone
fenoprofen
gold
halothane

isoniazid
methyldopa
penicillin
pentachlorophenol
phenobarbital
phenylbutazone
phenytoin
pyrimethamine

sulfasalazine
sulfathiazide
sulfonamides*
sulfonylureas*
thiamphenicol
tolbutamide
trimethoprim/sulfamethox-
    azole

Drugs that may significantly *reduce granulocyte cell counts* (various mechanisms)

acetaminophen
acetazolamide
allopurinol
amitriptyline
amodiaquine
benzodiazepines*
captopril
carbamazepine
carbimazole
cephalosporins*
chloramphenicol
chloroquine
chlorothiazide
chlorpromazine
chlorpropamide
chlorthalidone
cimetidine
clindamycin
dapsone
desipramine

disopyramide
ethacrynic acid
fansidar
gentamicin
gold
hydralazine
hydrochlorothiazide
imipramine
indomethacin
isoniazid
levamisole
meprobamate
methimazole
methyldopa
oxyphenbutazone
penicillamine
penicillins*
pentazocine
phenacetin
phenothiazines*

phenylbutazone
phenytoin
procainamide
propranolol
propylthiouracil
pyrimethamine
quinidine
quinine
ranitidine
rifampin
sodium aminosalicylate
streptomycin
sulfadoxime
sulfonamides*
tetracyclines*
tocainide
tolbutamide
trimethoprim/sulfamethox-
    azole
vancomycin

Drugs that may significantly *reduce blood platelet counts*

acetazolamide
actinomycin
allopurinol
alpha-interferon
amiodarone
ampicillin
aspirin
carbamazepine
carbenicillin
cephalosporins*
chenodeoxycholic acid
chloroquine
chlorothiazide
chlorpheniramine
chlorpropamide
chlorthalidone
cimetidine
cyclophosphamide
danazol
desferrioxamine

diazepam
diazoxide
diclofenac
digoxin
diltiazem
furosemide
gentamicin
gold
hydrochlorothiazide
imipramine
isoniazid
isotretinoin
levamisole
meprobamate
methyldopa
mianserin
minoxidil
morphine
nitrofurantoin
oxprenolol

oxyphenbutazone
penicillamine
penicillin
phenylbutazone
phenytoin
piroxicam
procainamide
quinidine
quinine
ranitidine
rifampin
sodium aminosalicylate
sulfasalazine
sulfonamides*
thioguanine
trimethoprim/sulfamethox-
    azole
valproate
vancomycin

*See Drug Class, Section Four.

Drugs that cause significant *hemolytic anemia* due to glucose-6-phosphate dehydrogenase (G6PD) deficiency of red blood cells

acetanilid	pamaquine	sulfanilamide
methylene blue	phenazopyridine	sulfapyridine
nalidixic acid	phenylhydrazine	thiazosulfone
naphthalene	primaquine	toluidine blue
niridazole	sulfacetamide	
nitrofurantoin	sulfamethoxazole	

Drugs that may cause *hemolytic anemia* by other mechanisms

antimony	methotrexate	quinidine
chlorpropamide	para-aminosalicylic acid	quinine
cisplatin	penicillamine	rifampin
mephenesin	phenazopyridine	sulfasalazine

Drugs that may cause *megaloblastic anemia*

acyclovir	metformin	primidone
alcohol	methotrexate	pyrimethamine
aminopterin	neomycin	sulfasalazine
azathioprine	nitrofurantoin	tetracycline
colchicine	nitrous oxide	thioguanine
cycloserine	oral contraceptives	triamterene
cytarabine	para-aminosalicylic acid	trimethoprim
floxuridine	pentamidine	vinblastine
fluorouracil	phenformin	vitamin A
hydroxyurea	phenobarbital	vitamin C (large doses)
mercaptopurine	phenytoin	zidovudine

Drugs that may cause *sideroblastic anemia*

alcohol	isoniazid	pyrazinamide
chloramphenicol	penicillamine	
cycloserine	phenacetin	

TABLE 6

Drugs That May Cause Heart Dysfunction or Damage

Drugs of very diverse classes can adversely affect both the function and structure of the heart. Disorders of the heart (that require drug therapy) often determine the nature of adverse effects induced by drugs. Some adverse effects are due to direct pharmacological actions of a drug on heart tissues (as with antiarrhythmic drugs); while other reactions are caused indirectly by altering biochemical balances that influence heart function (as with excessive loss of potassium due to diuretics resulting in abnormal heart rhythms and digitalis toxicity).

Drugs that may cause or contribute to *abnormal heart rhythms* (arrhythmias)

aminophylline	beta-adrenergic blocking	chlorpromazine
amiodarone	drugs*	cimetidine
amitriptyline	beta-adrenergic	digitoxin
antiarrythmic drugs*	bronchodilators*	digoxin
bepridil	carbamazepine	diltiazem

*See Drug Class, Section Four.

Drugs that may cause or contribute to *abnormal heart rhythms* (arrhythmias) (cont.)

disopyramide	maprotiline	sotalol
diuretics*	methyldopa	terbutaline
doxepin	mexiletine	theophylline
encainide	milrinone	thiazide diuretics*
fentolterol	phenothiazines*	thioridazine
flecainide	prenylamine	trazodone
isoproterenol	procainamide	tricyclic antidepressants*
ketanserin	quinidine	verapamil
lidocaine	ranitidine	

Drugs that may *depress heart function* (reduce pumping efficiency)

beta-adrenergic blocking drugs*	disopyramide	isoproterenol
	doxorubicin	nifedipine
cocaine	epinephrine	verapamil
daunorubicin	flecainide	
diltiazem	fluorouracil	

Drugs that may *reduce coronary artery blood flow* (reduce oxygen supply to heart muscle)

amphetamines*	ergotamine	vasopressin
beta-adrenergic blocking drugs* (abrupt withdrawal)	fluorouracil	vinblastine
	nifedipine	vincristine
	oral contraceptives	
cocaine	ritodrine	

Drugs that may *impair healing of heart muscle* following heart attack (myocardial infarction)

adrenocortical steroids*	anti-inflammatory drugs
nonsteroidal	(NSAIDs)*

Drugs that may cause *heart valve damage*

ergotamine	minocycline (blue-black
methysergide	pigmentation)

Drugs that may cause *pericardial disease*

actinomycin D	cytarabine	phenylbutazone
anthracyclines	fluorouracil	practolol
bleomycin	hydralazine	procainamide
cisplatin	methysergide	sulfasalazine
cyclophosphamide	minoxidil	

TABLE 7

Drugs That May Cause Lung Dysfunction or Damage

Adverse drug reactions that directly affect the lung are often difficult to distinguish from natural diseases or disorders that involve lung function or structure. As with other organ systems, the lung is subject to both principal types of drug reactions: Type

*See Drug Class, Section Four.

A—those due to known and expected pharmacological drug actions; Type B—those due to unexpected and unpredictable allergic or idiosyncratic reactions on the part of the drug user.

Drugs that may adversely affect *blood vessels of the lung*

Drugs that may cause thrombo-embolism

estrogens*
oral contraceptives (high
  estrogen type)

Drugs that may cause pulmonary hypertension

amphetamines*	oral contraceptives
fenfluramine	tryptophan

Drugs that may cause vasculitis (blood vessel damage) with or without hemorrhage

aminoglutethimide	febarbamate	phenytoin
amphotericin	nitrofurantoin	
cocaine	penicillamine	

Drugs that may cause adult respiratory distress syndrome (ARDS)

bleomycin	heroin	naloxone
codeine	hydrochlorothiazide	ritodrine
cyclophosphamide	methadone	terbutaline
dextropropoxyphene	mitomycin	vinblastine

Drugs that may adversely affect the *bronchial tubes*

Drugs that may cause bronchoconstriction (asthma)

acetaminophen	griseofulvin	anti-inflammatory
aspirin	maprotiline	drugs*
beta-adrenergic blocking	methacholine	penicillins*
drugs*	methoxypsoralen	pilocarpine
carbachol	metoclopramide	propafenone
cephalosporins*	morphine	pyridostigmine
chloramphenicol	neomycin	streptomycin
deanol	neostigmine	tartrazine (coloring agent)
demeclocycline	nitrofurantoin	
erythromycin	nonsteroidal	

Drugs that may cause bronchiolitis (with permanent obstruction of small bronchioles)

penicillamine	sulfasalazine

Drugs that may *damage lung tissues*

Drugs that may cause acute allergic-type pneumonitis

ampicillin	cephalexin	gold
bleomycin	chlorpropamide	imipramine

*See Drug Class, Section Four.

Drugs that may cause acute allergic-type pneumonitis (cont.)

mephenesin	nitrofurantoin	penicillin
mercaptopurine	nomifensine	phenylbutazone
metformin	nonsteroidal	phenytoin
methotrexate	anti-inflammatory	procarbazine
metronidazole	drugs*	sulfonamides*
mitomycin	para-aminosalicylic acid	tetracycline
nalidixic acid	penicillamine	vinblastine

Drugs that may cause chronic pneumonitis and fibrosis (scarring)

amiodarone	ergotamine	pentolinium
bleomycin	gold	practolol
bromocriptine	hexamethonium	sulfasalazine
busulfan	mecamylamine	tocainide
carmustine	melphalan	tolfenamic acid
chlorambucil	methysergide	
cyclophosphamide	nitrofurantoin	

Drugs that may *damage the pleura*

bromocriptine	methysergide	practolol

TABLE 8

Drugs That May Cause Liver Dysfunction or Damage

The liver is the principal organ that converts drugs into forms that can be readily eliminated from the body. Given the diversity of drugs in use today and the complex burdens
they impose upon the liver, it is not surprising that a broad spectrum of adverse drug
effects on liver functions and structures has been documented. The reactions range
from mild and transient changes in the results of liver function tests to complete liver
failure and death. Many drugs may affect the liver adversely in more than one way, as
cited below in several listings. The use of the following drugs requires careful monitoring of their effects on the liver during the entire course of treatment.

Drugs that may cause *acute dose-dependent liver damage* (resembling acute viral hepatitis)

acetaminophen (overdose)
salicylates (doses over 2 grams daily)

Drugs that may cause *acute dose-independent liver damage* (resembling acute viral hepatitis)

acebutolol	enflurane	maprotiline
allopurinol	ethambutol	metoprolol
atenolol	ethionamide	mianserin
carbamazepine	halothane	naproxen
cimetidine	ibuprofen	nifedipine
dantrolene	indomethacin	para-aminosalicylic acid
diclofenac	isoniazid	penicillins*
diltiazem	ketoconazole	phenelzine
disulfiram	labetalol	phenindione

*See Drug Class, Section Four.

Drugs that may cause *acute dose-independent liver damage* (resembling acute viral hepatitis) (cont.)

phenobarbital
phenylbutazone
phenytoin
piroxicam
probenecid

pyrazinamide
quinidine
quinine
ranitidine
rifampin

sulfonamides*
sulindac
tricyclic antidepressants*
valproic acid
verapamil

Drugs that may cause *acute fatty infiltration of the liver*

adrenocortical steroids*
antithyroid drugs
isoniazid
methotrexate

phenothiazines*
phenytoin
salicylates*
sulfonamides*

tetracyclines*
valproic acid

Drugs that may cause *cholestatic jaundice*

actinomycin D
amoxicillin/clavulanate
azathioprine
captopril
carbamazepine
carbimazole
cephalosporins*
chlordiazepoxide
chlorpropamide
cloxacillin
cyclophosphamide
cyclosporine
danazol
diazepam
disopyramide
enalapril

erythromycin
flecainide
flurazepam
flutamide
glyburide
gold
griseofulvin
haloperidol
ketoconazole
mercaptopurine
methyltestosterone
nifedipine
nitrofurantoin
nonsteroidal
   anti-inflammatory
   drugs*

norethandrolone
oral contraceptives
oxacillin
penicillamine
phenothiazines*
phenytoin
propoxyphene
propylthiouracil
sulfonamides*
tamoxifen
thiabendazole
tolbutamide
tricyclic antidepressants*
troleandomycin
verapamil

Drugs that may cause *liver granulomas* (chronic inflammatory nodules)

allopurinol
aspirin
carbamazepine
chlorpromazine
chlorpropamide
diltiazem
disopyramide

gold
hydralazine
isoniazid
methyldopa
nitrofurantoin
penicillin
phenylbutazone

phenytoin
procainamide
quinidine
ranitidine
sulfonamides*
tolbutamide

Drugs that may cause *chronic liver disease*

Drugs that may cause active chronic hepatitis

acetaminophen (chronic
   use, large doses)

dantrolene
isoniazid

methyldopa
nitrofurantoin

Drugs that may cause liver cirrhosis or fibrosis (scarring)

methotrexate   nicotinic acid

*See Drug Class, Section Four.

Drugs that may cause chronic cholestasis (resembling primary biliary cirrhosis)

chlorpromazine/valproic acid (combination)	imipramine	tolbutamide
chlorpropamide/erythromycin (combination)	phenothiazines*	
	phenytoin	
	thiabendazole	

Drugs that may cause *liver tumors* (benign and malignant)

anabolic steroids	oral contraceptives	thorotrast
danazol	testosterone	

Drugs that may cause *damage to liver blood vessels*

adriamycin	dacarbazine	vincristine
anabolic steroids	mercaptopurine	vitamin A (excessive doses)
azathioprine	methotrexate	
carmustine	mitomycin	
cyclophosphamide/cyclosporine (combination)	oral contraceptives	
	thioguanine	

TABLE 9
Drugs That May Cause Kidney Dysfunction or Damage

With regard to medicinal drugs, the kidneys perform two major functions: (1) the alteration (biotransformation) of the drug to facilitate its processing; (2) the elimination of the drug from the body via the excretion of urine. As with drug effects on the liver, many drugs may adversely affect the kidneys in several ways. This is illustrated in the following tables by the appearance of some drug names in more than one listing. The kidneys are quite sensitive to the toxic effects of medicinal drugs. Vigilance and careful monitoring are always advisable during the course of treatment with any of the drugs cited below.

Drugs that may primarily *impair kidney function* (without damage)

amphotericin	demeclocycline	nifedipine
angiotensin converting enzyme inhibitors* (with renal artery stenosis; with congestive heart failure)	diuretics/NSAIDs* (avoid this combination)	nitroprusside
	glyburide	nonsteroidal anti-inflammatory drugs*
	isofosfamide	
beta-adrenergic blocking drugs*	lithium/tricyclic antidepressants* (avoid this combination)	rifampin
		vinblastine
colchicine	methoxyflurane	

Drugs that may cause *acute kidney failure* (due to kidney damage)

Drugs that may damage the kidney filtration unit (the nephron)

acetaminophen (excessive dosage)	bismuth thiosulfate	hydralazine
	carbamazepine	metronidazole
allopurinol	cisplatin	mitomycin
aminoglycoside antibiotics*	cyclosporine	oral contraceptives
	enalapril	penicillamine
amphotericin	ergometrine	phenytoin

*See Drug Class, Section Four.

Drugs that may damage the kidney filtration unit (the nephron) (cont.)

quinidine	streptokinase	thiazide diuretics*
rifampin	sulfonamides*	

Drugs that may cause acute interstitial nephritis

allopurinol	diclofenac	phenindione
amoxicillin	diflunisal	phenobarbital
ampicillin	fenoprofen	phenylbutazone
aspirin	foscarnet	phenytoin
azathioprine	furosemide	piroxicam
aztreonam	gentamicin	pirprofen
captopril	glafenine	pyrazinamide
carbamazepine	ibuprofen	rifampin
carbenicillin	indomethacin	sodium valproate
cefaclor	ketoprofen	sulfamethoxazole
cefoxitin	mefenamate	sulfinpyrazone
cephalexin	methicillin	sulfonamides*
cephalothin	methyldopa	sulindac
cephapirin	mezlocillin	thiazide diuretics*
cephradine	minocycline	tolmetin
cimetidine	nafcillin	trimethoprim
ciprofloxacin	naproxen	vancomycin
clofibrate	oxacillin	warfarin
cloxacillin	penicillamine	
diazepam	penicillin	

Drugs that may cause muscle destruction and associated acute kidney failure

adrenocortical steroids*	cocaine	opioid analgesics*
alcohol	cytarabine	pentamidine
amphetamines*	fenofibrate	phenothiazines*
amphotericin	haloperidol	streptokinase
carbenoxolone	halothane	suxamethonium
chlorthalidone	heroin	
clofibrate	lovastatin	

Drugs that may cause *kidney damage resembling glomerulonephritis or nephrosis*

captopril	lithium	practolol
fenoprofen	mesalamine	probenecid
gold	penicillamine	quinidine
ketoprofen	phenytoin	

Drugs that may cause *chronic interstitial nephritis and papillary necrosis* (analgesic kidney damage)

acetaminophen	phenacetin (all with
aspirin	long-term use)

Drugs that may cause or contribute to *urinary tract crystal or stone formation*

acetazolamide	cytotoxic drugs	magnesium trisilicate
acyclovir	dihydroxyadenine	mercaptopurine

*See Drug Class, Section Four.

Drugs that may cause or contribute to *urinary tract crystal or stone formation* (cont.)

methotrexate	sulfonamides*	vitamin C
methoxyflurane	thiazide diuretics*	vitamin D
phenylbutazone	triamterene	warfarin
probenecid	uricosuric drugs	zoxazolamine
salicylates*	vitamin A	

TABLE 10

Drugs That May Cause Nerve Dysfunction or Damage

Medicinal drugs may adversely affect any segment of the nervous system from the brain to peripheral nerves. There is wide variability in the patterns of response to drugs among people—in both therapeutic effects and unwanted adverse effects. Individual variability is determined largely by genetic programming of drug metabolism and responsiveness. The following scheme of classification groups drugs according to the familiar clinical syndromes that represent drug-induced neurological disorders.

Drugs that may cause *significant headache*

amyl nitrate	indomethacin	sulindac
bromocriptine	labetalol	terbutaline
clonidine	naproxen	tetracyclines*
ergotamine (prolonged use)	nifedipine	theophylline
etretinate	nitrofurantoin	tolmetin
hydralazine	nitroglycerin	trimethoprim/sulfamethoxazole
ibuprofen	perhexilene	
	propranolol	

Drugs that may cause *seizures* (convulsions)

ampicillin	ether	penicillins* (synthetic)
atenolol	halothane	phenothiazines*
carbenicillin	indomethacin	pyrimethamine
cephalosporins*	isoniazid	terbutaline
chloroquine	lidocaine	theophylline
cimetidine	lithium	ticarcillin
ciprofloxacin	mefenamic acid	tricyclic antidepressants*
cycloserine	nalidixic acid	vincristine
disopyramide	oxacillin	

Drugs that may cause *stroke*

anabolic steroids	oral contraceptives
cocaine	phenylpropanolamine

Drugs that may cause features of *parkinsonism*

amitriptyline	droperidol	phenothiazines*
amodiaquine	haloperidol	reserpine
chloroquine	imipramine	thiothixene
chlorprothixene	levodopa	trifluoperidol
desipramine	lithium	
diazoxide	methyldopa	
diphenhydramine	metoclopramide	

*See Drug Class, Section Four.

Drugs that may cause *acute dystonias* (acute involuntary movement syndromes—AIMS)

carbamazepine	metoclopramide	propranolol
chlorzoxazone	phenothiazines*	tricyclic antidepressants*
haloperidol	phenytoin	

Drugs that may cause *tardive dyskinesia* (see Glossary)

haloperidol	phenothiazines*	thiothixene

Drugs that may cause *neuroleptic malignant syndrome (NMS)*. See this term in the Glossary for a list of causative drugs.

Drugs that may cause *peripheral neuropathy* (see Glossary)

amiodarone	disulfiram	perhexiline
amitriptyline	ergotamine	phenelzine
amphetamines*	ethambutol	phenylbutazone
amphotericin	glutethimide	phenytoin
anticoagulants*	gold	podophyllin
carbutamide	hydralazine	procarbazine
chlorambucil	imipramine	propranolol
chloramphenicol	indomethacin	propylthiouracil
chloroquine	isoniazid	stavudine
chlorpropamide	methaqualone	streptomycin
cimetidine	methimazole	sulfonamides*
clioquinol	methysergide	sulfoxone
clofibrate	metronidazole	thalidomide
colchicine	nalidixic acid	tolbutamide
colistin	nitrofurantoin	vinblastine
cytarabine	nitrofurazone	vincristine
dapsone	penicillamine	
disopyramide	penicillin	

Drugs that may cause a *myasthenia gravis* syndrome

aminoglycoside antibiotics*	penicillamine
	phenytoin
beta-adrenergic blocking drugs*	polymyxin B
	trihexyphenidyl

TABLE 11

Drugs That May Adversely Affect Sexuality

It is well established that certain drugs have the potential for affecting sexual functions in a variety of unintended ways. Many commonly prescribed drugs can cause both obvious and subtle effects on one or more aspects of sexual expression. Patients are usually unaware that changes in sexual performance or response may be related to medications they are taking. If they suspect it, they are often reluctant to discuss the possible association with their physician. In some situations, the sexual dysfunction may be a natural consequence of the disorder under treatment or of a concurrent and undetected disorder, possibilities often overlooked by both practitioner and patient. It is well known that disorders such as diabetes, kidney failure, hypertension, depression and alcoholism may reduce libido and cause failure of erection. In

*See Drug Class, Section Four.

addition, many of the drugs used to treat these conditions may have the ability to augment a subclinical sexual dysfunction through unavoidable pharmacological activity. Such situations require the closest cooperation between therapist and patient in order to correctly assess the possible cause-and-effect relationships and to change therapy appropriately.

Possible Drug Effects on Male Sexuality

1. Increased libido
   androgens (replacement therapy in deficiency states)
   baclofen (Lioresal)
   chlordiazepoxide (Librium) (antianxiety effect)
   diazepam (Valium) (antianxiety effect)
   haloperidol (Haldol)
   levodopa (Larodopa, Sinemet) (may be an indirect effect due to improved sense
   of well-being)

2. Decreased libido
   antihistamines
   barbiturates
   chlordiazepoxide (Librium) (sedative effect)
   chlorpromazine (Thorazine) 10% to 20% of users
   cimetidine (Tagamet)
   clofibrate (Atromid-S)
   clonidine (Catapres), 10% to 20% of users
   danazol (Danocrine)
   diazepam (Valium) (sedative effect)
   disulfiram (Antabuse)
   estrogens (therapy for prostatic cancer)
   fenfluramine (Pondimin)
   heroin
   licorice
   medroxyprogesterone (Provera)
   methyldopa (Aldomet), 10% to 15% of users
   metoclopramide (Reglan), 80% of users
   perhexilene (Pexid)
   prazosin (Minipress), 15% of users
   propranolol (Inderal), rarely
   reserpine (Serpasil, Ser-Ap-Es)
   spironolactone (Aldactone)
   tricyclic antidepressants (TAD's)

3. Impaired erection (impotence)
   anticholinergics
   antihistamines
   baclofen (Lioresal)
   barbiturates (when abused)
   beta blockers (see Drug Class, Section Four)
   chlordiazepoxide (Librium) (in high dosage)
   chlorpromazine (Thorazine)
   cimetidine (Tagamet)
   clofibrate (Atromid-S)
   clonidine (Catapres), 10% to 20% of users
   cocaine
   diazepam (Valium) (in high dosage)
   digitalis and its glycosides
   disopyramide (Norpace)
   disulfiram (Antabuse) (uncertain)
   estrogens (therapy for prostatic cancer)

ethacrynic acid (Edecrin), 5% of users
ethionamide (Trecator-SC)
fenfluramine (Pondimin)
furosemide (Lasix), 5% of users
guanethidine (Ismelin)
haloperidol (Haldol) 10% to 20% of users
heroin
hydroxyprogesterone (therapy for prostatic cancer)
licorice
lithium (Lithonate)
marijuana
mesoridazine (Serentil)
methantheline (Banthine)
methyldopa (Aldomet), 10% to 15% of users
metoclopramide (Reglan), 60% of users
monoamine oxidase (MAO) type A inhibitors, 10% to 15% of users
perhexilene (Pexid)
prazosin (Minipres) infrequently
reserpine (Serpasil, Ser-Ap-Es)
spironolactone (Aldactone)
thiazide diuretics, 5% of users
thioridazine (Mellaril)
tricyclic antidepressants (TAD's)

4. Impaired ejaculation
anticholinergics
barbiturates (when abused)
chlorpromazine (Thorazine)
clonidine (Catapres)
estrogens (therapy for prostatic cancer)
guanethidine (Ismelin)
heroin
mesoridazine (Serentil)
methyldopa (Aldomet)
monoamine oxidase (MAO) type A inhibitors
phenoxybenzamine (Dibenzyline)
phentolamine (Regitine)
reserpine (Serpasil, Ser-Ap-Es)
thiazide diuretics
thioridazine (Mellaril)
tricyclic antidepressants (TAD's)

5. Decreased testosterone
adrenocorticotropic hormone (ACTH)
barbiturates
digoxin (Lanoxin)
haloperidol (Haldol)
—increased testosterone with low dosage
—decreased testosterone with high dosage
lithium (Lithonate)
marijuana
medroxyprogesterone (Provera)
monoamine oxidase (MAO) type A inhibitors
spironolactone (Aldactone)

6. Impaired spermatogenesis (reduced fertility)
adrenocorticosteroids (prednisone, etc.)
androgens (moderate to high dosage, extended use)
antimalarials

aspirin (abusive, chronic use)
chlorambucil (Leukeran)
cimetidine (Tagamet)
colchicine
co-trimoxazole (Bactrim, Septra)
cyclophosphamide (Cytoxan)
estrogens (therapy for prostatic cancer)
marijuana
medroxyprogesterone (Provera)
methotrexate
metoclopramide (Reglan)
monoamine oxidase (MAO) type A inhibitors
niridazole (Ambilhar)
nitrofurantoin (Furadantin)
spironolactone (Aldactone)
sulfasalazine (Azulfidine)
testosterone (moderate to high dosage, extended use)
vitamin C (in doses of 1 gram or more)

7. Testicular disorders
   Swelling
   —tricyclic antidepressants (TAD's)
   Inflammation
   —oxyphenbutazone (Tandearil)
   Atrophy
   —androgens (moderate to high dosage, extended use)
   —chlorpromazine (Thorazine)
   —cyclophosphamide (Cytoxan) (in prepubescent boys)
   —spironolactone (Aldactone)

8. Penile disorders
   Priapism (see Glossary)
   —anabolic steroids (male hormonelike drugs)
   —chlorpromazine (Thorazine)
   —cocaine
   —guanethidine (Ismelin)
   —haloperidol (Haldol)
   —heparin
   —levodopa (Sinemet)
   —molindone (Moban)
   —prazosin (Minipress)
   —prochlorperazine (Compazine)
   —trazodone (Desyrel)
   —trifluoperazine (Stelazine)
   —warfarin (Coumadin)
   Peyronie's disease (see Glossary)
   —beta blocker drugs (see Drug Class, Section Four)
   —phenytoin (Dilantin, etc.)

9. Gynecomastia (excessive development of the male breast)
   androgens (partial conversion to estrogen)
   BCNU
   busulfan (Myleran)
   chlormadinone
   chlorpromazine (Thorazine)
   chlortetracycline (Aureomycin)
   cimetidine (Tagamet)
   clonidine (Catapres) (infrequently)
   diethylstilbestrol (DES)

      digitalis and its glycosides
      estrogens (therapy for prostatic cancer)
      ethionamide (Trecator-SC)
      griseofulvin (Fulvicin, etc.)
      haloperidol (Haldol)
      heroin
      human chorionic gonadotropin
      isoniazid (INH, Nydrazid)
      marijuana
      mestranol
      methyldopa (Aldomet)
      metoclopramide (Reglan)
      phenelzine (Nardil)
      reserpine (Serpasil, Ser-Ap-Es)
      spironolactone (Aldactone)
      thioridazine (Mellaril)
      tricyclic antidepressants (TAD's)
      vincristine (Oncovin)

10. Feminization (loss of libido, impotence, gynecomastia, testicular atrophy)
      conjugated estrogens (Premarin, etc.)

11. Precocious puberty
      anabolic steroids
      androgens
      isoniazid (INH)

Possible Drug Effects on Female Sexuality

1. Increased libido
      androgens
      chlordiazepoxide (Librium) (antianxiety effect)
      diazepam (Valium) (antianxiety effect)
      mazindol (Sanorex)
      oral contraceptives (freedom from fear of pregnancy)

2. Decreased libido
      See list of drug effects on male sexuality. Some of these *may* have potential for
      reducing libido in the female. The literature is sparse on this subject.

3. Impaired arousal and orgasm
      anticholinergics
      clonidine (Catapres)
      methyldopa (Aldomet)
      monoamine oxidase inhibitors (MAOI's)
      tricyclic antidepressants (TAD's)

4. Breast enlargement
      penicillamine
      tricyclic antidepressants (TAD's)

5. Galactorrhea (spontaneous flow of milk)
      amphetamine
      chlorpromazine (Thorazine)
      cimetidine (Tagamet)
      haloperidol (Haldol)
      heroin
      methyldopa (Aldomet)
      metoclopramide (Reglan)
      oral contraceptives

    phenothiazines
    reserpine (Serpasil, Ser-Ap-Es)
    sulpiride (Equilid)
    tricyclic antidepressants (TAD's)

6. Ovarian failure (reduced fertility)
    anesthetic gases (operating room staff)
    cyclophosphamide (Cytoxan)
    cytostatic drugs
    danazol (Danacrine)
    medroxyprogesterone (Provera)

7. Altered menstruation (menstrual disorders)
    adrenocorticosteroids (prednisone, etc.)
    androgens
    barbiturates (when abused)
    chlorambucil (Leukeran)
    chlorpromazine (Thorazine)
    cyclophosphamide (Cytoxan)
    danazol (Danocrine)
    estrogens
    ethionamide (Trecator-SC)
    haloperidol (Haldol)
    heroin
    isoniazid (INH, Nydrazid)
    marijuana
    medroxprogesterone (Provera)
    metoclopramide (Reglan)
    oral contraceptives
    phenothiazines
    progestins
    radioisotopes
    rifampin (Rifadin, Rifamate, Rimactane)
    spironolactone (Aldactone)
    testosterone
    thioridazine (Mellaril)
    vitamin A (in excessive dosage)

8. Virilization (acne, hirsutism, lowering of voice, enlargement of clitoris)
    anabolic drugs
    androgens
    haloperidol (Haldol)
    oral contraceptives (lowering of voice)

9. Precocious puberty
    estrogens (in hair lotions)
    isoniazid (INH, Nydrazid)

TABLE 12

Drugs That May Interact With Alcohol

Beverages containing alcohol may interact unfavorably with a wide variety of drugs. The most important (and most familiar) interaction occurs when the depressant action on the brain of sedatives, sleep-inducing drugs, tranquilizers and narcotic drugs is intensified by alcohol. Alcohol may also reduce the effectiveness of some drugs, and it can interact with certain other drugs to produce toxic effects. Some drugs may increase the intoxicating effects of alcohol, producing further impairment of mental alertness, judgment, physical coordination and reaction time.

While drug interactions with alcohol are generally predictable, the intensity and significance of these interactions can vary greatly from one person to another and from one occasion to another. This is because many factors influence what happens when drugs and alcohol interact. These factors include individual variations in sensitivity to drugs (including alcohol), the chemistry and quantity of the drug, the type and amount of alcohol consumed and the sequence in which drug and alcohol are taken. If you need to use any of the drugs listed in the following tables, you should ask your physician for help concerning the use of alcohol.

Drugs with which it is advisable to avoid alcohol completely

Drug name or class	Possible interaction with alcohol
amphetamines	excessive rise in blood pressure with alcoholic beverages containing tyramine**
antidepressants*	excessive sedation, increased intoxication
barbiturates*	excessive sedation
bromides	confusion, delirium, increased intoxication
calcium carbamide	disulfiramlike reaction**
carbamazepine	excessive sedation
chlorprothixene	excessive sedation
chlorzoxazone	excessive sedation
disulfiram	disulfiram reaction**
ergotamine	reduced effectiveness of ergotamine
fenfluramine	excessive stimulation of nervous system with some beers and wines
furazolidone	disulfiramlike reaction**
haloperidol	excessive sedation
MAO inhibitor drugs*	excessive rise in blood pressure with alcoholic beverages containing tyramine**
meperidine	excessive sedation
meprobamate	excessive sedation
methotrexate	increased liver toxicity and excessive sedation
metronidazole	disulfiramlike reaction**
narcotic drugs	excessive sedation
oxyphenbutazone	increased stomach irritation and/or bleeding
pentazocine	excessive sedation
pethidine	excessive sedation
phenothiazines*	excessive sedation
phenylbutazone	increased stomach irritation and/or bleeding
procarbazine	disulfiramlike reaction**
propoxyphene	excessive sedation
reserpine	excessive sedation, orthostatic hypotension**
sleep-inducing drugs (hypnotics) —carbromal —chloral hydrate	excessive sedation

*See Drug Class, Section Four.
**See Glossary.

Drug name or class	Possible interaction with alcohol
—ethchlorvynol	
—ethinamate	
—glutethimide	
—flurazepam	
—methaqualone	
—methyprylon	
—temazepam	
—triazolam	
thiothixene	excessive sedation
tricyclic antidepressants*	excessive sedation, increased intoxication
trimethobenzamide	excessive sedation

Drugs with which alcohol should be used only in small amounts (use cautiously until combined effects have been determined)

Drug name or class	Possible interaction with alcohol
acetaminophen (Tylenol, etc.)	increased liver toxicity
amantadine	excessive lowering of blood pressure
antiarthritic/anti-inflammatory drugs	increased stomach irritation and/or bleeding
anticoagulants (coumarins)*	increased anticoagulant effect
antidiabetic drugs (sulfonylureas)*	increased antidiabetic effect, excessive hypoglycemia**
antihistamines*	excessive sedation
antihypertensives*	excessive orthostatic hypotension**
aspirin (large doses or continuous use)	increased stomach irritation and/or bleeding
benzodiazepines*	excessive sedation
carisoprodol	increased alcoholic intoxication
diethylpropion	excessive nervous system stimulation with alcoholic beverages containing tyramine**
dihydroergotoxine	excessive lowering of blood pressure
diphenoxylate	excessive sedation
dipyridamole	excessive lowering of blood pressure
diuretics*	excessive orthostatic hypotension**
ethionamide	confusion, delirium, psychotic behavior
fenoprofen	increased stomach irritation and/or bleeding
griseofulvin	flushing and rapid heart action
ibuprofen	increased stomach irritation and/or bleeding
indomethacin	increased stomach irritation and/or bleeding
insulin	excessive hypoglycemia**
iron	excessive absorption of iron
isoniazid	decreased effectiveness of isoniazid, increased incidence of hepatitis
lithium	increased confusion and delirium (avoid all alcohol if any indication of lithium overdosage)
methocarbamol	excessive sedation
methotrimeprazine	excessive sedation

*See Drug Class, Section Four.
**See Glossary.

Drug name or class	Possible interaction with alcohol
methylphenidate	excessive nervous system stimulation with alcoholic beverages containing tyramine**
metoprolol	excessive orthostatic hypotension**
nalidixic acid	increased alcoholic intoxication
naproxen	increased stomach irritation and/or bleeding
nicotinic acid	possible orthostatic hypotension**
nitrates* (vasodilators)	possible orthostatic hypotension**
nylidrin	increased stomach irritation
orphenadrine	excessive sedation
phenelzine	increased alcoholic intoxication
phenoxybenzamine	possible orthostatic hypotension**
phentermine	excessive nervous system stimulation with alcoholic beverages containing tyramine**
phenytoin	decreased effect of phenytoin
pilocarpine	prolongation of alcohol effect
prazosin	excessive lowering of blood pressure
primidone	excessive sedation
propranolol	excessive orthostatic hypotension**
sulfonamides*	increased alcoholic intoxication
sulindac	increased stomach irritation and/or bleeding
tolmetin	increased stomach irritation and/or bleeding
tranquilizers (mild) —chlordiazepoxide —clorazepate —diazepam —hydroxyzine —meprobamate —oxazepam —phenaglycodol —tybamate	excessive sedation
tranylcypromine	increased alcoholic intoxication

Drugs capable of producing a disulfiramlike reaction** when used concurrently with alcohol

antidiabetic drugs (sulfonylureas)*	disulfiram	procarbazine
calcium carbamide	furazolidone	quinacrine
chloral hydrate	metronidazole	sulfonamides*
chloramphenicol	nifuroxine	tinidazole
	nitrofurantoin	tolazoline

TABLE 13

High-Potassium Foods

Diuretic drugs that cause loss of potassium from the body are often used to treat conditions that also require a reduced intake of sodium. The high-potassium foods listed

*See Drug Class, Section Four.
**See Glossary.

below have been selected for their compatibility with a sodium restricted diet (500 to 1000 mg of sodium daily).

Beverages

orange juice	skim milk	tomato juice
prune juice	tea	whole milk

Breads and Cereals

brown rice	muffins	waffles
cornbread	oatmeal	
griddle cakes	shredded wheat	

Fruits

apricot	fig	orange
avocado	honeydew melon	papaya
banana	mango	prune

Meats

beef	haddock	rockfish
chicken	halibut	salmon
codfish	liver	turkey
flounder	pork	veal

Vegetables

baked beans	parsnips	tomato
lima beans	radishes	white potato
mushrooms	squash	
navy beans	sweet potato	

TABLE 14
Your Personal Drug Profile

Knowing as much as possible about your body and your medicines can save your life. Please take the time to fill out this profile with the latest information.

Name:

Age:

Weight in kilograms: (pounds divided by 2.2)

Height in inches:

Prescription drug allergies:

Nonprescription drug allergies:

Food allergies:

My kidneys* are: normal_____

mildly_____   moderately_____   severely_____   compromised.

My liver* is: normal_____

mildly_____   moderately_____   severely_____   compromised.

Conditions or diseases that I have or have had:

Prescription and nonprescription medications I take regularly:

Make certain your dose is decreased if the drug is eliminated by an organ (such as the liver or kidneys) with which you have a problem. To determine which organs are involved, refer to the drug profile and "Conditions Requiring Dosing Adjustments" section for each medication you are taking.

Prescription and nonprescription medications I take periodically:

I find it very difficult_____
                     to remember to take medicines.
I find it very easy_____

I become constipated rarely_____   occasionally_____   never_____ .

Urination is usually easy_____   rather difficult_____   difficult_____ .

The phone number of the nearest Poison Control Center is _____ .

I sleep well_____   OK_____   poorly_____   little_____   on most nights.

I have_____   have never_____   had blood problems in the past.

I am considering becoming_____   might be_____   am_____   pregnant.

   I want the medications which offer the best balance of **price** and **outcomes** for my specific medical history and present conditions.

Sources

The following sources were consulted in the compilation and revision of this book:

Adverse Drug Reaction Bulletin. Edited by D. M. Davies. Meditext, Weybridge, Surrey, United Kingdom, 1992.

AMA Department of Drugs, *AMA Drug Evaluations*, Chicago: American Medical Association, 1992.

Andreoli, T. E., Carpenter, C. C. J., Plum, F., Smith, L. H., eds., *Cecil Essentials of Medicine.* Philadelphia: W. B. Saunders Co., 1986.

Arndt, K. A., *Manual of Dermatologic Therapeutics*, 4th ed. Boston: Little, Brown and Co., 1989.

Atkinson, A. J., Ambre, J. J., *Kalman and Clark's Drug Assay, The Strategy of Therapeutic Drug Monitoring*, 2nd ed. New York: Masson Publishing USA, 1985.

Avery, G. S., ed., *Drug Treatment*, 2nd ed. Sydney, Australia: ADIS Press, 1980.

Bartlett, John, *Medical Management of HIV*, 1996

Berkow, R., ed., *The Merck Manual*, 15th ed. Rahway, New Jersey: Merck Sharp & Dohme Research Laboratories, 1987.

Billups, N. F., ed., *American Drug Index 1992*, 36th ed. St. Louis: Facts and Comparisons, 1992.

Branch, W. T., *Office Practice of Medicine*, 2nd ed. Philadelphia: W. B. Saunders Co., 1987.

Briggs, G. G., Bodendorfer, T. W., Freeman, R. K., Yaffee, S. J., *Drugs in Pregnancy and Lactation.* Baltimore: Williams & Wilkins, 1983.

Brooke, M. H., *A Clinician's View of Neuromuscular Diseases*, 2nd ed. Baltimore: Williams & Wilkins, 1986.

Canadian Pharmaceutical Association, St. Paul's Hospital British Columbia Center of Excellence for HIV—AIDS, 1996.

Canadian Pharmaceutical Association, *Compendium of Pharmaceuticals and Specialties*, 26th ed. Ottawa: Canadian Pharmaceutical Association, 1991.

Cape, Ronald, *Aging: Its Complex Management.* Hagerstown, Maryland: Harper & Row, 1978.

Clin-Alert. Medford, New Jersey: Clin-Alert, Inc., 1989–1992.

Davies, D. M., ed., *Textbook of Adverse Drug Reactions*, 4th ed. New York: Oxford University Press, 1991.

Diamond, S., Dalessio, D. J., eds., *The Practicing Physician's Approach to Headache*, 4th ed. Baltimore: Williams & Wilkins, 1986.

DrugDex, CD-ROM 1996 edition.

Drug Interaction Facts. Edited by D. S. Tatro. St. Louis: Facts and Comparisons Division, J. B. Lippincott Co., 1995.

Drug Interactions Newsletter. Edited by P. D. Hansten, J. R. Horn. Spokane, Washington: Applied Therapeutics, Inc., 1996.

Drug Newsletter. Edited by B. R. Olin. St. Louis: Facts and Comparisons Division, J. B. Lippincott Co., 1996.

Drug Therapy, Physicians Prescribing Update. Lawrenceville, NJ: Excerpta Medica, 1992.

Dukes, M. N. G., ed., *Meyler's Side Effects of Drugs*, 11th ed. Amsterdam: Excerpta Medica, 1988.

Encyclopedia of Associations, 26th ed., Vol. 1, Part 2, Section 8. Detroit: Gale Research, Inc., 1992.

Facts and Comparisons. Edited by B. R. Olin. St. Louis: Facts and Comparisons Division, J. B. Lippincott Co., 1996.

F.D.A. Drug Bulletin. Rockville, Maryland: Department of Health and Human Services, Food and Drug Administration.

Fraunfelder, F. T., *Drug-Induced Ocular Side Effects and Drug Interactions*, 3rd ed. Philadelphia: Lea & Febiger, 1989.

Goodman, L. S., Gilman, A., eds., *The Pharmacological Basis of Therapeutics*, 8th ed. New York: Macmillan, 1990.

Greenberger, N. J., Arvanitakis, C., Hurwitz, A., *Drug Treatment of Gastrointestinal Disorders*. New York: Churchill Livingstone, 1978.

Handbook of Clinical Pharmacy, 1995.

Hansten, P. D., *Drug Interactions*, 6th ed. Philadelphia: Lea & Febiger, 1992.

Heinonen, O. P., Slone, D., Shapiro, S., *Birth Defects and Drugs in Pregnancy*. Littleton, Massachusetts: PSG Publishing Co., 1977.

Hollister, L. E., *Clinical Pharmacology of Psychotherapeutic Drugs*, 2nd ed. New York: Churchill Livingstone, 1983.

Huff, B. B., ed., *The Physicians' Desk Reference*, 46th ed. Oradell, New Jersey: Medical Economics Company, 1996.

International Drug Therapy Newsletter. Edited by F. J. Ayd. Baltimore: Ayd Medical Communications, 1995.

Jefferson, J. W., Greist, J. H., *Primer of Lithium Therapy*. Baltimore: Williams & Wilkens, 1977.

Journal of the American Medical Association. Edited by G. D. Lundberg. Chicago: American Medical Association, 1995.

Klippel, J. H., ed., Systemic Lupus Erythematosus. *Rheumatic Disease Clinics of North America*, Vol. 14, No. 1, April, 1988. Philadelphia: W. B. Saunders Co.

Koda-Kimbal, *Rational Therapeutics* 1994

Koller, W. C., ed., *Handbook of Parkinson's Disease*. New York: Marcel Dekker, 1987.

Kolodny, R. C., Masters, W. H., Johnson, V. E., *Textbook of Sexual Medicine*. Boston: Little, Brown and Co., 1979.

Lawrence, R. A., *Breast-Feeding*. St. Louis: Mosby, 1980.

Lieberman, M. L., *The Sexual Pharmacy*. New York: New American Library, 1988.

Long, J. W., *Clinical Management of Prescription Drugs*. Philadelphia: Harper & Row, 1984.

McEvoy, G. K., ed., *American Hospital Formulary Service, Drug Information 1995*. Bethesda, Maryland: American Society of Hospital Pharmacists, 1995.

Maddin, S., ed., *Current Dermatologic Therapy*. Philadelphia: W. B. Saunders Co., 1982.

The Medical Letter on Drugs and Therapeutics. Edited by H. Aaron. New Rochelle, New York: The Medical Letter, Inc., 1996.

Melmon, K. L., Morrelli, H. F., *Clinical Pharmacology*, 2nd ed. New York: Macmillan, 1978.

Messerli, F. H., ed., *Current Clinical Practice*. Philadelphia: W. B. Saunders Co., 1987.

Mohler, S. R., *Medication and Flying: A Pilot's Guide*. Boston: Boston Publishing Co., 1982.

The New England Journal of Medicine. Edited by J. P. Kassirer. Boston: The Massachusetts Medical Society, 1996.

Patient Drug Facts. Edited by B. R. Olin. St. Louis: Facts and Comparisons Division, J. B. Lippincott Co., 1992.

Postgraduate Medicine, The Journal of Applied Medicine for the Primary Care Physician. Minneapolis: McGraw-Hill, Inc., 1992.

Raj, P. P., *Practical Management of Pain.* Chicago: Year Book Medical Publishers, Inc., 1986.

Rakel, R. E., ed., *Conn's Current Therapy 1992.* Philadelphia: W. B. Saunders Co., 1992.

Rational Drug Therapy, Pharmacology for Physicians. Bethesda, Maryland: American Society for Pharmacology and Experimental Therapeutics, 1990.

Reynolds, J. E. F., ed., *Martindale, The Extra Pharmacopoeia,* 29th ed. London: The Pharmaceutical Press, 1995.

Rodman, M. J., Smith, D. W., *Clinical Pharmacology in Nursing.* Philadelphia: J. B. Lippincott Co., 1984.

Rogers, C. S., McCue, J. D., eds., *Managing Chronic Disease.* Oradell, New Jersey: Medical Economics Books, 1987.

Sauer, G. C., *Manual of Skin Diseases,* 5th ed. Philadelphia: J. B. Lippincott Co., 1985.

Schardein, J. L., *Drugs As Teratogens.* Cleveland: CRC Press, 1976.

Scientific American Medicine, CD-ROM edition 1996.

Shepard, T. H., *Catalog of Teratogenic Agents,* 6th ed. Baltimore: Johns Hopkins University Press, 1989.

Smith, L. H., Thier, S. O., *Pathophysiology, The Biological Principles of Disease,* 2nd ed. Philadelphia: W. B. Saunders Co., 1985.

Speight, T. M., ed., *Avery's Drug Treatment,* 3rd ed. Auckland: ADIS Press, 1987.

Swash, M., Schwartz, M. S., *Neuromuscular Diseases,* 2nd ed. Berlin: Springer-Verlag, 1988.

Tuchmann-Duplessis, H., *Drug Effects on the Fetus.* Sydney, Australia: ADIS Press, 1975.

USAN 1989 and the USP Dictionary of Drug Names. Edited by M. C. Griffiths. Rockville, Maryland: United States Pharmacopeial Convention, Inc., 1988.

USP Dispensing Information 1995, 12th ed., Vol. 1, *Drug Information for the Health Care Provider.* Rockville, Maryland: United States Pharmacopeial Convention, 1995.

Utian, W. H., *Menopause in Modern Perspective.* New York: Appleton-Century-Crofts, 1980.

Wallach, J., *Interpretation of Diagnostic Tests,* 5th ed. Boston: Little, Brown & Co., 1992.

Wartak, J., *Drug Dosage and Administration.* Baltimore: University Park Press, 1983.

Worley, R. J., ed., *Clinical Obstetrics and Gynecology,* Vol. 24, No. 1: *Menopause.* Hagerstown, Maryland: Harper & Row, 1981.

Young, D. S., *Effects of Drugs on Clinical Laboratory Tests, 1991 Supplement.* Washington: AACC Press, 1991.

Index

This index contains all the brand and generic drug names included in Section Two.

Brand names of drugs appear in italic type and are capitalized.

Each brand name is followed by its generic name, the generic name is the name under which you'll find the drug profile in Section Two.

The symbol [CD] indicates that the brand name represents a combination drug that contains the generic drug components listed below it. To be fully familiar with any combination drug [CD], it is necessary to read the Drug Profile of each of the components listed. The brand name of a combination drug *may* or *may not* appear in the brand name list of each Drug Profile that is cited in the index as a component of a particular combination drug. The index listing of component drugs for any combination drug product represents the manufacturer's formulation of that brand at the time this information was compiled for publication.

The symbol ✤ before the brand name of a combination drug indicates that the brand name is used in both the United States and Canada, but that the ingredients in the combination product in each country differ. The Canadian drug is marked with the symbol ✤ to distinguish it from the American drug which has the same name.

A generic name with no page designation indicates an active component of a combination drug for which there is no Profile in Section Two. It is included to alert you to its presence, should you wish to consult your physician regarding its significance.

A & D with prednisolone
 [CD]:
 prednisolone, 0.5%, 824
 Vitamin A, 1,500 units/G*
 Vitamin D, 200 units/G*
A.B.C. compound with
 codeine [CD]:
 codeine, 258
Abitrexate, methotrexate, 626
acarbose, 22, 27
AC & C [CD]:
 aspirin,98
 codeine, 258
Accopain, codeine, 258
Accupril, quinapril, 875
Accurbron, theophylline, 964
Accutane, isotretinoin, 533
acebutolol, 31
Acetaminophen-PM,
 diphenhydramine, 314
♣*Acet-Am,* theophylline, 964
♣*Acetazolam,* acetazolamide,
 35
acetazolamide, 35
acetic acids, 39
acetylsalicylic acid. *See*
 aspirin, 22, 98.
Aches-N-Pain, ibuprofen, 499,
 848
Achromycin, tetracycline, 959
Achromycin V, tetracycline,
 959
♣*Acrocidin,* tetracycline, 959
Acroseb-Dex, dexamethasone,
 286
Actagen-C [CD]:
 codeine, 258
 pseudoephedrine*
 triprolidine*

Actifed w/Codeine [CD]:
 codeine, 258
 pseudoephdrine*
 triprolidine*
♣*Actiprofen,* ibuprofen, 499,
 848
Actisite, tetracycline, 959
Actron, ketoprofen, 544, 848
Acular, ketorolac ophthalmic,
 39
acycloguanosin. *See*
 acyclovir,45.
acyclovir, 45
Adalat, nifedipine, 713
Adalat CC, nifedipine, 713
♣*Adalat FT,* nifedipine, 713
♣*Adalat P.A.,* nifedipine, 713
Adapin, doxepin, 333
Adrenaline, epinephrine,
 345
Adreno-Mist, epinephrine,
 345
Adsorbocarpine, pilocarpine,
 806
Advil, ibuprofen, 499, 848
A.E.A., theophylline, 964
Aerobid, flunisolide, 412
Aerobid-M, flunisolide, 412
Aerolate, theophylline, 964
Aeromax, salmeterol, 900
Afed-C [CD]:
 codeine, 258
 guifenesin*
 pseudoephedrine*
 triprolidine*
Akarpine, pilocarpine, 806
Ak-Chlor, chloramphenicol,
 200
♣*Ak-Cide [CD]:*

 prednisolone, 824
 sulfacetamide*
♣*Ak-Dex,* dexamethasone, 286
AK-Mycin Ophthalmic,
 erythromycin, 353
Akne-Mycin, erythromycin,
 353
♣*Ak-Pred,* prednisolone, 824
♣*Ak-Tate,* prednisolone, 824
Ak-Trol [CD]:
 dexamethasone, 286
 neomycin*
 polymixin B*
Ak-Zol, acetazolamide, 35
Alamine-C [CD]:
 chlorpheniramine*
 codeine, 258
 phenylpropanolamine*
Alamine Expectorant [CD]:
 codeine, 258
Alatone, spironolactone, 914
Alazine, hydralazine, 486
♣*Albert Furosemide,* 444
♣*Albert-Glyburide,* 464
albuterol, 48
alcohol. *See* ethanol, 366.
Aldactazide [CD]:
 hydrochlorothiazide, 487,
 970
 spironolactone, 914
Aldactone, spironolactone,
 914
Aldochlor [CD]:
 chlorothiazide, 208, 970
 methyldopa*
Aldoril-15/25 [CD]:
 hydrochlorothiazide, 487,
 970
 methyldopa*

*The symbol [CD] indicates that the brand name given is a combination drug consisting of generic drug
components listed below it. If there is no page numbering following the name of the generic drug component, there is no Drug Profile for that ingredient in this book.

*The symbol [CD] indicates that the brand name given is a combination drug consisting of generic drug components listed below it. If there is no page numbering following the name of the generic drug component, there is no Drug Profile for that ingredient in this book.

---

*The symbol [CD] indicates that the brand name given is a combination drug consisting of generic drug components listed below it. If there is no page numbering following the name of the generic drug component, there is no Drug Profile for that ingredient in this book.

---

*The symbol [CD] indicates that the brand name given is a combination drug consisting of generic drug components listed below it. If there is no page numbering following the name of the generic drug component, there is no Drug Profile for that ingredient in this book.

*The symbol [CD] indicates that the brand name given is a combination drug consisting of generic drug components listed below it. If there is no page numbering following the name of the generic drug component, there is no Drug Profile for that ingredient in this book.

*The symbol [CD] indicates that the brand name given is a combination drug consisting of generic drug components listed below it. If there is no page numbering following the name of the generic drug component, there is no Drug Profile for that ingredient in this book.

*The symbol [CD] indicates that the brand name given is a combination drug consisting of generic drug components listed below it. If there is no page numbering following the name of the generic drug component, there is no Drug Profile for that ingredient in this book.

---

*The symbol [CD] indicates that the brand name given is a combination drug consisting of generic drug components listed below it. If there is no page numbering following the name of the generic drug component, there is no Drug Profile for that ingredient in this book.

---

*The symbol [CD] indicates that the brand name given is a combination drug consisting of generic drug components listed below it. If there is no page numbering following the name of the generic drug component, there is no Drug Profile for that ingredient in this book.

About the Authors

JAMES J. RYBACKI, Pharm. D., was born in Oneonta, New York. He received his prepharmacy education at Creighton University, and his Doctor of Pharmacy degree from the University of Nebraska Medical Center, College of Pharmacy, in Omaha. More than 24 years of hospital experience have included early efforts in gas-liquid chromatography research characterizing human drug metabolites, and data collection for the College of American Pathologists to establish normal values for laboratory studies. He is a member of the clinical faculty at the University of Maryland School of Pharmacy and has provided clinical rounding and hospital experience for Pharm. D. and Bachelor students at Dorchester General Hospital. He presently teaches a Drug Information rotation for Pharm. D. students at The Clearwater Group. He is board certified in pain management at the Diplomat level by the American Academy of Pain Management, and provides ongoing clinical pain management consulting. Dr. Rybacki is actively involved in the postmarketing monitoring of medicines via The Drug Surveillance Network, a nationwide association of clinical pharmacists, and he is an approved External New Drug Application reviewer for the Canadian Drug Ministry. He lives in Easton, Maryland.

Dr. Rybacki's efforts in drug information and clinical pharmacy include eight years of active practice, which were at Dorchester General Hospital in Cambridge, Maryland, including infectious disease, pharmacokinetic, nutrition support, pain management, and pharmacological consultations at Dorchester General Hospital. Through the Occupational Health Unit, he has offered independent pain management and pharmacological consultations nationwide. He has also advised the World Health Organization's Expert Committee regarding revisions as well as selection of drugs to be listed in the next edition of *The Use of Essential Drugs* and is an assistant editor for the Drugdex drug information system. His past role as Vice President Clinical Services has bought him added expertise in overseeing Occupational Health, Physical Medicines, Laboratory Services, Imaging, Cardiology, Respiratory Therapy, Cancer Programs, and Continuing Medical Education. He has served as conference coordinator for the first and second annual Dorchester General Hospital Pain conferences, and served as seminar coordinator for the Eastern Shore of Maryland for the "Take Control" physician and public pain education programs with Johns Hopkins.

Dr. Rybacki is president of The Clearwater Group, and provides drug information support and clinical pharmacy rounding to physician groups and employers; holds seminars on medical cost containment, infectious disease, pain management, and therapeutics; provides information support to insuranc companies, HMOs, and the legal profession; produces educational tapes on me cines; and conducts independent pharmacological evaluations. He was sele for full membership in the American College of Clinical Pharmacy, and is a fied Densitometrist through the Society for Clinical Densitometry and a ' certified Forensic Examiner. He is a lifetime member of Who's Who i Business. Dr. Rybacki provides clinical pharmacy support and serves a of clinical therapeutics and outcomes of The BCD Densitometry Grou disciplinary osteoporosis screening and consulting group based in Cambridge, Maryland.

Dr. Rybacki has been a guest and guest host on numerous radio and television shows, and participates in numerous medical speakers bureaus, including Merck, Miles, Dupont Pharma, and Glaxo. He has been a member of the Bristol Myers Distinguished Speakers in HIV faculty since 1994. He has jointly authored several articles in professional journals on use of medicines in infectious diseases, critical care, therapeutics, and cost containment. *The Essential Guide to Prescription Drugs*, first published in 1977, was co-authored by Dr. Rybacki since 1994 before he assumed full authorship in 1996. In 1995 he developed and then subsequently produced and hosted "The Medicine Man," a nationwide live radio show. He is currently the writer and host of The American Pharmaceutical Association's *The Pharmacist Minute* radio program, sponsored by a grant from Johnson and Johnson Merck (Pepcid AC®). This program is heard on more than 1,300 radio stations nationwide, was the largest launch of a radio program, and is now heard in 140 countries worldwide. Dr. Rybacki believes that the new art of prescribing medicines lies in cost by containment without sacrifice of clinical outcomes.

JAMES W. LONG, M.D., was born in Allentown, Pennsylvania. He received his premedical education from the University of Maryland and his medical degree from the George Washington University School of Medicine in Washington, D.C. For 20 years he was in private practice of internal medicine in the Washington, D.C., metropolitan area, and for over 35 years he was a member of the faculty of the George Washington University School of Medicine. He has served with the Food and Drug Administration, the National Library of Medicine, and the Bureau of Health Manpower of the National Institutes of Health. Prior to his retirement, Dr. Long was director of Health Services for the National Science Foundation in Washington. He lives in Oxford, Maryland.

Dr. Long's involvement in drug information activities includes service on the HEW Task Force on Prescription Drugs, on the FDA Task Force on Adverse Drug Reactions, as a delegate-at-large to the U.S. Pharmacopeial Convention, as editorial consultant for *Hospital Formulary*, as a director of the Drug Information Association, and as a member of the Toxicology Information Program Committee of the National Research Council/National Academy of Sciences. He was consultant he Food and Drug Administration, serving as adviser to their staff on the devel- of patient package inserts. He is also the author of numerous articles in al journals. *The Essential Guide to Prescription Drugs* is an outgrowth of that the general public needs and is entitled to practical drug infor- he equivalent of the professional "package insert." He believes sonably certain of using medications with the least risk and n the patient has all the relevant information about the

Controlled Drug Schedules

Schedule I: These medicines are those with a high abuse and dependence potential. Typically, the only use for these substances are for research purposes. Examples include LSD and heroin. A prescription cannot be legally written for these drugs for medicinal use.

Schedule II: These medicines have therapeutic uses and have the highest abuse and dependence potential for drugs with medicinal purposes. Examples include analgesics such as morphine (MS Contin) and meperidene (Demerol). A written prescription is required and refills are **not** allowed.

Schedule III: Medicines in this schedule have an abuse and dependence potential that is less than those in schedule II, but greater than those in schedule IV. These medicines have clear medicinal uses and include such medicines as hydrocodone, codeine, and paregoric in combination. Common names include Tylenol number three with codeine and Tenuate. A telephone prescription is permitted for medications in this class; however, it must be converted to a written form by a pharmacist. Prescriptions for these medicines may be refilled, but only five times in six months.

Schedule IV: This schedule contains medicines with less abuse and dependence potential than those in schedule III. Examples of medicines in this schedule include propoxyphene (Darvon), diazepam (Valium), and chlordiazepoxide (Librium). Prescriptions for these medicines may be refilled, but only five times in six months.

Schedule V: These medicines have the lowest abuse and dependence potential. Medicines in this class include diphenoxylate (Lomotil) and loperamide (Imodium). Drugs in this class which require a prescription are handled the same as any nonscheduled prescription medicine. Some drugs in this class do not require a prescription, and can be sold only with the approval of a pharmacist. The buyer is required to sign a log book when the drug is dispensed. Examples include codeine and hydrocodone in combination with other active nonnarcotic drugs sold in preparations that have limited quantities of codeine or hydrocodone for control of diarrhea or cough.

Pregnancy Risk Categories

Definitions of FDA Pregnancy Categories

Category A: Adequate and well-controlled studies in pregnant women are **negative** for fetal abnormalities. Risk to the fetus is remote.

Category B: Animal reproduction studies are **negative** for fetal abnormalities, and data from adequate and well-controlled studies in pregnant women are not available.

OR

Animal reproduction studies are **positive** for fetal abnormalities. Adequate and well-controlled studies in pregnant women are **negative** for fetal abnormalities, and fail to show a risk to the fetus.

Category C: Animal reproduction studies are **positive** for fetal abnormalities. Information from adequate and well-controlled studies in pregnant women is not available.

OR

Information from animal reproduction studies **and** from adequate and well-controlled studies in pregnant women is not available.

Category D: Studies in pregnant women and/or premarketing (investigational) or postmarketing uses show **positive** evidence of human fetal risk. The drug is only used in serious disease or in life-threatening situations where safer medicines will not work or cannot be used. These situations may make the medicine acceptable despite its risks.

Category X: Animal reproduction studies and/or human pregnancy studies are **positive** for fetal abnormalities.

OR

Studies in pregnant women and/or premarketing (investigational) or postmarketing (phase four) experience shows **positive** evidence of human fetal risk.

AND

Potential fetal risks outweigh possible benefits of the drug. These medicines **should never** be used in pregnancy.

The FDA is currently evaluating these pregnancy categories, and may opt to modify them.